W9-AVI-905

Oncology Nursing

Oncology
Nursing

FOURTH EDITION

Shirley E. Otto, MSN, CRNI, AOCN
Clinical Nurse Specialist
Via Christi Regional Medical Center: St. Francis Campus
Wichita, Kansas

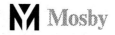 Mosby

A Harcourt Health Sciences Company
St. Louis London Philadelphia Sydney Toronto

LIBRARY

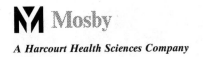

JAMES P. ADAMS
LIBRARY
RHODE ISLAND COLLEGE

Vice President and Publishing Director, Nursing: Sally Schrefer
Executive Editor: Barbara Nelson Cullen
Managing Editor: Sandra Clark Brown
Developmental Editor: Adrienne Simon
Production Manager: Donna L. Morrissey

Library of Congress Cataloging-in-Publication Data

Oncology nursing / [edited by] Shirley E. Otto—4th ed.
    p. ; cm.
    Includes bibliographical references and index.
    ISBN 0–323–01217–5
    1. Cancer—Nursing. I. Otto, Shirley E.
    [DNLM: 1. Neoplasms—nursing.
    2. Neoplasms—therapy. WY 156 O5748 2001]
RC266.O53 2001
610.73′698—dc21

                        00-049545

FOURTH EDITION

Copyright © 2001, 1997, 1994, 1991 by Mosby, Inc.   ISBN 0–323–01217–5

RC 266 O53 2001

All rights reserved. No part of this publication may be reproduced or transmitted in any form or by any means, electronic or mechanical, including photocopy, recording, or any information storage and retrieval system, without permission in writing from the publisher.

Permission to photocopy or reproduce solely for internal or personal use is permitted for libraries or other users registered with the Copyright Clearance Center, provided that the base fee of $4.00 per chapter plus $.10 per page is paid directly to the Copyright Clearance Center, 222 Rosewood Drive, Danvers, Massachusetts 01923. This consent does not extend to other kinds of copying, such as copying for general distribution, for advertising or promotional purposes, for creating new collected works, or for resale.

Mosby, Inc.
A Harcourt Health Sciences Company
11830 Westline Industrial Drive
St. Louis, Missouri 63146

Printed in the United States of America

Last digit is print number: 9   8   7   6   5   4   3   2   1

To all the current and previous contributors of Oncology Nursing *who have made a difference in the quality of life for many patients and families with cancer.*

Contributors

Joyce Alexander, MSN, RN, AOCN
(Chapter 5)
Clinical Nurse Specialist
Oncology/Bone Marrow Transplant
Halifax Medical Center
Daytona Beach, Florida

Carol Pappas Appel, MSN, RN, CNP, AOCN
(Chapters 2 and 24)
Oncology Nurse Practitioner
Barbara Ann Karmanos Cancer Institute
Detroit, Michigan

Margaret L. Barnett, MSN, ARNP, AOCN
(Chapter 27)
Cancer Care Clinical Nurse Specialist
Department of Nursing
University of Kansas Medical Center
Kansas City, Kansas

Cynthia F. Brogdon, MSN, RN, AOCN
(Chapter 13)
Clinical Nurse Specialist
Amgen
Thousand Oaks, California

Rebecca Crane-Okada, PhD, RN, AOCN
(Chapter 7)
Oncology Clinical Nurse Specialist
Joyce Eisenberg Keefer Breast Center
John Wayne Cancer Institute
Saint John's Health Center
Santa Monica, California

Betty Thomas Daniel, MS, RN, AOCN
(Chapters 9 and 16)
Clinical Nurse Specialist
The University of Texas M.D. Anderson
  Cancer Center
Houston, Texas

Mary Magee Gullatte, MN, RN, ANP, AOCN, FAAMA
(Chapters 4 and 26)
Director of Nursing, Oncology Services
Winship Cancer Institute
Emory University Hospital and Crawford Long
  Hospital
Atlanta, Georgia
Adult Nurse Practitioner
Primary Care
Marietta, Georgia

Andrea Sampson Haggood, MSN, RN, ANP, CS
(Chapter 12)
Hematology/Oncology Nurse Practitioner
Barbara Ann Karmanos Cancer Institute
Detroit, Michigan

Ryan Iwamoto, MN, ARNP, AOCN
(Chapter 22)
Oncology Clinical Specialist
NexCura, Inc.
Seattle, Washington
Nurse Practitioner, Department of Radiation
  Oncology
Virginia Mason Medical Center
Seattle, Washington
Clinical Instructor
Department of Biobehavioral Nursing and Health
  Systems
University of Washington
Seattle, Washington

Leslie A. Metivier Johnston, MSN, RN, CS, AOCN
(Chapter 28)
Clinical Manager Home Care Program
Barbara Ann Karmanos Cancer Institute
Detroit, Michigan

Claire Keller, MN, RN, OCN
(Chapter 25)
Bone Marrow Transplant Clinical Nurse Specialist
Barbara Ann Karmanos Cancer Institute
Detroit, Michigan

Suzanne Kirsch, MS
(Chapter 32)
Medical Family Therapist
Northwest Cancer Resource Center
Seattle, Washington

Martha Langhorne, MSN, RN, FNP, AOCN
(Chapter 18)
Oncology Advanced Practice Nurse
Clinical Nurse Specialist Oncology Services
United Health Services Hospitals and Cancer Center
Johnson City, New York

Mary E. Murphy, MS, RN, OCN, CHPN
(Chapters 6 and 8)
Home Care Team Manager
Hospice of Dayton
Dayton, Ohio

Jamie S. Myers, MN, RN, AOCN
(Chapter 20)
Oncology Clinical Nurse Specialist/Head Nurse
Research Medical Center
Kansas City, Missouri

Maureen E. O'Rourke, RN, PhD
(Chapter 10)
Assistant Professor, Nursing
University of North Carolina School of Nursing,
    Greensboro
Greensboro, North Carolina
Adjunct Assistant Professor of Medicine
Hematology/Oncology
Wake Forest University School of Medicine
Winston-Salem, North Carolina

Rosanne Eble Ososki, MSN, RN, CS
(Chapter 14)
Nurse Practitioner
Barbara Ann Karmanos Cancer Institute
Detroit, Michigan

Shirley E. Otto, MSN, CRNI, AOCN
(Chapters 11, 15, 17, 19, 23, 26, 28, 31, Appendices A, B,
    and C)
Clinical Nurse Specialist
Via Christi Regional Medical Center
Wichita, Kansas

Karen A. Pfeifer, PhD, RN, CNA
(Chapters 1 and 21)
Parish Nurse/Health Ministry Coordinator
St. Joseph Catholic Community
Waxahachie, Texas

Lisa Schulmeister, MN, RN, CS, OCN
(Chapters 3 and 29)
Oncology Nursing Consultant
Adjunct Assistant Professor of Nursing
Louisiana State University Health Sciences Center
New Orleans, Louisiana
Editor of *Clinical Journal of Oncology Nursing*

Judith A. Shell, PhDc, RN, AOCN
(Chapters 32 and 33)
Medical Family Therapist
Central Florida Cancer Centers
Kissimmee, Florida

Carol J. Swenson, MS, RN, OCN
(Chapter 30)
Administrative Director
Regional Cancer Center
Swedish American Health System
Rockford, Illinois

Preface

Oncology Nursing's previous editions were designed to provide the most current and relevant information needed for nursing care of patients with cancer. The books' strong clinical focus made them valuable resources for nurses in a variety of settings, including major cancer centers, local hospitals, clinics, physicians' offices, and patients' homes. Based on the many excellent comments received, the books met the varied practice needs:

"Someone wrote an oncology book with the staff nurse in mind. I can read, interpret, and incorporate the concepts into my nursing practice."

"It was the book of choice to prepare/review for the oncology nursing certification exam."

"The book is an excellent resource for the clinical nurse specialist, nurse practitioner, academia, or advanced practice nurse preparing informal/formal educational programs."

Other health care professionals stated that they found the book to be an excellent resource, enabling them to become more knowledgeable in cancer care.

The *fourth edition* of *Oncology Nursing* could be subtitled *Continuing to Make a Difference*. Multiple positive comments have been received from the previous editions. The consistent theme of comments is: "*Oncology Nursing* has made a difference for my oncology practice and me." These comments and suggestions, such as "have you thought about adding a chapter on *genetics*," have been added to this fourth edition. The original formula for all previous editions has stayed the same for this edition. Multiple choice questions appear at the end of each chapter, and all answers are at the back of the book.

Each chapter received major revisions, and features such as geriatric considerations, patient teaching priorities, expected patient outcome goals, disease- and treatment-related complications, future directions, and advances in therapy were incorporated throughout all chapters.

Unit I opens with a chapter on cancer pathophysiology that gives a fundamental explanation of carcinogenesis, neoplastic classification systems, cell cycle proper-

ties, hereditary and genetic issues, and the metastatic process. Chapters covering genetics, epidemiology; prevention, screening, and detection; and diagnosis and staging complete the unit. The most recent guidelines, recommendations, and statistics from the National Cancer Institute, the American Cancer Society, and the American Joint Committee on Cancer Staging are incorporated throughout the book. Updated information regarding chemoprevention trials for prevention of breast, prostate, and colorectal cancer; environmental and hereditary cancers and genetics in cancer prediction; and socioeconomic factors of poor, underserved, and uninsured Americans will be of interest to many nurses.

The chapters in Unit II cover clinical management of the most common cancers (brain/CNS, breast, colorectal, gastrointestinal, genitourinary, gynecologic, head and neck, HIV-related cancers, leukemia, lung, lymphoma, myeloma, and skin cancers) and oncologic complications, as well as pediatric cancers. This chapter features the most common pediatric cancers and the specific issues and concerns related to the pediatric population. All the disease chapters examine the epidemiology, etiology, prevention, screening, and detection of the particular type of cancer being discussed. Information on how the disease is classified, diagnosed, and staged, its clinical features, and the metastatic process precedes sections that explain the most prevalent treatments and prognosis for each type of cancer. Nursing diagnoses, interventions, and patient expected outcomes are presented in nursing management sections incorporated into each chapter. Additional features include geriatric considerations, patient teaching priorities, and disease- and treatment-related complications.

The chapter on oncologic complications defines the major complications that may occur as a result of cancer or its treatment. Etiology, incidence and risk factors, pathophysiology, clinical features, diagnostic evaluation, treatment modalities, and nursing management are covered for each of the following complications: anaphylaxis and hypersensitivity reactions, disseminated intravascular coagulation, hypercalcemia, malignant pleural effusion, neoplastic cardiac tamponade, septic shock, spinal cord compression, superior vena cava syndrome, syndrome of inappropriate antidiuretic hormone secretion, and tumor lysis syndrome. Algorithms for decision tree assessment and management are included for all oncologic emergencies. All of the varied oncologic complications assessment and interventions have been updated.

Unit III, which discusses cancer treatment modalities, includes chapters on surgery, radiation therapy, chemotherapy, biotherapy, bone marrow and stem cell transplantation, and cancer clinical trials. These chapters examine the principles and roles of each therapy. The surgery chapter explores preoperative, perioperative, and postoperative nursing assessment and interventions. The most recent concepts related to laser therapy options, sentinel lymph node biopsy and/or dissection, videothoroscopy, and intraoperative surgery with radiation therapy have been added to this chapter. Radiation therapy issues such as whole body, fractionated dose schedule, hyperthermia, radiation implants, intensity modulation radiation therapy (IMRT), photodynamic therapy, radiation sensitizers, and intraoperative therapies are included. The chapters on biotherapy and chemotherapy detail what the agents are and how they work, provide administrative guidelines, and explain safe handling, storage, and disposal. Factors that influence chemotherapy selection and administration such as the blood brain barrier, circadian rhythms, chemoprevention, chemoprotectants, liposomal agents, multidrug resistance, prophylactic therapies, and radiosensitizers have been updated and expanded. The bone marrow transplantation chapter provides pretransplant and posttransplant conditioning, dose-intensity regimens, transplantation options, intervention, and follow-up medical/nursing treatment protocols. Peripheral blood stem cell transplantation issues include catheter placement, pheresis process, costs, diseases most commonly treated, and survivorship issues. The cancer clinical trials chapter contains updates on all the current and upcoming disease prevention and treatment trials. Additional information includes ambulatory care setting and home care considerations and future directions and advances in all these therapies.

Unit IV, which features chapters on fatigue, home care and cancer resources, nutrition, pain management, protective mechanisms, and psychosocial/survivorship and sexuality issues, is intended to equip the nurse to better support and care for the patient and family regardless of the type of cancer or method of treatment. Fatigue, the most frequently experienced symptom of cancer and cancer treatment, has become an oncology practice priority. Definition, pathophysiology, etiology, and cancer therapies with nursing assessment and interventions for fatigue are addressed. The home care/cancer resources chapter provides many resources and guidelines to assist the nurse in discharging the patient from the acute care, ambulatory care, and/or extended care setting to the patient's home. Checklists for caregiver and home care/extended care assessment are provided. Multiple professional and public national and local resources are profiled (e.g., indigent patient drug resources, wound and skin management resources). An excellent table describing the ambulatory infusion pump's features used in multiple settings has been added. Guidelines regarding medicare clients receiving home health nursing care are included.

The nutrition chapter addresses the impact of cancer on nutritional status; assessment parameters are identified; and interventions for oral, enteral, and parenteral nutrition are suggested. Additional features include geriatric and ethical considerations. The chapter on pain management discusses analgesics, nonanalgesics, and nonsteroidal drugs, as well as administration principles specific to route dose titration, schedule, and side effects. Noninvasive pain management strategies are presented. Invasive pain management modalities are defined; rationales for the procedures are given; and potential outcomes are discussed. New pain management guidelines from the American Pain Society, American Geriatrics Society, Agency for Health Care Policy and Research—Cancer Pain Management, and Joint Commission on Accreditation for Healthcare Organizations 2000 standards (pain as the fifth vital sign) have been incorporated throughout the chapter, and multiple professional and pain management resources are listed.

Protective mechanisms, such as skin, mucous membrane, and bone marrow, are defined, and parameters of nursing assessment with effective interventions are provided. Information regarding Clinical Practice Guidelines on Pressure Ulcers in Adults: Prediction and Prevention from the Agency for Health Care Policy and Research and specialty bed placement/reimbursement issues are discussed. The psychosocial chapter has incorporated these timely topics, including quality of life, disability issues, hospice care, survivorship, ethics, advance directives, right-to-die legislation information, and the well-being of the professional and lay caregiver. The sexuality chapter discusses the impact of cancer and its therapy on sexuality. Many sensitive issues are explored, and strategies intended to help the patient enhance self and sexual images are provided.

In 2001, an estimated 1,268,000 new cases of invasive cancer will be diagnosed and 553,400 Americans (more than 1,500 people a day) are expected to die of cancer. Additionally, the current population is turning age 50 at the rate of 8 per minute, which translates to more than 80,640 people weekly. The impact of an "aged population" with designated oncology health care needs will be both an opportunity and a challenge for oncology nurses working in the varied oncology practice settings.

With the soon-to-be-completed human genome mapping, cancer prevention, detection, and treatment will have an entirely new approach. Successful treatments of pediatric cancers with multimodality therapies have resulted in an estimated 1 in every 900 individuals aged 16 to 44 years who will survive childhood cancer. Quality of life, psychosocial issues, and survivorship remain the major concerns of patients with cancer and their families. Because we believe the nurse is vital in providing high-quality care for patients with cancer, the nurse's role is interwoven throughout the content of each chapter, and then focused on in nursing management sections. These sections include nursing diagnoses, interventions, and expected patient outcomes to provide the nurse with concrete guidelines to ensure the best quality care throughout the course of the disease. Now, more than ever, during all the changing practices in cancer care, compassionate, competent, and conscientious nursing care is the right of the patient and family with cancer. What we say and do can make a difference in the quality of life for these individuals.

Shirley E. Otto

Acknowledgments

I wish to express my sincere appreciation to the many people who made this publication possible: the contributing authors, Karen, Carol A., Lisa, Mary G., Joyce, Mary M., Becky, Betty, Maureen, Andrea, Cynthia, Rosanne, Martha, Jamie, Ryan, Claire, Marge, Leslie, Carol S., Judy, and Suzanne, who, **one more time,** despite their personal, family, educational, and/or professional responsibilities, consulted and critiqued many credible resources to provide an excellent clinical practice and theory resource for oncology nursing; to Robert M. Fulcher, RPh, for his review of dosages; to all the Harcourt Health Sciences staff; and to all my oncology peers who continually encourage and support me.

Contents in Brief

NOTICE

Nursing is an ever-changing field. Standard safety precautions must be followed, but as new research and clinical experience broaden our knowledge, changes in treatment and drug therapy become necessary and appropriate. Readers are advised to check the product information currently provided by the manufacturer of each drug to be administered to verify the recommended dose, the method and duration of administration, and the contraindications. It is the responsibility of the treating licensed prescriber, relying on experience and knowledge of the patient, to determine dosages and the best treatment for the patient. Neither the publisher nor the editor assumes any responsibility for any injury and/or damage to persons or property.

The Publisher

Contents

UNIT III
Cancer Treatment Modalities

Clinical Aspects of the Cancer Diagnosis

Pathophysiology

Karen A. Pfeifer

Cancer is an important public health concern in the United States and throughout the world.[19] It is estimated that 1,220,100 new cases of invasive cancer will be diagnosed in the United States in the year 2000.[1] Among men, the most common cancers in 2000 are expected to be cancers of the prostate, lung and bronchus, and colon and rectum. Prostate cancer, the leading site for cancer incidence in men, will account for 29% of new cancer cases. Among women, the three most common cancers in 2000 are expected to be cancers of the breast, lung and bronchus, and colon and rectum. These sites are expected to account for over 50% of new cancer cases in women. Breast cancer alone will account for 182,800 (30%) of new cancer cases in 2000.[19] Approximately 8600 new cases of cancer are expected to occur among children aged 0 to 14 in 2000. Common sites in children include the blood and bone marrow, bone, lymph nodes, brain, sympathetic nervous system, kidneys, and soft tissues. The incidence rate of all childhood cancers increased from the early 1970s until 1991, leveling off and declining slightly through 1996.[1]

Cancer, the second most common cause of death in the United States, will kill approximately 552,000 persons in 2000. Most cancer deaths in men (52%) are expected to be from cancers of the lung and bronchus, prostate, and colon and rectum. In women, cancers of the lung and bronchus, breast, and colon and rectum are expected to account for more than half of all cancer deaths. In 1987, lung cancer surpassed breast cancer as the leading cause of cancer death in women. It is expected to account for 25% of all female cancer deaths in 2000.[19] Despite steady advances in treatment of children, 2300 children will die of cancer in the year 2000. Although cancer is only a minor cause of death in children under age 1 year, it is the leading cause of death from disease in children and young people aged 1 to 19.[1]

THE NORMAL CELL

Medical researchers have identified approximately 100 different types of cancers. Each cancer cell within these various diseases has an altered morphology and biochemistry from the normal cell. Cancer is not a disorderly growth of immature cells, but rather a logical, coordinated process in which a normal cell undergoes changes and acquires special capabilities.[28] It is important, then, to understand the morphology and biochemistry of the normal cell.

The basic unit of structure and function in all living things is the *cell*. Approximately 60,000 billion cells are in the adult human body, and although there are many different types of cells, all of them have certain common characteristics. For example, all cells need nourishment to maintain life, and all cells use almost identical nutrients. All cells use oxygen (O_2); the O_2 combines with fat, protein, or carbohydrates (CHO) to release the energy needed for cells to function. The mechanisms for changing nutrients into energy are generally the same in all cells, and all cells deliver their end-products of chemical reactions into nearby fluids. Most cells have the ability to reproduce. Whenever cells are destroyed, the remaining cells of the same type reproduce until the correct number has been replenished. This orderly replacement of cells is governed by a control mechanism that stops when the loss or damage has been corrected. Dynamic, active, and orderly, the healthy cell is a small powerhouse, laboratory, factory, and duplicating machine—perfectly copying itself over and over.[5, 20] Figure 1–1 shows the phases and characteristics of *mitosis* (cell division).

PROLIFERATIVE GROWTH PATTERNS

Cancer cells are not subject to the usual restrictions placed by the host on cell proliferation. However, proliferation is not always indicative of cancer. Abnormal cellular growth is classified as *nonneoplastic* and *neoplastic*.[12, 20, 32, 38, 42]

Nonneoplastic Growth Patterns

The four common nonneoplastic growth patterns are hypertrophy, hyperplasia, metaplasia, and dysplasia.[12, 20, 32, 38, 42]

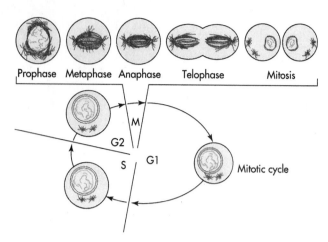

FIGURE 1–1 The cell cycle. (From Phipps WJ, Sands JK, Marek JF, editors: *Medical-surgical nursing: concepts and clinical practice,* ed 6, St Louis, Mosby, 1999.)

Hypertrophy is an increase in cell size. It commonly results from increased workload, hormonal stimulation, or compensation directly related to the functional loss of other tissue.[42]

Hyperplasia is a reversible increase in the number of cells of a certain tissue type, resulting in increased tissue mass. Hyperplasia commonly occurs as a normal physiologic response at times of rapid growth and development (e.g., pregnancy, adolescence). It is abnormal when the volume of cells produced exceeds the normal physiologic demand.[12, 20, 38, 42]

In *metaplasia,* one adult cell type is substituted for another type not usually found in the involved tissue (e.g., glandular for squamous). The process is reversible if the stimulus is removed, or metaplasia may progress to dysplasia if the stimulus persists. Metaplasia can be induced by inflammation, vitamin deficiencies, irritation, and various chemical agents. A common area for metaplasia to occur is the uterine cervix.[12, 20, 38, 42]

Dysplasia is characterized by alterations in normal adult cells in which the cell varies from its normal size, shape, or organization or one mature cell type is replaced with a less mature cell type. The common stimulus creating a dysplasia is usually an external one (e.g., radiation, inflammation, toxic chemicals, chronic irritation). Dysplasia is possibly reversible if the stimulus is removed.[20, 38, 42]

Hyperplasia, metaplasia, and dysplasia are not neoplastic conditions but may precede the development of cancer.[42]

Neoplastic Growth Patterns

Anaplasia means "without form" and is an irreversible change in which the structures of adult cells regress to more primitive levels. It is a hallmark of cancer. Anaplastic cells lose the capacity for specialized functions and are positionally and cytologically disorganized.[18, 20, 21, 31, 38, 42]

Neoplasm means "new growth" and describes an abnormal tissue mass that extends beyond the boundaries of normal tissue, failing to fulfill the normal function of cells in that tissue. Neoplasms are characterized by uncontrolled functioning, unregulated division and growth, and abnormal motility. Some neoplasms are potentially harmful to the host because they occupy space and compete for essential nutrients. Neoplastic growths are referred to as *benign neoplasms* or *malignant neoplasms.* Benign neoplasms include papillomas or warts. Malignant neoplasms include solid tumors and leukemia; these have the ability to destroy the host. *Cancer* is the common term for all malignant neoplasms.[12, 20, 21, 24, 41, 42] Table 1–1 summarizes the differences between benign and malignant growths.

CHARACTERISTICS OF CANCER CELLS

Microscopic Properties

Microscopic examination of cancer cells shows certain structural changes that are described in pathologic terms, as follows[21, 42, 44]:

TABLE 1–1
Comparison of Benign and Malignant Tumors

Characteristic	Malignant Tumor	Benign Tumor
Encapsulated	Rarely	Usually
Differentiated	Poorly	Partially
Metastasis	Frequently present	Absent
Recurrence	Frequent	Rare
Vascularity	Moderate to marked	Slight
Mode of growth	Infiltrative and expansive	Expansive
Cell characteristics	Cells abnormal and become more unlike parent cells	Fairly normal; similar to parent cells

From Bender CM, Yasko JM, Strohl RA: Cancer. In Lewis SM, Collier IC, Heitkemper MM, editors: Medical-surgical nursing: assessment and management of clinical problems, *ed 4, St Louis, Mosby, 1996.*

- *Pleomorphism.* Cancer cells vary in size and shape. Some are unusually large, whereas others are too small to be detected microscopically. Multiple nuclei may be seen.
- *Hyperchromatism.* Nuclear chromatin, the major component of genes, is more pronounced on staining.
- *Polymorphism.* The nucleus is larger and varies in shape.
- *Aneuploidy.* Unusual numbers of chromosomes are seen.
- *Abnormal chromosome arrangements.* A variety of possibilities exist, including translocations, the exchange of material between chromosomes, deletions, loss of chromosome sections, additions, extra chromosomes, and *fragile sites,* weak sections on chromosomes.

Kinetic Properties

Cancer cells possess certain kinetic characteristics, as follows:

- *Loss of proliferative control.* All cancer cells possess this characteristic. The need for cell renewal or replacement is the usual stimulus for cell proliferation. Cell production stops when the stimulus is gone, producing a balance between cell production and cell loss. In cancer, proliferation continues once the stimulus initiates the process, and cancer cells progress in continued, uncontrolled growth. The host's normal control mechanisms fail to stop this proliferation.[12, 20]
- *Loss of capacity to differentiate.* Differentiation is the process by which cells diversify and acquire specific structural and functional characteristics. In cancer, *differentiation* refers to the extent to which cancer cells resemble comparable normal cells. Cancer cells vary in their ability to retain the morphologic and functional traits of the original tissue. Cells that closely resemble the normal cell but form slow-growing, usually encapsulated tumors are *well differentiated.* These cells have recognizable specialized structures and functions. Cells that grow rapidly and do not have the original tissue's morphologic characteristics and specialized cell functions are termed *undifferentiated.* These cells have lost the capacity for specialized functions. The process by which cells lose characteristics of normal cells is called *dedifferentiation.* The more undifferentiated a malignant cell, the more virulent it is believed to be. It is possible to cause cells at one level of differentiation to transform into less well-differentiated cells by exposing them to cancer-causing agents.[12, 20, 21, 38, 42]
- *Altered biochemical properties.* Because of the cancer cell's loss of the capacity to differentiate, certain biochemical properties may be missing because of the cell's new immature state, or cells may acquire new properties because of enzyme pattern changes or alterations in deoxyribonucleic acid (DNA). Examples of these altered biochemical properties include production of tumor-associated antigens marking the cancer cell as "nonself"; continued reproduction despite diminished concentrations of growth hormones; higher rates of anaerobic glycolysis, making the cell less dependent on O_2; loss of cell-to-cell cohesiveness and adhesiveness; and abnormal production of hormones or hormone-like substances that induce paraneoplastic syndromes. In the latter, cancer cells may inappropriately secrete hormones in an organ or tissue that does not normally produce or release those hormones, resulting in signs and symptoms not directly related to the local effects of the tumor. For example, in small-cell carcinoma of the lung, antidiuretic hormone (ADH) is produced, resulting in hyponatremia[10, 12, 21, 42] (Table 1–2).
- *Chromosomal instability.* Cancer cells are less genetically stable than normal cells because of the development of abnormal chromosome arrangements. Chromosomal instability results in new, increasingly malignant mutants as cancer cells proliferate. These mutant cells can create a surviving subpopulation of advanced neoplasms with unique biologic and cytogenetic characteristics that are highly resistant to therapy.[11, 12, 16, 22, 42, 44]
- *Capacity to metastasize. Metastasis,* the spread of cancer cells from a *primary* (parent) site to distant secondary sites, is aided by the production of enzymes on the surface of the cancer cell. Cancer cells become increasingly malignant with each mutation, and an association exists between a cell's degree of malignancy and its ability to metastasize.[12, 20, 21, 42]

CELLULAR KINETICS

The field of *cellular kinetics* is the study of the quantitative growth and division of cells.[7, 12, 42]

Cell Cycle

The *cell cycle* is the sequence of events involved in replication and distribution of DNA to the daughter cells produced by cell division. All cells, nonmalignant and malignant, progress through the five phases of the cell cycle: G_0, G_1, S, G_2, and M[3, 12, 20, 42] (see Fig. 1–1).

G_0 Phase (Postmitotic Resting Phase). The G_0 phase encompasses that period of the cell cycle when normal renewable tissue is not actively proliferating. In this phase, cells perform all functions except those related to proliferation. This category includes nondividing cells and resting cells. Normal cells in the G_0 phase are

TABLE 1–2
Paraneoplastic Syndromes

Clinical Syndromes	Major Forms of Underlying Cancer	Causal Mechanism
ENDOCRINOPATHIES		
Cushing syndrome	Small-cell carcinoma of lung Pancreatic carcinoma Neural tumors	ACTH or ACTH-like substance
Syndrome of inappropriate antidiuretic hormone secretion	Small-cell carcinoma of lung; intracranial neoplasms	Antidiuretic hormone or atrial natriuretic hormones
Hypercalcemia	Squamous cell carcinoma of lung Breast carcinoma Renal carcinoma Adult T-cell leukemia/lymphoma Ovarian carcinoma	Parathyroid hormone-related peptide, TGF-α, TNF-α, IL-1
Hypoglycemia	Fibrosarcoma Other mesenchymal sarcomas Hepatocellular carcinoma	Insulin or insulin-like substance
Carcinoid syndrome	Bronchial adenoma (carcinoid) Pancreatic carcinoma Gastric carcinoma	Serotonin, bradykinin, (?)histamine
Polycythemia	Renal carcinoma Cerebellar hemangioma Hepatocellular carcinoma	Erythropoietin
NERVE AND MUSCLE SYNDROMES		
Myasthenia	Bronchogenic carcinoma	Immunologic
Disorders of the central and peripheral nervous systems	Breast carcinoma	
DERMATOLOGIC DISORDERS		
Acanthosis nigricans	Gastric carcinoma Lung carcinoma Uterine carcinoma	(?)Immunologic, (?)secretion of epidermal growth factor
Dermatomyositis	Bronchogenic, breast carcinoma	(?)Immunologic
OSSEOUS, ARTICULAR, AND SOFT TISSUE CHANGES		
Hypertrophic osteoarthropathy and clubbing of the fingers	Bronchogenic carcinoma	Unknown
VASCULAR AND HEMATOLOGIC CHANGES		
Venous thrombosis (Trousseau phenomenon)	Pancreatic carcinoma Bronchogenic carcinoma Other cancers	Tumor products (mucins that activate clotting)
Nonbacterial thrombotic endocarditis	Advanced cancers	Hypercoagulability
Anemia	Thymic neoplasms	Unknown
OTHERS		
Nephrotic syndrome	Various cancers	Tumor antigens, immune complexes

ACTH, adrenocorticotropic hormone; TGF, transforming growth factor; TNF, tumor necrosis factor; IL, interleukin.

From Cotran RS, Kumar V, Collins T, Robbins SL, editors: Robbins pathologic basis of disease, ed 6, Philadelphia, Saunders, 1999.

activated to reenter the reproductive cycle only by certain stimuli, such as the death of a cell of the same type.[3, 12, 20, 21, 38, 42]

G$_1$ Phase (Growth or Postmitotic/Presynthesis Period). The G$_1$ phase, which lasts from 12 to 14 hours, extends from the completion of the previous cell division to the beginning of chromosome replication. This is a period of decreased metabolic activity. Cells carry out their designated physiologic functions, synthesizing proteins needed in the formation of ribonucleic acid (RNA). The G$_1$ phase is primarily a stage of readiness, as cells prepare for entry into the S phase.[3, 12, 20, 21, 38, 42]

S Phase (Synthesis). In the S phase, which lasts approximately 7 to 20 hours, RNA is synthesized, which is essential for the synthesis of DNA. DNA synthesis is limited exclusively to this phase. *Histones,* the basic protein of chromatin, are also synthesized in the S phase. Cells are most vulnerable to damage during the S phase.[3, 12, 20, 21, 38, 42]

G$_2$ Phase (Postsynthetic/Premitotic Phase). The G$_2$ phase, which lasts from 1 to 4 hours, is one of relative hypoactivity, as the cells await entry into the mitotic phase. This phase encompasses the interval from the termination of DNA synthesis to the beginning of cell division. Some additional protein synthesis occurs during G$_2$, but it is mostly synthesis of structural proteins versus enzymes. Some additional RNA synthesis also occurs.[3, 12, 20, 21, 38, 42]

M Phase (Mitosis). In the M phase, which lasts from 40 minutes to 2 hours, mitosis and cell division occur. Protein synthesis continues but is drastically reduced. Duplication of DNA must be complete before cells enter the mitotic cycle. This phase is further subdivided into four stages: *prophase, metaphase, anaphase,* and *telophase* (see Fig. 1–1). *Interphase* encompasses all events before mitosis (i.e., G$_1$, S, and G$_2$). After mitosis the daughter cells either return to the G$_0$ phase and stop dividing or, if a stimulus for cell division exists, enter the G$_1$ phase and begin the cell reproductive cycle again.[3, 12, 20, 21, 38, 42]

Cancer cells are able to complete the cell cycle more quickly by decreasing the length of time spent in the G$_1$ phase. They are also much less likely to enter or remain in the G$_0$ phase of the cell cycle than are normal cells; thus cancer cells divide continuously.[3, 12, 28, 38]

The number of cells in the body "in cycle" is only a small fraction of the total number of cells, and this is true of cancer cells as well. The duration of the M, G$_2$, and S phases is relatively constant, whereas the time a cell spends in G$_1$ varies from a few hours to several days. This determines the overall length of the cell cycle. The *cell cycle time* (T$_c$) is the sum of M, G$_1$, S, and G$_2$:

$$T_c = TM + TG_1 + TS + TG_2$$

Those cells in the late G$_1$ or early S phase of the cell cycle are the most vulnerable to dedifferentiation.[3, 12, 20, 21, 42]

TUMOR GROWTH

In normal cell proliferation, cell birth approximates cell death. The body's demand for an increase in the number of cells and for cell replacement is initiated by loss of cells of the same type or by extra tissue function demands. All elements of normal tissue growth are found in cancer cell growth and reproduction. However, progressive failure of intrinsic normal growth mechanisms produces the growth common to cancer.[32, 33, 38]

A common misconception is that cancer is a population of cells that reproduces much faster than normal cells. In fact, many cancers are rather slow growing compared with some normal cells (e.g., cells of the epithelial lining, bone marrow cells). Not all cancer cells can proliferate indefinitely, but every neoplasm contains cells that fail to abide by the restraints placed on proliferation. This results in cell growth beyond normal margins and pressure on other organs and may contribute to the tendency of cancer cells to invade neighboring tissues and structures.[21]

Tumor Growth Properties

In general, cancer cells possess the following properties[24, 34–36]:

*   *Immortality of transformed cells.* Cancer cells are capable of passing through an infinite number of population doublings if sufficient nutrition and growth factors are available.[24]
*   *Decreased contact inhibition of movement.* Normal cells adjust to the proximity of neighboring cells by halting growth. They arrest movement when another cell is encountered and symmetrically arrange themselves around each other. Cancer cells invade others without respect to these constraints.[21, 24]
*   *Decreased contact inhibition of cell division.* Normal cells stop dividing because of full contact with other cells, not because nutrients become depleted or because of accumulated wastes. When normal cells are surrounded, they simply stop dividing. Cancer cells lack or exhibit decreased contact inhibition of growth, continuing to divide and even piling atop one another.[21, 24]
*   *Decreased adhesiveness.* Cancer cells are less adhesive, resulting in increased cell mobility. This is possibly caused by the loss of extracellular fibronectin. *Fibronectin,* a large external *transformation-sensitive* (LETS) glycoprotein, facilitates intercellular adhesion by collagen and elastin links.[23, 25, 28, 42]
*   *Loss of anchorage dependence.* Cancer cells do not need a surface on which to attach and proliferate. This property affects cells' shape and adhesiveness because the cell assumes a more rotund shape.[23]
*   *Loss of restrictive point control.* In the normal cell, several environmental growth conditions (e.g., high cell density or depletion of essential amino acids, glucose, and lipids) cause the cell to be blocked in G$_1$. This is called the *restriction point of G$_1$*, or the point where the cell is blocked from continuing the cell cycle. Cancer cells lose this stringent restriction point control and continue to proliferate despite suboptimal nutrition and high cell density.[23]

Tumor Growth Concepts

Normal cells are divided into three major categories of cell growth: *static* (nondividing), *expanding* (resting), and *renewing* (continuously dividing). Static cells do not continue to divide after the postembryonic period. If these cells are damaged or destroyed, they cannot be replaced. Examples are nerve and brain cells. Expanding cells temporarily stop reproduction on reaching normal size, but they can reenter the cell cycle and divide during times of physiologic need. Examples are liver, kidney, and endocrine gland cells. Renewing cells have the highest level of reproductive activity. These cells have a finite life span and continuously replicate to replace dying cells. Examples are germ cells, epithelial cells of the gastrointestinal mucosa, and blood cells. Likewise, not all cancer cells participate in active proliferation. Tumors are composed of mixtures of nondividing, resting, and continuously dividing cells.[12, 20]

In the simplest model for cell growth, a cell divides to produce two daughter cells, each of which then divides, producing four cells, eight cells, and so on. Thus, cell numbers increase in powers of two, called *exponential growth.*[7, 42]

The growth rate of tumors is expressed in doubling time. *Tumor volume-doubling time* (DT) is the time needed for a tumor mass to double its volume. Tumor cells undergo a series of doublings as the tumor increases in size. The average DT of most primary solid tumors is approximately 2 to 3 months, with a range of 11 to 90 weeks. In general, a tumor must progress through approximately 30 doublings before becoming palpable. The minimum clinically detectable body burden of tumor (*tumor volume*) is 10 billion cells (1 g). Tumor masses are usually 100 billion cells or 10 g at detection. Death of the host usually occurs when the body burden of tumor equals or exceeds 1 trillion cells or 1 kg of tumor. This growth from 1 g to 1 kg of tumor requires only 10 more doublings.[7, 12, 20, 33, 42]

Because not all tumor cells divide simultaneously, *growth fraction* (GF) is an important concept in the determination of DT. GF is the ratio of the total number of cells to the number of proliferating cells. Tumors with larger GFs increase their tumor mass more quickly.[12, 21, 42] As tumor volume increases, GF decreases. In the latter stages of tumor growth, the tumor usually has only a small proportion of actively proliferating cells. The tumor loses cells by differentiation, death, or desquamation. Cell growth usually continues only at the periphery of the tumor, with the center becoming increasingly dormant and eventually turning necrotic. Finally, the tumor reaches a point where cell death approximates cell birth, and a plateau is reached. The rapid proliferation of tumor cells followed by this continuous, but slowed, proliferation is called the *Gompertz*

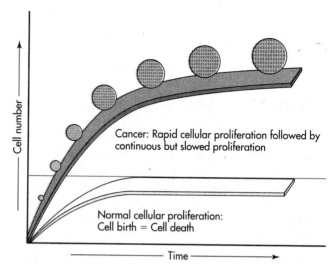

FIGURE 1 – 2 Gompertzian function. (From Phipps WJ, Sands JK, Marek JF, editors: *Medical-surgical nursing: concepts and clinical practice,* ed 6, St Louis, Mosby, 1999.)

function. The Gompertz function can be expressed by the *Gompertz growth curve* (Fig. 1–2). The growth curve illustrates the initial exponential growth of cancer cells, followed by the steady and progressive decrease in the GF because of a decrease in the fraction of proliferating cells and an increase in the rate of cell death.[7, 12, 20, 29, 33, 42]

CARCINOGENESIS

Carcinogenesis is the process by which normal cells are transformed into cancer cells. Although numerous theories have been proposed to explain it, no single unifying hypothesis has been offered or accepted. The exact cause of most human cancers is still unknown.[12, 21, 42]

An understanding of the following terms is necessary before theories of carcinogenesis can be discussed:

- *Initiating agent (carcinogen).* An initiating agent is a chemical, biologic, or physical agent capable of permanently, directly, and irreversibly changing the molecular structure of the genetic component (DNA) of a cell. This predisposes the cell to transformation when exposed to a prolonged or continuous promoting agent. An initiating agent may cause (1) complete division of the DNA chain in one or more places, (2) elimination of one of the component parts of the DNA chain (e.g., sugars, bases), or (3) errors in DNA repair. It may act at the initial point of contact, in the organ where carcinogens have accumulated, or at the site of metabolism or excretion. *Viral, environmental or life-style,* and *genetic factors* have all been identified as initiators of carcinogenesis.[37, 38, 42]
- *Promoting agent (cocarcinogen).* A promoting agent alters the expression of genetic information of the

cell, thereby enhancing cellular transformation. Examples include hormones, plant products, and drugs. Promoting agents do not directly react with a cell's genetic material and cannot mutate DNA by themselves. Although they work in conjunction with initiating agents to promote neoplastic change, promoting agents themselves do not cause cancer. The effects of promoting agents are temporary and reversible.[12, 38, 42]

- *Complete carcinogen.* A complete carcinogen possesses both initiating and promoting properties and is capable of inducing cancer on its own. The ability to act as a complete carcinogen may be dose related. Radiation is an example of a dose-related complete carcinogen.[12, 21, 28, 37]

- *Reversing agent.* A revising agent inhibits the effects of promoting agents by stimulating metabolic pathways in the cell that destroy carcinogens or altering the initiating potency of chemical carcinogens. Examples include drugs, enzymes, and vitamins.[21, 42]

- *Oncogene.* An oncogene is a gene that has evolved to control growth and repair of tissues. It is the genetic code that functions as the "off" and "on" signals that cells send and receive to control reproduction. Oncogenes include *proto-oncogenes,* the portion of DNA that regulates normal cell proliferation and repair, and *antioncogenes,* the portion of DNA that stops cell division. Oncogenes are the targets of carcinogens, producing mutations that may leave proto-oncogenes permanently in the "on" position and prevent antioncogenes from exerting the "off" signal at the appropriate time.[21, 42]

- *Progression.* As tumor cells proliferate, they undergo changes in their microscopic structures. This is referred to as *progression,* or the change in a tumor from a preneoplastic state, or low degree of malignancy, to a rapidly growing, virulent tumor. Tumor progression may be characterized by changes in growth rate, invasive potential, metastatic frequency, morphologic traits, and responsiveness to therapy. Progression occurs as a result of a cell type that grows more rapidly or metabolizes at a faster rate than other cells in the tumor mass. This cell then becomes the dominant cell type. Also, cytotoxic treatments may enhance tumor progression by their mutagenic effects, hastening the appearance of increasingly malignant variants.[12]

- *Heterogeneity.* The concept of heterogeneity is closely related to progression. It refers to differences among individual cells within a tumor. Cancer cells have a higher frequency of random mutation because of their genetic instability. These mutations produce clones whose acquired genetic variability results in heterogeneity within a tumor. Cells within a tumor can be heterogeneous with respect to the ability to invade surrounding tissue, genetic composition, growth rate, metastatic potential, hormone receptors, and susceptibility to antineoplastic therapy. The degree of heterogeneity increases as the tumor increases in size.[11, 12, 15, 22]

- *Transformation.* Transformation is a multistep process by which cells become progressively dedifferentiated after exposure to an initiating agent. There is probably more than one way to transform a cell. Transformation, however, generally results from a genetic alteration in the cell, which deregulates the control of cell proliferation. The controversy centers around the question of what stimuli induce the needed transformation in a cell's DNA. Many authorities believe that as many as 80% of known human cancers are the direct result of an individual's exposure to environmental carcinogens.[12, 21, 42]

Theories of Carcinogenesis

Carcinogenesis is believed to involve two or more steps. The *Berenblum theory,* first proposed in 1947, states that cancer occurs as the result of two distinct events: *initiation* and *promotion.* Initiation occurs first and is usually believed to be rapid and mutational. The change is brought about by an initating agent (e.g., a chemical substance). The second event involves a promoting agent, and its effect is generally believed to include changes in cell growth, transport, and metabolism. Without promotion, initiation will not result in a truly transformed cell. Promotion may occur shortly after initiation or much later in an individual's life. Initiation produces a change in the cell, but cancer will not develop until the cell is affected by one or several promoting agents[4] (Fig. 1–3).

Over the years, Berenblum's theory has evolved into the *three-stage theory of carcinogenesis.* This theory proposes that the process of transforming a normal cell into a cancer cell consists of three distinct phases with several substages, all of which occur in the cell's DNA.[21, 42]

In the first stage, *initiation,* a carcinogen damages DNA by altering a specific gene. This gene (1) undergoes repair, and no cancer results, (2) permanently changes but causes no cancer unless subsequently exposed to the action of a cocarcinogen at a later date, or (3) transforms and produces a cancer cell if the initiator is a complete carcinogen.[21, 42]

In the second stage, *promotion,* cocarcinogens are subsequently introduced, resulting in either reversible or irreversible damage to the proliferating mechanism of the cell. Irreversible damage results in cancer cell transformation. The effects of cocarcinogens may be inhibited by certain cancer-reversing agents (e.g., vitamin C) or certain host characteristics or both.[21, 42]

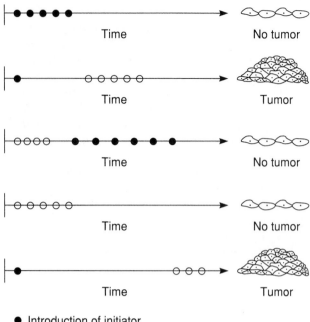

● Introduction of initiator

○ Introduction of promoter

FIGURE 1–3 Interactions of initiation and promotion.

In the final stage, *progression,* both mutagenic and nonmutagenic events occur, leading to morphologic changes within the cell and increased grades of malignant behavior (e.g., invasion, metastasis, drug resistance). This process is irreversible.[21, 42]

Carcinogenesis is a process that can occupy the better part of a person's life. In humans, carcinogenesis is more complex than any researcher-induced laboratory model. The distinction between the three stages is often blurred and complicated by the presence of a *latent period* between the initial exposure to a carcinogen and the actual development of a clinically detectable malignancy. This latent period is not characterized by particular clinical or subjective signs or symptoms, and no tests have been developed to detect latent transformed cells. It is, therefore, impossible to predict whether certain segments of a population are at risk for developing cancer. Tumors might not appear for 20, 30, or 40 years in these at-risk groups. Also, most persons diagnosed with cancer have no obvious history of exposure to a carcinogen. This phenomenon, known as the *multiple factor effect,* plays a significant role in human carcinogenesis.[12, 42]

Medical researchers have not been able to prove definitively that the initial event in carcinogenesis is a mutation. Whatever causes cancer, the final result is an irreversible change in the cellular genetic code. This leads to cell clones that eventually give rise to clinically detectable cancer.[12, 28, 42]

Hormonal Carcinogenesis

Changes in a person's hormonal environment most likely result from an overproduction of endogenous hormones or an excessive administration of exogenous hormones. Four main types of human cancer (i.e., cancer of the prostate, brain, breast, and endometrium) occur in hormone-responsive tissues (*target tissues*). Although target tissues require hormones for normal growth and function, there is little evidence that hormones produce any direct carcinogenic effects. Hormones do not interact with or exert an effect on nucleic acid. Rather, hormones promote the carcinogenic process by sensitizing a cell to the carcinogenic insult or modifying the growth of an established tumor.[20]

Chemical Carcinogenesis

Despite more than 6 million chemicals having been identified and registered with the Chemical Abstracts Service and more than 50,000 estimated to be used regularly in business and industry, probably fewer than 1000 chemicals or exposures have been examined for their potential to cause cancer. Even so, the literature for even this small fraction of known exposures is massive. Since the early 1970s, an extensive effort has been made to systematize available data on cancer risk attributed to chemical carcinogens.[39]

Chemical carcinogens include compounds or elements that alter DNA. The relationship between chemical carcinogens and cancer has been documented for several centuries, beginning with the high incidence of scrotal cancer observed among chimneysweeps. However, chemical carcinogens are not confined solely to the occupational arena. Environmental chemical carcinogens range from food preservatives to atmospheric pollution. The list of known human chemical carcinogens is short; the list of suspected human chemical carcinogens is longer and grows yearly. Table 1–3 provides examples of known chemicals that act as carcinogens.[10, 21, 28, 42]

The International Agency for Research on Cancer (IARC) has developed a comprehensive method for assessment of human cancer risks as related to chemical carcinogens. The IARC classifies chemical exposures into four categories: sufficient, limited, inadequate evidence of carcinogenicity, or evidence suggesting lack of carcinogenicity. *Sufficient evidence* of carcinogenicity implies that a causal relationship has been established between exposure to the chemical and human cancer and that chance, bias, and confounding evidence have been ruled out with reasonable confidence. *Limited evidence* implies that a positive association has been observed between exposure to the chemical and cancer for which a causal interpretation is considered to be

TABLE 1–3
Major Chemical Carcinogens

DIRECT-ACTING CARCINOGENS

Alkylating Agents
β-Propiolactone
Dimethyl sulfate
Diepoxybutane
Anticancer drugs (cyclophosphamide, chlorambucil, nitrosoureas, and others)

Acylating Agents
1-Acetyl-imidazole
Dimethylcarbamyl chloride

PROCARCINOGENS THAT REQUIRE METABOLIC ACTIVATION

Polycyclic and Heterocyclic Aromatic Hydrocarbons
Benz(a)anthracene
Benzo(a)pyrene
Dibenz(a,h)anthracene
3-Methylcholanthrene
7,12-Dimethylbenz(a)anthracene

Aromatic Amines, Amides, Azo Dyes
2-Naphthylamine (β-naphthylamine)
Benzidine
2-Acetylaminofluorene
Dimethylaminoazobenzene (butter yellow)

Natural Plant and Microbial Products
Aflatoxin B_1
Griseofulvin
Cycasin
Safrole
Betel nuts

Others
Nitrosamine and amides
Vinyl chloride, nickel, chromium
Insecticides, fungicides
Polychlorinated biphenyls

From Cotran RS, Kumar V, Collins T, Robbins SL, editors: Robbins pathologic basis of disease, ed 6, Philadelphia, Saunders, 1999.

credible, but chance, bias, or confounding evidence cannot be ruled out with reasonable confidence. *Inadequate evidence* of carcinogenicity means that the available research is of insufficient quality, consistency, or statistical power to permit a conclusion regarding causal association or that no data on cancer in humans are available. *Evidence suggesting lack of carcinogenicity* means that several adequate studies have covered the full range of exposure levels in humans and are mutually consistent in not showing a positive association between exposure to the chemical and the studied cancer at any observed level of exposure.[39]

Chemical carcinogens may be divided into two categories regardless of origin. The first category, *direct-acting chemical carcinogens,* acts directly on nucleic acids and proteins. These carcinogens form reactive ions that mutate DNA and do not require metabolic activation by the host. Examples include busulfan and nitrogen mustard. The second category involves *procarcinogens,* which are not directly effective as carcinogens but can mutate DNA after metabolic activation. These must be activated by carcinogen-activating enzymes attached to cells. Most chemical carcinogens are procarcinogens. Examples include soot, coal tar products, and cigarette smoke. Once metabolized, procarcinogens become *ultimate carcinogens.*[20, 21, 42]

Viral Carcinogenesis

Although evidence of viral carcinogenesis in animals has existed for many years, the connection between viruses and human cancers has been a fairly recent development. Viruses are thought to contribute to human carcinogenesis by infecting the host DNA, resulting in proto-oncogenic changes and cell mutation. Viral carcinogens may be *slow acting* (adenoviruses, herpesviruses) or *fast acting* (human T-cell leukemia/lymphoma [lymphotrophic] virus, or HTLV) and are *tissue specific,* infecting tissue selectively. Age and immunocompetence are believed to interact with and affect a person's vulnerability to viral carcinogens.[12, 21, 38, 42]

The link between the Epstein-Barr virus (EBV) and Burkitt's lymphoma and nasopharyngeal cancer as well as the association between hepatitis B virus (HBV) and hepatocellular cancer has been firmly established. The herpes simplex type 2 virus (HSV-2) is believed to be linked to the development of cervical cancer, but the evidence is inconclusive. Cytomegaloviruses (CMVs) have been linked to Kaposi's sarcoma and are found in the tissues of persons with different cancers.[20, 28, 38] Table 1–4 provides additional information on oncogenic viruses.

Time-space clusters of persons with leukemia and Hodgkin's disease suggest an infectious etiology. However, other environmental factors may be equally significant in both these conditions. In the past, the importance of viruses in carcinogenesis was considered minimal; however, as more information is uncovered about these relationships, this is changing.[20, 28]

Radiation Carcinogenesis

Radiation is a carcinogen and has the potential to be a complete carcinogen. Damage to the cell by this source may give rise to cancer when damage affects proto-oncogenes or antioncogenes. The first documented evidence of radiation carcinogenesis was shown when skin cancer occurred as a result of chronic exposure to radioactive chemicals, x-rays, and other radioactive materials (e.g., paints). Radiation appears to initiate carcinogenesis by damaging susceptible DNA, producing changes in the DNA structure. These changes may be single- and

TABLE 1-4
Viruses Associated with Human Cancer

Virus*	Benign Proliferation	Associated Malignancies	Percentage of Tumors Containing Virus	Latency Period (Years)
EBV	Infectious mononucleosis Hairy leukoplakia	High-grade B-cell lymphoma	100	0.1–10
		Endemic Burkitt's lymphoma	>95	3–10
		Nasopharyngeal carcinoma	100	30–40
		Hodgkin's disease	40–50	10–30
		Peripheral T-cell lymphoma	30–40	10–30
HBV/HCV	Focal liver hyperplasia	Hepatocellular carcinoma (HCC)	>80	20–50
HPV-16,18	Neoplasia in situ	Cervical squamous cell cancer	>75	5–30
		Anorectal squamous cell cancer	>50 (in setting of HIV-1)	5–30
HPV-5,8/others	Papillomas	Squamous cell cancers (in the setting of epidermodysplasia verruciformis)	> 90	5–30
HTLV-1	Smouldering leukemia	Adult T-cell leukemia/lymphoma (ATLL)	100	20–50
HTLV-II		Chronic T-cell lymphoproliferative disorders	Anecdotal	20–50
HIV-1		Kaposi's sarcoma (KS)	0[†]	>10
		Non-Hodgkin's lymphoma (NHL)	0[†]	
		Anogenital carcinoma (HPV-associated)	0[†]	
			0[‡]	
		Hodgkin's disease (HD)		

* EBV, Epstein-Barr virus; HBV/HCV, hepatitis B/C viruses; HPV, human papilloma virus; HTLV, human T-cell leukemia virus; HIV, human immunodeficiency virus.
[†] 25–100× increased incidence in association with HIV seropositivity.
[‡] Severalfold increased risk in association with HIV seropositivity.
From Kurzrock R, Talpaz M, editors: Molecular biology in cancer medicine, ed 2, London, Martin Dunitz, 1999.

double-strand breaks or cross-linking of spiral changes. Cell death may result, or the cells may become permanently altered and escape normal control mechanisms.[12, 20, 28, 42]

Both *ionizing radiation* and *electromagnetic radiation* have been known to cause cancer in animals and humans. Sources of ionizing radiation exposure include radioactive ground minerals, diagnostic or therapeutic x-rays, and synthetic radioactive materials (e.g., radioisotopes). Less than 3% of human cancers have been related to ionizing radiation. Factors that apparently influence the risk of carcinogenesis by ionizing radiation include the following[12, 28, 38, 42]:

- Host characteristics—these include level of tissue oxygenation, genetic makeup, age, and degree of stress.
- Cell cycle phase—cells in G_2 phase are more sensitive than cells in S or G_1 phase.
- Degree of differentiation—immature cells are most vulnerable.
- Cellular proliferation rate—cells with high mitotic rates are most vulnerable.

- Tissue type—gastrointestinal and hematopoietic tissues are extremely sensitive to radiation.
- Rate of dose and total dose—the higher the dose rate and total dose, the greater is the chance for mutation to occur.

Sources of *ultraviolet light* (UVL) radiation include the sun and certain industrial sources (e.g., welding arcs, germicidal lights). The risk of developing skin cancer from sunlight is well documented. Sunlight is responsible for most cases of squamous and basal cell carcinomas of the skin. UVL from the sun has little ability to penetrate body tissues, leaving the skin most vulnerable to its effects. The longer and more intense the exposure to the sun, the greater is the chance of developing skin cancer. Persons at greatest risk are fair-skinned white individuals (Irish, Scotch, Welsh, albinos, those with xeroderma pigmentosum) and those who work outdoors. UVL increases the risk of basal cell epithelioma and melanoma.[20, 28, 38, 42]

The long latency period between exposure and tumor growth has hindered the evaluation of radiation as a carcinogen, but several types of human cancers have been associated with previous exposure to radiation. Leukemia, particularly acute myelogenous leukemia (AML) and chronic myelogenous leukemia (CML), lymphoma, skin cancer, osteosarcoma, and cancers of the lung, thyroid, and breast have all been shown to occur at varying lengths of time after radiation exposure.[21, 42]

Immune System in Carcinogenesis

The immune system normally controls the proliferation of potential cancer cells. Potentially cancerous cells constantly arise within the human body but are continously screened by the immune system and eliminated before a tumor can be established. Human immunity to malignant disease is a function of *humoral factors* (tumor-specific antibodies) and *cellular factors* (sensitized lymphocytes and macrophages). Cancer cells often possess antigens that differ from the person's own antigens and therefore are recognized as foreign cells by the immune system and are destroyed.[38]

Cancer should arise only when the immune system is overwhelmed, as in malnutrition, chronic disease, advancing age, and stress. Support for this theory comes from the recognition that immunosuppressed or immunodeficient persons have a much higher chance of developing cancer than persons with normal immune system function. When evaluated at the time of initial diagnosis, persons with cancer often have abnormal immune function. However, not all types of cancer are increased by immunodeficiency.[38]

Heredity and Carcinogenesis

Knowledge about the role of genetics in the process of carcinogenesis is expanding at a rapid rate, partly because of the worldwide *Human Genome Project.* This project, which began in 1990 and is scheduled to be completed before the end of 2000, seeks to locate, map, and sequence the more than 100,000 genes that comprise the human genome. The number of genetic markers available for clinical use to identify individuals and families with a potential hereditary predisposition to cancer (otherwise known as *hereditary cancer syndrome* or HCS) is growing due, in large part, to the Human Genome Project.[13, 31]

It is estimated that 5% to 10% of all cancers result from hereditary predisposition. An inherited predisposition to cancer may be suspected when families have more cases of cancer than one would expect to occur by chance. HCS is characterized by diagnosis of the same cancer in multiple family members across multiple generations, an earlier age of onset than one would expect, unique tumor site combinations, an increased number of bilateral cancers in paired organs, and the presence of precancerous syndromes and rare cancers.[31] For more information on genetics and cancer, see Chapter 2.

TUMOR NOMENCLATURE

Histogenetic Classification System

Tumors are grouped according to the tissue from which they originate and are described by the *histogenetic classification system.* In this classification system, tumors are described by Latin and Greek terms[5] (Table 1–5).

Benign tumors usually end in the suffix *oma,* the Greek root for *tumor.* When the suffix *oma* follows a prefix designating a specific tissue, a benign tumor can be identified. For example, fibromas and adenomas are benign tumors of fibrous and glandular tissue, respectively. Exceptions to this rule include hepatomas and melanomas. By name, these cancers should be benign. However, melanomas are malignant neoplasias of melanocytes, and hepatomas are malignant neoplasias of the liver.[18, 21, 37, 42]

Malignant tumors also use the suffix *oma* to designate the presence of a tumor. However, malignant tumors of epithelial origin are designated by the root *carcin,* crablike, and those of connective tissue origin are designated by the root *sarc,* flesh.[37, 42] *Sarcomas* comprise about 10% of human cancers. Prefixes that describe specific connective tissue sarcomas include the following[5, 20, 21, 37, 42]:

Osteo—sarcomas arising in the bone
Chondro—sarcomas arising from cartilage
Lipo—sarcomas arising from fat
Rhabdo—sarcomas arising from skeletal muscle
Leiomyo—sarcomas arising from smooth muscle

Carcinomas comprise about 80% of human cancers. Certain prefixes are used to describe the type of epithelial tissue from which carcinomas originate. For example, *adeno* describes tumors originating from glandular (columnar) epithelium. *Squamous* describes tumors arising from squamous epithelial tissue.[21, 37, 42]

Blastoma is a suffix used for neoplasms with histologic features suggesting origin in embryonal tissue. Examples include neuroblastoma, hepatoblastoma, nephroblastoma, and retinoblastoma (i.e., tumors that arise in the adrenal gland, liver, kidney, and retina, respectively). *Mixed tumors* contain more than one neoplastic cell type. *Teratomas* are a special type of mixed tumor and may be benign or malignant. These tumors arise from totipotential (germ) cells and may be composed of several differentiated tissue types. Teratomas arise from three germ layers: endoderm, ectoderm, and mesoderm.[18, 21, 42]

T A B L E   1 – 5
Classification of Neoplasms

Parent Tissue	Benign Tumor	Malignant Tumor
EPITHELIUM		
Skin and mucous membrane	Papilloma	Squamous cell carcinoma
	Polyp	Basal cell carcinoma
		Transitional cell carcinoma
Glands	Adenoma	Adenocarcinoma
	Cystadenoma	
ENDOTHELIUM		
Blood vessels	Hemangioma	Hemangiosarcoma
		Angiosarcoma
Lymph vessels	Lymphangioma	Lymphangiosarcoma
Bone marrow		Multiple myeloma
		Ewing's sarcoma
		Leukemia
		Lymphosarcoma
		Lymphangioendothelioma
Lymphoid tissue		Reticular cell sarcoma (difficult to classify because of cell embryology)
		Lymphatic leukemia
		Malignant lymphoma
CONNECTIVE TISSUE		
Embryonic fibrous tissue	Myxoma	Myxosarcoma
Fibrous tissue	Fibroma	Fibrosarcoma
Adipose tissue	Lipoma	Liposarcoma
Cartilage	Chondroma	Chondrosarcoma
Bone	Osteoma	Osteogenic sarcoma
Synovial membrane	Synovioma	Synovial sarcoma
MUSCLE TISSUE		
Smooth muscle	Leiomyoma	Leiomyosarcoma
Striated muscle	Rhabdomyoma	Rhabdomyosarcoma
NERVE TISSUE		
Nerve fibers and sheaths	Neuroma	Neurogenic sarcoma
	Neurinoma (neurilemoma)	
		Neurofibrosarcoma
Ganglion cells	Neurofibroma	Neuroblastoma
Glial cells	Ganglioneuroma	Glioblastoma
	Glioma	Spongioblastoma
Meninges	Meningioma	
PIGMENTED NEOPLASMS		
Melanoblasts	Pigmented nevus	Malignant melanoma
		Melanocarcinoma
MISCELLANEOUS		
Placenta	Hydatidiform mole	Chorion-epithelioma (choriocarcinoma)
	Dermoid cyst	Embryonal carcinoma
		Embryonal sarcoma
		Teratocarcinoma

From Phipps WJ, Sands JK, Marek JF, editors: Medical-surgical nursing: concepts and clinical practice, *ed 6, St Louis, Mosby, 1999.*

Hematologic Malignancies

Leukemia is a cancer of the hematologic system and is a diffuse rather than a solid tumor. This disease is characterized by the abnormal proliferation and release of leukocyte (white blood cell [WBC]) precursors. Leukemia is classified as either *lymphoid* or *myeloid* according to the predominant cell type and as *acute* or *chronic* according to the level of maturity shown by the predominant cell. Acute leukemia is characterized by the proliferation of primitive WBCs; chronic leukemia is characterized by the proliferation of mature cells. The prefix *lympho* describes a leukemia of lymphoid (lymphatic system) origin. The prefix *myelo* or *granulo* describes a leukemia of myeloid (bone marrow) origin. The suffix *blastic* describes immature WBCs, whereas the suffix *cystic* describes the presence of more mature cells. For example, acute lymphoblastic leukemia describes a WBC disease that involves immature cells of lymphoid origin.[38, 42] For additional information on leukemia, see Chapter 14.

Malignant lymphoma is a cancer of the lymphoid tissue. Both non-Hodgkin's lymphoma and Hodgkin's disease are classified according to four primary features: cell type, degree of differentiation, type of reaction elicited by tumor cells, and growth patterns. If a nodular growth pattern is observed, the term *nodular* is used after the cell type. If no mention of growth pattern is made, the lymphoma is of a *diffuse* type.[38, 42] For additional information on lymphoma, see Chapter 16.

Multiple myeloma is a cancerous proliferation of plasma cells (B lymphocytes). It is characterized by bone marrow involvement, bone destruction, and the presence of a homogeneous immunoglobulin in the urine or serum.[21, 42] For additional information on multiple myeloma, see Chapter 17.

ROUTES OF TUMOR SPREAD

Cancer may remain a locally invasive process, or it may spread to nonadjacent areas by hematogenous or lymphatic channels. Some tumors exhibit an orderly pattern of progression. Initially, they grow locally, and as tumor growth continues, tumor cells spread to and colonize regional nodes. Finally, distant metastases occur. Other tumors metastasize to distant organs before or with their spread to regional nodes. Because there are different patterns of tumor spread, it is important to determine the extent of disease in the patient with cancer.[22]

The spread of cancer depends on a series of events that occur at the surface of the tumor cell and in the vascular bed of the person with cancer. The spread of cancer cells from a primary tumor occurs by two major processes: *direct spread* to contiguous areas or *metastatic spread* to nonadjacent tissues. Dissemination of cancer cells may not be limited to only one process because spread by one route may permit entry into another.[12, 23, 43]

Direct Spread

Direct invasion is the ability of a tumor to penetrate and destroy adjoining tissue.[12, 21, 42] Factors believed to enhance this process include:

- *Tumor angiogenesis factor.* This substance, when secreted by cancer cells, stimulates new capillary formation. Once a tumor becomes vascularized, its growth rate increases and its ability to invade local tissue is enhanced.[12, 23]
- *Mechanical pressure and rate of tumor growth.* Rapid tumor growth creates an intratumor pressure that forces finger-like projections of cancer cells into adjacent tissues. Uncontrolled replication produces densely packed and expanding tumor masses that exert pressure on adjacent tissues. Tumors extend into normal tissue along natural fracture lines that part in response to mechanical pressure.[11, 23]
- *Cell motility and loss of cellular adhesiveness.* Cancer cells have a propensity for locomotion, and this, coupled with the slippery nature of cancer cells, promotes tumor cell dispersion.[20]
- *Tumor-secreted enzymes.* Recent research documents a strong association between the invasive potential of some tumor cells and the intracellular levels of specific enzymes (e.g., *plasminogen activator*). These enzymes may play a role in the destruction of normal tissue barriers, allowing invasion of cancer cells.[21]

Direct spread of tumor cells also occurs by *serosal seeding.* After tumor cells spread locally into tissue and penetrate body cavities, these cells can embolize, attaching to the serosal surfaces of organs within the cavity. Serosal seeding commonly occurs with lung and ovarian tumors. Although tumor cells implant on the surface of organs in the pleural and peritoneal cavities, tumor cell infiltration into the parenchyma of the organ is uncommon.[12]

Surgical instrumentation also provides a direct pathway for the spread of cancer cells. Contamination of normal tissue can occur during the course of surgical procedures (e.g., diagnostic biopsy, paracentesis). Tumor cells may be seeded by needles as the needles are withdrawn, or manipulation of the tumor during surgery may release cells into the circulation.[12]

Metastatic Spread

Metastasis is derived from the Greek prefix *meta*, indicating a change. This process permits the release of cells from the primary site and subsequent spread and attachment to structures in distant sites (Fig. 1–4). A cancer cell's ability to invade adjacent tissues and metastasize to distant sites is its most virulent property. This is an important characteristic of cancer. Benign tumors do not metastasize. Approximately 30% of patients with solid tumors have clinically detectable metastasis at the time of initial diagnosis. An additional 20% to 30% of patients have occult micrometastases at the time of

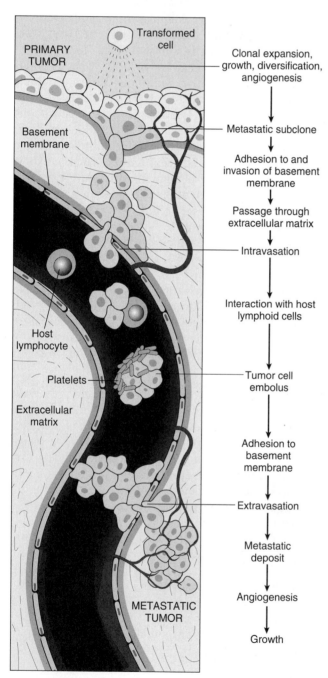

FIGURE 1–4 The metastatic cascade. (From Cotran RS, Kumar V, Collins T, Robbins SL, editors: *Robbins pathologic basis of disease,* ed 6, Philadelphia, Saunders, 1999.)

initial treatment of the primary tumor. As many as 75% of those persons with cancer who die have metastatic lesions in the liver, and it is estimated that liver failure is the direct cause of death in 40% of persons with liver involvement. Anorexia and cachexia secondary to metastatic disease are also frequent causes of death.[12, 20, 26, 30, 38, 43]

The sequence of events in the metastatic process by *hematogenous channels* (dissemination of tumor cells through veins or arteries) is as follows:

- *Growth and progression of the primary tumor.* The first requirement for metastasis is rapid growth of the primary tumor. Most tumors must reach 10 billion cells or 1 cm in size before metastasis is possible.[20, 24]
- *Angiogenesis at the primary site.* As in direct invasion, release of tumor angiogenesis factor stimulates new capillary formation. An avascular tumor is rarely metastatic. It has been shown experimentally that tumor cells do not enter the bloodstream until after the primary tumor has been vascularized.[2, 23]
- *Detachment.* Cancer cells are more motile than normal cells. The period of least cellular adhesiveness is during mitosis; a tumor with a high mitotic index might be able to detach more cells than normal tissue. In the advancing tips of a tumor's capillaries, wide gaps exist between these endothelial cells, and there is no basement membrane in the foremost part of the capillaries. This may explain the apparent ease with which tumor cells can enter the bloodstream from a vascularized tumor.[2, 23]
- *Circulation of tumor cells.* Tumor cells have been found in the bloodstream of patients and animals with vascularized tumors. In some animal tumors, cancer cells are shed into the circulation continuously—as many as 1 million cells per day. However, most of these cells usually die. Only about 1% or fewer survive to become a viable metastatic lesion. It seems that the circulatory system itself is cytotoxic. The longer tumor cells circulate in the bloodstream, the higher their death rate. Factors that inhibit coagulation also keep tumor cells circulating and reduce the number of tumor emboli that attach to the vascular bed. Other causes of cell death have been proposed, such as immunologic destruction of circulating tumor cells.[6, 9, 20, 23]
- *Arrest of tumor cells on vascular endothelium.* After entering the bloodstream, tumor cells aggregate with lymphocytes, platelets, or other tumor cells and form a fibrin-platelet clot. This protects the tumor cells from the hostile environment and promotes metastasis by enhancing their ability to adhere to the capillary walls of the target organ.[12]
- *Site predilection.* Site predilection does not depend on the anatomy of the circulation as previously believed.

In the figure labels (Fig. 1–4):
- Transformed cell
- PRIMARY TUMOR
- Basement membrane
- Host lymphocyte
- Platelets
- Extracellular matrix
- METASTATIC TUMOR
- Clonal expansion, growth, diversification, angiogenesis
- Metastatic subclone
- Adhesion to and invasion of basement membrane
- Passage through extracellular matrix
- Intravasation
- Interaction with host lymphoid cells
- Tumor cell embolus
- Adhesion to basement membrane
- Extravasation
- Metastatic deposit
- Angiogenesis
- Growth

Tumor cells flow through the circulatory system based on venous drainage from the primary tumor. However, the site and survival of disseminated tumor cells depend on the *qualities* and *properties unique to the tumor cell* itself. Certain tumor cells possess an affinity for specific organs. The metastatic process is not random.[14, 20, 23, 27, 33]

- *Escape from the circulation.* Once implanted into the vessel wall of the chosen organ, tumor cells must exit the organ's circulation and penetrate its tissue to proliferate (*extravasation*). This process is complex. Arrested tumor cells appear to damage the intact endothelium of the blood vessel by compression. Once the endothelium is damaged, tumor cells escape through the vessel wall and invade the organ tissue itself[8, 12, 23] (Fig. 1–5).

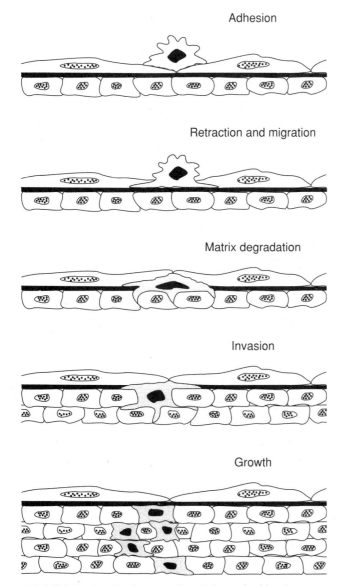

Adhesion

Retraction and migration

Matrix degradation

Invasion

Growth

FIGURE 1 – 5 Cancer cells exit from the bloodstream.

- *Angiogenesis of metastatic implant.* Once tumor cells arrive in the extravascular tissue, they continue to grow as a small cluster up to about 10 million cells. Continued growth, however, requires the induction of new capillaries. Without an adequate blood supply, tumor cells remain dormant and harmless, receiving only enough diffused nutrition to maintain viability. New blood vessels, induced again by the tumor's release of tumor angiogenesis factor, are needed for the continued growth of the new metastatic lesion.[12, 17, 23]

Lymphatic spread occurs when the cancer cells penetrate lymphatic channels draining the affected site. Much less is known about this mechanism versus spread of cancer cells by hematogenous channels. In many cancers the first evidence of spread of disease is a mass in the lymph nodes that drain the area or region of the body carrying the tumor. Previously it was thought that the filtering action of lymph nodes was responsible for nodal metastasis, but recent research shows that filtration is a relatively minor factor. The physiochemical changes on the cancer cell's surface and lymph node interaction may also be important in determining whether and where cancer cells become lodged in lymph nodes. Conventional thinking also asserts that lymph nodes become positive primarily for anatomic reasons, because the lymph nodes that drain the primary tumor are often positive first. This is a naive assumption, however, for the same reason it is now realized that hematogenous metastases are not random or completely directed by anatomy. In some instances, metastatic tumor cells bypass local lymph nodes and seed in more distant nodes in the lymph chain.[21, 42]

Several outcomes await those cancer cells that do become lodged in lymph nodes. They may die as a result of local inflammation or the encountered environment; they can grow into a lump; or they can remain dormant for unknown reasons. A significant feature of the lymphatic system is that the main lymphatic trunk enters the venous system just before the veins enter the heart. Therefore the lymphatic and circulatory systems are interconnected, and cancer cells that enter the lymphatic system are able to enter the bloodstream as well.[21, 42]

Carcinomatosis, the extensive dissemination of tumor cells by gravity, may also be a causal factor of metastasis. During the spread of cancer over the serous membranes of larger cavities (e.g., pleural, peritoneal), cancer cells may break away and gravitate to the lower reaches of the cavity.[21]

Host and Treatment Factors as Modifiers of Metastasis

Several factors and conditions modify the frequency of metastasis. Factors known to *increase* the likelihood of metastasis include a primary tumor of long duration; a high mitotic rate; trauma, including biopsy and tumor massage; heat; radiation; and chemotherapy. Factors known to *decrease* the likelihood of metastasis include those that reduce tumor cell adherence to endothelial cells, retard intravascular coagulation, and kill tumor cells.[21]

Although the search continues for the key cellular factors that determine metastatic potential, all that is known to date in regard to clinical application is that undifferentiated tumors are more likely to metastasize than differentiated tumors. Even with histologically similar tumors, however, individuals can exhibit different metastatic disease patterns. This suggests that host factors, such as hormonal environment and age, are important in determining how, and whether, tumors will metastasize.[21]

Other Aspects of the Metastatic Process

Metastases from Metastasis. Because a metastatic tumor is penetrated by new blood vessels in the same manner as a primary tumor, the secondary implant itself may release cells in the circulation, leading to tertiary implants. This is an important clinical concern. The decision about when, or whether, to remove metastatic lesions surgically depends partly on the threat of further metastases from a metastasis.[21, 23]

Inhibitory Effect of Primary Tumors. Remarkable evidence indicates that a primary tumor can inhibit the growth of already established metastatic lesions and in some cases can inhibit implantation. The strength of this inhibition is directly related to tumor mass. This may explain the increased growth rate of existing metastatic lesions observed after a primary tumor is removed. It also provides further substantiation for initiating adjuvant chemotherapy after surgical resection of an advanced primary tumor instead of waiting for the first metastasis to appear.[21, 24, 40]

Dormancy. Metastatic growth may appear in persons many years after apparent cure of a primary tumor. For example, in breast cancer, metastases can appear in the vertebrae 30 years after the original diagnosis. Presumably, metastatic tumor cells remain dormant for periods far beyond what would be expected based on logarithmic division of cells. Investigators do not know what causes metastatic tumor cells to go into a dormant stage and remain dormant or what causes them to eventually reemerge. Of all aspects of metastasis, this is the least understood.[21, 24]

CONCLUSION

The essential features of the cancer cell that distinguish it from the normal cell are its ability to reproduce uncon-

trollably, invade normal tissue, disseminate to distant body sites, and destroy the host. These factors constitute the essence of the transformed cell.[20]

The nurse involved in the care of patients with cancer must comprehend the principles of normal and abnormal cellular physiology.[42] These principles form the basis for defining the essential concepts related to the nursing care of the individual with cancer (e.g., teaching about health promotion and prevention, diagnosis, treatment, and follow-up) and determining implications for the professional development of the oncology nurse (e.g., use of appropriate terminology and nomenclature necessary for teaching and interdisciplinary communication; understanding rationale for treatment protocols, timing of treatment, follow-up, intensity of initial treatment protocols, current research and trends in care, and disease prognoses; initiating cancer nursing research; enhancing participation in discussion of ethical issues related to cancer and treatment).

CASE STUDY

Your patient, Mrs. W., a 65-year-old white woman, is admitted for a right lobectomy for stage II non–small-cell lung cancer. Mrs. W. has never smoked in her life. She did, however, work as a waitress in various diners during the 1960s and 1970s, and her husband has smoked two packs of cigarettes per day for 40 years (80 pack-years). Mrs. W. does not have a family history of lung cancer. During your preoperative evaluation of Mrs. W., she asks, "Why has this happened to me? I never smoked a day in my life!" Discuss how you would respond to her question and statement.

Chapter Questions

1. A *rhabdosarcoma* arises from:
   a. Bone
   b. Smooth muscle
   c. Skeletal muscle
   d. Cartilage
2. *Polymorphism* means that many cancer cells:
   a. Contain unusual numbers of chromosomes
   b. Have large nuclei
   c. Vary in size and shape
   d. Contain abnormal chromosome arrangements
3. The five *phases of the cell cycle* are:
   a. G_1, S_1, G_2, S_2, and M
   b. G_0, S_1, G_1, S_2, and M
   c. G_0, G_1, S, G_2, and M
   d. G_1, G_2, S_1, S_2, and M
4. *Decreased contact inhibition of movement* allows a cancer cell to:
   a. Invade neighboring tissues
   b. Adhere to other cancer cells

c. Assume a more rotund shape

d. Continue to divide

5. Death usually occurs when the body burden of tumor equals or exceeds:

    a. 1 g

    b. 10 g

    c. 0.1 g

    d. 1 kg

6. *Growth fraction* is:

    a. The time needed for a tumor mass to double its volume

    b. The minimum clinically detectable body burden of tumor

    c. Cell numbers increasing in powers of two

    d. The ratio of the total number of cells in a tumor to the number of proliferating cells

7. A malignant tumor that originates in connective tissue is a:

    a. Sarcoma

    b. Adenoma

    c. Carcinoma

    d. Fibroma

8. Hyperplasia:

    a. Is an increase in the number of cells of a certain tissue type

    b. Is an increase in cell size

    c. Occurs when one cell type is substituted for another not usually found in the involved tissue

    d. Occurs when a mature cell is replaced with a cell that is less mature

9. In cancer, *complete carciogens*:

    a. Alter the expression of genetic information of a cell

    b. Inhibit the effects of promoting agents

    c. Are capable of inducing cancer on their own

    d. Control the growth and repair of tissues

10. Factors influencing the risk of cancer by ionizing radiation include:

    a. Tissue type

    b. Host characteristics

    c. Cell cycle phase

    d. All of the above

BIBLIOGRAPHY

1. American Cancer Society: *Cancer facts and figures—2000,* Atlanta, The Society, 2000.

2. Ausprunk DH, Folkman J: Migration and proliferation of endothelial cells in preformed and newly formed blood vessels during tumor angiogenesis, *Microvasc Res* 14:53, 1977.

3. Bender C: Implications of antineoplastic therapy for nursing. In Clark JC, McGee RF, editors: *Core curriculum for oncology nursing,* ed 2, Philadelphia, Saunders, 1992.

4. Berenblum I: Established principles and unresolved problems in carcinogenesis, *J Natl Cancer Inst* 60:723, 1978.

5. Black JM, Matassarin-Jacobs E, editors: *Luckmann and Sorensen's medical-surgical nursing: a psychophysiologic approach,* ed 4, Philadelphia, Saunders, 1993.

6. Butler TP, Gullino PM: Quantitation of cell shedding into efferent blood of mammary adenocarcinoma, *Cancer Res* 35:512, 1975.

7. Calabresi P, Schein PS, Rosenberg SA, editors: *Medical oncology: basic principles and clinical management of cancer,* ed 2, New York, McGraw-Hill, 1993.

8. Chew EC, Josephson RL, Wallace AC: Morphologic aspects of the arrest of circulating cancer cells. In Weiss L, editor: *Fundamental aspects of metastasis,* Amsterdam, North-Holland, 1975.

9. Clifton EE, Agostino D: The effects of fibrin formation and alterations in the clotting mechanism on the development of metastases, *Vasc Dis* 2:43, 1965.

10. DeVita VT Jr, Hellman S, Rosenberg SA, editors: *Cancer: principles and practice of oncology,* ed 5, Philadelphia, Lippincott, 1997.

11. Dexter DL, Calabresi P: Intraneoplastic diversity, *Biochim Biophys Acta* 695:97, 1982.

12. Donehower MG: The behavior of malignancies. In Johnson BL, Gross J, editors: *Handbook of oncology nursing,* New York, Wiley, 1985.

13. Engelking C: The human genome exposed: a glimpse of promise, predicament, and impact on practice, *Oncol Nurs Forum* 22(2 suppl):3, 1995.

14. Fidler IJ: Selection of successive tumor lives for metastases, *Nature New Biol* 242:148, 1973.

15. Fidler IJ: The evolution of biological heterogeneity in metastatic neoplasms. In Nicholson GL, Miles L, editors: *Cancer invasion and metastasis: biologic and therapeutic aspects,* New York, Raven, 1984.

16. Fidler IJ, Hart IR: Biological diversity in metastatic neoplasms: origins and implications, *Science* 217:998, 1982.

17. Folkman J, Cotran RS: Relation of vascular proliferation to tumor growth. In Richter GW, Epstein MA, editors: *International review of experimental pathology,* New York, Academic, 1976.

18. Goldfarb S: Pathology of neoplasia. In Kahn SB and others, editors: *Concepts in cancer medicine,* New York, Grune & Stratton, 1983.

19. Greenlee RT, Murray T, Bolden S, Wingo PA: Cancer Statistics, 2000. *CA Cancer J Clin* 50(1):7, 2000.

20. Griffiths MJ, Murray KH, Russo PC: *Oncology nursing: pathophysiology, assessment, and intervention,* New York, Macmillan, 1984.

21. Groenwald SL and others, editors: *Cancer nursing: principles and practice,* ed 4, Boston, Jones & Bartlett, 1997.

22. Haskell CM, editor: *Cancer treatment,* ed 4, Philadelphia, Saunders, 1995.

23. Holland G: Pathophysiological features of cancer: clinical knowledge for nurses. In McIntire SN, Cioppa AL, editors: *Cancer nursing: a developmental approach,* New York, Wiley, 1984.

24. Holland JF, editor: *Cancer medicine,* ed 4, Philadelphia, Williams & Wilkins, 1997.

25. Jordan VC: Hormones. In Kahn SB and others, editors: *Concepts in cancer medicine,* New York, Grune & Stratton, 1983.

26. Kinsey DL: An experimental study of preferential metastases, *Cancer* 13:674, 1960.

27. Kirkpatrick CS: *Nurse's guide to cancer care,* Totowa, NJ, Rowman, 1986.

28. Laishes BA: Local growth of neoplasms. In Kahn SB and others, editors: *Concepts in cancer medicine.* New York, Grune & Stratton, 1983.

29. Lydon J: Metastasis. Part I. Biology and prevention, *Oncol Nurs* 2(5):1, 1995.

30. Mahon SM, Casperson DS: Hereditary cancer syndrome. Part 1. Clinical and educational issues, *Oncol Nurs Forum* 22(5):763, 1995.

31. Marx J: Cell growth control takes balance, *Science* 239:975, 1988.

32. Nicolson G: Organ specificity of tumor metastasis: role of preferential adhesion, invasion and growth of malignant cells at specific secondary sites, *Cancer Metastasis Rev* 7:143, 1988.

33. Otto SE: *Pocket guide to intravenous therapy,* ed 4, St Louis, Mosby, 2001.

34. Potter VR: The cancer cell. In Kahn SB and others, editors: *Concepts in cancer medicine,* New York, Grune & Stratton, 1983.

35. Ruddon R: *Cancer biology,* New York, Oxford University Press, 1981.

36. Sirica AE: Pathogenesis. In Kahn SB and others, editors: *Concepts in cancer medicine,* New York, Grune & Stratton, 1983.

37. Sirica AE: Classification of neoplasms. In Sirica AE, editor: *The pathobiology of neoplasia,* New York, Plenum, 1989.

38. Snyder CC: *Oncology nursing,* Boston, Little, Brown, 1986.

39. Stellman JM, Stellman SD: Cancer and the workplace, *CA Cancer J Clin* 46(2):70, 1996.

40. Sugarbaker EV, Thornthwaite J, Ketcham AS: Inhibitory effect of primary tumor on metastasis. In Day SB, editor: *Cancer invasion and metastasis,* New York, Raven, 1977.

41. Thompson JM and others: *Mosby's clinical nursing,* ed 3, St Louis, Mosby, 1993.

42. Volker DL: Pathophysiology of cancer. In Clark JC, McGee RF, editors: *Core curriculum for oncology nursing,* ed 2, Philadelphia, Saunders, 1992.

43. Wolberg WH: Metastasis. In Kahn SB and others, editors: *Concepts in cancer medicine,* New York, Grune & Stratton, 1983.

44. Yunis JJ, Hoffman WR: Fragile sites as a mechanism in carcinogenesis, *Cancer Bull* 41:283, 1989.

Genetics

CHAPTER 2

Carol Pappas Appel

The last decade has seen an explosion in the field of genetics and its role in the development of cancer. The knowledge that cancer is a genetic disease, the discovery of oncogenes, proto-oncogenes, and tumor suppressor genes, the identification of cancer predisposition genes, and the ability to test individuals at high risk for specific mutations in these cancer-causing genes are but a few of the strides made in cancer genetics. We are heading into the new millenium with the assurance that new discoveries affecting the care of cancer patients and their families will rapidly occur. As oncology nurses, we will play an active role in the education and support of patients related to their cancer risks, their options for screening, testing, and treatment, and the impact of hereditary predisposition on their lives and those of their families.

As part of the multidisciplinary cancer genetics team, the oncology nurse must possess the knowledge and understanding of basic genetics, the components of a cancer risk assessment, the purpose and process of genetic counseling, and the options for prevention and screening available to individuals at increased risk of developing cancer.[17]

OVERVIEW OF GENETICS

To understand the relationship between genetics and cancer development, it is helpful to review the basic components, such as chromosomes, genes, DNA, and the principles of inheritance.

Chromosomes are packages of genes and are located within the cell nucleus. Human cells contain 46 chromosomes, 23 inherited from each parent. Forty-four chromosomes (or 22 pairs) are autosomes and two are sex chromosomes. Each chromosome has a long arm "q" and a short arm "p." These arms are separated by the *centromere*. Each gene has a specific location on the chromosome known as its *genetic locus*. The genetic locus is identified first by the number of the chromosome, next by its location on the chromosome arm (ei-

ther p or q), and finally, by its position on the arm with respect to the centromere. The lower the number the closer the gene is to the centromere.[88, 89, 104]

Genes are the fundamental units of heredity. There are approximately 50,000 to 100,000 genes in the human genome. Each gene is composed of DNA that carries the instructions for protein formation. DNA is made up of sugar phosphate molecules and nucleotide bases. A base from one DNA strand pairs with a specific base from the other DNA strand within the DNA spiral, double helix. Together, they form one of the approximately 3 billion base pairs within the DNA. The base pairs form patterns that make up specific genetic codes for sequences of amino acids that form proteins.[88, 89] Proteins synthesized by cells are determined by the specific sequence of amino acids. Twenty different amino acids make up proteins. These proteins then exert their effects on the cells. They can act as enzymes or hormones, or determine the physical structure of cells, organs, and so on.[49, 104]

Specific regions within genes are responsible for the coding of proteins. These areas are known as *exons*. The large noncoding areas between exons are the *introns*. Introns are sometimes referred to as junk DNA because they have no specific coding function. Introns compose about 70% of DNA. During protein synthesis, the genetic code is copied from the exon regions of the DNA to the messenger RNA (mRNA). The intron regions are not copied to mRNA. The mRNA leaves the nucleus with the compacted genetic code and enters the ribosomes within the cellular cytoplasm (Fig. 2-1). Here, transfer RNA (tRNA) converts the genetic code into a chain of amino acids to form proteins.[88, 89]

Any change in the normal DNA base pair sequencing results in a *mutation* (Fig. 2-2). Changes can occur as a result of copying errors during DNA synthesis or injuries to the cell by outside carcinogens. Under normal circumstances, cells have the capability to correct these mistakes or to program cell death in the event that the errors cannot be corrected. Some mutations have no

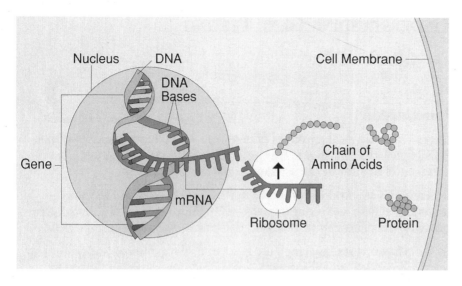

FIGURE 2–1 Protein synthesis. (From National Institutes of Health, National Cancer Institute. Understanding gene testing. Rockville, MD, U.S. Department of Health and Human Services, NIH Publication no. 96-3905, 1995.)

significant effect on protein function. Disease-associated mutations do alter protein function and can result in genetic instability, unregulated cell growth, and tumorigenesis.[49, 104]

There are a variety of mutation types. The most frequently seen mutation is the misspelling of a single DNA base. This *missense mutation* occurs when the wrong base is substituted. A *nonsense mutation* occurs when a base pair is completely lost. A *frameshift mutation* can result when one base is lost (frameshift deletion) or added (frameshift insertion), shifting the reading of subsequent bases. This causes a change in the amino acid that is supposed to be coded for and, thus, a change in the protein formed.[6, 66] Mutations may be inherited or acquired. Inherited or *"germline" mutations,* occur in germ cells (ova and sperm). The mutation is then passed on to offspring in all the body cells (Fig. 2–3). Germline mutations make up only a small percentage of all cancers.[18, 54]

Acquired or *somatic mutations* occur after birth and, therefore, are not inherited. An alteration in DNA occurs as a result of chance or exposure to cancer-causing agents. The mutations are found in the tumor cells of the affected organ, not in all body cells, as seen with germline mutations. Most cancers are thought to occur in this manner. A single exposure or genetic change is usually not sufficient to cause a cancer to occur. Rather, multiple changes and multiple exposures over many years result in the development of cancer.[18, 54, 55]

Knudsen's *two-hit hypothesis* describes a model for carcinogenesis in which two genetic events occur, resulting in the loss of both copies of a tumor suppressor

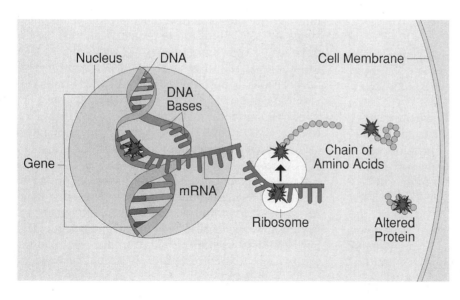

FIGURE 2–2 Gene mutation resulting in altered protein. (From National Institutes of Health, National Cancer Institute. Understanding gene testing. Rockville, MD, U.S. Department of Health and Human Services, NIH Publication no. 96-3905, 1995.)

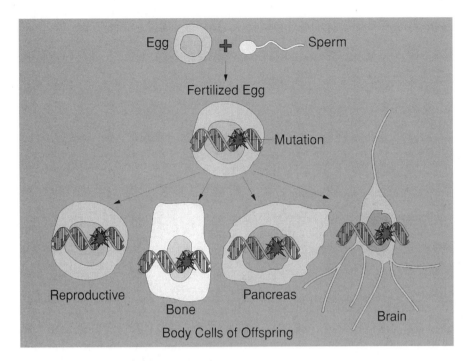

FIGURE 2 – 3 Hereditary mutation. (From National Institutes of Health, National Cancer Institute. Understanding gene testing. Rockville, MD, U.S. Department of Health and Human Services, NIH Publication no. 96-3905, 1995.)

Egg + Sperm

Fertilized Egg

Mutation

Reproductive

Bone

Pancreas

Brain

Body Cells of Offspring

gene. Without this "off switch," unregulated cell growth leads to cancer. In the individual who has inherited a mutated copy of a tumor suppressor gene (the first "hit"), there is only one functional copy remaining. This individual is at greater risk of developing a cancer than someone without an inherited mutation. Only one additional genetic event or somatic mutation (the second "hit") is needed to eliminate the remaining functional copy of the tumor suppressor gene resulting in tumorigenesis.[18, 24] (Refer to Chapter 1 for a complete review of the multistep process of carcinogenesis.)

Mutations are inherited in a dominant or recessive pattern. With *autosomal dominant inheritance,* only one parent is needed to donate a copy of a mutated gene for a disease to be expressed. The disease is seen in males and females, over several generations (a vertical pattern of inheritance), and is usually considered highly penetrant (the frequency of disease occurrence), meaning the risk of developing cancer is high. There is a 50% chance that each offspring of a mutation carrier will inherit a copy of the mutated gene.[24, 66, 84]

Autosomal recessive inheritance occurs when both parents carry a single gene mutation. As carriers, the parents do not actually have the disease. Their offspring have a 50% chance of inheriting a single copy of the mutated gene and, thus, becoming a carrier, a 25% chance of inheriting a copy of the mutated gene from each parent and expressing the disease, and a 25% chance of not inheriting a mutated gene copy from either parent, thus, not becoming a carrier or expressing the disease. Often several members of the same generation

are affected (horizontal pattern of inheritance) and both genders can be affected.[24, 66]

X-linked inheritance is caused by genetic mutations on the X chromosome. The mutations are passed through the mother and can be either dominant or recessive. With X-linked dominant inheritance, both genders have a 50% chance of inheriting a copy of the mutated gene and expressing the disease and a 50% chance of not inheriting the mutation or the disease. With X-linked recessive inheritance, there is a 50% chance of a woman passing a mutation to a son (who would express the disease) or a daughter (who would be a carrier) and a 50% chance of passing a normal copy of the gene to her offspring.[24, 66]

GENETICS AND CANCER DEVELOPMENT

Whether a mutation is inherited or acquired, cancer develops when sufficient damage is done to DNA to cause cells to transform from normal to malignant. Normally, cells are regulated by keeping growth-promoting genes and growth-suppressing genes evenly balanced. If there is a mutation in one of these key regulator genes, cell growth continues unchecked, leading to cancer development.[18, 89]

Oncogenes are the mutated form of proto-oncogenes. *Proto-oncogenes* are the normal growth-promoting genes. When a mutation occurs in a proto-oncogene, the resulting oncogene causes excessive production of growth factors responsible for tumorigenesis. Oncogenes can be activated when only one allele of each gene pair has mutated.[2, 16, 18, 53]

Antioncogenes, or *tumor suppressor genes,* are the normal growth-suppressing genes. They function by encoding proteins that block growth-promoting proteins. When a mutation occurs in a tumor suppressor gene, the cell loses its "off switch," allowing cell growth to proceed unabated. The most common tumor suppressor gene mutation is found in the p53 gene. Mutations in p53 are seen in half of all cancers. Normally, p53 functions by halting the cell cycle in the G_1 phase, allowing DNA repair genes to correct mistakes in DNA copying. In the event that the mistakes cannot be corrected, p53 induces *apoptosis,* or programmed cell death. When the p53 gene is mutated, cells are able to replicate without repairing DNA damage, resulting in uncontrolled abnormal cell growth. Tumor suppressor genes must have mutations in both copies of the gene to cause tumorigenesis.[16, 49, 53]

Mutations can also occur in the genes responsible for the repair of DNA mistakes. When these mismatch repair genes are damaged, corrections are not made in the DNA copy, allowing these errors to be propagated. In essence, the cell loses its "spell check" capabilities, causing mutations to accumulate at thousands of sites.[49, 66]

THE HUMAN GENOME PROJECT

The Human Genome Project is an international effort, begun in 1990, coordinated by the National Institutes of Health and the U.S. Department of Energy. The goals of the project are to:

1. Develop a genetic map
2. Develop a physical map
3. Sequence the entire genome
4. Develop technologies
5. Investigate the ethical, legal, and social implications of the project

This project was originally expected to conclude in 2005, but due to the continuing advances in technology, the project was completed in June 2000. The information obtained from this project will affect cancer prevention, early detection and treatment in the short term, and hopefully, eradication of cancer in the long run.[13, 79]

HEREDITARY AND SPORADIC CANCERS

About 90% of cancers are not inherited. Hereditary cancers are those cancers that arise from germline mutations. They exhibit certain features that distinguish them from sporadic or familial cancers. Hereditary cancers are diagnosed at an earlier age, usually 15 to 20 years earlier than cancers that are not inherited. Often, several relatives have the same or related cancers, they are more likely to be bilateral, and multiple cancers are seen in single individuals. These multiple cancers are often seen in unusual organ combinations, such as breast and sarcoma, breast and thyroid, leukemia and brain tumors. Hereditary cancers are characterized by the presence of precursor lesions, such as polyps in colorectal cancer and dysplastic nevi in melanoma.[24, 97]

Sporadic cancers are those seen in the general population and, therefore, make up the majority of all cancers diagnosed. Their incidence increases with age, usually beyond the sixth decade of life. There are few cancers in the family, they are rarely bilateral, and rarely are associated with a precursor lesion.[24, 49]

Familial cancers can also occur that do not appear to be inherited. A number of family members may have cancer, but they are usually diagnosed at the same age as the general population. The cancers may be the result of a shared life-style or environmental exposure. As with sporadic cancers, there is no autosomal dominant pattern of inheritance, bilaterality, or multiple cancers in individual family members. This is an important distinction, for although the cancers occur within families, they are sporadic in nature and not the result of an inherited mutation in a cancer-susceptibility gene.[24]

CANCER RISK ASSESSMENT

When an individual or family is suspected of having a mutation in a cancer-causing gene, a cancer risk assessment is performed. This is the first step toward identifying hereditary cancer predisposition. The process of risk assessment begins with a comprehensive family history. Information is obtained from the individual (the "proband") regarding his or her first-, second-, and third-degree relatives. First-degree relatives include the person's parents, siblings, and children. Second-degree relatives are maternal and paternal grandparents, aunts and uncles (parents' siblings), nieces and nephews. Third-degree relatives include first cousins, grandparents' siblings, and great grandparents. Information is collected on all relatives, regardless of whether or not they are affected with cancer. It is essential to identify all unaffected relatives, because this is important information when assessing a family for potential inheritance patterns. Each individual's name, date of birth, and date and cause of death (when applicable) are recorded. In family members affected with cancer, additional information regarding type of cancer(s) and age when diagnosed, is obtained, along with information on any known environmental or occupational exposures. The family's ethnic background is determined because there are known mutations seen with increased frequency among certain ethnic groups, such specific BRCA-1 and BRCA-2 mutations in individuals of Ashkenazi Jewish descent.[35] It is also important to determine if any family member has already been found to have a mutation in an autosomal dominant cancer-susceptibility gene. This would confer a 50% risk of such a mutation being passed to the individual's first-degree relatives, 25% risk of mutation to second-degree relatives, and 12.5% risk of mutation in third-degree relatives.[18, 42, 44, 84]

Once the detailed family history is completed, medical records are obtained. These records are necessary to confirm the cancer diagnoses identified in the family history. Confirmation is a critical step in the risk assessment process. In some instances, family members who were thought to have cancer actually are found to have benign or premalignant conditions on review of the medical records. Conversely, family members who were not known to have a malignancy have in fact been found to have a cancer diagnosis that increases the family's risk for genetic mutation. The records usually requested include pathology reports, autopsy reports, death certificates, and discharge summaries from hospitalizations. Confirmation of cancer diagnoses through medical record analysis provides the client with the most accurate risk analysis possible.[24]

Physical examination is another component of the risk assessment. In certain suspected inherited conditions, specific physical findings may be manifest. A directed physical examination would be important to identify these findings for further evaluation and recommendations.[42]

During the cancer risk assessment process, it is helpful to identify the individual's perception of the risk of inheriting a mutation in a cancer-susceptibility gene, as well as the risk of developing cancer. Individuals both under- and overestimate their risk, depending on a number of factors. Previous experiences with cancer in a family member, perceptions that cancer is a "death sentence," individual personality traits and coping behaviors, and cultural and religious beliefs play a role in the client's ability to process information learned during risk assessment and genetic counseling.[42, 78, 85, 103]

CANCER GENETIC COUNSELING

Genetic counseling is an essential component of the genetic evaluation. It is comprehensive in its approach to provide education, health promotion, informed consent, and support to individuals and families facing the uncertainty of hereditary cancer and cancer syndromes.[72, 73, 78, 85]

The education component of genetic counseling is accomplished using a variety of teaching methods, including one-on-one discussions, videotapes, and educational booklets and articles. Whatever method is used, it is imperative that there is ample opportunity for questions to be answered. Genetic information is complex and technical in nature. The basic principles of medical genetics, patterns of heredity, and risk calculations can

be presented in a clear and concise manner. It is also helpful to provide basic information about cancer epidemiology, carcinogenesis, disease presentation, diagnosis, and treatment. All information is tailored to the specific cancer risks of the individual and family. The education component lays the foundation for decision-making regarding genetic testing, surveillance, and treatment options.[72, 73, 78, 85]

Genetic counseling is the term used to describe the process of psychosocial assessment, anxiety reduction, grief counseling, and decision-making about genetic testing. Information about benefits, risks, and limitations of testing are discussed in detail. It is crucial to the process that the counselor understands the individual's perception of risk and cancer development. The person's fears, previous encounters with a family member with cancer, and individual coping abilities shape the ability to process the information and make an informed decision. Family members present for the education and counseling can assist in supporting the individual's decisions. However, it is important to be sure that the individual is truly making his own decisions and not being coerced by the family. This can be difficult because testing of an individual has implications for the entire family. The counselor discusses with the person whether or not he plans to inform the family members of the test results. Genetic counseling is provided before and after genetic testing is offered.[6, 50, 56, 72, 73, 78, 85]

Informed consent is a mandatory component of genetic testing. There are a number of ramifications to genetic testing and it is imperative that individuals be made aware of all the issues before undergoing testing. In addition to the psychosocial issues already addressed, a detailed discussion regarding the benefits, risks, and limitations of testing must be provided. The potential benefits to testing include:

- Identifying individuals with mutations in cancer-susceptibility genes so they may take advantage of more intensive screening programs and prevention options
- Identifying individuals who do not carry mutations so that they are not put through unnecessary intensive surveillance and surgeries
- Relieving the uncertainty for individuals
- Determining a more accurate risk status of individual and family members[52]

The potential risks of genetic testing include:

- Severe psychological reactions. Individuals who learn they carry a mutation in a cancer-susceptibility gene may experience anger, fear, guilt, and depression. Individuals who learn they do not carry a mutation may experience "survivor's guilt," particularly if they are the only member of their family who is not a mutation carrier.[3, 43, 57]

- Interpreting a negative test result as having no risk of developing cancer. Individuals may use this as an excuse not to undergo regular population screening recommendations.
- Workplace or insurance discrimination. As a result of the 1997 enactment of the Health Insurance Portability Accountability Act, group health plans cannot consider genetic information a preexisting condition.[40]
- Family disruptions. Not all family members want to know test results. In some instances, test results could confirm that the individual is not biologically related to other "family" members. The knowledge of having a mutation in a cancer-susceptibility gene could deter an individual from having children or even getting married.

The limitations of genetic testing include:

- Accuracy of the test. A mutation may be present but technology does not exist to identify it. Therefore, the test is negative for known mutations, but inconclusive for unknown mutations. Sometimes, testing reveals the presence of a variant in a gene, the significance of which is unknown at this time.
- A negative test result is only informative if a mutation has been identified in the family and it is not found in the individual tested. This is why an affected family member is the ideal candidate to be tested first.
- Medical management of a positive test result. There are no effective screening or cancer prevention measures for many cancers, so why do testing if there is no proven preventive treatment available. In some instances, a positive test result only indicates a *probability* of developing cancer; it does not indicate a *certainty*.[1, 3, 6, 39, 41, 53, 85]

Informed consent must also include a discussion regarding the cost of testing, how the test is to be performed, and who in the family is the most appropriate member to test first. The cost of testing varies. Some insurance plans pay for testing, others pay a portion of the cost, and some pay nothing at all. Some individuals wish to self-pay for testing to avoid alerting their insurance company to their mutation status, for fear of discrimination.[39, 41, 53]

In determining the most appropriate person in the family to test first, generally it is best to test an affected family member. If a mutation is identified in a person with cancer, it is more likely to have caused the cancer. Then, subsequent family members can be tested for the specific mutation and testing is most informative.[11, 39, 53, 77]

In 1997, the Oncology Nursing Society published its position on Cancer Genetic Testing and Risk Assessment Counseling (Fig. 2–4). It outlines the necessary components to counseling and informed consent.

CANCER GENETIC TESTING

Genetic testing is offered to individuals who are likely to carry a mutation in a cancer-susceptibility gene in which a test exists to identify the mutation. The results of testing must be interpretable and affect medical management.[1, 45] Genetic testing is not a screening test for people with the general population risk of developing cancer.

Testing is done through DNA analysis of a blood specimen. There are four methods of testing blood for gene mutations. DNA sequencing is the gold standard and is the most sensitive method for identifying mutations. It looks at every nucleotide base pair on both copies of the gene being tested. Allele-specific oligonucleotides (ASO) probes only detect specific known mutations. Conformation-sensitive DNA screening tests are not as sensitive as DNA sequencing and they can miss some coding region mutations. Protein truncation assay is sensitive for specific mutations in which shortened proteins are produced. It cannot detect missense mutations.[6, 53, 100]

GENETIC CANCER SYNDROMES

A number of known cancer-causing mutations in several genes result in the development of cancers. They exhibit different patterns of inheritance and ranges of risk for developing cancer. Although some of these syndromes are rare, the cancers that develop as the result of these inherited mutations are familiar to the oncology nurse.

Hereditary Breast and Ovarian Cancer

Hereditary breast and ovarian cancers are those cancers caused by germline mutations in specific cancer-susceptibility genes. In total, these cancers comprise only 5% to 10% of all breast cancers. The most common known mutations occur in the BRCA-1, BRCA-2, p53, and PTEN genes. Together they account for about 80% of all hereditary breast cancers. The remaining 20% of these breast cancers are due to undiscovered genetic mutations.[15, 20, 22]

BRCA-1. In 1990, BRCA-1 was identified as the first major cancer-susceptibility gene. It was localized to chromosome 17, specifically the long arm, 17q. By 1994, this large gene was sequenced. Extensive research into families with multiple breast cancer cases revealed that a mutation in the BRCA-1 gene was implicated in 45%

ONCOLOGY NURSING SOCIETY POSITION

Cancer Genetic Testing and Risk Assessment Counseling

The ability to identify individuals and families who potentially are at high risk for developing a malignancy because of inheritance of a cancer predisposition gene is possible through genetic testing. However, while providing the capability to target those individuals who might best benefit from intensive screening and preventive services, genetic testing also creates a spectrum of dilemmas inherent in identifying one's genetic makeup.

IT IS THE POSITION OF ONS THAT

- Genetic testing must include informed consent and pre- and post-test counseling by qualified individuals (e.g., certified genetic counselors, advanced practice oncology nurses with specialized education in genetics).
- Ethical principles must form the foundation of providing counseling services, guide the development of standards of care in cancer genetic counseling, and address potential ethical issues inherent in genetic testing.
- Counseling must occur in a manner consistent with the individual's cultural and healthcare beliefs.
- Legislation to provide protection from genetic discrimination in both employment and insurance and to provide reimbursement of and access to genetic counseling, genetic testing services, and appropriate medical management must be introduced and implemented.
- Educational resources for healthcare providers, those individuals at high risk, and the lay public must be developed.
- A research plan related to all aspects of cancer genetics, including the efficacy of prevention/early de-

tection strategies, the psychologic impact of predisposition testing, and long-term outcomes of testing must be developed.
- Efforts to standardize and regulate laboratories that provide cancer genetic testing must be undertaken.

Background

The rapid evolution of genetic testing technologies has led to an increased number of individuals and laboratories involved in predisposition testing. Although genetic testing currently is available commercially, as well as through investigative research settings, access to testing and counseling services is limited because of cost and reimbursement issues. Limited data are available regarding the psychosocial and behavioral impact of testing as well as the best screening, preventive, and surveillance measures for individuals with a hereditary predisposition to cancer. Informed consent is crucial in understanding the ramifications of predisposition testing, and pre- and post-test counseling is essential for comprehensive patient care.

ONS Board of Directiors Approved 8/97

To obtain copies of the ONS position "Cancer Genetic Testing and Risk Assessment Counseling," contact the Customer Service Center at the ONS National Office at 501 Holiday Drive, Pittsburgh, PA 15220-2749 (412-921-7373). Positions also may be downloaded from ONS Online (www.ons.org).

FIGURE 2–4 ONS position statement. (From Oncology Nursing Society Position Statement. Cancer genetic testing and risk assessment counseling. *Oncol Nurs Forum* 25(3):464, 1998.)

---

of their cancers. If the families had both breast and ovarian cancers, the BRCA-1 gene mutation was responsible up to 90% of the time.[34, 71] Research has continued during the ensuing years and over 500 different mutations in the BRCA-1 gene have been reported. Over 70% of these mutations are frameshift mutations.[15, 93, 94]

BRCA-1 mutations account for about 45% of all inherited breast cancer. The mutations are transmitted by an autosomal dominant pattern of inheritance. They are

highly penetrant, though not completely so. The lifetime risk of developing breast cancer in a woman with a BRCA-1 mutation is 56% to 85%, compared to the general population risk of 12%. There is also a lifetime risk of developing ovarian cancer of 15% to 45%, again compared to the general population risk of 1% to 2%. The difference in risk, from 56% to 85% and from 15% to 45%, is due to the fact that the earliest studies were conducted with severely affected families with multiple breast and ovarian cancers. Subsequent studies included women from unselected families, with less compelling family histories, hence the lower lifetime risks.[12, 14, 19, 34, 48, 70, 71]

Features of hereditary breast and ovarian cancers associated with BRCA-1 mutations include an early onset of breast or ovarian cancer or both. Fifty percent of women with a BRCA-1 mutation are diagnosed with cancer by age 41. Bilateral disease is not uncommon, with 40% to 60% of women diagnosed with a second primary breast cancer. It is also not uncommon to see breast cancer and ovarian cancer diagnosed in the same woman. Families with BRCA-1 mutations are also at higher risk of developing colon and prostate cancers.[48, 70, 71, 102]

Researchers have discovered two BRCA-1 founder mutations prevalent in the Ashkenazi Jewish population. *Founder mutations* are those mutations that are seen with high frequency in a population founded by a small ancestral group, where one or more of the founders were carriers of the mutation.[71] These two founder mutations in the Ashkenazi Jewish population are the 185delAG and the 5382insC mutations. The 185delAG mutation has been detected in about 1% of Ashkenazi Jews. Approximately 20% of Ashkenazi Jewish women who develop breast cancer before the age of 40 carry this mutation, compared to 10% of the non-Ashkenazi Jewish, white, American women. The 5382insC mutation is found in 0.15% of Ashkenazi Jewish women, as well as others of Eastern European heritage. Each of these founder mutations accounts for 10% of the all identified BRCA-1 mutations.[30, 35, 46, 48, 95]

Panguluri and coworkers[76] studied 45 high-risk, African American families for BRCA-1 founder mutations. They found two frameshift mutations designated 943ins10 and 345del14, resulting in protein truncation. The first mutation was observed in five families with a common distant African ancestor. The second mutation was reported in a Norwegian and two Canadian families, reinforcing the genetic diversity among individuals of African descent.

BRCA-2. The BRCA-2 gene was isolated in 1995 and localized to the long arm of chromosome 13 (13q). Mutations in the BRCA-2 gene are responsible for a high risk of early onset breast cancer and about 15% of all male breast cancer.[96] More than 100 different BRCA-2 mutations have been identified on this very large gene. BRCA-2 mutations are responsible for about 35% of all inherited breast cancers. As with BRCA-1, BRCA-2 is also a tumor suppressor gene and is inherited in an autosomal dominant fashion. The lifetime risk of developing breast cancer in a woman with a BRCA-2 mutation is 50% to 85%. However, the lifetime risk of developing ovarian cancer is 10% to 20%, somewhat lower than with BRCA-1 mutations. BRCA-2 muta-

tions confer a 6% lifetime risk of male breast cancer, significantly higher than the general population risk. Families with BRCA-2 mutations also have a higher risk of developing prostate, pancreatic, and laryngeal cancers.[8, 23, 71, 92, 101]

There are two known BRCA-2 founder mutations, 6174delT and 999del5. The first of these mutations was identified in 8% of Ashkenazi Jewish women diagnosed with breast cancer before age 42 and in 1.5% of all Ashkenazim. However, it is only thought to be associated with a 25% lifetime risk of breast cancer. The 999del5 founder mutation appears to be responsible for more than 50% of all inherited breast and ovarian cancer in Iceland.[30, 35, 68, 71, 95]

BRCA-1 and BRCA-2 mutations are found only in individuals with inherited cancers. They have not been identified in people with sporadic cancers, which may indicate the molecular differences in germline versus sporadic cancers.[33]

p53. Li-Fraumeni syndrome is a rare genetic condition caused by germline mutations in the p53 gene, identified in 1990. It is responsible for cancers of the breast, brain, soft tissue sarcomas, leukemias, and adrenocortical carcinomas, all within the same family. This very important tumor suppressor gene is located on chromosome 17. It encodes for a protein that stops cell divison when DNA damage is detected, allowing DNA repair to occur. It also codes for programmed cell death in the event that the DNA damage is too extensive to repair. A mutation in the p53 gene allows cell division to continue without repairing damaged DNA.

Persons with known p53 mutations have a 50% risk of developing cancer by age 35, with 30% of cancers occurring before age 15. By age 70, 90% of women and 70% of men with Li-Fraumeni syndrome have been diagnosed with a cancer. Breast cancer is the most common of the adult-onset cancers associated with this syndrome; sarcomas (bone and soft tissue) are most frequently seen in children with the mutation. Li-Fraumeni syndrome accounts for approximately 1% of all inherited breast cancers.[71, 104]

PTEN. Cowden disease is another rare condition caused by germline mutations in the PTEN gene. The PTEN gene is located on chromosome 10 and 81% of the mutations associated with Cowden disease are found at 10q23.3. Features of this condition include mucocutaneous lesions, thyroid abnormalities (including cancer), fibrocystic disease, breast cancer, gastrointestinal hamartomas, and macrocephaly. Breast cancers associated with Cowden disease comprise less than 1% of all inherited breast cancers. Women with a PTEN mutation have a 25% to 50% lifetime risk of developing breast cancer, usually before age 40. They frequently have bilateral breast cancers.[21]

Risk Prediction Models for Hereditary Breast and Ovarian Cancers. A number of models are available to assess the breast and ovarian cancer risk among individuals based on their family and personal histories. These models are used to predict the risk of developing breast and ovarian cancer and the risk of having a mutation in a breast cancer susceptibility gene. They were developed from epidemiologic studies in families with high risk of breast and ovarian cancer. These models are used when mutation carrier status is unknown. Once genetic testing is done and results are informative, they are no longer useful. The most commonly used models include the Gail model and the Claus model. A number of tables are also used to predict the probability of carrying a mutation in BRCA-1 or BRCA-2 (or both). These include the Couch and Frank tables.[14, 23]

Gail Model. The Gail model was based on data from the Breast Cancer Detection and Demonstration Project (BCDDP) and was used in the NSABP Breast Cancer Prevention Trial (BCPT) to estimate breast cancer risk. This model is now available to health care providers in several formats, from flip chart to computer diskette to handheld calculator. The calculation of risk is based on several personal and family history factors including, race, current age, age at menarche, age at first live birth, number of maternal first-degree relatives with breast cancer, number of breast biopsies, and whether atypical hyperplasia was present in any biopsy specimen. The Gail model calculates the 5-year and lifetime risks of developing breast cancer. According to the Gail model, a 45-year-old, nulliparous, white woman who had menarche at 11 and two breast biopsies, with a mother and sister with breast cancer, would have an 8.2% risk of developing breast cancer within the next 5 years and a 45.5% chance of developing breast cancer in her lifetime.[25]

The application of this model in hereditary breast cancer is limited and most often underestimates risk. Because of the autosomal dominant pattern of inheritance of hereditary breast cancers, both the maternal and paternal family history must be considered. This model calculates risk based on maternal family history alone and does not factor in the age at diagnosis, a significant factor in hereditary breast and ovarian cancers. Also, only first-degree relatives with breast cancer are included in the Gail model, leaving significant second-degree relatives with breast cancer from the calculation. Finally, the Gail model does not account for male breast cancers or ovarian cancers in either the maternal or paternal family history. Using our previous example, if the same woman had a paternal grandmother and a paternal aunt with breast cancer instead of a mother and sister with breast cancer, the Gail model would calculate her 5-year risk as 2.7%, with a 17.8% lifetime risk. This would clearly underestimate her risk of hereditary breast and ovarian cancers by not incorporating the risk she has on the paternal side of her family.

Claus Model. The Claus model was developed based on data from the CASH (Cancer and Steroid Hormone) Study evaluating 5000 breast cancer patients, aged 20 to 54, and 5000 age-matched controls. In this model, the predicted cumulative probability of developing breast cancer is calculated using the current age and the age at onset of various first- and second-degree relatives with either breast or ovarian cancer. The model predicts that although most individuals with breast cancer are not mutation carriers, the likelihood of having a mutation increases by the number of relatives with the disease, especially when these relatives were diagnosed at an early age. Unlike the Gail model, the Claus model considers both maternal and paternal family history.[12] Using the Claus model, our earlier example of the 45-year-old woman with the mother (diagnosed at age 39) and sister (diagnosed at age 27) with breast cancer, her lifetime risk of developing breast cancer is 46%. With the paternal grandmother and aunt diagnosed at the same ages (39 and 27), her lifetime risk of breast cancer is 26%.

Although the Claus model has greater applicability with inherited breast and ovarian cancers than the Gail model, it too has limitations. It is more likely to underestimate the risk of developing breast cancer among individuals with gene mutations, whereas it overestimates the risk in those who do not have mutations in cancer-susceptibility genes. Also, because this model was developed before the knowledge that Ashkenazi Jewish heritage significantly increased the risk of hereditary breast cancer, this population's risk would be underestimated using the Claus model.

Couch Tables. The Couch tables were developed from a study of women with breast cancer and a strong family history of breast cancer, who were evaluated in breast cancer clinics for high-risk women and in general practice clinics. The 263 women were tested for BRCA-1 mutations and the resultant tables predict the probability of detecting a BRCA-1 mutation in families with breast and ovarian cancer. These tables are useful in families with multiple members with breast and ovarian cancer. The Couch tables consider the average age at diagnosis of breast cancer among all affected relatives, and both breast and ovarian cancer, as well as breast and ovarian cancer in a single individual family member. There are separate tables for individuals of Ashkenazi Jewish heritage.[14] To continue with our example of the 45-year-old woman, according to the Couch tables, her probability of having a BRCA-1 mutation with either maternal or paternal affected relatives is 17.4% (the average age of diagnosis is 33) if she is not Ashkenazi Jewish and 48% if she is Ashkenazi Jewish.

Limitations of the Couch tables include the small sample size (263 women versus 10,000 women in Claus model), all women in the study were white and, because average age of diagnosis is used, may underestimate risk in families with sporadic cases of breast cancer (over age 60) among inherited cases. In this same example, if the woman also had a grandmother with breast cancer diagnosed at 80, the average age at diagnosis in her family would be 49 and her probability would fall to 5% if she is not Ashkenazi Jewish and 19% if she is Ashkenazi Jewish. If the grandmother's breast cancer was sporadic, the woman's probability of mutation is clearly underestimated.

Frank Table. The Frank table was developed from a study of 238 women with early onset breast cancer or ovarian cancer (at any age), with at least one first- or second-degree relative with either breast or ovarian cancer. It predicts the probability of carrying a BRCA-1 or BRCA-2 mutation. This table accounts for early age of onset and the presence of both breast and ovarian cancer in the family. Bilateral breast or ovarian cancer is also a factor in the risk analysis, as is male breast cancer.[23] Using the Frank table, the 45-year-old woman's probability of having a BRCA-1 or BRCA-2 mutation is 20% (her mother and sister have a 40% probability of mutation in either BRCA-1 or BRCA-2). The limitations of the Frank table include the small sample size and the lack of ethnic diversity among study participants.

Individuals undergoing cancer risk assessment and genetic counseling, who have a greater than 10% probability of having a mutation in BRCA-1 or BRCA-2 are eligible for genetic testing. Even when eligible for testing, the ultimate decision to have blood testing lies with the individual.

Genetic Testing for BRCA-1 and BRCA-2 Mutations. The process of genetic testing for BRCA-1 and BRCA-2 gene mutations involves DNA sequencing of the nucleotides on both copies of the genes. Complete sequencing is the most sensitive technique available to detect coding region mutations. It can miss large insertions or deletions or noncoding mutations, however. The process is labor intensive and costly. Therefore, an affected member of the family is tested first, as the most likely candidate for having a mutation. If a mutation is identified, testing of other family members can be limited to the small portion of the gene where a previously identified mutation has occurred. This is much less labor intensive and, consequently, less costly than complete gene sequencing.[7]

Individuals of Ashkenazi Jewish heritage may undergo common mutation testing in which sequencing of the areas of the three common Ashkenazi mutations (185delAG, 5582insC, and 6174delT) alone is performed. If one of these mutations is not identified, complete sequencing of BRCA-1 and BRCA-2 may then be carried out, if the individual so chooses.

BRCA-1 and BRCA-2 mutation testing is commercially available. Results are usually available in 4 to 6 weeks. Insurance companies may pay all or part of the cost of testing. Genetic testing is also available to eligible individuals in the research setting. There is usually no cost for research testing; however, results are not usually available for years, if ever. The purpose of research testing is less for clinical management than it is for furthering our knowledge about mutations and mutation carriers in families.[27]

Genetic testing is undertaken when the results will affect the medical management of the patient. A negative test result in a family with a known BRCA-1 or BRCA-2 mutation is considered confirmatory. This individual would not be at high risk for breast or ovarian cancer and would not require heightened surveillance or other strategies used to manage high-risk individuals. It is very important to remember that a negative test result does not completely eliminate the risk of breast or ovarian cancer. Rather, the individual has the population risk for these diseases due to sporadic cancers and would still need to undergo age-appropriate screening according to American Cancer Society guidelines. A positive result, on the other hand, would identify that individual as someone in need of heightened surveillance. A negative test result in a family with no known BRCA-1 or BRCA-2 mutation is not informative because there could be an undetected mutation in BRCA-1 or BRCA-2, or they may have a mutation in another cancer-susceptibility gene.[10, 64]

Financial expense is not the only "cost" of BRCA-1 or BRCA-2 testing. The psychological costs can be tremendous. In families in which all but one sibling is found to carry a mutation, the "survivor's guilt" experienced by the sole noncarrier can be as difficult to handle as the news of being positive for the mutation. It can be devastating for a parent to learn that she passed a mutation to her child, especially if the child (as an adult) develops breast or ovarian cancer and the parent does not. For these reasons as well as others, it is critical that individuals receive genetic couseling before having actual blood testing. The psychological ramifications of testing are discussed with individuals and families as part of the genetic counseling process.[15, 39, 44, 50, 51]

Clinical Management of the BRCA Mutation-Positive Patient. Individuals who are found to have a mutation in BRCA-1 or BRCA-2, or individuals who have not been tested but are from a family in which a mutation in BRCA-1 or BRCA-2 has been identified, are provided a number of options for management. These options can be categorized into primary prevention and secondary prevention strategies.

Primary Prevention. The primary prevention strategies available to mutation-positive individuals include chemoprevention and prophylactic surgeries. Chemoprevention is an option for people who have not yet been diagnosed with breast or ovarian cancer; prophylactic surgeries may be an option for both affected and nonaffected individuals. It is important to remember that these strategies do not completely eliminate the risk of breast or ovarian cancers.

The chemoprevention of breast cancer has become an option after results of the BCPT demonstrated a 49% reduction in incidence of invasive breast cancers among high-risk women with the use of tamoxifen. It is likely that some mutation carriers were among the high-risk women in the trial. The exact reduction in risk afforded by the use of tamoxifen in mutation carriers is not known at this time. However, because the reduction of invasive breast cancers was identified in almost every subgroup, it is likely that tamoxifen therapy was of some benefit to women with mutations in BRCA-1 and BRCA-2. Further research regarding mutation carriers and tamoxifen therapy may help to confirm its role as an effective chemoprevention agent.[91]

Chemoprevention in ovarian cancer involves the use of oral contraceptives (OCP). It is now known that long-term use (10 years) of OCP reduces the population risk of ovarian cancer by 80%. Even using OCP for 3 years can reduce ovarian cancer risk in the general population by 40% to 50%. This may be a favorable option for women with BRCA-1 mutations who still want to have children and are not interested in a surgical approach to risk reduction. The exact reduction in risk that OCP afford mutation carriers is not known at this time. There may also be an increased risk of breast cancer among this subset of women. More research is needed in this area to effectively answer the questions about chemoprevention of both breast and ovarian cancers.[9, 67]

Prophylactic surgical procedures, including mastectomy and oophorectomy, have been shown to significantly reduce the incidence of breast and ovarian cancers. They are an option for women who have already had cancer, as well as mutation carriers who are at high-risk for developing breast and ovarian cancers.

Schrag and colleagues[90] calculated the effect of prophylactic mastectomy and oophorectomy on risk of breast and ovarian cancers in women with known BRCA-1 or BRCA-2 mutations. They reported a substantial reduction in risk of cancer and gain in life expectancy especially among younger women. Grann and coworkers[29] reported that among women testing positive for BRCA-1 or BRCA-2 mutations, prophylactic mastectomy and oophorectomy substantially improved survival, particularly when the surgeries were done at a young age.

Hartmann and associates[36] conducted a retrospective study of women with a family history of breast cancer who underwent bilateral prophylactic mastectomy at the Mayo Clinic between 1960 and 1993. These were not women who were known mutation carriers. Of the 639 women studied, 214 had features suggestive of having a BRCA-1 or BRCA-2 mutation. The remaining 425 women were considered at moderate risk for breast cancer with most having at least one first-degree relative with the diagnosis. The Gail model was used to predict who was considered high risk and who was moderate risk. They concluded that breast cancer incidence with prophylactic mastectomy had been reduced by at least 90%. This reduction in risk persisted through a median 14 years of follow-up.

Schrag and coworkers,[91] in a study examining the life expectancy gains of a variety of prevention strategies for BRCA-1 and BRCA-2 mutation carriers with breast cancer, found that prophylactic mastectomy offered young women with early disease a substantial gain in life expectancy.

Berchuck and colleagues[4] identified the benefits of prophylactic oophorectomy in young, mutation-positive women at risk for ovarian cancer. In addition to a decrease in ovarian cancer incidence, they found oophorectomy was more easily tolerated with less body image changes than with mastectomy, especially when the procedure was done laproscopically. Menopausal symptoms could be managed with hormone replacement therapy, although there may be an increased risk of breast cancer in mutation carriers. The negatives to undergoing oophorectomy included the potential costs of the surgery, both financial and in morbidity. There is still no proven reduction in ovarian cancer incidence. There have been reported cases of peritoneal cancers similar to ovarian cancer in women who underwent prophylactic oophorectomy, though the true incidence of this in mutation-positive women is not known.

Rebbeck and associates reported a statistically significant reduction in breast cancer risk after prophylactic oophorectomy in BRCA-1 mutation carriers.[82, 83] This reduction persisted 5 to 10 years after surgery and was not negated by the postoperative use of hormone replacement therapy.

Secondary Prevention. Many BRCA-1 and BRCA-2 mutation carriers are reluctant to pursue the primary prevention strategies previously discussed. They prefer to undergo increased surveillance instead. These secondary prevention strategies are familiar to most oncology nurses. They include breast self-examination (BSE), clinical breast examination (CBE), mammography, pelvic examination, transvaginal ultrasound, and CA-125. Though the recommendations have not been studied in mutation carriers, there is a presumed benefit to heightened surveillance. BSE continues to be an important recommendation for all women from at least age 18 on through adulthood. In mutation carriers as in the general population, this should be practiced monthly. This is particularly important in younger women in whom mammograms are of reduced efficacy. The oncology nurse is the ideal practitioner to provide women with known BRCA-1 or BRCA-2 mutations the education and training necessary to develop confidence in their BSE technique. CBE is recommended every 6 to 12 months in mutation carriers, beginning at least 10 years before the cancer diagnosis of first-degree relatives with breast cancer. As with BSE, in young women with dense breasts, CBE may be more sensitive than mammography, but the benefit has not been proven. Mammograms are recommended to begin at age 25 in women with BRCA-1 or BRCA-2 mutations. Randomized clinical trials have not reported a substantial benefit to mammograms before the age of 50; however, these were screening trials done in women without mutations in cancer susceptibility genes.[84, 91]

Breast Cancer in BRCA-1 and BRCA-2 Mutation Carriers—Implications for Management. A number of investigators are looking at the relationship between breast cancer and mutation-positive status with regard to prognosis and treatment implications. If a BRCA-1 or BRCA-2 mutation carrier is diagnosed with breast cancer, should she receive a different or more intensive chemotherapy? Should she receive radiation therapy regardless of surgical decision? Is she a candidate for breast conservation or must bilateral mastectomies be performed? Is her breast cancer more likely to locally recur or distantly metastasize? Is the prognosis for a mutation-positive breast cancer worse? These questions have been posed and retrospective analyses done to try to identify exactly what role a BRCA-1 or BRCA-2 mutation plays in treatment and prognosis of breast cancer.[38]

Robson and colleagues[86] studied 91 Ashkenazi Jewish women with early onset breast cancer and found 33% had a BRCA-1 or BRCA-2 mutation. These mutation carriers were less likely to have stage I disease and more likely to have nodal involvement at diagnosis than women without mutations. Mutation carriers also had higher grade tumors and were more likely to be estrogen receptor (ER) negative. They were more likely to develop contralateral breast cancers. These differences did not appear to significantly affect relapse-free survival or overall survival.

Phillips and coworkers reviewed studies of breast cancer patients and a variety of known prognostic factors.[81] There appeared to be certain characteristics of breast cancers diagnosed in BRCA-1 mutation carriers. They were more likely to have medullary or atypical medullary features; they were more likely to be high-grade tumors, and were more often ER negative and progesterone receptor (PR) negative than the breast cancers of women without mutations. These characteris-

tics were not as consistently seen among BRCA-2 mutation carriers. Further review was done of 14 trials evaluating overall survival in BRCA-1 and BRCA-2 mutation carriers with breast cancer and matched controls. Of the seven trials involving BRCA-1 mutation carriers with breast cancer, overall survival was better among mutation carriers compared with controls in four studies, worse in two studies, and the same in one study. Of the three trials involving BRCA-2 mutation carriers with breast cancer, overall survival was better in two studies and worse in one study. Many of these studies were methodologically flawed and the results conflicting. Therefore, it is difficult to draw useful conclusions regarding the impact of mutation carrier status on prognosis in breast cancer.

Turner and associates[99] studied women with breast cancer who underwent breast-conserving therapy and experienced ipsilateral breast recurrence. Median time to disease recurrence was 7.8 years in BRCA-1 and BRCA-2 mutation carriers and 4.7 years in noncarriers. These mutation-positive women appeared to have developed a new primary breast cancer, as opposed to a recurrent breast cancer. This study points out that knowledge of mutation status before definitive surgery might assist women in the process of making a decision between mastectomy and breast conservation.[26]

Hereditary Colorectal Cancer Syndromes

Hereditary colorectal cancers are the result of germline mutations in specific cancer-susceptibility genes. They comprise 15% of all colorectal cancers. There are a number of well-characterized inherited predispositions to colorectal cancer, including hereditary nonpolyposis colorectal cancer (HNPCC), familial adenomatous polyposis (FAP), juvenile polyposis, Peutz-Jeghers syndrome, Muir-Torre syndrome, and Turcot syndrome. An individual with a mutation in the mismatch repair genes that lead to HNPCC has an 80% lifetime risk of developing colorectal cancer. In FAP, the lifetime risk is over 95%. When compared to the population risk of 5%, the hereditary colorectal cancer syndromes confer substantially higher risks of colorectal cancer than even a personal history of colorectal cancer, with a 15% to 20% lifetime risk of developing a subsequent colorectal cancer.[59, 61, 69, 80]

Hereditary Nonpolyposis Colorectal Cancer. Hereditary nonpolyposis colorectal cancer (HNPCC), or Lynch syndrome, is the most common of the hereditary colorectal cancer syndromes. It comprises 5% of all colorectal cancers, or about 6600 cases annually. Lynch syndrome was described in the 1960s, before the discovery of the genetic mutations responsible for its manifestations. In 1993, the MSH2 gene was localized on the short arm of chromosome 2. At this time, there are five known genetic mutations in mismatch repair genes causing susceptibility to HNPCC, including MLH6, PMS1 (also found on chromosome 2), PMS2 (located on chromosome 7), and MLH1 (located on chromosome 3). They are transmitted via an autosomal dominant pattern of inheritance and confer a risk of developing colorectal cancer of about 80%. Approximately 90% of all HNPCC cases are due to MSH2 and MLH1 gene mutations.[59, 61, 62, 80]

During DNA transcription, incorrect base substitutions occur. Mismatch repair genes are responsible for making corrections in the nucleotide sequences. Mutations in mismatch repair genes allow mistakes to propagate, resulting in genetic instability at repeat sequences (*microsatellites*) within the gene. This is known as *microsatellite instability* and leads to an accumulation of additional mutations, unregulated cell growth, and, eventually, cancer. High-frequency microsatellite instability has been found in 95% of HNPCC cases and in approximately 15% of sporadic cases of colorectal cancer.[32, 62]

Clinical features of HNPCC include early age of onset, with the average age at diagnosis of 45 years, (range, 13–74 years). Affected individuals have no polyps and only one or two adenomas. In HNPCC cases, the progression from adenoma to carcinoma is accelerated over that of sporadic cancers. At least 70% of the cancers involve the right colon, proximal to the splenic flexure. The presence of synchronous and metachronous colorectal cancers is not uncommon. A number of extracolonic cancers are associated with HNPCC. These include endometrial, ovarian, urinary tract, stomach, small bowel, and bile duct cancers. They occur more frequently in HNPCC families than within the general population.[59, 61] Indeed, the lifetime risk of endometrial cancer among mutation carriers is 45% to 60%, compared to the general population risk of 3%.

A subset of HNPCC patients has a rare variant known as Muir-Torre syndrome. Individuals with this syndrome have the typical features of HNPCC as well as sebaceous gland tumors and keratoacanthomas. Genetic testing has identified MSH2 and MLH1 as the mutations most closely associated with Muir-Torre syndrome.[59, 61]

In 1991, the International Collaborative Group on HNPCC established the "Amsterdam criteria" for identifying HNPCC families. The criteria include three or more relatives with colorectal cancer, one case being a first-degree relative of the others. The cancers must occur within two or more generations and have one diagnosis by the age of 50. Colorectal cancer cases due to FAP are not included in the Amsterdam criteria.[62] The Amsterdam criteria are conservative and are limited in their utility because they fail to address extracolonic cancers so often seen in HNPCC families.

Genetic Testing for HNPCC Susceptibility. The process of genetic testing for the mismatch repair gene mutations associated with HNPCC begins with denaturing gradiant gel electropheresis (DGGE). If a mutation is identified, DNA sequencing is performed. Full DNA sequencing is available for MSH2 and MLH1 only, because these are the most common mutations found in HNPCC. Protein truncation testing is available commercially for MSH2 and MLH1. Although this is less labor intensive and less costly than full sequencing, there is a higher false-negative rate.[80]

As with hereditary breast and ovarian cancers, genetic testing for HNPCC mutations should ideally begin with an affected family member. If the family meets Amsterdam criteria, or an affected family member was diagnosed at a very early age, genetic testing is an option. If a mutation is identified in this affected individual, other family members are then eligible for genetic testing. If a mutation is not identified in an individual within a known HNPCC mutation family, the individual would be at population risk for the development of colorectal cancer and would not require heightened surveillance. It is important to remember that the individual would still require general population screening, because a negative mutation test does not eliminate the risk of sporadic colorectal cancers.[58, 59, 61, 65]

If a mutation is not identified in the affected individual, the results are considered inconclusive. The individual may not have an HNPCC mutation or may have a mutation that is not detectable. In this situation, genetic testing would not be offered to other family members. The family would still be considered high risk and would require intensive screening and surveillance.

Clinical Management of the HNPCC Mutation Carrier. A number of primary and secondary prevention options are available for individuals who are carriers of mutations associated with HNPCC. These options include surgery, chemoprevention, and surveillance strategies.

Primary Prevention. Individuals with germline mutations in mismatch repair genes are at high risk for more than just colorectal cancers. Because of this risk, primary disease prevention through use of pharmacologic agents to inhibit or reverse the process of carcinogenesis before the development of cancer has been studied at length. Current research trials are evaluating the activity of a cyclooxygenase inhibitor (COX-2) against adenoma and mucosa biomarkers. Another trial is investigating whether aspirin and resistant starch can reduce the incidence of colon adenomas (CAPP-2). Ideally, these chemoprevention agents will also have an impact on the development of extracolonic cancers as well.[37, 62]

The role of prophylactic surgery in the prevention of colorectal cancers in HNPCC families is not clear-cut. There is no evidence that prophylactic subtotal colectomy with ileorectal anastomosis is beneficial. It may be an option only in individuals who are unable to follow recommended surveillance by colonoscopy. For women with mutations in HNPCC-associated genes, prophylactic hysterectomy and bilateral oophorectomy is also an option. As with hereditary breast and ovarian cancers, prophylactic surgeries in no way eliminate all risk of developing cancer. There is still a risk of cancers developing in the tissue left behind, particularly intraperitoneal carcinomatosis.[41, 59, 61, 62]

Secondary Prevention. Because there are no proven benefits to the above primary prevention strategies, heightened surveillance provides secondary prevention options for HNPCC-associated mutation carriers. The National Human Genome Research Institute convened a task force to develop recommendations for screening of high-risk individuals with known mutations in cancer susceptibility genes. The recommendations regarding screening for colorectal cancer include full colonoscopy every 1 to 2 years, beginning at 20 to 25 years of age. The frequency of examinations is due to the high incidence of interval colorectal cancers that develop between colonoscopies done every 3 years. Flexible sigmoidoscopy is not recommended in this high-risk group in light of the high incidence of right-sided colon cancers.[59, 61, 62] In women with HNPCC-associated mutations, screening for endometrial cancer should also be recommended. There has been no proven benefit to annual endometrial cancer screening. However, the recommendations for this high-risk group include annual endometrial aspirate.[9] In addition, annual ovarian cancer screening in known mutation carriers can be done, including CA-125 and transvaginal ultrasound.

Familial Adenomatous Polyposis. Familial adenomatous polyposis is a hereditary colorectal cancer syndrome that is responsible for approximately 1% of all colorectal cancers. The lifetime risk of developing colorectal cancer in FAP families is greater than 95% (compared to the population risk of about 5%).[59, 61] FAP results from germline mutations in the adenomatous polyposis coli (APC) gene located on the long arm of chromosome 5. The APC gene functions as a tumor suppressor and requires both alleles to be mutated before function is lost. In most FAP families there appear to be separate, distinct mutations of the APC gene. There are over 700 known APC gene mutations, most leading to truncation of the APC protein. Nonsense and frameshift mutations are the most common types of mutations seen in FAP.[80] APC gene mutations are seen in 30% of individuals with no family history of colorectal cancer. This is known as a *de novo mutation* and arises in the sperm or ovum of an unaffected individual. It is then passed on to their offspring, who, with no family history of colorectal cancer, develop FAP and colorectal cancer.

A founder mutation in the APC gene has been identified in individuals of Ashkenazi Jewish heritage. The mutation, I1307K, is a missense mutation that, unlike other FAP mutations that truncate the APC protein, instead causes the creation of an unstable DNA sequence. This leads to the development of somatic mutations that result in familial colorectal cancer. The I1307K mutation is associated with a high lifetime risk of colorectal cancer among Ashkenazi Jews. It has been identified in 28% of Ashkenazi Jewish individuals with a personal as well as a family history of colorectal cancer (compared to 6% of all Ashkenazi Jewish individuals and nearly 0% of the non-Jewish population).[47]

A number of clinical features are associated with FAP, none more distinct than the hundreds to thousands of adenomatous polyps found in the colon of affected individuals, usually at a very young age. The diagnosis of FAP is made on the basis of having at least 100 adenomatous polyps throughout the colon. These polyps can be found in children as young as 10 years of age. If left untreated, there is virtually a 100% chance of developing colorectal cancer, usually before age 40.[80]

Another clinical feature associated with FAP is congenital hypertrophy of the retinal pigment epithelium (CHRPE). These pigmented lesions are visible on funduscopic examination of the retina. CHRPE is a benign finding and was used as a marker for FAP before genetic testing was available. Individuals with mutations in the APC gene are also at risk for extracolonic tumors such as upper gastrointestinal, brain, and thyroid carcinomas, desmoid tumors, osteomas, hepatoblastomas, and hepatopancreatic tumors.[59, 61]

There is a variant of FAP known as Gardner's syndrome. Individuals with Gardner's syndrome exhibit the same clinical features common to individuals with FAP plus additional distinct features, including epidermal cysts, osteomas, desmoid tumors, and supernumary teeth. These additional features are usually benign.

Attenuated FAP is another variation of FAP also known as "hereditary flat adenoma syndrome." This syndrome is characterized by a smaller number of adenomas throughout the colon. Attenuated FAP occurs later in life, usually over the age of 50, but is still associated with a high risk of colorectal cancer, as well as a higher risk of upper cancers. Individuals with attenuated FAP do not exhibit CHRPE. Mutations associated with attenuated FAP are found on the same APC gene, but appear to be located at either end of the gene.[59, 61]

Genetic Testing for FAP. Genetic testing for APC gene mutations is commercially available and is indicated in individuals who have known polyposis or the presence of over 100 adenomatous polyps throughout the colon. There need not be a family history of colorectal cancer because the incidence of de novo mutations in FAP is about 30%. Testing is also indicated for relatives of known APC gene mutation carriers, as well as individuals suspected of having attenuated FAP. The most common method of testing is the protein truncation assay. This test is virtually 100% accurate in identifying mutation carriers, once a mutation has been found in a family member.[59, 60, 80]

There are a number of benefits to testing for FAP. First, identification of individuals with a mutation before the development of colorectal cancer can improve morbidity and mortality from colorectal cancer. These individuals would be screened more diligently than the general population. Secondly, by identifying individuals in the family who are not mutation carriers, heightened surveillance would not be necessary.

There is clearly a psychological component to learning of a mutation-positive status. With FAP, there is an almost certainty regarding the development of cancer, particularly at a young age. Adolescents and young adults are going through developmental stages in which body image is important. Reluctance to undergo colonoscopic surveillance due to embarrassment and fear is not uncommon. Also, the fear of undergoing colectomy and possibly colostomy is very real to these individuals.[80]

Unfortunately, there remain certain limitations to testing for FAP. Testing unaffected individuals without prior knowledge of an identified mutation in the family could result in uninformative results. For individuals suspected of having attenuated FAP, mutations on the extreme ends of the gene can go undetected, leading to false-negative test results.[80]

Clinical Management of the APC Mutation-Positive Patient. Individuals who are found to have a mutation in the APC gene are provided with options for managing their high risk for colorectal cancer. These options can be categorized into primary and secondary prevention strategies.

Primary Prevention. The primary prevention strategies available to mutation-positive individuals include prophylactic surgery and chemoprevention. Surgical interventions are indicated when there are confirmed polyps in the colon. Children can begin to develop polyps as early as 10 years of age, though every attempt is made to delay surgery until after puberty, if at all possible. Surgical procedures performed include subtotal colectomy with ileorectal anastomosis and rectal mucosectomy with ileal pouch and anal anastomosis. The latter option would be appropriate for individuals who have adenomatous polyps involving the rectum or in those who are unwilling or unable to be compliant with annual surveillance guidelines. Individuals with mutations in the APC gene are prone to develop desmoid tumors and sometimes the preventive surgery itself can cause these tumors to form. These desmoids are the most

common cause of death among patients with FAP who undergo prophylactic surgery. Investigation is underway to determine the genetic mechanism for desmoid development.[97] Mutation carriers are also at risk for upper gastrointestinal cancers.

A number of chemoprevention studies are underway for individuals with known germline mutations in the APC gene. The goals of these prevention trials are to prevent polyp formation and to cause regression of existing polyps before they undergo malignant transformation. Based on evidence that regular use of aspirin or other nonsteroidal anti-inflammatory drugs reduced mortality from colorectal cancer by 40%, studies were developed to explore their use in individuals with FAP. The anti-inflammatory agents inhibit COX enzymes, which catalyze steps in the conversion of arachidonic acid to prostaglandins. Prior research has identified an increased COX-2 expression in human colorectal adenocarcinomas and intestinal tumors. It has been theorized that increased COX-2 levels have a disruptive effect on the APC gene and act as a tumor promoter in the intestine. A number of trials have investigated the use of nonselective COX-1 or COX-2 inhibitors (such as aspirin, sulindac, and piroxicam) and selective COX-2 inhibitors (celecoxib) on intestinal tumor growth.[37, 87]

Sulindac was one of the first drugs studied and was reported to cause the regression of rectal adenomas in four patients with FAP. Several follow-up sulindac trials confirmed the resolution of adenomas in patients with FAP. Giarelli and coworkers[28] reported the results of a randomized, double-blinded, placebo-controlled trial of 40 patients with FAP receiving oral sulindac or placebo. There was a 44% decrease in the number of polyps in the sulindac arm after 9 months of treatment, as well as a 35% decrease in the size of the polyps from baseline.

Other agents under investigation in prevention trials include vitamin C, calcium carbonate, and 5-fluorouracil. Studies suggest these agents reduce the size and quantity of colonic polyps.[37]

Secondary Prevention. Surveillance strategies for individuals with a mutation in the APC gene include a baseline flexible sigmoidoscopy beginning at age 10 to 12 years, with annual flexible sigmoidoscopies thereafter. Upper endoscopies are preformed every 1 to 3 years, beginning when colonic polyps appear. Once subtotal colectomy has been done, annual screening of the rectal remnant is necessary.[59, 61]

Multiple Endocrine Neoplasia

Multiple endocrine neoplasia (MEN) is a hereditary disorder characterized by the occurrence of tumors involving endocrine glands. MEN can be further divided into clinically and genetically distinct syndromes known as MEN1 and MEN2.

MEN1. MEN1, also known as Wermer's syndrome, is an autosomal dominant inherited syndrome associated with germline mutations in the MEN1 gene located on the long arm of chromosome 11 (11q13). The syndrome is characterized by tumors of the pituitary and parathyroid glands, as well as the pancreatic islet cells. Tumors can also involve the adrenal cortex and the thyroid gland.[28]

MEN2. MEN2 is also an autosomal dominant inherited syndrome associated with germline mutations of the RET gene, located on the long arm of chromosome 10 (10q11.2). MEN2 is subdivided into three categories known as MEN2A, MEN2B, and familial medullary thyroid carcinoma (FMTC). Each of these syndromes has its own distinct features, but the one feature common to all three is the presence of medullary thyroid carcinoma (MTC).

Hereditary MTC affects the C cells, which are responsible for the production of calcitonin. These cells develop hyperplasia, which is the precursor for the hereditary form of MTC. An abnormally elevated calcitonin level can be identified as early as 5 years of age. MTC comprises 10% of all thyroid cancers. Of all MTCs, 75% are sporadic and the remaining 25% are due to MEN2. Hereditary MTC is distinctly different from sporadic MTC in that most hereditary cases are bilateral, with an earlier age of onset than sporadic cases. This is not unlike other hereditary cancer syndromes. Of all hereditary MTC cases, 90% are due to MEN2A and 5% each are due to MEN2B and FMTC.[28, 31]

MEN2A is an autosomal inherited disorder that is comprised of MTC, pheochromocytoma, and parathyroid hyperplasia. Distinct skin lesions, known as cutaneous lichen amyloidosis, are also associated with this disorder in some families. Individuals who develop clinical manifestations of MEN2A have a 100% lifetime risk of developing MTC and a 50% risk of developing pheochromocytoma, of which only about 4% are malignant. There is also a 15% to 30% risk of developing hyperparathyroidism, which is usually not symptomatic. In MEN2A families, the diagnosis of MTC is made early in life. The average age of diagnosis is 15 years of age.

MEN2B is also an autosomal dominant inherited disorder characterized by MTCs diagnosed at an earlier age than seen with MEN2A. This is a more aggressive form of MTC with an average age of diagnosis of 5 years of age. Pheochromocytoma is also present but hyperparathyroidism is not. MEN2B is also characterized by developmental abnormalities including mucosal neuromas, ganglioneuromatosis, Marfan-like features, and the presence of megacolon. Individuals with MEN2B have a number of clinical features including thick lips, lumpy tongues, elongated faces, and thick eyelids.[28]

Familial MTC is an autosomal dominant inherited disorder characterized by the diagnosis of MTC in four or more family members. Pheochromocytoma and hyperparathyroidism are not associated with FMTC. The cases of MTC in this syndrome are usually of later age of onset and are slower growing than those associated with MEN2A and MEN2B.[31]

Genetic Testing for MEN2 Syndromes. The MEN2 syndromes are all associated with germline mutations in the RET gene on the long arm of chromosome 10. The RET (rearranged during transfection) gene is a proto-oncogene that encodes a cell surface glycoprotein within the receptor tyrosine kinase family. These receptor tyrosine kinases transduce signals for cell growth and differentiation. When there is a mutation in the RET proto-oncogene, it remains activated, leading to unchecked cell growth and tumorigenesis.[28]

Testing for the RET mutation has become a standard of care and is recommended for all individuals with MTC. Even though approximately 75% of all MTC is considered sporadic, at least 50% of all MEN2B cases have no family history and most likely have de novo mutations. If germline mutations are found in individuals with suspected sporadic MTC, the diagnosis of MEN2 is made and the patient and family are managed accordingly.

Two types of tests are used to screen for RET mutations. Direct DNA sequencing is done for families with known RET mutations. If the mutation is found, the individual is diagnosed with MEN2. If the mutation is not found, the individual has no hereditary risk of MTC. Mutation testing for MEN2A and MEN2B is highly predictive. In individuals with MTC and either pheochromocytoma or hyperparathyroidism or both, a germline mutation in the RET gene is present 97% to 100% of the time. In individuals with MTC and the previously described developmental abnormalities, there is a 95% probability of a RET gene mutation.[31]

Testing for MEN2 can also be done through biochemical screening of blood for calcitonin, calcium, and parathormone levels, and urine for catecholamines and metabolites. This was the gold standard before the availability of DNA testing. At this time, studies have confirmed that DNA sequencing is more sensitive and specific than biochemical screening.

There are definite benefits to RET mutation testing. By identifying mutation carriers very early, before the development of MTC, there is a substantial reduction in morbidity and mortality from the disease. Also, by identifying mutation-negative individuals, they are spared unnecessary screening and evaluation. Testing is very reliable in MEN2A and MEN2B families. Unfortunately, some families have no detectable mutation, despite the presence of clinical features of MEN2. This is most likely due to FMTC, but occasionally it is due to MEN2A or MEN2B.[28, 31]

Clinical Management of the RET Mutation Carrier. Individuals with known RET mutations have a 100% risk of developing MTC. Therefore, prophylactic thyroidectomy is recommended for all mutation carriers. This is usually done between the ages of 5 and 10 years in MEN2A families and in as early as infancy in MEN2B families. Surgery can be delayed in FMTC families because the onset of disease is later and the course often less aggressive.

Postoperatively, individuals are placed on thyroid replacement hormone. Biochemical screening can be done to monitor for residual or metastatic MTC and for the development of pheochromocytoma or hyperparathyroidism. Blood and urine screening is done annually or biannually.[28, 31]

CONCLUSION

Cancer genetics is the latest frontier where war is being waged against a dreaded enemy. As the human genome is mapped and the discovery of new genetic mutations continues, the entire approach to the diagnosis and treatment of cancer is likely to occur. We will move closer to the reality of cancer prevention before disease manifestation. Although the eradication of cancer is the goal, it will not come without a price. There is much to do with regard to the social, legal, and ethical implications of this genetic information. The oncology nurse as educator, caregiver, and advocate can capably provide patients and families with the knowledge and support necessary to make the potentially difficult decisions that must be made in the face of hereditary cancers.[5, 54, 55, 63, 74, 75, 98]

Nursing Management

There are tremendous implications related to genetic testing and risk assessment counseling. This is truly a family process and is therefore affected by family issues and relationships. At the same time, individual issues and concerns must be at the forefront of the decision-making process. Informed consent is an essential component to the process. Information is critical for the individual to make the decisions that have lasting impact on the person and the family. The oncology nurse is an integral part of the cancer genetics multidisciplinary team. With the background in cancer development, diagnosis, treatment, and symptom management, the oncology nurse can participate in the education process, informing the individual and the family about the fundamental principles of carcinogenesis and basic genetics. The oncology nurse creates an atmosphere conducive to educating the family about complex and often emotionally charged subject matter. Privacy is maintained and adult principles of learning are used to optimize the learning experience. The oncology nurse develops a rapport with the individual and family to help reduce anxiety and create a comfortable learning environment that allows individuals and their family members to feel free to ask questions. The oncology nurse must be cognizant of the family dynamics during the counseling and risk assessment session to ensure that pressure and coercion are not applied to the individual undergoing testing. The oncology nurse provides resources in the form of written materials, videotapes, and Internet support and arranges follow-up consultations to assist the individual and the family in the decision-making process. With expanded education in cancer genetics, the oncology nurse can provide care and support in the form of risk assessment and counseling. In 1997, the Oncology Nursing Society developed and approved a position regarding the role of the oncology nurse in cancer genetic counseling.

Nursing Diagnosis

- *Ineffective Family Coping related to mutation status*
- *Ineffective Individual Coping related to mutation status*

Outcome Goal

- Patient and family will be able to use effective coping strategies.

Assessments

- Present coping behaviors
- Family communication patterns
- Current support systems
- Family expectations

Interventions

- Identify and encourage effective coping strategies.
- Encourage effective family communication.

- Encourage use of support systems.
- Consult therapist, social worker, chaplain to assist as needed.

Nursing Diagnosis

- *Anxiety related to perceived risk of cancer*
- *Fear related to perceived risk of cancer*

Outcome Goals

- Patient and family will be able to acknowledge the validity of their feelings.
- Patient and family will be able to use effective skills for dealing with their fears and anxiety.

Assessments

- Perception of cancer risk
- Knowledge of risk factors for hereditary cancers
- Misconceptions related to cancer risk
- Emotional responses
- Psychosocial response
- Physical responses (sweating, flushing, shortness of breath, elevated heart rate, elevated blood pressure)
- Support systems

Interventions

- Establish rapport.
- Provide information about basic genetics, carcinogenesis, personal risk factors, screening guidelines.
- Acknowledge validity of feelings.
- Encourage verbalization of feelings.

- Encourage use of support systems.
- Teach anxiety reduction techniques (relaxation, diversional activities, massage, etc.).

Nursing Diagnosis

- *Knowledge Deficit related to genetic testing*
- *Decisional Conflict related to genetic testing, recommendations*

Outcome Goals

- Patient and family will be able to discuss their risk of having a genetic mutation.
- Patient and family will be able to describe surveillance recommendations.
- Patient and family will be able to identify benefits and limitations of genetic testing.

Assessments

- Knowledge of mutation risk
- Knowledge of surveillance recommendations
- Knowledge of benefits and limitations of genetic testing

Interventions

- Provide information about the probability of having a genetic mutation in a cancer-susceptibility gene.
- Provide surveillance recommendation information.
- Provide information regarding the current benefits and limitations of genetic testing.
- Provide a list of available resources to assist in coping with their cancer risks.

Chapter Questions

1. All of the following are included in a three-generational pedigree *except:*
   a. Mother
   b. Spouse
   c. Brothers
   d. Grandparents
2. All of the following are examples of autosomal dominant pattern of inheritance *except:*
   a. Hereditary nonpolyposis colorectal cancer (HNPCC)
   b. Hereditary breast cancer
   c. Multiple endocrine neoplasia (MEN)
   d. Sporadic ovarian cancer syndrome
3. Which of the following gene mutations leads to an increased risk for breast cancer?
   a. APC
   b. BRCA-2

   c. HNPCC
   d. p15
4. All of the following are risk prediction models for *hereditary* breast cancer *except:*
   a. Frank tables
   b. Claus model
   c. Gail model
   d. Couch tables
5. Screening recommendations for an individual with a mutation in the APC gene would include:
   a. Biannual mammogram
   b. Annual sigmoidoscopy
   c. Annual CA-125
   d. Annual thyroid function studies
6. Multiple endocrine neoplasia type 2b (MEN2B) is comprised of all of the following *except:*
   a. Pheochromocytoma
   b. Medullary thyroid carcinoma
   c. Developmental abnormalities
   d. Hyperparathyroidism

7. An individual with a mutation in the RET gene is a candidate for which prophylactic surgery?
  a. Bilateral mastectomy
  b. Thyroidectomy
  c. Bilateral oophorectomy
  d. Subtotal colectomy

8. The elements of informed consent for genetic testing include all *except:*
  a. Treatment options
  b. Benefits of testing
  c. Limitations of testing
  d. Risks of testing

9. A genetic test result is considered confirmatory if:
  a. It involves complete gene sequencing
  b. It is negative in an unaffected individual who is tested first in the family
  c. It is positive for a individual in a family with a known inherited mutation
  d. It is negative in an affected individual who is tested last in the family

10. The goals of the Human Genome Project include all of the following *except:*
  a. Sequencing the entire genome
  b. Investigating the ethical, legal, and social implications of the project
  c. Developing a genetic map
  d. Developing chemoprevention agents for each identified cancer-causing mutation

BIBLIOGRAPHY

1. American Society of Clinical Oncology Subcommittee: Statement of the American Society of Clinical Oncology: Genetic testing for cancer susceptibility, *J Clin Oncol* 14(5):1730, 1996.
2. Bale AE, Li FP: Principles of cancer management: cancer genetics. In DeVita VT, Hellman S, Rosenberg SA, editors: *Cancer: principles and practice of oncology,* ed. 5, Philadelphia, Lippincott, 1997.
3. Baron RH, Borgen PI: Genetic susceptibility for breast cancer: testing and primary prevention options, *Oncol Nurs Forum* 24(3):461, 1997.
4. Berchuck A and others: Managing hereditary ovarian cancer risk, *Cancer* 86(11)Suppl:2517, 1999.
5. Bernhardt BA and others: Evaluation of nurses and genetic counselors as providers of education about breast cancer susceptibility testing, *Oncol Nurs Forum* 27(1):33, 2000.
6. Biesecker BB: Programmed instruction: cancer genetics: genetic testing for cancer predisposition, *Cancer Nurs* 20(4):285, 1997.
7. Blackwood MA, Weber BL: BRCA1 and BRCA2: from molecular genetics to clinical medicine, *J Clin Oncol* 16(5):1969, 1998.
8. Breast Cancer Linkage Consortium: Cancer risks in BRCA2 mutation carriers, *J Natl Cancer Inst* 91(15): 1310, 1999.
9. Burke W and others: Recommendations for follow-up care of individuals with an inherited predisposition to cancer: II. BRCA1 and BRCA2, *JAMA* 277(12):997, 1997.
10. Cho MK and others: Commercialization of BRCA1/2 testing: practitioner awareness and use of a new genetic test, *Am J Med Genet* 83:157, 1999.
11. Clark BA and others: Genetic testing for cancer, *Patient Care for the Nurse Practitioner* 3(2):46, 2000.
12. Claus EB, Risch N, Thompson WD: Autosomal dominant inheritance of early-onset breast cancer, *Cancer* 73(3):643, 1994.
13. Collins FS: Shattuck Lecture: medical and societal consequences of the human genome project, *N Engl J Med* 341(1):28, 1999.
14. Couch FJ and others: BRCA1 mutations in women attending clinics that evaluate the risk of breast cancer, *N Engl J Med* 336(20):1409, 1997.
15. Cummings S, Olopade O: Predisposition testing for inherited breast cancer, *Oncology* 12(8):1227, 1998.
16. Daly M: New perspectives in breast cancer: the genetic revolution, *Oncol Nurs Updates* 1(6):1, 1994.
17. Dimond E and others: Programmed instruction: cancer genetics: the role of the nurse in cancer genetics, *Cancer Nurs* 21(1):57, 1998.
18. Dimond E, Peters J, Jenkins J: Programmed instruction: human genetics: the genetic basis of cancer, *Cancer Nurs* 20(3):213, 1997.
19. Easton DF and others: Breast and ovarian cancer incidence in BRCA1-mutation carriers, *Am J Hum Genet* 56:265, 1995.
20. Easton DF, Steele L, Fields PEA: Cancer risks in two large breast cancer families linked to BRCA2 on chromosome 13q12–13, *Am J Hum Genet* 61:120, 1997.
21. Eng C: Genetics of Cowden syndrome: through the looking glass of oncology, *Int J Oncol* 12:701, 1998.
22. Ford D: Genetic heterogeneity and penetrance analysis of the BRCA1 and BRCA2 genes in breast cancer families, *Am J Hum Genet* 62:676, 1998.
23. Frank TS and others: Sequence analysis of BRCA1 and BRCA2: correlation of mutations with family history and ovarian cancer risk, *J Clin Oncol* 16(7):2417, 1998.
24. Fraser MC, Calzone KA, Goldstein AM: Familial cancers: evolving challenges for nursing practice, *Oncol Nurs Updates* 4(3):1, 1997.
25. Gail MH and others: Projecting individualized probabilities of developing breast cancer for white females who are being examined annually, *J Natl Cancer Inst* 81:1879, 1989.
26. Garber J: Inherited breast cancer: increasingly familiar territory, *J Clin Oncol* 16(5):1639, 1998.
27. Garber J: A 40-year-old woman with a strong family history of breast cancer, *JAMA* 282(20):1953, 1999.
28. Giarelli E: Medullary thyroid carcinoma: one component of the inherited disorder multiple endocrine neoplasia, type 2A, *Oncol Nurs Forum* 24(6):1007, 1997.
29. Grann VR and others: Decision analysis of prophylactic mastectomy and oophorectomy in BRCA1-positive or BRCA2-positive patients, *J Clin Oncol* 16(3):979, 1998.
30. Grann VR et al: Benefits and costs of screening Ashkenazi Jewish women for BRCA1 and BRCA2, *J Clin Oncol* 17(2):494, 1999.

31. Grosfeld FJM and others: Psychosocial consequences of DNA analysis for MEN type 2, *Oncology* 10(2):141, 1996.

32. Gryfe R and others: Tumor microsatellite instability and clinical outcome in young patients with colorectal cancer, *N Engl J Med* 342(2):69, 2000.

33. Haber D: Breast cancer in carriers of BRCA1 and BRCA2 mutations: tackling a molecular and clinical conundrum, *J Clin Oncol* 17(11):3367, 1999.

34. Hall J and others: Linkage of early-onset familial breast cancer to chromosome 17q21, *Science* 250:1684, 1990.

35. Hartge P and others: The prevalence of common BRCA1 and BRCA2 mutations among Ashkenazi Jews, *Am J Hum Genet* 64:963, 1999.

36. Hartmann LC and others: Efficacy of bilateral prophylactic mastectomy in women with a family history of breast cancer, *N Engl J Med* 340(2):77, 1999.

37. Hawk E, Lubet R, Limburg P: Chemoprevention in hereditary colorectal cancer, *Cancer* 86(11) Suppl:2551, 1999.

38. Healy B: BRCA genes: bookmaking, fortune-telling, and medical care, *N Engl J Med* 336(20):1448, 1997.

39. Holtzman NA: Are we ready to screen for inherited susceptibility to cancer? *Oncology* 10(1):55, 1996.

40. Jacobs LA: At-risk for cancer: genetic discrimination in the workplace, *Oncol Nurs Forum* 25(3):475, 1998.

41. Jacobs LA: Hereditary nonpolyposis colon cancer: genetic basis, testing, and patient-care issues, *Oncol Nurs Forum* 25(4):719, 1998.

42. Jenkins J, Lea DH: Cancer genetics for nurses, part II: integrating genetics into oncology nursing practice, *Oncol Nurs Updates* 4(6):1, 1997.

43. Kelly PT: Breast cancer risk assessment and counseling: a clinician's guide, *Breast J* 3(6):311, 1997.

44. Kelly PT: Hereditary breast cancer: risk assessment is the easy part, *Breast J* 5(1):52, 1999.

45. Koenig BA and others: Genetic testing for BRCA1 and BRCA2: recommendations of the Stanford program in genomics, ethics, and society, *J Womens Health* 7(5):531, 1998.

46. Krainer M and others: Differential contributions of BRCA1 and BRCA2 to early-onset breast cancer, *N Engl J Med* 336(20):1416, 1997.

47. Laken SJ and others: Familial colorectal cancer in Ashkenazim due to a hypermutable tract in APC, *Nat Genet* 17:79, 1997.

48. Langston A and others: BRCA1 mutations in a population-based sample of young women with breast cancer, *N Engl J Med* 334:137, 1996.

49. Lea DH, Jenkins J: Cancer genetics for nurses: part I. The genetic basis of cancer, *Oncol Nurs Updates* 4(5):1, 1997.

50. Lerman C, Croyle RT: Emotional and behavioral responses to genetic testing for susceptibility to cancer, *Oncology* 10(2):191, 1996.

51. Lerman C and others: What you don't know can hurt you: adverse psychologic effects in members of BRCA1-linked and BRCA2-linked families who decline genetic testing, *J Clin Oncol* 16(5):1650, 1998.

52. Li FP: Cancer control in susceptible groups: opportunities and challenges, *J Clin Oncol* 17(2):719, 1999.

53. Loescher LJ: DNA testing for cancer predisposition, *Oncol Nurs Forum* 25(8):1317, 1998.

54. Loescher LJ: Genetics in cancer prediction, screening and counseling: part 1, genetics in cancer prediction and screening, *Oncol Nurs Forum* 22(2) Suppl:10, 1995.

55. Loescher LJ: Genetics in cancer prediction, screening, and counseling: part II, the nurse's role in genetic counseling, *Oncol Nurs Forum* 22(2) Suppl:16, 1995.

56. Lynch HT: Genetic counseling in cancer: a status report, *Oncology* 10(1):23, 1996.

57. Lynch HT: Genetic counseling in cancer: a status report—part 2, *Oncology* 10(2):131, 1996.

58. Lynch HT, Lynch J: Genetic counseling for hereditary cancer, *Oncology* 10(1):27, 1996.

59. Lynch HT, Shaw TG, Lynch JF: The genetics of colorectal cancer, *Prim Care Cancer* 19(6):27, 1999.

60. Lynch HT, Smyrk T, Lynch JF: Molecular genetics and clinical-pathology features of hereditary nonpolyposis colorectal carcinoma (Lynch syndrome), *Oncology* 55:103, 1995.

61. Lynch HT and others: Clinical impact of molecular genetic diagnosis, genetic counseling, and management of hereditary cancer, part II: hereditary nonpolyposis colorectal carcinoma as a model, *Cancer* 86(11) Suppl:2457, 1999.

62. Lynch PM: Clinical challenges in management of familial adenomatous polyposis and hereditary nonpolyposis colorectal cancer, *Cancer* 86(11) Suppl:2533, 1999.

63. MacDonald DJ: Ethical, legal, and social issues related to predisposition testing for breast cancer risk: what nurses need to know, *Genetics: Implications for Practice in Quality of Life, A Nursing Challenge* 6(1):8, 1997.

64. Matloff ET, Peshkin BN: Complexities in cancer genetic counseling: breast and ovarian cancer, *Principles and Practice of Oncology Updates* 12(1):1, 1998.

65. Menko FH and others: Genetic counseling in hereditary nonpolyposis colorectal cancer, *Oncology* 10(1):71, 1996.

66. Middelton LA, Peters KF, Helmbold EA: Programmed instruction: genetics and gene therapy: genes and inheritance, *Cancer Nurs* 20(2):129, 1997.

67. Narod SA and others: Oral contraceptives and the risk of hereditary ovarian cancer, *N Engl J Med* 339:424, 1998.

68. Neuhausen S and others: Recurrent BRCA-2 6174delT mutations in Ashkenazi Jewish women affected by breast cancer, *Nat Genet* 13:126, 1996.

69. Offit, K: Genetic prognostic markers for colorectal cancer, *N Engl J Med* 342(2):124, 2000.

70. Olopade OI, Weber BL: Breast cancer genetics: toward molecular characterization of individuals at increased risk for breast cancer: part I, *Principles and Practice of Oncology Updates* 12(10):1, 1998.

71. Olopade OI, Weber BL: Breast cancer genetics: toward molecular characterization of individuals at increased risk for breast cancer: part II, *Principles and Practice of Oncology Updates* 12(11):1, 1998.

72. Olopade OI, Cummings S: Genetic counseling for cancer: part I, *Principles and Practice of Oncology Updates* 10(1):1, 1996.

73. Olopade OI, Cummings S: Genetic counseling for cancer: part II, *Principles and Practice of Oncology Updates* 10(2):1, 1996.

74. Oncology Nursing Society: ONS position statement: cancer genetic testing and risk assessment counseling, *Oncol Nurs Forum* 25(3):463, 1998.

75. Oncology Nursing Society: ONS position: the role of the oncology nurse in cancer genetic counseling, *Oncol Nurs Forum* 25(3):464, 1998.

76. Panguluri RCK and others: BRCA1 mutations in African Americans, *Hum Genet* 105:28, 1999.

77. Peters J, Dimond E, Jenkins J: Programmed instruction: cancer genetics: clinical applications of genetic technologies to cancer care, *Cancer Nurs* 20(5):359, 1997.

78. Peters JA, Stopfer JE: Role of the genetic counselor in familial cancer, *Oncology* 10(2):159, 1996.

79. Peters KF, Hadley DW: Programmed instruction: the human genome project, *Cancer Nurs* 20(1):62, 1997.

80. Petersen GM, Brensinger JD: Genetic testing and counseling in familial adenomatous polyposis, *Oncology* 10(1):89, 1996.

81. Phillips K, Andrulis I, Goodwin P: Breast carcinomas arising in carriers of mutations in BRCA1 or BRCA2: are they prognostically different? *J Clin Oncol* 17(11): 3653, 1999. ·

82. Rebbeck TR: Inherited genetic predisposition in breast cancer, *Cancer* 86(11) Suppl:2493, 1999.

83. Rebbeck TR and others: Breast cancer risk after bilateral prophylactic oophorectomy in BRCA1 mutation carriers, *J Natl Cancer Inst* 91(17):1475, 1999.

84. Rieger PT: The impact of cancer genetics on oncology nursing practice, *Nurs Interventions Oncol* 9:15, 1997.

85. Rieger PT, Pentz RD: Genetic testing and informed consent, *Semin Oncol Nurs* 15(2):104, 1999.

86. Robson M and others: BRCA-associated breast cancer in young women, *J Clin Oncol* 16(5):1642, 1998.

87. Rosenblum DS, Shiff SJ: Chemoprevention of colorectal cancer: a practical approach, *Prim Care Cancer* 19(6): 22, 1999.

88. Rosenthal N: Molecular medicine: DNA and the genetic code, *N Engl J Med* 331(1):39, 1994.

89. Sack GH: *Medical genetics,* New York, McGraw-Hill, 1999.

90. Schrag D and others: Decision analysis—effects of prophylactic mastectomy and oophorectomy on life expectancy among women with BRCA1 or BRCA2 mutations, *N Engl J Med* 336(20):1465, 1997.

91. Schrag D and others: Life expectancy gains from cancer prevention strategies for women with breast cancer and BRCA1 or BRCA2 mutations, *JAMA* 283(5):617, 2000.

92. Schubert EL and others: BRCA2 in American families with 4 or more cases of breast or ovarian cancer: recurrent and novel mutations, variable expression, penetrance, and the possibility of families whose cancer is not attributable to BRCA1 or BRCA2, *Am J Hum Genet* 60:1031, 1997.

93. Shattuck-Eidens D and others: A collaborative survey of 80 mutations in the BRCA1 breast and ovarian cancer susceptibility genes, *JAMA* 273(7):535, 1995.

94. Shattuck-Eidens D and others: BRCA1 sequence analysis in women at high risk for susceptibility mutations: risk factor analysis and implications for genetic testing, *JAMA* 278:1242, 1997.

95. Struewing JP and others: The risk of cancer associated with specific mutations of BRCA1 and BRCA2 among Ashkenazi Jews, *N Engl J Med* 336(20):1401, 1997.

96. Szabo C, King M: Inherited breast and ovarian cancer, *Hum Genet* 4:1811, 1995.

97. Tinley ST, Lynch HT: Integration of family history and medical management of patients with hereditary cancers, *Cancer* 86(11) Suppl:2525, 1999.

98. Tranin AS: Cancer genetic counseling: exemplars from oncology nursing, *Genetics: Implications for Practice in Quality of Life, A Nursing Challenge* 6(1):17, 1997.

99. Turner BC and others: BRCA1/BRCA2 germline mutations in locally recurrent breast cancer patients after lumpectomy and radiation therapy: implications for breast-conserving management in patients with BRCA1/BRCA2 mutations, *J Clin Oncol* 17(10):3017, 1999.

100. U.S. Department of Health and Human Services: Understanding gene testing, National Cancer Institute Publication 96-3905, 1995.

101. Verhoog L and others: Survival in hereditary breast cancer associated with germline mutations of BRCA2, *J Clin Oncol* 17(11):3396, 1999.

102. Weber BL and others: Familial breast cancer, *Cancer* 72:1013, 1994.

103. Weitzel JN: Genetic cancer risk assessment, *Cancer* 86(11):2483, 1999.

104. Williams JK: Principles of genetics and cancer, *Semin Oncol Nurs* 13(2):68, 1997.

Epidemiology

3 CHAPTER

Lisa Schulmeister

The science of *epidemiology* studies the variations in disease frequencies among human population groups and the factors influencing these variations. The goal of epidemiology is to identify the cause of disease so that the causative agent may be removed and ultimately that the disease can be prevented. Unlike basic research, the emphasis of epidemiology is on humans rather than animals, and unlike clinical medicine, epidemiology studies groups or populations rather than individuals. In addition, epidemiology focuses on the events occurring before the illness rather than the treatment after disease diagnosis. The endpoint of therapeutic research is to discover the cure for cancer; the endpoint of epidemiologic research is to prevent cancer.[30]

Epidemiology was initially associated with the study of infectious diseases. In the 1940s, however, scientists began to notice an increasing number of deaths from chronic causes, such as cancer and heart disease. One of the earliest and best known cancer epidemiologic studies was performed by the British surgeon Percival Pott in 1775. Pott first described occupational carcinogens by noting the high incidence of scrotal cancer in chimneysweeps. The astute observation of Dr. Pott preceded the laboratory discovery of the carcinogenic properties of polycyclic hydrocarbons, such as coal and soot, by decades. Cancer epidemiology became a refined research discipline partly as a result of oncology becoming a distinct subspecialty and the beginning of the computer age.

In addition to epidemiologic principles, demography and the natural and social sciences are used to help discover causes of cancer. Examples of these fields include geographic variations in the occurrence of cancer, the relationship of cancer incidence to social habits and environmental agents, the comparison of populations with and without cancer, and results after removal of suspected cancer-causing agents.

A basic understanding of epidemiologic terminology and techniques assists oncology nurses to interpret literature about cancer patterns and causation. This knowledge is useful in targeting populations for education, prevention, and screening programs.

TERMINOLOGY

Many terms are associated with the science of epidemiology. This chapter limits discussion to four terms that help to describe the cancer problem and are commonly used in cancer literature: incidence, prevalence, mortality, and survival.

Incidence

The number of newly diagnosed cases of cancer in a specified period of time in a defined population is called the cancer *incidence*. It is defined as follows:

Number of persons developing cancer in a specified period of time/Total population living at that time

Usually the period is 1 year and the rates are expressed per 100,000 persons.[14] For example, in 1999 for the Metropolitan Detroit tricounty female population of 2,006,867, there were 2564 cases of invasive breast cancer diagnosed. Using the formula, the incidence rate for breast cancer is 127.76:

$$2564/2,006,867 \times 100,000 = 127.76$$

In the United States in 1999, there were 175,000 newly diagnosed cases of breast cancer in women and the incident rate was 113.2/100,000.[21] The advantage of expressing incidence as a rate is that it allows comparison of rates among different populations. The fact that in 1999 Utah had 800 new cases of breast cancer and California had 16,900 new cases of breast cancer has little meaning because of their population differences. If the rate of incidence per 100,000 population in Utah was 72.3 and in California it was 93.8, however, one could investigate what differences were responsible for the higher incidence rate in California. In addition, when the incidence rate is adjusted for age, it also takes into account population age differences, which can influence the rate. Important epidemiologic questions may arise when comparing incidence rates around the United States and around the world. For the year 2000, the estimated new cancer cases in the United States will be 1,220,100.[14]

The longest ongoing population-based resource is the Connecticut Tumor Registry, which has been collecting incidence data since 1935. Before 1973, cancer incidence data were collected through several periodic surveys in selected U.S. areas. These surveys, coordinated by the National Cancer Institute (NCI), were conducted in 1937–1939, 1947–1948, and 1969–1971. In 1973 the NCI established and funded the Surveillance, Epidemiology, and End-Results Program (SEER) to gather information on cancer incidence, mortality, and survival. The registries located in Atlanta; Detroit; San Francisco/Oakland; Seattle/Puget Sound; the entire states of Connecticut, Hawaii, Iowa, New Mexico, and Utah; and Puerto Rico represent about 10% of the U.S. population with considerable geographic and ethnic variations.

In addition to SEER data, incidence information is also collected in individual hospital cancer registries. Individual tumor registries are certified by the American College of Surgeons (ACS). These registries abstract demographic and disease-related information from the charts of patients with newly diagnosed cancer. All patients are followed for survival data. The registries also conduct disease-specific studies as requested by the ACS. Incidence data collection focuses on two specific areas: demographic and medical. *Demographic* information extrapolates age, gender, race, marital status, and place of residence. *Medical* data on the same individual report onset of illness, location of tumor, stage, histology, treatment, and survival over time. These data assist epidemiologists in describing the current cancer problem in terms of geographic distribution, age and race of patients, and increase or decrease in specific types of cancer.

Care must be exercised when deriving conclusions from incidence data. For example, there has been a slight but steady increase in the overall cancer incidence over the past decade. This information does not necessarily mean cancer is on the rise. Consider this hypothesis: more than half of all cancers are diagnosed after age 65; with the "graying of America," a greater portion of the population is over 65, and therefore this expanding aged population accounts for some of the increase in new cases. Apply this theory to these data: there were 142,900 new cases of breast cancer in 1989 compared with 175,000 in 1999. These figures would seem to indicate an increasing rate of breast cancer incidence, but, in fact, they reflect population growth because there were more women alive over the age of 50 in 1999 with the potential to develop breast cancer. Concomitantly,

marked increases in use of mammography, allowing for early detection of breast cancers, have also influenced the rising incidence rate.

Prevalence

The measurement of all cancer cases, both old and new, at a *designated point in time,* is called cancer *prevalence.*[22] The prevalence rate is defined as follows:

Number of persons with cancer at a given point in time/Total population living at that time

These data are not routinely collected by the SEER registries and must be determined by conducting a special survey. This is expensive and is further prohibited by the difficulty in determining who actually has been cured of the disease and should not be counted in the prevalence survey. Also, any cancer therapy that improves survival would actually increase the prevalence of cancer.

The prevalence rate provides useful information for health care planning, including physical facilities, manpower, and the design and implementation of screening programs.[29]

Mortality

The number of deaths attributed to cancer in a specified time period and in a defined population is the cancer *mortality.*[22] The mortality rate is defined as follows:

Number of persons dying of cancer in a specified period of time/Total population living at that time

The 2000 estimated number of cancer deaths in the United States is 552,200 persons.[14] Unlike incidence data, mortality data have routinely been collected in the United States since 1930. The National Death Index is a centralized source for death information and can be accessed by investigators. Mortality data of comparable quality are available throughout the world and can be used for comparison of death rates. The shortcoming of mortality data, however, is accuracy. Death certificates routinely assign a single cause of death to each patient. A patient with colon cancer that metastasized to the liver may be reported to have died from liver failure rather than colon cancer.

Mortality figures are actually only a variable reflection of the cancer incidence. Therefore, when epidemiologists try to determine causes of cancer, the incidence figures are usually more helpful. Mortality data enable us to determine trends over time in the magnitude of cancer as a cause of death among members of the U.S. population. It is also useful in evaluating the impact of advances in cancer treatment.

Survival

The link between incidence and mortality data is *survival analysis,* the observation over time of persons with cancer and the calculation of their probability of dying over several time periods.[29] Survival data are a useful measure of the end result of cancer treatment and can indicate improvements over time in the management of cancer. Survival data can provide a baseline for individual institutions to compare their local survival rates with national rates. Major discrepancies may indicate the need for education of community physicians regarding cancer management or more intense community education regarding early detection. The disadvantage of survival data, however, is that the data are influenced by the statistical methods used as well as measures unrelated to treatment efficacy, such as earlier detection and changes in disease classification systems. Some researchers advocate basing survival statistics on conditional survival and annual hazard calculations; these techniques consider the fact that long-term prognosis for cancer is influenced by the number of years that individuals have already survived cancer.[25, 46] Factors unrelated to treatment efficacy appear to lengthen survival without actually changing the natural course of the disease. Some studies of survival take these factors into account; for instance, differences in cervical cancer survival among African American and white women were analyzed using a comprehensive model that included demographic factors such as age, stage of disease, other tumor characteristics, and treatment. Despite analysis of these factors, race remained an independent predictor of survival; 7-year survival was greater among the white women.[17] Racial differences in breast cancer survival between African America and white women also have been identified. Race has been shown to be an independent predictor of breast cancer survival, and these findings suggest that racial differences exist in the molecular biology of breast cancer.[19] Recent survival studies also are including the additional factor of health care access. In a study of a group of women in a managed care population, African American women were diagnosed with breast cancer at a later stage than other women and had a significantly lower 5-year survival. Although all of the women in the study adhered to standardized breast cancer screening, ethnic differences in stage of breast cancer at diagnosis occurred.[48]

The 5-year survival rate has become almost a standard term, although there is no specific biologic significance about having survived 5 years. Some statisticians have suggested that median survival times are better indicators of survival than 5-year relative survival rates when survival times are short.[31]

Data about long-term survival of cancer is beginning to be reported. Relative survival after diagnosis of breast and prostate cancer has been found to decline up to 15 years after diagnosis, whereas survival after diagnosis of lung and colon cancer remain approximately constant after 5 and 10 years. Among patients with localized breast and prostate cancer, women younger than age 45 and men 75 years old and older had the poorest survival rates.[20, 26, 45]

Identification of Trends

The ultimate value of incidence, prevalence, mortality, and survival data is the identification of trends. This is the root of epidemiologic studies. A particular trend is identified that raises the question "why?" From that point, a study is designed to determine the possible cause of the trend. Why have lung cancer deaths exceeded breast cancer deaths in women? Why has the incidence of melanoma increased 1000% over the past 50 years?[9]

The trends found in monitoring cancer incidence and mortality statistics have significant implications for cancer education and prevention. For example, the incidence of lung cancer in women increased dramatically every year this past decade. Epidemiologic studies reveal this was caused by the acceptance of and subsequent increase in women smoking after World War II. This was an impetus for education and smoking cessation interventions targeting women. Likewise, the alarming increase in the incidence of malignant melanoma resulted in nationwide public education about the risks of sun exposure. Industry responded to both medical research and public concern by marketing more effective sunscreen products and including "sun-sense" education in their advertising campaigns.

Box 3–1 lists some examples of current trends in cancer incidence, mortality, and survival.

TYPES OF STUDIES

The epidemiologic method is composed of an orderly progression of three types of studies: descriptive, analytic, and experimental. *Descriptive studies* are observational in nature and record the existing patterns of disease. Identified trends generate a hypothesis as to the possible cause of the cancer trend. The intermediate step, the *analytic study,* tests the hypothesis and tries to identify the causal relationship. The final step, the *experimental study,* removes the suspected cause and evaluates the effect on the population (Fig. 3–1).

Descriptive Studies

Descriptive studies form the body of data within which the hypothesis may be sought. The disease of cancer can be described in many ways. One method of description

BOX 3-1

Current Trends in Cancer Incidence, Mortality, and Survival

INCIDENCE

Approximately 1,220,100 new cases of invasive cancer were diagnosed in the United States in 2000.

Higher rate of incidence is seen in men than women.

Overall incidence is highest in African Americans and lowest in Native Americans.

Prostate cancer incidence rates are 49% higher for African American men than white men.

Leading sites of incidence in men are prostate, lung, and colon.

Leading sites of incidence in women are breast, lung, and colon.

Melanoma incidence has increased 1000% in the past 50 years.

MORTALITY

More than 552,200 cancer-related deaths occurred in the United States in 2000.

Lung cancer accounts for 31% of male cancer deaths.

Lung cancer accounts for 25% of female cancer deaths.

Risks of dying of lung cancer are 22 times higher for male smokers and 12 times higher for female smokers.

Leading causes of male death are cancers of the lung, prostate, colon, and pancreas and non-Hodgkin's lymphoma.

Leading causes of female death are cancers of the lung, breast, colon, pancreas, and ovary.

Cancer is the leading cause of death in women from ages 40 to 79.

For all ages, cancer is the second most common cause of death, following heart disease.

For children under age 15, cancer is the second most common cause of death.

African Americans are 45% more likely to die of cancer than are whites.

After significant increases for the past 70 years, cancer mortality rates for all cancers combined began to decline in the 1990s.

SURVIVAL

Overall 5-year relative survival rate for all cancer is 60%.

Data from references 11, 14, 27, and 33.

might be evaluating the *frequency* of a cancer. This is the purpose of incidence, prevalence, and mortality data. Specific methods are available to describe the *classification* of the cancer: site of the tumor, morphology and grade, and the stage of the disease. This information is found in the medical record at the time of diagnosis and can be extrapolated by the epidemiologist. Person, place, and time are classic descriptive epidemiologic variables that serve as a major source of clues to cancer etiology.

Person. Age, gender, and racial differences account for fundamental differences in cancer rates.

Age. With a few exceptions, cancer becomes more prevalent in older individuals. Sixty percent of all cancers occur in persons age 65 or older[47] and cancer is the second most common cause of death in persons older than 65.[3] Epidemiologists previously explained the increase of cancer incidence with advancing age as an increased susceptibility problem or perhaps an impaired immune system. It is now believed, however, that the increased incidence reflects the importance of duration of carcinogen exposure and of long induction periods of some cancers.[43] Population predictions indicate that the elderly population is the fastest growing segment of the population and that by 2030, one in five Americans will be 65 years old or older.[47] Therefore, a rise in cancer incidence among the elderly is expected. Also, with the decline in deaths related to cardiovascular disease, cancer will become an even more prominent cause of death among those over age 65.[3]

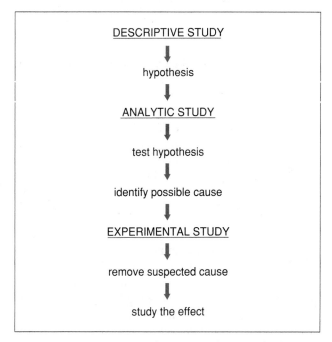

FIGURE 3-1 The epidemiologic method.

Cancer incidence among infants also is increasing. Many cancers in infants demonstrate unique epidemiologic, clinical, and genetic characteristics compared with cancers in older children. From 1973 to 1992, the average annual increase in rates of cancer among infants was 2.9%. Increasing trends were greatest for retinoblastoma, central nervous system cancers, and neuroblastoma.[15, 21]

Gender. More men develop cancer than do women, and more men die from cancer than do women. As women adopt roles and habits in society similar to men, the rates of non–gender-linked cancers would become similar, if the current differences are related to environmental and occupational causes.[29]

Race. There are striking racial and ethnic variations in cancer incidence. The incidence of cancer in men is highest in African Americans, followed by whites, Hispanics, and Asian/Pacific Islanders. In women, the incidence of cancer is highest in whites, followed by African Americans, Hispanics, and Asian/Pacific Islanders.[14] There also is a significant variation in the kinds of cancer seen in different races. Compared with other races, whites have especially high rates of melanoma, Hodgkin's disease, non-Hodgkin's lymphomas, and leukemia. African Americans have elevated rates of multiple myeloma and cancers of the oral cavity, esophagus, and colon. Prostate cancer incidence is greatest among African American men.[14] Vietnamese women have high rates of cervical cancer,[32] and Native Americans have a remarkable prevalence of stomach cancer. Hawaiian women develop lung, breast, and ovarian cancer more frequently than others.[6, 14] Lung cancer rates among Alaska Native men is very high, and although tobacco is believed to play a central role, other factors, such as genetic predisposition and radiation exposure, may play a role.[5] Racial and ethnic populations present unique opportunities for studying environmental and host differences.

Other factors. Other "person" or host factors such as general health and wellness status—including nutritional status, cultural and socioeconomic variables, marital status, psychological factors, and susceptibility factors—help to describe the cancer situation. These variables add to the body of information and may help define the hypothesis of a particular cancer cause.

Place. The evaluation of incidence and mortality statistics for various geographic locales has led to the identification of major international differences in the cancer burden. Japan exemplifies a unique cancer spectrum when compared with 24 other countries. The Japanese population has a low international incidence rate of breast cancer and the highest international incidence of stomach cancer.[33] Differing genetic constitutions and social habits may be possible explanations. Japanese women who migrate to Hawaii or California and adopt new habits develop cancer risks similar to American women, with an increase in their breast cancer incidence and a decrease in stomach cancers.

In addition to a specific location, the category of place in descriptive studies also involves physical and biologic environmental variables such as geologic structure, water sources, flora, weather, climate, plants, and animals. For instance, a positive correlation has been observed between geographic latitude and mortality of pancreatic cancer; mortality is higher in northern countries, such as Denmark and Sweden, than in countries closer to the equator.[42] "Place" descriptions also include the socioeconomic environment: urban versus rural, waste disposal systems, industrialization, pollution, and so forth. Epidemiologists may study changes in the environment that coincide with changes in cancer incidence to develop a hypothesis about the potential causative agent.

Time. Evaluating the incidence of cancer over time may indicate significant trends. The increased incidence of mesothelioma throughout the 1970s and early 1980s has been attributed to occupational exposure to asbestos during World War II.[35] Epidemiologic studies also have found an association between a history of sunburn and sun exposure and the increasing incidence of cutaneous melanoma.[9] The well-recognized time trend of mounting lung cancer deaths led to the extensive series of studies that ultimately incriminated cigarette smoking as a principal cause.

Studying descriptive data and incidence trends raises obvious questions regarding environmental, geographic, dietary, and sociocultural variables of affected populations. Sources of variability and even sources of nonvariability may serve as an element of hypothesis formulation. Box 3–2 lists factors used in descriptive epidemiologic study.

Analytic Studies

Descriptive epidemiologic studies generate possible causes of disease. These etiologic hypotheses are then tested in the second investigative phase, the analytic study. Analytic epidemiology also assists in further defining risk factors. This type of study is observational in nature, and its purpose is to elucidate which type of exposure causes which kind(s) of cancer.[29] The three types of analytic studies are cross-sectional studies, case-control studies, and cohort studies. The element of *time* distinguishes these types of studies. A cross-sectional study occurs in the present, case-control studies are based on subjects with past exposure (*retrospective*), and cohort studies examine populations who have been exposed to see if they develop the disease in the future (*prospective*).

BOX 3-2

Descriptive Epidemiology Factors

FREQUENCY

Incidence
Prevalence
Mortality

DISEASE

Site
Morphology
Grade
Stage

PERSON

Age
Gender
Race
Marital status
Nutritional status
Cultural differences
Socioeconomic variables
Psychologic factors
Susceptibility factors

PLACE

Physical environment
Biologic environment
Geographic location

TIME

Changes in frequency patterns over specified periods
of time

Cross-sectional Studies. These studies may also be called *prevalence surveys*. The purpose is to canvas a population of subjects to ascertain a relationship between the disease and variables of interest as they exist in the group at a specific time. The drawback of such a survey is that the causal nature of a relationship cannot be established because the design does not allow accounting for the time sequence of events.[22]

Cohort Design. This type of study examines over time a population or group of individuals with or without a specific exposure to determine their disease incident rate or health outcome or both. When the study is conducted prospectively, it may also be referred to as a *concurrent study*. People selected for a cohort study all have been exposed to the suspected cancer-causing factor. These subjects are followed into the future to evaluate the possible development of cancer. For example, to test the hypothesis that tanning in a tanning parlor causes skin cancer, two groups of people are followed: a group who tanned in parlors and a group who did not. All subjects are followed over a period of years to determine if the exposed group had a higher incidence of skin cancer. The disease incidence or mortality rates for various levels of exposure (high, medium, low, none) are then compared. If a causal relationship exists between tanning booths and skin cancer, one would expect to see the highest incidence of skin cancer in the sample with the most frequent exposure to tanning beds.

A second type of cohort study is the *historical cohort design,* also called the *historical prospective study.* This design is frequently used in occupational studies because both the exposure and the onset of cancer have already occurred. Information is collected by reviewing records of the sample under study and reconstructing the disease history. It is important in a cohort or prospective study that the time the study begins is clearly identified, that all of the participants are free of cancer when enrolled in the study, and that all participants are followed the same way. Complete long-term follow-up of all the participants in a cohort study, using medical records, death certificates, and other available resources, is crucial. Prospective studies have the disadvantage of being very large and expensive trials that take an extended period of time to complete.

A third type of cohort study is a *migrant study.* Migrant studies take advantage of the wide geographic variation in cancer risk and incidence. Cancer rates from migrants, obtained from routinely collected incidence and mortality statistics, are compared with those in the host country or country of origin; the rate of change with time since migration (or age at migration) and in subsequent generations is assessed, and the results are interpreted in the light of differences in socioeconomic status and degree of cultural assimilation. Rapid changes in cancer risk and incidence following migration imply that life-style or environmental factors are of overriding importance in cancer etiology.[24]

Case-Control Design. This method evaluates a case group of persons diagnosed with the cancer under study who have exposure to the suspected cancer-causing agent. This group is compared with a control group chosen from the general population. The case-control design is a retrospective study that evaluates the outcome of past events. This type of study is frequently used because it is quickly implemented and can be performed with even small numbers of cases.[29]

An example of a case-control study is the evaluation of two groups of women—one group with a diagnosis of endometrial cancer and one group without. Both groups are interviewed to determine prior use of estrogens to test the hypothesis that estrogen use causes endometrial cancer. The percentage of women with endometrial cancer who used estrogens is referred to as the exposure frequency. If the exposure frequency is greater in the case group than the control group, the incidence of endometrial cancer after estrogen use is greater than the incidence of endometrial cancer without estrogen use.

Study Analysis. The endpoint of an analytic study is the determination of risk. *Risk* refers to the likelihood that people who are without a disease but who come in contact with certain factors thought to increase the disease risk will acquire the disease.[22] Factors associated with an increased risk of acquiring cancer are *risk factors*. Risk factors may be associated with the environment (e.g., ultraviolet radiation, toxins), personal behavior (e.g., tobacco and alcohol use, sexual practices), or personal history (e.g., genetic changes).

Risk can be calculated as either relative or attributable. *Relative risk* estimates how much the risk of acquiring cancer increases with exposure to a risk factor.[22] Relative risk can also be thought of as the ratio of the rate of cancer between exposed and unexposed individuals. The higher the relative risk, the stronger is the association between the risk factor and the cancer. A relative risk of 1.0 means the risk is the same for both groups. Thus a relative risk factor of 10 implies that the risk of acquiring cancer is 10 times greater for an exposed person than an unexposed person. Relative risk ratios are a useful tool for identifying factors that increase risk for developing a particular kind of cancer. Early age of sexual intercourse, multiple sexual partners, and cigarette smoking are known risk factors for developing cervical cancer; women with these behaviors show several times the rate of cervical cancer than women without these behaviors.

Attributable risk describes the expected or normal number of unexposed people who acquire cancer, such as the number of nonsmokers expected to develop lung cancer in a year. Attributable risk is calculated by simply subtracting the rate of incidence in the exposed population from the rate of incidence in the nonexposed population. If a nonsmoking population develops lung cancer at a rate of 200/100,000 and a smoking population develops lung cancer at a rate of 543/100,000, then 343 cases of lung cancer per 100,000 population were caused by smoking and could have been prevented.

Experimental Studies

An experimental study modifies host characteristics, makes life-style changes, or uses screening to prevent disease. Experimental studies are prospective and often take the form of a randomized clinical trial. Experimental studies may also be *called intervention studies, clinical trials,* or *prophylactic studies. A randomized clinical trial* is an experiment involving volunteers that determines which intervention is superior among various alternatives. An example of the experimental study design is the chemoprevention trial, in which an agent is given to achieve regression of a precursor lesion, to prevent cancer recurrence, or to prevent the development of cancer in a high-risk population. The Breast Cancer Prevention Trial, initiated in 1992 by the NCI and the National Surgical Adjuvant Breast and Bowel Project (NSABP), showed that tamoxifen was effective in significantly reducing the incidence of both invasive and noninvasive breast cancer in women at high risk for the disease.[10] A second chemoprevention study was initiated in 1999 by the NCI and NSABP. The Study of Tamoxifen and Raloxifene (STAR) will include 22,000 postmenopausal women at increased risk of developing breast cancer to determine whether the osteoporosis-prevention drug raloxifene is as effective in reducing the chance of breast cancer as tamoxifen.[40]

CAUSES OF CANCER

Because one of the primary purposes of epidemiology is to discover the causes of cancer, the concept of "cause" must be understood. *Sufficient cause* is one that produces the effect.[22] In other words, if sufficient cause existed and were removed, the event would not occur. Because cancer is a complex and multifactorial disease, there is no single sufficient cause, the removal of which will prevent the disease. What must be examined then are various components of sufficient causes. The presence of a component increases the probability of the effect but requires other components to produce it. Components may be active or passive. Personal susceptibility factors (e.g., genetics, environment, immunity) are *passive components;* carcinogens are *active components.* Each of these component causes is not "complete"; blocking the action of a component cause can make an otherwise sufficient cause become insufficient to produce the effect.[22, 29] See Box 3-2 for a list of descriptive epidemiology factors.

The various theories of carcinogenesis are discussed extensively in Chapter 1. To review, initiators are early stage sequences of limited exposure and are irreversible, whereas promoters occur at a later stage, involve repeated exposures at frequent intervals, and are reversible. Therefore limiting or eliminating the promoter may prevent the occurrence of cancer or reverse malignant changes. The promoter, or carcinogen, may be the active component cause. By removing this agent, sufficient cause cannot exist. Chapter 1 also describes the various groups of carcinogens: chemicals, hormones, viruses, and radiation. In addition, specific cancer etiologies are presented in Chapter 4 and each of the disease chapters. This chapter does not repeat a discussion of these agents, but Table 3–1 lists a number of environmental causes of cancer, the type of exposure, and the kind of resulting cancer. Some of these carcinogenic agents were identified by laboratory research; others were identified by the epidemiologic methods detailed in this chapter.

TABLE 3-1
Environmental Causes of Human Cancer

Agent	Type of Exposure	Site of Cancer
Aflatoxin	Contaminated foodstuffs	Liver
Alkylating agents (melphalan, cyclophosphamide, chlorambucil, semustine)	Medication	Leukemia
Androgen-anabolic steroids	Medication	Liver
Aromatic amines (benzidine, 2-naphthylamine, 4-aminobiphenyl)	Manufacturing of dyes and other chemicals	Bladder
Arsenic (inorganic)	Mining and smelting of certain ores, pesticide manufacturing and use, medication, drinking water	Bladder, lung, skin, liver (angiosarcoma), soft tissue sarcoma
Arylamines	Manufacturing	Bladder
Asbestos	Manufacturing and use	Lung, pleura, peritoneum, renal cell
Benzene	Leather, petroleum, rubber and other industries	Leukemia
Bis(chloromethyl)ether	Manufacturing	Lung (small cell)
Chlornaphazine	Medication	Bladder
Chromium compounds	Manufacturing	Lung
Dioxin	Leather industry	Soft tissue sarcoma
Ionizing radiation	Atomic bomb explosions, treatment and diagnosis, radium dial painting, uranium and metal mining	Most sites
Isopropyl alcohol production	Manufacturing by strong acid process	Nasal sinuses
Mustard gas	Manufacturing	Lung, larynx, nasal sinuses
Nickel dust	Refining	Lung, nasal sinuses
Parasites	Infection	
Schistosoma haematobium		Bladder (squamous carcinoma)
Clonorchis (Opisthorchis) sinensis		Liver (cholangiocarcinoma)
Pesticides	Application	Non-Hodgkin's lymphoma, lung
Phenacetin-containing analgesics	Medication	Renal pelvis
Phenoxyherbicides	Application	Soft-tissue sarcoma, non-Hodgkin's lymphoma
Polycyclic hydrocarbons	Coal carbonization products and some mineral oils	Lung, skin (squamous carcinoma)
Silica	Manufacturing	Lung
Tobacco smoke	Secondhand ("passive smoking")	Lung
Ultraviolet radiation	Sunlight	Skin (including melanoma), lip
Viruses	Infection	
Epstein-Barr virus		Burkitt's lymphoma, nasopharyngeal carcinoma, Hodgkin's disease
Hepatitis B and C viruses		Hepatocellular carcinoma
Human immunodeficiency virus		Kaposi's sarcoma, non-Hodgkin's lymphoma, Hodgkin's disease, squamous cell carcinoma of conjunctiva, small bowel lymphoma, leiomyosarcoma
Human papillomavirus		Cervix, other anogenital tumors
Human T-cell leukemia/lymphoma (lymphotrophic) virus type I		T-cell leukemia/lymphoma
Vinyl chloride	Manufacturing of polyvinyl chloride	Liver (angiosarcoma), soft tissue sarcoma
Wood dusts	Furniture manufacturing (hardwood)	Nasal sinuses (adenocarcinoma)

Data from references 1, 2, 4, 7, 8, 12, 13, 16, 18, 23, 28, 34, 36, 37, 38, 39, 41, 44, 49.

An excellent historic example of an epidemiologic study is the Argonne Radium Study. In the 1920s, many people worked as "luminators" in watch factories. Their job was to apply radium paint to the numerals on watch dials. This obviously detailed work required a paintbrush with a very fine tip. This pointed tip was achieved by touching the end of the brush to the lips or tongue. This practice transferred a considerable amount of the sticky radium paint to the mouth. In a few years a luminator may have ingested 5 mg or more of radioactive substances, which would be deposited in their bones, spleen, and liver. It would remain in these organs, emitting a steady stream of radioactivity to the surrounding tissues.

By 1924, nine young women working in the same New Jersey factory died within 3 years. Other workers developed gingivitis, osteomyelitis, and anemia. The Argonne Radium Study was initiated to study the luminators as well as chemists and patients treated with radium. This became one of the largest epidemiologic studies to evaluate the health effects of ionizing radiation on humans. The Argonne study produced an undeniable link between radiation exposure and certain forms of cancer, including osteosarcomas, paranasal sinus cancers, and mastoid cancers.[29, 43] Even more than 65 years later, this study continues as epidemiologists identify, interview, and even arrange for the exhumation of additional subjects. An impressive contribution of the Argonne study is that it served as a basis for plutonium exposure guidelines during the Manhattan Project of the World War II era.

CONCLUSION

Examples of cancer-causing agents highlight the role of epidemiology in the cancer problem. Once a cancer-causing agent is identified, steps must be taken to eliminate or limit exposure. This involves public health and government agencies at the local, state, and national levels. Nurses must be knowledgeable about environmental carcinogens not only to answer patients' questions but also to take more accurate health histories and adequately assess high-risk exposures. Oncology nurses can use their knowledge of epidemiology, cancer patterns, and trends to develop educational programs to increase awareness and prevention activity. Screening and detection efforts can be targeted to populations that are at great risk for specific cancers. Familiarity with terminology and epidemiologic methods enables the nurse to interpret medical literature more accurately; new information can be more easily understood and therefore integrated into the personal knowledge base. Nurses can develop a more acute awareness in their practice setting, allowing possible observations of clusters or trends. Curiosity and observation may lead to nursing research questions.

Chapter Questions

1. The endpoint of epidemiologic research is to:
   a. Prevent cancer
   b. Detect cancer
   c. Cure cancer
   d. Delay the development of cancer
2. The number of newly diagnosed cases of cancer in a specified period of time in a defined population is the definition of cancer:
   a. Incidence
   b. Prevalence
   c. Mortality
   d. Survival
3. A survey reports that 7000 new cases of breast cancer are found in upstate New York, whereas 23,000 are found in New York City. The large difference in numbers of cases can be attributed to differences in:
   a. Life-style
   b. Population
   c. Environment
   d. Screening programs
4. Relative risk estimates:
   a. How much the risk of acquiring cancer increases with exposure to a risk factor
   b. The number of unexposed people who acquire cancer
   c. Cancer incidence
   d. Survival statistics categorized by each type of cancer and its risk factors
5. Which of the following is an active component that can cause cancer?
   a. Genetics
   b. Environment
   c. Immunity
   d. Carcinogens
6. To prevent investigator biases, a study design may be:
   a. Experimental
   b. Cohort design
   c. Random selection
   d. Double blind
7. The advantage of a retrospective study is:
   a. Study is usually less expensive
   b. Medical records are used for data collection
   c. The study uses a previously defined cohort
   d. All the above are correct

8. Cancer prevalence is defined as:
   a. Likelihood cancer will occur in a lifetime
   b. Number of persons with cancer at a given point in time
   c. Number of new cancers in a year
   d. All cancer cases over 5 years old
9. Individuals participating in a cohort study:
   a. Are of similar age, race, and economic status
   b. Must have already been diagnosed with cancer
   c. Must be related
   d. Have all been exposed to a certain factor
10. The science of epidemiology focuses on:
   a. Curing cancer
   b. Natural progression of the cancer
   c. Groups or populations
   d. Delineation of cancer risk factors

BIBLIOGRAPHY

1. Aboulafia D: Epidemiology and pathogenesis of AIDS-related lymphomas, *Oncology* 12:1068, 1998.
2. Armstrong AA and others: Epstein-Barr virus and Hodgkin's disease: further evidence for the three disease hypothesis, *Leukemia* 12:1272, 1998.
3. Balducci L, Lyman GH: Cancer in the elderly. Epidemiologic and clinical implications, *Clin Geriatr Med* 13(1):1, 1997.
4. Beral V, Newton R: Overview of the epidemiology of immunodeficiency-associated cancers, *J Natl Cancer Inst Monographs* 23:1, 1998.
5. Bowerman RJ: Alaska Native cancer epidemiology in the Arctic, *Public Health* 112(1):7, 1998.
6. Daly M, Obrams GI: Epidemiology and risk assessment for ovarian cancer, *Semin Oncol* 25:255, 1998.
7. Dosemeci M, Posemeci M, Rothman N, Yin SN, Li-GL, Linet M, Wacholder S, Chow WH, and Hayes RB: Validation of benzene exposure assessment, *Ann NY Acad Sci* 837:114, 1997.
8. Duffus JH: Epidemiology and the identification of metals as human carcinogens, *Sci Prog* 79(Pt 4):311, 1996.
9. Elwood JM: Melanoma and sun exposure, *Semin Oncol* 23:650, 1996.
10. Fisher B: Highlights from recent National Surgical Adjuvant Breast and Bowel Project studies in the treatment and prevention of breast cancer, *CA Cancer J Clin* 49:159, 1999.
11. Fremgen AM, Bland KI, McGinnis Jr. LS, Eyre HJ, McDonald CJ, Menck HR, and Murphy GP: Clinical highlights from the National Cancer Data Base, 1999, *CA Cancer J Clin* 49:145, 1999.
12. Friedberg JS, Kaiser LR: Epidemiology of lung cancer, *Semin Thorac Cardiovasc Surg* 9(1):56, 1997.
13. Goldsmith DF: Evidence for silica's neoplastic risk among workers and derivation of cancer risk assessment, *J Exposure Anal Environ Epidemiol* 7:291, 1997.
14. Greenlee RT, Murray J, Bolden S, and Wingo PA: Cancer Statistics, 2000, *CA Cancer J Clin* 50:7, 2000.
15. Gurney JG and others: Infant cancer in the U.S.: histology-specific incidence and trends, 1973–1992, *J Pediatr Hematol Oncol* 19:428, 1997.
16. Herrero R: Epidemiology of cervical cancer, *J Natl Cancer Inst Monographs* 21:1, 1996.
17. Howell EA and others: Differences in cervical cancer mortality among black and white women, *Obstet Gynecol* 94:509, 1999.
18. Johansson SL, Cohen SM: Epidemiology and etiology of bladder cancer, *Semin Surg Oncol* 13:291, 1997.
19. Joslyn SA, West MM: Racial differences in breast cancer survival? *Cancer* 88:114, 2000.
20. Keller DM, Peterson EA, and Silberman G: Survival rates for four forms of cancer in the United States and Ontario, *Am J Public Health* 87:1164, 1997.
21. Kenney LB, Miller BA, Gloeckler LA, Nicholson HS, Byrne J, and Reaman GH: Increased incidence of cancer in infants in the U.S.: 1980–1990, *Cancer* 82:1396, 1998.
22. Li FP, Kantor AF: Cancer epidemiology. In Holland JF and others, editors: *Cancer medicine,* ed 4, Baltimore, Williams & Wilkins, 1997.
23. Magrath IT: Non-Hodgkin's lymphomas: epidemiology and treatment, *Ann NY Acad Sci* 824:91, 1997.
24. McCredie M: Cancer epidemiology in migrant populations, *Recent Results Cancer Res* 154:298, 1998.
25. Merrill RM, Henson DE, and Ries LA: Conditional survival estimates in 34,963 patients with invasive carcinoma of the colon, *Dis Colon Rectum* 41:1097, 1998.
26. Merrill RM and others: Conditional survival among patients with carcinoma of the lung, *Chest* 116:697, 1999.
27. Mettlin C: Global cancer mortality statistics, *CA Cancer J Clin* 49:139, 1999.
28. Neugut AI, Jacobson JS, Suh S, Mukherjee R, and Arber N: The epidemiology of cancer of the small bowel, *Cancer Epidemiol Biomarkers Prev* 7:243, 1998.
29. Oleske DM: Epidemiologic principles for cancer nursing practice. In McCorkle R and others, editors: *Cancer nursing: a comprehensive textbook,* ed 2, Philadelphia, Saunders, 1996.
30. Oliveria SA, Miranda A, Albericio F, Andreu D, Paiva AC, Nakaie CR, and Tominaga M: The role of epidemiology in cancer prevention, *Proc Soc Exp Biol Med* 216(2):142, 1997.
31. Papworth DG, Lloyd RA: Cancer survival in the USA, 1973–1990: a statistical analysis, *Br J Cancer* 78:1514, 1998.
32. Parker SL, Davis KJ, Wingo PA, Ries LAG, and Heath CW: Cancer statistics by race and ethnicity, *CA Cancer J Clin* 48:31, 1998.
33. Parkin DM, Pisani P, and Ferlay J: Global cancer statistics, *CA Cancer J Clin* 49:33, 1999.
34. Persson B: Occupational exposure and malignant lymphoma, *Int J Occup Med Environ Health* 9:309, 1996.
35. Price B: Analysis of current trends in United States mesothelioma incidence, *Am J Epidemiol* 145:211, 1997.
36. Ross RK, James PA, Yu MC: Bladder cancer epidemiology and pathogenesis, *Semin Oncol* 23:536, 1996.
37. Salasche SJ: Epidemiology of actinic keratoses and squamous cell carcinoma, *J Am Acad Dermatol* 42(1 Pt 2):4, 2000.

38. Sandler DP, Ross JA: Epidemiology of acute leukemia in children and adults, *Semin Oncol* 24:3, 1997.

39. Stadltander DT, Waterbor JW: Molecular epidemiology, pathogenesis and prevention of gastric cancer, *Carcinogenesis* 20:2195, 1999.

40. STAR Update. Tamoxifen and raloxifene study needs volunteers, *Clin J Oncol Nurs* 3:144, 1999.

41. Tavani A, La Vecchia C: Epidemiology of renal-cell carcinoma, *J Nephrol* 10(2):93, 1997.

42. Tominaga S, Kuroishi T: Epidemiology of pancreatic cancer, *Semin Surg Oncol* 15:3, 1998.

43. Trichopoulous D, Lipworth L, Petridou E, and Adami Hans-Olov HO: Epidemiology of cancer. In DeVita VT, Hellman S, Rosenberg SA, editors: *Cancer: principles and practice of oncology,* ed 5, Philadelphia, Lippincott-Raven, 1997.

44. Wilmink AB: Overview of the epidemiology of colorectal cancer, *Dis Colon Rectum* 40:483, 1997.

45. Wingo PA, Landis SH, Murray T, and Bolden S: Long-term cancer patient survival in the United States, *Cancer Epidemiol Biomarkers Prev* 7:271, 1998.

46. Wun LM, Merrill RM, and Feuer EJ: Estimating lifetime and age-conditional probabilities of developing cancer, *Lifetime Data Anal* 4:169, 1998.

47. Yancik R: Cancer burden in the aged: an epidemiologic and demographic overview, *Cancer* 80:1273, 1997.

48. Yood MU, Johnson CC, Blount A, Abrams J, Wolman E, McCarthy BD, Raju U, Nathanson DS, Worsham M, and Wolman SR: Race and differences in breast cancer survival in a managed care population, *J Natl Cancer Inst* 91:1487, 1999.

49. Zahm SH, Fraumeni JF: The epidemiology of soft tissue sarcoma, *Semin Oncol* 24:504, 1997.

Prevention, Screening, and Detection

CHAPTER 4

Mary Magee Gullatte

Cancer continues to be second only to cardiovascular disease as a leading cause of death in the United States. Regularly scheduled cancer screenings by health care professionals can result in early detection of cancers of the breast, colon, rectum, cervix, prostate, testis, oral cavity, and skin at an earlier stage when the outcomes are likely to be more positive for the patient. The American Cancer Society (ACS) estimates that 1,220,100 new cancer cases will be diagnosed in 2000.[11] The number of deaths from cancer is estimated to exceed 500,000 Americans in 2000. The ACS estimates of cancer incidence and mortality for 2000 are outlined in Figure 4–1.

Prevention, screening, and early detection are among the best strategies available in the quest to conquer cancer. The U.S. Department of Health and Human Services (DHHS) *Healthy People 2010* objectives identified two overarching goals: increase quality and years of healthy life and eliminate health disparities.[59] Within the context of these goals DHHS has identified 28 focus areas of which cancer is the third. The goal of the cancer focus area is to reduce the number of cancer cases as well as the illness, disability, and death caused by cancer. These reductions can be achieved by smoking cessation, diet modification, early detection through screening programs, and state-of-the art cancer treatments. Further reductions may be achieved through elimination of occupational and environmental risks and changes in life-style, focusing on healthy choices in diet and exercise. Early diagnosis is crucial to reducing the morbidity and mortality associated with cancer. Table 4–1 shows the positive impact of early detection on survival for the four most prevalent cancers.

Prevention of human cancers is a major focus in education and research as America embraces the new millennium. Despite advances in the treatment of cancers, overall mortality statistics greatly exceed desired outcomes. There continues to be wide disparities in cancer care outcomes among women, the underserved, and minorities. Neoplastic transformation is a multistep process in the development of human cancers involving three sequences of events: initiation, promotion, and progression. Goals of prevention, risk reduction, and early detection are aimed at eliminating or modifying neoplastic transformation of human cells.

The ACS and National Cancer Institute (NCI) are promoting nationwide cancer education, screening, and early detection initiatives, targeting African American, Hispanic, Asian/Pacific Islanders, and American Indians and the underserved or socioeconomically disadvantaged (SED) populations. The differences in cancer incidence, mortality, and survival among minority Americans are disproportionately high for most sites when compared with the majority of Americans. Tables 4–2 and 4–3 list the cancer incidence, mortality, and survival rates by race and ethnic group. The rates presented in each table show differences in neoplastic growth that appear to result from ethnic, cultural, environmental, economic, or hereditary differences within each group.

Cancer incidence rates are nearly twice as high or higher for African Americans compared with whites for cancers of the esophagus, uterus, cervix, liver, stomach, prostate, and multiple myeloma.[27] Cancer mortality is higher in African Americans than in all races for several reasons, including higher rates of new disease, later stage at diagnosis, and poor survival experience.[11, 55]

CANCER PREVENTION GUIDELINES

The focus of prevention of cancer in this chapter is two dimensional: *primary prevention* aimed at measures to ensure that the cancer never develops and *secondary prevention* aimed at detecting and treating the cancer early while in its most curable stage.

The ACS estimates that 80% of all cancers may be associated with environmental exposures and are potentially preventable. Smoking accounts for the highest overall health risk in the United States. Cigarette smoking is the major cause of lung cancer and is estimated

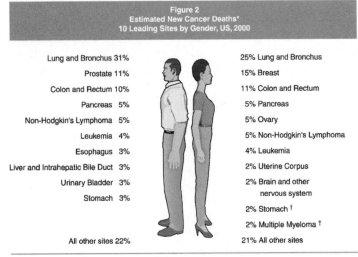

Figure 1
Estimated New Cancer Cases*
10 Leading Sites by Gender, US, 2000

Prostate 29%	30% Breast
Lung and Bronchus 14%	12% Lung and Bronchus
Colon and Rectum 10%	11% Colon and Rectum
Urinary Bladder 6%	6% Uterine Corpus
Non-Hodgkin's Lymphoma 5%	4% Ovary
Melonoma of Skin 4%	4% Non-Hodgkin's Lymphoma
Oral Cavity and Pharynx 3%	3% Melanoma of Skin
Kidney and Renal Pelvis 3%	2% Urinary Bladder
Leukemia 3%	2% Pancreas
Pancreas 2%	2% Thyroid
All other sites 19%	22% All other sites

* Excludes basal and squamous cell skin cancers and in situ carcinomas except urinary bladder.
  Percentages may not total 100% due to rounding.

Figure 2
Estimated New Cancer Deaths*
10 Leading Sites by Gender, US, 2000

Lung and Bronchus 31%	25% Lung and Bronchus
Prostate 11%	15% Breast
Colon and Rectum 10%	11% Colon and Rectum
Pancreas 5%	5% Pancreas
Non-Hodgkin's Lymphoma 5%	5% Ovary
Leukemia 4%	5% Non-Hodgkin's Lymphoma
Esophagus 3%	4% Leukemia
Liver and Intrahepatic Bile Duct 3%	2% Uterine Corpus
Urinary Bladder 3%	2% Brain and other nervous system
Stomach 3%	2% Stomach †
	2% Multiple Myeloma †
All other sites 22%	21% All other sites

* Excludes in situ carcinomas except urinary bladder.
†These two cancers both receive a ranking of 10; they have the same projected number of deaths and contribute the same percentage. Percentages may not total 100% due to rounding.

FIGURE 4–1 Estimated new cancer cases and cancer deaths for 10 leading sites by gender, 2000. (Used with permission from Greenlee RT, Murray J, Bolden S, Wingo PA: Cancer Statistics, 2000, *CA Cancer J Clin* 50(1):16, 2000.)

to cause 87% of lung cancer deaths and 30% of all cancer deaths.[59]

Major factors placing humans at risk for developing cancer include tobacco, high-fat diet, life-style, and occupational and environmental exposures. Table 4–4 presents site-specific guidelines related to cancer risk factors, signs and symptoms, screening, and early detection. Health promotion, cancer prevention, and risk reduction guidelines of selected life-style, occupational, socioeconomic status (SES), and environmental factors are reviewed next.

TOBACCO

A reported 90% of all lung cancer is caused by tobacco smoke from pipes, cigarettes, cigars, and sidestream or second-hand smoke.[38, 52, 63] The link between cigarette smoking and lung cancer was first suspected in the 1920s and 1930s.[13] The ACS estimates that cigarette smoking is responsible for 87% of lung cancer deaths among men and 75% among women.[10] Over the past decade the gap between the number of lung cancer deaths caused by smoking in men and women has narrowed. Lung cancer now exceeds breast cancer as the leading cause of cancer death in women. Passive exposure to cigarette smoke (sidestream and exhaled smoke) appears to increase the risk of lung cancer in nonsmokers who live with smokers.[32] Smoking is associated with cancers of the mouth, pharynx, larynx, esophagus, pancreas, uterine cervix, kidney, and bladder.[10]

The DHHS released the *Healthy People 2010* objectives in January 2000. The 467 objectives cover 28 focus

Text continued on page 65

TABLE 4 – 1
Five-Year Relative Survival Rates* by Stage at Diagnosis, 1989–1995

Site	All Stages %	Local %	Regional %	Distant %	Site	All Stages %	Local %	Regional %	Distant %
Breast (female)	85	96	77	21	Ovary	50	95	79	28
Colon, rectum	61	90	65	8	Pancreas	4	18	6	1
Esophagus	12	25	13	2	Prostate†	92	100	—	32
Kidney	60	88	61	10	Stomach	21	60	21	2
Larynx	65	81	53	41	Testis	95	99	97	74
Liver	5	15	5	1	Thyroid	95	100	92	43
Lung, bronchus	14	49	20	2	Urinary bladder	81	93	49	6
Melanoma	88	95	58	13	Uterine cervix	70	91	48	13
Oral	53	81	43	22	Uterine corpus	84	95	64	25

* Rates are adjusted for normal life expectancy and are based on cases diagnosed from 1989–1995, followed through 1996.

† The rate for local stage represents local and regional stages combined.

Local: An invasive malignant cancer confined entirely to the organ of origin. Regional: A malignant cancer that (1) has extended beyond the limits of the organ of origin directly into surrounding organs or tissues; (2) involves regional lymph nodes by way of lymphatic system; or (3) has both regional extension and involvement of regional lymph nodes. Distant: A malignant cancer that has spread to parts of the body remote from the primary tumor either by direct extension or by discontinuous metastasis to distant organs, tissues, or via the lymphatic system to distant lymph nodes.

From Surveillance, Epidemiology, and End Results Program, 1973–1996, Division of Cancer Control and Population Sciences, National Cancer Institute. Used with permission from Cancer facts and figures, 2000 (p. 14). Atlanta, American Cancer Society.

TABLE 4–2

Cancer Incidence and Death Rates* by Site, Sex, and Race/Ethnicity, United States, 1990–1995

	All Sites	Lung and Bronchus	Female Breast	Prostate	Colon and Rectum
INCIDENCE					
All Races					
Male	487.9	75.8	—	154.5	54.0
Female	343.1	41.7	108.9	—	37.6
White					
Male	485.6	74.3	—	150.3	53.8
Female	352.0	43.3	113.2	—	37.2
African American					
Male	605.1	114.4	—	224.3	59.4
Female	336.1	46.4	99.0	—	45.5
Asian/Pacific Islander					
Male	324.1	52.4	—	82.2	47.2
Female	243.4	22.4	71.4	—	31.2
American Indian					
Male	180.1	25.1	—	46.4	21.9
Female	135.9	14.1	31.9	—	‡
Hispanic†					
Male	331.2	40.0	—	104.4	35.6
Female	244.9	19.8	69.3	—	24.3
MORTALITY					
All Races					
Male	216.5	72.5	—	26.2	22.1
Female	141.5	33.1	26.2	—	15.0
White					
Male	210.1	70.7	—	24.1	21.8
Female	140.1	33.6	26.0	—	14.6
African American					
Male	311.4	102.0	—	55.0	28.0
Female	168.8	32.7	31.5	—	20.1
Asian/Pacific Islander					
Male	129.9	35.1	—	10.9	13.6
Female	83.9	15.0	11.6	—	9.0
American Indian					
Male	122.8	40.0	—	14.2	10.5
Female	88.8	19.6	11.7	—	8.7
Hispanic†					
Male	132.6	32.4	—	16.8	13.2
Female	86.5	11.0	15.3	—	8.5

* Rates are per 100,000 and are age-adjusted to the 1970 US standard population.

† Hispanic is not mutually exclusive from whites, African Americans, Asian/Pacific Islanders, and Native Americans.

‡ Statistic not shown. Rate is based on fewer than 10 cases per year within the time interval.

From NCI Surveillance, Epidemiology, and End Results Program, 1998. Used with permission from Cancer facts and figures for African Americans, 1998–1999 (p. 16). Atlanta, American Cancer Society.

T A B L E   4 – 3

Trends in 5-Year Relative Survival Rates* by Race and Year of Diagnosis, United States, 1974–1995

Site	White			Black			All Races		
	Relative 5-Year Survival Rate (%)			Relative 5-Year Survival Rate (%)			Relative 5-Year Survival Rate (%)		
	1974–76	1980–82	1989–95	1974–76	1980–82	1989–95	1974–76	1980–82	1989–95
All Sites	51	52	61†	39	40	48†	50	51	59†
Brain	22	25	30†	27	31	39†	22	25	30†
Breast (female)	75	77	86†	63	66	71†	75	76	85†
Colon	51	56	62†	46	49	52†	50	55	62†
Esophagus	5	7	13†	4	5	9†	5	7	12†
Hodgkin's disease	72	75	83†	69	72	76	71	75	82†
Kidney	52	51	61†	49	55	58†	52	52	60†
Larynx	66	69	66	60	58	53	66	68	65
Leukemia	35	39	44†	31	33	34	34	39	43†
Liver	4	4	6†	2	2	3	4	4	5†
Lung, bronchus	13	14	14†	12	12	11	13	13	14†
Melanoma	80	83	88†	67‡	61§	68‡	80	83	88†
Multiple myeloma	24	28	28†	28	29	31	24	28	28†
Non-Hodgkin's lymphoma	48	52	52†	48	50	41†	47	51	51†
Oral cavity	55	55	56	36	31	34	53	53	53
Ovary	37	39	50†	41	39	47†	37	39	50†
Pancreas	3	3	4†	3	5	4†	3	3	4†
Prostate	68	75	93†	58	65	84†	67	73	92†
Rectum	49	53	60†	42	38	51†	49	52	60†
Stomach	15	17	19†	17	19	22	15	18	21†
Testis	79	92	96†	76‡	90‡	88	79	92	95†
Thyroid	92	94	95†	88	94	89	92	94	95†
Urinary bladder	74	79	82†	48	58	62†	73	78	81†
Uterine cervix	70	68	71†	64	61	59	69	67	70
Uterine corpus	89	83	86†	61	54	56	88	82	84†

* Rates are adjusted for normal life expectancy and are based on cases diagnosed from 1989–1995, followed through 1996.

† The difference in rates between 1974–76 and 1989–95 is statistically significant (P < .05).

‡ The standard error of the survival rate is between 5 and 10 percentage points.

§ The standard error of the survival rate is greater than 10 percentage points.

From Surveillance, Epidemiology, and End Results Program, 1973–1996, Division of Cancer Control and Population Sciences, National Cancer Institute. Used with permission from Cancer facts and figures, 2000 (p. 16). Atlanta, American Cancer Society.

T A B L E 4 – 4

Site-Specific Cancer Risk, Screening, and Early Detection Guidelines

Site	Associated Risk Factors	Signs and Symptoms	Screening and Detection
Biliary tract (gallbladder and bile ducts)	Older Americans (ages 60s–70s) Female predominance Higher in white women than African American women Chronic infection with liver parasites (*Clonorchis sinensis*) Eating raw or pickled freshwater fish from Southeast Asia Chronic ulcerative colitis	Pruritus Jaundice Abdominal pain Nausea and vomiting Fever Malaise Enlarged liver Palpable mass in upper right quadrant Lower extremity edema Ascites	Physical examination Ultrasound
Bladder	Occupational exposure (e.g., textile, rubber) Cigarette smoking Chronic bladder infections	Microscopic or gross hematuria Dysuria Bladder irritability Urinary urgency, frequency, and hesitancy	Urinalysis Urine cytology Physical examination
Brain	Environmental exposures (e.g., vinyl chlorides) Epstein-Barr virus	Persistent generalized headache Vomiting Seizures Loss of fine motor control Unsteady gait Change in personality Lethargy Slurring of speech Loss of memory Impaired vision	Physical examination Prompt follow-up with onset of signs and symptoms
Breast	Previous history of cancer (colon, thyroid, endometrial, ovary, breast) Obesity High fat intake Family history of breast cancer Exposure to ionizing radiation before age 35 Early menarche Late menopause Nulliparity First pregnancy after age 30	Painless mass or thickening in breast or axilla Skin dimpling, puckering, or nipple retraction Nipple discharge or scaliness Edema (peau d'orange) Erythema, ulceration Change in size, contour, or shape of breast	Consist of three modalities[21]: 1. *Breast self-examination* monthly at age 20 and older 2. *Clinical examination* ages 20–40: every 3 years; over 40: every year 3. *Mammography* ages 40–49: every 1–2 years; ages 50 and over: every year Baseline mammogram at age 25 recommended for genetically predisposed women Fine-needle aspiration Ultrasound Genetic Testing: BRCA genes

Site	Risk factors	Signs and symptoms	Detection/Screening

Central nervous system	Unknown etiology
	Speculation related to genetic disorders
		Headache
		Nausea and vomiting
		Edema
		Loss of fine motor coordination
		Unsteady gait
		Seizures
		Vision and speech problems
			No effective screening measures
			Family history
			Computed tomography scan of brain
			Magnetic resonance imaging
			Cerebrospinal fluid analysis
			Tumor markers
			  α-Fetoprotein
			  β-Human chorionic gonadotropin

Cervix	Early age at first intercourse (before age 20) Multiple sex partners Smoking Human papillomavirus infection (condylomata acuminata, warts) Herpes simplex virus type 2 Diet	Abnormal vaginal bleeding Persistent postcoital spotting	Papanicolaou (Pap) test Pelvic examination

Colon and rectum	Colorectal polyps(s)
	Diets high in fat
	Diets low in fiber
	Genetic component:
	  Familial polyposis
	  Gardner's syndrome
	  Peutz-Jeghers syndrome
	Inflammatory bowel disease
	Crohn's disease
	Ulcerative colitis
		Depend on location of tumor:
		Right colon
		  Anemia
		  Gastrointestinal bleeding
		  Persistent lower abdominal pain
		  Right lower quadrant mass
		Left colon
		  Gross blood in stool
		  Decrease in stool caliber
		  Change in bowel habits, constipation, diarrhea
		Rectum
		  Hematochezia
		  Tenesmus
		  Feeling of incomplete evacuation
		  Rectal pain (late sign)
		  Prolapse of tumor
			Digital rectal examination, annually after age 40
			Stool occult blood testing, annually age 50 and older
			Flexible sigmoidoscopy
			(See Table 4–12 for frequency of these tests/procedures)

Endometrium	Postmenopause
	High socioeconomic status
	Nulliparity
	Obesity: >50 pounds over ideal body weight
	Prolonged use of exogenous estrogen without supplemental progesterone
	High fat intake
	Diabetes
	Hypertension
	Stein-Leventhal syndrome (failure to ovulate and infertility—polycystic ovaries)
	Menstrual aberration
		Early sign
		  Abnormal vaginal bleeding
		Late signs
		  Pain in pelvis, legs, or back
		  General weakness
		  Weight loss
			Annual pelvic examination ages 40–49
			Aspiration curettage
			At menopause, endometrial tissue in high-risk women

Table continued on following page

TABLE 4-4

Site-Specific Cancer Risk, Screening, and Early Detection Guidelines *Continued*

Site	Associated Risk Factors	Signs and Symptoms	Screening and Detection
Esophagus	Elderly men (70–80 years old) Nitrosamines and ethanol consumption Cigarette smoking Precancerous lesions Achalasia (failure of lower esophagus to relax with swallowing) Combined smoking and drinking Barrett's esophagus (chronic gastric reflux)	*Early* 　Dysphagia 　Weight loss 　Regurgitation 　Aspiration 　Odynophagia (pain on swallowing) 　Gastroesophageal reflux *Advanced* 　Cervical adenopathy 　Chronic cough 　Choking after eating 　Massive hemoptysis 　Hematemesis 　Hoarseness	Esophagoscopy with staining techniques Brush biopsy Radioisotopes in tumor scanning
Head and neck	Tobacco (inhaled or chewed) Ethyl alcohol Combination of tobacco and alcohol Poor oral hygiene Wood dust inhalation Nickel exposure Leukoplakia	*Mouth and oral cavity* 　Swelling 　Ulcer that does not heal *Nose and sinuses* 　Pain 　Swelling 　Bloody nasal discharge 　Nasal obstruction *Salivary glands* 　Painless swelling 　Unilateral facial paralysis *Hypopharynx* 　Dysphagia 　Persistent earache 　Lymphadenopathy *Nasopharynx* 　Double vision 　Hearing loss 　Loss of smell 　Hoarseness 　Adenopathy *Larynx* 　Hoarseness 　Difficulty breathing	Semiannual dental/oral examination Awareness of signs and symptoms (cancer's seven warning signs)
Human immunodeficiency virus/acquired immunodeficiency syndrome (HIV/AIDS) related (Kaposi's sarcoma [KS])	All age-groups Homosexual or bisexual men highest risk Intravenous drug users Unprotected sexual contact Multiple sex partners	Multifocal, widespread lesions on skin (face, extremities, torso) Persistent intermittent fever Weight loss, diarrhea Malaise, fatigue Severe cellular immune deficiency	High-risk group Appearance of skin lesions HIV serum testing Oral examination

Type	Risk factors	Signs and symptoms	Detection
Leukemia			

Acute	Men higher risk than women
	Whites higher risk than African Americans
	Exposure to radiation
	Exposure to toxic organic chemicals (e.g., benzene)
	Drugs (e.g., alkylating agents, chloramphenicol)
		Generalized lymphadenopathy
		Respiratory infections:
		  Pneumocystis carinii
		  Tuberculosis
		Difficulty breathing
		Oral lesions
		Enlarged liver and spleen
		Low-grade fever
		Anemia, pallor
		Lymphadenopathy
		Generalized weakness
		Frequent infections
		Easy bruising
		Bleeding (nose, gums)
		Petechiae on lower extremities
		Bone and joint pain
			Complete blood count
			Platelet count
			Physical examination

Chronic	Benzene exposure High-dose radiation Philadelphia chromosome	Lymphadenopathy Splenomegaly Weight loss Night sweats Malaise, weakness Recurrent infections, fever Early satiety	

Liver	Exposure to aflatoxin
	Environmental exposures
	Viral hepatitis
	More frequent in males
	Alcoholic cirrhosis
	Parasitic infestation
	Chronic venous obstruction
	Paraneoplastic syndromes
	Anabolic steroid use
		Early
		  Bloating
		  Abdominal pain
		  Fever
		  Weight loss
		  Decreased appetite
		  Nausea
		Advanced
		  Jaundice
		  Ascites
		  Extreme weight loss
		  Anorexia
			Annual physical examination
			Awareness of risk factors
			Ultrasound

Lung	Cigarette smoking (active, passive) Increase in age Asbestos Occupational exposure among miners Air pollution (e.g., benzopyrenes, hydrocarbons) Genetic predisposition Vitamin A deficiency	Nagging cough Dull ache in the chest Recurrent or persistent upper respiratory infection Wheezing Dyspnea Hemoptysis Change in volume, color, and odor of sputum	Chest x-ray Computed tomography scan Positron emission tomography scan

Table continued on following page

TABLE 4-4

Site-Specific Cancer Risk, Screening, and Early Detection Guidelines *Continued*

Site	Associated Risk Factors	Signs and Symptoms	Screening and Detection
Lymphoma *Hodgkin's*	Epstein-Barr virus Higher socioeconomic status Small family	Persistent swelling or painless lymph nodes (neck, axilla) Recurrent fevers Night sweats Weight loss Pruritus Cough, shortness of breath Leukocytosis	Physical examination Complete blood count
Non-Hodgkin's	Occupational exposure (flour and agricultural industries) Abnormalities of immune system HIV Exposure to radiation or chemotherapy	Lymphadenopathy Fatigue Fever, chills Night sweats Decreased appetite Weight loss	
Multiple myeloma	Older Americans High levels of immunoglobulin (B cells) African Americans at significantly increased risk than whites (14:1)	*Early* Anemia Fatigue Bone pain (back, legs) Weakness Unexplained bleeding (nose, gums) Recurrent upper respiratory infection *Advanced* Hypercalcemia Pathologic fractures	Annual physical examination Radiologic tests
Ovary	Familial disposition Late menopause Nulliparity First pregnancy after age 30	*Early* Vague abdominal discomfort Dyspepsia Flatulence Bloating Digestive disturbance *Advanced* Abdominal distention Pain Abdominal and pelvic masses Ascites Lower extremity edema	Genetic testing: BRCA genes Pelvic ultrasonography (with vaginal probe) Elevated serum markers: Carcinoembryonic antigen (CEA) CA-125 antigen

Pancreas	Older men Smoking Chronic pancreatitis Ethanol consumption Diabetes	*Early* Hypoglycemia Weight loss, anorexia Abdominal pain Cramping pain associated with diarrhea Pruritus *Advanced* Jaundice Ascites Lower extremity edema	Blood glucose test Physical examination
Prostate	Occupational exposure Cadmium, heavy metals, chemicals Age (median age of incidence, 70 years) Increased fat intake African American median age 45	*Early* Difficult starting urinary stream Unexplained cystitis Urinary bleeding Dribbling Bladder retention *Advanced* Bladder outlet obstruction Urinary retention Ureteral obstruction with anuria Azotemia Uremia Anorexia Hematuria Bone pain	Digital rectal examination (DRE) Biochemical markers Prostate-specific antigen (PSA) Transrectal ultrasound (TRUS)
Skin (nonmelanoma)	Fair-skinned, freckles Blonde hair, blue eyes Sun exposure Severe sunburn in childhood Familial conditions Previous skin cancers History of dysplastic nevi	Changes in wart or mole Sore that does not heal *ABCDs* of skin cancer: A—Asymmetry (change in size and shape) B—Border irregularity C—Color (change in color) D—Diameter (> than 6 mm)	Extensive skin examination Mole mapping
Soft-tissue sarcoma (bone or muscle)	Familial and genetic syndromes (e.g., von Recklinghausen's disease) High-dose radiation Toxic chemical exposure (e.g., Agent Orange)	Swelling of extremity Painless mass Fever Malaise Weight loss Occasionally hypoglycemia Functional difficulty or pain in joints Pathologic fractures	Annual physical examination Awareness of cancer's early warning signs

Table continued on following page

T A B L E 4 – 4
Site-Specific Cancer Risk, Screening, and Early Detection Guidelines *Continued*

Site	Associated Risk Factors	Signs and Symptoms	Screening and Detection
Stomach	Dietary carcinogens (e.g., smoked, salt-cured and charcoal-cooked foods) Familial and genetic disposition Persons with type A blood (15–20% increase incidence) Benign gastric ulcers	Feeling of fullness Weight loss Loss of appetite Anemia (iron deficiency) Malaise Complaints of indigestion Gastrointestinal bleeding Abdominal pain Persistent epigastric distress	Occult blood testing Complete blood count
Testis	Cryptorchid testes Young white men have rate four times that of African Americans	*Early* Painless mass Gynecomastia Heavy sensation in scrotum *Advanced* Ureteral obstruction Abdominal mass Pulmonary symptoms Elevated human chorionic gonadotropin	Testicular self-examination (monthly) beginning in adolescence Testicular ultrasound
Vulva	Postmenopausal History of genital warts Human papillomavirus Other sexually transmitted diseases Lower socioeconomic status Multiple sex partners Precancerous or cancerous lesions of cervix	Lump or ulcer Itching Pain Burning Bleeding Discharge	Visual and manual inspection of external genitalia Colposcopic exam in women with human papillomavirus

Data from references 8, 10, 11, 14–16, 19, 26, 35, 44, 50.

TABLE 4-5
Healthy People 2010 Focus Areas

1. Access to Quality Health Services
2. Arthritis, Osteoporosis, and Chronic Back Conditions
3. Cancer
4. Chronic Kidney Disease
5. Diabetes
6. Disability and Secondary Conditions
7. Educational and Community-Based Programs
8. Environmental Health
9. Family Planning
10. Food Safety
11. Health Communication
12. Heart Disease and Stroke
13. HIV
14. Immunization and Infectious Diseases
15. Injury and Violence Prevention
16. Maternal, Infant, and Child Health
17. Medical Product Safety
18. Mental Health and Mental Disorders
19. Nutrition and Overweight
20. Occupational Safety and Health
21. Oral Health
22. Physical Activity and Fitness
23. Public Health Infrastructure
24. Respiratory Diseases
25. Sexually Transmitted Diseases
26. Substance Abuse
27. Tobacco Use
28. Vision and Hearing

From Healthy people 2010: understanding treatment options. *U.S. Department of Health and Human Services, January 2000.*

areas aimed at improving the health of each individual, the health of communities, and the health of the nation. Table 4–5 identifies the 28 focus areas of *Healthy People 2010.* Cancer has been identified as the third area of focus, following access to health services and chronic conditions such as arthritis and back conditions.[59] Several of the focus areas have a direct implication for cancer prevention, screening, and early detection. The second goal of the 2010 objectives is targeted at eliminating health disparities among different segments of the population. Current information exploring the biologic and genetic characteristics of African Americans, Hispanics, American Indians, Alaska Natives, Asians, Native Hawaiians, and Pacific Islanders does not explain the health disparities experienced by these groups when compared to whites in the United States. Presently these disparities are believed the result of complex interaction among genetic variation, environmental factors, and specific health behaviors.[59] Racial, age, and gender differences in smoking habits between African Americans and whites in the United States have also been identified. African American adolescents are less likely than white adolescents to smoke; however, African American adults are more likely than white adults to begin smoking after adolescence.[10, 11, 34] Tables 4–6 through 4–10 depict differences in smoking trends by age and race. The data in these tables correlate with recent studies that indicate an overall decline in cigarette smoking in the United States.

One of the national health objectives for the year 2010 is to reduce the initiation of cigarette smoking among adolescents and adults. Among current smokers, more than 80% started smoking before age 21 and about half started before age 18.[11, 51, 54] Racial and gender disparities exist among adolescent smokers. In 1997, 40% of white high school students smoked compared to 34% of Hispanic and 23% of African Americans.[13] Gender comparisons between white and Hispanic high school girls versus boys are not statistically different, as depicted in Figure 4–2. The same report for adults indicated that American Indians, Alaska Natives, blue-

TABLE 4-6
Cigarette Use,* Adults 18 and Older, United States, 1995

Characteristic	Men (%)	Women (%)	Total (%)
AGE GROUP (YEARS)			
18–24	27.8	21.8	24.8
25–44	30.5	26.8	28.6
45–64	27.1	24.0	25.5
65 or older	14.3	11.5	13.0
RACE/ETHNICITY			
White (non-Hispanic)	27.1	24.1	25.6
African American (non-Hispanic)	28.8	23.5	25.8
Hispanic	21.7	14.9	18.3
American Indian/ Alaskan Native†	37.3	35.4	36.2
Asian/Pacific Islander	29.4	4.3	16.6
EDUCATION (YEARS)‡			
8 or fewer	28.4	17.8	22.6
9–11	41.9	33.7	37.5
12	33.7	26.2	29.5
13–15	25.0	22.5	23.6
16 or more	14.3	13.7	14.0
TOTAL	27.0	22.6	24.7

* Persons who reported having smoked ≥100 cigarettes and who reported now smoking every day or on some days.

† Estimates should be interpreted with caution because of the small sample sizes.

‡ Persons aged ≥25 years.

From National Health Interview Survey, 1995. Used with permission from Cancer risk report—prevention and control, 1998 (p. 4). Atlanta, American Cancer Society.

TABLE 4–7
Tobacco Use, High School Students, United States, 1997

Characteristic	Cigarette Use		Current Smokeless Tobacco‡	Current Cigar Use§
	Ever Tried*	Frequent†		
SEX				
Male	70.9	17.6	15.8	31.2
Female	69.3	15.7	1.5	10.8
RACE/ETHNICITY				
White (non-Hispanic)	70.4	19.9	12.2	22.5
Male	70.4	19.8	20.6	32.5
Female	70.3	20.1	1.6	9.6
African American (non-Hispanic)	68.4	7.2	2.2	19.4
Male	70.1	10.1	3.2	28.1
Female	66.8	4.3	1.3	11.0
Hispanic	75.0	10.9	5.1	20.3
Male	76.9	13.2	8.4	26.3
Female	72.7	8.1	1.2	13.0
GRADE				
9	67.7	13.1	9.7	17.3
10	70.0	15.0	6.8	22.3
11	68.8	18.9	10.0	24.2
12	73.7	19.4	10.5	23.8
TOTAL	70.2	16.7	9.3	22.0

* Ever tried cigarette smoking, even one or two puffs.

† Smoked cigarettes on ≥20 of the 30 days preceding the survey.

‡ Used smokeless tobacco on ≥1 of the 30 days preceding the survey.

§ Smoked cigars on ≥1 of the 30 days preceding the survey.

From Youth Risk Behavior Survey, 1997. Used with permission from Cancer risk report—prevention and control, 1998 (p. 2). Atlanta, American Cancer Society.

TABLE 4–8
Tobacco Use Among African American* High School Students, United States, 1997

	Females (%)		Males (%)		Total (%)	
	African American	White	African American	White	African American	White
Cigarette use						
Current†	17.4	39.9	28.2	39.6	22.7	39.7
Frequent‡	4.3	20.1	10.1	19.8	7.2	19.9
Smokeless tobacco use§	1.3	1.6	3.2	20.6	2.2	12.2
Current cigar use	11.0	9.6	28.1	32.5	19.4	22.5

* Non-Hispanic, African Americans.

† Smoked cigarettes on ≥1 of the 30 days preceding the survey.

‡ Smoked cigarettes on ≥20 of the 30 days preceding the survey.

§ Used chewing tobacco or snuff during the 30 days preceding the survey.

From Youth Risk Behavior Survey, CDC, 1997. Used with permission from Cancer facts and figures for African Americans, 1998–1999 (p. 16). Atlanta, American Cancer Society, 1998.

TABLE 4-9

Trends in the Percentage of Current Cigarette Smokers,* African American Adults 18+, United States, 1978-1995

	1978–1980	1987–1988	1992–1993	1994–1995
GENDER				
Men	45.0	37.6	32.4	31.4
Women	31.4	28.0	22.6	22.7
AGE (YEARS)				
18–34	38.7	32.0	22.1	21.0
35–54	43.9	37.2	35.9	34.2
55+	26.5	26.1	22.3	23.5
EDUCATION†				
Less than high school	36.4	36.3	34.2	34.8
High school	42.1	38.8	31.9	31.3
Some college	36.7	33.0	27.5	26.4
College	34.6	19.7	18.2	16.7

* For 1978–1991, current cigarette smokers include persons who reported smoking at least 100 cigarettes in their lives and who reported at the time of the survey that they currently smoked; for 1991–1995, current smokers include persons who reported smoking at least 100 cigarettes in their lives and who reported at the time of the survey that they currently smoked every day or on some days. Data exclude African Americans who reported Hispanic origin.

† Includes persons aged 25 years and older.

From National Center for Health Statistics, 1978–1995. Used with permission from Cancer facts and figures for African Americans, 1998–1999 (p. 15). Atlanta, American Cancer Society.

TABLE 4-10

Status: Tobacco Use, American Cancer Society Measures of Success

	Baseline 1987 (%)	1994 (%)	1995 (%)	Year 2000 Goal (%)
CIGARETTE SMOKING PREVALENCE AMONG ADULTS*				
Adults 18 years and older	29	26	25	15
Blue collar workers, 18 years and older	41	39	36	20
African Americans, 18 years and older	33	27	26	18
Hispanics, 18 years and older	24	20	18	15
Women of reproductive age, 18–44 years	29	27	26	12
High school education or less, 20 years and older	34	31	30	20

	Baseline 1991 (%)	1995 (%)	1997 (%)	Year 2000 Goal (%)
TOBACCO USE AMONG HIGH SCHOOL STUDENTS†				
Tried smoking				
9th grade students	65	63	68	42
12th grade students	75	74	74	48
Frequent cigarette user				
9th grade students	8	10	13	4
12th grade students	16	21	19	8
Smokeless tobacco users				
Male	19	20	16	12

* From National Health Interview Survey, 1987, 1994, 1995; Healthy People 2000 Review.[11]

† From Youth Risk Behavior Survey, 1991, 1995, 1997. Used with permission from Cancer risk report—prevention and control, 1998 (p. 4). American Cancer Society.

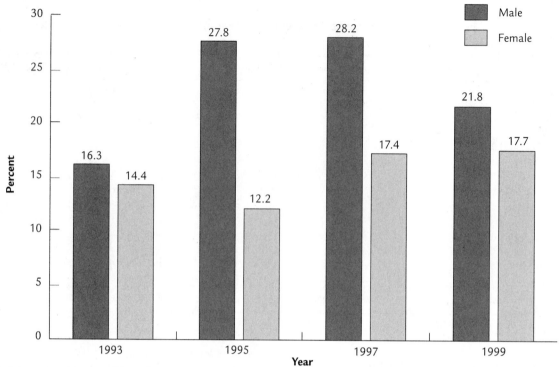

*Smoked cigarettes on 1 or more of the 30 days preceding the survey.
Source: Youth Risk Behavior Surveillance Survey, 1993, 1995, 1997, 1999.
National Center for Chronic Disease Prevention and Health Promotion, Centers for Disease
Control and Prevention.

American Cancer Society, Surveillance Research, 2000.

FIGURE 4 – 2 Trends in the percentage of current cigarette smokers,* non-Hispanic African-American high school students, United States, 1993–1999. (Used with permission from *Cancer facts and figures for African Americans, 2000–2001* (p. 9). Atlanta, American Cancer Society.)

collar workers, and military personnel had the highest smoking rates.[13] There also seems to be a correlation between lack of formal education and the smoking rate among adults. The percentage of people 25 years of age and older who report less than 12 years of education is three times higher than those persons reporting 16 years or more of education.[13]

A number of organizations offer smoking cessation programs and are reporting successes in the campaign toward a smoke-free America. Cessation of smoking reduces the risk of death from lung cancer; after 15 years, former smokers have lung cancer death rates only about two times greater than nonsmokers.[13] The ACS has identified comprehensive school health education as a priority initiative to help the youth develop and practice health habits that reduce cancer risk.

The 1990s saw a surge of legal actions initiated by lung cancer victims or families on their behalf to sue for damages and health-related claims from loss of health or life from lung cancer induced by smoking. States also began to file suits against the tobacco companies to reimburse state Medicaid programs for expenses incurred to treat past and future tobacco-related diseases.

In 1997, David Kessler, the commissioner of the Food and Drug Administration (FDA), and former U.S. Surgeon General C. Everett Koop, MD, led a committee to develop recommendations to guide national tobacco policy.[39] The Kessler-Koop Advisory Committee proposed a blueprint for the future of tobacco policy and public health. In November 1998, the tobacco industry negotiated a national settlement for $206 billion dollars, over 25 years, to settle all state lawsuits.[39] The final settlement included 46 states and four territories. Beyond monetary gains, the settlement also included removing billboards and financing education initiatives and research aimed at preventing smoking and encouraging smoking cessation among youth.

DIET

Research continues into the connection between diet, cancer causation, and cancer prevention. At this time the only consensus recommendations related to cancer, diet, and nutrition are to reduce the intake of fat, both saturated and unsaturated, and to increase the amount of daily intake of natural fiber (components that are not broken down during the digestive process) in the diet. An estimated 107 million adults in the United States are overweight or obese.[59] Adolescents and adults from poor households are twice as likely to be overweight than those from middle and high income households.[13, 59]

Healthy People 2010 included nutrition and overweight objectives aimed at reducing the proportion of children, adolescents, and adults who are overweight or obese. These conditions substantially increase the risk of illness from hypertension, cardiovascular disease, diabetes, arthritis, gallbladder disease, sleep disturbances, and breathing problems, as well as cancers of the endometrium, breast, prostate, and colon.[59] Scientific evidence suggests that one third of the 552,200 estimated cancer deaths in 2000 will be related to nutrition and other preventable life-style factors.[10, 25]

Specific dietary recommendations, related to macronutrients and micronutrients, chemoprevention, and sources of mutagenic and carcinogenic chemicals used to preserve, protect, or cultivate food sources, remain clouded in uncertainty. Estimates are that 30% to 60% of all cancers in men and women, respectively, are related to diet.[46, 50] Foods high in fat have been associated with an increased incidence of colon, prostate, and breast cancer. Dietary fat acts as a cancer promoter. As

much as 40% of food energy in the American diet is provided by fat.[37, 46] Studies indicate that obesity (40% or more overweight) is a risk factor in the development of cancer of the colon, breast, endometrium, and prostate.[13, 35] In a cancer prevention study conducted by the ACS from 1960 to 1972, women 40% over their ideal body weight had a 55% greater mortality from cancer than those of normal weight; overweight men had a 33% greater mortality.[4, 27] Figures 4–3 and 4–4 show trends in the percent of overweight adults and the percent by state.

Although the exact mechanism(s) of action is unknown, dietary fiber appears to offer a protective effect in relation to colon cancer. Fiber can be found in fresh fruits and vegetables, legumes, and whole-grain breads and cereals. Several functions are believed to account for the protective effect of dietary fiber. Fiber reduces the concentration of fecal bile acids, dilutes colonic content, reduces the level of fecal mutagens, and decreases transient time of fecal material in the gut.[28, 30, 66] In the mid 1990s a national campaign was launched to encourage Americans to include more fruits and vegetables in their diet. The "5 a day" initiative to change eating habits and behaviors of Americans by including at least five servings of fruits and vegetables a day in the diet continues. The DHHS estimates that as much

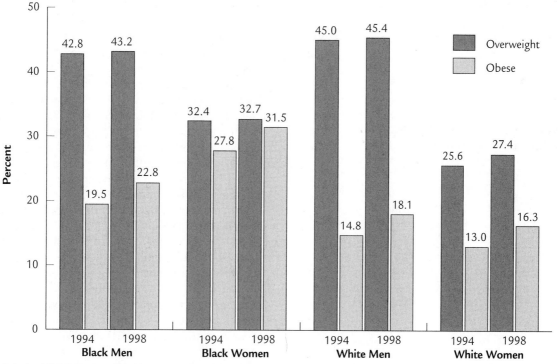

Source: Behavioral Risk Factor Surveillance System, 1994, 1998, National Center for Chronic Disease Prevention and Health Promotion, Centers for Disease Control and Prevention.

American Cancer Society, Surveillance Research, 2000.

FIGURE 4 – 3 Trends in the percentage of overweight and obese adults, by sex and race, 1994, 1998. (Used with permission from *Cancer facts and figures for African Americans, 1998–1999* (p. 10). Atlanta, American Cancer Society.)

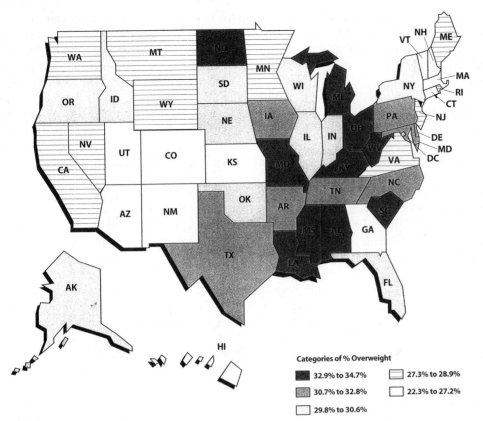

FIGURE 4 – 4 Overweight adults, 18 and older. (Used with permission from *Cancer risk report—prevention and control, 1998.* Atlanta, American Cancer Society.)

Categories of % Overweight

- 32.9% to 34.7%
- 30.7% to 32.8%
- 29.8% to 30.6%
- 27.3% to 28.9%
- 22.3% to 27.2%

as 40% of a family's food budget is spent in restaurants and take-out meals. Foods eaten away from home are usually higher in fat, cholesterol, and sodium and lower in fiber (containing fewer vegetables and fruits) than meals prepared at home. Table 4–11 depicts dietary

TABLE 4 – 11
Dietary Behaviors Among High School Students, by Race, United States, 1997

	Fruits and Vegetables ≥ 5 Servings†		High-fat Foods ≤ 2 Servings‡	
	African American (%)	White* (%)	African American* (%)	White* (%)
Sex				
Male	31.9	31.0	47.0	54.9
Female	23.7	25.7	62.5	73.0
Total	27.7	28.8	54.9	62.9

* Non-Hispanic.

† Had eaten ≥5 servings of fruit, fruit juice, green salad, and cooked vegetables on the day preceding the survey.

‡ Had eaten ≤2 servings of hamburgers, hot dogs, sausage, french fries, potato chips, cookies, doughnuts, pie, or cake on the day preceding the survey.

From Youth Risk Behavior Survey, CDC, 1995. Used with permission from Cancer facts and figures for African Americans, 1998–1999. Atlanta, American Cancer Society.

behaviors among high-school students in the United States.

The *Food Guide Pyramid* (Fig. 4–5) is now widely used to increase public awareness about healthier eating. The pyramid reinforces the principles of good nutrition, balance, and variety in daily food choices. The Food Guide Pyramid is also consistent with the dietary guidelines from both the ACS and NCI.[4]

Several micronutrients have been profiled as having a protective effect in reducing cancer risk. Naturally occurring vitamin A in the form of *β-carotene*, found in yellow and green vegetables and fruits, and *retinol*, occurring in foods of animal origin, dairy products, eggs, and liver, are associated with a protective effect against cancer. Inverse associations have been found in studies relating vitamin A precursors and cancers of the lung, larynx, esophagus, stomach, and prostate.[17, 29, 46]

The protective action of vitamin C hinders the formation of nitrosamines by blocking the reaction between nitrite and amines. Historic studies have shown an inverse association between vitamin C and cancers of the stomach, esophagus, larynx, and cervix.

Another micronutrient is *selenium*. Animal studies involving selenium indicate a protective role against chemically induced cancers. A fine line exists between therapeutic and toxic levels of selenium, however, and the evidence does not support its use as an anticancer compound.[13, 46]

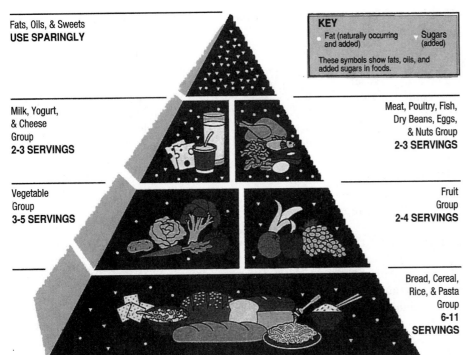

Fats, Oils, & Sweets
USE SPARINGLY

KEY
• Fat (naturally occurring and added)   ▽ Sugars (added)
These symbols show fats, oils, and added sugars in foods.

Milk, Yogurt, & Cheese Group
2-3 SERVINGS

Meat, Poultry, Fish, Dry Beans, Eggs, & Nuts Group
2-3 SERVINGS

Vegetable Group
3-5 SERVINGS

Fruit Group
2-4 SERVINGS

Bread, Cereal, Rice, & Pasta Group
6-11 SERVINGS

FIGURE 4–5 A guide to daily food choices. (From U.S. Department of Agriculture: *USDA's food guide pyramid,* USDA Human Nutrition Information Publication No. 249, Washington, DC, 1992, U.S. Government Printing Office. In Potter PA, Perry AG: *Fundamentals of nursing: concepts, process, and practice,* ed 4, St Louis, Mosby, 1997.)

The NCI continues to sponsor human chemoprevention and diet and nutrition trials in an effort to answer questions and update earlier studies related to the diet and cancer connection. Cancer prevention trials are aimed at behavior modification or deliberate and planned intervention designed to interfere with carcinogenesis. These trials may be either nutritive or nonnutritive. The ACS, NCI, and other organizations with an interest in health promotion through dietary modifications have developed dietary guidelines to reduce cancer and other health risks. Based on review of scientific literature the ACS revised its nutrition guidelines in 1999. These guidelines are consistent with the principles from the 1992 U.S. Department of Agriculture Food Guide Pyramid and the 1995 Dietary Guidelines for Americans and other agencies promoting a healthier America. The ACS has identified the following four dietary guidelines:

1. Choose most of the foods you eat from plant sources.
2. Limit your intake of high-fat foods, particularly from animal sources.
3. Be physically active; achieve and maintain a healthy weight.
4. Limit consumption of alcoholic beverages if you smoke.[10]

The Centers for Disease Control and Prevention (CDC) and the American College of Sports Medicine issued the following physical fitness guidelines in 1995: Every U.S. adult accumulate 30 minutes or more of moderate-intensity physical activity (e.g., brisk walking or exercise at a perceived rate of exertion of 60–63%) on most, preferably all, days of the week to promote health, prevent disease, and maintain a healthy weight.[13] The *Healthy People 2010* objectives for physical activity and fitness are aimed at increasing the proportion of adolescents who engage in vigorous physical activity that promotes cardiorespiratory fitness three or more days per week for 20 minutes or more minutes per occasion and increasing the proportion of adults who engage regularly, preferably daily, in moderate physical activity at least 30 minutes per day. Regular physical activity is associated with a decreased risk of colon cancer.[47, 48, 59]

ALCOHOL

Excessive consumption of ethyl alcohol can lead to cancers in the head and neck, larynx, and possibly the liver and pancreas.[10, 18, 35, 50] The synergistic effects of alcohol and tobacco can be a lethal combination. The lethal effects of alcohol and tobacco may involve the direct action of alcohol on epithelial tissues or the ability of alcohol as a solvent to increase the delivery of smoke-derived chemicals, including formaldehyde, arsenic, tar, and many others, to cause cancer.

GENETIC RISK AND TESTING

The genetic or family factor associated with cancer risk and causation is recognized but not well understood.

Two approaches are used in the study of familial clustering: epidemiologic and genetic. The *epidemiologic approach* examines the frequency of the disease among relatives; the *genetic approach* studies the pattern of disease expression among relatives.[20, 26, 41] These approaches help to provide evidence of familial aggregation but do not answer why a particular cancer expresses itself. The greatest known cancer risk exists when there is a primary relative of a patient with an autosomal dominant inherited cancer.[8, 32, 41] A thorough and complete family history can be invaluable in identifying relative risks and traits within a family aggregate. The relative risk measures the strength of the relationship between risk factors and the specific cancer.

Studies in the 1930s revealed that the relative risk for developing breast cancer if a first-degree relative had the disease was twofold to threefold. Although the role of genetics is not completely clear in human oncogenesis, it is certain that the environmental carcinogens in the tissue are modified by the host genetic makeup.[23, 32] No known genetic basis exists to explain the major racial differences in cancer incidence and outcome.[22, 49, 55] Continued research into the genetic/hereditary factor in the development of human cancers represents another edge in the fight toward cancer prevention and risk reduction.

The development of breast and ovarian cancer is believed to be caused by changes in certain genes and mutations. The increased risk of breast and ovarian cancer is caused by an alteration or mutation of two genes—BRCA-1 and BRCA-2. Having an inherited BRCA mutation increases cancer risk. The genetic screen for the mutated BRCA gene is obtained from a venous blood sample. In 1996 the American Society of Clinical Oncology recommended that genetic testing be only offered to individuals with a strong family history of cancer. Extensive counseling must occur before an individual consents to genetic testing. The true value of genetic testing in cancer screening, as a predictor of an individual who will definitely develop a cancer, is still in the developmental stages of the science. Cost for genetic testing can range from $200 to $2000 dollars. The risk of loss of insurance coverage and other financial risks are part of the individual counseling. Another dilemma for the individual considering genetic testing is what to do with the information, if the test results are positive. In the case of women and men at risk for breast cancer, should they have a prophylactic mastectomy, on the basis of a positive BRCA gene? Women with a mutation of either the BRCA-1 or BRCA-2 gene have a 33% to 50% risk of developing breast cancer before age 50, and a 56% to 80% risk by age 80. The presence of the BRCA-1 gene increases the risk of ovarian cancer to 20% to 60% by age 70 years and the BRCA-2 gene

ovarian cancer risk is between 18% and 27% by age 80 years.[23]

SOCIOECONOMIC FACTORS

Issues related to barriers to primary prevention and health care access have been reported as major factors in the differences in cancer incidence, delayed diagnosis, poor survival statistics, and increased mortality from cancer in minority and SED populations. Figure 4–6 reviews the incidence and mortality estimates for 1999 by site and sex of cancers among African Americans. A comparison of the 5-year relative survival rate for major cancer sites diagnosed between 1989 and 1994 is highlighted in Figure 4–7. There is a marked difference in overall survival for African Americans and whites; the rate is 58% for whites and 42% for African Americans.[9, 11, 12, 27] Regardless of the age at the time of diagnosis, between 1989 and 1994, whites experienced a higher 5-year survival rate than African Americans.[11] The ACS, in collaboration with the NCI and the CDC, in May and June 1989 sponsored national hearings on cancer and the poor. The objective of the hearings was to determine the magnitude of unmet cancer prevention and control needs among poor and underserved Americans. The most profound findings came from the ACS report to the nation in June 1989. Freeman,[22] then president of the ACS, reported the following five critical issues related to cancer and the poor:

1. Poor people endure greater pain and suffering from cancer than other Americans.
2. Poor people and their families must make extraordinary personal sacrifices to obtain and pay for health care.
3. Poor people face substantial obstacles in obtaining and using health insurance and often do not seek care if they cannot pay for it.
4. Current cancer education programs are culturally insensitive and irrelevant to many poor Americans.
5. Fatalism about cancer is prevalent among the poor and prevents them from seeking health care.

Freeman further reported other findings about the poor. There are 39 million poor Americans (living below the poverty level of $11,200 a year for a family of four). Two thirds of the poor are white, nearly one third are African American, and a total of 37 million Americans have no health insurance.[22] Poverty is a proxy for other elements of living, including lack of education, unemployment, substandard housing, inadequate nutrition, risk-promoting behaviors and life-style, and limited or no access to health care.[5, 10, 11, 22, 45, 59, 61] Freeman remarked that to be poor and African American and to have cancer is a double-jeopardy situation.[22] Differ-

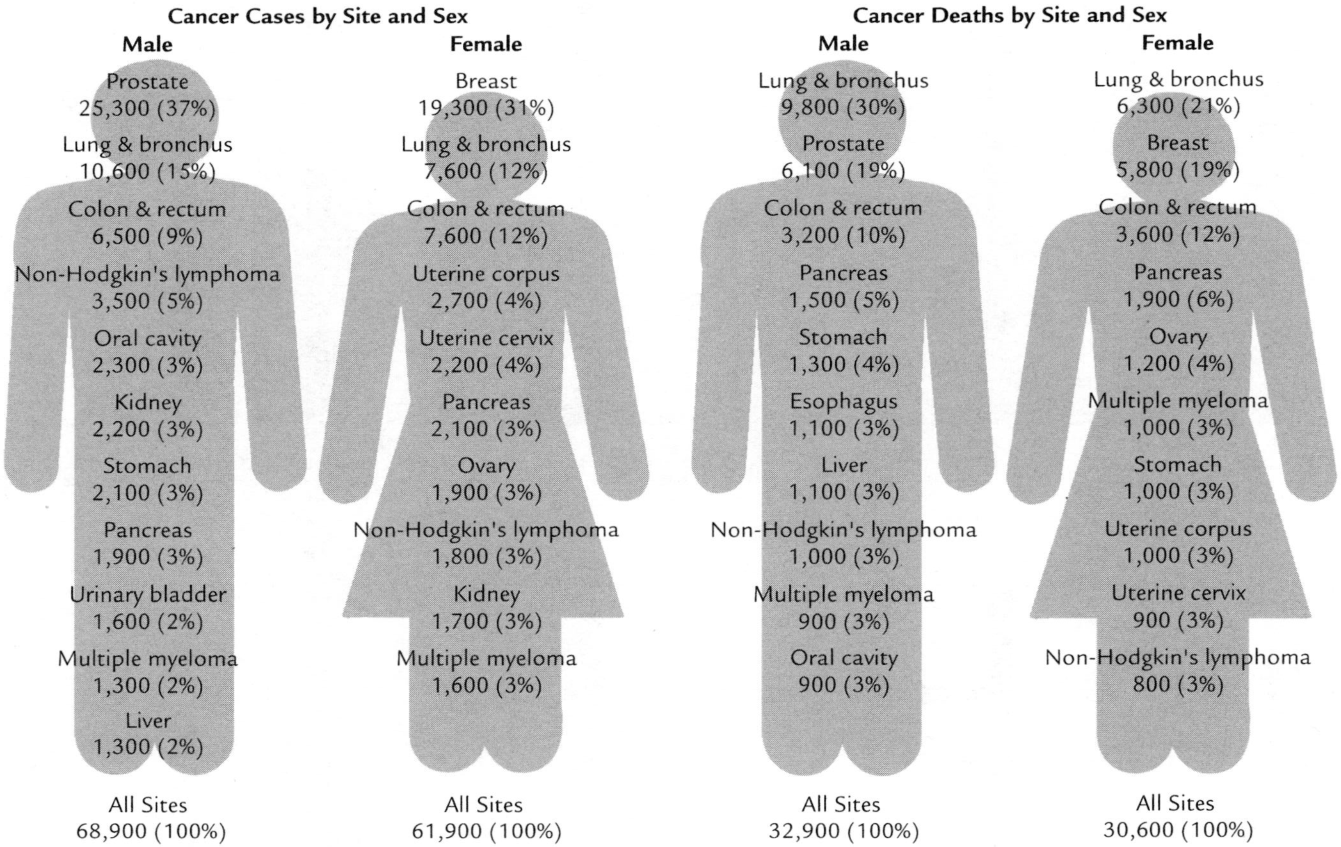

Cancer Cases by Site and Sex

Male

Prostate
25,300 (37%)

Lung & bronchus
10,600 (15%)

Colon & rectum
6,500 (9%)

Non-Hodgkin's lymphoma
3,500 (5%)

Oral cavity
2,300 (3%)

Kidney
2,200 (3%)

Stomach
2,100 (3%)

Pancreas
1,900 (3%)

Urinary bladder
1,600 (2%)

Multiple myeloma
1,300 (2%)

Liver
1,300 (2%)

All Sites
68,900 (100%)

Female

Breast
19,300 (31%)

Lung & bronchus
7,600 (12%)

Colon & rectum
7,600 (12%)

Uterine corpus
2,700 (4%)

Uterine cervix
2,200 (4%)

Pancreas
2,100 (3%)

Ovary
1,900 (3%)

Non-Hodgkin's lymphoma
1,800 (3%)

Kidney
1,700 (3%)

Multiple myeloma
1,600 (3%)

All Sites
61,900 (100%)

Cancer Deaths by Site and Sex

Male

Lung & bronchus
9,800 (30%)

Prostate
6,100 (19%)

Colon & rectum
3,200 (10%)

Pancreas
1,500 (5%)

Stomach
1,300 (4%)

Esophagus
1,100 (3%)

Liver
1,100 (3%)

Non-Hodgkin's lymphoma
1,000 (3%)

Multiple myeloma
900 (3%)

Oral cavity
900 (3%)

All Sites
32,900 (100%)

Female

Lung & bronchus
6,300 (21%)

Breast
5,800 (19%)

Colon & rectum
3,600 (12%)

Pancreas
1,900 (6%)

Ovary
1,200 (4%)

Multiple myeloma
1,000 (3%)

Stomach
1,000 (3%)

Uterine corpus
1,000 (3%)

Uterine cervix
900 (3%)

Non-Hodgkin's lymphoma
800 (3%)

All Sites
30,600 (100%)

American Cancer Society, Surveillance Research, 2000.

*Excludes basal and squamous cell skin cancer and in situ carcinomas except urinary bladder.
†Estimates are rounded to the nearest 100.
Estimates of new cases are projected based on incidence rates from the National Cancer
Institute, Surveillance, Epidemiology, and End Results Program, 1979–1997.

FIGURE 4-6 Leading sites of new cancer cases* and deaths among African Americans, 2001 estimates.† (Used with permission from *Cancer facts and figures for African Americans,* 2000–2001. Atlanta, American Cancer Society.)

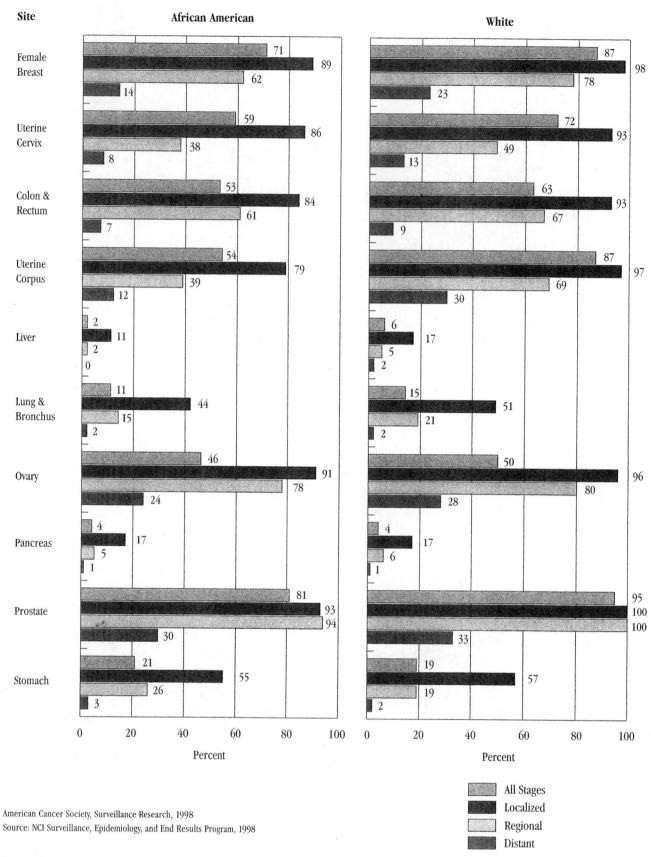

American Cancer Society, Surveillance Research, 1998

Source: NCI Surveillance, Epidemiology, and End Results Program, 1998

FIGURE 4 – 7   Five-year relative survival rates by race and stage at diagnosis, United States, 1989–1994. (Used with permission from *Cancer facts and figures for African Americans, 1989–1994,* Atlanta, American Cancer Society.)

ences in survival for African American and SED (poor) populations largely result from the late stage of cancer diagnosis.

In a study of socioeconomic factors and cancer incidence among African Americans and whites, Baquet and others[5] found that when age-adjusted incidence data were correlated with SES, the comparative risks changed: whites showed an elevated risk of cancer at all sites combined. The disproportionate distribution of African Americans at lower socioeconomic levels accounts for a large percentage of their excess cancer burden. It is, therefore, imperative for health care professionals to target SED and minority populations with culturally sensitive and relevant educational information on cancer prevention, risk reduction, and early detection and to legislate for changes in health care policies to facilitate access to health care for all Americans. In the words of the great civil rights leader, the Reverend Martin Luther King, Jr, "Of all the forms of inequality, injustice in health is the most shocking and inhumane."[22]

ELECTROMAGNETIC FIELDS

The public continues to express concern about cancer risk and exposure to electromagnetic fields (EMFs). The presence of electric power lines, running through and surrounding residential and industrial areas where one lives and works, is the basis of this growing concern. Epidemiologic studies have been in progress since the late 1970s attempting to document a possible link between EMF exposure over time and the development of certain cancers in humans. In a review of the literature by Heath,[33] at present no form of electromagnetic energy at frequency levels below those of ionizing radiation (x-rays) and ultraviolet (UV) radiation has been shown to cause cancer.

SUNLIGHT

The sun is the primary source of natural UV light exposure that is known to cause skin cancer. The three types of skin cancers are basal cell, squamous cell, and melanoma. Of the three types of skin cancer, *melanoma* is the most potentially lethal and is increasing in incidence at a rate of 4% per year.[10]

The ACS estimates that 56,900 new cases of skin cancer (excluding basal and squamous cell) will occur in 2000, with an estimated 9600 deaths. Approximately 1.3 million cases of basal or squamous cell cancers will occur in 2000.[10]

Skin cancer rates are 10 times higher in whites than in African Americans.[10] At highest risk for developing skin cancer are persons who work outdoors, who are fair-skinned, and who have occupational exposure to coal tar, arsenic compounds, and radium. Among African Americans the incidence of skin cancer development is low because of heavy skin pigmentation. The UV rays of the sun are strongest between 10 AM and 3 PM. Sun exposure should be limited during those hours and protective clothing (hats, scarves, long sleeves) worn to offer some protection from the UV rays. Children should be especially protected because of the possible link between severe sunburn in childhood and greatly increased risk of melanoma in later life.[10] Sunscreens should be worn when deliberate sun exposure is expected (i.e., when pool side or on the beach). A sunscreen with a sun protection factor (SPF) of 15 or higher should be worn on all sun-exposed skin surfaces. Sunscreens protect against a spectra of UV rays and should be applied before sun exposure and reapplied after being in the water. Sun tanning parlors, which are increasing in popularity among Americans, should be avoided.

Early detection of skin cancers is crucial to saving lives and reducing the extent of surgical intervention. Basal and squamous cell cancers of the skin usually appear over areas of the body chronically exposed to the sun, including the nose, cheeks, and ears. These cancers appear as pale, waxlike nodules or a red, scaly patch that tends to bleed. Melanomas are small, molelike eruptions on the skin that can appear anywhere on the body, including the soles of the feet and palms of the hand. Melanomas change in color, shape, and size and can ulcerate and bleed.

A simple *ABCD* rule outlines the warning signs of melanoma: *A* is for asymmetry; *B* is for border irregularity; *C* is for change in color or pigmentation; and *D* is for diameter greater than 6 mm. Adults should practice skin self-examination and mole mapping monthly and report any suspicious indicators to a member of the health care team.

SEXUAL LIFE-STYLES

Sexual beliefs, attitudes, and practices are no longer private and unassuming. The sexual mores of the 1980s and 1990s have thrust the association between sexual activity and cancer risk from obscurity to the front lines. The advertising slogan "sex sells" has almost prompted an attitude of "anything goes." Sexually transmitted diseases (STDs), genital cancers, human immunodeficiency virus (HIV), and acquired immunodeficiency syndrome (AIDS) have a documented direct relationship to sexual life-styles and practices. The association between sex and genital cancer has been known for more than 150 years.[36] Research indicates an association between sexual life-styles and AIDS and cancer of the cervix, vulva, and vagina. Risk factors common in women with cervical cancer include a high rate of STDs, early age at first coitus, multiple sexual partners, and exposure to high-risk sexual partners. Several viruses have been implicated in the etiology of cervical neoplasia, including herpes simplex virus (HSV) and human papillomavirus (HPV). Penile HPV (genital wart or condyloma acuminatum) infection in a male partner places the woman at risk of cervical cancer.

The incurable and deadly diseases, HIV and AIDS, have cast a shadow over the American sexual revolution and sexual freedom as have no other diseases or health threats. Sexual behaviors considered to be high-risk factors associated with HIV and AIDS include unprotected vaginal or anal intercourse, internal "water sports" (urinating into a body cavity such as the vagina or anus), "fisting" (inserting a finger, fingers, or fist into the anus), and oral-anal sex, also known as "rimming."[36] Sharing of dirty needles by intravenous (IV) drug users is also a high-risk factor. Male homosexuals and IV drug users are at greatest risk for acquiring HIV and AIDS and other related neoplasms; however, the CDC reports a growing rate of HIV and AIDS cases among the heterosexual population.[63] The mortality rate for HIV and AIDS is greater than 40% within the first year of diagnosis.[36, 53] Reducing the cancer risk related to sexual life-styles can be effected by safe sexual practices.

EARLY DETECTION AND SCREENING RECOMMENDATIONS

Most Americans are adopting more health-conscious behaviors, including diet modification, physical fitness, smoking cessation, and overall healthier life-styles. Heightened awareness of health-promoting activities and early detection techniques related to cancer continue to be a focus of many cancer information agencies (e.g., ACS, NCI) and professional organizations (e.g., Oncology Nursing Society). The ACS has updated the screening and early detection guidelines as outlined in Table 4–12. Socioeconomic barriers to screening and early detection include: lack of health insurance, poverty, unemployment, and lack of education. Overall cancer survival can be increased through early detection. Regular breast, cervical, and prostate screening techniques are validated by scientific evidence of their effec-

T A B L E   4 – 1 2
Summary of American Cancer Society Recommendations for the Early Detection of Cancer in Asymptomatic People

Site	Recommendation
Cancer-related checkup	A cancer-related checkup is recommended every 3 years for people aged 20–40 and every year for people age 40 and older. This exam should include health counseling and depending on a person's age, might include examinations for cancers of the thyroid, oral cavity, skin, lymph nodes, testes, and ovaries, as well as for some nonmalignant diseases.
Breast	Women 40 and older should have an annual mammogram, an annual clinical breast examination (CBE) by a health care professional, and should perform monthly breast self-examination. The CBE should be conducted close to the scheduled mammogram. Women ages 20–39 should have a CBE by a health care professional every 3 years and should perform monthly breast self-examination.
Colon and rectum	Beginning at age 50, men and women should follow *one* of the examination schedules below: A fecal occult blood test every year and a flexible sigmoidoscopy every 5 years.* A colonoscopy every 10 years.* A double-contrast barium enema every 5–10 years.*
Prostate	The ACS recommends that both the prostate–specific antigen (PSA) blood test and the digital rectal examination be offered annually, beginning at age 50, to men who have a life expectancy of at least 10 years and to younger men who are at high risk. Men in high-risk groups, such as those with a strong familial predisposition (i.e., two or more affected first-degree relatives), or African Americans may begin at a younger age (i.e., 45 years).
Uterus	**Cervix:** All women who are or have been sexually active or who are 18 and older should have an annual Pap test and pelvic examination. After three or more consecutive satisfactory examinations with normal findings, the Pap test may be performed less frequently. Discuss the matter with your physician. **Endometrium:** Women at high risk for cancer of the uterus should have a sample of endometrial tissue examined when menopause begins.

* A digital rectal exam should be done at the same time as sigmoidoscopy, colonoscopy, or double-contrast barium enema. People who are at moderate or high risk for colorectal cancer should talk with a doctor about a different testing schedule.

Used with permission from Cancer facts and figures, 2000 (p. 34). Atlanta, American Cancer Society.

tiveness in detecting cancers early. The public should be educated to individual risk factors, prevention strategies and screening recommendations.[16, 21, 24, 31, 42]

CONCLUSION

Cancer mortality will not be reduced without heightened public awareness and a multidisciplinary approach involving health care professionals, epidemiologists, and researchers. Agencies such as the ACS, Leukemia Society, and NCI play a vital role in cancer control efforts through funding and support of all aspects of cancer research and public and professional education. These agencies and organizations also must increase activity and involvement in social and political decisions influencing health care policy, cancer research, and treatment. A positive example of such efforts by the American public and support agencies is the ban on cigarette smoking on all domestic airline flights.

Because cancer is predominantly a disease of older adults, many signs and symptoms can mimic the normal aging process and are ignored and undetected by older persons and their significant others. Nurses can play a vital role in cancer prevention, screening, and risk reduction by identifying high-risk individuals and assessing life-style, personal and family history, and occupational or environmental exposure to carcinogens. Nurses' efforts should also include promoting follow-up and surveillance of those identified as high risk.

Minority and underserved Americans offer the greatest challenge to nurses and other health care professionals. The underserved and SED populations make up a significant percentage of the American public and often bear the greatest burden of cancer risk and mortality. This is reflected in poorer overall survival, most frequently because of a later stage at which the cancer is detected. In excess of 40 million Americans are uninsured or underinsured, and this number is escalating. Another barrier for this population is limited access to health care because of lack of health insurance, unemployment, homelessness, transportation issues, and inability to wait 6 to 8 hours in a overcrowded health care facility because of family and job responsibilities. Screening and early detection have little significance but to imply a "death sentence" to someone who has no access to health care intervention and follow-up and for whom the situation seems hopeless.[21, 57, 58, 60–62]

To offer public health teaching and support, the nurse and other health care professionals must be sensitive to social, cultural, ethnic, and religious beliefs, values, and attitudes that can affect an individual's receptivity to health promotion and disease prevention strategies. Nurses can best prepare to meet the public education needs through sensitivity training sessions, development of printed materials that reflect cultural diversity and are at an appropriate literacy level, and thorough "train-the-trainer" programs for volunteers. Train-the-trainer programs facilitate contact with previously difficult-to-reach groups by training a volunteer from within the community or group to deliver the message of cancer prevention, risk reduction, and health promotion. Cancer prevention efforts should be aimed at improved agricultural and grain storage techniques, safe sexual practices, reduced occupational and environmental exposure to carcinogens, health promotion activities, and education.[56, 62]

Nursing Management

Patient and family education in the prevention, screening, and early detection of cancer lays the foundation for overcoming ignorance and fear of cancer related to health beliefs, practices, and attitudes. Nurses can take active roles in sharing knowledge, skills, and expertise with Americans who have limited access to health care and who are at a higher risk for developing certain cancers. Nurses can work through neighborhood outreach groups and legislators to advocate for reduced-cost or no-cost cancer screening tests for the underserved and high-risk population. Nurses can involve at-risk youth by facilitating health education programs, conducting risk appraisals, and providing information on nutrition and life-style choices and changes for health promotion and disease prevention. Overall, professional nurses can have the greatest impact on the public by "walking the talk," that is, by practicing good health habits, weight reduction, smoking cessation, and self-examination and by facilitating public and professional education programs. The nurse can take a proactive role by coordinating screening projects and participating in health fairs.[46, 64, 65]

By eliciting the aid of church, social, and civic organizations, nurses can reach many of those individuals who have limited or no access to health care and who are at greatest risk for cancer morbidity and mortality.[30]

Nursing Diagnosis

- *Knowledge deficit related to prevention and early detection of site-specific cancers* (see Table 4–4)

Outcome Goals

The individual will be able to:

- State the seven warning signals of cancer.
- Demonstrate site-related self-examination related to breast, oral, skin, vulva, penile, and testicular cancers.
- Recognize cancer-related signs and symptoms that require follow-up in the health care system.
- Identify cancer information sources (e.g., ACS, Leukemia Society, NCI).
- Identify his or her relative risk for cancer development.

Assessments

Assess the following:

- Patient education level
- Literacy level
- Cultural and ethnic needs related to cancer education
- Beliefs and attitudes toward cancer
- Individual history and relative risk of cancer development

Interventions

- Discuss site-specific cancer risk factors.
- Identify signs and symptoms of site-specific cancer.
- Implement health teaching related to diet, nutrition, and life-style choices and desired modifications.
- Provide appropriate and culturally sensitive, literacy and linguistically appropriate printed information.
- Provide a list of cancer information and support agencies.
- Instruct individual in self-examination of breast, mouth, skin, cervix, vulva, penis, and testes, as appropriate.
- Review ACS screening guidelines.[6, 16, 20]

- Assist patient with access to health care issues for cancer screening and early detection.
- Identify signs and symptoms that warrant access to the health care system.
- Identify community resources available for smoking cessation, stress reduction, weight management and and diet control.
- Identify occupational and environmental risk factors and reporting agencies: OSHA (Occupational Safety and Health Administration), EPA (Environmental Protection Agency), NRC (Nuclear Regulatory Commission), and FDA (Food and Drug Administration).
- Provide mechanism for necessary referral and follow-up.

PATIENT TEACHING PRIORITIES

Cancer

Ensure that printed teaching materials are literacy appropriate at or below the fifth-grade reading level.

Include culturally sensitive and relevant content and visual aids with printed materials and presentations.

Seek out or develop translated printed materials appropriate to the target population.

In reaching out to diverse communities with cancer prevention, screening, and detection strategies, consider the following:

- Assessment of cultural and community needs
- Involve community volunteers in the program planning process
- Collaboration with community volunteers on content, time, location, and length of the program
- Ease of access by the target population
- Partnerships with community leaders and other organizations with similar health promotion and disease prevention goals to maximize resources

---

Chapter Questions

1. Initiatives to decrease smoking prevalence should be targeted to which of the following groups?
   a. High school graduates
   b. High school drop outs
   c. College graduates
   d. Persons with some college
2. More that 75% of all prostate cancers occur in which of the following groups?
   a. African American men
   b. Men over the age of 65
   c. Asian/Pacific Islanders
   d. Men between the age of 45 and 50

3. Neoplastic transformation in human cancers involves the following sequence of events:
   a. Stimulus, response, and initiation
   b. Risk, exposure, and progression
   c. Initiation, promotion, and progression
   d. Irritation, promotion, and susceptibility
4. According to the American Cancer Society guidelines, for optimal breast health, asymptomatic women should do which of the following?
   a. Annual breast self-examination (BSE) and mammography starting at age 50
   b. Clinical breast examination (CBE) and BSE, monthly, starting at age 40
   c. Monthly BSE and annual CBE and mammogram starting at age 40
   d. Annual CBE and mammogram every 3 years starting at age 50
5. Poor survival statistics, delayed diagnosis, and increased mortality among minority populations stem from barriers related to:
   a. Primary prevention and lack of access
   b. Socioeconomic status and secondary prevention
   c. Lack of access and illiteracy
   d. Secondary and tertiary prevention
6. A 45-year-old African American man is seen by an advance practice nurse for a routine physical. Which of the following would be the most appropriate screening test for his race and age?
   a. DRE and PSA
   b. Colonoscopy
   c. Ultrasound of the bladder
   d. Stool for occult blood
7. Reducing cancer risk related to sexual life-styles can most *realistically* be accomplished by:
   a. Avoiding homosexuality
   b. Engaging in safe sexual practices
   c. Practicing abstinence
   d. Avoiding intravenous drug use
8. The overall *incidence* of cancers can best be reduced by:
   a. Early detection
   b. Screening
   c. Prevention
   d. Early treatment
9. The American Cancer Society estimates that 80% of all cancers are associated with which of the following:
   a. Genetic predisposition
   b. Racial and ethnic factors
   c. Socioeconomic factors
   d. Environmental exposures
10. *Healthy People 2010* focus areas identify cancer as the _____ area of focus:
    a. Fifth
    b. Fourth
    c. Second
    d. Third

BIBLIOGRAPHY

1. Albright LA and others: Genetic predisposition to cancer. In DeVita VT Jr, Hellman S, Rosenberg SA, editors: *Important advances in oncology,* Philadelphia, Lippincott, 1991.
2. American Cancer Society: *Official position on the tobacco settlement, part XII: Restrictions on marketing and advertising.* Atlanta, The Society, 1997.
3. *Annotated bibliography of cancer-related literature on black populations,* NIH Publication No. 89-3024, Public Health Service, US Department of Health and Human Services.
4. Bal DG, Nixon DW, Foerster SB, Brownson RC: Cancer prevention. In Murphy G, Lawrence W, Lenhard R, editors: *ACS textbook of clinical oncology,* ed 2, Atlanta, American Cancer Society, 1995.
5. Baquet CR and others: Socioeconomic factors and cancer incidence among blacks and whites, *J Natl Cancer Inst* 83:551, 1991.
6. Bell I: Testicular self-examination, *Nurs Times* 86:38, 1990.
7. *Black and minority health: report of the secretary's task force,* Washington, DC, 1985, US Department of Health and Human Services.
8. Burke W, Daly M, Garber J, Botkin J, Kahn MJE, Lynch P, McTiernan A, Offitt K, Perlman J, Petersen G, Thornson E, Varricchio C: Recommendations for follow-up care of individuals with an inherited predisposition to cancer. II. BRCA1 and BRCA2. Cancer genetics cancer consortium, *JAMA* 277:997, 1997.
9. *Cancer among blacks and other minorities: statistical profiles,* NIH Publication No. 86-2785, Washington, DC, 1986, Public Health Service, US Department of Health and Human Services.
10. *Cancer facts and figures—2000,* Atlanta, American Cancer Society, 2000.
11. *Cancer facts and figures for African Americans—1998–1999,* Atlanta, American Cancer Society, 1998.
12. *Cancer prevention and detection,* Atlanta, American Cancer Society, 1989.
13. *Cancer risk report: prevention and control,* Atlanta, American Cancer Society, 1998.
14. Cookson MS, Smith JA: PSA testing: To screen or not to screen? *Primary Care Consultant* 40:4, 670, 2000.
15. Cuzick J: Human papillomavirus testing for primary cervical cancer screening, *JAMA,* 283:108, 2000.
16. Dodd GD: American Cancer Society guidelines on screening for breast cancer: an overview, *CA Cancer J Clin* 42:177, 1992.
17. Drago JR: The role of new modalities in the early detection and diagnosis of prostate cancer, *CA Cancer J Clin* 39:326, 1989.
18. Faulkenberry JE: Cancer in men: a case for cancer prevention and early detection, *Dimens Oncol Nurs* 2:17, 1988.
19. Fink DJ, Mettlin CJ: Cancer detection: the cancer related checkup guidelines. In Murphy G, Lawrence W, Lenhard

R, editors: *ACS textbook of clinical oncology,* ed 2, Atlanta, American Cancer Society, 1995.

20. Fitzsimmons ML and others: Hereditary cancer syndromes: nursing's role in identification and education, *Oncol Nurs Forum* 16:87, 1989.

21. Frank-Stromborg, M: Cancer screening and early detection. In Varricchio C, editor: *A cancer source book for nurses,* ed 7, Atlanta, American Cancer Society, 1997.

22. Freeman HP: Cancer in the socioeconomically disadvantaged, *CA Cancer J Clin* 39:266, 1989.

23. Gene testing for breast and ovarian cancer (monograph): American Medical Association, 1–8, 1999.

24. Goolsby MJ: Screening, diagnosis, and management of prostate cancer: improving primary cancer outcomes, *Nurse Pract* 23:3, 1998.

25. Gorman C: Colon cancer: Katie's crusade. *Time,* 70–76, March 13, 2000.

26. Graves PL, Thomas CB, Mead LA: Familial and psychological predictors of cancer, *Cancer Detect Prev* 15:59, 1991.

27. Greenlee RT, Murray J, Bolden S, Wingo PA: Cancer statistics, 2000, *CA Cancer J Clin* 50:1, 2000.

28. Griffiths EK, Schapira DV: Serum ferritin and stool occult blood and colon cancer screening, *Cancer Detect Prev* 15:303, 1991.

29. Gullatte MM: Cancer prevention and early detection in black Americans: prostate, *In Touch* 9:4, 1988.

30. Gullatte MM: Cancer prevention and early detection in black Americans: colon and rectum, *J Natl Black Nurses Assoc* 3:49, 1989.

31. Held-Warmkessel J: *Contemporary issues in prostate cancer: a nursing perspective,* Boston, Jones & Bartlett, 2000.

32. Heath CW: Cancer prevention. In Holleb AI, Fink DJ, Murphy GP, editors: *ACS textbook of clinical oncology,* Atlanta, American Cancer Society, 1991.

33. Heath CW: Electromagnetic field exposure and cancer: a review of epidemiologic evidence, *CA Cancer J Clin* 46:29, 1996.

34. Hescock HR, Richman E: Common solid malignancies: a primary care perspective, *Clin Rev* 9:5, 55, 1999.

35. Heusinkveld KB: Cancer prevention and risk assessment. In Varricchio C, editor: *A cancer source book for nurses,* Atlanta, American Cancer Society, 1997.

36. Holmes BC: *Sexual lifestyles and cancer risk,* Atlanta, American Cancer Society, 1988.

37. Holmes MD, Hunter DJ, Colditz GA, Stampfer MJ, Hankinson SE, Speizer FE, Rosner B, Willett WC: Association of dietary intake of fat and fatty acids with risk of breast cancer, *JAMA* 281:914, 1999.

38. Iribarren C and others: Effect of cigar smoking on the risk of cardiovascular diseases, chronic obstructive pulmonary disease and cancer in men, *N Engl J Med* 340:1773, 1999.

39. Kessler-Koop Advisory Committee: Report of the Kessler-Koop Advisory Committee on tobacco policy and public health, July, 1999. (online) www.tobaccofreekids.org/html/koop_kessler_report.html.

40. Levin VA, Palitz A, Grossman S, Conell C, Finkler L, Ackerson L, Rumore G, Selby JV: Predicting advanced proximal colonic neoplasia with screening sigmoidoscopy, *JAMA* 281:1611, 1999.

41. Lynch HT, Lynch JF: Familial factors and genetic predisposition to cancer: population studies, *Cancer Detect Prev* 15:49, 1991.

42. Marshall JR: Chemoprevention of prostate cancer in a high-risk population, *Oncology Economics* 1:40, 2000.

43. Miller AB: Role of early diagnosis and screening: biomarkers, *Cancer Detect Prev* 15:21, 1991.

44. Murphy GP, Lawrence W, Lenhard RE: *ACS textbook of clinical oncology,* ed 2, Atlanta, American Cancer Society, 1995.

45. Noel L and others: The cost effectiveness of tamoxifen in the prevention of breast cancer, *Oncology Economics* 1:45, 2000.

46. *Nutrition and cancer prevention: guidelines on diet, nutrition, and cancer prevention: Reducing the risk of cancer with healthy food choices and physical activity,* Atlanta, American Cancer Society, 1999.

47. Pate RR, Pratt M, Blair SN, Haskell WL, Macera CA, Bouchard C, Buchner D, Ettinger W, Heath GW, King AC, Kriska A, Leon AS, Marcus BH, Morris J, Paffenberger Jr. RS, Patrick K, Pollock ML, Rippe JM, Sallis J, Wilmore JH: Physical activity and public health: a recommendation from the Centers for Disease Control and Prevention and the American College of Sports Medicine, *JAMA* 273:402, 1995.

48. Pazdur R, Royce M: *Myths and facts about colorectal cancer,* New York, PRR, 1999.

49. Phillips J, Belcher A, O'Neil A: Special populations. In Varricchio C, editor: *A cancer source book for nurses,* ed 7, pp. 56–66, Atlanta, American Cancer Society, 1997.

50. Rosenbaum EH, Dollinger M, Newell GR: *Risk assessment, cancer screening and prevention: everyone's guide to cancer therapy,* Kansas City, Somerville House, 1991.

51. Ruckdeschel JC: *Myths and facts about lung cancer: what you need to know,* New York, 1999, PRR.

52. Satcher D: Cigars and public health, *N Engl J Med* 340:1829, 1999.

53. Schiffman M and others: HPV DNA testing in cervical cancer screening: results from women in a high-risk province of Costa Rica, *JAMA* 283:87, 2000.

54. Smoking—attributable mortality and years of potential life lost—United States, 1988, *MMWR* 40:62, 1991.

55. Stromborg MF, Olsen SJ: *Cancer prevention in minority populations: cultural implications for health care professionals,* St Louis, Mosby, 1993.

56. Tubiana M: Trends in primary and secondary prevention, *Cancer Detect Prev* 15:1, 1991.

57. Underwood SM: African-American men: perceptual determinants of early cancer detection and cancer risk reduction, *Cancer Nurs* 14:281, 1991.

58. Underwood SM: Cancer risk reduction and early detection behaviors among black men: focus on learned helplessness, *J Community Health Nurs* 9:21, 1992.

59. US Department of Health and Human Services. *Healthy people 2010: Understanding and improving health.* US Government Printing Office, Washington, DC, No. 012-00-00543-6, ISBN 0-16-050260-8. www.health.gov/healthypeople/. January, 2000.

60. Vainio H, Hemminki K: Use of exposure information and animal cancer data in the prevention of environmental and occupational cancer, *Cancer Detect Prev* 15:7, 1991.

61. Vernon SW and others: Early detection of breast cancer among women veterans: a study to determine the effectiveness and efficiency of methods to improve compliance with mammography screening guidelines, *Oncology Economics* 1:32, 2000.

62. Watkins MC: Computerized cancer information sources, *J Med Assoc Ga* 81:143, 1992.

63. Wingo PA, Ries LAG, Giovino GA, et al: Annual report on the status of cancer, 1973–1996, *J Natl Cancer Inst* 91:675, 1999.

64. Wholihan DJ: Incorporating cancer prevention interventions into the home health visit, *Home Healthcare Nurse* 9:19, 1991.

65. Willis MA and others: Inter-agency collaboration: teaching breast self-examination to black women, *Oncol Nurs Forum* 16:171, 1989.

66. Ziegler RG, Devesa SS, Fravmeni JF Jr: Epidemiologic patterns of colorectal cancer. In DeVita VT Jr, Hellman S, Rosenberg SA, editors: *Important advances in oncology*, Philadelphia, Lippincott, 1991.

Diagnosis and Staging

Joyce Alexander

The diagnosis of cancer requires a multidisciplinary team, including the attending physician, specialists, radiologists, surgeons, oncologists, pathologists, technicians, and nurses. Treatment decisions are based on the histology (tumor type) and the assessed extent of disease. New techniques to diagnose and stage cancers have facilitated development of sophisticated plans of treatment, which have produced improved patient survival rates, as well as cures for some malignancies.

DIAGNOSIS

History and Physical Examination

Although for some patients an early cancer is detected through screening (see Chapter 4), for many the diagnosis begins with a visit to the physician's office. The patient, or a family member, may have noted symptoms that caused concern, or a wellness examination may detect disconcerting symptoms. A nursing history and systems assessment adds valuable data to a thorough history and physical performed by the physician. Carefully listening to the patient's experience of symptoms provides vital information. In young children parents often report behavior changes that become important clues. A review of cancer risk factors may increase the suspicion of malignancy. From the initial database, potential diagnoses are developed and testing initiated to rule out or confirm the more likely possibilities.

The physical examination is a systematic assessment of major body sites: head, ears, nose, throat, cardiovascular system, chest, abdomen, genitourinary system, extremities, lymph nodes, and nervous system. Positive and negative findings are documented and evaluated in terms of the patient's medical history. An enlarged liver, for example, may lead to suspicion of metastatic disease in the patient with a past history of colon or breast cancer.

Following the history and physical examination, a diagnostic work-up is planned. Even though the diagnostic work-up yields evidence of malignancy, that diagnosis must be confirmed through histologic and cytologic examination. Staging completes the necessary information for planning treatment.

Diagnostic Work-up

A diagnostic work-up is initiated to determine the diagnosis. A wide range of diagnostic procedures may be used in the individualized work-up for each patient. Testing begins with less invasive procedures but may include highly technical innovations. After the diagnosis of malignancy is established, further diagnostic tests may be done to determine the stage of the cancer. Knowledge of symptoms, a high index of suspicion for malignancy, and knowledge of biologic behavior of a particular cancer are all useful in reaching a diagnosis.

Radiologic Studies. Examinations generally begin with the least invasive and expensive study that may provide the information needed for diagnosis. A work-up often begins with a basic chest x-ray. A mammogram, flat plate of the abdomen, or x-ray films of the extremities may also add information.

Computed tomography (CT) scans use serial radiologic views. A computer analyzes the information and produces multiple cross-sectional images of internal structures. CT detects differences in tissue density and is most useful for tissue not surrounded by bone. Contrast solutions containing iodine may be used to improve CT images. CT scans are often used to guide biopsy procedures.

Barium, a radiopaque, nonabsorbable substance, may be given orally or by enema to reveal changes in the lumen of the gastrointestinal tract. An intravenous pyelogram (IVP) follows excretion of an intravenous contrast through the urinary tract. Myelogram, a study using intrathecal injection of contrast, may be enhanced with CT for diagnosis of pathology of the spinal column.[22]

Magnetic Resonance Imaging (MRI). MRI provides sensitive images of soft tissues without interference from bone. Images are produced by placing the patient within a strong magnetic field, causing alignment of certain atoms within cellular molecules. Pulsed radio waves cause absorption and release of energy as the atomic nuclei change orientation. Energy differences are detected and measured by antennae, and the information is used by the MRI computer to produce images. MRI is superior for visualization of tissues obscured by bone in other diagnostic techniques, including central nervous system, mediastinal, and hilar areas. MRI has recently been used to determine tumor extent in nasopharyngeal cancer.[10]

Ultrasonography. Ultrasonagraphy is the use of echoes of high-frequency sound waves to visualize internal structures. Abdominal, pelvic, or peritoneal masses may be detected by ultrasound. Lesions identified in the breast through mammography are often evaluated using ultrasonagraphy. Transrectal ultrasound is useful in evaluation of prostate cancer.

Nuclear Medicine Scans. Radioactive isotopes may be injected and tracked to those tissues for which the isotope has an affinity. Concentrations of the isotope in focal points indicate greater activity of cells, which may be caused by disease, infection, or malignancy. Areas of decreased uptake may also be significant in tissues that normally take up an isotope. A bone scan provides a low-cost, whole body image, which is highly sensitive for detection of malignancy[25] and is often used to detect metastatic bone disease. Scans of the thyroid, brain, and liver are done to evaluate possible primary or metastatic disease in those organs.

Positron Emission Tomography (PET). Unlike radiographic studies relying on density and size of tissues and lymph nodes to determine abnormalities, PET scans reveal differences in metabolic processes. The image in PET scanning is produced by detection of positron emissions from radionuclides. Flourine-18–labeled deoxyglucose (FDG) is the most commonly used positron emitter. The deoxyglucose molecule is taken up by cells in place of glucose, creating an accumulation of FDG in metabolically active cells. Tumors have an accelerated glycolysis compared to the tissues of origin and, therefore, produce concentrations of FDG.[1] Akhurst and Larson[1] recommend the use of FDG PET scanning in colon cancer for staging, assessing elevated tumor markers in patients with otherwise negative or indeterminate conventional imaging, determination of operability of potentially resectable tumor, and monitoring response to therapy. FDG PET scanning has also been recommended to improve accuracy of preoperative lung cancer staging through improved detection of lymph node abnormalities.[3, 8] Usefulness has also been demonstrated in esophageal cancer,[12] head and neck cancer,[23]

and cervical cancer.[22] Recently, the chemotherapeutic agent, 5-fluorouracil has been tagged with the ^{18}F isotope and followed by PET scan to assess delivery of the chemotherapy to tumor.[1]

Immunoscintigraphy. Immunoscintigraphy, a form of nuclear imaging, uses monoclonal antibodies specific to tumor antigens. These antibodies, tagged with tracer amounts of radioisotopes, are injected intravenously. The antibody binds to antigen on tumor cells, creating concentrations of the tracer isotope. The gamma camera then produces images revealing sites of malignancy or metastasis.[18] *Scintimammography* has shown value in detection of breast malignancy and metastasis. Used as an adjunct to mammography, this process may reduce the incidence of surgery for suspicious but nonmalignant lesions.[19] Immunoscintography has also shown promise in imaging of non–small-cell lung cancer,[11] detection of prostate cancer lymph node metastases,[13] to guide the surgeon in colorectal cancer,[16] and in detection of recurrence in colorectal and ovarian cancer.[20]

Visualization. Advances in endoscopy techniques have made visual examination of many tissues possible. Colonoscopy and flexible sigmoidoscopy are used in the diagnosis of colorectal cancer; bronchoscopy is often useful in diagnosis of cancer of bronchogenic or lung origin; gastroscopy can differentiate causes of gastric symptoms; and laparoscopy is now being used to view and biopsy abdominal tissues. These techniques are used not only to visualize the tissues, but also to obtain samples for pathologic examination.

Laboratory Studies. Each patient's work-up includes a battery of common laboratory procedures, such as complete blood count with differential analysis of white blood cells, blood chemistries, liver function tests, renal function tests, and urinalysis. Additional laboratory studies, such as serum electrophoresis, calcium and magnesium levels, and levels of tumor markers, are ordered as indicated by the patient's symptoms. Table 5–1 lists some common laboratory studies used in a diagnostic work-up.

Tumor Markers. Tumor markers are hormones, enzymes, or antigens produced by tumor cells and measurable in the blood of persons with malignancies. Tumor markers are measurable by chemical analysis or more recently by monoclonal antibodies designed to identify specific antigens in a sample of blood. *Bence-Jones protein*, produced by myeloma cells, was the first known tumor marker. Hormonal tumor markers include *human chorionic gonadotropin* (HCG) and *α-fetoprotein* (AFP) produced by germ cell tumors.

Usefulness of a tumor marker in diagnosis and tracking of malignancy depends on the marker's *sensitivity* and *specificity*. The most sensitive marker would always

T A B L E 5 – 1
Selected Laboratory Studies

Examination	Detects or Assesses
Bone marrow aspiration/biopsy	Hematologic abnormalities
Blood chemistries and hepatic function studies	Abnormalities of the liver, kidneys, and bone related to cancer or its therapy. These may be used to monitor response to treatment.
Complete blood count	Bone marrow abnormalities or treatment toxicity
Creatinine clearance	Kidney function; especially important prior to administration of nephrotoxic drugs.
Hemoccult test	Presence of blood in stool; screening but not specific for cancer
Pap smear	Cervical cancer or premalignant changes
Serum electrophoresis	Serum protein and immunoglobulin levels (multiple myeloma)
Urine catecholamines	Neuroblastoma, pheochromocytoma

Refer to Appendix B for more specific information on laboratory studies.

be identifiable in the presence of a malignancy. The most specific marker would never be positive in the absence of disease. Tumor markers vary in sensitivity and specificity. Recent data has shown the marker CA27.29 to have both higher sensitivity and specificity in detection of breast cancer than the previously used CA15.3.[6] However, because of the relatively low sensitivity of both markers for early stage disease neither is recommended for screening. Combinations of tumor markers are sometimes used to overcome sensitivity and specificity problems. *Carcinoembryonic antigen* (CEA) is an antigen identified in colorectal, lung, and breast cancer. The addition of a second marker, *CA-72-4,* produces a more sensitive test. Tumor marker results must be evaluated for each patient in terms of symptoms and history. *Prostate-specific antigen* (PSA) is the first tumor marker to prove useful for screening. Although eleva-

tions of PSA may occur in benign prostatic disease, such elevations do indicate a need to evaluate for the presence of prostate cancer. Table 5–2 lists some commonly used tumor markers.

Pathology

Actual tumor cells must be obtained and examined by the pathologist before a clinical diagnosis of cancer or a determination of the grade of the malignancy can be made. Cells may be obtained by cytologic examination techniques, biopsy, or surgical excision of a suspected mass.

Cytology. *Cytology* is the examination of cells obtained from tissue scrapings, body fluids, secretions, or washings. *Pap smears* (named for Dr. George Papanicolaou,

T A B L E 5 – 2
Commonly Used Tumor Markers

Marker	Elevations May Indicate	Useful For
PSA (prostate-specific antigen)	Prostate cancer, benign prostate enlargement	Screening for prostate cancer in at-risk populations Monitoring response of patients to treatment
CEA (carcinoembryonic antigen)	Breast cancer, colorectal cancer, lung cancer	Monitoring or management of patients with known disease
HCG (human chorionic gonadotropin)	Germ cell tumors (testicular, certain types ovarian, others), pregnancy	Differentiation of germ cell tumors
AFP (α-fetoprotein)	Germ cell tumors, liver cancer, benign liver disease, pregnancy	Differentiation of germ cell tumors
CA-125 (antigen)	Ovarian cancer, also elevated in some nonmalignant conditions and in some nongynecologic cancers	Monitoring response
CA 27.29	Breast and ovarian cancer (replacing CA 15-3)	Monitoring of metastatic disease
CA 72-4	Ovarian, colorectal, and gastric cancers	Detection of primary disease and monitoring of treatment progress
CA 19-9	Pancreatic, colorectal, gastric cancer and inflammatory bowel or biliary disease	Monitoring response to treatment

who developed the technique) use scrapings from the cervix to identify abnormal cervical cells. A new reporting scheme, the *Bethesda system*, provides improved Pap smear reporting. The Bethesda system reports infectious or reactive changes as benign cellular changes. Epithelial cell abnormalities include squamous or glandular cells, ranging from atypical cells to carcinoma. Fluids aspirated by thoracentesis, paracentesis, or lumbar puncture may yield cells for examination. Fine-needle aspiration may also be used to obtain cells for evaluation. Once procured, cytology specimens must be evaluated by a skilled pathologist. False-positive results are possible, and negative results indicate only that no cancer cells were found in the sample.

Biopsy. A portion of tissue, generally obtained by surgical procedure, is examined in a biopsy specimen. Biopsy is often done as part of an endoscopic procedure or under the guidance of CT to ensure that suspicious areas are sampled. *Bone marrow biopsy,* which uses a special needle to aspirate bone marrow tissue, is included in the work-up for hematologic disorders, including lymphomas, and when bone marrow metastasis is suspected.

Excision. Excision is the surgical removal of a lesion. Whenever a mass is surgically removed, whether or not a definitive diagnosis has been made, the tissue removed must be examined by a pathologist.

Tissue Analysis. The pathologist uses a number of techniques to determine the tissue type and the degree of differentiation (grade) of the tumor. *Frozen section* is a procedure by which a small amount of tissue is quickly frozen, thinly sliced, and stained for immediate examination. A permanent section is prepared using tissue preserved in formalin, thinly sliced, stained, and prepared for microscopic examination. The pathologist begins the examination of the tissues with an overview and measurement of the gross specimen and then examines prepared slides using light microscopy. Careful attention is paid to the margins of the excised specimen to determine if margins are free of malignancy.

Immunoperoxidase staining identifies specific cell types using monoclonal or polyclonal antibodies against cellular antigens. PSA can be stained using a mono-clonal antibody and suggests that tissue is of prostatic origin. Leukocyte common antigen can be used to identify non-Hodgkin's lymphomas. Electron microscopy may be used when light microscopy and special stains fail to differentiate the cell type.

Receptor status is important in certain malignancies. Estrogen and progesterone receptor status must be determined for breast malignancy. The epidermal growth factor gene (HER2/*neu*) is overexpressed in at least a quarter of human breast cancers, and at a high frequency in ovarian, lung, gastric, and oral cancers. Overexpression of HER2/*neu* results in increased HER2 receptors on the cell surface, which can be identified using monoclonal antibodies. HercepTest is a kit for determining HER2 receptor status, which has been approved by the Food and Drug Administration (FDA). Although overexpression of HER2/*neu* may have significant prognostic implications,[15] current recommendations are for use in breast cancer when treatment with Herceptin (transtuzumab) is indicated.[21] Recently, evidence of increased risk of subsequent breast cancer has been shown to be associated with HER-2/*neu* amplification in benign biopsy.[15, 24]

Polymerase chain reaction (PCR) identifies specific genetic changes or chromosomal abnormalities. PCR can be used to determine risk of certain inherited cancers but is more often used in the identification of malignant cells in tissue, blood, or body fluid. Hematologic and other malignancies can be differentiated on the basis of PCR data; effectiveness of therapy can be tracked; and early relapse can be identified.

In addition to determining the definitive diagnosis of cancer and the tissue of origin, the pathologist must determine the grade. As noted, grade is a classification based on the differentiation of the malignancy. The more unlike normal tissue and less differentiated or less mature the cells, the higher is the grade. Behavior of a malignancy can be predicted on the basis of grade. Table 5–3 lists grade classifications.

Classification of Hematologic Malignancies. Hematologic malignancies are not graded following the grade classifications for solid tumors. In the past, leukemias

TABLE 5–3
Pathological Grade

Grade	Differentiation	Definition
X	Cannot be assessed	
I	Well differentiated	Mature cells; look very much like normal tissue.
II	Moderately differentiated	Cells have some immaturity; vary from normal tissue.
III	Poorly differentiated	Immature cells; do not look like normal cells.
IV	Undifferentiated	Cells are very immature; look nothing at all like normal tissue, often difficult to determine tissue of origin.

were classified as acute or chronic, lymphocytic or myeloid. Lymphomas have been classified by a number of
conflicting systems. In 1982, these were replaced by *The
Working Formulation*. The Working Formulation subdivided three grades of lymphoma (low grade, intermediate grade, and high grade) into specific cell types based
on the microscopic appearance of the cells (morphology) and clinical response to treatment regimens used
at that time. The Working Formulation did not include
information from immunologic and cytogenetic testing.
The *Revised European-American Classification of
Lymphoid Neoplasms* (REAL), published in 1994, was
devised to combine immunophenotyping, histologic,
clinical, and genetic information as well as the postulated cell of origin.[9] Lymphoid leukemias were included.
The REAL system is now being refined by the World
Health Organization into *The World Health Organization Classification of Hematopoietic and Lymphoid
Malignancies,* which includes all leukemias as well as
lymphomas. Within the WHO classification, as well as
the REAL system on which it is based, there is no
clinical grouping such as the low, intermediate, and high
grade found in the Working Formulation. Each hematopoietic and lymphoid malignancy in the extensive listing
is considered a unique disease, with specific features.
Prognostic factors are applied within the disease category, rather than to groups of diseases.[9]

STAGING

Once a cancer diagnosis is confirmed by pathology, information from previous tests and scans is combined
with additional work-up studies to determine the stage
of the malignancy. *Stage* is a classification system based
on the apparent anatomic extent of the malignancy. A
universal system of staging allows comparison of cancers
of similar cellular origin. Classification assists in determination of a treatment plan and prognosis for the individual patient, evaluation of research, comparison of
treatment results between institutions, and comparison
of worldwide statistics.

A comprehensive staging system was developed by
the American Joint Committee on Cancer (AJCC), a
coalition sponsored by the American Cancer Society
(ACS), National Cancer Institute (NCI), College of
American Pathologists, American College of Physicians, American College of Radiology, and American
College of Surgeons (ACS). This group published the
first staging manual in 1977. The International Union
Against Cancer later joined the group, and the system
became international. The fifth edition of the staging
manual was published in 1997.

The *TNM system* outlined by AJCC involves assessment of three basic components: the size of the *primary
tumor* (*T*), the absence or presence of regional *lymph
nodes* (*N*), and the absence or presence of distant *meta-

static disease* (*M*). General definitions used throughout
the system are included in Table 5–4.[5]

Information from the TNM classification is combined
to define the stage. Stage classifications have been determined for most cancer sites and are published in the
Manual for Staging of Cancer.[5] The stage is determined
before beginning treatment and is the basis for treatment decisions. The stage is often changed after surgery,
however, when pathologic measurements more accurately define tumor size and nodal involvement. Stage
determined before treatment is termed the *clinical stage*
(cTNM or TNM). When stage is changed after surgery,
the term *pathologic stage* (pTNM) is used. Refer to
Tables 5–5 and 5–6 for breast cancer staging, as an
illustration of the TNM system.

Surgical regional lymph node dissection is required
for determination of the "N" portion of staging. In
breast cancer and in melanoma, axillary or groin node
dissection has been the standard for determining stage.
Recently, *lymphatic mapping* and *sentinel lymph node
biopsy* have been used in both breast cancer and melanoma.[4] The sentinel lymph node is the first node receiving lymphatic drainage from the area of disease. The
sentinel node is identified by injection of a radioisotope
into the region, often accompanied by a dye. The passage of the isotope and dye are tracked and the identified
node is removed and examined for disease. For melanoma patients sentinel node biopsy allows accurate
identification of patients who will benefit from lymph
node dissection without subjecting those with negative
nodes to increased morbidity caused by lymph node
dissection.[4] In breast cancer, the ACS Oncology Group

T A B L E   5 – 4
TNM System

PRIMARY TUMOR (T)

TX	Primary tumor cannot be assessed.
T0	No evidence of primary tumor
Tis	Carcinoma in situ
T1, T2, T3, T4	Increasing size and/or local extent of the primary tumor

REGIONAL LYMPH NODES (N)

NX	Regional lymph nodes cannot be assessed
N0	No regional lymph node metastasis
N1, N2, N3	Increasing involvement of regional lymph nodes.

DISTANT METASTASIS (M)

MX	Distant metastasis cannot be assessed
M0	No distant metastasis
M1	Distant metastasis

*Used with the permission of the American Joint Committee on Cancer (AJCC®),
Chicago, Illinois. The original source for this material is the AJCC® Cancer
Staging Manual, 5th edition (1997) published by Lippincott-Raven Publishers,
Philadelphia, Pennsylvania.*

TABLE 5-5
Staging of Breast Cancer

Stage Grouping

Stage 0	Tis	N0	M0
Stage I	T1	N0	M0
Stage IIA	T0	N1	M0
	T1	N1	M0
	T2	N0	M0
Stage IIB	T2	N1	M0
	T3	N0	M0
Stage IIIA	T0	N2	M0
	T1	N2	M0
	T2	N2	M0
	T3	N1	M0
	T3	N2	M0
Stage IIIB	T4	Any N	M0
	Any T	N3	M0
Stage IV	Any T	Any N	M1

Used with the permission of the American Joint Committee on Cancer (AJCC®), Chicago, Illinois. The original source for this material is the AJCC® Cancer Staging Manual, 5th edition (1997) published by Lippincott-Raven Publishers, Philadelphia, Pennsylvania.

and the National Surgical Adjuvant Breast and Bowel Project (NSABP) are conducting ongoing clinical trials.[4] A large trial is needed to determine the prognostic significance of the sentinel node and to determine the proper positioning of this technique in the breast cancer treatment arsenal.

Before 1992, gynecologic cancers were typically classified using a separate system developed by the Federation of International Gynecology and Obstetrics (FIGO). Information from the FIGO system has been incorporated into the staging system published in the *Manual for Staging of Cancer.*

Staging of cancers of the central nervous system (CNS) varies from that for other disease sites. Important prognostic indicators in brain cancer are the biologic behavior, or rate of growth, and the location and size of the tumor (see Chapter 6). Staging for brain cancer, therefore, considers grade (*G*) and tumor size and location (*T*). A higher grade is a more malignant tumor; a grade 3 tumor (*G3*) is classified stage *III* unless the tumor crosses the midline. Any tumor that crosses the midline (*T4*) or any CNS tumor with metastasis is classi-

TABLE 5-6
Definitions of TNM (Breast)

PRIMARY TUMOR (T)

TX		Primary tumor cannot be assessed.
T0		No evidence of primary tumor
Tis		Carcinoma in situ: Intraductal carcinoma, lobular carcinoma in situ, or Paget's disease of the nipple with no tumor
T1		Tumor 2 cm or less in greatest dimension
	T1mic	Microinvasion 0.1 cm or less in greatest dimension
	T1a	Tumor more than 0.1 but not more than 0.5 cm in greatest dimension
	T1b	Tumor more than 0.5 cm but not more than 1 cm in greatest dimension
	T1c	Tumor more than 1 cm but not more than 2 cm in greatest dimension
T2		Tumor more than 2 cm but not more than 5 cm in greatest dimension
T3		Tumor more than 5 cm in greatest dimension
T4		Tumor of any size with direct extension to (a) chest wall or (b) skin, only as described below
	T4a	Extension to chest wall
	T4b	Edema (including peau d'orange) or ulceration of the skin of the breast or sattelite skin nodules confined to the same breast
	T4c	Both (T4a and T4b)
	T4d	Inflammatory carcinoma
		Note: Paget's disease associated with a tumor is classified according to the size of the tumor.

REGIONAL LYMPH NODES*

NX	Regional lymph nodes cannot be assessed (e.g., previously removed).
N0	No regional lymph node metastasis
N1	Metastasis to movable ipsilateral axillary lymph node(s)
N2	Metastasis to ipsilateral axillary lymph node(s) fixed to one another or to other structures
N3	Metastasis to ipsilateral internal mammary lymph node(s)

DISTANT METASTASIS

MX	Distant metastasis cannot be assessed.
M0	No distant metastasis
M1	Distant metastasis (includes metastasis to ipsilateral supraclavicular lymph node[s])

* Refer to AJCC staging manual for pathologic classification (pN)

Used with the permission of the American Joint Committee on Cancer (AJCC®), Chicago, Illinois. The original source for this material is the AJCC® Cancer Staging Manual, 5th edition (1997) published by Lippincott-Raven Publishers, Philadelphia, Pennsylvania.

fied *stage IV*. The brain is not supplied with lymphatic drainage; therefore "N" is not used.

Hematologic malignancies cannot be classified using the TNM system. Leukemias are classified according to cell type as described previously. Prognosis for leukemias is affected by cell type, genetic features, percentage of marrow involvement, and relapse status. Myeloma may be staged on the basis of clinical manifestations, including hemoglobin, serum calcium, presence of lytic bone lesions, and serum protein levels. The clinical features used in classification serve as indicators of tumor burden.[2] After pathologic classification, lymphomas, both Hodgkin's disease and non-Hodgkin's lymphoma, are staged according to the Ann Arbor system. Under the *Ann Arbor system*, lymphomas are staged *I, II, III,* or *IV* based on the area or region of lymph nodes involved. Stages are subdivided into A or B with *A* indicating absence of systemic symptoms and *B* indicating presence of systemic symptoms.[5]

In addition to TNM staging, colorectal tumors may also be classified by the *Dukes system,* which is compared to the TNM stage in the fifth edition of the AJCC cancer staging manual (Table 5–7).

The prognosis for patients with malignant melanoma largely depends on the depth of penetration of the original lesion. Two classification systems, *Clark's* and *Breslow's,* have been used to classify melanomas on the basis of depth of penetration. Information from these systems

TABLE 5–7
Colon Cancer Staging

Stage Grouping

AJCC/UICC				DUKES
Stage 0	Tis	N0	M0	—
Stage I	T1	N0	M0	A
	T2	N0	M0	—
Stage II	T3	N0	M0	B
	T4	N0	M0	—
Stage III	Any T	N1	M0	C
	Any T	N2	M0	—
Stage IV	Any T	Any N	M1	—

Used with the permission of the American Joint Committee on Cancer (AJCC®), Chicago, Illinois. The original source for this material is the AJCC® Cancer Staging Manual, 5th edition (1997) published by Lippincott-Raven Publishers, Philadelphia, Pennsylvania.

has been incorporated into the TNM system, using a pathologic (after-excision) T staging.[5]

CONCLUSION

The diagnostic period can be confusing and frightening for both the patient and the family. Overwhelmed patients and family ultimately look to the nurse to be both advocate and educator. Competent and confident delivery of nursing care can help reduce the anxiety experienced during this period.

Nursing Management

The word *cancer* has frightening connotations for individuals who may associate a diagnosis of cancer with death or pain. Virtually all diagnostic work-ups involve periods of waiting for information. Time may be perceived as endless and may provoke extreme anxiety for the patient and family awaiting an unknown or feared diagnosis. The family of a child with a potential cancer diagnosis may find this time especially stressful. Regardless of the patient's age, the family shares this experience with the patient and frequently is the patient's major support system. Families must be an integral part of the care of oncology patients, especially during the stressful time of diagnosis and staging. Responses of the patient and family are influenced by social and cultural factors, which must also be considered. This section describes nursing assessments, diagnoses, and interventions for both patients and families during the difficult period of diagnosis and staging.

Initial nursing assessments during the diagnosis and staging phase include assessment of the patient's and family's feelings and beliefs about the diagnostic process and about cancer; cultural and social influences on beliefs about cancer and healing and on coping styles; knowledge of the diagnostic process; ability to understand information presented; support systems available and used in past crisis situations; and effectiveness of coping styles. The nurse must establish rapport before the patient and family can feel comfortable sharing this information. Sitting with them, maintaining eye contact when eye contact is culturally appropriate, demonstrating respect for the individual, listening, and arranging uninterrupted time can be helpful in establishing rapport. The following responses may be experienced by the patient and family during this phase and may be identified as nursing diagnoses from a successful interview: (1) Fear related to a possible diagnosis of cancer; (2) Anxiety related to uncertainty about a diagnosis of cancer; (3) Ineffective individual coping; (4) Ineffective family coping; (5) Spiritual distress; (6) Knowledge deficit regarding procedures; (7) Knowledge deficit regarding cancer, disease, and treatment; (8) Anticipatory grieving; and (9) Health-seeking behaviors.[17] Other nursing diagnoses may be identified depending on presenting symptoms, prior conditions, and individual and family responses.

One result of recent changes in health care is the movement of most diagnostic and staging procedures to the outpatient setting. In addition to the previously described responses, patients and families experience problems unique to the outpatient setting. There is an increased potential for delays in diagnosis, staging, and treatment because appointments may be scheduled weeks rather than days apart, appointments may be missed, or results may be lost within the system. The nurse can advocate for the patient by coordinating scheduling and following up on tests and evaluations. Transportation may also present a problem and should be included in the nursing assessment. The nurse must also contribute to development of systems that facilitate procedures and allow time for patient and family assessment, questions, teaching, and support. Nursing input in the development of *care maps* for outpatient diagnosis and staging is one means of accomplishing this goal.

Nursing interventions depend on identified nursing diagnoses. Basic information about the diagnostic process, what test is to be done (do not assume the patient understood the physician's explanation), what may be learned, and how that information fits into the total picture is needed by most patients and families. When providing patient teaching materials, the nurse should evaluate and select material that is appropriate to the patient's reading level and that is culturally sensitive. Nurses can also correct misconceptions and provide reassurance. Some cancers can be cured and others can be controlled for many years, with treatment based on appropriate staging information. The nurse can present information about the treatment plan once a diagnosis has been determined. The patient and family will be asked to participate in the decision-making process at this point. Patients often feel pressured and turn to the nurse for assistance. Further clarification of options and potential outcomes is one possible intervention. The nurse should show respect for individual and cultural decision-making styles in any intervention at this time. Information about support groups and interaction with cancer survivors may also be helpful after a diagnosis has been confirmed.

Nursing Diagnosis

- *Fear related to possible cancer diagnosis*

Outcome Goals

Patient/significant others will be able to:
- Acknowledge validity of feelings.
- Identify effective means of dealing with diagnosis and treatment.

Assessments

- Emotional response
- Knowledge base and misconceptions, support systems

Interventions

- Establish rapport.
- Acknowledge validity of feelings.
- Correct misconceptions and provide information.
- Encourage use of support systems.

Nursing Diagnosis

- *Anxiety related to uncertainty/diagnosis of cancer*

Outcome Goals

Patient/significant others will be able to:

- Identify source of anxiety.
- Use effective skills for dealing with the perceived threat.

Assessments

- Uncertainty of diagnosis, situation, or prognosis
- Perceptions of individual about the situation
- Psychosocial responses to the situation
- Physical responses (sweating, flushing, hyperactivity, sighing respirations or shortness of breath, rapid heart rate, elevated blood pressure)
- Speech patterns (pressured speech, blaming, returning to a single topic, refusing to talk about cancer)

Interventions

- Limit time waiting for information.
- Provide information about disease and treatment.
- Explain diagnostic procedures, including sensations likely to be experienced.
- Encourage exploration and verbalization of feelings.
- Explore previous effective responses.
- Encourage use of effective responses.
- Teach behavioral interventions, including relaxation and distraction.[7]

Nursing Diagnosis

- *Knowledge deficit related to procedure*

Outcome Goal

Patient/significant others will be able to:

- Verbalize knowledge of procedure, rationale, and information to be obtained.

Assessments

- Knowledge of procedure
- Cognitive level and reading ability
- Stress level

Interventions

- Explain procedure and rationale.
- Provide simple written instructions for preparation, appointment time, and location.
- Explain what information may be gained.
- Provide culturally sensitive, written information appropriate to patient's cognitive and reading level.
- Repeat and simplify information for those persons under stress.

Nursing Diagnosis

- *Ineffective family coping*

Outcome Goal

Family/patient will be able to:

- Use effective coping strategies.

Assessments

- Coping styles
- Family communication patterns

- Family strengths
- Vulnerability of the family to a crisis event[14]
- Support systems

Interventions

- Identify and encourage effective coping strategies.
- Encourage effective family communication.
- Encourage use of support systems, including community support.
- Consult social worker, chaplain, and other support services as appropriate.

Nursing Diagnosis

- *Health-seeking behaviors*

Outcome Goal

Patient/significant others will be able to:

- Identify effective health-seeking behaviors.

Assessments

- Behaviors and questions aimed at seeking health
- Effectiveness of those behaviors
- Cultural beliefs about health

Interventions

- Encourage behaviors that are effective in prevention of cancer or maintenance of a healthy lifestyle (stopping smoking, low-fat diet, increased exercise).
- Answer questions openly and provide information.

Chapter Questions

1. Mr. Y., a heavy smoker, presents to his family physician with a complaint of a nagging cough continuing for several months. Which of the following examinations is Mr Y.'s physician most likely to order first?
   a. A CT scan of the chest
   b. A blood PSA level
   c. A chest X-ray
   d. An MRI of the chest
2. In preparing Mr. Y. for tests, patient reaching should include:
   a. Information presented at a level Mr. Y. and his family can understand.
   b. Simple written instructions for preparation, time and location of testing.
   c. Reinforcement of information as needed.
   d. All of the above.

3. Mr. Y. has completed a series of exams that indicate a lung mass in the right lower lobe. He is scheduled for a CT guided biopsy. Mr. Y.'s daughter asks, "Why must my father go through further tests? Why don't you just go ahead and treat this? You know it's a cancer!" The nurse's most appropriate response would be:
   a. We have to be absolutely certain it is cancer before we can treat. The only way to be certain is to have the pathologist look at a sample of the tissue.
   b. This institution participates in clinical trials. We are required to document a tissue diagnosis prior to initiation of treatment.
   c. This test is a part of his work-up. It's really not that big a deal; we do them every day. Don't worry.
   d. Perhaps you would like to discuss that question with your father's physician. Are you making a list of questions for the next time he comes in?

4. Mrs. S., a patient with breast cancer, has complained of back pain and is being evaluated for bone metastasis. Which of the following tests is most likely to be used to evaluate bone metastasis?
   a. Abdominal ultrasound
   b. Myelogram
   c. Intravenous pyelogram
   d. Bone scan

5. In planning a community screening program, which of the following would be appropriate to include as a screening examination?
   a. CEA
   b. CA 29.27
   c. AFP
   d. PSA

6. Grade is a classification system based on:
   a. Anatomic location of a tumor
   b. Size of the original tumor
   c. Resectability and location of a malignancy
   d. Differentiation of the cells

7. Staging is necessary for:
   a. Comparison of treatment results and research data among facilities
   b. Planning of treatment and prognosis for the individual patient
   c. Comparison of worldwide statistics
   d. All of the above

8. A reference on a patient's chart to a "T1-N0-M0" stage malignancy means the patient:
   a. Has a small tumor with negative lymph nodes and no metastases
   b. Has a large tumor and status of lymph nodes and metastases is unknown
   c. Has expressed a wish that NO one be told about the malignancy
   d. Has a small tumor with multiple lymph nodes involved and widespread metastases

9. Mrs. Y. tells the nurse that she is fearful of the outcome of her breast biopsy. The nurse should:
   a. Tell Mrs. Y. that there is nothing to be afraid of; everything will be all right.
   b. Acknowledge the validity of Mrs. Y.'s feelings and allow her to verbalize them further.
   c. Tell Mrs. Y. that since 80% of breast cancer biopsies are negative, she has nothing to fear.
   d. Provide Mrs. Y. with printed information about breast cancer, the various forms of treatment, and the side effects of treatment.

10. PET scan is likely to be most useful for tumors that have:
    a. A large tumor mass
    b. A high metabolic rate
    c. A poor blood supply
    d. Metastasis to bone.

BIBLIOGRAPHY

1. Akhurst T, Larson S: Positron emission tomography imaging of colorectal cancer, *Semin Oncol* 26:577, 1999.
2. Cassady S, Salmon S: Plasma cell neoplasms. In DeVita V, Hellman S, Rosenberg S, editors: *Cancer: principles and practice of oncology,* ed 5, Philadelphia, Lippincott-Raven, 1997.
3. Coates G, Skehan S: Emerging role of PET in the diagnosis and staging of lung cancer, *Can Respir J* 6:145, 1999.
4. Evans D: Surgical oncology, *J Am Coll Surg* 190:215, 2000.
5. Fleming I and others: *AJCC cancer staging manual,* ed 5, Philadelphia, Lippincott-Raven, 1997.
6. Gion M and others: Comparison of the diagnostic accuracy of CA27.29 and CA15.3 in primary breast cancer, *Clin Chem* 45:630, 1999.
7. Grim P: Coping: psychosocial issues. In Itano J, Taoka K, editors: *Core curriculum for oncology nursing,* ed 3, Philadelphia, Saunders, 1998.
8. Gupta N and others: Comparative efficacy of positron emission tomography with FDG and computed tomographic scanning in preoperative staging of non-small cell lung cancer, *Ann Surg* 229:286, 1999.
9. Jaffe E, Harris NL, Diebold J, and Muller-Hermelnik HK: World Health Organization classification of neoplastic diseases of the hematopoietic and lymphoid tissues: a progress report, *Am J Clin Pathol* 111(suppl 1):S8, 1999.
10. King A and others: MRI of local disease in nasopharyngeal carcinoma: tumour extent vs tumour stage, *Br J Radiol* 72:734, 1999.
11. Lau S, Johnson D, Coel M: Imaging of non-small-cell lung cancer with indium-111 pentetreotide, *Clin Nucl Med* 25:24, 2000.
12. Luketich J and others: Evaluation of distant metastases in esophageal cancer: 100 consecutive positron emission tomography scans, *Ann Thoracic Surg* 68:1133, 1999.
13. Manyak M and others: Immunoscintigraphy with indium-11-capromab pendetide: evaluation before definitive therapy in patients with prostate cancer, *Urology* 54:1058, 1999.
14. McNally J: Home care. In Groenwald S, Frogge MH, Goodman M, Yarbro CH, editors: *Cancer nursing: principles and practice,* ed 4, Sudbury, MA, Jones and Bartlett, 1997.
15. Mitchell M, Press M: The role of immunohistochemistry and fluorescence in situ hybridization for HER-2/*neu* in assessing the prognosis of breast cancer, *Semin Oncol* 26(4, suppl 12):108, 1999.
16. Muxi A and others: Radioimmunoguided surgery of colorectal carcinoma with an ^{111}In-labelled anti-TAG72 monoclonal antibody, *Nucl Med Commun* 20:123, 1999.
17. NANDA Staff (editors): *NANDA nursing diagnoses: definitions and classification, 1999–2000,* Philadelphia, Nursecom, 1999.
18. O'Mary S: Diagnostic evaluation, classification, and staging. In Groenwald S, Frogge MH, Goodman M, Yarbro CH, editors: *Cancer nursing: principles and practice,* ed 4, Sudbury, MA, Jones and Bartlett, 1997, p. 175.

19. Ortapamuk H and others: Role of technetium tetrofosmin scintimammography in the diagnosis of malignant breast masses and axillary lymph node involvement: a comparative study with mammography and histopathology, *Eur J Surg* 165:1147, 1999.

20. Pinkas L and others: Clinical experience with radiolabelled monoclonal antibodies in the detection of colorectal and ovarian carcinoma recurrence and review of the literature, *Nucl Med Commun* 20:689, 1999.

21. Ravdin P: Should HER2 status be routinely measured for all breast cancer patients? *Semin Oncol* 26(4, suppl 12):117, 1999.

22. Shafaie F and others: Comparison of computed tomography myelography and magnetic resonance imaging in the evaluation of cervical spondylotic myelopathy and radiculopathy, *Spin* 24:1781, 1999.

23. Slevin N and others: The diagnostic value of positron emission tomography (PET) with radiolabelled fluoro-deoxyglucose (^{18}F-FDG) in head and neck cancer, *J Laryngol Otol* 113:548, 1999.

24. Stark A and others: HER-2/*neu* amplification in benign breast disease and the risk of subsequent breast cancer, *J Clin Oncol* 18:267, 2000.

25. Tryciecky E, Gottschalk A, Ludema K: Oncologic imaging: interactions of nuclear medicine with CT and MRI using the bone scan as a model, *Semin Nucl Med* 27:142, 1997.

Clinical Management of
Major Cancer Diseases

Cancers of the Brain and Central Nervous System

Mary E. Murphy

Cancer of the central nervous system (CNS) includes primary and metastatic tumors of the brain and spinal cord. Despite a relatively high ratio of primary tumors in the pediatric population, adult CNS tumors represent only 2.4% of all cancer deaths. Metastatic lesions continue to present symptom and treatment management concerns. This chapter will deal with adult CNS tumors. Additional readings are recommended for the pediatric population.[1, 14, 34, 61]

EPIDEMIOLOGY

Cancer of the CNS accounts for less than 1.4% of all malignancies, with 16,500 diagnosed cases in 2000. Peak incidence occurs from birth to 6 years and after age 45. CNS tumors are the fourth leading cause of cancer death in persons ages 15 to 34. Peak incidence occurs before age 10 and after age 50. Current evidence shows a rapid increase in the population over 70 years of age. CNS tumors are more common in the white population than African Americans with men having a higher mortality rate. CNS cancers account for 13,000 deaths each year. Metastatic brain lesions represent 20% to 40% of all CNS neoplasms and commonly arise from the lung, breast, melanoma, and kidney.[1, 2, 10, 38, 39, 49]

ETIOLOGY AND RISK FACTORS

Specific causes and risk factors have not been identified. Chemical carcinogens and some oncologic viruses have induced CNS tumors in laboratory animals. Genetic factors have been linked with neurofibromatosis, tuberous sclerosis, familial polyposis, von Hippel-Lindau disease, Turcot syndrome, and family syndromes of breast cancer, soft-tissue sarcoma, leukemia, and chromosomal abnormalities such as the p53 gene (chromosome 17p) have been linked to aggressive astrocytomas in families with Le-Fraumen syndrome (LFS).[4]

Chemical exposures that have been implicated include vinyl chloride, radiation, petrochemicals, inks, acrylonitrile, lubricating oils, solvents, and aspartame (a sugar substitute). Viruses have also been implicated, including the Epstein-Barr virus genome. In addition, it is also noted that immunosuppressed patients have a higher incidence of CNS lymphoma. Traumatic causes and environmental carcinogens have not been implicated at this time. Ongoing investigation is in progress to evaluate the relationship to brain tumor formation and exposure to electromagnetic fields from cellular telephones, high-tension wire exposure, meningitis, tick-flea pesticides, and diets high in N-nitroso compounds and cured foods and low in vitamin C. To date head injuries of any type have not been indicated as a cause of disease.[8, 12, 15, 62]

PREVENTION AND SCREENING DETECTION

At this time, no screening or prevention methods exist for CNS and brain cancer. Symptoms appear gradually and do not lend themselves to diagnostic prescreening methods.

CLASSIFICATION

Tumors of the CNS include both brain and spinal cord tumors. CNS tumors are classified as primary and metastatic in nature. *Primary tumors* may exist as intracerebral or extracerebral. Major *intracerebral tumors* include those within the brain, neuroglia, neurons, and cells of the blood vessels of the connective tissue (Fig. 6–1). *Extracerebral tumors* originate outside of the brain and include meningiomas and acoustic nerve, pituitary, and pineal gland tumors. *Metastatic tumors* may exist either inside or outside the brain, CNS, or elsewhere in the body. The classification of benign versus malignant is

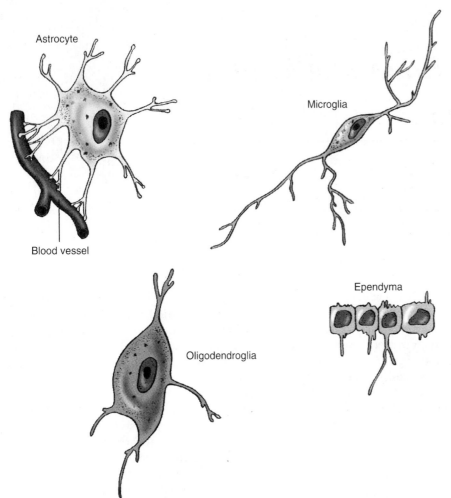

Astrocyte

Microglia

Blood vessel

Oligodendroglia

Ependyma

FIGURE 6-1 Types of neuroglial cells. (From Monahan FD: *Medical-surgical nursing: foundations of clinical practice*, ed 2, Philadelphia, Saunders, 1998.)

not differentiated, because surgical accessibility determines the ultimate prognosis.

Classification of CNS tumors is based on a variety of methods according to the preferences of the physician and pathologist. Common prognostic factors included in all systems include cell type, grade, and location. Some tumors also are evaluated by metastatic spread into the cerebrospinal fluid. Table 6–1 lists tumor classifications by location, characteristic, and cell origin. The most common cell type is the astrocytic, which makes up over 50% of all types of primary brain tumors. Glioblastoma multiforme, which represents 20% of all tumors in this category, has the poorest prognosis.[58]

Because primary brain tumors rarely if ever metastasize outside of the CNS, the standard TNM system is of little benefit as a staging system. The most commonly used are the Kernohan (a four-grade system) and the World Health Organization (WHO) three-grade system to stage glial neoplasms.* Table 6–2 compares these

two systems. Table 6–3 shows the standard TMN classification system.[6, 32, 34, 38]

Glial tumors represent two thirds of all types of CNS tumors, with glioblastomas representing the largest subclass. *Schwannomas* and *meningiomas* represent the largest classification of spinal cord tumors. CNS *lymphomas* are seen among immunosuppressed patients, particularly patients diagnosed with acquired immunodeficiency syndrome (AIDS). Metastatic brain tumors may be present in as many as 20% to 40% of all cancer patients, with the largest representation among patients with lung tumors.

CLINICAL FEATURES

The clinical features manifested by CNS tumors vary according to their size and specific location. The most common symptoms are headache and seizure activity. Headaches are typically bifrontal and bioccipital and occur on awakening; they occur in 50% of all patients. Episodes of nausea and vomiting may also appear with the complaints of headache. Seizure activity is seen in

---

* References 3, 8, 12, 13, 32, 34, 38.

T A B L E   6 – 1
Brain and Spinal Cord Tumors

Neoplasm	Percent of Tumors	Location	Characteristics	Cell of Origin
GLIOMAS				
Astrocytoma	20	Anywhere in brain or spinal cord	Grade I and II Slow growing, invasive	Supportive tissue, astrocytes, glial cells
Glioblastoma multiforme	30	Common in cerebral hemispheres	Grade III, IV Highly invasive and malignant	Thought to arise from mature astrocytes
Oligodendrocytoma	4	Common in frontal lobes deep in white matter; may arise in brain stem, cerebellum, and spinal cord	Avascular, tends to be encapsulated; more malignant form called oligodendroblastoma	Oligodendrites, glial cells
Ependymoma	5	Intramedullary; wall of ventricles; may arise in caudal tail of spinal cord	Common in children, variable growth rates; more malignant, invasive form called ependymoblastoma; may extend into ventricle or invade brain tissue	Ependymal cells
Neurilemoma	4	Cranial nerves (most often vestibular division of cranial nerve VIII)	Slow growing	Schwann cells
Neurofibroma		Extramedullary: spinal cord	Slow growing	Neurilemma, Schwann cells
PITUITARY TUMORS	8	Pituitary gland; may extend to or invade floor of third ventricle	Age linked, several types slow growing, macroadenomas and microadenomas may be secreting or nonsecreting	Pituitary cells, pituitary chromophobes, basophils, eosinophils
PINEAL REGION TUMORS	1	Pineal region; pineal parenchyma, posterior or third ventricle	Several types (e.g., germinoma, pineocytoma, teratoma)	Several types with different cell origin
BLOOD VESSEL TUMORS				
Angioma	3	Predominantly in posterior cerebral hemispheres	Slow growing	Arising from congenitally malformed arteriovenous connections
NEURONAL CELL TUMORS				
Medulloblastoma	1	Posterior cerebellar vermis, roof of fourth ventricle	Well demarcated, rapid growing, fills fourth ventricle	Embryonic cells
MESODERMAL TISSUE TUMORS				
Meningioma	20	Intradural, extramedullary; sylvian fissure region, superior parasagittal surface of frontal and parietal lobes, olfactory groove, wing of sphenoid bone, superior surface of cerebellum, cerebellopontine angle, spinal cord	Slow growing, circumscribed, encapsulated, sharply demarcated from normal tissues, compressive in nature	

Table continued on following page

TABLE 6-1
Brain and Spinal Cord Tumors *Continued*

Neoplasm	Percent of Tumors	Location	Characteristics	Cell of Origin
CHOROID PLEXUS TUMORS				
Papilloma	1	Choroid plexus of ventricular system; lateral ventricle in children, fourth ventricle in adults	Usually benign; slow in expansion, inducing hemorrhage and hydrocephalus; malignant tumor is rare	Epithelial cells
CRANIAL NERVE AND SPINAL NERVE ROOT TUMORS				
Hemangioblastoma	2	Arises from blood vessels, predominant in cerebellum	Benign, slow growing	Embryonic vascular tissue
Lymphoma	1	Cerebral hemispheres	Metastasis common	B cells
METASTATIC TUMORS	35 of all cancer patients	Cerebral cortex diencephalon	Malignant spread	From lung, breast, colon, kidney, thyroid, prostate

From Monahan FD: Medical-surgical nursing: foundations of clinical practice, ed 2, Philadelphia, Saunders, 1998.

20% to 50% of all patients with brain tumors and is most common in parietal and temporal tumors. As tumor bulk increases in size, cerebral edema accumulates and increased intracranial pressure (ICP) and brain tissue hemorrhages may be seen. Displacement of cerebral structures may result in brain herniation, an emergency and frequently lethal complication of increased tumor size and local invasion.[22, 32, 33, 46]

Structural changes, memory defects, and speech, motor, and visual changes are also displayed and vary depending on tumor location and size. Figure 6-2 demonstrates the principal functional subdivisions of the cerebral hemisphere and the functions of specific cortical areas. Figure 6-3 illustrates common sites of intracranial tumors. Tumor-related side effects result from tumor type, location, and approximate size of the tumor at diagnosis.

Spinal cord tumors are also related to the site and size of the lesion. Pain is the most common presenting symptom. Weakness, sensory loss, muscle spasms, and loss of bowel and bladder control occur as the tumor invades local tissue causing nerve destruction.[13, 14, 38, 42, 61, 62]

DIAGNOSTIC AND PATHOLOGIC STAGING

Initial assessment of a suspected CNS tumor should include a physical and neurologic assessment. Pertinent data on emotional and physical changes may need to be obtained from family members because the patient may already be experiencing significant cognitive defects.

TABLE 6-2
Comparison of Kernohan and WHO Classifications

Kernohan Classification	WHO Classification
Grade I and II	Astrocytoma
Grade III	Anaplastic Astrocytoma
Grade IV	Glioblastoma multiforme

Modified from Armstrong T, Gilbert M: Glial neoplasms: classification, treatment, and pathways for the future, Oncol Nurs Forum 23:615-627, 1996.

CLINICAL FEATURES
Central Nervous System Tumors

Very early	Late
Headache	Impaired cognitive skills
Seizures	Personality changes
Nausea	Short-term memory loss
Vomiting	Aphasia
	Sensory/motor defects
	Visual changes
	Loss of sphincter control

TABLE 6–3
TNM Classification of Brain Tumors

PRIMARY TUMOR(T)
TX: primary tumor cannot be assessed
T0: no evidence of primary tumor

SUPRATENTORIAL TUMOR
T1: tumor 5 cm or less in greatest dimension; limited to one side
T2: tumor more than 5 cm in greatest dimension; limited to one side
T3: tumor invades or encroaches on ventricular system
T4: tumor crosses midline, invades opposite hemisphere, or invades infratentorially

INFRATENTORIAL TUMOR
T1: tumor 3 cm or less in greatest dimension; limited to one side
T2: tumor more than 3 cm in greatest dimension; limited to one side
T3: tumor invades or encroaches on the ventricular system
T4: tumor crosses midline, invades opposite hemisphere, or invades supratentorially

REGIONAL LYMPH NODES (N)
This category does not apply to this site.

DISTANT METASTASIS (M)
MX: presence of distant metastasis cannot be assessed
M0: no distant metastasis
M1: distant metastasis

HISTOPATHOLOGIC GRADE (G)
GX: grade cannot be assessed
G1: well differentiated
G2: moderately well differentiated
G3: poorly differentiated
G4: undifferentiated

STAGE GROUPING
Stage IA: G1-T1-M0
Stage IB: G1-T2-M0
            G1-T3-M0
Stage IIA: G2-T1-M0
Stage IIB: G2-T2-M0
            G2-T3-M0
Stage IIIA: G3-T1-M0
Stage IIIB: G3-T2-M0
            G3-T3-M0
Stage IV: G1, G2, G3-T4-M0
            G4-any T-M0
            Any G-any T-M1

Used with the permission of the American Joint Committee on Cancer (AJCC®), Chicago, Illinois. The original source for this material is the AJCC® Manual for Staging of Cancer, 4th edition (1992) published by Lippincott-Raven Publishers, Philadelphia.

Magnetic resonance imaging (MRI) is the most common diagnostic tool used to evaluate suspected malignancies of the CNS due to its ability to perform multiplanar images and ease of instillation of contrast media such as gadolinium, which has minimal allergic or renal complications. A computed tomography (CT) scan may still be used in patients with smaller tumors, spinal cord tumors, and imaging calcification. Several MRI techniques are now available including spin-echo, gradient-echo, fast spin-echo, and three-gradient echo techniques, all of which demonstrate unique specificity for particular tumors and their complications. This variety of MRIs has enhanced the surgical capabilities of surgical biopsy. Newer open models have assisted patients with the claustrophobic episodes that have required sedation techniques.

Limitations exist even with CT scan and MRI despite their improvements. Evaluation of tumor biology and tumoral response to therapeutic treatment require the use of positron emission tomography (PET), single photon emission computed tomography (SPECT), and magnetic resonance spectroscopy (MRS). All techniques assist with the evaluation of late radiation injury, necrosis, and recurrent tumor growth. Figure 6–4 demonstrates the use of SPECT versus MRI to distinguish this occurrence. Additional tests used include angiography, spinal films, and electroencephalography (EEG). Spinal taps are seldom used unless CNS lymphoma is suspected.

Definitive diagnosis may require tumor biopsy or resection using computer-assisted stereotactic tumor removal. The role of functional MRI is to assist with visualization of the tumor during surgery. Functional MRI provides increased contrast to the motor/sensory cortex and language area so damage to these areas is minimized. Figure 6–5 demonstrates the use of diagnostic technique to visualize biopsy and remove tumor using stereotactic technique. Craniotomy may also be used when tumor burden is large and debulking may assist in increased survival.*

Diagnostic examinations can only be tentative unless the tumor size or location is easily identified. Biopsy is the true diagnosis for all stages of CNS tumors. This is accomplished using an open biopsy, such as a craniotomy, or through stereotactic needle biopsy. Additional treatment modalities such as radiation, chemotherapy, or implants may also be accomplished at the time of the tumor removal or debulking. Metastatic tumors are diagnosed based on symptoms and disease progression.

Staging varies with institutions and pathologists. The most common staging is the Kernohan and the WHO

---

* References 5, 8, 12, 17, 19, 22, 33, 38, 45.

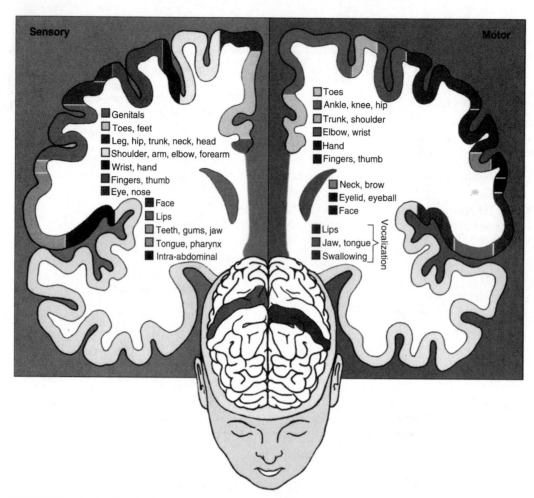

FIGURE 6-2 Cerebral cortex (From Monahan FD: *Medical-surgical nursing: foundations of clinical practice*, ed 2, Philadelphia, Saunders, 1998.)

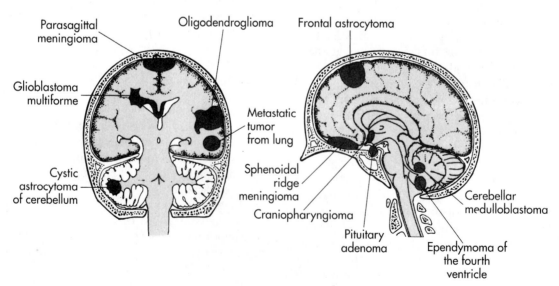

FIGURE 6-3 Common sites of intracranial tumors. (From McCance KL, Huether SE: *Pathophysiology: the biologic basis for disease in adults and children*, ed 3, St Louis, Mosby, 1998.)

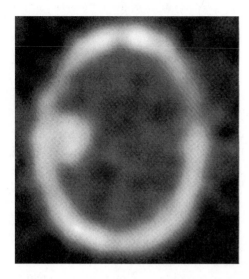

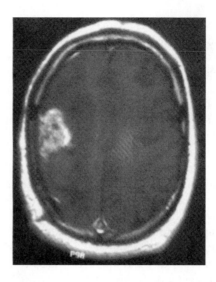

FIGURE 6–4 Thallium 201 SPECT image. (From Berger MS, Wilson CB, editors: *The gliomas,* Philadelphia, Saunders, 1999.)

classification used for astrocytoma classification (Table 6–2). The TNM system has been used but lacks the ability to clearly classify tumor staging because metastases from primary brain tumors are uncommon (Table 6–3).

METASTASIS

The spread of primary CNS tumors beyond the brain and spinal cord is rare. Seeding is the most common method of spread within the CNS and spinal cord. Medulloblastoma tumors have the greatest potential to develop metastatic lesions within the CNS.[24, 46, 61]

TREATMENT MODALITIES

Surgery

In most cases surgery serves as a diagnostic and treatment modality. Surgical intervention provides tissue sampling for histology, decreases the tumor burden for further treatment, and can provide a cure for low-grade tumors. The ability for complete resection varies with size and tumor location. Various types of surgical procedures may be performed depending on the ability to access the tumor and the patient's overall ability to tolerate the surgical procedure without gross neurologic

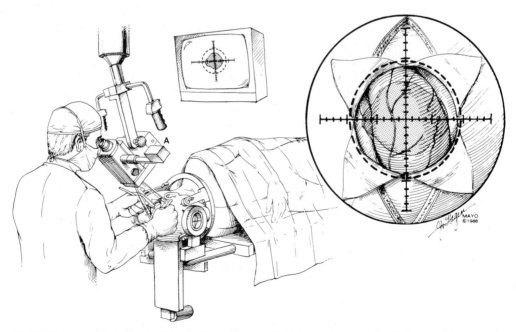

FIGURE 6–5 Stereotactic resection of a superficial tumor (From Kelly PJ: Volumetric stereotactic surgical resection of intra-axial brain mass lesions, *Mayo Clin Proc,* 63:1186–1198, 1988.)

defects. A craniotomy is the most common surgical procedure performed to remove tumor mass or debulk the largest portion of the tumor thus assisting with clinical improvement of symptoms related to tumor pressure or edema. Surgical debulking and placement of wafers impregnated with chemotherapy may also be done at this time or intraoperative radiation may be administered. In almost all cases, resection prolongs the ultimate prognosis except when the tumor is infiltrating or difficult to dissect or the patient is a poor surgical candidate. Additional surgical procedures may include stereotactic biopsy for removal of small tumors.[5, 7]

Pretreatment techniques involve use of steroids such as dexamethasone (Decadron) that are administered to assist with the reduction of cerebral edema, which may cause personality changes, altered level of consciousness, and sensorimotor defects. Anticonvulsant therapy may also be administered for patients with focal changes that result in seizure activity. Steroid and anticonvulsant therapy may be continued after surgery or radiation to minimize potential side effects.[11, 21]

Metastatic tumors may also lend themselves to surgical removal if benign lesions exist or favorable prognosis from the original primary tumor exists.

Radiation Therapy

Tumors that are inoperable or have only partial tumor resection may respond to radiation therapy if the tumor histology is radiosensitive. Tumors that are radiosensitive include medulloblastomas, high-grade astrocytomas, metastatic brain tumors of the breast and lung, and sarcomas.[14, 18, 35, 37]

Radiation treatments may be administered in a variety of doses and methods. Conventional dose therapy is usually given over a series of weeks, allowing normal tissue to heal. Other methods of delivery may be a modified linear accelerator and particle charged beams. Patients are placed under local anesthesia and intravenous sedation is given. The stereotactic frame is anchored to the skull and the treatment is administered. Patients must be monitored for perilesional edema. Other radiation variations include intensity modulator radiation therapy (IMRT), which delivers a controlled intense beam to one target site with increased radiation to multiple sites in the tumor itself.[63]

Particle therapy uses a cyclotron to administer high-energy fast neutron beam to the tumor providing greater tumor kill. This method is also useful in hypoxic areas. Various combinations of proton and neutron radiotherapy delivery and combined interstitial brachytherapy have also been attempted.

Additional treatment options include hyperfactional treatments, which permit two or three treatments delivered daily, thus increasing the overall effect to the tu-

mor. Brachytherapy or interstitial therapy may be used alone or with the use of hyperthermia to deliver radiation to a specific area. Under local anesthesia and using a computer guide, radioactive seeds such as iodine-125 or iridium-1-192 are placed at the tumor site. Seeds will remain in place for several days. Permanent seed placement of ^{125}I and ^{198}Au is also being evaluated. Hyperthermia has also been added to interstitial therapy to moderate the effect by causing further damage to tumor cells.[18, 24, 30, 53]

Radiation may also be given at the time of surgery and includes interstitial implants of radioactive seeds directly to the tumor. Radiation may also be administered via the stereotactic route during surgery. This method allows a single dose of radiation to be administered to one area of the brain.[1, 5]

Other methods of radiation administration include *hyperthermia,* a local treatment done during surgery that uses catheters implanted into the tumor. These catheters administer heat throughout the tumor. Tumor cells are more sensitive to heat, and therefore hyperthermia may enhance radiation therapy to the tumor site.

Radiosurgery

When the tumor mass is small or surgical debulking is not indicated, radiosurgery may be performed by applying a stereotactic frame. A radioactive source such as cobalt 60 is used to deliver radiation to the tumor.

Stereotactic Therapy

Therapy is delivered with the use of a gamma knife, linear accelerator, and heavy beam particles. Heavy beam particles are used because they can be adjusted without causing damage to surrounding tissues. Stereotactic surgery offers alternatives to craniotomy surgery for tumors under 30 mm in size. Complications include nausea and vomiting, radiation necrosis, and intracranial neuropathies. Use of this technique is limited because of the complexity of medical knowledge needed to provide treatment, technical considerations, and added cost for treatment and equipment. As technology develops, the future of stereotactic surgery remains hopeful as an alternative to current therapy.[1, 2, 7] Table 6–4 summarizes various treatment modalities used for treatment of CNS tumors and include radioactive sensitizers, hyperfractionation, heavy particle radiation therapy, and neutron capture therapy.[1, 6, 8, 9, 27]

Photodynamic Therapy

Photodynamic therapy (PDT) is an oxygen-dependent, photochemical oxidative process in which retention of the photosensitizing agents in the tumor tissue results

TABLE 6–4
Types of Radiation Therapy

Type	Definition
Radiosensitizer	Uses radiosensitized drugs to substitute ingredient to repair cells
Hyperfractional radiation therapy	Doses of radiation are given in fractional increments closer together to allow for cell cycle vulnerability
Heavy particle therapy	Charged particles are superior to external rays by decreasing damage and increasing tumor cell kill
Neutron capture therapy	Nonionizing radiation with a drug concentrates in tumor cells; radiation activates tumor cells and kills them
Brachytherapy	Use of radioactive seeds instilled at tumor site
Hyperthermia	Application of heat to tumor site with or without brachytherapy
Stereotactic surgery	Use of head immobilizer with a fixed screw to skull, includes gamma knife modified linear accelerator of charged particles
Standard therapy	Delivered in fractional doses or total dose, usually for metastatic disease
Intensity modulated radiation therapy	Controlled intense beam to target site with increased radiation at different sites in tumor

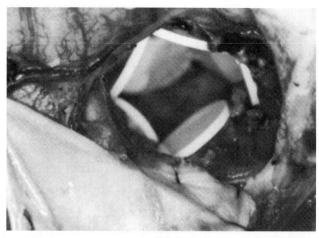

FIGURE 6–6 Intraoperative carmustine-polymer disks (From Berger MS, Wilson CB, editors: *The gliomas,* Philadelphia, Saunders, 1999.)

in entrapment because of the inability to eliminate the chemical. Photofrin is the most commonly used agent. Forty to fifty hours after intravenous administration of the photoactive drug Photofrin, light in the form of a laser is used to activate the drug within the cancer cells to promote cellular destruction.[18, 43]

Chemotherapy

Chemotherapy may be used in combination with surgery and radiation for the treatment of gliomas and medulloblastomas. Response rate remains as low as 20% to 40% because of the blood–brain barrier mechanism.[6] The most frequently used drugs are the nitrosoureas (BCNU, CCNU). Additional agents are the alkylating (cisplatin, cyclophosphamide, nitrogen mustard) and antitumor antibiotics (bleomycin), plant alkaloids (vincristine, etoposide), antimetabolites (methotrexate), and procarbazine. When used with radiation they are termed radiosensitizers and serve to enhance radiation response and tumor kill.

Common routes of administration include oral and intravenous. Additional methods include intra-arterial into the carotid or vertebral artery. Intra-arterial car-

mustine, cisplatin, and methotrexate have been used for chemotherapy administration after an infusion of mannitol, which shrinks the blood–brain barrier. Another new method is the use of the Gliadel wafer to deliver carmustine directly into the resected cavity. Medication will slowly be dispensed over a 3-week period. Figure 6–6 demonstrates wafer insertion. Another new medication released by the Food and Drug Administration is Temodar (temozolomide), which is in a new class named idazotetazines to treat refractory anoplastic astrocytomas.* Table 6–4 summarizes types of radiation therapy. Box 6–1 indicates area of ongoing investigations.

Metastatic Brain Tumors

Brain metastases represent a continued concern because of the frequency of a majority of cancer metastases occurring to the brain from the "end-artery" pattern, where 20% of the blood flow from the heart allows trapped cancer cells to multiply and form metastatic deposits. Thirty percent of all brain tumors are the result of metastatic disease. Common sites of metastasis include lung, breast, melanomas, colon, and kidney. Treatment is based on location, size, and prognostic factors. The standard treatment remains radiation and steroid therapy. Surgery is indicated only if there is a single lesion and the patient has a high performance status. Prognosis for survival is 3 to 6 months from time of metastatic diagnosis. Table 6–5 lists the clinical features of patients with brain tumors.

---

* References 9, 16, 19, 23, 26, 27, 44, 50, 57, 59.

B O X   6 - 1

Areas of Investigation

Intracavity immunotherapy
Lak cells
Peripheral blood lymphocytes
Lymphokine-activated killer cells
Tumor infiltration lymphocytes
Cytokines
Interleukin 2
Interferon
Monoclonal antibodies
Boron neutron capture therapy (BNET)
Polymines
Radiosentizers using BUdR and IUdR
High-dose BCNU with autologus bone marrow
   rescue
Intramural administration with surgery intervention
Antigenetic drugs with thalidomide and TNP-470
Gene therapy with TK gene and administration of
   Cytovene

SPINAL CORD TUMORS

Primary spinal cord tumors represent a rare primary malignancy and only 2% of all cancers. Secondary tumors from metastatic disease are documented as high as 40%. Spinal tumors are classified by cell type and origin. Tumors may grow in or around the spinal column, with neurilemomas, meningiomas, and sarcomas representing the major histologic types. Presentation

---

T A B L E   6 - 5
Characteristics of Patients with Brain Tumors

Clinical Features	Nursing Management
Headache	Note time, duration, and location of headache; medicate per orders.
Weakness	Monitor for increased intracranial pressure (wide pulse pressure, irregular respirations, bradycardia); elevate head of bed.
Seizure activity	Institute seizure precautions (note time, duration, and site of seizure).
Blurred vision	Monitor for altered level of consciousness; orient; perform cranial checks.
Gait disturbance	Institute safety precautions with ambulation; assist with activities of daily living.
Altered sensorium	Explain tests, procedures, and treatment modalities.
Personality changes	Offer support to patient/caregiver if terminal prognosis.

of tumor is highest in the thoracic and cervical areas. Metastasis is likely to occur from primary sites of breast, lung, thyroid, kidney, and prostate and multiple myeloma.

The patient's chief complaints are back pain, weakness, and sensorimotor alterations as well as bowel and bladder dysfunction. The diagnosis is made using enhanced MRI, myelography, and CT. Treatment modalities include steroid therapy, partial or complete resection of the tumor followed by radiation therapy, and hormonal therapy for patients with breast and prostate cancer.

Nursing management is similar to the preoperative and postoperative care of the patient experiencing a brain tumor, with a focus on early detection and management of complications. Rehabilitation is indicated in individuals with residual neurologic deficits.[19, 22, 23, 41]

DISEASE-RELATED COMPLICATIONS

Major disease-related complications include increased ICP from cerebral edema and displaced brain structures resulting in brain herniation. A major complication of spinal cord tumors is spinal cord compression.

Elevated ICP is caused by an increase in intracellular volume from the expanding tumor mass and edema. Clinical features of increased ICP and brain steam herniation are listed in the Clinical Features box. Cerebral edema results in tissue hypoxia and acidosis. If left to progress, brain stem compression occurs and herniation of the brain results. Ultimately, respiratory arrest will follow. Management includes surgical removal and supportive therapy with diuretics and corticosteriods. Close nursing observation is required to monitor a potentially fatal outcome.

TREATMENT-RELATED COMPLICATIONS

Radiation Therapy

Radiation treatment-related side effects are based on the dose and location of treatment. Local and long-term

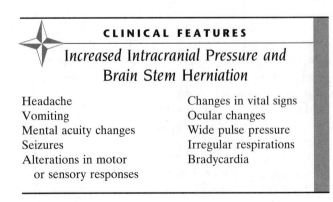

CLINICAL FEATURES

Increased Intracranial Pressure and Brain Stem Herniation

Headache	Changes in vital signs
Vomiting	Ocular changes
Mental acuity changes	Wide pulse pressure
Seizures	Irregular respirations
Alterations in motor	Bradycardia
or sensory responses	

BOX 6-2

Radiation Therapy Side Effects

EARLY

Hair loss
Skin changes (redness, darkness, itching)
Nausea
Inflammation around the ear
Edema (increased intracranial pressure)
Anorexia
Lethargy
Fatigue
Radiation somulence syndrome 4–6 weeks after radiation

LONG TERM

Decreased intellect
Altered motor and sensory functions
Pituitary dysfunction
Radiation Necrosis

SPINAL CORD

Radiation myelopathy

TABLE 6-6
Chemotherapy Drugs and Related Side Effects

Drug	Side Effects
BCNU	Bone marrow suppression
CCNU	Nausea, alopecia, pulmonary fibrosis
Cisplatin	Ototoxicity, renal dysfunction, bone marrow depression, anorexia, nausea/vomiting
Cyclophosphamide	Nausea/vomiting, diarrhea, alopecia, bone marrow suppression
Nitrogen mustard	Nausea/vomiting, anorexia, alopecia, diarrhea, bone marrow suppression, hepatic/neurologic dysfunction
Bleomycin	Nausea/vomiting, stomatitis, hepatic/neurologic dysfunction, pulmonary fibrosis
Vincristine	Nausea/vomiting, anorexia, alopecia, neurologic dysfunction
Etoposide	Nausea/vomiting, anorexia, hypotension, bone marrow suppression
Methotrexate	Bone marrow suppression, renal tubular necrosis, stomatitis, diarrhea, hepatic dysfunction
Procarbazine	Nausea/vomiting, diarrhea, alopecia, myelosuppression, hepatic and neurologic dysfunction
Temodar	Mild nausea, fatigue, no hair loss

---

side effects can be experienced (Box 6–2). Most side effects are temporary and related to local irritation or disruption of myelin formation. Radiation doses are cumulative, and re-treatment in the same manner is not recommended.[14, 21, 33]

Chemotherapy

Major side effects related to chemotherapy are based on the combination of drugs and their specific dose. Major areas that are affected include the bone marrow, hair follicles, and gastrointestinal tract. Table 6–6 lists major side effects of common drugs used in CNS tumors.[6, 18]

Biotherapy

Side effects of biotherapy are related to dose and combined modality (Box 6–3).

Surgery

Size and location of tumor and the overall preoperative state of the patient enhance the potential for complications.

Radiosurgery

Side effects include perilesional edema, radiation necrosis, and pain at fixation of screw device.

BOX 6-3

Biotherapy Side Effects

Flulike symptoms (headache, fever, chills, arthralgia, myalgia)
Nausea/vomiting (varies with individual and amount of dose)
Weight loss (amount depends on amount of side effects)
Altered neurologic functioning (decreased short-term memory concentration and attention)
Alopecia (partial)
Skin changes (erythema, rash, pruritus)
Fluid and electrolyte imbalances (hypocalcemia, hypomagnesemia)
Bone marrow suppression (pancytopenia)

COMPLICATIONS

CNS Tumor Surgery

Intracranial bleeding	Neuromotor deficits
Cerebral edema	Thrombosis
Infection	Hydrocephalus

Steroid Therapy

Use of steroids preoperatively and postoperatively can also lead to a variety of treatment side effects that can produce local and systemic effects. Steriods are administered to produce an anti-inflammatory response and reduce cerebral swelling. Steroid therapy may begin after an initial dose of mannitol, which may be used before, during, or after surgery to reduce immediate cerebral edema. Postoperative management with titration is performed with steroids such as dexamethasone. Box 6–4 lists the side effects of steroid therapy.

POSTOPERATIVE CARE

Surgery

Surgery for CNS tumors may be done by standard craniotomy or use of laser surgery. Use of laser surgery is limited but it has two main advantages:

1. It decreases the amount of dissection to surrounding tissue.
2. It has the ability to reach tumors that were formerly inaccessible.

Spinal tumors can also be removed by laser surgery or standard decompression laminectomy. Surgery is always indicated to assist with histologic typing and debulking of tumor mass. Inoperable tumors may respond by the relief of general symptoms of compression and intracranial pressure.

BOX 6–4

Steroid Therapy Side Effects

Hyperglycemia
Irritability
Insomnia
Psychotic reactions, mood swings
Hypokalemia
Hypernatremia
Depressed immune response
Elevated lipid and cholesterol levels
Fluid retention
Cataract formation
Osteoporosis
Thrombophlebitis
Steroid-induced gastric ulcers
Relocation of fat deposits (round face and thick trunk)
Cutaneous striae
Withdrawal symptoms (doses must be reduced from intravenous to oral and then in amount and frequency)

PATIENT TEACHING PRIORITIES

Radiation Therapy

Knowledge of treatment schedule
Knowledge of skin care routine
   Marks are not to be washed off
   No creams or lotions to treatment site
Knowledge of radiation complications

Radiation Therapy

If the tumor excision has been incomplete and the histologic report reveals a radiosensitive tumor, a patient may receive radiation therapy treatments after postoperative healing has occurred. The patient and family will need information on the length of treatment and expected side effects.

Spinal cord tumors are also treated with radiation, although the dose and treatment time may vary. The most serious consequence of spinal cord radiation is radiation myelopathy, which results in paraplegia and loss of bowel and bladder control. This is usually a late occurrence (6–15 months after therapy). Family and patients need to be instructed to notify their physician if any symptoms occur. Symptoms of therapy complications may also manifest tumor recurrence. Constant anxiety exists even for those patients with better prognostic factors. Assessment of the emotional stability of the family and patient is ongoing and a critical nursing factor.

Chemotherapy and Biotherapy

Nursing management of patients receiving chemotherapy and biotherapy treatments includes providing knowledge about drugs and their expected side effects. Monitoring side effects and appropriate treatment can ensure patient comfort and safety.

GERIATRIC CONSIDERATIONS

The normal age-related changes in the geriatric population may lead to a delay or misdiagnosis of CNS tumors.

PATIENT TEACHING PRIORITIES

Chemotherapy and Biotherapy

Knowledge of drug administration route and schedule
Knowledge of side effects and supportive measures:
   Weight changes and loss of appetite
   Nausea
   Bruising and bleeding episodes
   Temperature changes
   Oral hygiene routine

Altered ambulation patterns, sensory impairment, decreased visual and hearing acuity, and changes in cognition are similar to CNS tumor changes. Once diagnosed, these normal physiologic changes will also interfere with adequate postoperative assessment and the speed of recovery. Response to extensive surgery and treatment modalities may also produce increased side effects in elderly persons. Rehabilitation needs and expanded home care referrals are required to assist the expansion needs of the geriatric population. These specific concerns are listed in the Geriatric Considerations box.[31, 35, 36]

PROGNOSIS

The ultimate prognosis of CNS tumors is determined by the following factors: histologic type, tumor grade, size and extent of tumor, patient's age, performance status, and residual tumor.[11] Survival rates range from complete cure to rapid deterioration and death. Glioblastoma multiforme (grade IV) has the poorest prognosis and a life expectancy of 9 to 12 months. Younger individuals who are neurologically intact survive longer than the geriatric patient.

Metastatic lesions present a different prognosis and vary depending on whether the tumor is a single lesion or disseminated, size and cell type of primary tumor,

---

GERIATRIC CONSIDERATIONS

CNS *Tumors*

Diagnostic difficulties
Increased assessment (preoperatively and postoperatively)
Treatment modality complications
Rehabilitation
Home care referral

---

other metastatic lesions, patient age, performance status, and the time from the treatment of the primary lesions until the start of the metastasis.[8, 10, 11, 19]

A summary of the clinical features of patients with brain tumor is given in Table 6–5.

CONCLUSION

Despite the low incidence of CNS tumors, they continue to produce rapid deterioration, debilitation, and higher mortality than most primary cancers. Metastatic CNS tumors represent a continued challenge to the medical community. New clinical trials involving combination therapies and surgical modalities are under investigation in the hopes of providing relief of symptoms and increased survival rates.

Nursing Management

The diagnosis of cancer produces high levels of anxiety and fear in most patients and families; of particular concern are those patients diagnosed with CNS tumors. Emotional distress is brought on by the rapid onset of debilitation, physical and emotional changes, and the ultimate poor prognostic factors. Preparation time from the onset of symptoms to diagnosis and surgery is limited and often allows little time for emotional support and education. Most information on the treatment course will be provided after surgery and is based on tumor size, type, and location and ability to remove tumor mass.

Lack of past experience with hospitalization and surgery further increases the anxiety and fear patterns. Paralysis, coma, neurologic defects, and altered body image from surgery and steroid therapy may all be a postoperative reality. For patients with metastatic disease who have already undergone treatment, the knowledge of cancer recurrences can be devastating.

Nursing Diagnoses

- *Fear and anxiety related to diagnosis and postoperative outcomes*

- *Knowledge deficit related to limited experience with diagnostic preoperative and postoperative routines*

Outcome Goals

Patient will be able to:

- Verbalize expression of concerns (fears and anxiety) related to diagnoses and postoperative outcomes.
- State knowledge of preoperative and postoperative routines.

Interventions

Interventions are based on providing emotional support through information and teaching on expected outcomes. Assessment of past coping mechanisms and support systems within the family structure are needed. Education should be based on teaching learning principles and include visual information. A basic review of the anatomy and physiology of the CNS system will assist in the understanding of tumor locations and causes of present symptoms. Discussion should include an explanation of tests and procedures, their diagnostic indications, postoperative routines, monitoring devices, potential postoperative complications, and expected body image alterations including preoperative site preparation. Patients with altered cognition from extensive CNS involvement may not be able to participate. These families will need additional support systems of family, clergy, or other hospital supports that may be available. The inclusion of a clinical nurse specialist in neurology is helpful and can provide additional information on postoperative concerns. The box on the right summarizes patient/family education needs related to surgery.

PATIENT TEACHING PRIORITIES

CNS Tumor Surgery

Explanation of surgical diagnostic procedures
Basic review of anatomy and physiology of
    CNS system
    Tumor location
    Expected signs/symptoms
    Preoperative procedures
Postoperative monitoring
    Equipment
Postoperative nursing care routines
Postoperative complications
Body image concerns

Nursing Management

The postoperative course requires complex monitoring for complications. Further treatment is based on operative results, tumor histology, and patient complications. Families continue to need intense emotional support during the postoperative course. For those patients with inoperable tumors, a referral for home care or hospice is appropriate.

Nursing Diagnoses

- *Self-care deficit related to postoperative procedure*
- *Body image disturbance related to altered physical status*
- *Sensory/perceptual alterations related to neurologic deficits*
- *Injury, risk for, related to altered cognition and side effect of medications*
- *Pain related to surgical procedure*
- *Coping, ineffective family: compromised, and coping, ineffective individual, related to prognostic factors*

Outcome Goals

Patient will be able to:

- Demonstrate ability to increase self-care deficits.
- Express concerns related to altered body image.
- Maintain sensory and perceptual abilities during postoperative period.
- Demonstrate effective coping skills during postoperative period.

Interventions

Postoperative care of the patient with a craniotomy includes frequent neurologic examinations, measurement of vital signs, supportive nursing care of positioning, and administration of medications, including pain, steroids, and anticonvulsant therapy. Observation of increased ICP and brain herniation is a critical factor in the postoperative course. Patients with infratentorial versus supratentorial incisions will require increased observation for complications and have a longer postoperative course. Common postoperative complications are included in the Complications box.

Neurologic examinations should include measurement of the level of consciousness, orientation, emotional response to surgery, and motor and sensory perception, particularly swallowing ability from damage to the vagus and glossopharyngeal nerves. Pupils are observed for inequality. Vital signs should be observed for decreased respirations and pulse and widened pulse pressure. The patient should be placed in a quiet, nonstimulating environment and positioned according to physician protocol. The most common position is with the head of the bed at a 30-degree angle to reduce cerebral edema and stress on the suture line. Dressings and drains are monitored for the type and amount of drainage. Coughing, deep-breathing techniques, and suctioning are done in a nonaggressive manner to reduce increased ICP.

The patient will experience a self-care deficit for several days and require skin and mouth care as well as maintenance of bowel and urinary function. Assessment of the patient's comfort level is done during administration of care. Restlessness and moaning or increased head movement may indicate pain. Positioning, maintenance of a quiet environment, and low doses of mild pain medication are provided. Safety measures for those patients with potential seizure activity may include seizure pads and the administration of anticonvulsant therapy.

Management of increased ICP is through administration of mannitol and corticosteroids such as dexamethasone.[21, 31, 34] Long-term use of steroids to reduce edema can cause serious side effects (see Box 6–4) and therefore requires a titration schedule to reduce the amount and frequency of the drug.

After the immediate postoperative care the patient and family need further evaluation and continued support. Postoperative changes such as hair loss, edema, and generalized weight loss can cause extreme depression because of altered body image. Patients left with residual neurologic deficits may require nutritional supplements, tube feedings, or hyperalimentation depending on the ultimate prognosis. Rehabilitation and supportive equipment may also assist in caring for the patient at home.

Patients with primary spinal cord tumors experience a similar but less aggressive postoperative course. Nursing observations include observation of neurologic function and level of motor and sensory function. Bowel and bladder control may be altered depending on the location of the tumor. Paralysis or motor deficits require additional rehabilitative consults. Prognostic factors and the amount of deficit will determine the amount of aggressive rehabilitative therapy. Support and follow-up are needed to assist patients and families during this critical period.

Metastatic spinal cord tumors represent a potential oncology emergency that requires immediate medical intervention. Early signs include neck and back pain, motor weakness, and loss of sensation. Treatment includes radiation therapy followed by surgery if the tumor does not respond to radiation and use of steroids.

Nursing Management

Nursing Diagnoses

- *Knowledge deficit related to lack of experience with chemotherapy routine and side effects*
- *Nutrition, altered: less than body requirements related to chemotherapy-induced nausea*
- *Oral mucous membrane, altered, related to chemotherapy administration*
- *Infection, risk for, related to altered immune status*
- *Self-esteem disturbance related to chemotherapy-induced side effects*

Outcome Goals

Patient will be able to:

- Express knowledge of chemotherapy routine and side effects.
- Maintain nutritional status and maintain body weight within 10% of prechemotherapy state.
- Maintain oral mucous membranes through chemotherapy regimen.
- Demonstrate no evidence of signs or symptoms of infection throughout chemotherapy regimen.

Interventions

Knowledge of the limited use and experimental nature of chemotherapy, experimental issues, and other modalities is important for patients and family. Because of the blood–brain barrier, a limited number of drugs are considered effective therapy for CNS tumors. Patients need to understand drug treatment schedules, follow-up blood work, and expected side effects.[34]

Nursing interventions include assessment of the patient's nutritional status, administration or antiemetics, small frequent bland feedings, monitoring intake and output, weight checks, and providing nutritional consultations.

Blood counts assist with monitoring the hematologic and immune status alterations produced by chemotherapy treatments. Limiting visitors with colds, vigilant handwashing, monitoring changes in temperature, and observation of signs and symptoms of infection all are critical for those patients with lowered leukocyte counts. Reduction of hemoglobin and platelets may produce cellular damage. Patients should be observed for shortness of breath, weakness, fatigue, bruises, petechiae, and signs of active bleeding. Applying pressure to injection sites and limited use of rectal medications are also methods of controlling increased trauma and induction of bleeding.

Oral hygiene is essential to reduce risk of infection and to promote cleanliness and comfort. Oral assessment for evidence of yeast infections or lesions should be done daily. Specific mouth care protocols should follow physician's routine.

The administration of steroids is a common occurrence for many chemotherapy protocols, particularly CNS tumors. Common side effects from steroidal therapy can be found in Box 6–4. The nurse monitors the patient's response to steroid therapy by continued observation of vital signs, blood sugars, changes in emotional state, and potential gastrointestinal bleeding. Administration of antacids or gastric antagonists assists with potential gastric complications. Body image changes from steroidal therapy, hair loss, or residual neurologic deficits may cause increased depression and withdrawal. Supportive care is required for both patients and family.

Patients receiving experimental treatments who experience increased symptoms may require removal from treatment because of an effort to keep data collection complete. Patients and families may experience anger and frustration over removal from the last hope of treatment.

Nursing Management

Nursing Diagnoses

- *Knowledge deficit related to lack of experience with radiation routine and side effects*
- *Skin integrity, impaired, related to radiation treatment modality*
- *Self-esteem disturbance related to change in physical appearance/therapy markings, skin changes, and hair loss*
- *Sensory/perceptual alterations related to postradiation damage and cerebral edema*
- *Fatigue related radiation treatments and concurrent therapies*

Outcome Goals

Patient will be able to:

- Verbalize knowledge of radiation routine and side effects.
- Maintain skin integrity.
- Verbalize alterations in self-esteem related to body image change.

- Identify neurologic changes and report symptoms
- Verbalize methods to minimize fatigue

Interventions

Patients and family should be informed of the number of treatments that will be required. Normal treatments are daily for 4 to 8 weeks. Transportation arrangements may be indicated if mobility limitations are present. A brief introduction to the radiation department and an explanation of the use of radiation therapy helps to eliminate additional anxieties.

Included in teaching of side effects is knowledge of skin markings, hair loss, and skin changes near the radiation site. Instructions on skin care include not washing marks off and no application of creams near treatment sites. If treatments are given near the ear or in a visual field, hearing and vision may become impaired. Radiation treatments may also cause an increase in ICP and may require additional steroid therapy. Reporting signs and symptoms of headache or changes in personality is an important consideration. Emotional support is needed to deal with additional self-esteem concerns.

Chapter Questions

1. All of the following are possible chemotherapy drugs used to treat CNS tumors except:
   a. Adriamycin
   b. BCNU
   c. Cisplatin
   d. Temodar
2. Complications of steroid therapy include all except:
   a. Relocation of fat deposits
   b. Fluid retention
   c. Hyperkalemia
   d. Hyperglycemia
3. Possible causes of CNS tumors include all except:
   a. Li-Fraumen syndrome (LFS)
   b. Chemical exposures to petrochemicals

   c. Epstein-Barr virus
   d. Head injuries
4. Common diagnostic assessments used to diagnose CNS tumors include all except:
   a. Computed tomography
   b. Lumbar puncture
   c. Positron emission tomography
   d. Single photon emission computed tomography
5. The most common clinical feature of a CNS tumor is:
   a. Personality change
   b. Sensory and motor defects
   c. Headache
   d. Seizures
6. Signs of increased ICP include all except:
   a. Headache
   b. Nausea and vomiting

c. Narrow pulse pressure

d. Irregular respiration

7. The treatment of choice for CNS tumors is:

a. Dexamethasone therapy

b. Surgery

c. Radiation therapy

d. Chemotherapy

8. Lowered drug response in CNS tumor management is a result of:

a. Late diagnosis

b. Existence of multiple metastatic lesions

c. Poor patient tolerance for chemotherapy-related side effects

d. Blood–brain barrier mechanism

9. Mr. Smith was diagnosed with prostate cancer 1 year ago and now complains of numbness in both legs. A likely cause would be:

a. Hypocalcemia

b. Spinal metastasis

c. Phlebitis

d. Postradiation complications

10. A possible side effect of radiation is:

a. Radiation myelopathy

b. Pain

c. Hypersensitivity reaction

d. Personality change

BIBLIOGRAPHY

1. American Cancer Society: *Cancer facts and figures—2000,* Atlanta, The Society, 2000.
2. Armstrong T: *Clinical trials for brain tumors—a fact sheet,* San Francisco, National Brain Tumor Association.
3. Armstrong T, Gilbert T: Glial neoplasms: classifications, treatment, and pathways to the future, *Oncol Nurs Forum* 23:615, 1996.
4. Bale A, Li F: Principles of cancer management—cancer genetics. In DeVita V, Hellman S, Rosenburg S, editors: *Cancer principles and practice of oncology,* ed 5, Philadelphia, Lippincott-Raven, 1997.
5. Baker I, Gutin P: Surgical approaches to gliomas. In Berger M, Wilson C, editors: *The gliomas,* Philadelphia, Saunders, 1999.
6. Beahrs OH, Henson DE, Huttler RV, Kennedy BJ: *American Joint Commission on Cancer—manual for staging of cancer,* ed 4, Philadelphia, Lippincott-Raven, 1998.
7. Berger D, Roslyn J: Cancer surgery in the elderly, *Clin Geriatr Med* 13:119, 1997.
8. Berger M, Wilson C, editors: *The gliomas,* Philadelphia, Saunders, 1999.
9. Berkery R, Cleri L, Skarin A: *Oncology pocket guide to chemotherapy,* ed 3, St Louis, Mosby, 1997.
10. Bieford K: Central nervous system cancers. In Groenwalds S, Groenwald SL, Frogge MH, Goodman M, Yorbo CH, editors: *Cancer nursing: principles and practice,* ed 4, Boston, Jones and Bartlett, 1997.
11. Bohen M: Nursing care of the client with cancer of the neurology system. In Itano J, Taoka K, editors: *Core curriculum for oncology nursing,* ed 3, Philadelphia, Saunders, 1998.
12. Bronstein K: Epidemiology and classification of brain tumors. *Crit Care Nurs Clin North Am* 7:79, 1995.
13. *Brain tumor: a guide.* San Francisco, National Brain Tumor Foundation, 1999.
14. Buchholtz J: Central nervous system tumors. In Dow KH, Bucholtz JD, Iwamoto I, Fieler V, Hilderley L, editors: *Nursing care in radiation oncology,* ed 2, Philadelphia, Saunders, 1997.
15. Clinton S, Giovannucci E: Chemoprevention, nutrition in the etiology and prevention of cancer. In Holland J and others, editors: *Cancer medicine,* Baltimore, Williams & Wilkins, 1997.
16. Cokger I, Friedman H, Friedman A: Chemotherapy with malignant glioma, *Cancer Invest* 17:264, 1999.
17. Copstead L, Banaski J: *Pathophysiology biological and behaviorial perspectives,* ed 2, Philadelphia, Saunders, 2000.
18. Daley N: New strategies in radiation therapy, *New Therapies Symposia Highlights* 4:4, 1999.
19. DeVita V: Principles of cancer management: chemotherapy. In DeVita V, Hellman S, Rosenburg S, editors: *Cancer principles and practice,* ed 5, Philadelphia, Lippincott-Raven, 1997.
20. Devroom H: *Gene therapy: a new experimental treatment for brain tumors,* San Francisco, National Brain Tumor Foundation, 1999.
21. Doenges M, Moorehouse M, Geissler A: *Nursing care plans,* ed 4, Philadelphia, Davis, 1997.
22. Doilinger M and others: Brain tumors. In *Everyone's guide to cancer therapy,* ed 3, Kansas City, Andrews McMeel, 1997.
23. Dropcho E: Intra-arterial chemotherapy for malignant gliomas. In Berger M, Wilson C, editors: *The gliomas,* Philadelphia, Saunders, 1999.
24. Dunne-Daley C: Principles of radiation therapy. In Dow KH, Bucholtz JD, Iwamoto D, Fieler V, Hilderley L, editors: *Nursing care in radiation oncology,* ed 2, Philadelphia, Saunders, 1997.
25. Dunkel I, Finlay J: High-dose chemotherapy followed by autologous bone marrow rescue for high-grade gliomas. In Berger M, Wilson C, editors: *The gliomas,* Philadelphia, Saunders, 1999.
26. Englehard H, Groothuis D: The blood-brain barrier: structure, function and response to neoplasia. In Berger M, Wilson C, editors: *The gliomas,* Philadelphia, Saunders, 1999.
27. Eriken S, Hall W: Chemotherapy delivered blood-brain barrier disruption offers new option for treating malignant brain tumors, *Cope* 11:38, 1996.
28. Exterman M: Assessment of the Older Cancer Patient Proceedings from the 35th American Geriatric Society meeting, p 353, Washington, DC, 1999.
29. Fernandez P, Brems S: Malignant brain tumors in the elderly, *Clin Geriatr Med* 13:327, 1997.
30. Fontanesi J, Clark WC, Weir A, Barry A, Kumar P, Miller A, Eddy T, Tai D, Kum LE: Interstital iodine-125 and concomitant cisplatin followed by hyperfractionated external beam irradiation for malignant supratentorial gliomas, *Am J Clin Oncol* 16:412, 1993.

31. Grimaldi PL: Can Medicare beneficiaries pay outpatient drug bills? *J Nurs Management* 30(1):11, 2000.

32. Heideman R and others: Tumors of the central nervous system. In Pizzo P, Poplack D, editors: *Principles and practice of pediatric oncology,* ed 4, Philadelphia, Lippincott-Raven, 1997.

33. Hickey J: *The clinical practice of neurological and neurosurgical nursing,* ed 4, Philadelphia, Lippincott Williams & Wilkins, 1999.

34. Key J, Armstrong T: Brain tumors. In Hickey J, editor: *The clinical practice of neurological and neurosurgical nursing,* ed 4th, Philadelphia, Lippincott Williams & Wilkins, 1999.

35. Lamb M: Alterations in sexuality and sexual functioning, In McCorkle R, Grant M, Baird SB, editors: *Cancer nursing: a comprehensive textbook,* ed 2, Philadelphia, Saunders, 1997.

36. Lamb S: Radiation therapy options for management of the brain tumor patient. *Crit Care Nurs Clin North Am* 7:103, 1995.

37. Larson D, Shrieve D, Gutin P: Radiosurgery. In Berger M, Wilson C, editors: *The gliomas,* Philadelphia, Saunders, 1999.

38. Levin V, Leibel S, Gutin P: Neoplasms of the central nervous systems. In DeVita V, Hellman S, Rosenburg S, editors: *Cancer: principles and practice of oncology,* ed 5, Philadelphia, Lippincott-Raven, 1997.

39. Martin-Preston S: Epidemiology. In Berger M, Wilson C, editors: *The gliomas,* Philadelphia, Saunders, 1999.

40. Meeker M, Rothrock J: *Alexanders care of the patient in surgery,* St Louis, Mosby, 1999.

41. Monahan DF: *Medical-surgical nursing: foundations for clinical practice,* ed 2, Philadelphia, Saunders, 1998.

42. National Brain Foundation: Understanding brain tumors glioblastoma multiforme, 1999.

43. Nguyen A: Photodynamic therapy with porfimer sodium (Photofrin), *Highlights in Oncology Practice* 15:21, 1997.

44. Page M: *New chemotherapy drugs for brain tumor patients—a fact sheet,* San Francisco, National Brain Tumor Foundation, 1999.

45. Pardos M, Berger M, Wilson C: Primary central nervous system tumors: advances in knowledge and treatments, *CA Cancer J Clin* 48:331, 1998.

46. PDQ Data Base: *Adult brain tumor,* Bethesda, MD, National Cancer Institute, 2000.

47. Pizzo P, Poplack S, editors: *Principles and practice of pediatric oncology,* Philadelphia, Lippincott-Raven, 1997.

48. Poindexter B, Armstrong T: Caring for the patient with malignant brain tumors, *Am J Nurs Suppl* May 9–17, 1997.

49. Preston-Martin S, Navidi W, Thomas D, Lee PJ, Bowman J, Pogoda J: Epidemiology of primary CNS neoplasm, *Neurol Clin* 14:1, 1996.

50. Reuters Medical News: *FDA approves temozolomide for refractory anaplastic strocytoma,* pp 1–2, 1999.

51. Riese N, Noll L: Chemical modifers of radiation therapy. In Dow K and others, editors: *Nursing care in radiation oncology,* ed 2, Philadelphia, Saunders, 1997.

52. Rosenburg S: Principles of cancer management: biologic therapy. In DeVita V, Hellman S, Rosenburg S, editors: *Cancer principles and practice of oncology,* ed 5, Philadelphia, Lippincott-Raven, 1997.

53. Scharfren C and others: High activity iodine-125 interstitial implant for glioma, *Int J Radiat Oncol Biol Physics* 24:538, 1992.

54. Sitton E: Managing side effects of skin changes and fatigue. In Dow KH, Bucholtz JD, Iwamoto I, Fieler V, Hilderley L, editors: *Nursing care in radiation oncology,* ed 2, Philadelphia, Saunders, 1997.

55. Sneed P, Gutin P: Interstitial radiation and hyphertheria. In Berger M, Wilson C, editors: *The gliomas,* Philadelphia, Saunders, 1999.

56. Stelzen K, Laramore G: Particle beam therapy. In Berger M, Wilson C, editors: *The gliomas,* Philadelphia, Saunders, 1999.

57. Stewart D: Hyperosmolar disruption of the blood-brain barrier as a chemotherapy potentation in the treatment of brain tumors. In Berger M, Wilson C, editors: *The gliomas,* Philadelphia, Saunders, 1999.

58. Surawicz T and others: Brain tumor survival; results from the National Cancer Data Base. *J Neuro-Oncol* 40:151, 1998.

59. Thompson R, Brem H: Treatment of gliomas using polymer-drug delivery. In Berger M, Wilson C, editors: *The gliomas,* Philadelphia, Saunders, 1999.

60. Welsh D: Hyperthermia treatment of malignant brain tumors. *Crit Care Nurs Clin North Am* 7:115, 1995.

61. Wilson C, Prados M: Neoplasms of the central nervous system. In Holland JF, Bast RC, Morton DL, editors: *Cancer medicine: principles of radiation therapy oncology,* Baltimore, Williams & Wilkins, 1997.

62. Wrensh M: *Who gets brain tumors and why.* San Francisco, National Brain Tumor Foundation Fact Sheet, pp 1–3, 1999.

63. Young R: The role of the gamma knife in the treatment of malignant primary and metastatic brain tumors, *CA Cancer J Clin* 48:3, 1998.

Breast Cancers

Rebecca Crane-Okada

Breast cancer is the third most frequent cancer in the world, the most common cancer and the leading cause of cancer deaths in women throughout the world, and a major public health concern.[294] The incidence of breast cancer is increasing throughout the world for reasons not fully understood. Although higher age-specific incidence rates for female breast cancer occur in developed countries, nearly half of the cases of breast cancer diagnosed in the next year will be in developing countries.[127]

In the United States, public awareness of breast cancer has grown considerably in recent years. Women in the public eye have spoken out about their experiences with breast cancer; media coverage has expanded to include breast health as well as breast cancer care information; legislative efforts have made screening mammography more available under insurance coverage; and grass-roots movements have placed women's health care issues into the forefront in the competition for research dollars.[346]

It has been only in the past 30 years that the Halsted radical mastectomy has been replaced with more conservative surgery.[384] The "one-step" procedure (biopsy with frozen-section diagnosis and immediate surgery) has been replaced with the two-step procedure. Women are expected to be involved in their treatment planning. The knowledge that breast cancer needed to be considered a systemic disease at the time of diagnosis led to increasing justification for the use of chemotherapy and hormonal manipulation as adjuncts to surgery to improve survival. Several questions regarding such adjuvant therapy continue to be addressed in ongoing national clinical trials:

1. Which women with negative nodes and smaller tumors should receive systemic treatment?
2. What is the optimal timing for initiation of treatment?
3. What is the optimal combination of drugs, the dose size, and intensity to be used?
4. What is the optimal duration of treatment?

Randomized clinical trials continue to assess the value of more dose intensive and combination therapies in the treatment of women with breast cancer at high risk for recurrence and with advanced disease. New technologies in molecular genetics have led to the localization of two breast cancer susceptibility genes, BRCA-1 and BRCA-2.[264, 398] Researchers continue to study tumor suppressor genes and oncogenes to understand better their effects on breast cancer initiation and development and their role as prognostic variables. Results of the Breast Cancer Prevention Trial, begun in 1992, led to approval by the Food and Drug Administration (FDA) in late 1998 of tamoxifen for use as a preventive agent in women at increased risk for breast cancer.[120, 122] A subsequent prevention trial will compare the toxicity, benefits, and risks of tamoxifen and raloxifene in the prevention of breast cancer in postmenopausal women who are at increased risk for the disease.[120] In addition, other clinical trials are addressing questions about the effects of a reduced-fat diet on breast cancer: the Women's Health Initiative (WHI) and the Women's Intervention Nutrition Study (WINS).[63, 263] Each of these endeavors lends hope that new and better methods for the prevention and treatment of breast cancer will lead to reductions in mortality.

Early detection remains the key to breast cancer control. Breast cancer screening guidelines continue to come under discussion.[9, 114, 354, 355] Mammography remains the mainstay for finding breast cancer before it has become clinically detectable. Coupled with regular and thorough breast self-examination (BSE) and regular periodic examination of the breasts by a professional, breast cancer can be found early, when it is more likely to be cured, often with conservative surgical management. Studies of socioeconomic and cultural differences in the practice of breast cancer control activities as well as stage at diagnosis and survival have pointed out the need for more attention to these factors in all phases of the breast care continuum.* As the population of women in the United States ages, more consideration

---
* References 21, 64, 105, 130, 253, 299.

must also be given to the needs of an elderly population of women at risk for, diagnosed with, or followed after treatment for breast cancer.

The psychosocial impact of breast cancer screening, diagnosis, and treatment on the individual or family remains a major clinical and research responsibility for nursing, particularly in such challenging arenas as socioeconomic and ethnic diversity, the aging female population, and pregnancy after breast cancer. Because research results are at times confusing, conflicting, and controversial, women need help in integrating the information they are given, whether regarding risk of developing breast cancer or treatment options after the diagnosis. Nurses have a key role in advocating for women, whether in the political arena or at the bedside. Nurses need to be knowledgeable about current trends in breast cancer management so they can assist women throughout their treatment process. Nurses are also vital to public education efforts directed at breast cancer screening, teaching BSE and guidelines for mammography and professional breast examinations, and portraying the hope of breast cancer cure with early detection.

EPIDEMIOLOGY

The average American woman's risk for ever developing invasive breast cancer is 1 in 8.[163] This translates into 182,800 newly diagnosed female cases in the United States during 2000. Men rarely develop breast cancer by comparison, accounting for only 1400 new cases during the same year. It is predicted that 40,800 women and 400 men will die from the disease in 2000—fewer women than in prior years.[163] These numbers reflect cases of invasive breast cancer. Carcinoma in situ (CIS) (discussed later in this chapter) will account for about 42,600 additional new cases of breast cancer in women in 2000, increased significantly from the 30,000 cases estimated for 1996.[9, 163]

Overall, breast cancer incidence rates in women in the United States continued to increase by about 4% per year in the 1980s, but leveled off in the 1990s.[9] This is probably due to increased use of screening programs, particularly mammography, and therefore earlier detection.[8] Mortality rates remained essentially unchanged for the past 50 years, despite improvements in treatment and earlier detection.[8] In some parts of the world, such as Japan, breast cancer mortality rates continue to increase. Yet in other countries, such as the United States, Canada, Germany, and the United Kingdom, a decline in breast cancer deaths was noted beginning in the 1990s.[261] The greatest decline in the United States has been for younger and white women.[8, 261] Since 1987, more American women have died each year from lung cancer than breast cancer.[9] Breast cancer remains the most common site of cancer in American women.

The highest incidence rates of breast cancer in the world are in North America, followed next by Australia and New Zealand, temperate South America, Northern and Western Europe.[294] In the United States women who are white have a higher incidence rate than other ethnic groups, but African American women have the highest mortality rate.[8, 93] African American women in the United States are more likely to be diagnosed with breast cancer at a later stage, and subsequently have a 5-year relative survival rate that is nearly 15% lower than that for white women.[93, 163, 204] A disproportionate number of African Americans in the United States are at lower socioeconomic levels; associated with an inadequate social and physical environment, inadequate information and education, a risk-promoting life-style, and impaired access to health care, this most likely accounts for more of the differences in cancer survival than race.[4, 130]

ETIOLOGY AND RISK FACTORS

Research has shown that there is no known single cause of breast cancer. It is a heterogeneous disease, most likely developing as a result of many different factors that are not the same from woman to woman and most of which are yet unknown. Several characteristics, or *risk factors,* appear to increase the probability of a woman developing breast cancer.[181] Women diagnosed with breast cancer may or may not have any of the risk factors. In fact, in one large prospective study by the American Cancer Society (ACS), 75% of the breast cancers detected occurred in women who had none of the most widely recognized higher risk factors.[339] It is therefore understandable that the concept of risk in breast cancer is often confusing and frequently fear inducing. Many women overestimate their risk of developing breast cancer.[209] This can lead to extremes of reaction from that of avoidance of health care to that of the opposite—worry and seeking of unnecessary repeated evaluations. Health care providers who do not understand risk may reinforce such fears. It is important for women and their nurses to understand the concept of risk and current knowledge of risk factors to develop individualized breast health plans of care.

Understanding Breast Cancer Risk

Breast cancer risk can be expressed as risk of development or risk of death from the disease. This chapter emphasizes risk as it relates to the development of breast cancer. *Absolute risk* is the number of breast cancer cases in a given population divided by the number of women in the population, expressed as an *average risk* for every woman in that population.[286] For white women in the United States today, this comes out to be about a 12.6% chance of developing breast cancer, most commonly expressed as the often-quoted "1 in 8" statistic.[163] This can be deceiving. This percentage is a cumulative lifetime risk based on the sum of risks at different ages (*age-specific risks*) for all women from birth to about 100 years of age.[8, 286] This does not take into account an individual woman's situation (her estimated life span, her current age, or the presence of other potentially high-risk factors). Absolute risk is sometimes expressed as age-specific risk for women in different age brackets. For example, American women ages 40 to 59 have a risk of developing breast cancer of approximately 4.1% (1 in 25), whereas at ages 60 to 79 they have a 7% (1 in 15) age-specific risk of developing breast cancer.[163] The risk is higher for older women because breast cancer occurs more frequently as age increases. The cumulative lifetime risk for white women 35 years of age (to age of 100) is 10%, whereas at age 65 there is a 6.3% risk of developing breast cancer by the age of 100.[181] The cumulative lifetime risk is lower for the 65-year-old woman because she has fewer years left to be at risk (even if she did live to be 100, because it is still a comparison based on years of life remaining). This risk for developing breast cancer is also lower for nonwhite women in both age groups because their overall incidence is lower.[9] Because absolute risk can be presented in different ways and does not consider individual situations, it may be difficult to derive personal meaning from such numbers. Absolute risk may underestimate the risk for some women (e.g., those with a family history of breast cancer) and overestimate the risk for others (e.g., nonwhite women).[244] However, absolute risk is a very meaningful statistic when addressing the magnitude of the breast cancer problem in the United States or for a very specific population.[8, 209]

Relative risk is the incidence rate of breast cancer in a population of women with a known or suspected risk factor divided by the incidence rate of breast cancer in a population of women without that risk factor.[8, 181, 209] Summary tables often categorize risk factors by relative risk, based on results of epidemiologic studies of breast cancer.[8, 181] A woman with no risk factors would have a relative risk of 1.0; a relative risk greater than 1.0 indicates a greater likelihood of developing breast cancer than individuals without the risk factors.[8, 244] For example, if the relative risk for a woman with a given risk factor is 2.0, she is two times more likely than the population to develop breast cancer. Relative risk allows for quantification of additional risk due to the given risk factor. The relative risk will potentially increase as the number of risk factors increases. To determine individual risk, one cannot multiply the cumulative lifetime risk (absolute risk) by the relative risk and obtain a meaningful number. However, *multiplying the age-specific risk by the relative risk* will give a percent

risk, for example, for the next 10 years of life; that is, the woman age 40 with an age-specific risk of 4.1% between the ages of 40 and 59 and a relative risk of 2.0 would have about an 8.2% chance of developing breast cancer over the next 19 years.[163, 209, 244, 286]

Attributable risk is the number of cancer cases in a population that are associated with given risk factors and that could potentially be prevented by alteration or removal of those factors.[244, 339] It is most useful in public health policy and planning for cancer prevention and control. Unlike lung cancer, where there is a clear causal link with smoking, there are no such factors in breast cancer. Attributable risk does not account for the majority of breast cancer cases.[339] Where a known associated risk exists for some women, the factors involved (e.g., family history, nulliparity, or late age at first birth) are ones over which they generally have little or no control.[8, 212]

Risk Factors

The following information covers those risk factors most widely acknowledged or suspected to increase the probability of a woman developing breast cancer.

Gender. Women are more likely than men to develop breast cancer. In the United States, breast cancer accounts for 30% of all invasive cancers in women and less than 1% of the cancers in men.[163]

Age. The incidence of breast cancer increases with age. Most breast cancer cases are diagnosed in women 40 years of age and older, but the majority of cases occur in women over age 50.[8] Most women who develop breast cancer will have no known risk factors other than being female and over 40 years of age.

Personal History of Cancer. A previous diagnosis of breast cancer increases a woman's lifetime risk for developing a second breast cancer in the opposite (contralateral) breast. Estimates are that this lifetime risk is approximately 1% per year, or a relative risk of 2.1 to 4.0 or greater.[8, 71] The risk has been shown to be even higher in women who also have a family history of breast cancer.[8, 71] In addition, a previous history of primary ovarian, endometrial, or colon cancer has been associated with an increased risk of breast cancer (relative risk under 1.1–2.0).[8]

Family History of Cancer and Genetics. Women with a family history of breast cancer in a first-degree relative (mother, sister, or daughter) have a relative risk of 2.1 to 4.0.[8] This is a risk two to four times that of the general population. Risk increases further if both the mother and sister have had breast cancer (relative risk > 4.0).[8, 212] Risk is greatest when the occurrence of breast cancer was premenopausal and bilateral.[8, 31] In some families this clustering of breast cancer may be accounted for only by chance or possibly from interactions among shared environmental, cultural, or socioeconomic factors that are less well understood.[388]

In other families, *genetics* may be a critical factor. Clinical features of possible hereditary breast cancer include a younger age at diagnosis, bilateral occurrence, multiple family members (maternal *or* paternal) affected over three or more generations, and the occurrence of cancers in other sites (e.g., colon, ovary, uterus).[181, 388] The presence of these features warrants cancer risk counseling and consideration of genetic susceptibility testing. Recent advances in molecular technology have enabled scientists to study in great detail the genetic structure of individual chromosomes and thus some of the mechanisms by which tumor suppressor genes and growth factors work to produce cancer. In 1990, the discovery was made of the tumor suppressor gene (oncogene) p53 on the short arm of chromosome 17.[250] Mutations of this tumor suppressor gene are found in patients with Li-Fraumeni familial syndrome, a rare syndrome associated with a high incidence of familial cancers, including breast cancer.[250, 388] Mutations of p53 may account for only 1% of all breast cancers in women under age 40.[31]

In 1994, the BRCA-1 tumor suppressor gene was isolated on the long arm of chromosome 17.[264] Female carriers of a mutation of this gene are at great risk of developing breast cancer or ovarian cancer. Also in 1994, the second tumor suppressor gene, BRCA-2, was localized on the long arm of chromosome 13.[397, 398] It appears that BRCA-2 mutations confer a high risk of breast cancer but not the same high risk of ovarian cancer as BRCA-1.[398] Such inherited genetic mutations are estimated to account for only 5% to 10% of breast cancer cases.[8, 402] However, in women who are carriers of either mutation, the lifetime risk of breast cancer to age 80 can reach 87%.[388] It is possible that the presence of mutations in BRCA-1 or BRCA-2 may also occur in noninherited or sporadic breast cancer cases.[225, 402]

This is perhaps the most exciting area of research, with the hope of improved understanding of breast cancer inheritance and development, diagnosis, prevention, and treatment.[230] Commercial testing for the presence of mutations in the BRCA-1 or BRCA-2 genes has become available only recently. Testing can reveal the presence of a mutation that in turn may guide a patient and her health care team in planning careful screening or preventive measures. Test results may be indeterminate, when a mutation of unknown significance is discovered. Test results may also be negative, when no mutation is found. Because most women at risk do not have the inherited gene mutation but a series of genetically determined factors that interact with life-style and environmental factors to predispose them to the development

of breast cancer, widespread genetic testing in the absence of a family history is not indicated at this time.[181] The American Society of Clinical Oncology (ASCO) has recommended that cancer predisposition testing should be considered only in cases where there is a strong family history of cancer with early age at onset, test results can be adequately interpreted, and results of such testing will guide the medical management of the patient.[15] In families with a high incidence of cancer, risk counseling should include a thorough family cancer history, a review of environmental and life-style risk factors, personal medical history, and an individualized plan of screening and follow-up.[15, 209, 230] (For more information on genetics and cancer, see Chapter 2.)

Early Menarche and Late Menopause. The exact role of hormones in the etiology of breast cancer has not been precisely determined. *Early onset of menarche* (before age 12), *late menopause* (at 55 or above), and greater total duration of years of regular menses are associated with an increased risk of breast cancer.[8, 31, 166] This is thought to be due to the total lifetime exposure of the breast to estrogen and progesterone, with fluctuations in cell growth and change in the breast tissues with each ovulatory cycle. In countries such as the United States, better nutrition is one factor contributing to a lowering of the average age at menarche and menstrual cycle length.[211] Surgically induced menopause (bilateral oophorectomy) reduces breast cancer risk, perhaps slightly greater than with natural menopause.[212, 305]

Reproductive History. Having no children (*nulliparity*) or the *first full-term pregnancy after age 30* places a woman at increased risk.[166, 181] The relative risk is higher for the woman who delays childbirth than for the nulliparous woman.[166] Childbirth at an early age may have some protective effect, although the mechanism is unclear and probably a combination of factors that alter the hormonal and cellular environment in the breast tissues.[305] Some studies have also shown that as the number of months of breastfeeding increases, an associated reduction occurs in the risk of developing breast cancer, particularly for premenopausal women.[166] The trend for some American women to delay childbearing until a later age, and to have a shorter duration of breastfeeding, may account for some of the variation in breast cancer incidence rates in the United States.

Benign Breast Disease. The term *benign breast disease* is frequently misunderstood in discussions of risk.[209] The term encompasses a broad array of histopathologic diagnoses women typically experience clinically at some time in their lives but that are never biopsied. Some question why such a common condition should be termed a "disease." Many of these so-called diseases are not associated with any increased risk of breast cancer. "Fibrocystic disease" is a catchall phrase to describe clinical symptoms and findings of local or generalized lumpiness, pain, or cystic changes. *Fibrocystic changes* may be a more appropriate term to describe these often normal breast changes.

Benign breast lesions, when pathologic diagnosis is made, are classified into three groups. *Nonproliferative lesions,* when found alone, are not associated with any increased risk of breast cancer. These include histologically diagnosed cysts, apocrine metaplasia, papillary apocrine change, epithelial-related calcifications, fibroadenomas, and mild hyperplasia.[99, 140] The presence of gross cysts in women with a family history of breast cancer has been shown to be associated with increased risk.[99, 292]

Proliferative lesions without atypia include moderate or florid ductal epithelial hyperplasias of the usual (common) type, sclerosing adenosis, and intraductal papillomas.[99, 140, 292] Some evidence indicates that multiple as opposed to single papillomas, occurring peripherally rather than centrally, are more susceptible to breast cancer development.[140] Occurring as increased growth of epithelial cells in the ductal or lobular tissue of the breast, proliferative lesions without atypia have been associated with a slightly increased risk (1.5–2.0) of breast cancer during the 10 to 20 years after biopsy.[99, 140, 292]

Proliferative lesions with atypia, or *atypical hyperplasia,* constitute the third category of benign breast disease and are most associated with increased breast cancer risk.[99, 140, 292] Less than 5% of benign breast disease biopsies are found to have atypical cells.[100] Atypical hyperplasia can be found in either ductal or lobular tissue. It is a proliferation of abnormal-looking cells within the duct or lobule. The diagnosis by biopsy of atypical ductal or lobular hyperplasia is associated with a relative risk of 4.0 to 5.0 during the 10 to 20 years after biopsy.[99, 100, 140, 292] This risk is greater in women who also have a family history of breast cancer.[100]

The presence of cells in the ductal or lobular tissue that are proliferating abnormally, have characteristics of cancer cells, and are within the ductal or lobular structure, are defined as *carcinoma in situ* (CIS), or cancer confined to the site of origin. The presence of CIS is associated with a relative risk of 8.0 to 10.0 of developing invasive breast cancer during the 10 to 20 years after biopsy.[224, 292] Treatment of women with this diagnosis is discussed later in this chapter.

Obesity and Dietary Fat. *Obesity* has been shown to be associated with increased risk of developing breast cancer in postmenopausal women.[8, 190, 212, 305, 358] Excess adipose tissue is rich in the necessary enzyme to convert precursors into circulating estrogen.[197, 212] Consequently, obese women may have increased levels of circulating estrogens, which can affect hormone-dependent breast cancer cells.[197, 212, 305] Another observation has been that obesity is associated with decreased levels of sex hormone-n-binding globulin (SHBG), which normally binds estradiol and would prevent stimulation of breast cancer cells.[197, 212]

Incidence of breast cancer is increased in industrialized countries with a high socioeconomic status and an increased consumption of *dietary fat,* suggesting a relationship. Migrant studies evaluating first- and second-generation immigrants from Japan, China, or Mexico (where incidence of breast cancer is low and dietary fat consumption is low) to the United States have shown rates of breast cancer much higher than in their country of origin and, in some cases, approaching rates for American white women.[166, 211] Dietary factors said to be associated with these variations in breast cancer incidence are likely different for premenopausal and postmenopausal women, and perhaps influenced by dietary fat intake during childhood and adolescence.[166] The studies to date do not give a clear picture of the relationship between obesity, weight change, and dietary fat intake and increased breast cancer risk. Recent studies of the influence of obesity have measured weight gain, body mass index, waist/hip ratio, waist circumference, and weight gain at specific times in the life cycle.* Studies of the influence of dietary fat intake have considered fat consumption ranging from 20% or less to 35% or more of total calories from fat, different types of fat intake, and fat intake at specific times in the life cycle.[185, 399] The U.S. per capita fat intake was about 33% of total calories in the mid 1990s.[10] A reduction in fat intake to 20% to 30% of total calories and the addition of high-fiber foods have been suggested as healthy dietary habits because of the potential for cancer risk reduction as well as risk reduction in other illnesses such as heart disease.[10, 181] Two major studies were initiated in the 1990s to address the relationship between dietary factors and estrogen, other hormones and breast cancer risk in several thousand women across the country (WHI and WINS).[63, 263, 320]

Radiation Exposure. A greater than expected incidence of breast cancer has been seen in women exposed to ionizing radiation for the treatment of tuberculosis or postpartum mastitis, in survivors of the atomic bombs at Hiroshima and Nagasaki, and in survivors of Hodgkin's disease.[35, 170, 259, 265] Sensitivity of the breast tissue to the damaging effects of radiation is greatest during childhood (ages 10–14) and decreased to almost negligible by age 40.[265] The current availability of low-dose mammography coupled with regular use in women *over 40*

* References 190, 203, 296, 358, 365.

years of age makes the risk from radiation exposure with screening mammography almost negligible.[265]

Exogenous Hormones. Because breast cancers are thought to be hormone related, numerous studies have evaluated the risk associated with the use of *oral contraceptives* (OCs) or *estrogen replacement therapy* (ERT). The majority of these studies have shown no increased risk for most women who have ever used OCs or taken ERT.[76, 307] However, further analyses of women who have ever used OCs or ERT have distinguished subgroups at possible increased risk based on the age at onset of use, duration and recency of use, and dosing regimen.

In January 1989, the Fertility and Maternal Health Drugs Advisory Committee of the FDA concluded no relationship exists between OC use and breast cancer and recommended further studies. In fall 1989, the Committee on the Relationship Between Oral Contraceptives and Breast Cancer within the Institute of Medicine was assembled to examine the etiology of breast cancer as related to OCs.[198] Its report recommended that no fundamental change in clinical practice with respect to the use of OCs is supported by the knowledge to date about OCs and risk of breast cancer.[198] It also recommended that women seeking contraception be given adequate information and counseling as to the current ambiguities in the knowledge to date of the relationship between OCs and breast cancer.[198] Recent studies have suggested an increased risk associated with early onset and long-term use of OCs, particularly for younger women,[42, 76, 181, 318, 390] but not for women over 40 years of age with past long-term use,[171] or for Asian American women.[376]

Estrogen replacement therapy for postmenopausal women has been available in the United States since 1942, with widespread use since the 1960s.[209] With new concern about the risk of endometrial cancer risk in women taking unopposed estrogens, progesterone was added to the ERT regimen in the late 1970s. In postmenopausal women, ERT has been used to manage the menopausal symptoms of hot flashes and dyspareunia secondary to atrophic vaginitis. In recent years, ERT has also been used to prevent osteoporosis and reduce the risk of cardiovascular disease. Some aspects of the relationship between ERT and breast cancer remain unclear, as in the type of estrogen taken,[77] or whether there is no increased risk for women with a family history of breast cancer[340] or personal history of proliferative breast disease.[98] Several studies have shown an increased risk for breast cancer when a progestin is added to estrogen (combination hormone replacement therapy),[72, 319, 328] or when use is prolonged (more than 5 years).[72, 77, 181, 307, 319] Until further studies better address all of these issues, women should be advised of the

current knowledge in the field and be guided in weighing the potential benefits and risks of undertaking ERT.[72, 244]

Alcohol Consumption. Several studies have shown an increased risk of breast cancer (relative risk of 1.1–2.0) associated with alcohol consumption of 2 or more drinks per day.* The age at which drinking begins, amount and type of alcohol consumed, and duration and recency of consumption, each appear to be important variables in fully understanding the risk that can be attributed to alcohol.† One theory about the mechanisms of the risk associated with alcohol suggests that premenopausal breast tissue is more susceptible to injury. Another theory proposes an intricate relationship between alcohol metabolism and estrogen levels that might stimulate cancerous cell growth.[364] Heavy alcohol consumption may also be associated with poor nutrition or other social and environmental factors that may affect general health, access to care, and stage at diagnosis. Further study is needed of each of these variables.

Other Factors. Certain mammographic parenchymal (tissue) patterns have been associated with an increased risk of breast cancer.[39] Higher socioeconomic status is associated with a higher risk of developing breast cancer, but lower socioeconomic status is associated with a greater risk of dying from the disease.[8, 130] Ethnicity also is associated with risk, with nonwhite women being less at risk of developing breast cancer but at greater risk of dying from the disease.[8] No clear associations with increased risk of breast cancer have been found for cigarette smoking, stress, personality type, psychiatric diagnosis, lack of physical activity, exposure to electromagnetic fields, silicone breast implants, caffeine, or hair dyes.‡

For the woman who appears to have an increased risk based on family history or other factors, a detailed assessment should be conducted to determine actual individual risk. *Cancer risk assessment* programs are available in many cancer centers throughout the United States.[52] A cancer risk assessment can be initiated in any setting, however (see Chapter 2). In addition to the assessment of specific risk factors associated with breast cancer, the assessment should thoroughly explore a woman's perceptions of risk, her attitudes toward and beliefs about early detection methods (BSE, clinical breast examination [CBE], mammography) as well as her participation in each, and her need for information. Women and their family members may need help in understanding that risk estimates based on such assess-

---

* References 8, 116, 138, 356, 367, 382, 383.

† References 38, 116, 147, 241, 242, 382, 383.

‡ References 34, 43, 78, 141, 142, 184, 209, 212, 315.

ments are projections about the *possibility* of developing breast cancer in the future, and do not tell if a woman will ever develop the disease. Screening guidelines for the early detection of breast cancer in asymptomatic women need to be followed. The National Comprehensive Cancer Network (NCCN) has recommended that women with a known deleterious mutation should begin annual mammography, annual or semiannual CBE, and proficient BSE at age 25.[83] Others have suggested annual mammography and CBE beginning at age 25 to 35.[47] Women whose histories indicate a strong possibility of the presence of a deleterious mutation (e.g., family history of premenopausal breast cancer and multiple cases of breast and ovarian cancer) should also consider following these guidelines.[83]

There is no clear preventive intervention. Reduction in alcohol and dietary fat intake, and weight loss if postmenopausal and obese, are some measures that the individual can take, but none has a clear association with breast cancer prevention. Prophylactic mastectomy (discussed later in this chapter) may reduce the incidence of breast cancer by as much as 90%, and increase life expectancy, for women at high risk of breast cancer, but should only be considered for women who have a clearly increased risk of breast cancer, or with clinical conditions that make evaluation extremely difficult.[31, 162, 173, 334, 357]

There remains much to learn about risk factors for breast cancer and the effects of combinations of risk factors now known or suspected. New risk factors need to be identified, risk quantified, and control measures studied. Most women who will be diagnosed with breast cancer have no known risk factors. Current knowledge about risk factors in breast cancer will help the nurse guide the patient in obtaining personally meaningful information. In most cases, interventions will need to be focused less on risk factor reduction and more on developing a plan of care for the early detection of breast cancer when it occurs.

PREVENTION, SCREENING, AND DETECTION

It is not known what causes breast cancer or how to prevent the disease. Breast cancer is a *heterogeneous disease;* in other words, it is a disease of many characteristics, varying from woman to woman in its potential for development, growth, and metastasis. The epidemiology of the disease indicates that it is hormonally influenced, with the duration of exposure to elevated levels of circulating estrogens being a primary factor in the promotion of cancer cell development over several years. This period of cell promotion is characterized by reversibility. If this exposure could be reduced or if the adverse effects of the exposure could be prevented, breast cancer might be prevented.

The Breast Cancer Prevention Trial, begun in 1992, evaluated the effectiveness of tamoxifen in preventing the occurrence of invasive breast cancer in a group of women at higher risk for breast cancer development. As a placebo-controlled trial, women who consented to participate in the study were randomized to receive either the tamoxifen or a placebo. To participate in the study, women were 60 years of age or older, or 35 to 59 years of age with a 5-year predicted risk for breast cancer of 1.67% or higher, or with a history of lobular carcinoma in situ (LCIS).[122] Women who participated took the medication (tamoxifen or placebo) for 5 years and were followed regularly. Because tamoxifen has been associated with an increased risk of endometrial cancer, and because estrogens are known to have an important role in reducing rates of coronary heart disease and osteoporosis in postmenopausal women, these were also closely monitored as part of the study. More than 13,000 women participated. This study demonstrated that tamoxifen reduced the risk of invasive breast cancer by 49% and the risk of noninvasive breast cancer by 50%, for women at increased risk for breast cancer, with low toxicity.[120, 122] As a result, in October 1998, the FDA approved tamoxifen for use in preventing breast cancer in women at high risk for the disease. A subsequent prevention trial, the Study of Tamoxifen and Raloxifene (STAR), will compare the effectiveness of tamoxifen and raloxifene in preventing breast cancer in 22,000 postmenopausal women 35 years and older who are at increased risk of the disease, as well as evaluate toxicities.[120] The results of these and other studies evaluating prevention will, in the next decade, give us clearer direction in the prevention and treatment of breast cancer.

Early detection is therefore the most important means for control of breast cancer. Research has shown that survival is directly related to the stage of the disease at diagnosis. The ACS maintains *screening guidelines* for asymptomatic women that incorporate the following three methods of early detection[9, 355]:

1. *Breast self-examination* (*BSE*) should be performed monthly by all women beginning at age 20.
2. *Clinical breast examination* (*CBE*) by a health professional should be done every 3 years for women ages 20 to 39 and annually beginning at age 40.
3. *Mammography* (routine screening mammography) should be performed every year beginning at age 40.

The Cancer Genetics Consortium has recommended that women who are known to carry a BRCA-1 or BRCA-2 mutation, or who have a high likelihood of being a carrier, should begin annual or semiannual CBE and annual mammography at the age of 25 to 35.[47] A woman with known risk factors (e.g., family history) or

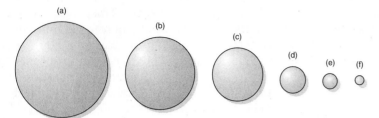

(a) 3.6 cm = discovered by accident
(b) 2.5 cm = conventional BSE practiced less than once a month
(c) 2.0 cm = conventional BSE practiced once a month
(d) 1.0 cm = clinical breast examination
(e) 0.5 cm = MammaCare® technique practiced regularly
(f) 0.3 cm = MammaCare® technique practiced expertly

FIGURE 7–1 (a) Average-sized lump found by accident. (b) Average-sized lump found by women practicing BSE less than once a month. (c) Average-sized lump found by women practicing monthly BSE. (d) Average-size lump found on CBE. (e) Average-size lump found by MammaCare® practiced regularly. (f) Average-sized lump found by MammaCare® practiced expertly. (Data source courtesy of Mammatech Corporation, ©1990.)

chronic symptomatology should be advised to consult with her physician or nurse practitioner regarding the frequency and specificity of CBEs and mammography for her situation. Nurses have a major role in teaching these potentially lifesaving guidelines to all women. For greatest effectiveness, frequency (regular and periodic) and proficiency (skill and thoroughness) are key concepts to consider in each screening method.

Mammography

Mammography is the only proven means of detecting breast cancer before it can be discovered by CBE or BSE. Screening mammography is used to detect cancer in *asymptomatic* women. By the time a lesion is 1 cm in diameter and can be felt, it is estimated that it may have been present for 8 or more years.[180] Figure 7–1 depicts the average-sized lump detected with BSE and mammography. Since the Health Insurance Plan of Greater New York (HIP) study in the early 1960s and the Breast Cancer Detection Demonstration Project (BCDDP) in the 1970s, screening mammography has repeatedly been shown to be effective in reducing the number of deaths associated with breast cancer through the detection of clinically occult lesions as small as 1 to 2 mm in size.* Mammography is also useful in evaluating high-risk women and women with breasts difficult to palpate (e.g., breasts that are large and pendulous or with severe fibrocystic changes). Xeromammography was popular for several years beginning in the early 1970s. However, refinements in technology have made film-screen mammography the preferred breast imaging method because of its higher image contrast, lower radiation dose, and less equipment downtime.[379] Digital mammography, which involves the translation of film-screen images into a computer-generated image, holds promise for breast imaging of the future.

Ultrasound is helpful in conjunction with mammography to help differentiate a fluid-filled cyst from a solid mass. Other methods for imaging the breasts, such as thermography, diaphonography (transillumination), and magnetic resonance imaging (MRI), have been evaluated but have not been shown to be effective in screening for breast cancer.[181] MRI may be useful in evaluating the augmented breast, evaluating the extent of disease in the breast, or in searching for a primary cancer.[220] Scintimammography, which involves injection of a radioisotope (technetium-99m sestamibi) followed by a nuclear medicine scan of the breasts, has been studied as an adjunct to mammography in differentiating benign from malignant lesions, but preliminary results are inconclusive.[220, 374] Positron emission tomographic (PET) scanning, may be useful in evaluating the breast and axilla. The radioisotope used in PET has an affinity for tissues with increased metabolic activity, which may be associated with many breast cancers.[220]

Screening mammography generally consists of two views of each breast: one from side to side that includes the axilla and upper outer quadrant of the breast (mediolateral oblique) and one from top to bottom (craniocaudal).[24, 379] For each view the breast is compressed to decrease the thickness of the breast and enable better visualization of the structures of the tissue, also reducing the amount of radiation. It may be uncomfortable, but an explanation that proper breast compression is one of the most important factors in a quality mammogram may help women understand the importance of that momentary discomfort.[379] It is also helpful if premenstrual women avoid having their screening mammogram immediately before their menses because of the potential for increased breast tenderness at that time of the month. *Diagnostic mammography* consists of additional views of the breast to help delineate an area of concern

---

* References 24, 114, 194, 221, 279, 353, 354, 368.

found on a screening mammogram or a palpable mass. For example, spot compression allows for greater compression of an isolated area and may be used in conjunction with magnification to enlarge an area of calcifications or asymmetry.[24]

When properly performed, mammography can effectively detect 85% to 90% of breast cancers. It is possible for 10% to 15% of malignant lesions to be undetected.[220] Therefore, in women with clinical symptoms, a negative mammogram does not rule out the need for a biopsy. Dense breast tissue, lesions that cannot be seen on mammogram, the skill of the technologist, the experience of the radiologist, and the quality of the equipment may all contribute to false-negative readings. To address the quality of care issues, the Mammography Quality Standards Act (MQSA) was passed by Congress in 1992, effective October 1, 1994, and renewed by Congress in 1998 (Mammography Quality Standards Reauthorization Act). The MQSA sets federal quality standards for equipment, personnel, and record keeping at all mammography facilities. By law a facility must be certified by the FDA as providing quality mammography services, and to be certified it must be accredited by a federally approved private nonprofit or state accreditation body and inspected annually.[379, 381] The MQSA quality standards require that the following are present[379]:

- Dedicated mammographic equipment with regular monitoring to ensure that the minimum necessary radiation dose is administered and that the quality of films processed is maintained
- Radiologic technologists who are specially trained and experienced in mammography
- Radiologists with demonstrated experience and competence in mammography
- Records of mammography that include comparisons with prior films, findings, and recommendations

Despite its value, many women do not get regular mammograms. Although approximately 84% of U.S. women in 1997 reported having ever had a mammogram, less than 65% of women 40 to 49 years of age had completed a mammogram within 2 years, and less than 58% of women 50 years of age and older had completed a mammogram within the past year.[10] Some women are concerned about radiation exposure from mammograms. The radiation dose delivered has been significantly lowered since the 1960s, and with equipment dedicated solely to mammography, the risk is negligible. Cost can prohibit some women from obtaining screening mammograms. The cost for a screening mammogram can range from $10 for a copayment to over $100, with a national average of $100. Through efforts of the ACS, National Cancer Institute (NCI), and other organizations, costs for screening mammography have

declined and insurance coverage has improved for many women in the United States. Many centers offer low cost mammograms at different times of the year. In 1991, the U.S. Congress established the National Breast and Cervical Cancer Early Detection Program (NB-CCEDP) (reauthorized in 1998), to bring breast and cervical cancer screening to underserved women. Federal and state matching funds have established programs in all 50 states, U.S. territories, and American Indian and Alaska Native organizations. As of 1998, close to 1 million underserved women had received a mammogram as a result of this program.[58] Women have reported additional reasons for not getting a mammogram including fear of discomfort, embarrassment, fear that cancer will be found, a belief that one is not at risk, that other tests (e.g., CBE) are adequate, that the test takes too much time, not having incorporated the mammogram into their health care routine, and difficult access.[60, 62, 237, 379] Women who are more likely to complete a mammogram may have stronger beliefs in the benefits of the examination, the seriousness of breast cancer if diagnosed, and of personal susceptibility to the disease, with lowered perceptions of barriers.[60, 62]

One additional reason that mammography has been underutilized has been physician disagreement or poor compliance with following screening guidelines for mammography and recommending the procedure to patients. A 1989 survey of more than 1000 U.S. physicians revealed that although physicians reported a greater inclination (since 5 years previously) to order screening mammography in asymptomatic women, reasons given for not ordering a mammogram included concerns about affordability and cost, reliability of the test, availability of a qualified radiologist or equipment, doubt of need if no symptoms or family history, and radiation risk.[6] Physician referral or recommendation does encourage women to get a mammogram.[237, 257] One study demonstrated that the specialty of the referring physician also influenced mammography participation by women 65 years of age and older, with the highest participation by patients (78%) when the primary care physician was a gynecologist.[119] More confusion on the part of consumers and health care providers, as demonstrated in the debate in the late 1990s about the value of screening mammography in women ages 40 to 49, can make mammography participation difficult.[354] However, increasing evidence has supported the value of annual mammography for women ages 40 to 49.[115, 194, 349, 355, 368] The ACS and the American College of Radiology (ACR) have maintained a commitment to the benefits of annual screening mammography in women ages 40 and over, with no upper age limit for the discontinuation of regular mammograms.[114, 355] *Healthy People 2010* goals include increasing the proportion of primary care providers who counsel patients about mammograms, from 37% in 1988 to 85% in 2010.[378] Ongoing health care provider and public education and health care advocacy efforts remain critical to minimizing each of these known barriers.

Breast Self-Examination

Breast self-examination is a free, private, and relatively simple examination, part of the breast cancer detection triad.[9, 181] In areas of the world where mammography or professional health care examinations are not consistently available, BSE may have even greater importance in the early detection of breast cancer. For women under 40 years of age, regular BSE increases awareness of one's normal anatomy and may help identify changes that would not otherwise be noticed. For women over age 40, BSE provides an additional safety net for the limitations of mammography,[354] and may aid in the prompt seeking of care for a newly detected abnormality. The majority of palpable breast lumps *are* discovered by a woman herself. There is some evidence in the research literature that women who perform BSE sometimes or regularly are more likely to discover smaller tumors and to have a smaller number of positive lymph nodes at diagnosis compared with women whose cancer is discovered accidentally.* It has been estimated that regular practice of BSE could reduce the overall breast cancer mortality by approximately 19%.[164] Other reports suggest that instruction and proficiency in, and frequency of performance of BSE, may be important factors influencing the relationship between BSE and breast cancer survival, and thus further study is needed.[19, 108, 343] More than 120,000 women ages 40 to 64 years participated in the first prospective, randomized, controlled trial to evaluate the effectiveness of BSE, begun in 1985 in Moscow and St. Petersburg with the World Health Organization (WHO).[341, 342] Interim results indicate that women taught BSE were more likely to seek care for breast problems but were no different from the women not taught BSE in terms of breast cancer incidence or stage at diagnosis.[341]

Most women in the United States know about BSE, but only 19% to 40% of them report practicing BSE on a regular basis.[73] Many women who practice BSE do not do it thoroughly (proficiently).[1, 61, 69] Compliance may be poor for a variety of reasons, such as inadequate knowledge of how to do BSE, lack of confidence in ability to perform BSE and to detect abnormalities, fear of finding something, discomfort with touching breasts, lack of confidence in BSE as a means of detecting changes, forgetfulness, lack of motivation, lack of physician recommendation, or lack of access to services.†

How effective will a woman be if she performs BSE monthly but poorly, or thoroughly but less often? Through one-on-one education that is repeated at intervals, monthly reminders, and encouragement by health professionals, compliance rates may improve. Studies have shown that education needs to include factual information about normal breast changes, breast cancer, and early detection and should promote positive attitudes or values.[61, 69, 73] Pamphlets and video instruction are passive teaching methods that have not been shown to be effective when used alone.[17] Cultural and age sensitivity, language, and reading level should also be considered when selecting educational methods and materials. BSE is a motor skill that entails coordination of palpation, movement, and sensation.[69, 208] Opportunities for women to practice on silicone breast models and on themselves with feedback during the practice are crucial and may also enhance self-confidence in BSE performance.[7, 17, 61, 69, 73, 74, 271]

Women should be advised to perform BSE monthly. Premenopausal women should examine their breasts 5 to 7 days after their menstrual period begins. At this time their breasts may be less engorged and tender, thus allowing a more thorough and less distorted examination. Nonmenstruating or postmenopausal women should select the same day each month to do BSE. Selecting an anniversary or birth date is one suggestion to encourage women to remember. Women who are pregnant or breastfeeding should still examine themselves monthly, but the breastfeeding mother should do so soon after her breasts have been emptied. Women who have had breast cancer surgery should still perform BSE, with special attention to any surgical scar area and to the chest wall (postmastectomy).

Breast self-examination includes inspection and palpation of the breasts in both standing and lying positions. Attention is focused on evaluating for change. It is best done in an atmosphere that is unhurried and most comfortable for the individual woman. A thorough BSE will usually take 20 to 30 minutes. The ACS and NCI are two sources of patient and professional educational materials on BSE. The MammaCare® Personal Learning System is perhaps the most comprehensive and researched program, emphasizing proficiency through individualized instruction, the use of specially designed breast palpation models, an instruction manual, and a video program for self-learning.[251] Use of this system as well as other reviews of BSE proficiency are in the literature.* The components of BSE for proficiency in practice include *inspection* of the breasts in front of a mirror, *palpation* of the entire area of the breast using the flat *pads of the fingers* at different levels

---

*References 22, 73, 128, 150, 192, 219, 222, 348.
†References 7, 17, 61, 69, 110, 133, 134.

---

*References 7, 69, 73, 125, 287, 297, 325.

of *pressure,* in a specific *pattern* and *motion* within that pattern (i.e., small dime-sized circles in a vertical strip, wedge, or circular pattern), most easily done when in a flat or partial side-lying (upper body turned at 45-degree angle) *position* (Fig. 7–2).[7, 325]

Inspection of the breasts is best conducted standing in front of a mirror, with the arms at the sides and both breasts exposed for complete visualization of the skin surface, nipple/areola complex, and breast contour. Turning slightly side to side, the breasts are inspected

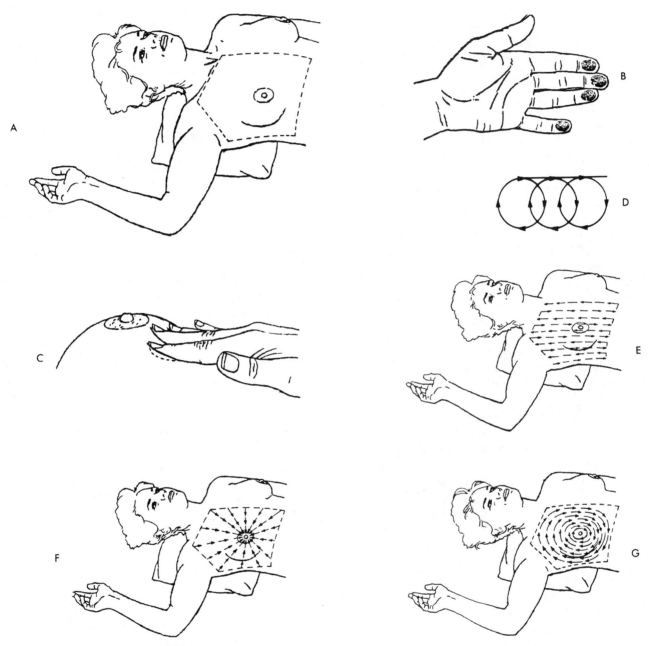

FIGURE 7–2 Breast self-examination (BSE). **A,** Perimeter of area to be examined should include all breast tissue. This area is bounded by a line that extends vertically from middle of axilla (armpit) to rib just beneath breast and continues horizontally along underside of breast to midsternum (middle of breastbone). It continues up midsternum to clavicle (collarbone) and along lower border of clavicle to shoulder and back to midaxilla. **B,** Palpation is performed with pads of fingers. **C** and **D,** Move your fingers (three or four) in small circles about the size of a dime. Varying levels of pressure (light, medium, and firm) should be applied to each spot palpated. Moderate pressure is illustrated. The following patterns can be used for the examination: **E,** vertical strip; **F,** wedge; and **G,** circle. (Courtesy American Cancer Society, California Division.)

for any evidence of skin retraction, puckering, dimpling, erythema, vein prominence, and presence of other characteristics such as nevi. The nipples should be noted as everted or inverted. Women with pendulous breasts should lift the breast on either side to inspect the skin on the lower side of the breasts and the chest area. It is normal that one breast may be slightly larger than the other. With hands on the hips pressing in and down, the same observation is repeated. This is further repeated with the arms over the head and with the arms in front while leaning forward.

Palpation is then performed lying down as previously described. Lotion can be applied to the flat pads of the fingers to smooth the skin. With respect to areas of the breast that may warrant additional attention, the upper outer quadrant of the breast is the most common location of most types of breast cancer, followed by the central area of the breast around the nipple.[180] Common errors in technique include *not palpating at different levels of pressure, not palpating the entire breast tissue area including behind the nipple,* and *using the fingertips for palpation rather than the flat pads of the three middle fingers.* Palpation needs to be done at three levels of pressure: light, medium, and firm. The light pressure will detect any changes in the skin that too-firm pressure might push away. Medium pressure will enable a woman to feel the glandular and fatty tissue of the breast. Firm pressure allows examination of the breast tissue close to the underlying ribs and muscle. The fingertips should be avoided because they are less sensitive than the finger pads. Women should be reminded not to do the examination too hurriedly. Beginning at the axilla or in the upper outer quadrant, the entire breast, axilla, and supraclavicular areas need to be examined. This area extends from the axilla to the bra line, over to the sternum, up to the supraclavicular notch, along the clavicle to the shoulder, and back to the axilla.[325] This completed pattern is followed by an additional palpation in the axilla. Some women may also want to repeat the entire BSE in the shower. Though no longer included in all BSE instruction, many women have been taught in the past to also gently check the nipple for discharge.

It is crucial to emphasize that when first performing BSE, a woman is learning her normal breast characteristics so that any future variations or changes can be recognized and evaluated. If she notices a change on one breast, she may want to check the other breast for symmetry. She should be encouraged to have a plan of action should she detect a change that needs evaluation. This might be to call her health care provider for an appointment. Prompt medical attention should be sought if any of the clinical features or common symptoms of breast cancer are present. Although fear is a common feeling experienced when a new change or symptom is discovered, women can be encouraged when told that most breast lumps discovered are benign.[7, 9]

Clinical Breast Examination

Next to mammography, CBE is the most commonly used screening technique for breast cancer today.[6, 10] In the HIP study previously described, CBE contributed significantly to reductions in breast cancer mortality.[266] The importance of the BCDDP findings was that each of the screening measures (mammography, CBE, BSE) detected breast cancer cases not initially found by the other.[7] Studies have estimated that a lump of 0.3 cm can be detected by palpation in silicone breast models.[124] For CBE to be as effective as possible, the professional performing the examination needs to be proficient. Research suggests, however, that health professionals vary considerably in their confidence in and ability to perform CBE,[124, 231] and may not be as effective as women proficient in BSE.[199] One study of registered nurses found an association between high confidence in their own BSE and use of CBE in elderly women.[246] Unfortunately, many women relegate the examination of their breasts solely to their health care providers. A physician or other health professional does not have the advantage of being familiar with a woman's normal monthly breast

CLINICAL FEATURES

Breast Cancer

MOST COMMON SYMPTOMS AT PRESENTATION

Mass (particularly if hard, irregular, nontender) or thickening in breast or axilla

Spontaneous, persistent, unilateral nipple discharge that is serosanguineous, bloody, or watery in character

Nipple retraction or inversion

Change in size, shape, or texture of breast (asymmetry)

Dimpling or puckering of skin

Scaly skin around nipple

Symptoms of local or regional spread

Redness, ulceration, edema, or dilated veins

Peau d'orange skin changes

Enlargement of lymph nodes in axilla

Evidence of metastatic disease

Enlargement of lymph nodes in supraclavicular (collarbone) cervical area

Abnormal chest x-ray film with or without pleural effusion

Elevated alkaline phosphatase, elevated calcium, positive bone scan, and/or bone pain related to bone involvement

Abnormal liver function tests

irregularities when examinations are performed only yearly. The California Division of the ACS developed a program to help health professionals become more proficient in their performance of CBE, outlined in a publication describing seven areas of proficiency, modeled after those for BSE (see Fig. 7–2).[5] The Mamma-Care® Professional Learning System is a commercially available program, similar to that for BSE, but geared to the health care professional who will be performing regular CBEs.[252] Clinical competence in CBE requires training to proficiency and regular practice.[298]

During CBE the health professional can demonstrate BSE technique, explain the rationale for each step, and encourage women to be partners in their care by continuing monthly BSE at home. In addition, a woman's particular normal anatomic variations can be pointed out. Signs and symptoms of breast abnormalities can be discussed and risk factors for breast cancer reviewed, with particular attention to what that means to the individual woman. The establishment of a relationship of trust between the health professional and the patient may lead to improved participation in breast cancer screening activities.

It is hoped that by the end of the year 2010, 80% of U.S. women ages 40 and over will have ever received a CBE and mammogram, and 70% of women ages 40 and over will have received a mammogram within the prior 2 years.[377, 378] This is increased from 36% in 1987 and 79.9% in 1997 for both exams, and 68% in 1998 for the mammogram alone.[10, 377] Particular attention needs to be paid to special populations for all aspects of breast cancer screening. Problems in access, knowledge, and priorities are evident in medically underserved women, with resultant higher mortality.* Reports of cancer screening practices of women in urban[131, 226, 254, 316] or rural settings,[351, 359] and studies of mammography utilization[129, 249] and BSE practice by nonwhite,[64, 95, 133, 299, 303] low income[133, 172, 249] elderly,[26, 239, 271, 396] or higher-risk women,[18, 28, 40, 82, 109] graphically demonstrate the need to find improved ways of reaching these populations with breast cancer screening.

Regular mammograms for eligible women, regular physical examinations, and monthly BSE can detect early breast cancers. All three components must be included in breast cancer screening. None of them is as effective individually as when combined. Early detection provides the opportunity for women and their physicians to select treatment options for managing small breast cancers and results in improved survival. These breast cancer detection recommendations are to be taught to all women, and women should be encouraged to incorporate these behaviors into their individual life-styles.

CLASSIFICATION

Knowledge of the anatomy of the breast helps in understanding the classification of breast cancer. The breast is a gland located on the chest wall (Fig. 7–3). The overlying skin contains hair follicles and sweat and sebaceous glands. The pigmented area surrounding the nipple is known as the *areola,* and this has sebaceous glands that secrete a lubricant during breastfeeding. Fibrous strands called *Cooper's ligaments* pass through the glandular and fatty tissues from the skin to the underlying muscle, giving the breast support. The glandular tissue is made up of 15 to 20 lobes arranged in a radial pattern, capable of producing milk and connecting with ducts that drain into the nipple. An extensive lymphatic and vascular supply is present. Breast tissue extends to the clavicle, sternum, latissimus dorsi muscles, and up into the axilla. The axillary lymph nodes are thought to drain between 75% and 97% of the lymph fluid from the breast.[290, 317] The rest of the lymph fluid goes to the internal mammary chain, behind the sternum. The axillary nodes are distributed from low in the armpit, at the lateral border of the pectoralis minor muscle (level I), to midway behind the pectoralis minor muscle (level II), and above at the medial border of the pectoralis minor (level III). Lymph nodes located between the pectoralis major and minor muscles are known as *Rotter's nodes.* The remainder of the lymph is drained from the internal mammary nodes.[290, 317]

Primary breast cancers are grouped as invasive or noninvasive. A malignancy confined to the ducts or lobules is classified as noninvasive, or *carcinoma in situ* (CIS). If it arose in the ductal system, it is referred to as *ductal carcinoma in situ* (DCIS); in the lobule system it is called *lobular carcinoma in situ* (LCIS). Once the malignant cells penetrate the tissue outside the ducts or lobules, the cancer is described as *infiltrating* or *invasive.* Most breast malignancies are carcinomas and classified as ductal or lobular, with a small number of sarcomas and metastatic tumors reported. *Infiltrating ductal carcinoma* accounts for approximately 80% of all breast carcinomas and *infiltrating lobular carcinomas* about 10%.[181] Less common are *inflammatory carcinoma,* which is characterized by swelling, erythema, and invasion of the dermal lymphatics (giving the classic peau d'orange, or orange peel, appearance), *medullary, papillary,* and *tubular carcinoma. Paget's disease* of the nipple, a *presentation* of breast cancer, occurs infrequently (2% of all cases) and is most often associated with an underlying in situ or invasive carcinoma.[224] When noninvasive cancer is found with invasive cancer, the staging and treat-

---

* References 4, 48, 110, 130, 163, 378.

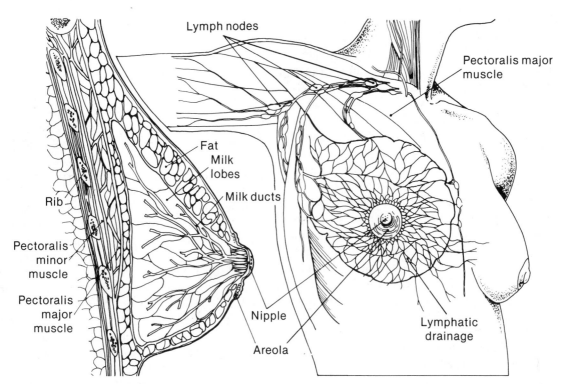

FIGURE 7 – 3 Anatomy of the female breast. (From DiSaia PJ and Creasman WT: *Clinical gynecologic oncology*, ed 5, St. Louis, Mosby, 1997.)

ment planning are based on the characteristics of the invasive carcinoma.

CLINICAL FEATURES

In asymptomatic women, mammography serves to detect microscopic changes indicative of cancer, such as a small, irregular mass, indistinct or speculated margins, microcalcifications, skin thickening, architectural distortion of the ductal or ligament structures, or asymmetric density.[24] Palpable breast masses may also have these characteristics, as well as nipple or skin retraction when underlying structures are involved.[24] The Clinical Features box lists additional clinical signs and symptoms of breast cancer at presentation.

DIAGNOSIS AND STAGING

Tissue Diagnosis

Breast cancer can be diagnosed with cytologic (cells) or histologic (tissue) evaluation. Examination of tissue will give a definitive diagnosis. *Fine-needle aspiration* (FNA) *biopsy* for cytology is the preferred technique when dominant masses are palpable. It is a relatively simple procedure involving the aspiration of material from the mass using a syringe and 21- to 23-gauge needle.[293] The

content of the aspiration is mounted on slides and processed for review. In skilled hands it is highly accurate; false-negative and false-positive results are rare. A negative result in the presence of a suspicious mass warrants further evaluation. Although FNA can lead to the diagnosis of carcinoma, it cannot distinguish whether it is invasive or noninvasive.[121] Some advantages of the FNA are the ease with which it can be done in the office setting, use of minimal local anesthesia, and the low incidence of damage to surrounding tissue. When the results are cancer, it also prevents the necessity of surgical biopsy before treatment planning for definitive surgery.[293]

Core needle biopsy provides a core of tissue from a dominant mass. Insertion of a specially designed 14-gauge needle into the palpable mass is accomplished either manually or with the aid of an automated device.[293] This procedure requires some local anesthesia and has been associated with more bleeding and pain than the FNA, especially when deeper lesions are involved. False-positive results may be a greater problem than with FNA, although they are still low in incidence. A core needle biopsy may be helpful after a nondiagnostic or suspicious FNA. Because it provides a larger sample of tissue, core needle biopsy can differentiate in situ from invasive cancer.[293] *Incisional biopsy* is performed when the mass is large; it involves removal of only a portion of the mass. *Excisional biopsy* involves removal of the entire mass and a margin of normal tissue around it. It is used for palpable and nonpalpable lesions.

Nonpalpable abnormalities detected only on mammogram need to be evaluated under radiographic guidance. The *needle localization biopsy* requires that a radiologist localize the suspicious area under mammography guidance by directing a small wire with a hook on the end, or a needle, into the lesion. The wire (or needle) is then taped to the patient's skin, the patient is transferred to the operating room, and the abnormality at the tip of the wire is excised by the surgeon. The tissue removed is radiographed to verify removal of the suspicious area (or to direct further excision). The tissue is then examined microscopically in permanent sections. Although this is not a difficult procedure, it is not an exact procedure and more tissue than necessary may be removed.[51, 330]

Stereotactic FNA or core needle biopsy is intended to improve on the needle localization biopsy procedure both in accuracy and in patient comfort. It can be performed on most nonpalpable, suspicious abnormalities found on mammogram,[25] and is available in most breast centers. For this procedure, patients are positioned prone on an examination table, with their affected breast suspended through an opening in the table. The breast is compressed as for mammography, films are taken, the skin anesthetized, and the biopsy needle mechanically and precisely aligned by radiograph and computer to the area of abnormality.[330] Two major advantages of the stereotactic needle biopsy are the precision of the technique and the possible elimination of some unnecessary excisional biopsies for benign lesions.[330] Contraindications to the procedure may include lesions close to the chest wall or skin, obesity, and other medical conditions that would prohibit appropriate positioning on the exam table, or being on anticoagulant therapy.[25] *Ultrasound-guided biopsy* is also used in some settings. In this case the woman is positioned supine, the lesion localized with ultrasound, and the biopsy needle guided manually by the physician.

It is rare today that any woman would have a definitive surgical procedure for breast cancer without first learning she has cancer through some preliminary diagnostic test such as an FNA or some type of tissue biopsy.[121] For women who have already had an FNA or core needle biopsy diagnosis of carcinoma, a biopsy is usually performed intraoperatively to reconfirm the diagnosis just before the definitive surgical procedure. These procedures enable the determination of a definitive diagnosis of cancer and the opportunity for a woman to be involved in her treatment plan. Women need to be assured that the interval between diagnosis and definitive treatment, to obtain recommendations regarding management options, does not adversely affect survival.

Staging

Breast cancer is most frequently staged according to the *TNM classification* system, which evaluates the tumor size (*T*), involvement of regional lymph nodes (*N*), and distant spread of the disease or metastases (*M*) (discussed in detail in Chapter 1). The stages may be simply classified as follows[11]:

Stage 0 — Carcinoma in situ (Tis-N0-M0)

Stage I — Tumor under 2 cm with negative nodes (T1-N0-M0) (includes microinvasive T1, < 0.1 cm)

Stage IIA — Tumor 0 to 2 cm with positive nodes (including micrometastasis N1, or < 0.2 cm), or 2 to 5 cm with negative nodes (T0-N1, T1-N1, T2-N0, all M0)

Stage IIB — Tumor 2 to 5 cm with positive nodes or greater than 5 cm with negative nodes (T2-N1, T3-N0, all M0)

Stage IIIA — No evidence of primary tumor or tumor less than 2 cm with involved fixed lymph nodes, or tumor greater than 5 cm with involved movable or nonmovable nodes (T0-N2, T1-N2, T2-N2, T3-N1, T3-N2, all M0)

Stage IIIB — Tumor of any size with direct extension to chest wall or skin, with or without involved lymph nodes, or any size tumor with involved internal mammary lymph nodes (T4-any N, any T-N3, all M0)

Stage IV — Any distant metastasis (includes ipsilateral supraclavicular nodes) (all M1)

The historical classification of stage, still seen in national statistical reports, classifies stage as *local* (no lymph nodes involved), *regional,* and *distant.* Of breast cancer patients diagnosed between 1989 and 1995 in the United States, 62% had local disease, 29% regional disease, and 6% distant (metastatic) disease at diagnosis.[8] African American women (51%) were less likely than white women (63%) to have their breast cancer diagnosed at a local stage from 1989 to 1995,[163] and had a poorer 5-year relative survival during that same time period than white women (89% versus 97%) (Table 7–1). More than half (56.2%) of all breast cancers diagnosed in 1995 were stage 0 (CIS) or stage I (< 2 centimeters and no involved lymph nodes), an improvement over

TABLE 7-1
Survival According to the Number of Nodes Involved and Stage of Disease

Number of Nodes	10-Year Relative Survival (%)
0	65–70
1–3	48–63
4–9	28
>10	18

Stage	10-Year Relative Survival (%)
0	95
I	88
II	66
III	36
IV	7

Stage	5-Year Relative Survival (%)	
	White	African American
All stages	86	71
Localized	97	89
Regional	78	63
Distant	22	14

Data from: Fremgen A, et al: Clinical highlights from the National Cancer Data Base, 1999, CA Cancer J Clin 49:145–158, 1999. Greenlee R, Murray T, Bolden S, Wingo P: Cancer statistics, 2000, CA Cancer J Clin 50:7–33, 2000. Henderson IC: Breast cancer. In Murphy GP, et al: American Cancer Society textbook of clinical oncology, ed 2, p. 209, Atlanta, American Cancer Society, 1995.

the 42.5% recorded for 1985.[132] However, in 1996 white women were more likely than African American women to be diagnosed with stage 0 or stage I breast cancer (57% versus 44.8%).[93] One researcher has predicted, based on these trends, that during the 21st century the median diameter of invasive breast cancer will be 1 cm or less.[51]

Evaluating the extent of disease allows appropriate therapy to be planned, determines the overall prognosis, and permits comparison of research results related to treatment.[181] The clinical staging process routinely begins preoperatively with a thorough history and physical examination, bilateral mammography, complete blood count, liver function tests, alkaline phosphatase, and calcium. Pathologic staging is based on the histologic review of the primary tumor from surgical specimens (type, size, and margins) and, when invasive carcinoma is present, the lymph nodes. Evaluation of a patient's bony structure, chest, liver, and brain are individualized according to the patient's specific symptoms, laboratory test results, clinical evidence of enlarged axillary nodes, or stage III disease.[24] For example, elevated liver enzymes with or without hepatomegaly might warrant a computed tomography (CT) scan of the abdomen or

liver to rule out liver metastases. Specific complaints of bone pain or an elevated alkaline phosphatase or calcium level would be evaluated with a bone scan or bone survey. A woman with clinical or pathologic stage III breast carcinoma may have a bone scan and a CT of the chest, abdomen, and pelvis to rule out metastatic disease. Extensive local surgery might be contraindicated if distant metastases are discovered at the initial diagnosis.

Tumor markers are substances secreted by some cancers, which can be detected in the circulating blood. In breast cancer a tumor marker may be useful in monitoring response to systemic therapy for metastatic disease and in monitoring for recurrence of disease. Serial levels that show a pattern of continued increase over time are evidence of metastasis.[176] For this reason a baseline test is often requested prior to beginning definitive treatment. Three of these tumor markers with some value in breast cancer are *carcinoembryonic antigen* (CEA), *CA15-3,* and *CA27.29.* CEA has been the most widely studied marker.[176] This marker, however, is limited in its value because it can be elevated with other conditions, such as benign breast disease or smoking. Also, less than half of all patients with known breast cancer recurrence show an elevation in the CEA.[175]

CA15-3 and CA27.29 may also be elevated in benign breast conditions but are not elevated in smokers. They may also be elevated in other inflammatory or malignant conditions of epithelial organs (e.g., ovary).[175] From studies to date, these appear to be more sensitive markers for breast cancer metastases than CEA, with elevated levels in 65% to 90% and 58% to 83%, respectively, of such patients.[362] In patients with *primary* early stage breast cancer, CA15-3 levels are elevated in 5% to 30% of patients, compared with only 10% to 15% of patients who will have an elevated CEA.[362] Neither test is specific enough to be routinely used for staging and follow-up.

PROGNOSTIC FACTORS

Tumor size and lymph node status, incorporated into the staging system, have long been recognized as pathologic characteristics that alone have value in predicting survival. The staging system provides direction for treatment, but does not provide the means by which to predict which women in a particular stage group will have disease recurrence and which will not. Unfortunately 20% to 30% of women with negative lymph nodes at the time of breast cancer diagnosis will develop a recurrence within 10 years.[180] Adjuvant therapy would be most appropriately directed to those women if one could somehow identify them by additional pathologic studies of the tumor. Several pathologic characteristics have been studied for their ability to determine risk of local recurrence, metastasis, response to therapy, and overall prognosis. These are known as *prognostic factors,* shown in Box 7–1.

Tumor Size

The smaller the tumor size, the less likely there will be axillary lymph node involvement at diagnosis and the less likely the cancer will recur within the breast or axilla. Additionally with a small tumor there is greater likelihood of eligibility for breast-conserving surgery. Tumor size is directly related to prognosis. The 5-year survival rate for women with small tumors and negative lymph nodes is 99% when tumor size is less than 0.5 cm, 90.6% to 84.6% for tumors 2 to 4.9 cm, and 82.2% for tumors greater than 5 cm.[56]

Axillary Lymph Node Status

The most important predictor of disease recurrence and survival is the presence of axillary lymph node metastasis. The larger the tumor, the greater is the likelihood that lymph nodes will be involved. The more lymph nodes that are involved, the greater is the risk that distant micrometastases are present. Survival is directly related to the number of lymph nodes involved (see Table 7–1). Women with negative lymph nodes have a higher rate of survival than women with involved lymph nodes. U.S. white women diagnosed between 1989 and 1995 with localized disease (no lymph node involvement) have 5-year relative survival rates of 97% versus 78% for those with regional disease (any lymph node involvement).[163] Similarly, women with one to three involved lymph nodes do better than women with four or more involved lymph nodes.[180] Surgical evaluation of the nodes is important because clinically negative nodes will be pathologically involved in about 30%.[180] Newer laboratory techniques, which involve immunohistochemistry, can detect even smaller deposits of cancer cells in lymph nodes (micrometastatic disease) than has been previously possible.[66, 70, 189] However, the significance of these findings is unclear and remains under investigation.

Bone Marrow

Bone marrow aspiration and biopsy are not routinely performed in the staging of early breast cancer. Some evidence suggests that the presence of metastatic breast cancer cells in bone marrow, detected with immunohistochemical techniques, may be a better marker than lymph node status in predicting risk of recurrence and survival, and might be useful in determining which

---

BOX 7–1

Key Prognostic Factors in Breast Cancer

Prognostic Factor	Favorable Range
Tumor size	Noninvasive or <1 cm invasive
Axillary lymph node status	Negative
Estrogen receptors	Positive
Progesterone receptors	Positive
Histologic grade	Well differentiated
Nuclear grade	Low grade
DNA content	
Ploidy	Diploid (DNA = 1.00%)
S-phase fraction	Low ($\leq$4%)
Oncogenes	
her-2/*neu*	Low expression
Tumor suppressor genes	
p53	Low expression
Lymphatic and blood vessel invasion	None

Other factors with value in predicting response to therapy, or local or distant recurrence[68]:
Heat shock stress response proteins
Tumor necrosis
Inflammatory response
Extensive intraductal component (EIC)
Demographic characteristics (e.g., age, ethnicity, socioeconomic status)

women with negative lymph nodes would benefit from adjuvant chemotherapy.[91, 139, 291] The significance of this finding remains unclear and is under investigation.

Estrogen and Progesterone Receptors

The effects of estrogen and progesterone on human breast cancer cells are mediated by steroid receptors known as estrogen and progesterone receptors (ER/PR).[106] Both normal and cancer cells have these receptors, but they are frequently overexpressed in breast cancer.[106, 394] These receptors are located in the nucleus or on the surface of the cell and bind to circulating steroid hormones. The receptor-hormone complex then works within the cell nucleus to promote cellular growth and division. A biochemical or immunohistochemical analysis of breast cancer cells removed at the time of tissue diagnosis can quantify the presence of these receptors in noninvasive or invasive breast cancers. Patients are said to be positive or negative for ER and PR based on the level of binding receptors present. It should be routine at the time of biopsy or definitive surgery that a representative sample of the suspicious or malignant tissue is processed appropriately for ER and PR measurement.[394] Approximately 60% to 65% of primary breast cancers are ER positive, and fewer are PR positive.[394]

The presence of ER and PR in breast cancer tissue is a predictor of responsiveness to hormonal therapy, to adjuvant therapy, and of survival.[106] The greatest likelihood of response to hormonal therapy is related to high levels of both ER and PR. Tumors that are ER

negative and PR positive have shown more responsiveness to hormone treatment than ER-negative and PR-negative tumors.[394] In addition, receptor status correlates with a variety of clinical and biologic parameters, some of which are also noted as prognostic factors (Table 7–2). PR may be a better determinant of prognosis and ER a better predictor of endocrine response.[207] ER-positive cancers are seen more frequently in postmenopausal women, are associated with other good prognostic factors (e.g., lower grade, lower S phase, and diploid), and usually have a lower recurrence rate and better overall prognosis.[106] PR-positive cancers are more common in premenopausal women, and PR status is less useful as a prognostic factor.[106]

Histologic and Nuclear Grade

The *histologic grade* generally refers to the cellular arrangement, or structure of the tumor, and defines the tumor as well differentiated (grade I), moderately well differentiated (grade II), or poorly differentiated (grade III).[207] *Nuclear grade* refers to the differentiation of the tumor cell nuclei, the shape and size of the nuclei, and the number of mitoses, or *mitotic index*.[68] Nuclear grade is considered to be more important than histologic grade as a prognostic factor. The Scarf-Bloom-Richardson grading system combines assessments of the structure of the tumor, the mitotic index, and other features of the nuclei.[68] A low number refers to a well-differentiated tumor (and better prognosis), whereas a score of 9 at the other end of the scale reflects a poorly differentiated tumor (and poorer prognosis).[181] Poorly differenti-

TABLE 7–2
Clinical and Biologic Differences between ER-Positive and ER-Negative Tumors

Biologic Parameter	ER Positive	ER Negative
Histologic grade	Well differentiated (low grade)	Poorly differentiated (high grade)
Nuclear grade	Cell nuclei well differentiated	Poorly differentiated cell nuclei (high grade)
DNA content	Normal (diploid)	Abnormal (aneuploid)
S-phase fraction	Low percentage of cells in S phase	High percentage of cells in S phase
her-2/*neu*	Low expression	High expression
p53	Low expression	High expression
Age/menopausal status	≥50 postmenopausal	<50 premenopausal
Clinical course of disease	Prolonged disease-free and overall survival	Shorter time to recurrence and shorter overall survival
Type of metastases	Bone, soft tissue, reproductive organs	Visceral involvement (liver, brain)
Response to and benefit from endocrine therapy	More likely	Less likely
Response to and benefit from chemotherapy	Less likely	More likely

Data from Clark G: Prognostic and predictive factors. In Harris J, Lippman M, Morrow M, Osborne C, editors: Diseases of the breast, ed 2, pp. 489–514, Philadelphia, Lippincott Williams & Wilkins 2000. Early Breast Cancer Trialists' Collaborative Group: Tamoxifen for early breast cancer: an overview of the randomized trials, Lancet 351:1451–1467, 1998. Elledge R, Fuqua S: Estrogen and progesterone receptors. In Harris J, Lippman M, Morrow M, Osborne C, editors: Diseases of the breast, ed 2, pp. 471–488, Philadelphia, Lippincott Williams & Wilkins, 2000.

ated tumors (with high mitotic rate) are generally considered to be associated with a poorer prognosis.

DNA Content

Breast cancer cells are also evaluated for their potential to proliferate. *Flow cytometry* evaluates the aggressiveness of a cancer by analyzing the cellular deoxyribonucleic acid (DNA) content (*ploidy*) of the cells, and the percentage of cells in the S phase of cellular division (*S-phase fraction,* or SPF). Tumors are classified as *diploid* (normal DNA content) or *aneuploid* (abnormal DNA content) and with high or low SPF based on numerical values.[62, 181] Cutoff values for high versus low SPF (and higher or lower risk groups) are not standardized and have varied in studies to date.[68] In general, a greater risk of recurrence and worse prognosis are associated with aneuploid tumors and cells with a high SPF, but studies in progress continue to evaluate these in relation to other prognostic factors.[68] This information may be most useful in defining which subsets of node-negative breast cancer patients need systemic adjuvant therapy. Another method of measuring cell proliferation is the *thymidine labeling index* (TLI). Its value as a prognostic factor is less well understood.

Oncogenes

Proto-oncogenes are normally involved in regulating cell growth and differentiation. When altered in the cell (*somatic mutation*), they become known as *oncogenes,* the genes responsible for cancer.[151] Abnormalities of amplification (multiple copies) or overexpression (multiple quantities) of the proto-oncogene her-2/*neu* (or c-*erb*B-2) in the DNA of some breast cancers has been associated with tumor growth, more aggressive cancers, local or distant recurrence, and poorer overall survival; they may also aid in the prediction of response to chemotherapy and endocrine therapy.[68, 151] Other proto-oncogenes under investigation are c-*myc* and Ha-*ras.* *Tumor suppressor genes,* or *antioncogenes,* may be absent or not functional. Normally inhibiting cancer growth, their absence has significance in cancer cell growth. Currently under study are p53, Rb-1, and nm23.[68, 151] High expression of p53 is associated with aneuploidy, high SPF, and ER- and PR-negative tumors.[151] As discussed earlier in this chapter, a *germline* (inherited) mutation in either the BRCA-1 or BRCA-2 gene significantly increases a woman's risk of developing breast cancer. The study of oncogenes will greatly enhance our understanding of the biology of breast cancer and lead to the development of new diagnostic and therapeutic techniques.

Lymphatic and Blood Vessel Invasion

The presence of lymphatic and blood vessel invasion by tumor cells is generally associated with a greater incidence of disease recurrence and a worse prognosis.[332] No specific, completely objective laboratory method is available to identify lymphatic or blood vessel invasion.[332]

Epidermal Growth Factor Receptor

Epidermal growth factor receptor (EGFR) influences breast cancer growth by binding with receptors. The presence of increased EGFR has been associated with more aggressive tumors, recurrence, poorer prognosis, and resistance to endocrine therapy.[68] Therapeutic trials of monoclonal antibodies to EGFR, to block growth signals to breast cancer cells, are underway.[68, 151]

Cathepsin D

Cathepsin D, a glycoprotein, may promote cancer cell growth and invasion by destroying the basement membrane, the extracellular structure, and connective tissues.[151] Therefore high values of cathepsin D could be associated with greater risk of distant spread of disease and decreased survival.[68] However, further study is needed.

Other Factors

Many other factors are under investigation for their role independently and with each other in predicting cancer cell growth and regulation, response to systemic treatment, or risk of local recurrence and metastasis. Tumor size, axillary lymph node status, ER and PR levels, grade, DNA ploidy, SPF, and her-2/*neu* are the most prominent prognostic factors considered when projecting risk of recurrence and response to systemic therapy. The heterogeneity of breast cancer makes precise determinations of prognosis and response to treatment impossible. Yet further study of these and other potential prognostic factors will enable refinement in laboratory measurement techniques, reporting of results, and analyses of interactions among prognostic factors. Nearly two thirds of all cases of invasive breast cancer diagnosed today will not involve axillary nodes (localized disease).[163] Approximately 70% of those patients will be cured without adjuvant therapy, but the remaining 30% will not be.[180] The study of prognostic factors will be most helpful if additional tools are discovered that aid in the identification of the women at greatest risk of recurrence, who would only be cured with adjuvant therapy.

METASTASIS

Adjuvant systemic therapy has been shown to improve overall survival and prevent or delay the development of metastatic disease. Distant metastases can develop as long as 10 or more years after the initial diagnosis.[180] Once metastatic disease develops, the goal of treatment is palliation. Breast cancer spreads by direct invasion of surrounding tissues, along mammary ducts, or by way of lymphatic or blood vessels. The major site of regional spread is the axillary lymph nodes. These nodes are positive in approximately 50% of patients who have cancers that are 3 to 4 cm at diagnosis.[180] Systemic or distant spread of the disease can occur in a variety of organs and tissues. The most frequent sites are bone, lung, pleura, liver, and adrenals. Other less common sites are the brain, thyroid, leptomeninges, eye, pericardium, and ovary.[180] Symptoms that may be associated with metastasis include bone pain, shortness of breath, loss of weight, or neurologic changes. Elevated serum alkaline phosphatase, calcium, or liver function tests may be indicative of site-specific metastases, when seen in combination with clinical and radiographic findings (see Clinical Features box).

Two serious complications of metastatic disease, considered oncologic emergencies, are *spinal cord compression* and *hypercalcemia.* Metastatic tumor compressing the spinal cord results in motor weakness and progresses to autonomic or sensory deficits and paralysis. Preservation of neurologic function depends on early diagnosis and prompt treatment. Therapeutic options include radiotherapy alone or in combination with surgical decompression. Further palliative systemic treatment may be added. Hypercalcemia is generally a reversible metabolic problem. The symptoms are nonspecific: nausea, constipation, weakness, confusion, and lethargy. This problem may be the result of progressive bone metastases or compromised renal function or part of a "flare reaction." Another complication associated with breast cancer metastasis is *malignant pleural effusion.* Gradual to acute onset of increasing respiratory distress, particularly dyspnea on exertion, is the most common sign. (Chapter 20 presents further information on oncologic complications.)

The 5-year relative survival rate for women diagnosed between 1989 and 1995 with metastatic breast cancer is 21%.[9] The average survival when breast cancer recurs as metastatic disease is about 2 years, although some patients (10–20%) may live for 5 years or more, and another small percentage (2–5%) may be long-term survivors (>10 years).[13, 107, 178, 181, 352] Patients who were diagnosed with metastases a longer time after their initial breast cancer diagnosis and who have metastases to the bone or soft-tissue areas have a longer survival.[352] Metastatic breast cancer is not considered curable, but

therapies are usually available that will control or perhaps alleviate the symptoms altogether and prolong life.

TREATMENT MODALITIES

Surgery

Surgical management of breast cancer is noted in writings from the first century AD.[137] The use of general anesthesia and understanding of principles of asepsis did not occur until the late 1800s.[137] The primary goal of surgery has always been to achieve local and regional control of the disease. It has only been within the past century that surgical intervention has shown survival benefits. The view that breast cancer spreads in an orderly fashion from the breast to the lymph nodes prompted surgeon William Stewart Halsted (1852–1922) to perform what is now known as the radical mastectomy, removal of the pectoralis major along with the axillary lymph nodes and entire breast.[137] Newer views that breast cancer is a systemic disease at diagnosis, and that lymph nodes do not serve as a barrier to metastasis, prompted further investigation into less extensive surgery and the addition of radiation therapy in the early to mid-1900s.[137] By the mid 1970s the modified radical mastectomy was replacing the radical mastectomy, and by the 1980s breast-conserving surgery with radiation therapy was replacing modified radical mastectomy for many women with early invasive breast cancer. Removal of regional lymph nodes at levels I and II has long been considered the best method for determining nodal status in patients undergoing mastectomy or breast-conserving surgery for invasive breast cancer.[350] Axillary node sampling, which removes lymph nodes in the lower axilla without following a defined anatomic boundary, is not recommended.[369] Sentinel lymph node biopsy, a new technique to identify the lymph node that receives drainage from the primary site of breast cancer, is allowing preservation of lymph nodes for some women. (This will be discussed later in this section.) Box 7–2 describes surgical procedures in the treatment of breast cancer.

Primary Therapy. The type of surgery selected is based on clinical stage of the disease (tumor size, fixation, histology, nodes, metastases), mammographic findings (including evidence of cancer cells in other areas of the breast separate from the primary), the tumor location, patient history, available surgical and radiotherapeutic expertise, breast size and shape, and patient preference.

Some research has suggested timing of breast cancer surgery during the menstrual cycle may influence recurrence and survival.[79, 157, 188, 234] The hypothesis that surgery is associated with the highest curability when performed in midcycle is based on animal studies that demonstrated this was a time of greater cellular immune

---

BOX 7-2

Surgical Procedures in Treatment of Breast Cancer

Modified radical mastectomy (also referred to as *total mastectomy with axillary node dissection*). The entire breast is removed along with axillary lymph nodes and the lining over the pectoralis major muscle. The pectoralis major muscle is not removed. The pectoralis minor muscle may or may not be removed.

Total mastectomy (also referred to as *simple mastectomy*). All the breast tissue, including the nipple-areolar complex and the lining over the pectoralis major muscle, is removed. There is no axillary node dissection. Chest wall muscles are not removed.

Lumpectomy (or excision: *tumorectomy*). The tumor is removed and the major portion of the breast is left. A *tylectomy* refers to a wide excision with at least 3 cm of normal breast tissue around the tumor.

Wide excision (*limited resection, partial mastectomy*). Excision of the tumor with grossly clean margins of normal breast tissue.[277]

Quadrantectomy (also referred to as *partial mastectomy*). The entire quadrant of the breast containing the tumor is removed along with the overlying skin and the lining over the pectoralis major muscle.

Note: In each of the breast-conserving surgical procedures (lumpectomy, wide excision, and quadrantectomy) axillary node dissection is usually performed through a separate incision, and surgical intervention is followed by radiation therapy to the remaining breast tissue to treat any undetected cancer and achieve local control.[277]

Data from reference 350.

---

response.[188] Problems with the research to date and possible reasons for conflicting results include the retrospective nature of most studies, lack of control for other variables that might influence outcome, such as individual variability in tumor characteristics or immune function, irregular menstrual cycles, having had other procedures before definitive surgery (e.g., FNA or excisional biopsy), and lack of measurement of hormone levels at the time of surgery. Although the timing of breast cancer surgery during the menstrual cycle may have some clinical application in the future, further study is needed.[169, 344] Patients who desire scheduling of surgery in accord with their menstrual cycle should be encouraged to discuss this option with their physician.

Nearly all patients with operable breast cancer are candidates for the *modified radical mastectomy*. In large tumors this procedure allows for local control and pathologic staging. For most women with smaller tumors (stages I and II disease), *breast-conserving treatment* is now recognized as appropriate therapy with proven equivalence to modified radical mastectomy in terms of overall and relapse-free survival rates.[65, 123, 156] Breast-conserving surgery without axillary node dissection is also the preferred treatment for most cases of noninvasive breast cancer. Adequate time should be allowed in all cases for full discussion with the patient as to her options, and the advantages and disadvantages of each. Although patients will differ in their desire for and seeking of information, their involvement in the decision-making process is essential.[87, 276, 361, 366, 386] Also critical to the success of breast-conserving surgery is appropriate patient selection and a multidisciplinary approach. Patients are selected for breast-conserving treatment based on the factors noted in Box 7–3.[181, 391]

Studies of utilization patterns of breast-conserving surgery in women with stage I or II disease have been undertaken to assess implementation of guidelines originally released in 1990.[165, 177, 229] Some studies indicate that in certain areas of the United States, breast-conserving treatment is not being applied appropriately.[229] This has also been shown in Canada.[177] Studies have also shown differences in the treatment of young and elderly women.[20, 33] Availability of radiation facilities and of surgeons and radiation oncologists who specialize in the management of breast cancer is important for optimal results. Lack of such expertise may be one factor in underutilization of breast-conserving surgery. Professional and public knowledge, beliefs, and education may be greater barriers. Continued attention needs to be given on solutions to these disparities.

To prevent breast cancer in certain high-risk women, *prophylactic mastectomy* (unilateral or bilateral removal of the normal breast), with or without reconstruction, may be considered after careful discussion of potential risks and benefits. Skin-sparing total mastectomy is the preferred surgical procedure because more complete excision of breast tissue is possible.[104, 196] Women for whom this procedure may be appropriate include those with the following[31, 357]:

1. Strong family history of breast cancer (e.g., premenopausal bilateral breast cancer)
2. Biopsy-proven DCIS or LCIS or proliferative benign breast disease (atypical hyperplasia) with a family history of breast cancer
3. Personal history of contralateral multicentric CIS or invasive breast cancer
4. Women with an identified mutation in BRCA-1 or BRCA-2[173]

When accompanied by any of these risk factors, the presence of extremely nodular or dense breasts that make clinical or mammographic examination difficult might be the strongest medical indication for prophylactic mastectomy.[31] In women with a moderate to high risk of breast cancer, bilateral prophylactic mastectomies may reduce the risk of breast cancer by as much as 90%.[173] Reductions in risk will never reach 100%, as

---

BOX 7-3

Considerations in Patient Selection for Breast-Conserving Treatment

1. *Tumor size.* Local control is best with relatively small tumors. Most published experience in treating patients has been with tumors a maximum of 4 to 5 cm in diameter. *Contraindications* include stage III or IV disease or the inability to obtain clear margins after repeated attempts at excision of remaining invasive breast cancer.

2. *Tumor location.* The location is not a factor in choosing breast-conserving treatment, although tumors located centrally in the breast, beneath the nipple area, usually require removal of the entire nipple-areolar complex and cosmesis is then a consideration. *Contraindications* include two or more gross malignancies in other quadrants of the breast or mammographic indications of suspicious calcifications throughout the breast (multicentric disease).

3. *Breast size.* The tumor/breast size ratio influences the cosmetic results. If lumpectomy will result in a large surgical defect, a mastectomy followed by breast reconstruction may be more appropriate. A *contraindication* may be large pendulous breasts because of difficulties encountered with radiation therapy: reproducing the positioning of the patient and availability of equipment to provide dose homogeneity.

4. *Patient preference and attitude, and access to radiation facility.* A woman's desire to save her breast and a willingness to undergo 5 to 6 weeks of daily outpatient radiation therapy are important factors. A short hospital stay may also be required if interstitial implants are used. Some women might consider this extended treatment an unacceptable cost and inconvenience, or they may achieve greater peace of mind with the physical certainty of surgical removal. Living a great distance from a radiation treatment facility may cause additional hardship on some women and their families. Nurses can be supportive of patients in this decision-making process by facilitating communications, providing information, and helping them explore their personal values, relationships, and resources.* Many studies to date have shown no significant differences for general measures of emotional distress or overall quality of life in women undergoing mastectomy or breast-conserving surgery.[94, 333, 347, 386] However, studies have shown that women undergoing breast-conserving surgery may have a more positive sexual and body image and fewer problems with clothing than women undergoing a total mastectomy.[†]

5. Other *contraindications* are prior radiation to the chest (e.g., in Hodgkin's lymphoma) that would limit therapeutic dosing to the breast; a history of collagen vascular disorder, which has been associated with poor tolerance of radiation; and pregnancy. Women in first or second trimester of pregnancy would be unable to undergo radiation therapy; women in their third trimester could feasibly begin radiation after delivery.

Data from references 123, 181, and 391.

* References 87, 268, 276, 304, 361, 366, 387.

† References 144, 201, 216, 309, 333, 386.

---

all of the breast tissue cannot be removed. Anxiety and worry about cancer, confidence in breast cancer screening methods (i.e., BSE, CBE, mammography), and perceptions of cancer risk are each important to consider when supporting women who are considering this option.[269, 363]

Subcutaneous mastectomy, consisting of removal of breast tissue through an inframammary incision,[196] removes 90% to 95% of the tissue, retaining the skin and nipple-areolar complex. Because of the difficulty removing all the breast tissue and problems with cosmesis, it is not recommended for primary surgical treatment of invasive breast cancer.

Ductal and lobular carcinoma in situ (DCIS and LCIS), referred to earlier in this chapter, are noninvasive. In the past these were rarely seen. It is estimated that 15% to 20% of all breast cancers found on mammography are in situ.[126] Incidence rates of DCIS have increased by 28% per year between 1982 and 1988, and

6% between 1988 and 1996, a direct result of increased mammography use, because DCIS is primarily discovered on mammography.[8]

Lobular CIS is found *incidentally* in biopsies of suspicious lesions or masses, accounts for only 13% of in situ cancers, and has not increased in incidence since 1988.[8] DCIS is associated with a high risk of development of invasive ductal carcinoma at or near the biopsy site, whereas LCIS appears to be an indicator of the possible future development of invasive cancer anywhere in either breast. The management of each is different and can be controversial.[120, 136, 181, 392]

Ductal CIS is frequently associated with suspicious clustered microcalcifications found on mammogram.[136] This type of abnormality could be biopsied via a stereotactic core biopsy or a needle localization excision. It is not known whether all DCIS will progress to an invasive cancer or when. DCIS may also be found incidentally near an invasive cancer. When found outside the area of the primary tumor, DCIS is referred to as *multicentric foci* (sites outside the quadrant of the breast where the primary tumor was found) or *multifocal* (sites within the same quadrant as the primary tumor).[274] True multicentricity is rare.[274] Microinvasion, or occult invasion, refers to the presence of a microscopic focus (<1 mm) of invasive breast cancer in a specimen containing DCIS. The larger the DCIS, the greater the risk of microinvasion.[274] Involvement of the axillary lymph nodes is rare with DCIS but has been reported, usually in association with extensive DCIS of high nuclear grade or with microinvasion.[392, 403]

Mastectomy has been the primary treatment for DCIS, with a cure rate of nearly 100%.[392] Low axillary node dissection is usually included in a mastectomy. This degree of surgery may be overtreatment for many women with DCIS.[392] Several studies have demonstrated that, for most women with DCIS, breast-conserving surgery (complete removal of DCIS with clear margins of normal tissue) followed by radiation therapy to the remaining breast tissue reduces the risk of local recurrence of DCIS or invasive cancer.[120, 392] Results of the Breast Cancer Prevention Trial[120] have given support for considering tamoxifen in women with DCIS, for the prevention of invasive breast cancer.[274]

Lobular CIS, when found incidentally on a biopsy specimen, presents different management problems. It is not truly a precancerous lesion but an indicator of the risk of future invasive cancer in either breast, most often invasive ductal carcinoma.[272] It occurs primarily in premenopausal women and may be found diffusely in both breasts.[181, 272] Treatment options for LCIS include no further surgery and close follow-up, tamoxifen, or bilateral total mastectomy with reconstruction.[272] Neither axillary node dissection or radiation therapy is indicated for LCIS.[272] Tamoxifen significantly reduces the risk of invasive breast cancer in these women.[120, 122, 272]

Sentinel lymph node biopsy (SLNB) refers to the removal of the lymph node first to receive drainage from the site of a breast cancer. It is based on the hypothesis that cancer cells drain first to the sentinel lymph node before spreading to other lymph nodes.[70] Lymphatic mapping provides the means of identifying the sentinel lymph node. Preoperatively the location of the sentinel lymph node may be identified by means of a nuclear medicine scan. A radioactive isotope is injected into the breast at the site of the cancer and a scan of the breast, supraclavicular and axillary lymph node, and inner chest areas (lymphoscintigraphy) identifies its location. Intraoperatively a blue dye may be injected into the breast at the site of the cancer. An incision is made in the axilla (usually near the top of the bra line under the arm), and the sentinel lymph node is identified by use of a handheld probe to detect radioactivity or by visual identification of the blue lymphatic channel and blue-stained lymph node[155] (Fig. 7–4).

Research to date suggests this technique may be most useful for women with small invasive breast cancers who are at lowest risk of having involved lymph nodes and for whom a complete axillary lymph node dissection may be unnecessary surgery. The most experienced surgeons have demonstrated that identification of a negative sentinel lymph node is predictive that the remaining lymph nodes are also negative.[70, 155, 375] If the sentinel lymph node is positive for cancer, standard axillary lymph node dissection is indicated unless the patient is participating in a clinical trial.[70] When no sentinel lymph node can be identified, standard axillary lymph node dissection should be performed.[70] SLNB may be most appropriate for women with invasive breast cancers 1 cm or less. Contraindications to SLNB include tumors greater than 5 cm in greatest dimension or in multiple sites in the breast, a large biopsy cavity, presence of a

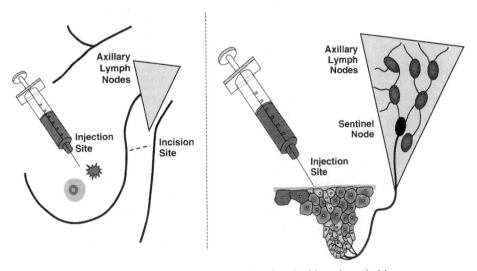

FIGURE 7 – 4 Lymphatic mapping/sentinel lymph node biopsy.

large hematoma or seroma, or the presence of palpable lymph nodes.[273] Surgeons offering SLNB must establish their competency in the technique, that their identification of the sentinel lymph node is truly predictive of the remaining lymph nodes. This is done by first performing standard axillary lymph node dissection along with SLNB on a minimum of 20 to 30 patients (but possibly as many as 60).[23, 81, 275]

Metastatic Disease. Surgery also has a role in the management of metastatic disease. Examples include procedures to excise a local skin recurrence, drain pleural effusions, debulk and decompress spinal cord metastasis, and oophorectomy (removal of ovaries to eliminate that source of endogenous estrogen).

Breast Reconstruction. The disfigurement and loss associated with a mastectomy can be devastating for many women and their sexual partners. A woman's breasts are equated with femininity, sexual attractiveness, and nurturing behavior.[322, 401] Health care providers and patients now increasingly recognize the psychosexual consequences related to breast cancer surgery.* Consequently, reconstruction has become an important element in a woman's rehabilitation after breast cancer surgery. Improved reconstructive techniques offer women hope for a more unaltered body image. The goal of breast reconstruction is to replace lost breast tissue and skin, rebuilding the breast mound to symmetry, with or without formation of a nipple and areola. A well-informed patient and a coordinated treatment approach by the surgeon, medical oncologist, and plastic surgeon will increase the likelihood of achieving the desired results.

Whether reconstruction is immediate (at the time of the mastectomy) or delayed to some future date until other treatments have been completed has been the subject of much debate. Perhaps the strongest argument against immediate reconstruction has been the concern that adjuvant chemotherapy would be delayed, particularly in women with stage III disease, because of prolonged recovery. This has not been supported. Neither has the argument that breast reconstruction would hide or delay diagnosis of local recurrence.[118] Another reason given for delaying reconstruction has been the belief that women needed first to adjust to the mastectomy and diagnosis before making a decision about reconstruction, as if this might somehow enable them to make a better decision and thus better appreciate the reconstructed breast.[118] These beliefs have been unfounded.[31, 118] Patients undergoing immediate reconstruction have been found to experience less overall trauma with their mastectomy.[2, 327]

Another advantage of immediate reconstruction is the elimination of one other hospitalization and anesthesia for the first stage of reconstruction. Immediate reconstruction may be more preferable because scar tissue has not yet formed and the tissues are more pliable at the time of mastectomy.[118] For most women undergoing mastectomy, particularly those with stage 0 (in situ) or stage I or IIa breast cancer, there is no scientific justification for not offering immediate reconstruction.[258]

Delayed reconstruction is a reasonable choice for some women, and sometimes it is medically preferred. For some women who delayed reconstruction, the desire to have reconstructive surgery diminishes over time. Schain described possible reasons for not pursuing reconstruction including fear of additional surgery, fear of recurrence of cancer, adjustment to their physical change, guilt feelings related to the desire to restore their breast, and reluctance to separate from their prosthesis.[326] Cost may be another factor. Costs for reconstruction vary based on the type of procedure, geographic area, and insurance. Federal and state laws have provided support to ensure that many insurance providers will include coverage for reconstruction, as well as symmetry procedures on the opposite breast, if they cover mastectomy.[118] Women considering these procedures will need to inquire with their individual insurance plans regarding coverage. Some cost savings may occur when hospitalization for mastectomy and reconstruction are combined.[213] Advanced age is not a contraindication for reconstruction as long as the woman is in sufficient health to tolerate the effects of surgery. Women who are obese, are smokers, or have a history of diabetes or debilitating disease have the highest rates of complications, all factors that are also relative contraindications to the more extensive tissue flap procedures.[118]

Treatment of breast cancer must remain the priority; thus treatment planning within the team will help clarify timing of reconstruction and adjuvant therapies. A thoughtful discussion of the options for reconstruction ideally should be incorporated within the initial treatment planning period. Every effort should be made to coordinate scheduling of surgery with the general or oncologic surgeon and the plastic surgeon in a timely manner, when the patient is fully informed about the treatment options and made her decision. The amount of information about the diagnosis and treatment options, potential for adjuvant therapy, clinical trial participation, and the discussion of reconstruction can be overwhelming for the patient as she sifts through the details while experiencing distress over the diagnosis and potential losses. Whether or not she chooses to undergo reconstruction, having that information can inspire hope and show support that she does have options.

---

* References 201, 216, 235, 262, 309, 386.

Most women with breast cancer preparing to have a mastectomy, particularly those with stage I or II disease, are candidates for reconstruction.[36] The patient's motivation and desire for a restored breast is one of the most important indicators for reconstruction.[36] The reasons women seek breast reconstruction, whether immediate or at a later date, are varied and may include a desire to feel whole again, to maintain a sense of femininity and positive body image, to eliminate an external prosthesis and to have a lasting result, or to reestablish physical symmetry and a sense of balance.[258] Some women will choose mastectomy with reconstruction over breast-conserving surgery because of a desire not to worry about remaining breast tissue or having to undergo radiation therapy. Patients with unrealistic expectations that reconstruction will eliminate the physical and psychological effects of mastectomy for a breast cancer diagnosis or will result in a perfect replication of the lost breast are more likely to be dissatisfied with the results.

Considerations in the type of reconstructive surgery include the quality and amount of skin, the size and shape of the opposite breast, the initial surgical procedure for cancer, and the patient's goals and general health.[118, 258] Table 7-3 lists breast reconstructive surgery procedures.

Silicone gel-filled breast *implants* were first developed in the early 1960s. By 1989 over 1 million implants had been placed in women, with over 80% of these in women for elective breast augmentation and only 20% in women who underwent reconstruction for breast cancer.[118] In response to concerns that silicone gel-filled implants were associated with autoimmune disease, in 1992 the FDA[380] restricted use of silicone gel-filled implants to prospective controlled clinical studies for women who have a medically related need for the implant (e.g., breast cancer, rupture of old implant). Although these concerns have not been substantiated, the restrictions continue.[118] Saline-filled silicone implants, not restricted by the FDA, are available for any woman seeking reconstruction, and currently account for the majority of implants placed today. *Tissue expanders* consist of an elastomer or silicone shell liner and a valve or port through which the shell is inflated with saline gradually over several weeks. These are useful in stretching the skin to accommodate a full-size prosthesis. Some expanders once fully filled will remain in the tissue as the permanent prosthesis. Others require a second operation for removal and replacement with a permanent implant.

The most common complication of implants is *capsular contracture,* or hardening of the scar tissue, resulting in firmness of the breast tissue and sometimes distortion of shape. Mechanical problems with inflation or deflation can occur with the tissue expanders but are uncommon. The potential also exists for a missed cancer on mammography, although a knowledgeable and skilled

TABLE 7-3
Breast Reconstructive Surgery Procedures in Breast Cancer

Procedure	Method

Implant (with or without tissue expander)
  Silicone gel filled (use is limited to controlled clinical trials)
  Saline-filled silicone shells
  Saline-filled tissue expanders
	Surgically placed under skin and muscle of chest
	
	Valve under skin allows adjustments in saline until ideal size reached

Permanent Temporary	Expander becomes permanent implant Implant is surgically replaced with permanent implant

Myocutaneous flaps
  Latissimus dorsi
  Transverse rectus abdominis (TRAM)
	Transfer of skin and underlying muscle with its intact blood supply to breast area

Free flap transfer
  Gluteus maximus
  Transverse rectus abdominis (TRAM)
	Transfer of skin, muscle, and blood vessels to breast area, with microsurgical reconnection of blood vessels to those in chest and axilla

Nipple-areolar complex	Areola: transfer of skin from lateral chest, inner thigh, or opposite areola and/or intradermal tattoo for color symmetry Nipple: skin flap raised from skin of breast mound, or graft used from opposite nipple
Symmetry	Augmentation Mastopexy (breast lift) Reduction

Data from references 36, 118, 154, and 258

mammography technician will be able to displace the implant and maximize the breast tissue captured in the mammogram. Until further information is available on the safety of implants, breast reconstruction with implants in women with breast cancer should continue to be preceded by a full discussion of the available options, risks, and benefits.

The *latissimus dorsi myocutaneous flap* from the upper back is useful in women after modified radical mastectomy or after lumpectomy/segmental mastectomy.[258] It involves the transfer of fat on the surface of the latissimus dorsi, and overlying skin, to the anterior chest wall mastectomy site.[118, 258] It may be supplemented with an implant for full symmetry. The *transverse rectus abdominis myocutaneous (pedicled or tunneled) flap* (TRAM) from the lower abdomen accomplishes a simultaneous abdominoplasty (similar to a "tummy tuck") and does not require the use of an implant. The rectus abdominis muscle and its blood supply, with overlying fat and skin, is used in the building of the breast mound. Complications with either of these procedures include flap loss from damage to the blood supply, skin necrosis, infection, hematoma, delayed wound healing, and fat necrosis or fibrosis.[36, 118, 258] Hernias at the donor site have occurred with the TRAM flap but should be rare.[258] In either procedure an additional scar is left, but the scar from the TRAM procedure is usually hidden within an acceptable "bikini" line. The TRAM flap can also be performed bilaterally. The TRAM procedure carries greater risk for the woman who has a history of smoking or obesity or is in otherwise compromised health.[36, 118] In the *transverse rectus abdominis myocutaneous (free) flap* (TRAM) transfer, a segment of the rectus abdominis muscle, overlying fat and skin is taken, and its blood supply microsurgically anastomosed to vessels at the site of implantation (e.g., internal mammary vessels).[118, 154] Advantages of this procedure include its successful use in smokers, greater ease of mobility then with conventional pedicled TRAM, and usefulness in patients needing bilateral reconstruction.[118] There is potentially a greater risk of loss of the flap with this procedure, but advancements in microsurgical technique and skill of the surgical team has made this the preferred procedure of many surgeons.[118, 154] The added expense of extended operating room time and hospitalization for the TRAM procedures, over other types of reconstruction, may be offset to an extent with defined clinical pathways that facilitate optimum care for patients,[195] and high patient satisfaction with these procedures.

Augmentation, mastopexy (breast lift), or *reduction* of the remaining breast is sometimes necessary to achieve *symmetry*. This and any further refinements in the reconstructed breast often are completed before or concurrently with the nipple-areolar complex reconstruction.[118] Saving the nipple-areolar complex at the time

of mastectomy for later reconstruction is not recommended. *Skin transfers* (see Table 7–3) have been the primary means of nipple and areola reconstruction. However, newer and more satisfactory techniques involve the raising of a flap of skin from the reconstructed breast mound and folding back sections of the flap to create the projecting nipple.[36, 118, 154] In all patients, *tattooing* of the nipple-areolar complex usually follows to achieve color symmetry.[36, 118] Figure 7–5 illustrates optimal reconstructive results.

Radiation Therapy

Radiation therapy has localized effects on breast cancer. As such it has a role in combination with other therapies, or sometimes alone, as adjuvant treatment of local/regional disease, and for local/regional advanced or metastatic disease. In the past, radiotherapy was routinely used after a modified radical mastectomy to decrease the risk of local/regional disease recurrence. Now this is primarily reserved for patients who have a high risk for local recurrence of the disease, specifically those women whose deep surgical margin of resection is involved, or those with tumors greater than 5 cm in size with four or more positive nodes.[156, 168]

Radiation therapy in conjunction with breast-conserving surgery is administered to achieve local control of disease, or reduce the risk of local recurrence, in women with early stage (I or II) invasive breast cancer. Multiple randomized clinical trials comparing mastectomy with breast-conserving surgery followed by radiation to the whole breast have demonstrated equivalence in terms of overall survival.[101, 123, 391] In stage IIIA disease, preoperative chemotherapy often shrinks the primary tumor enough to allow these women to undergo breast-conserving surgery and radiation. For women with DCIS, radiation has been shown to reduce the risk of subsequent invasive tumor growth.[121, 156, 392]

External beam radiotherapy usually begins by 2 to 4 weeks, and no later than 12 weeks, after surgery.[156, 391, 392] However, some women with invasive breast cancer will be advised to have adjuvant chemotherapy prior to radiation. Treatment planning for radiotherapy is done to ensure homogeneity of dose through consistent reproducible positioning of the patient and the use of supervoltage equipment.[391] Each field is treated daily, Monday through Friday, to a total whole-breast dose of 4500 to 5000 centigrays (cGy), or rads, at 180 to 200 cGy per fraction, over 4 to 5 weeks.[391, 392] A radiation boost to the original tumor site is given when surgical margins are involved or close after segmental mastectomy for invasive breast cancer,[391] and often for women with DCIS. This remains controversial, however, particularly for women with DCIS.[391, 392] The boost dose can be delivered by two methods: electron beam (external

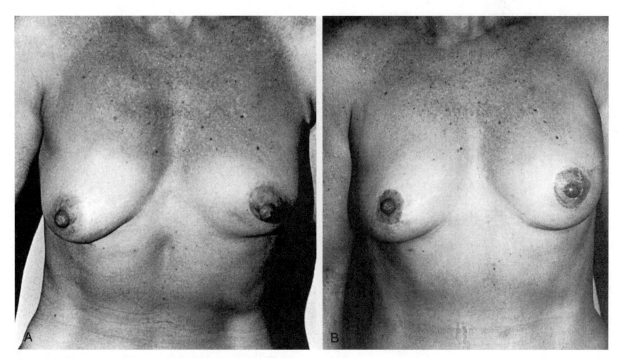

FIGURE 7–5   Breast reconstruction results. (From: McCraw JB and others: Breast reconstruction following mastectomy. In Bland KI and Copeland EM, editors: *The breast: comprehensive management of benign and malignant diseases,* ed 2, vol 2, p. 989, Philadelphia, WB Saunders, 1998.)

boost) or interstitial implants. The latter requires a short hospital stay. The external boost is generally preferred because of cost, convenience, and cosmesis. The boost increases the total dose to the primary tumor site to 6000 to 6600 cGy.[391, 392] Radiation to the axilla is not given after a diagnosis of DCIS, or to women with a diagnosis of invasive breast cancer if a level I and II axillary node dissection or sentinel lymph node biopsy has been done.[391, 392] Radiotherapy to the supraclavicular area is recommended after breast-conserving surgery when four or more lymph nodes are involved.[391] Further research is needed to determine if there are subgroups of women who do not need postoperative radiotherapy and/or a boost dose.[273]

For patients with locally advanced disease or unable to undergo a surgical procedure, radiotherapy may be used alone or in conjunction with chemotherapy and hormone therapy. In metastatic cancer, radiation therapy is palliative for painful bony metastases, shrinks metastatic brain lesions or tumors compressing the spinal cord, and relieves the symptoms of superior vena cava syndrome.

The toxicities associated with radiation therapy are generally mild and reversible. They include local skin changes, generalized fatigue, pain related to temporary inflammation of the nerves or the pectoral muscles in the radiation field, and occasionally sore throat. Extended axillary irradiation can aggravate lymphedema and range-of-motion difficulties. (For a more detailed dis-

cussion of the radiation-associated toxicities and specific nursing interventions, see Chapter 22 and the Complications box).

Systemic Therapy

Systemic treatment of breast cancer involves the use of chemotherapy or endocrine manipulation to treat patients with (1) axillary node involvement, (2) poor prognosis, node-negative disease, (3) advanced local/regional disease, or (4) distant metastases. The specific therapy recommended is influenced by the prognostic factors discussed earlier and the patient's general medical condition. Dosages used and the duration of therapy vary. Table 7–4 lists some common chemotherapy regimens used in adjuvant therapy, as well as individual drugs active in metastatic disease.

Adjuvant Chemotherapy. Breast cancer can spread not only to axillary nodes but also to distant sites through the bloodstream. A percentage of women will therefore have micrometastases at diagnosis. Adjuvant chemotherapy or hormone therapy (or both) to prevent or delay the development of metastatic disease has been in clinical use and studied in clinical trials for the past 30 years. It is given after the definitive surgical treatment while the tumor burden is small (suspected micrometastases) and the cells are least likely to become drug resistant. Clinical trials have clearly demonstrated that adju-

COMPLICATIONS

Breast Cancer Disease and Treatment

Disease Related	Treatment Related
Local/Regional Recurrence	**Surgery**
	Impaired wound healing/ seroma
Ulceration	Nerve injury
Lymphedema	Lymphedema
Brachial plexopathy	Shoulder dysfunction
Distant Recurrence	**Radiation Therapy**
Spinal cord compression	Skin reactions
Brain/leptomeningeal metastases	Lymphedema
Hypercalcemia	Shoulder dysfunction
Pathologic fractures	Marrow suppression
Pleural effusion	Fatigue
Lymphangitic spread	
Pericardial effusion/tamponade	**Chemotherapy**
Superior vena cava syndrome	Marrow suppression (bleeding/sepsis)
	Stomatitis
	Anorexia/nausea/ vomiting
	Extravasation/skin necrosis
	Hemorrhagic cystitis

vant chemotherapy delays recurrence and improves disease-free and overall survival in women with early stage disease, particularly those under age 50 but also those 50 to 69 years of age, those with estrogen negative tumors, and those with higher-risk tumors and negative lymph nodes.*

There is no one optimal drug combination, treatment schedule, or duration of therapy for all patients, although some general guidelines have been established. Since 1985, the National Institutes of Health (NIH) has gathered panels of experts to evaluate the results of adjuvant clinical trials and to make treatment recommendations.[277, 278] For example, clinical trials to date have resulted in a gradual decrease in the total length of time recommended for adjuvant chemotherapy, to the current duration of 4 to 6 months as suitable for most patients.[102, 181, 289] The regimens most often used in adjuvant therapy contain a combination of *cyclophosphamide* (C), *methotrexate* (M) or an anthracycline such as *doxorubicin* (A), and *5-fluorouracil* (F).[102, 289] (see Table 7–4). Studies in progress will determine if the

---

* References 102, 156, 181, 278, 289, 404.

addition of a taxane (*paclitaxel* or *docetaxel*) to traditional adjuvant chemotherapy regimens, such as AC (doxorubicin and cyclophosphamide), enhances the disease-free and overall survival.[50, 156, 191, 289, 312] Trastuzumab (Herceptin), useful in the treatment of women with metastatic breast cancer whose tumors overexpress the her-2/*neu* protein, is not indicated in adjuvant therapy outside of a clinical trial.[289] Dose intensity of traditional adjuvant chemotherapy regimens and the optimum scheduling of adjuvant therapy remain under investigation.[57, 102, 156, 289]

In general, panel recommendations are made for treatment of patients not enrolled in a clinical trial. Consensus panel reports for treatment of early stage breast cancer in 1998 and prior years have addressed adjuvant therapy for subsets of women.[156, 277, 278, 404] Table 7–5 summarizes current standard practice recommendations for women not registered in a clinical trial. These recommendations primarily consider menopausal status, lymph nodes, and ER status, although for women with node-negative disease histologic or nuclear grade as well as age and possibly lymphatic or vascular inva-

TABLE 7–4
Major Chemotherapy Regimens for Breast Cancer

ADJUVANT THERAPY Acronym (usual duration)	Drugs
CMF (~6 mo)	cyclophosphamide (Cytoxan) methotrexate 5-fluorouracil (5-FU)
AC (~3–4 mo)	doxorubicin (Adriamycin) cyclophosphamide (Cytoxan)
CAF or FAC (~4–6 mo)	cyclophosphamide (Cytoxan) doxorubicin (Adriamycin) 5-fluorouracil (5-FU)
AC + T (~6–8 mo)	doxorubicin and cyclophosphamide followed by paclitaxel (Taxol)

RECURRENT OR METASTATIC DISEASE

In addition to those listed under Adjuvant Therapy, the following drugs have proven activity in breast cancer alone or in combination for recurrent or metastatic disease, or in high-dose therapy with peripheral blood stem cell transplant:

capecitabine	gemcitabine
carboplatin	mitomycin C
carmustine	mitoxantrone
cisplatin	thiotepa
docetaxel (Taxotere)	trastuzumab (Herceptin)
epirubicin	vinblastine
etoposide	vinorelbine

Note: Concurrent or sequential tamoxifen may also be recommended as adjuvant therapy or for treatment of recurrent or metastatic disease.

Data from references 57, 102, 103, 107, 156, 181, 289, and 290.

TABLE 7–5

Summary of Recommendations for Adjuvant Breast Cancer Therapy for Patients Not Enrolled in Clinical Trials (Invasive Cancer)

NODE NEGATIVE

Menopausal Status	Hormone Receptor Status	Adjuvant Treatment
Low Risk (≤1 cm, receptor positive, low grade, age > 35 y)		
Premenopausal	Positive	None or tamoxifen
Postmenopausal	Positive	None or tamoxifen
Elderly	Positive or negative	None or tamoxifen
Intermediate Risk (>1–2 cm, receptor positive, low to intermediate grade)		
Premenopausal	Positive	Tamoxifen ± chemotherapy
Postmenopausal	Positive	Tamoxifen ± chemotherapy
Elderly	Positive or negative	Tamoxifen (± chemotherapy*)
High Risk (>2 cm, or receptor negative, or intermediate to high grade, or age < 35 y)		
Premenopausal	Positive	Chemotherapy + tamoxifen
	Negative	Chemotherapy
Postmenopausal	Positive	Tamoxifen + chemotherapy
	Negative	Chemotherapy
Elderly	Positive or negative	Tamoxifen (vs. chemotherapy if no ER/PR expression)

NODE POSITIVE

Menopausal Status	Tumor Size	Hormone Receptor Status	Adjuvant Treatment
Premenopausal	Any	Positive	Chemotherapy + tamoxifen
	Any	Negative	Chemotherapy
Postmenopausal	Any	Positive	Tamoxifen alone, or with chemotherapy
	Any	Negative	Chemotherapy (± tamoxifen*)
Elderly	Any	Positive	Tamoxifen (vs. chemotherapy if no ER/PR expression)

* Area of controversy, under investigation. The above summary may be revised as more research data become available. Note that some physicians will determine treatment based on additional prognostic factors, such as DNA content (ploidy) and S phase (measure of cell division). For those situations when treatment is not well defined, patients should carefully review the risks and benefits of any treatment plan with their physician.

Data from references 102, 103, 156, 277, 278, and 289.

sion are important factors.[156] The value of using her-2/*neu* overexpression as a determinant of responsiveness to anthracyclines needs further study.[156]

In the past, patients with negative nodes were considered to have a good prognosis and no additional therapy after surgery was recommended. The report of the 1990 NIH Consensus Conference, in summarizing the knowledge to date, recommended that outside of participation in a clinical trial, women with negative lymph nodes should be made aware of the risks and benefits of adjuvant chemotherapy based on current knowledge so as to be able to make an informed decision about such treatment.[277] However, evidence now suggests that some of these patients will develop recurrent disease. The difficulty through the years has been determining who these women are, the long-term toxicities, and the risk/benefit ratio for these women.[181, 404] The International Consensus Panel on the Treatment of Primary Breast Cancer concluded that all women, including those with negative lymph nodes, who have a greater than 10% risk of relapse are candidates for adjuvant systemic therapy.[156, 404] Supplemental information to the earlier NIH consensus

statement suggests chemotherapy be considered in women with node-negative, ER-negative tumors, as well as in combination with tamoxifen for women with node-negative, ER-positive tumors.[278]

In general, women who will most clearly benefit from systemic chemotherapy with or without endocrine therapy are those with positive lymph nodes regardless of age and premenopausal women with larger tumors regardless of lymph node status.[102, 156, 181] Women at low risk of relapse, those with tumors less than 1 cm in diameter and negative lymph nodes, probably do not warrant adjuvant chemotherapy outside of a clinical trial. Further studies in progress will identify the specific subsets of patients who need adjuvant chemotherapy and the most appropriate regimen.[156, 181, 277, 278, 289]

The medical decision to recommend adjuvant therapy and the patient's decision to receive it can be complex and difficult. As with decisions about the type of surgical procedure, patients need help understanding the concept of adjuvant therapy and information about the benefits and risks.[308, 311, 313, 370] Although increased numbers of women have been given the opportunity to participate in clinical trials through the Community Clinical Oncology Programs (CCOP), emphasis should still be placed on participation by women and their physicians in clinical trials. Clinical trials continue to evaluate the benefits of perioperative chemotherapy (begun within hours after surgery), neoadjuvant therapy (administered for a period before surgery), short-course intensive chemotherapy, and high-dose chemotherapy with peripheral blood stem cell transplant (discussed later in this chapter).[57, 102, 120, 156, 289]

Adjuvant Endocrine Therapy. *Selective estrogen receptor modulators,* or *SERMs,* are those antiestrogen drugs that have both estrogen-like positive effects on some tissues (e.g., bone and cardiovascular tissues) and estrogen-blocking effects in other tissues (e.g., breast).[106, 107] Tamoxifen is the standard SERM used in adjuvant therapy today. Tamoxifen binds to ER sites in breast cancer cells, thereby blocking the uptake of estrogen necessary for cell proliferation. Tamoxifen delays recurrence in women who have had breast cancer, irrespective of menopausal status or age.[103] Tamoxifen also reduces the incidence of cancers in the opposite breast for all women with a history of breast cancer.[103] In the presence of ER-positive tumors, regardless of lymph node status, women have the greatest potential benefit from tamoxifen. This benefit is increased further when tamoxifen is combined with adjuvant chemotherapy, particularly for premenopausal women but also for older women.[278] The optimal duration and sequencing of treatment of tamoxifen has yet to be established, although current studies indicate the optimal duration of tamoxifen appears to be 5 years.[103, 156, 278] Continuing tamoxifen beyond 5 years is not currently recommended because it does not appear to give any additional benefit.[181, 278]

Tamoxifen is taken orally and has few toxicities. All patients receiving tamoxifen need to be monitored for side effects, which may be disruptive enough to cause a woman to discontinue therapy. Primarily these consist of hot flashes, gynecologic problems (e.g., vaginal discharge, irritation, or dryness), impaired sexual functioning and, more so for women over 50, an increased risk of uterine cancer and of thrombolytic events.[85, 103, 120, 122, 181] A potential benefit from tamoxifen use is an improvement in bone density for postmenopausal women and a reduction in low-density lipoproteins (LDLs).[103, 289]

Treatment of Advanced Disease. Certain patients with features of *locally advanced* disease may be considered inoperable at diagnosis. This includes tumors with direct extension to the chest wall or skin, large palpable axillary nodes, skin ulceration, and inflammatory changes (stage IIIB, some stage IIIA). Although potentially resectable with radical mastectomy, the local recurrence rate is high, and in most patients, overall survival is poor at 5 years even with additional therapy.[32] Some, but not all, of these patients will have distant metastases at the time of diagnosis and need laboratory and radiologic evaluation to rule this out. Patients with locally advanced disease benefit from preoperative combination chemotherapy, with or without endocrine therapy, followed by radiation therapy or surgical intervention or both for local control.[186] The presence of supraclavicular or infraclavicular nodes or large, nonmovable axillary nodes at the initial diagnosis, and response to chemotherapy will determine whether the subsequent treatment is radiation therapy alone, modified radical mastectomy with radiation therapy, or segmental mastectomy with radiation therapy. For many women with stage III disease, a good response to preoperative chemotherapy will enable breast-conserving surgery. Systemic therapy is usually resumed after surgery. The optimum therapy for locally advanced disease still has not been determined despite improved responses with this sequential therapy.[186]

The goal of therapy in metastatic disease is control of the disease and palliation of symptoms. Metastatic breast cancer is incurable with either chemotherapy or hormone manipulation. These modalities are able to achieve temporary regression of the disease in a majority of patients, but these responses rarely last a long time. Overall, the mean survival after the development of metastatic disease is less than 2 years.[107, 310] However, 5% to 10% of these patients may be alive at 5 years, and a smaller percentage will become long-term survivors and may be cured.[13, 107, 178]

Women with receptor-positive cancers have more potentially beneficial treatment options available to them than those with receptor-negative cancers. Those whose recurrence occurs 5 years or more after the initial diagnosis generally have a more favorable outcome from treatment.[107] Local/regional, soft-tissue, and bony recurrences that are not life-threatening are generally treated with endocrine therapy first. Radiation therapy may be used for local or symptomatic control. For more aggressive disease (liver, lymphangitic lung disease, and widespread, painful bony metastases), frontline treatment is chemotherapy. The regimen selected may be one of those listed in Table 7–4; selection is based on prior adjuvant treatment, prior response, and current physical condition.[107]

Chemotherapy. Responses to combination drug therapy occur in approximately 50% to 75% of patients.[107, 310] These responses generally last from 6 to 12 months.[352] Doxorubicin (Adriamycin) is the most effective single agent in the treatment of metastatic breast cancer.[107, 352] Other active single agents typically used initially in combination regimens may include cyclophosphamide, methotrexate, 5-fluorouracil, mitoxantrone, vinorelbine, or the taxanes (paclitaxel/Taxol, docitaxel/Taxotere), or the monoclonal antibody, trastuzamab (Herceptin), for women whose tumors overexpress her-2/*neu*.[107, 352] Once initial therapy for distant metastases fails, subsequent treatment regimens may include epirubicin, mitoxantrone, vinblastine, gemcitabine, mitomycin C, etoposide, and capecitabine.[107] Because there is no "standard" therapy for metastatic disease, new approaches are regularly being tested in phases II and III research. Examples include non–cross-resistant therapy, new phase II agents, standard versus intensified dose therapy, intensive chemotherapy and autologous bone marrow transplantation, chemoendocrine combinations, weekly low-dose chemotherapy, and continuous infusion regimens.

High-Dose Chemotherapy and Transplant. For women with locally advanced ($\geq$10 positive lymph nodes) or metastatic breast cancer, chemotherapy options are less effective and potentially associated with more myelosuppressive toxicity. This may be improved if the patient's own bone marrow is removed before high-dose treatment and reinfused after treatment, as with *autologous bone marrow transplant* (ABMT) or when the patient's peripheral blood stem cells are harvested and later reinfused (*peripheral stem cell transplant* [PSCT]). The addition of *granulocyte* and *granulocyte/macrophage colony-stimulating factors* (G-CSF and GM-CSF) to the treatment regimen has enabled more rapid recovery and reduced toxicities associated with myelosuppression. Based on initial studies that showed a favorable impact on disease-free survival in women with metastatic disease, several randomized phase III clinical trials have been initiated to evaluate the effectiveness of ABMT or PSCT in comparison with standard chemotherapy regimens in patients with metastatic disease, and in patients with several lymph nodes involved. PSCT is also being studied as initial adjuvant therapy in women with stage II or III disease in phase II studies. Preliminary results for studies of ABMT in metastatic disease or PSCT in metastatic or locally advanced disease have been too preliminary to draw firm conclusions about the benefits or limitations of either therapy in comparison with traditional treatments.[300] PSCT appears to have lower costs, morbidity, and mortality and thus may be preferred to ABMT for patients with locally advanced or metastatic disease.[14] Quality of life has been reported as relatively high for women undergoing PSCT,[393] but similar to that of women receiving traditional chemotherapy.[300] Problems in sexual functioning were commonly reported by women one year after PSCT.[393]

For PSCT, most treatment is conducted on an outpatient basis, with the patient and family closely involved in the procedures. The patient and significant other(s) need to remain close to the treatment facility. An experienced multidisciplinary transplant team that can ensure 24-hour access for patients is critical for the success of PSCT.[44, 49, 331] After a prescreening evaluation, medical evaluation, and insurance approval, the treatment begins with an alkylating agent followed by a series of self-injections of G-CSF or GM-CSF. These serve to "mobilize" the stem cells from the bone marrow into the peripheral circulation. Cells are harvested from the patient peripherally in a procedure known as *apheresis*. Several aphereses are performed over a projected number of days to achieve an adequate volume of cells.[44, 331] Dose-intensive chemotherapy is then administered, followed by the infusion of the PSCT. White blood cell and platelet counts usually return to normal within 2 weeks.[44] Patients are then monitored closely on an outpatient basis for possible complications in the 2 to 3 weeks after PSCT. Many patients will return to their primary care physician or oncologist for further follow-up. Until further research results are available, eligible patients should be informed about the availability of this treatment option only in the context of a randomized clinical trial.[156] As with adjuvant therapy, decisions about treatment for locally advanced and metastatic disease can be very difficult. In one study breast cancer survivors were asked to consider a hypothetical situation of having their disease recur and needing to decide about treatment. The women were given projections about toxicities and increases in life expectancies with each treatment. Only 10% of these breast cancer survivors said they would want to be in a clinical trial where they would be randomized to receive PSCT or traditional chemotherapy.[260] More information about transplantation can be found in Chapter 25.

Hormonal Manipulation. The ability to quantify ERs and PRs in breast cancer cells has allowed oncologists to predict with greater accuracy which women might respond to hormone manipulation. Patients with tumors that are both ER- and PR-positive respond to hormone manipulation about 75% of the time, whereas only 10% of receptor-negative patients will respond.[161] A variety of hormonal manipulation approaches are available, but most types of therapy require several weeks to be effective. Therefore in women with life-threatening liver, lung, or brain metastases, chemotherapy will likely be preferred. The dosage and duration of these therapies vary.

Tamoxifen is the primary SERM used as treatment for all women with metastatic disease, but particularly those with receptor-positive tumors. Newer SERMS under investigation for use in metastatic disease still do not appear to be as effective as tamoxifen. For premenopausal women, *ovarian ablation,* to reduce the level of circulating estrogens available to stimulate breast cancer cells, may be preferred initially or may follow tamoxifen.[107, 181, 215] This can be achieved with bilateral *oophorectomy* (removal of the ovaries) or with luteinizing hormone-releasing (LHRH) agonists (leuprolide, goserelin).[107] Recent studies have shown that tamoxifen and oophorectomy are equally effective in treating premenopausal women with distant metastases, but tamoxifen is perhaps safer and more tolerable.[107, 181] Therefore tamoxifen will usually be selected as first-line therapy for metastatic disease in premenopausal patients as well.[181]

Progression after tamoxifen or oophorectomy usually requires a sequential trial of other endocrine therapies. Metastatic tumors that have responded to one form of hormone therapy are more likely to respond to another type of hormone therapy if there is a recurrence or progression of disease.[161, 181] Simply discontinuing a form of therapy may result in a "withdrawal response," with subsequent shrinkage of a tumor or metastatic disease.[107, 181] For the postmenopausal woman who has progression of disease while on tamoxifen, the next treatment choice might be a *selective aromatase inhibitor (SAI)*. SAIs are drugs that suppress postmenopausal estrogen levels by inhibiting an enzyme, aromatase, necessary for estrogen production. This enzyme is more prevalent in breast tissue after menopause and in breast cancer tissue.[107] Nonsteroidal SAIs include anastrozole and letrozole. Exemestane and formestane are two examples of steroidal SAIs in clinical trials.[107] Side effects of SAIs include fatigue, nausea and vomiting, headache.[107, 160] Aminoglutethimide, one of the earlier SAIs, has proven effectiveness after progression of disease on tamoxifen, but has less selective action in the tissues and therefore more toxic side effects including glucocorticoid deficiency.[107] Other side effects include lethargy, dizziness, skin rash, nausea/vomiting, and cushingoid symptoms.[215] SAIs alone are contraindicated in premenopausal women with metastatic breast cancer, because the effect of inhibited estrogen production in the ovaries can lead to polycystic ovaries and masculinization from excess androgen production.[107]

Progestins might be the next step for premenopausal women whose disease has progressed after an initial response to tamoxifen and ovarian ablation.[107, 181, 215] Progestins are also used in postmenopausal women after failure on an aromatase inhibitor. The progestins most often used are megestrol acetate (Megace) and medroxyprogesterone acetate (Depo-Provera). Recent studies have shown these drugs to be as effective as other forms of hormone manipulation. The mechanism of action of progestins has not been established. Relatively few side effects are associated with their use; weight gain is the most frequently experienced side effect, but there is also an increased risk of thromboembolic events.[107, 215] *Estrogens* such as diethylstilbestrol (DES) can also re-

sult in tumor regressions in postmenopausal women. High doses of estrogen act at the level of the hypothalamus to inhibit the release of luteinizing hormone, which normally stimulates the ovaries to produce estrogen. These drugs may be as effective as tamoxifen but are associated with significant side effects (nausea, vomiting, anorexia, vaginal bleeding, breast engorgement, edema) and are contraindicated in patients with a cardiac or thromboembolic disorder.[107, 181, 215]

Androgens, or male hormones, are less effective than estrogens or tamoxifen.[181] Testosterone and fluoxymesterone (Halotestin) have been evaluated, but fluoxymesterone is preferred. The exact mechanism of action of androgens is unknown. Side effects are minimal, but the usefulness of these compounds is limited because of the unacceptability of masculinizing effects (facial and body hair, deepening of the voice, alopecia). The flare response and hypercalcemia have been associated more frequently with androgen therapy than with any other endocrine therapy.[215]

With any endocrine therapy, but primarily those with the positive effects of estrogen, "flare reaction" may occur during the first few days to weeks of treatment. The most frequent symptom of a flare reaction is abrupt onset of diffuse musculoskeletal aching, increased pain at sites of known disease, erythema at sites of skin metastases, or hypercalcemia.[107, 181] Hypercalcemia is the most serious manifestation of a flare reaction. This reaction should not be confused with progressive disease and is not an indication of therapeutic response. The endocrine therapy should be continued unless the calcium levels exceed 14 mg/dL. A transient elevation of tumor markers (e.g., CA15-3 or CA27.29) may also occur in the first month or two, in response to endocrine therapy.[107, 181] Women receiving all endocrine therapies as well as postablative therapies (e.g., adrenalectomy, hypophysectomy) must be monitored for this reaction, reassured, and provided treatment for their symptoms. *Bisphosphanates* (e.g., pamidronate, clodronate) for the treatment of metastasis to bone may provide symptomatic relief of pain and reduce the risk of pathologic fractures, hypercalcemia, spinal cord compression, or need for radiation therapy, but they do not independently affect overall survival and have no proven efficacy in prevention of bone metastasis.[182] Current trials of endocrine therapy in patients with metastatic disease include different agents alone or in combination with other therapies such as chemotherapy or biologic response modifiers.[107, 215]

CONCLUSION

Breast cancer presents nurses with many challenges along a continuum of prevention, early detection, treatment, and survival. The nurse must be knowledgeable about breast cancer and its ever-changing management; honest, realistic, and creative when providing support and care; skilled at symptom management; attentive to the patient's concerns within the context of the family or significant others; and ready to involve oneself in the professional and lay communities to promote breast health for all. Breast health care for elderly women will continue to be a particular concern as the female population ages. Early detection outreach to socioeconomically disadvantaged women will also be a focus of breast cancer control efforts, with potential for significant benefit in reducing the number of deaths from breast cancer. Nurses have a pivotal role in all these areas.

Nursing Management

This section discusses selected nursing diagnoses and interventions. Further nursing diagnoses and interventions are based on patient age, clinical history, specific problems and concerns, other current physical and psychosocial problems, visual or auditory deficits, educational level, cultural influences, language, coping strategies, prior experience with illness, social support, and specific treatment goals and options planned. The role of nursing along a continuum of health care experiences for the woman at risk for or diagnosed with breast cancer is described by Thomas[372] and is reflected here in the discussion of phases of care.

PREDIAGNOSTIC PHASE

Nurses who work in public health clinics or other ambulatory care settings have many opportunities to interact with women who are entering the health care system for routine screening procedures. A valuable role for nurses is to offer public education programs on breast health and to reinforce the positive health care maintenance behaviors of individual women. When a woman notices a change in her breast, when her health care provider finds a palpable mass, or when she receives a report of an abnormal mammogram, anxiety and fear are likely to follow.[88] Taking further action to learn the nature of the abnormality requires participation by the woman with her health care provider. Thomas[372] described many factors that might influence a woman's actions during this time, such as usual coping style, experience with the health care system, beliefs about cancer, and cultural background. Access to the health care system and the services necessary, a problem for elderly and socioeconomically disadvantaged persons, could result in a delay in diagnosis.* Denial or lack of understanding of the significance of a symptom,[12, 54, 111, 112, 372] fear or fatalistic beliefs[111, 303] may also be causes for delay. High optimism and expectations for positive outcomes may enhance care seeking for a breast problem.[228] Prior experience with breast problems or knowledge of other women who have had breast problems or breast cancer may also affect a woman's response, favorably or unfavorably. Nurses can be strong advocates for women seeking breast cancer screening or evaluation of a new symptom.

DIAGNOSTIC PHASE

When a procedure is indicated to evaluate an abnormality, a woman may experience anxiety, fear, and even anticipatory grieving over the threat of the diagnosis of cancer and loss of the breast. Diagnostic procedures and tests can be overwhelming and frightening.[29] Simply waiting for test results may seem unbearable. The stress at this time is also experienced by significant others.[280, 285] The main components of nursing care during this phase include (1) preparation of the patient for the procedures/tests, both physically and emotionally; (2) creation of a positive and supportive environment; and (3) provision of adequate information and resources to address patient and family concerns.[86, 210, 233, 285]

Nursing Diagnosis

- *Anxiety related to fear of diagnosis of breast cancer*

Outcome Goals

- Anxiety will be manageable so that patient will complete the diagnostic work-up.
- Patients without a cancer diagnosis will have a plan of care that prepares them for early detection of cancer and reduces anxiety as much as possible.
- Patients with a diagnosis of cancer will be supported in adjusting to the next phase of care.

Interventions

- Explain, in patient's primary language or with the aid of an interpreter, the purpose, preparation, and steps of procedures required for diagnosis (mam-

---

* References 110, 111, 130, 226, 227, 385.

mography, ultrasound, FNA, stereotactic or needle localization biopsy, excisional biopsy).[337] Include significant others as appropriate and as directed by patient.

- Provide literature that is culturally sensitive and at the appropriate reading level for the patient, as indicated.
- Allow patient (and significant other) to ventilate fears and concerns regarding possible malignant diagnosis.
- Explain postprocedural care.
- Encourage patient to bring spouse/significant other/friend when returning for test results.
- Be present, if possible, when patient is given test and biopsy results. Continuity of care and a relationship of trust established early in the treatment phase do much to allay anxieties about the health care system.
- Patients who do not have a diagnosis of cancer will need information about follow-up specific to their diagnosis. This may be an opportune time to reinforce instruction in BSE, provide guidelines for follow-up with mammography and CBE, and offer general information about a healthy life-style and cancer risk reduction.[30] Some may need an individualized plan for regular screening. Women with benign proliferative breast disease and/or a strong family history of breast cancer who have concerns about personal breast cancer risk should be referred to appropriate resources for counseling regarding risk.[209, 248]

PREOPERATIVE PERIOD

Patients who have been diagnosed with breast cancer are faced with an onslaught of information that ranges from the basic fact of the diagnosis of cancer to the complexity of choosing a type of surgical procedure with or without a second treatment (radiation therapy), with or without chemotherapy or hormonal therapy, and possibly within the context of a clinical research study. The decision about what to recommend to a patient and how that is subsequently explained to the patient can be equally complex for health care providers. It is important that patients are given adequate information from which they can make informed decisions. Many states now mandate that patients be given information on surgical treatment options. Some insurance providers require second surgical opinions before any elective surgery. Repeated discussions are often necessary to clarify information previously given, but forgotten or not heard because of the high stress levels experienced by women and their significant others during this time.

Responses of women at this time can be quite varied. Some will seek additional information, some will want to defer to the physician's opinion, some may defer to their family or significant other's opinion, and others may be in shock and immobilized temporarily. Most women benefit from some time to think over the information provided, discuss that information with significant others in their support network, and review again with the physician and treatment team.[321, 387] Continuity of care providers is important for the continuity of information provided. A coordinated approach by a multidisciplinary team, and specialized nurses may also be helpful.[3, 135, 371] Potential nursing diagnoses during this time can include (1) anticipatory grieving related to threatened changes in body image, work, or personal role relationships; (2) powerlessness related to inability to control diagnosis and perceived inability to make decisions; and (3) ineffective individual coping. Most women find their coping mechanisms challenged during this time but respond appropriately.

Nursing Diagnosis

- *Powerlessness related to decisional conflict and informational overload regarding breast cancer treatment options and plan of care*

Outcome Goal

Patient will be able to:

- Have adequate information and support to make an informed decision about treatment, involving her significant other(s) as appropriate

Interventions

- Be present with medical team, if possible, when the treatment plan is initially discussed and at subsequent discussions.
- Provide appropriate literature to supplement verbal discussion.
- Clarify information as appropriate.
- Act as liaison between the patient and the medical team.
- Anticipate patient and family concerns and questions and involve significant others as indicated by the patient and her situation.[214, 284, 314, 323] Women often need coaching or reassurance in their interactions with their children and young grandchildren about their diagnosis and treatment.[236, 345] Identification of the social support network of the patient will be helpful throughout treatment.[247, 321, 389]
- Clarify misinformation that women may have or may receive through other sources about breast cancer and its treatment.

- Assist decision-making by helping the patient review the pros and cons of her options and think through how each option would work for her.
- Allow the patient and her significant others to verbalize their concerns openly. Reinforce the normalcy of responses ranging from anger, exhaustion, information-seeking, sadness, fear, and even relief once a decision is made about treatment.
- Consider referral to recovered patients who have undergone a specific treatment, such as breast-conserving surgery with radiation. The Reach to Recovery program of the ACS is one resource.
- Consider referral to professional resources for additional support in coping and adjustment for patients who have unusual difficulty processing the information and who do not follow through with making a treatment decision.

OPERATIVE PHASE

When Thomas[372] described the periods of care in breast cancer in 1978, many women were still undergoing a one-step procedure, waking up after a biopsy only to discover that they had indeed undergone a mastectomy. Fortunately, today this is not the case and women admitted to the hospital for surgical treatment are better prepared. Hospitalization and surgery alone are associated with stressors, such as separation from family, disruption in sense of control, and general anesthesia. Inpatient care is focused on immediate physical care needs including wound and pain management, targeted psychosocial support, and discharge teaching and referrals (e.g., care of drains).[288] Feelings of sadness at the anticipated loss (whether part or all of the breast), a sense of readiness for the surgery, and relief (that the cancer will be removed) are often interspersed postoperatively with concern about the final pathology report and the involvement of lymph nodes.

Wound care and remobilization of the arm are physical tasks of this period.[16] Some controversy exists as to the best time to begin mobilization of the arm and shoulder postoperatively and differences between patients undergoing mastectomy or breast-conserving surgery.[84, 202, 243, 302, 335] Concerns about early mobilization (days 1–2 postoperatively) have been related to the potential for increased drain tube output, delay in drain removal, postdrain seroma formation, and potential for impaired wound healing and infection. Concerns about late mobilization are related to arm and shoulder motion difficulties that may occur when exercise is not begun sooner. Restricted mobility carries the potential risk of later development of a "frozen shoulder." Some postoperative exercise to include flexion and extension of the hand, wrist, and elbow and limited movement for simple activities (eating,

brushing teeth) seem reasonable immediately after surgery, gradually increasing exercises beginning within 3 to 5 days after surgery, designed to regain full range of motion (ROM) of the shoulder joint. Often such exercise programs are designed by a treatment team from nursing, surgery, occupational therapy, and physical therapy.[148] Because surgical admissions are of much shorter duration, much preoperative preparation takes place in the clinic or office setting along with postoperative education.[46] Nurses have an important role not only in educating but in promoting the expression and exploration of feelings by the patient and her spouse or significant other. It is important to include both individuals in the treatment planning and follow-up (see Complications box on page 140 and Patient Teaching Priorities box below).

 PATIENT TEACHING PRIORITIES

Breast Cancer

PREVENTION AND EARLY DETECTION

Risk factors
Breast self-examination
Clinical breast examination
Mammography
Signs and symptoms to report to health care professional (e.g., mass in breast or axilla; dimpling, puckering, and/or scaly skin; spontaneous, persistent nipple discharge)
Follow ACS guidelines for health care examination
Plan of action (appointments, who to call)

TREATMENT OPTIONS

Biopsy procedures
Surgery
    Breast-conserving treatment
    Breast reconstruction
Radiation therapy
Chemotherapy
Hormonal therapy
Clinical trials

DISEASE-RELATED AND TREATMENT-RELATED COMPLICATIONS

Disease recurrence, infection, impaired wound healing, lymphedema, shoulder dysfunction, marrow suppression, alopecia, stomatitis, hemorrhagic cystitis, weight gain, "flare reaction," pain, anorexia

OTHER

Prosthesis options
Support and advocacy groups
Recovery and long-term follow-up

Possible nursing diagnoses during this phase include (1) body image disturbance; (2) risk for infection related to surgical wound and axillary lymph node dissection; (3) impaired physical mobility related to imposed restriction, pain, or fatigue; and (4) anxiety regarding final pathology report.

Nursing Diagnosis

- *Risk for injury (infection, delayed wound healing, immobility), related to surgical wound and impaired lymph drainage secondary to breast cancer surgery, complicated by failure to view and care for wound/drains*

Outcome Goals

Patient will be able to:

- Be free of infection in the postoperative period, without delayed drain removal, excess fluid reaccumulation, or delayed wound healing, and care successfully for her wound at home.
- View her operative site and begin to integrate this into her body image and sense of self, involving her spouse and significant others as appropriate.
- Describe arm care and demonstrate beginning ROM exercises.

Interventions

- Inform patient and family about hospital and surgical routines.
- Describe postoperative activity (positioning and care of the arm on the operative side, drains, pain management, intravenous lines, ambulation) before surgery so that patient will be prepared to participate appropriately.
- Position arm on operative side slightly elevated with flat pillow or folded towel behind upper arm until patient is fully awake and ambulatory. Maintain position when reclining.
- Reinforce importance of early ambulation, coughing, and deep breathing.
- All intravenous access sites or venipunctures should be managed on the nonoperative side.
- Monitor wound for inflammation, tenderness, swelling, or purulent drainage. Change dressing when ordered using aseptic technique.
- Monitor drains and instruct patient simultaneously: intact, secured to the skin or clothing so as not to dangle, color and amount of fluid output.[92]
- Assess patient for level of pain or discomfort, and medicate as ordered.
- Provide information on normal sensory sensations patient will experience postoperatively, such as paresthesias of the inner aspect of the upper arm

and increased skin sensitivity.[223] Some women report that rolling up a small towel or washcloth and placing it in the axilla or between the arm and chest helps alleviate some of the discomfort from immediate postoperative paresthesias. "Phantom breast" experiences have also been reported by women after mastectomy.[223, 238]

- Assess readiness to look at incision, and offer support when patient decides to view the incision. Description of the wound appearance may be helpful to some patients before actual viewing. Discuss possible response of patient's spouse/partner toward viewing the incision and patient's readiness for this.
- Instruct patient in arm care and postsurgical arm exercises (see the box on page 149).[148, 153] This will usually require some type of follow-up in the outpatient setting for the first 6 weeks after surgery, although a program of exercise may need to be continued for up to 6 months for full recovery and flexibility. Examples of recommended exercises include squeezing a ball, brushing the hair, shoulder shrugs and circles, and finger climbing up a wall when facing the wall (standing about 6 inches away) and turned perpendicular to the wall. All exercises should begin gently without the sensation of pain. Gentle stretching of muscles, but not strain, is encouraged. Reach to Recovery volunteers also can demonstrate exercises. Referral to physical therapy may be necessary, if they were not initially involved in the patient's care or the patient's ROM recovery is not progressing.
- Instruct patient in avoidance of strenuous household tasks such as vacuuming, sweeping, moving heavy objects (i.e., more than 10 pounds) until ROM is improved and the surgical wound is healed.
- Instruct patients after mastectomy in the use of a temporary prosthesis, camisole, or bra, and options for symmetry and balance until able to be fitted for a weighted prosthesis or to have reconstruction.

Breast Reconstruction

Preoperative nursing care of the patient who is to undergo immediate or delayed reconstruction focuses on the woman's perceptions and expectations of the specific reconstructive approach chosen. Problems and dissatisfaction can be minimized if the woman has realistic expectations of the procedure. Important aspects to reinforce from the physician's discussions with the patient include the appearance of the reconstructed breast, the type of scar(s), the surgical dressing and wound suction, and the use of a bra. A preoperative or postoperative visit by a woman who has had a successful breast reconstruction can be beneficial.

Arm Exercises after Lymph Node Dissection (Goal: Return to Full Range of Motion)*

Remember: These exercises are to be done slowly, to stretch muscles *gently,* and to return you back to your normal movement. They are not intended to cause pain. However, your muscles in your arm and shoulder may be very tired, stiff, or achy. If you find that you have a lot of tightness or soreness after doing your exercises one day, take it a little easier the next day. Doing these regularly and faithfully is more important than pushing yourself too hard too fast. If you do not do your exercises, you may develop problems with movement that are very difficult to treat.

Do each *four times* a day.

Rest briefly between exercises. Take a slow, deep breath before starting again.

Don't forget to breathe while you are doing the exercises!

You can always use your other arm to assist your weaker arm.

1. Open and close the fingers of your hand on the side of your surgery (make a fist and then relax your fingers). Repeat as often as you like.
2. Sitting, crawl up and down your thigh with your fingers on the surgery side. This should be pretty easy. Repeat as often as you like.
3. Bend and extend your elbow with your arm down at your side. Repeat as often as you like.
4. With your arm extended down at your side, twist your hand/wrist/lower arm in and then out. Repeat three times.
5. Look in the mirror if you can, and shrug your shoulders. See if you are favoring the shoulder on the side of your surgery. Eventually you should be able to raise both shoulders together when you are fully recovered. Shrug your shoulders. Roll your shoulders forward. Relax your shoulders down. Stretch your shoulders back, like a soldier standing at attention. Repeat three times. You may try this in reverse (shoulders up, back, down, forward). You may try this in a rolling motion or circle up, back, down, forward.
6. On the side where you had your surgery, take that hand and put it on your shoulder, like you had a "wing." Draw small circles in the air with your elbow, forward or back. Repeat this three times.
7. Take the hand on the side of your surgery, and crawl up your opposite arm to your shoulder, over your head, and to your other shoulder. Go back the other way. If you get tired during this exercise, rest your hand on your head or shoulder. After a short pause you may be able to continue. If you feel discomfort or fatigue, use your "good" hand to help your weak arm down to your side.
8. Try to reach your hand on the surgery side behind your back at your waist. Bring it back around to the front.

After the drain tube(s) have been removed:
9. "Wall climbing": Always do a few warm-up exercises before you try these.
   a. *Facing the wall.* Face a wall and stand about a foot away from it. Using both hands for balance, crawl or slide with your fingers up the wall, going as far as you can without causing pain. Pause. Take a deep breath and notice how far you have climbed. Crawl or slide back down the wall. Rest a moment and repeat three times. **Caution:** If you get to the top of where you can go, *do not* drop your arms down. Always remember to crawl or slide back down. Goal: To reach all the way up, flat against the wall. You should notice gradual improvement every day.
   b. *With your side facing the wall.* Stand about a foot away from a wall, and crawl or slide your fingers (on the surgery side) up the wall, going as far as you can without causing pain. Pause. Take a deep breath and notice how far you have climbed. Crawl or slide back down the wall. Rest a moment and repeat three times. **Caution:** If you get to the top of where you can go, *do not* drop your arms down. Always remember to crawl or slide back down. Goal: To reach all the way up, flat against the wall. *This is the most difficult exercise and the most important.* You should notice gradual improvement every day.
10. With your hands behind your head, bring your elbows in toward your face, and then back. Repeat this three times.
11. Laying down on a flat surface, bring your arm on the surgery side straight up from your side, and reach over your head. Return your arm to your side. Swimming is a very good exercise to help your recovery. However, you should be able to do this exercise without much difficulty before you get into a pool. Check with your doctor about when you can begin this exercise.

Lifting anything over 10 pounds or vigorous and repeated movement that exerts strain on your arm should not be done until you have fully recovered from your surgery (4–6 weeks). This includes weight training. Ask your doctor about your recovery and if you want to know about beginning or returning to weight training.

If you notice any new swelling or redness in your arm on the side of your surgery and it lasts more than 24 hours, please contact the nurse or doctor's office.

* Note: Confirm with your physician before initiating these exercises.
Data from Harbor-UCLA Medical Center, Torrance, California.

Postoperative care will be dictated by the type of reconstructive procedure performed. Patients receiving breast implants will need to be taught wound care and bandaging, often inclusive of some type of external pressure support, eventual massage of the implants, and a restricted exercise routine (no heavy lifting or stretching for 4–6 weeks). Patients undergoing tissue flap reconstruction will have more critical wound care needs (e.g., major abdominal surgery with the TRAM flap) in the hospital. Attention to skin care is vital because mobility will be restricted in the immediate postoperative period. Further discharge teaching should include the specifics of exercise appropriate to the surgical procedure.

Lymphedema

Lymphedema after breast cancer surgery is the accumulation of lymph fluid in the tissues of the upper extremity, extending from the upper arm and potentially to the hand and fingers. It occurs in 15% to 20% of women who have had an axillary lymph node dissection,[148] although some studies have reported a higher incidence.[301] The risk of developing lymphedema is affected by the extent of lymph node dissection (levels I, II, and III or levels I and II, versus sentinel lymph node biopsy), and radiation therapy to the axilla, but may also be affected by factors such as obesity, poor nutritional status, increased age, and wound infection.[301] It may occur at any time after surgery. It is caused by the interruption or removal of lymph channels and nodes after axillary node dissection or radiation therapy. These procedures result in less efficient filtration of lymph fluid and a pooling of lymphatic fluid in the tissues. Prevention of cosmetic deformity, emotional distress, functional impairment, infection, and discomfort are the goals.[373] Nurses can teach the importance of reporting any swelling or red appearance of the affected arm, or new sensory changes.[80, 301] Intervention should be instituted as soon as lymphedema is noted so as to prevent or reduce the extent of further progression. This includes elevation of the arm, ROM exercises,

not carrying shoulder bags or heavy objects on the affected arm, and prompt attention to unavoidable injuries that break the skin surface (e.g., scratch or dry, irritated skin). Elevation of the arm at rest, complete digestive physiotherapy (which includes a gentle massage known as *manual lymph drainage,* and bandaging), compression garments, and mechanical decompression with a pneumatic pump and arm sleeve are all interventions that may be considered.[41, 193, 301] Once a reduction in the swelling has been achieved, the patient can be fitted for a compression sleeve and gauntlet that provides gradient pressure to the upper extremity from the hand to the shoulder. Assessment of patients with a new onset of lymphedema should also include evaluation for possible infection, injury, or obstructive problems (vein thrombosis or tumor recurrence). The box below lists specific arm care precautions for all patients to prevent trauma and infection in the arm on the operative side.

Arm Care Precautions After Axillary Lymph Node Dissection

Avoid sunburns or heavy sun exposure (and wear sunscreen).

Avoid burns while cooking, baking, or smoking. (Smoking is never a healthy habit!)

Wear protective gloves when gardening.

Use the *unaffected* arm for injections, blood samples, intravenous access, or blood pressure readings.

Use a thimble when sewing.

Watches, jewelry, and clothing should fit loosely on the arm and hand.

Use creams and lotions to keep cuticles soft; do not pull cuticles.

Treat cuts promptly and monitor for signs of infection.

No chemotherapy is to be given in the affected arm.

Consider wearing a compression sleeve and gauntlet with air travel.

Nursing Management

ADJUVANT TREATMENT PHASE

During this period, patients will need continued reinforcement of exercise routines so as to regain full shoulder function. Wound healing will be completed and final pathology reports discussed. Patients face new decisions about adjuvant chemotherapy or hormonal therapy, and additional information needs to be clarified. Making a decision about treatment that potentially has side effects when one feels well is not easy. The discussion earlier in this chapter regarding patient decision-making is also relevant here. Many women will be receiving chemotherapy after surgery, before having radiation therapy. Patients undergoing breast-conserving surgery who do not need chemotherapy will go on to radiation therapy. Some women will be starting on hormonal therapy with tamoxifen.

The transition to this therapy phase and its completion constitute another important intervention period for nurses.[96] Sociocultural and psychosocial factors continue to be important throughout a physical treatment phase.[149, 187] The impact of the diagnosis and treatment may be felt more fully during this time not only by the patient but also by her spouse/significant other and family members. The patient and her family may face new challenges to work and role relationships and to functioning.[183, 255, 270] Interventions during this time are directed toward reducing the psychological and physiologic distress these women experience.

Possible nursing diagnoses during this period include (1) risk for infection secondary to chemotherapy, (2) impaired skin integrity related to radiation therapy[306]; (3) fatigue related to radiation or chemotherapy treatments, limiting energy and usual exercise routine[37, 395]; (4) body image disturbance related to surgery, alopecia, weight gain or loss; (5) sexual dysfunction related to decreased/absent vaginal secretions related to chemotherapy-induced or hormone therapy-induced ovarian suppression; (6) altered role performance related to disruption in life and work patterns secondary to treatments; (7) knowledge deficit related to chemotherapy side effects; and (8) anxiety related to completion of adjuvant therapy and transition to a regular follow-up schedule.[240]

Nursing Diagnosis

- *Anxiety related to fear of side effects of additional treatment with chemotherapy or radiation therapy and to impact on resumption of usual activities in social and family life*

Outcome Goal

Patient will be able to:

- Complete adjuvant therapy as close to schedule as possible with successful management of side effects and changes in role or daily activities

Interventions

- Explain rationale for adjuvant systemic therapy.
- Promote participation in breast cancer treatment clinical trials as appropriate.
- Describe specific treatment regimen schedule, route(s) of administration, anticipated side effects, and prevention or management of side effects.[27, 146]
- For premenopausal women, discuss effects of chemotherapy on menstrual function: irregularities, amenorrhea, and potential for pregnancy, with options for birth control while undergoing treatment.[217]
- Provide postmenopausal women or premenopausal women undergoing tamoxifen therapy with information about potential side effects such as hot flashes and vaginal discharge and dryness.[295] Tell patients to report such symptoms and provide subsequent guidance on the management of these problems.
- Emphasize and monitor compliance with the proposed treatment regimen.
- Monitor for potential side effects of treatment and intervene appropriately.
- Monitor for potential shoulder dysfunction secondary to a decrease in exercises.[167, 205, 256] Also, assess involvement in other exercise activities. Weight gain is a common problem during standard adjuvant chemotherapy.[90, 158]
- Assist patient and her significant other in identifying real or imagined barriers that may influence resumption of normal sexual relations.[145]
- Assist patient in locating resources for support, such as specifically targeted breast cancer patient support groups,[113, 179, 321] resources for fitting for a breast prosthesis, or other programs in the community.[53, 202] The benefits of exercise during treatment have also been described.[267, 336, 338] Adjuvant treatment and onset of menopause predict weight gain after a breast cancer diagnosis.
- Encourage discussion of other psychosocial concerns, such as role functions in the home, return to work, vocational retraining, and family and social relationships.

- Patients may need assistance in identifying their emotional strengths, sources of support, and positive qualities separate from their appearance, at a time when they are feeling vulnerable, threatened, and undesirable. Facilitating open communication between the patient and her partner can be very helpful in the couple's adjustment to the cancer diagnosis and treatment. Referral to appropriate resources may be indicated.
- For other specific interventions for patients undergoing radiation therapy and chemotherapy, see Chapters 22 and 23, respectively.

RECOVERY, REHABILITATION, AND LONG-TERM FOLLOW-UP PHASE

During this period, the patient is adjusting to the completion of chemotherapy or radiation therapy and may still be receiving tamoxifen therapy. The patient often has feelings of loss and anxiety associated with stopping adjuvant therapy or the fear that stopping such therapy may somehow allow the cancer to return. The patient, now free from regular frequent medical visits and perhaps beginning to feel more physically well again, faces a potential return to more usual patterns of living. The majority of women who were employed before the diagnosis of breast cancer will return to work.[67, 324] This is usually not without some difficulty, however, including concerns about how coworkers will respond, her own ability to withstand work pressures, or physically being able to work the same schedule or type of work.[55, 67, 255] Loss of a job and loss of insurance benefits are of even greater concern now than in the past. Job discrimination is also a real fear for those seeking employment.[55, 67] Although discrimination against disabled persons is prohibited by The Federal Rehabilitation Act of 1973 and the Americans with Disabilities Act (ADA), some courts have decided that recovered cancer patients are not disabled (see Chapter 32). The ADA specifically addresses persons who had or have cancer, providing some legal protection for them against employment discrimination by any private employer with 15 or more employees.[148] However, discrimination is not always so obvious. *Reintegration* describes the process of assisting women with a history of breast cancer to return to work through a program with their employers and organizations that is directed to understanding the needs of each and how to work together.[55, 67] Women who find that new employment is necessary may find help in vocational rehabilitation, often available through state or private industry programs.

After standard adjuvant chemotherapy is completed, some premenopausal will not resume menstrual function. The older a woman's age, (35–40 years and older), the greater the risk of premature menopause.[159, 245] Some women who resume normal menstrual function after treatment will want to get pregnant. Most studies of women who became pregnant after successful treatment of breast cancer have found that pregnancy did not negatively influence survival. However, this topic has many issues that have been reviewed in the literature, including concern that the increased hormonal activity with pregnancy will cause a return of the breast cancer.[97, 152, 174] Reproductive techniques that assist conception (e.g., in vitro fertilization) may have similar risks but these are unknown.[152] Because the greatest risk for recurrence of breast cancer is in the first 1 to 2 years after diagnosis, some women may be advised to delay pregnancy until after that time. This solution may not be reasonable for older women. Issues related to quality of life for a woman and her partner considering this decision may include exploring: the desire for children, adoption as an alternative, determining the support available from the extended social network, confidence in the plan for monitoring both breasts during pregnancy for early detection of cancer, the risk of disease recurrence and implications for single parenthood for the surviving parent.[97, 174] The issue of pregnancy after breast cancer, with more women delaying childbirth, is likely to remain an integral aspect of the nursing care of premenopausal women with breast cancer.

Nursing Diagnosis

- *Impaired social interaction*

Outcome Goal

Patient will be able to:

- Effectively resume, reestablish, or begin anew personal and social relationships that are meaningful and rewarding and integrate the concept of survivorship.

Interventions

- Assist patient to verbalize fears and concerns.
- Provide supportive information regarding those concerns and to ease fears, as appropriate, such as plans for continued medical follow-up, positive appraisal of her strengths, and services for vocational rehabilitation.
- Encourage and facilitate discussion with appropriate medical resources for pregnancy planning.
- Encourage participation in survivorship activities or group support, if desired.
- Encourage patient and family to resume participation in activities previously enjoyed.

- Encourage healthy life-style behaviors (e.g., diet, exercise, stress reduction).[89]

RECURRENCE, METASTASIS, AND TERMINAL PHASE[235, 272]

Fortunately, many women diagnosed with breast cancer today will not die from their disease. The fear of recurrence continues long after diagnosis.[117] Unfortunately, some women will face a recurrence, and the experience may be much more traumatic than the initial diagnosis.[283] Local recurrences are often managed with local treatments, such as surgical resection or radiation therapy. For the woman experiencing a local recurrence after breast-conserving surgery, mastectomy may be recommended. Nursing care in such circumstances has been addressed previously.

The patient with metastatic recurrence (or disease at diagnosis) may exhibit physical signs or symptoms such as bone pain, hypercalcemia, dyspnea, or fatigue, or the recurrence may be suspected before symptoms present (e.g., elevated liver function tests, abnormal bone scan). This is a time when there is recognition that the previous treatment failed to control the disease completely. Coping strategies that worked well in the past may be stressed during this time. There is much uncertainty and anticipation of loss.[282, 283] The sense of hope may be challenged. It is a time when information about the next plan of action can give hope and direction. Many agents have demonstrated effectiveness against breast cancer, and although cure is no longer possible, palliation of symptoms and prolonged control of the disease are reasonable and worthwhile goals.

Nursing Diagnosis

- *Anticipatory grieving, related to possible losses, including death*

Outcome Goals

Patient will be able to:

- Effectively grieve the loss of the concept of cure and feel supported in resuming therapy, if indicated.
- Experience satisfactory control of side effects and complications of treatment.
- Come to some degree of acceptance of death in the terminal phase (see Chapter 32).

Interventions

- Provide support when patient is informed of diagnosis and treatment plan.

- Explain rationale for treatments and side effects to anticipate and their management.
- Encourage patient and her significant other(s) to discuss their quality of life concerns openly with the health care team.[45, 235, 280–282, 360]
- With the diagnosis of recurrence, or when conventional treatment fails or is difficult, patients may seek additional help from complementary or alternative therapies.[200, 232] Encourage patients to share this information with the health care team and facilitate patient access to accurate information[232] (see Chapter 26).
- Assist patient and family to manage symptoms or complications of disease and/or treatment, such as pain and hypercalcemia.
- Assess coping and support needs of patient and family. Assist patient and family in the terminal phase to verbalize feelings about the meaning of illness and death.
- Referrals to supportive resources may be indicated, such as home nursing care and hospice programs, support groups, pastoral care, and professional counselors for therapeutic intervention.[218]

FOLLOW-UP

All patients with breast cancer require periodic follow-up evaluations for the remainder of their life. These evaluations are performed to monitor for recurrent disease and complications of treatment (see Complications box, page 140). Long-term effects of adjuvant chemotherapy, stem cell or bone marrow transplant, or other therapies are not fully known. Regular evaluations also allow opportunity to assess the patient's level of coping and that of her partner/ significant other and family.

Because the risk for recurrence is highest during the first 2 years after diagnosis, physical examinations may be as often as every 6 months during the first 1 to 2 years, every 6 to 12 months during the next 2 to 3 years, and then annually. Some patients will choose to stagger visits to their different specialists so that they see one member of their health care team on a more frequent basis. Mammography may be performed every 6 months for the first 1 to 3 years, then annually thereafter. Serum chemistry tests are usually obtained annually, along with a tumor marker (e.g., CA 27.29). A chest x-ray may be done annually, and a bone or CT scan as indicated. Any signs or symptoms the patient has at the time of each evaluation will influence what additional tests or imaging studies are ordered, and their frequency.

Difficulties in psychosocial adjustment to breast cancer are not confined to the early phase of the illness but persist over time for both patients and family

GERIATRIC CONSIDERATIONS

Breast Cancer

PREVENTION AND DETECTION[26, 75, 114, 246, 329, 355]

Health assessments need to incorporate cognitive function, physical limitations/sensory deficits, and support network.

Education efforts should address knowledge, skill, and confidence in BSE, mammography, and CBE and benefits of early detection.

Continuity and participation may be enhanced when health care is coordinated by one or few providers (e.g., advocate, case manager).

Community-based breast cancer screening is beneficial.

Education of health care providers should emphasize that regularly scheduled screening of elderly women is still needed, and that the ACS and ACR recommend annual screening mammography beginning at age 40 with no upper age limit for discontinuing it.

DIAGNOSIS AND TREATMENT[206, 329, 400]

Importance of patient involvement in decision-making needs to be considered regardless of age.

Age alone should not determine type or extent of surgery or subsequent therapy.

Care throughout the operative phase includes careful preoperative assessment and intraoperative and postoperative physiologic monitoring.

Early *comprehensive discharge planning* should involve patient and significant other.

Side effects with radiation and chemotherapy may be enhanced or prolonged.

Most trials of systemic therapy have excluded women over 70 years of age.

REHABILITATION[143, 145, 400]

Return to or maintenance of precancer level of functioning is a reasonable goal.

Care should be taken to incorporate psychosexual assessment and intervention as appropriate for all ages.

Physical illness can impair developmental task completion.

Depression in elderly women may be masked by physical symptoms.

METASTATIC DISEASE

Differential diagnosis of symptoms must differentiate normal or pathologic changes of aging from signs of metastatic disease.

Chronic pain may be indirectly expressed through other physical changes (e.g., anorexia, irritability, aching, insomnia).

Recurrent disease may exacerbate other felt losses of elderly women.

members. Fear of disease recurrence, role adjustment-problems, resource depletion, toxicities of therapy, and changes in body image, self-esteem, and patterns of sexuality are problems the patient and partner experience.[235, 280, 282] Children are also affected and may need support.[235, 246] Emotional problems may require referrals to trained counselors or support groups available through the ACS, local hospitals, or community resources.

Partners or significant others should be encouraged to come to the follow-up evaluations with the patients. This allows them to be included in the discussion regarding concerns and problems they are experiencing individually and as a couple. Special consideration also needs to be given to the elderly woman, who may have a limited social support network, as outlined in the Geriatric Considerations box.

In addition to regular evaluations by a health professional, women must be encouraged to begin or continue monthly BSE and regular mammograms. It is also important to identify high-risk family members, to whom appropriate screening recommendations can be provided.[314]

Teaching priorities for the patient with breast cancer are summarized in the Patient Teaching Priorities box.

Chapter Questions

1. Which of the following statements about risk factors for breast cancer is *most* true?
   a. Dietary factors account for the greatest percentage of risk.
   b. Women develop breast cancer twice as often as men.
   c. Only a small percentage of cases of breast cancer are due to mutations in BRCA-1 or BRCA-2.
   d. Women of low socioeconomic status are at greater risk of developing breast cancer than women of high socioeconomic status.

2. *Absolute risk* is a term that refers to which of the following?
   a. Risk to relatives of a woman who has been diagnosed with breast cancer
   b. Average risk for every woman in a given population, such as in the United States (e.g., this is reported as 1 in 8)
   c. Risk related to one specific risk factor (e.g., absolute risk from alcohol)
   d. Number of cancer cases in a population associated with given risk factors that could be prevented

3. Which of the following types of benign breast disease have *not* been associated with an increased risk of breast cancer?
   a. Atypical ductal hyperplasia
   b. Intraductal papilloma
   c. Atypical lobular hyperplasia
   d. Fibroadenoma

4. A 42-year-old asymptomatic woman is thinking about having prophylactic mastectomies to prevent breast cancer because she is very fearful and untrusting of mammograms and uneasy about doing BSE because she has never received instruction in how to do it. Her mother had a mastectomy 1 year ago at age 68 for stage I breast cancer. As a member of her health care team, how would the nurse best address her concerns?
   a. Tell her to get a clinical breast examination (CBE) twice a year, an annual mammogram, and practice BSE monthly. There is no way to prevent breast cancer.
   b. Find out when she had her last CBE and mammogram, and when she last tried to do BSE. Assess her beliefs about how effective prophylactic mastectomy would be. Ask her about other cases of cancer in the family. Refer her to a therapist for behavioral modification.
   c. Tell her that prophylactic mastectomy does not completely eliminate the risk of breast cancer. If monthly BSE is difficult to perform, then annual CBE and annual mammography are adequate for her.
   d. Offer to provide instruction in BSE, and give her information about the safety and effectiveness of mammograms. Reassure her that annual mammography by an accredited facility, monthly BSE, and annual CBE together are the most effective in identifying breast changes that need to be investigated.

5. A 33-year-old patient, recently diagnosed with invasive breast cancer, has just met with her surgeon to discuss her surgical treatment options. She wants to know more about breast-conserving surgery and radiation. How would the nurse *best* approach the patient?
   a. Clarify what the patient's primary questions include, address those first, and give additional information about the surgical routines, recovery, the treatments, and self-care management. Arrange for an appointment with the radiation oncologist.
   b. Advise her about side effects of the radiation versus chemotherapy, and advise her strongly that she should not get pregnant.
   c. Share experiences of other patients, ask if she has further questions, and refer to a support group.
   d. Arrange for an appointment with the radiation oncologist, a medical oncologist, and tours of the radiation therapy unit and infusion clinic.

6. Which of the following *best* describes the purpose of giving standard adjuvant chemotherapy to women with invasive breast cancer?
   a. It is a systemic form of cancer treatment given to treat metastatic breast cancer after the primary site of breast cancer has been surgically removed.
   b. It is a systemic form of cancer treatment given to enhance the effects of antiestrogen therapy.
   c. It is a systemic form of cancer treatment given to treat micrometastases after surgical removal of the primary site of cancer for certain high-risk women, based on data from clinical trials.
   d. It is a systemic form of cancer treatment given before any other treatment.

7. A 78-year-old woman with metastatic breast cancer has recently begun taking tamoxifen. She calls the nurse at her physician's office with the complaint of aching all over and increased pain at her sites of bony metastases. What is the most likely explanation for her experience?
   a. Arthritis
   b. Progressive disease
   c. Flu or virus
   d. "Flare reaction" to endocrine therapy

8. A patient who is going to have a segmental mastectomy and sentinel lymph node biopsy returns to the office for a preoperative teaching session. She is accompanied by her husband. She verbalizes that they are having a disagreement about the purpose of the sentinel lymph node biopsy. He says it is to identify a lymph node that *might* contain cancer, and she says that finding it means there *is* cancer in the lymph node. How can the nurse *best* help clarify this couple's understanding of her surgical plan?

   a. They are both right. First one has to find the sentinel lymph node, and if one does, then it is highly probable that it contains cancer cells.

   b. The purpose of the sentinel lymph node biopsy is to identify and remove the lymph node in the axilla that contains cancer cells, based on lymphatic flow from the site of the breast cancer.

   c. The purpose of the sentinel lymph node biopsy is to identify and remove the lymph node in the axilla that is the first to receive lymphatic drainage from the site of the cancer, and therefore the one most likely to contain cancer if it has spread to the lymph nodes.

   d. The purpose of the sentinel lymph node biopsy is to identify and remove a portion of a lymph node that contains cancer cells, for further study in the laboratory.

9. For the elderly woman, which of the following does *not* accurately reflect barriers to breast health care?

   a. Social isolation and low income may decrease participation in health care programs.

   b. Sensory changes of aging may delay identification of symptoms or decrease touch sensitivity in BSE.

   c. Physical symptoms may mask underlying depression and associated lack of interest in self-care.

   d. Screening and breast cancer treatments are not effective after age 70.

10. A 41-year-old woman who was successfully treated for breast cancer a year ago reports to the nurse on her regular clinical follow-up that she is experiencing increasing stress at her work and frequently is in conflict with her husband and children. She has had new aches and pains that frighten her, but the physician said she was doing well. Her menstrual cycle has never returned after chemotherapy, but she has had no symptoms of menopause. The nurse could *best* help this patient by doing which of the following?

   a. Acknowledge her concerns and allow her to explore them further.

   b. Tell her this is a normal consequence of cancer treatment.

   c. Suggest she seek consultation with a gynecologist.

   d. Advise her to bring her husband and together talk further with her physician.

BIBLIOGRAPHY

1. Alagna S, Reddy D: Predictors of proficient technique in successful lesion detection in self breast examination, *Health Psychol* 3(2):113, 1984.
2. Al-Ghazal S, Sully L, Fallowfield L, Blamey R: The psychological impact of immediate rather than delayed breast reconstruction, *Eur J Surg Oncol* 26(1):17, 2000.
3. Ambler N and others: Specialist nurse counselor interventions at the time of diagnosis of breast cancer: comparing 'advocacy' with a conventional approach, *J Adv Nurs* 29(2):445, 1999.
4. American Cancer Society: *Special report on cancer in the economically disadvantaged*, New York, The Society, 1986.
5. American Cancer Society: *Clinical breast examination: proficiency criteria and guidelines*, Oakland, CA, The Society, California Division, 1998.
6. American Cancer Society: 1989 survey of physicians' attitudes and practices in early cancer detection, *CA Cancer J Clin* 40(2):77, 1990.
7. American Cancer Society: *Special touch breast health trainer's guide*, ed 3, Oakland, CA, The Society, California Division, 1995.
8. American Cancer Society: *Breast cancer facts and figures 1999–2000*, Atlanta, The Society, 1999.
9. American Cancer Society: *Cancer facts and figures 2000*, Atlanta, The Society, 2000.
10. American Cancer Society: *Cancer prevention and early detection. Cancer facts and figures 2000*, Atlanta, The Society, 2000.
11. American Joint Committee on Cancer: *AJCC cancer staging manual*, ed 5, Philadelphia, Lippincott-Raven, 1997.
12. Andersen B, Cacioppo J, Roberts D: Delay in seeking a cancer diagnosis: delay stages and psychophysiological comparison processes, *Br J Soc Psychol* 34:33, 1995.
13. Anderson W, Reeves J, Elias A, Berkel H: Outcome of patients with metastatic breast carcinoma treated at a private medical oncology clinic, *Cancer* 88(1):95, 2000.
14. Antman K and others: High-dose chemotherapy with autologous hematopoietic stem-cell support for breast cancer in North America, *J Clin Oncol* 15(5):1870, 1997.
15. ASCO Public Issues Committee: Statement of the American Society of Clinical Oncology: genetic testing for cancer susceptibility, *J Clin Oncology* 14(5):1730, 1996.
16. Ash C, Rodriguez C: Breast cancer: nursing management issues. In Bland K, Copeland E, editors: *The breast: comprehensive management of benign and malignant diseases*, ed 2, vol. 2, p. 1489, Philadelphia, Saunders, 1998.
17. Assaf AR and others: Comparison of three methods of teaching women how to perform breast self-examination, *Health Educ Q* 12:259, 1985.

18. Audrain J and others: The impact of a brief coping skills intervention on adherence to breast self-examination among first-degree relatives of newly diagnosed breast cancer patients, *Psychooncology* 8(3):220, 1999.

19. Auvinen A, Elovainio L, Hakama M: Breast self-examination and survival from breast cancer. A prospective follow-up study, *Breast Cancer Res Treat* 38(2): 161, 1996.

20. Ayanian J, Guadagnoli E: Variations in breast cancer treatment by patient and provider characteristics, *Breast Cancer Res Treat* 40(1):65, 1996.

21. Ayanian JZ and others: The relation between health insurance coverage and clinical outcomes among women with breast cancer, *N Engl J Med* 329(5):326, 1993.

22. Baines CJ: Breast self-examination, *Cancer* 69(7 Suppl):1942, 1992.

23. Bass S, Cox C, Reintgen D: Learning curves and certification for breast cancer lymphatic mapping, *Surg Oncol Clin N Am* 8(3):497, 1999.

24. Bassett L: Breast imaging. In Bland K, Copeland E, editors: *The breast: comprehensive management of benign and malignant diseases,* ed 2, vol. 1, p. 648, Philadelphia, Saunders, 1998.

25. Bassett L and others: Stereotactic core-needle biopsy of the breast: a report of the Joint Task Force of the American College of Radiology, American College of Surgeons, and College of American Pathologists, *CA Cancer J Clin* 47(3):171, 1997.

26. Baulch Y, Larson P, Dodd M, Deitrich C: The relationship of visual acuity, tactile sensitivity, and mobility of the upper extremities to proficient breast self-examination in women 65 and older, *Oncol Nurs Forum* 19(9):1367, 1992.

27. Beisecker A and others: Side effects of adjuvant chemotherapy: perceptions of node-negative breast cancer patients, *Psychooncology* 6(2):85, 1997.

28. Benedict S and others: Breast cancer detection by daughters of women with breast cancer, *Cancer Pract* 5(4): 213, 1997.

29. Benedict S, Williams R, Baron P: Recalled anxiety: from discovery to diagnosis of a benign breast mass, *Oncol Nurs Forum* 21(10):1723, 1994.

30. Benedict S, Williams R, Baron P: The effect of benign breast biopsy on subsequent breast cancer detection practices, *Oncol Nurs Forum* 21(9):1467, 1994.

31. Bilimoria M, Morrow M: The woman at increased risk for breast cancer: evaluation and management strategies, *CA Cancer J Clin* 45(5):263, 1995.

32. Bland K, McCraw J, Copeland E: General principles of mastectomy: evaluation and therapeutic options. In Bland K, Copeland E, editors: *The breast: comprehensive management of benign and malignant diseases,* ed 2, p. 817, Philadelphia, Saunders, 1998.

33. Bland K and others: Axillary dissection in breast-conserving surgery for stage I and II breast cancer: a National Cancer Data Base study of patterns of omission and implications for survival, *J Am Coll Surg* 188(6):586, 1999.

34. Bleiker E and others: Personality factors and breast cancer development: a prospective longitudinal study, *J Natl Cancer Inst* 88(20):1478, 1996.

35. Boice JD Jr, Monson RR: Breast cancer in women after repeated fluoroscopic examinations of the chest, *J Natl Cancer Inst* 59(3):823, 1977.

36. Bostwick J: Breast reconstruction following mastectomy, *CA Cancer J Clin* 45(5):289, 1995.

37. Bower J and others: Fatigue in breast cancer survivors: occurrence, correlates, and impact on quality of life, *J Clin Oncol* 18(4):743, 2000.

38. Bowlin S and others: Breast cancer risk and alcohol consumption: results from a large case-control study, *Int J Epidemiol* 26(5):915, 1997.

39. Boyd N and others: Mammographic densities and breast cancer risk, *Cancer Epidemiol Biomarkers Prev* 7(12): 1133, 1998.

40. Brain K, Norman P, Gray J, Mansel R: Anxiety and adherence to breast self-examination in women with a family history of breast cancer, *Psychosom Med* 61(2): 181, 1999.

41. Brennan M, Miller L: Overview of treatment options and review of the current role and use of compression garments, intermittent pumps, and exercise in the management of lymphedema, *Cancer* 83(12 Suppl):2821, 1998.

42. Brinton L and others: Oral contraceptives and breast cancer risk among younger women, *J Natl Cancer Inst* 87(11):827, 1995.

43. Bryla C: The relationship between stress and the development of breast cancer: a literature review, *Oncol Nurs Forum* 23(3):441, 1996.

44. Buchsel PC, Kapustay PM: Peripheral stem cell transplantation. In Hubbard SM, Goodman M, Knobf MT: *Oncology nursing: patient treatment and support,* Philadelphia, Lippincott, 1995.

45. Bull A and others: Quality of life in women with recurrent breast cancer, *Breast Cancer Res Treat* 54(1):47, 1999.

46. Burke C and others: Patient satisfaction with 23-hour "short-stay" observation following breast cancer surgery, *Oncol Nurs Forum* 24(4):645, 1997.

47. Burke W and others: Recommendations for follow-up care of individuals with an inherited predisposition to cancer. II. *BRCA1 and BRCA2, JAMA* 277(12):997, 1997.

48. Burnett C, Steakley C, Tefft M: Barriers to breast and cervical cancer screening in underserved women of the District of Columbia, *Oncol Nurs Forum* 22(10):1551, 1995.

49. Burns J and others: Critical pathway for administering high-dose chemotherapy followed by peripheral blood stem cell rescue in the outpatient setting, *Oncol Nurs Forum* 22(8):1219, 1995.

50. Buzdar A, Hortobagyi G: Recent advances in adjuvant therapy of breast cancer, *Semin Oncol* 26(4 Suppl 12): 21, 1999.

51. Cady B: Traditional and future management of nonpalpable breast cancer, *Am Surg* 63(1):55, 1997.

52. Calzone K and others: Establishing a cancer risk evaluation program, *Cancer Pract* 5(4):228, 1997.

53. Cameron C, Ashbury F, Iverson D: Perspectives on Reach to Recovery and CanSurmount: informing the evaluation model, *Cancer Prev Control* 1(2):102, 1997.

54. Caplan L and others: Reasons for delay in breast cancer diagnosis, *Prev Med* 25(2):218, 1996.

55. Carter B: Surviving breast cancer: a problematic work re-entry, *Cancer Pract* 2(2):135, 1994.

56. Carter C, Allen C, Henson D: Relation of tumor size, lymph node status, and survival in 24,740 breast cancer cases. The Surveillance, Epidemiology, End Result (SEER) program of the National Cancer Institute, *Cancer* 63(1):181, 1989.

57. Castiglione-Gertsch M, Gelber R, Goldhirsch A: Adjuvant systemic therapy: the issues of timing and sequence, *Recent Results Cancer Res* 140:201, 1996.

58. Centers for Disease Control and Prevention: The National Breast and Cervical Cancer Early Detection Program. At-a-glance 2000. Retrieved March 18, 2000 from the World Wide Web: http://www.cdc.gov/cancer/nbccedp/about.htm

59. Champion V: Beliefs about breast cancer and mammography by behavioral stage, *Oncol Nurs Forum* 21(6):1009, 1994.

60. Champion V: Development of a benefits and barriers scale for mammography utilization, *Cancer Nurs* 18(1):53, 1995.

61. Champion V: Results of a nurse-delivered intervention on proficiency and nodule detection with breast self-examination, *Oncol Nurs Forum* 22(5):819, 1995.

62. Champion V: Revised susceptibility, benefits, and barriers scale for mammography screening, *Res Nurs Health* 22(4):341, 1999.

63. Chlebowski R: Dietary fat intake reduction for patients with resected breast cancer, *Adv Exp Med Biol* 364:11, 1994.

64. Choudhry U, Srivastava R, Fitch M: Breast cancer detection practices of south Asian women: knowledge, attitudes, and beliefs, *Oncol Nurs Forum* 25(10):1693, 1998.

65. Christian M and others: The National Cancer Institute audit of the National Surgical Adjuvant Breast and Bowel Project protocol B-06, *N Engl J Med* 333(22):1469, 1995.

66. Chu K and others: Do all patients with sentinel node metastasis from breast carcinoma need complete axillary node dissection? *Ann Surg* 229(4):536, 1999.

67. Clark J, Landis L: Reintegration and maintenance of employees with breast cancer in the workplace, *Am Assoc Occup Health Nurses* 37(5):186, 1989.

68. Clark G: Prognostic and predictive factors. In Harris J, Lippman M, Morrow M, Osborne C, editors: *Diseases of the breast,* ed 2, p. 489, Philadelphia, Lippincott Williams & Wilkins, 2000.

69. Clarke V, Savage S: Breast self-examination training: a brief review, *Cancer Nurs* 22(4):320, 1999.

70. Cody H: Sentinel lymph node mapping breast cancer, *Oncology* 13(1):25, 1999.

71. Cody H, Borgen P: Bilateral breast cancer. In Bland K, Copeland E, editors: *The breast: comprehensive management of benign and malignant diseases,* ed 2, vol. 2, p. 1407, Philadelphia, Saunders, 1998.

72. Colditz G and others: The use of estrogens and progestins and the risk of breast cancer in postmenopausal women, *N Engl J Med* 332(24):1589, 1995.

73. Coleman E: Practice and effectiveness of breast self examination: a selective review of the literature (1977–1989), *J Cancer Educ* 6(2):83, 1991.

74. Coleman E, Pennypacker H: Measuring breast self-examination proficiency, *Cancer Nurs* 14(4):211, 1991.

75. Coleman E and others: Efficacy of breast self-examination teaching methods among older women, *Oncol Nurs Forum* 18(3):561, 1991.

76. Collaborative Group on Hormonal Factors in Breast Cancer: Breast cancer and hormonal contraceptives: collaborative reanalysis of individual data on 53,297 women with breast cancer and 100,239 women without breast cancer from 54 epidemiological studies. Collaborative Group on Hormonal Factors in Breast Cancer, *Lancet* 347(9017):1713, 1996.

77. Collaborative Group on Hormonal Factors in Breast Cancer: Breast cancer and hormone replacement therapy: collaborative reanalysis of data from 51 epidemiological studies of 52,705 women with breast cancer and 108,411 women without breast cancer. Collaborative Group on Hormonal Factors in Breast Cancer, *Lancet* 350(9084):1047, 1997.

78. Cook L and others: Hair product use and the risk of breast cancer in young women, *Cancer Causes Control* 10(6):551, 1999.

79. Cooper L and others: Survival of premenopausal breast carcinoma patients in relation to menstrual cycle timing of surgery and estrogen receptor/progesterone receptor status of the primary tumor, *Cancer* 86(10):2053, 1999.

80. Coward D: Lymphedema prevention and management knowledge in women treated for breast cancer, *Oncol Nurs Forum* 26(6):1047, 1999.

81. Cox C and others: Implementation of new surgical technology: outcome measures for lymphatic mapping of breast carcinoma, *Ann Surg Oncol* 6(6):553, 1999.

82. Daly M and others: Gail model breast cancer risk components are poor predictors of risk perception and screening behavior, *Breast Cancer Res Treat* 41(1):59, 1996.

83. Daly M: NCCN practice guidelines: Genetics/familial high-risk cancer screening, *Oncology* 13(11A):161, 1999.

84. Dawson I and others: Effect of shoulder immobilization on wound seroma and shoulder dysfunction following modified radical mastectomy: a randomized prospective clinical trial, *Br J Surg* 76(3):311, 1989.

85. Day R and others: Health-related quality of life and tamoxifen in breast cancer prevention: a report from the National Surgical Adjuvant Breast and Bowel Project P-1 study, *J Clin Oncol* 17(9):2659, 1999.

86. Deane K, Degner L: Information needs, uncertainty, and anxiety in women who had a breast biopsy with benign outcome, *Cancer Nurs* 21(2):117, 1998.

87. Degner L and others: Information needs and decisional preferences in women with breast cancer, *JAMA* 277(18):1485, 1997.

88. DeKeyser F and others: Distress, symptom distress, and immune function in women with suspected breast cancer, *Oncol Nurs Forum* 25(8):1415, 1998.

89. Demark-Wahnefried W and others: Current health behaviors and readiness to pursue life-style changes among

men and women diagnosed with early stage prostate and breast carcinomas, *Cancer* 88(3):674, 2000.

90. Demark-Wahnefried W, Winer E, Rimer B: Why women gain weight with adjuvant chemotherapy for breast cancer, *J Clin Oncol* 11(7):1418, 1993.

91. Diel I, Cote R: Bone marrow and lymph node assessment for minimal residual disease in patients with breast cancer, *Cancer Treat Rev* 26(1):53, 2000.

92. Dietrick-Gallagher M, Hyzinski M: Teaching patients to care for drains after breast surgery for malignancy, *Oncol Nurs Forum* 16(2):263, 1989.

93. Dignam J: Differences in breast cancer prognosis among African-American and Caucasian women, *CA Cancer J Clin* 50(1):50, 2000.

94. Dorval M, Maunsell E, Deschenes L, Brisson J: Type of mastectomy and quality of life for long term breast carcinoma survivors, *Cancer* 83(10):2130, 1998.

95. Douglass M and others: Breast cancer early detection: differences between African American and white women's health beliefs and detection practices, *Oncol Nurs Forum* 22(5):835, 1995.

96. Dow K, Kalinowski B: Nursing care in patient management and quality of life. In Harris J, Lippman M, Morrow M, Osborne C, editors: *Diseases of the breast,* ed 2, p. 985, Philadelphia, Lippincott Williams & Wilkins, 2000.

97. Dow K and others: Pregnancy after breast-conserving surgery and radiation therapy for breast cancer, *Monogr Natl Cancer Inst* 16:131, 1994.

98. Dupont W and others: Estrogen replacement therapy in women with a history of proliferative breast disease, *Cancer* 85(6):1277, 1999.

99. Dupont W, Page D: Risk factors for breast cancer in women with proliferative breast disease, *N Engl J Med* 312(3):146, 1985.

100. Dupont W, Page D: Risk factors for breast carcinoma in women with proliferative breast disease. In Bland K, Copeland E, editors: *The breast: comprehensive management of benign and malignant diseases,* ed 2, vol. 1, p. 427, Philadelphia, Saunders, 1998.

101. Early Breast Cancer Trialists' Collaborative Group: Effects of radiotherapy and surgery in early breast cancer: an overview of the randomized trials, *N Engl J Med* 333(22):1444, 1995.

102. Early Breast Cancer Trialists' Collaborative Group: Polychemotherapy for early breast cancer: an overview of the randomised trials, *Lancet* 352(9132):930, 1998.

103. Early Breast Cancer Trialists' Collaborative Group: Tamoxifen for early breast cancer: an overview of the randomised trials, *Lancet* 351(9114):1451, 1998.

104. Eisen A, Weber B: Prophylactic mastectomy—the price of fear [Editorial], *N Engl J Med* 340(2):137, 1999.

105. Eley J and others: Racial differences in survival from breast cancer: results of the National Cancer Institute Black/White Cancer Survival Study, *JAMA* 272(12):947, 1994.

106. Elledge R, Fuqua S: Estrogen and progesterone receptors. In Harris J, Lippman M, Morrow M, Osborne C,

editors: *Diseases of the breast,* ed 2, p. 471, Philadelphia, Lippincott Williams & Wilkins, 2000.

107. Ellis M, Hayes D, Lippman M: Treatment of metastatic breast cancer. In Harris J, Lippman M, Morrow M, Osborne C, editors: *Diseases of the breast,* ed 2, p. 749, Philadelphia, Lippincott Williams & Wilkins, 2000.

108. Ellman R and others: Breast self-examination programmes in the trial of early detection of breast cancer: ten year findings, *Br J Cancer* 68(1):208, 1993.

109. Epstein S and others: Excessive breast self-examination among first-degree relatives of newly diagnosed breast cancer patients. High-Risk Breast Cancer Consortium, *Psychosomatics* 38(3):253, 1997.

110. Facione N: Breast cancer screening in relation to access to health services, *Oncol Nurs Forum* 26(4):689, 1999.

111. Facione N: Delay versus help seeking for breast cancer symptoms: a critical review of the literature on patient and provider delay, *Soc Sci Med* 36(12):1521, 1993.

112. Facione N, Giancarlo C: Narratives of breast symptom discovery and cancer diagnosis: psychologic risk for advanced cancer at diagnosis, *Cancer Nurs* 21(6):430, 1998.

113. Fawzy F, Fawzy N: A structured psychoeducational intervention for cancer patients, *Gen Hosp Psychiatry* 16(3):149, 1994.

114. Feig S and others: American College of Radiology guidelines for breast cancer screening, *AJR Am J Roentgenol* 171(1):29, 1998.

115. Feig S: Increased benefit from shorter screening mammography intervals for women ages 40-49 years, *Cancer* 80(11):2035, 1997.

116. Ferraroni M and others: Alcohol consumption and risk of breast cancer: a multicentre Italian case-control study, *Eur J Cancer* 34(9):1403, 1998.

117. Ferrell B and others: Quality of life in breast cancer survivors: implications for developing support services, *Oncol Nurs Forum* 25(5):887, 1998.

118. Fine N, Mustoe T, Fenner G: Breast reconstruction. In Harris J, Lippman M, Morrow M, Osborne C, editors: *Diseases of the breast,* ed 2, p. 561, Philadelphia, Lippincott Williams & Wilkins, 2000.

119. Finison K and others: Screening mammography rates by specialty of the usual care physician, *Eff Clin Pract* 2(3):120, 1999.

120. Fisher B: Highlights from recent National Surgical Adjuvant Breast and Bowel Project studies in the treatment and prevention of breast cancer, *CA Cancer J Clin* 49(3):159, 1999.

121. Fisher B and others: Lumpectomy and radiation therapy for the treatment of intraductal breast cancer: findings from National Surgical Adjuvant Breast and Bowel Project B-17, *J Clin Oncol* 16(2):441, 1998.

122. Fisher B and others: Tamoxifen for prevention of breast cancer: report of the National Surgical Adjuvant Breast and Bowel Project P-1 study, *J Natl Cancer Inst* 90(18):1371, 1998.

123. Fisher B and others: Reanalysis and results after 12 years of follow-up in a randomized clinical trial comparing total mastectomy with lumpectomy with or without irradiation in the treatment of breast cancer, *N Engl J Med* 333(22):1456, 1995.

124. Fletcher S, O'Malley M, Bunce L: Physician's abilities to detect lumps in silicone breast models, *JAMA* 253(15):2224, 1985.

125. Fletcher S and others: How best to teach women breast self-examination: a randomized controlled trial, *Ann Intern Med* 112(10):772, 1990.

126. Forbes J: Screening for breast cancer and treatment of early lesions (ductal carcinoma in situ): summary, *Recent Results Cancer Res* 140:155, 1996.

127. Forbes J: The incidence of breast cancer: the global burden, public health considerations, *Semin Oncol* 24(1 Suppl 1):S1-20-S1-35, 1997.

128. Foster R and others: Breast self examination practices and breast cancer stage, *N Engl J Med* 299(6):265, 1978.

129. Frazier E, Jiles R, Mayberry R: Use of screening mammography and clinical breast examinations among black, Hispanic, and white women, *Prev Med* 25(2):118, 1996.

130. Freeman H: Cancer in the socioeconomically disadvantaged, *CA Cancer J Clin* 39(5):266, 1989.

131. Frelix G and others: Breast cancer screening in underserved women in the Bronx, *J Natl Med Assoc* 91(4):195, 1999.

132. Fremgen A and others: Clinical highlights from the National Cancer Data Base, 1999, *CA Cancer J Clin* 49(3):145, 1999.

133. Friedman L and others: Breast cancer screening among ethnically diverse low-income women in a general hospital psychiatry clinic, *Gen Hosp Psychiatry* 21(5):374, 1999.

134. Friedman L and others: Dispositional optimism, self-efficacy, and health beliefs as predictors of breast self-examination, *Am J Prev Med* 10(3):130, 1994.

135. Frost M and others: A multidisciplinary healthcare delivery model for women with breast cancer: patient satisfaction and physical and psychosocial adjustment, *Oncol Nurs Forum* 26(10):1673, 1999.

136. Frykberg E, Bland K: Current concepts on the biology and management of in situ (Tis, stage 0) breast carcinoma. In Bland K, Copeland E, editors: *The breast: comprehensive management of benign and malignant diseases,* ed 2, p. 1012, Philadelphia, Saunders, 1998.

137. Frykberg E, Bland K: Evolution of surgical principles and techniques for the management of breast cancer. In Bland K, Copeland E, editors: *The breast: comprehensive management of benign and malignant diseases,* ed 2, vol. 1, p. 766, Philadelphia, Saunders, 1998.

138. Fuchs C and others: Alcohol consumption and mortality among women, *N Engl J Med* 332(19):1245, 1995.

139. Funke I, Schraut W: Meta-analysis of studies on bone marrow micrometastases: an independent prognostic impact remains to be substantiated, *J Clin Oncol,* 16(2): 557, 1998.

140. Gadd M, Souba W: Evaluation and treatment of benign breast disorders. In Bland K, Copeland E, editors: *The breast: comprehensive management of benign and malignant diseases,* ed 2, vol. 1, p. 233, Philadelphia, Saunders, 1998.

141. Gammon M and others: Cigarette smoking and breast cancer risk among young women (United States), *Cancer Causes Control* 9(6):583, 1998.

142. Gammon M, John E: Recent etiologic hypotheses concerning breast cancer, *Epidemiol Rev*15(1):163, 1993.

143. Ganz P: Breast cancer in older women: quality-of-life considerations, *Cancer Control J Moffitt Cancer Ctr* 1: 372, 1994.

144. Ganz P and others: Breast conservation *versus* mastectomy. Is there a difference in psychological adjustment or quality of life in the year after surgery? *Cancer* 69(7): 1729, 1992.

145. Ganz P and others: Predictors of sexual health in women after a breast cancer diagnosis, *J Clin Oncol* 17(8):2371, 1999.

146. Ganz P and others: Impact of different adjuvant therapy strategies on quality of life in breast cancer survivors, *Recent Results Cancer Res* 152:396, 1998.

147. Garland M and others: Alcohol consumption in relation to breast cancer risk in a cohort of United States women 25–42 years of age, *Cancer Epidemiol Biomarkers Prev* 8(11):1017, 1999.

148. Gaskin T, Trammell L: Rehabilitation. In Bland K, Copeland E, editors: *The breast: comprehensive management of benign and malignant diseases,* ed 2, vol. 2, p. 1506, Philadelphia, Saunders, 1998.

149. Gaston-Johansson F and others: Pain, psychological distress, health status, and coping in patients with breast cancer scheduled for autotransplantation, *Oncol Nurs Forum* 26(8):1337, 1999.

150. Gastrin G and others: Incidence and mortality from breast cancer in the Mama Program for Breast Screening in Finland, 1973–1986, *Cancer* 73(8):2168, 1994.

151. Gelmann E: Oncogenes in human breast cancer. In Bland K, Copeland E, editors: *The breast: comprehensive management of benign and malignant diseases,* ed 2, vol. 1, p. 499, Philadelphia, Saunders, 1998.

152. Gemignani M, Petrek J: Pregnancy after breast cancer, *Cancer Control* 6(3):272, 1999.

153. Gerber L, Augustine E: Rehabilitation management: restoring fitness and return to functional activity. In Harris J, Lippman M, Morrow M, Osborne C, editors: *Diseases of the breast,* ed 2, p. 1001, Philadelphia, Lippincott Williams & Wilkins, 2000.

154. Giomuso C, Suster V: Free flap breast reconstruction, *Medsurg Nurs* 3(1):9, 1994.

155. Giuliano A and others: Sentinel lymphadenectomy in breast cancer, *J Clin Oncol* 15(6):2345, 1997.

156. Goldhirsch A and others: Meeting highlights: International Consensus Panel on the Treatment of Primary Breast Cancer, *J Natl Cancer Inst* 90(21):1601, 1998.

157. Goldhirsch A and others: Menstrual cycle and timing of breast surgery in premenopausal node-positive breast cancer: results of the International Breast Cancer Study Group, *Ann Oncol* 8(8):751, 1997.

158. Goodwin P and others: Adjuvant treatment and onset of menopause predict weight gain after breast cancer diagnosis, *J Clin Oncol* 17(1):120, 1999.

159. Goodwin P and others: Risk of menopause during the first year after breast cancer diagnosis, *J Clin Oncol* 17(8):2365, 1999.

160. Goss P: Risks versus benefits in the clinical application of aromatase inhibitors, *Endocr Relat Cancer* 6(2):325, 1999.

161. Gradishar W, Jordan V: Endocrine therapy of breast cancer. In Bland K, Copeland E, editors: *The breast: comprehensive management of benign and malignant diseases,* ed 2, vol. 2, p. 1350, Philadelphia, Saunders, 1998.

162. Grann V and others: Prevention with tamoxifen or other hormones versus prophylactic surgery in BRCA1/2-positive women: a decision analysis, *Cancer J Sci Am* 6(1):13, 2000.

163. Greenlee R, Murray T, Bolden S, Wingo P: Cancer statistics, 2000, *CA Cancer J Clin* 50(1):7, 2000.

164. Greenwald P and others: Estimated effect of breast self-examination and routine physician examination on breast cancer mortality, *N Engl J Med* 299(6):271, 1978.

165. Guadagnoli E and others: The quality of care for treatment of early stage breast carcinoma: is it consistent with national guidelines? *Cancer* 83(2):302, 1998.

166. Guinee V: Epidemiology of breast cancer. In Bland K, Copeland E, editors: *The breast: comprehensive management of benign and malignant diseases,* ed 2, vol. 1, p. 339, Philadelphia, Saunders, 1998.

167. Hack T and others: Physical and psychological morbidity after axillary lymph node dissection for breast cancer, *J Clin Oncol* 17(1):143, 1999.

168. Hagan M, Mendenhall N: Adjuvant radiotherapy after modified radical mastectomy. In Bland K, Copeland E, editors: *The breast: comprehensive management of benign and malignant diseases,* ed 2, p. 1160, Philadelphia, Saunders, 1998.

169. Hagen A, Hrushesky W: Menstrual timing of breast cancer surgery, *Am J Surg* 175(3):245, 1998.

170. Hancock S, Tucker M, Hoppe R: Breast cancer after treatment of Hodgkin's disease, *J Natl Cancer Inst* 85(1):25, 1993.

171. Hankinson S and others: A prospective study of oral contraceptive use and risk of breast cancer (Nurses' Health Study, United States), *Cancer Causes Control* 8(1):65, 1997.

172. Hardy R and others: Difficulty in reaching low-income women for screening mammography, *J Health Care Poor Underserved* 11(1):45, 2000.

173. Hartmann L and others: Efficacy of bilateral prophylactic mastectomy in women with a family history of breast cancer, *N Engl J Med* 340(2):77, 1999.

174. Hassey K: Pregnancy and parenthood after treatment for breast cancer, *Oncol Nurs Forum* 15(4):439, 1988.

175. Hayes D: Evaluation of patients after primary therapy. In Bland K, Copeland E, editors: *The breast: comprehensive management of benign and malignant diseases,* ed 2, vol. 1, p. 709, Philadelphia, Saunders, 1998.

176. Hayes D: Serum (circulating) tumor markers for breast cancer, *Recent Results Cancer Res* 140:101, 1996.

177. Hebert-Croteau N and others: Compliance with consensus recommendations for the treatment of early stage breast carcinoma in elderly women, *Cancer* 85(5):1104, 1999.

178. Heimann R, Hellman S: Clinical progression of breast cancer malignant behavior: what to expect and when to expect it, *J Clin Oncol* 18(3):591, 2000.

179. Helgeson V and others: Education and peer discussion group interventions and adjustment to breast cancer, *Arch Gen Psychiatry* 56(4):340, 1999.

180. Hellman S, Harris J: Natural history of breast cancer. In Harris J, Lippman M, Morrow M, Osborne C, editors: *Diseases of the breast,* ed 2, p. 407, Philadelphia, Lippincott Williams & Wilkins, 2000.

181. Henderson IC: Breast cancer. In Murphy GP and others: *American Cancer Society textbook of clinical oncology,* ed 2, Atlanta, American Cancer Society, 1995.

182. Hillner B and others: American Society of Clinical Oncology guideline on the role of bisphosphonates in breast cancer, *J Clin Oncol* 18(6):1378, 2000.

183. Hilton B: Getting back to normal: the family experience during early stage breast cancer, *Oncol Nurs Forum* 23(4):605, 1996.

184. Hjerl K and others: Breast cancer risk among women with psychiatric admission with affective or neurotic disorders: a nationwide cohort study in Denmark, *Br J Cancer* 81(5):907, 1999.

185. Holmes M and others: Association of dietary intake of fat and fatty acids with risk of breast cancer, *JAMA* 281(10):914, 1999.

186. Hortobagyi G, Singletary S, Strom E: Treatment of locally advanced and inflammatory breast cancer. In Harris J, Lippman M, Morrow M, Osborne C, editors: *Diseases of the breast,* ed 2, p. 645, Philadelphia, Lippincott Williams & Wilkins, 2000.

187. Hoskins C: Breast cancer treatment-related patterns in side effects, psychological distress, and perceived health status, *Oncol Nurs Forum* 24(9), 1575, 1997.

188. Hrushesky W: Menstrual cycle timing of breast cancer resection, *Recent Results Cancer Res* 140:27, 1996.

189. Hsueh E, Giuliano A: Sentinel lymph node technique for staging of breast cancer, *Oncologist,* 3(3):165, 1998.

190. Huang Z and others: Waist circumference, waist:hip ratio, and risk of breast cancer in the Nurses' Health Study, *Am J Epidemiol* 150(12):1316, 1999.

191. Hudis C: The current state of adjuvant therapy for breast cancer: focus on paclitaxel, *Semin Oncol* 26(1 Suppl 2):1, 1999.

192. Huguley CM Jr and others: Breast self-examination and survival from breast cancer, *Cancer* 62(7):1389, 1988.

193. Humble C: Lymphedema: incidence, pathophysiology, management, and nursing care, *Oncol Nurs Forum* 22(10):1503, 1995.

194. Hunt K, Rosen E, Sickles E: Outcome analysis for women undergoing annual versus biennial screening mammography: a review of 24,211 examinations, *Am J Roentgenol* 173(2):285, 1999.

195. Hwang T and others: Implementation and evaluation of a clinical pathway for TRAM breast reconstruction, *Plast Reconstr Surg* 105(2):541, 2000.

196. Iglehart J: Prophylactic mastectomy. In Harris J, Lippman M, Morrow M, Osborne C, editors: *Diseases of the breast,* ed 2, p. 225, Philadelphia, Lippincott Williams & Wilkins, 2000.

197. Ingram D and others: Obesity and breast disease: the role of the female sex hormones, *Cancer* 64(5):1049, 1989.

198. Institute of Medicine, Committee on the Relationship Between Oral Contraceptives and Breast Cancer, Division of Health Promotion and Disease Prevention: *Oral*

contraceptives and breast cancer, Washington, DC, National Academy Press, 1991.

199. Jacob T, Penn N, Giebink J, Bastien R: A comparison of breast self-examination and clinical examination, *J Natl Med Assoc* 86(1):40, 1994.

200. Jacobson J, Workman S, Kronenberg F: Research on complementary/alternative medicine for patients with breast cancer: a review of the biomedical literature, *J Clin Oncol* 18(3):668, 2000.

201. Jahkola T: Self-perceptions of women after early breast cancer surgery, *Eur J Surg Oncol* 24(1):9, 1998.

202. Jansen R and others: Immediate versus delayed shoulder exercises after axillary lymph node dissection, *Am J Surg* 160(5):481, 1990.

203. Jernstrom H, Barrett-Connor E: Obesity, weight change, fasting insulin, proinsulin, C-peptide, and insulin-like growth factor-1 levels in women with and without breast cancer: the Rancho Bernardo Study, *J Womens Health Gend Based Med* 8(10):1265, 1999.

204. Joslyn S, West M: Racial differences in breast carcinoma survival, *Cancer* 88(1):114, 2000.

205. Kakuda J and others: Objective assessment of axillary morbidity in breast cancer treatment, *Am Surg* 65(10):995, 1999.

206. Kantor D, Houldin A: Breast cancer in older women: treatment, psychosocial effects, interventions, and outcomes, *J Gerontol Nurs* 25(7):19, 1999.

207. Kaufmann M: Review of known prognostic variables, *Recent Results Cancer Res* 140:77, 1996.

208. Kegeles S: Education for breast self-examination: why, who, what, and how? *Prev Med* 14(6):702, 1985.

209. Kelly P: *Understanding breast cancer risk,* Philadelphia, Temple University Press, 1991.

210. Kelly P, Winslow E: Needle wire localization for nonpalpable breast lesions: sensations, anxiety levels, and informational needs, *Oncol Nurs Forum* 23(4):639, 1996.

211. Kelsey J, Horn-Ross P: Breast cancer: magnitude of the problem and descriptive epidemiology, *Epidemiol Rev* 15(1):7, 1993.

212. Kelsey J, Whittemore A: Epidemiology and primary prevention of cancers of the breast, endometrium, and ovary. A brief overview, *Ann Epidemiol* 4(2):89, 1994.

213. Khoo A and others: A comparison of resource costs of immediate and delayed breast reconstruction, *Plast Reconstr Surg* 101(4):964, 1998.

214. Kilpatrick M and others: Information needs of husbands of women with breast cancer, *Oncol Nurs Forum* 25(9):1595, 1998.

215. Kimmick G, Muss HB: Current status of endocrine therapy for metastatic breast cancer, *Oncology* 9(9):877, 1995.

216. Kissane D and others: Psychological morbidity and quality of life in Australian women with early-stage breast cancer: a cross-sectional survey, *Med J Aust* 169(4):192, 1998.

217. Knobf M: Natural menopause and ovarian toxicity associated with breast cancer therapy, *Oncol Nurs Forum* 25(9):1519, 1998.

218. Kogon M and others: Effects of medical and psychotherapeutic treatment on the survival of women with metastatic breast carcinoma, *Cancer* 80(2):225, 1997.

219. Koibuchi Y and others: The effect of mass screening by physical examination combined with regular breast self-examination on clinical stage and course of Japanese women with breast cancer, *Oncol Rep* 5(1):151, 1998.

220. Kopans D: Imaging analysis of breast lesions. In Harris J, Lippman M, Morrow M, Osborne C, editors: *Diseases of the breast,* ed 2, p. 123, Philadelphia, Lippincott Williams & Wilkins, 2000.

221. Kricker A and others: Breast cancer in New South Wales in 1972–1995: tumor size and the impact of mammographic screening, *Int J Cancer* 81(6):877, 1999.

222. Kurebayashi J, Shimozuma K, Sonoo H: The practice of breast self-examination results in the earlier detection and better clinical course of Japanese women with breast cancer, *Surg Today* 24(4):337, 1994.

223. Kwekkeboom K: Postmastectomy pain syndromes, *Cancer Nurs* 19(1):37, 1996.

224. Lagios M, Page D: In situ carcinomas of the breast: ductal carcinoma in situ, Paget's disease, lobular carcinoma in situ. In Bland K, Copeland E, editors: *The breast: comprehensive management of benign and malignant diseases,* ed 2, p. 261, Philadelphia, Saunders, 1998.

225. Langston AA and others: BRCA1 mutations in a population-based sample of young women with breast cancer, *N Engl J Med* 334(3):137, 1996.

226. Lauver D and others: Engagement in breast cancer screening behaviors, *Oncol Nurs Forum* 26(3):545, 1999.

227. Lauver D, Coyle M, Panchmatia B: Women's reasons for and barriers to seeking care for breast cancer symptoms, *Women's Health Issues* 5(1):27, 1995.

228. Lauver D, Tak Y: Optimism and coping with a breast cancer symptom, *Nurs Res* 44(4):202, 1995.

229. Lazovich D and others: Breast conservation therapy in the United States following the 1990 National Institutes of Health Consensus Development Conference on the treatment of patients with early stage invasive breast carcinoma, *Cancer* 86(4):628, 1999.

230. Lea D, Jenkins J, Francomano C: Genetics in clinical practice. New directions for nursing and health care, Sudbury, Mass, Jones and Bartlett, 1998.

231. Lee K, Dunlop D, Dolan N: Do clinical breast examination skills improve during medical school? *Acad Med* 73(9):1013, 1998.

232. Lee M and others: Alternative therapies used by women with breast cancer in four ethnic populations, *J Natl Cancer Inst* 92(1):42, 2000.

233. Lehto R, Cimprich B: Anxiety and directed attention in women awaiting breast cancer surgery, *Oncol Nurs Forum* 26(4):767, 1999.

234. Lemon H, Rodriguez-Sierra J: Timing of breast cancer surgery during the luteal menstrual phase may improve prognosis, *Nebr Med J* 81(4):110, 1996.

235. Lewis F, Deal L: Balancing our lives: a study of the married couple's experience with breast cancer recurrence, *Oncol Nurs Forum* 22(6):943, 1995.

236. Lewis F and others: The functioning of single women with breast cancer and their school-aged children, *Cancer Pract* 4(1):15, 1996.

237. Lewis M and others: Women's approaches to decision making about mammography, *Cancer Nurs* 22:380, 1999.

238. Lierman L: Phantom breast experiences after mastectomy, *Oncol Nurs Forum* 15(1):41, 1988.

239. Lierman L and others: Effects of education and support on breast self-examination in older women, *Nurs Res* 43(3):158, 1994.

240. Longman A, Braden C, Mishel M: Side-effects burden, psychological adjustment, and life quality in women with breast cancer: pattern of association over time, *Oncol Nurs Forum* 26(5):909, 1999.

241. Longnecker M, Paganini-Hill A, Ross R: Lifetime alcohol consumption and breast cancer risk among postmenopausal women in Los Angeles, *Cancer Epidemiol Biomarkers Prev* 4(7):721, 1995.

242. Longnecker M and others: Risk of breast cancer in relation to lifetime alcohol consumption, *J Natl Cancer Inst* 87(12):923, 1995.

243. Lotze M and others: Early versus delayed shoulder motion following axillary dissection, *Ann Surg* 193(3):288, 1981.

244. Love SM: Dr. *Susan Love's breast book,* ed 2, Reading, Mass, Addison-Wesley, 1995.

245. Lower E and others: The risk of premature menopause induced by chemotherapy for early breast cancer, *J Womens Health Gend Based Med* 8(7):949, 1999.

246. Ludwick R: Registered nurses' knowledge and practices of teaching and performing breast exams among elderly women, *Cancer Nurs* 15(1):61, 1992.

247. Lugton J: The nature of social support as experienced by women treated for breast cancer, *J Adv Nurs* 25(6):1184, 1997.

248. Mahon S: Cancer risk assessment: conceptual considerations for clinical practice, *Oncol Nurs Forum* 25(9):1535, 1998.

249. Makuc D, Breen N, Freid V: Low income, race, and the use of mammography, *Health Serv Res* 34(1 Pt 2):229, 1999.

250. Malkin D: Germline *p53* mutations and heritable cancer, *Annu Rev Genet* 28:443, 1994.

251. Mammatech Corporation: *MammaCare® personal learning system,* Gainesville, FL, Mammatech, 1990.

252. Mammatech Corporation: *MammaCare® professional learning system,* Gainesville, FL, Mammatech, 1990.

253. Mandelblatt J and others: Impact of access and social context on breast cancer stage at diagnosis, *J Health Care Poor Underserved* 6:342, 1995.

254. Mandelblatt J and others: The costs and effects of cervical and breast cancer screening in a public hospital emergency room. The Cancer Control Center of Harlem, *Am J Public Health* 87(7):1182, 1997.

255. Maunsell E and others: Work problems after breast cancer: an exploratory qualitative study, *Psychooncology* 8(6):467, 1999.

256. Maunsell E, Brisson J, Deschenes L: Arm problems and psychological distress after surgery for breast cancer, *Can J Surg* 36(4):315, 1993.

257. May D and others: Compliance with mammography guidelines: physician recommendation and patient adherence, *Prev Med* 28(4):386, 1999.

258. McCraw J and others: Breast reconstruction following mastectomy. In Bland K, Copeland E, editors: *The breast: comprehensive management of benign and malignant diseases,* ed 2, vol. 1, p. 962, Philadelphia, Saunders, 1998.

259. McGregor H and others: Breast cancer incidence among atomic bomb survivors, Hiroshima and Nagasaki, 1950–1969, *J Natl Cancer Inst* 59(3):799, 1977.

260. McQuellon R and others: Patient preferences for treatment of metastatic breast cancer: a study of women with early-stage breast cancer, *J Clin Oncol* 13(4):858, 1995.

261. Mettlin C: Global breast cancer mortality statistics, *CA Cancer J Clin* 49(3):138, 1999.

262. Meyerowitz B and others: Sexuality following breast cancer, *J Sex Marital Ther* 25(3):237, 1999.

263. Michels KB, Willett WC: The Women's Health Initiative: will it resolve the issues? *Recent Results Cancer Res* 140:295, 1996.

264. Miki Y and others: A strong candidate for the breast and ovarian cancer susceptibility gene BRCA1, *Science* 266(5182):66, 1994.

265. Miller A and others: Mortality from breast cancer after irradiation during fluoroscopic examinations in patients being treated for tuberculosis, *N Engl J Med* 321(19):1285, 1989.

266. Miller A: Screening and detection. In Bland K, Copeland E, editors: *The breast: comprehensive management of benign and malignant diseases,* ed 2, vol. 1, p. 625, Philadelphia, Saunders, 1998.

267. Mock V and others: Effects of exercise on fatigue, physical functioning, and emotional distress during radiation therapy for breast cancer, *Oncol Nurs Forum* 24(6):991, 1997.

268. Monson M, Harwood K: Helping women select primary breast cancer treatment, *Am J Nurs* 98(4 Suppl):3, 1998.

269. Montgomery L and others: Issues of regret in women with contralateral prophylactic mastectomies, *Ann Surg Oncol* 6(6):546, 1999.

270. Moore K: Breast cancer patients' out-of-pocket expenses, *Cancer Nurs* 22(5):389, 1999.

271. Morrison C: Determining crucial correlates of breast self-examination in older women with low incomes, *Oncol Nurs Forum* 23(1):83, 1996.

272. Morrow M, Schnitt S: Lobular carcinoma *in situ.* In Harris J, Lippman M, Morrow M, Osborne C, editors: *Diseases of the breast,* ed 2, p. 377, Philadelphia, Lippincott Williams & Wilkins, 2000.

273. Morrow M, Harris J: Local management of invasive breast cancer. In Harris J, Lippman M, Morrow M, Osborne C, editors: *Diseases of the breast,* ed 2, p. 515, Philadelphia, Lippincott Williams & Wilkins, 2000.

274. Morrow M, Schnitt S, Harris J: Ductal carcinoma *in situ* and microinvasive carcinoma. In Harris J, Lippman M, Morrow M, Osborne C, editors: *Diseases of the breast,* ed 2, p. 383, Philadelphia, Lippincott Williams & Wilkins, 2000.

275. Morton D: Intraoperative lymphatic mapping and sentinel lymphadenectomy: community standard care or clinical investigation? *Cancer J Sci Am* 3(6):328, 1997.

276. Moyer A, Salovey P: Patient participation in treatment decision making and the psychological consequences of breast cancer surgery, *Womens Health* 4(2):103, 1998.

277. National Institutes of Health Consensus Development Panel: Consensus statement: treatment of early-stage breast cancer. In Consensus Development Conference on the Treatment of Early-Stage Breast Cancer, *J Natl Cancer Inst Monogr* 11:1, NIH Publication No. 90-3187, Washington, DC, US Government Printing Office, 1992.

278. National Institutes of Health Consensus Development Panel: Supplemental information for NIH consensus statement on treatment of early-stage breast cancer. Retrieved April 9, 2000 from the World Wide Web: http://odp.od.nih.gov/consensus/cons/081/081_statement.htm

279. Niederhuber J: Interval breast cancer and the kinetics of neoplastic growth. In Bland K, Copeland E, editors: *The breast: comprehensive management of benign and malignant diseases,* ed 2, vol. 1, p. 634, Philadelphia, Saunders, 1998.

280. Northouse L and others: Emotional distress reported by women and husbands prior to a breast biopsy, *Nurs Res* 44(4):196, 1995.

281. Northouse L and others: The quality of life of African American women with breast cancer, *Res Nurs Health* 22(6):449, 1999.

282. Northouse L, Dorris G, Charron-Moore C: Factors affecting couples' adjustment to recurrent breast cancer, *Soc Sci Med* 41(1):69, 1995.

283. Northouse L, Laten D, Reddy P: Adjustment of women and their husbands to recurrent breast cancer, *Res Nurs Health* 18(6):515, 1995.

284. Northouse L and others: Couples' adjustment to breast cancer and benign breast disease: a longitudinal analysis, *Psychooncology* 7(1):37, 1998.

285. Northouse L, Tocco K, West P: Coping with a breast biopsy: how healthcare professionals can help women and their husbands, *Oncol Nurs Forum* 24(3):473, 1997.

286. O'Grady L, Rippon M: The high-risk patient. In O'Grady L, Lindfors K, Howell L, Rippon M, editors: *A practical approach to breast disease,* Boston, Little, Brown, 1995.

287. O'Malley MS: Cost-effectiveness of two nurse-led programs to teach breast self-examination, *Am J Prev Med* 9(3):139, 1993.

288. Oncology Nursing Society: *Short-stay surgery for breast cancer.* ONS Position Statement. Pittsburgh, Oncology Nursing Press, 1998. Available on-line at http://www.ons-.org/ons/library/ons/default2.htm

289. Osborne C: Adjuvant systemic therapy of primary breast cancer. In Harris J, Lippman M, Morrow M, Osborne C, editors: *Diseases of the breast,* ed 2, p. 599, Philadelphia, Lippincott Williams & Wilkins, 2000.

290. Osborne M: Breast anatomy and development. In Harris J, Lippman M, Morrow M, Osborne C, editors: *Diseases of the breast,* ed 2, p. 1, Philadelphia, Lippincott Williams & Wilkins, 2000.

291. Osborne M, Rosen P: Detection and management of bone marrow micrometastases in breast cancer, *Oncology* 8(8):25, 1994.

292. Page D, Simpson J: Benign, high-risk, and premalignant lesions of the breast. In Bland K, Copeland E, editors: *The breast: comprehensive management of benign and malignant diseases,* ed 2, vol. 1, p. 19, Philadelphia, Saunders, 1998.

293. Parker SH: Needle selection. In Parker SH, Jobe WE: *Percutaneous breast biopsy,* New York, Raven, 1993.

294. Parkin D, Pisani P, Ferlay J: Global cancer statistics, *CA Cancer J Clin* 49(1):64, 1999.

295. Pasacreta J, McCorkle R: Providing accurate information to women about tamoxifen therapy for breast cancer: current indications, effects, and controversies, *Oncol Nurs Forum* 25(9):1577, 1998.

296. Peacock S and others: Relation between obesity and breast cancer in young women, *Am J Epidemiol* 149(4):339, 1999.

297. Pennypacker H and others: Toward an effective technology of instruction in breast self-examination, *Int J Ment Health* 11(3):98, 1982.

298. Pennypacker H, Naylor L, Sander A, Goldstein M: Why can't we do better breast examinations? *Nurse Pract Forum* 10(3):122, 1999.

299. Peragallo N, Fox P, Alba M: Breast care among Latino immigrant women in the U.S., *Health Care Women Int* 19(2):165, 1998.

300. Peters W and others: High-dose chemotherapy and peripheral blood progenitor cell transplantation in the treatment of breast cancer, *Oncologist* 5(1):1, 2000.

301. Petrek J, Lerner R: Lymphedema. In Harris J, Lippman M, Morrow M, Osborne C, editors: *Diseases of the breast,* ed 2, p. 1033, Philadelphia, Lippincott Williams & Wilkins, 2000.

302. Petrek J and others: Axillary lymphadenectomy: a prospective, randomized trial of 13 factors influencing drainage, including early or delayed arm mobilization, *Arch Surg* 125(3):378, 1990.

303. Phillips J, Cohen M, Moses G: Breast cancer screening and African American women: fear, fatalism, and silence, *Oncol Nurs Forum* 26(3):561, 1999.

304. Pierce P: Deciding on breast cancer treatment: a description of decision behavior, *Nurs Res* 42(1):22, 1993.

305. Pike M and others: Estrogens, progestogens, normal breast cell proliferation, and breast cancer risk, *Epidemiol Rev* 15(1):17, 1993.

306. Porock D and others: Predicting the severity of radiation skin reactions in women with breast cancer, *Oncol Nurs Forum* 25(6):1019, 1998.

307. Pritchard K, Roy J-A, Sawka C: Sex hormones and breast cancer: the issue of hormone replacement, *Recent Results Cancer Res* 140:285, 1996.

308. Protiere C and others: Patient participation in medical decision-making: a French study in adjuvant radiochemotherapy for early breast cancer, *Ann Oncol* 11(1):39, 2000.

309. Pusic A and others: Surgical options for the early-stage breast cancer: factors associated with patient choice and postoperative quality of life, *Plast Reconstr Surg,* 104(5):1325, 1999.

310. Rahman Z and others: Results and long term follow-up for 1581 patients with metastatic breast carcinoma treated with standard dose doxorubicin-containing chemotherapy: a reference, *Cancer* 85(1):104, 1999.

311. Ravdin P: A computer based program to assist in adjuvant therapy decisions for individual breast cancer patients, *Bull Cancer* 82 (Suppl 5):561s, 1995.

312. Ravdin P: Emerging role of docetaxel (Taxotere) in the adjuvant therapy of breast cancer, *Semin Oncol* 26(3 Suppl 9):20, 1999.

313. Ravdin P, Siminoff I, Harvey J: Survey of breast cancer patients concerning their knowledge and expectations of adjuvant therapy, *J Clin Oncol* 16(2):515, 1998.

314. Rees C, Bath P: Meeting the information needs of adult daughters of women with early breast cancer. Patients and health care professionals as information providers, *Cancer Nurs* 23(1):71, 2000.

315. Roberts F and others: Self-reported stress and risk of breast cancer, *Cancer* 77(6):1089, 1996.

316. Rojas M and others: Barriers to follow-up of abnormal screening mammograms among low-income minority women, *Ethn Health* 1(3):221, 1996.

317. Romrell L, Bland K: Anatomy of the breast, axilla, chest wall, and related metastatic sites. In Bland K, Copeland E, editors: *The breast: comprehensive management of benign and malignant diseases,* ed 2, vol. 1, p. 19, Philadelphia, Saunders, 1998.

318. Rookus M, vanLeeuwen F: Oral contraceptives and risk of breast cancer in women aged 20–54 years. Netherlands Oral Contraceptives and Breast Cancer Study Group, *Lancet* 344(8926):844, 1994.

319. Ross R and others: Effect of hormone replacement therapy on breast cancer risk: estrogen versus estrogen plus progestin, *J Natl Cancer Inst* 92(4):328, 2000.

320. Rossouw J, Hurd S: The Women's Health Initiative: recruitment complete—looking back and looking forward [editorial], *J Womens Health* 8(1):3, 1999.

321. Rowland J, Massie M: Psychosocial issues and interventions. In Harris J, Lippman M, Morrow M, Osborne C, editors: *Diseases of the breast,* ed 2, p. 1009, Philadelphia, Lippincott Williams & Wilkins, 2000.

322. Sachs B: Breasts: sex symbols and releasers, *Dis Breast* 4(4):26, 1978.

323. Samms M: The husband's untold account of his wife's breast cancer: a chronologic analysis, *Oncol Nurs Forum* 26(8):1351, 1999.

324. Satariano W, DeLorenze G: The likelihood of returning to work after breast cancer, *Public Health Rep* 111(3):236, 1996.

325. Saunders K, Pilgrim C, Pennypacker H: Increased proficiency of search in breast self-examination, *Cancer* 58(11):2531, 1986.

326. Schain W, Jacobs E, Wellisch D: Psychosocial issues in breast reconstruction: intrapsychic, interpersonal and practical concerns, *Clin Plast Surg* 11(2):237, 1984.

327. Schain W and others: The sooner the better: a study of psychological factors in women undergoing immediate versus delayed breast reconstruction, *Am J Psychiatry* 142(1):40, 1985.

328. Schairer C and others: Menopausal estrogen and estrogen-progestin replacement therapy and breast cancer risk, *JAMA* 283(4):485, 2000.

329. Schapira M, McAuliffe T, Nattinger A: Underutilization of mammography in older breast cancer survivors, *Med Care* 38(3):281, 2000.

330. Schmidt RA: Stereotactic breast biopsy, *CA Cancer J Clin* 44(3):172, 1994.

331. Schmit-Pokorny, Hruska M, Ursick M: Peripheral blood stem cell transplantation: outpatient strategies, *Innov Breast Cancer Care* 3(3):52, 1998.

332. Schnitt S, Guidi A: Pathology of invasive breast cancer. In Harris J, Lippman M, Morrow M, Osborne C, editors: *Diseases of the breast,* ed 2, p. 425, Philadelphia, Lippincott Williams & Wilkins, 2000.

333. Schover L: The impact of breast cancer on sexuality, body image, and intimate relationships, *CA Cancer J Clin* 41(2):112, 1991.

334. Schrag D and others: Life expectancy gains from cancer prevention strategies for women with breast cancer and BRCA1 or BRCA2 mutations, *JAMA* 283(5):617, 2000.

335. Schultz I, Barholm M, Grondal S: Delayed shoulder exercises in reducing seroma frequency after modified radical mastectomy: a prospective randomized study, *Ann Surg Oncol* 4(4):293, 1997.

336. Schwartz A: Daily fatigue patterns and effect of exercise in women with breast cancer, *Cancer Pract* 8(1):16, 2000.

337. Sciartelli C: Using a clinical pathway approach to document patient teaching for breast cancer surgical procedures, *Oncol Nurs Forum* 22(1):131, 1995.

338. Segar M and others: The effect of aerobic exercise on self-esteem and depressive and anxiety symptoms among breast cancer survivors, *Oncol Nurs Forum* 25(1):107, 1998.

339. Seidman H, Stellman S, Mushinski M: A different perspective on breast cancer risk factors: some implications of the nonattributable risk, *CA Cancer J Clin* 32(5):301, 1982.

340. Sellers T and others: The role of hormone replacement therapy in the risk for breast cancer and total mortality in women with a family history of breast cancer, *Ann Intern Med* 127(11):973, 1997.

341. Semiglazov V and others: Interim results of a prospective randomized study of self-examination for early detection of breast cancer (Russia/St. Petersburg/WHO), *Vopr Onkol* 45(3):265, 1999.

342. Semiglazov V and others: Study of the role of breast self-examination in the reduction of mortality from breast cancer. The Russian Federation/World Health Organization Study, *Eur J Cancer* 29A(14):2039, 1993.

343. Senie R and others: Method of tumor detection influences disease-free survival of women with breast carcinoma, *Cancer* 73(6):1666, 1994.

344. Senie R, Tenser S: The timing of breast cancer surgery during the menstrual cycle, *Oncology* 11(10):1509, 1997.

345. Shands M, Lewis F, Zahlis E: Mother and child interactions about the mother's breast cancer: an interview study, *Oncol Nurs Forum* 27(1):77, 2000.

346. Sharp N: The politics of breast cancer, *Nurs Manage* 22(9):24, 1991.

347. Shimozuma K and others: Quality of life in the first year after breast cancer surgery: rehabilitation needs and patterns of recovery, *Breast Cancer Res Treat,* 56(1):45, 1999.

348. Shugg D and others: Practice of breast self-examination and the treatment of primary breast cancer, *Aust NZ J Surg* 60(6):455, 1990.

349. Sickles E: Breast cancer screening outcomes in women ages 40–49: clinical experience with service screening using modern mammography, *J Natl Cancer Inst Monogr* 22:99, 1997.

350. Singletary E: Techniques of surgery. In Harris J, Lippman M, Morrow M, Osborne C, editors: *Diseases of the breast,* ed 2, p. 577, Philadelphia, Lippincott Williams & Wilkins, 2000.

351. Skaer T and others: Cancer-screening determinants among Hispanic women using migrant health clinics, *J Health Care Poor Underserved* 7(4):338, 1996.

352. Sledge G: Chemotherapy for metastatic breast cancer. In Bland K, Copeland E, editors: *The breast: comprehensive management of benign and malignant diseases,* ed 2, p. 1324, Philadelphia, Saunders, 1998.

353. Smart C and others: Twenty-year follow-up of the breast cancers diagnosed during the Breast Cancer Detection Demonstration Project, *CA Cancer J Clin* 47(3):134, 1997.

354. Smith R, D'Orsi C: Screening for breast cancer. In Harris J, Lippman M, Morrow M, Osborne C, editors: *Diseases of the breast,* ed 2, p. 101, Philadelphia, Lippincott Williams & Wilkins, 2000.

355. Smith R and others: American Cancer Society guidelines for the early detection of cancer, *CA Cancer J Clin* 50(1):34, 2000.

356. Smith-Warner S and others: Alcohol and breast cancer in women: a pooled analysis of cohort studies, *JAMA* 279(7):535, 1998.

357. Society of Surgical Oncology: SSO develops position statement on prophylactic mastectomies, *SSO News,* Summer 1993, p 1.

358. Sonnenschein E and others: Body fat distribution and obesity in pre- and postmenopausal breast cancer, *Int J Epidemiol* 28(6):1026, 1999.

359. Sortet J, Banks S: Health beliefs of rural Appalachian women and the practice of breast self-examination, *Cancer Nurs* 20(4):231, 1997.

360. Spencer S and others: Concerns about breast cancer and relations to psychosocial well-being in a multiethnic sample of early-stage patients, *Health Psychol* 18(2):159, 1999.

361. Stanton A and others: Treatment decision making and adjustment to breast cancer: a longitudinal study, *J Consult Clin Psychol* 66(2):313, 1998.

362. Stearns V, Yamauchi H, Hayes D: Circulating tumor markers in breast cancer: accepted utilities and novel prospects, *Breast Cancer Res Treat* 52(1–3):239, 1998.

363. Stefanek M and others: Bilateral prophylactic mastectomy decision making: a vignette study, *Prev Med* 29(3):216, 1999.

364. Stoll B: Alcohol intake and late-stage promotion of breast cancer, *Eur J Cancer* 35(12):1653, 1999.

365. Stoll B: Perimenopausal weight gain and progression of breast cancer precursors, *Cancer Detect Prev* 23(1):31, 1999.

366. Street R and others: Increasing patient involvement in choosing treatment for early breast cancer, *Cancer* 76(11):2275, 1995.

367. Swanson C and others: Alcohol consumption and breast cancer risk among women under age 45 years, *Epidemiology* 8(3):231, 1997.

368. Tabar L and others: Efficacy of breast cancer screening by age. New results from the Swedish Two-County Trial, *Cancer* 75(10):2507, 1995.

369. Taneja C, Gardner B: Therapeutic value of axillary lymph node dissection for breast cancer. In Bland K, Copeland E, editors: *The breast: comprehensive management of benign and malignant diseases,* ed 2, vol. 2, p. 943, Philadelphia, Saunders, 1998.

370. Taylor J and others: The comprehensive health enhancement support system, *Qual Manag Health Care* 2(4):36, 1994.

371. Thijs-Boer F, de Kruif A, van de Wiel H: Supportive nursing care around breast cancer surgery: an evaluation of the 1997 status in The Netherlands, *Cancer Nurs* 22(2):172, 1999.

372. Thomas SG: Breast cancer: the psychosocial issues, *Cancer Nurs* 1(1):53, 1978.

373. Tobin M and others: The psychological morbidity of breast cancer-related arm swelling, *Cancer* 72(11):3248, 1993.

374. Tolmos J and others: Scintimammographic analysis of nonpalpable breast lesions previously identified by conventional mammography, *J Natl Cancer Inst* 90(11):846, 1998.

375. Turner R and others: Histopathologic validation of the sentinel lymph node hypothesis for breast carcinoma, *Ann Surg* 226(3):271, 1997.

376. Ursin G and others: Breast cancer and oral contraceptive use in Asian-American women, *Am J Epidemiol* 150(6):561, 1999.

377. US Department of Health and Human Services: *Healthy people 2000,* Publication No. 91-50212, Washington, DC, Public Health Service, 1991.

378. US Department of Health and Human Services. *Healthy people 2010* (Conference Edition, in Two Volumes). Washington, DC, 2000. Available On-Line from the World Wide Web: http://web.health.gov/healthypeople/default.htm *or* Limited number of copies available from ODPHP Communication Support Center, P.O. Box 37366, Washington, DC 20013-7366, (301) 468-5960. $22 (B0074). *or* on CD-ROM contains *Understanding and Improving Health, Objectives for Improving Health,* and *Tracking Healthy People 2010.* Available from ODPHP Communication Support Center, P.O. Box 37366, Washington, DC 20013-7366, (301) 468-5960. $5 (B0071).

379. US Department of Health and Human Services: *Quality determinants of mammography,* Publication No. 95-0632, Rockville, Md, Agency for Health Care Policy and Research, 1994.

380. US Food and Drug Administration: Chronology of FDA activities related to breast implants. Retrieved April 2, 2000 from the World Wide Web: http://www.fda.gov/cdrh/breastimplants/bichron.html

381. US Food and Drug Administration: FDA's mammography program. Retrieved March 18, 2000 from the World Wide Web: http://www.fda.gov/cdrh/mammography/consumers.html

382. van den Brandt P, Goldbohm R, van't Veer P: Alcohol and breast cancer: results from The Netherlands Cohort Study, *Am J Epidemiol* 141(10):907, 1995.

383. Viel J and others: Alcoholic calories, red wine consumption and breast cancer among premenopausal women, *Eur J Epidemiol* 13(6):639, 1997.

384. Wagner F, Martin R, Bland K: History of the therapy of breast disease. In Bland K, Copeland E, editors: *The breast: comprehensive management of benign and malignant diseases,* ed 2, vol. 1, p. 1, Philadelphia, Saunders, 1998.

385. Wall P and others: Diagnostic delay in breast disease. A system analysis of a public urban hospital, *Arch Surg* 133(6):662, 1998.

386. Wapnir I, Cody R, Greco R: Subtle differences in quality of life after breast cancer surgery, *Ann Surg Oncol* 6(4):359, 1999.

387. Ward S, Heidrich S, Wolberg W: Factors women take into account when deciding upon type of surgery for breast cancer, *Cancer Nurs* 12(6):344, 1989.

388. Weber B: Familial breast cancer, *Recent Results Cancer Res* 140:5, 1996.

389. Wellisch D and others: An exploratory study of social support: a cross-cultural comparison of Chinese-, Japanese-, and Anglo-American breast cancer patients, *Psychooncology* 8(3):207, 1999.

390. White E and others: Breast cancer among young U.S. women in relation to oral contraceptive use, *J Natl Cancer Inst* 86(7):505, 1994.

391. Winchester D, Cox J: Standards for diagnosis and management of invasive breast carcinoma. American College of Radiology. American College of Surgeons. College of American Pathologists. Society of Surgical Oncology, *CA Cancer J Clin* 48(2):83, 1998.

392. Winchester D, Strom E: Standards for diagnosis and management of ductal carcinoma in situ (DCIS) of the breast. American College of Radiology. American College of Surgeons. College of American Pathologists. Society of Surgical Oncology, *CA Cancer J Clin* 48(2):108, 1998.

393. Winer E and others: Quality of life in patients surviving at least 12 months following high dose chemotherapy with autologous bone marrow support, *Psychooncology* 8(2):167, 1999.

394. Witliff J, Pasic R, Bland K: Steroid and peptide hormone receptors: methods, quality control, and clinical use. In Bland K, Copeland E, editors: *The breast: comprehensive management of benign and malignant diseases,* ed 2, vol. 1, p. 458, Philadelphia, Saunders, 1998.

395. Woo B and others: Differences in fatigue by treatment methods in women with breast cancer, *Oncol Nurs Forum* 25(5):915, 1998.

396. Wood R: Breast self-examination proficiency in older women: measuring the efficacy of video self-instruction kits, *Cancer Nurs* 19(6):429, 1996.

397. Wooster R and others: Identification of the breast cancer susceptibility gene BRCA2, *Nature* 378(6559):789, 1995.

398. Wooster R and others: Localization of a breast cancer susceptibility gene, BRCA2, to chromosome 13q12-13, *Science* 265(5181):2088, 1994.

399. Wu A, Pike M, Stram D: Meta-analysis: dietary fat intake, serum estrogen levels, and the risk of breast cancer, *J Natl Cancer Inst* 91(6):529, 1999.

400. Wyatt G, Friedman L: Physical and psychosocial outcomes of midlife and older women following surgery and adjuvant therapy for breast cancer, *Oncol Nurs Forum* 25(4):761, 1998.

401. Yalom M: *A history of the breast.* New York, Alfred A. Knopf, 1997.

402. Yang X, Lippman M: BRCA1 and BRCA2 in breast cancer, *Breast Cancer Res Treat* 54(1):1, 1999.

403. Zavotsky J and others: Lymph node metastasis from ductal carcinoma in situ with microinvasion, *Cancer* 85(11):2439, 1999.

404. Zujewski J, Liu E: The 1998 St. Gallen's Consensus Conference: an assessment, *J Natl Cancer Inst* 90(21):1587, 1998.

8 Colorectal Cancers

CHAPTER

Mary E. Murphy

Colorectal cancer is the third most common malignant tumor in the United States, second only to lung cancer in its incidence and mortality. An estimated 130,500 new cases develop each year, with an annual death rate of 56,300. Mortality rates show a decline in both men and women and are most likely related to increased diagnostic screening, community awareness, and dietary modifications.[1, 8–10, 21, 22]

EPIDEMIOLOGY

Colorectal cancer affects both genders with a slight increase in the female population and with the incidence increasing significantly in persons over age 50. The mean age at the time of diagnosis is 62. The disease occurs most frequently in the industrialized countries of North America and northern Europe. Individuals from low-incidence countries who move to western countries develop colorectal cancer at the same rate as in western countries. The incidence among the African American population shows an increase in African American women with an increase in mortality among both men and women.*

ETIOLOGY AND RISK FACTORS

The cause of colorectal cancer is unknown, but recent research indicates that diet, genetics, and other predisposing factors such as bowel disorders may play an important role in its development.

Diet

The relationship between diet and colorectal cancer remains under investigation, but evidence shows that individuals with diets low in animal fats and high in fiber demonstrate a significantly lower incidence of disease. Research indicates that fats and meat products may alter the concentration of normal body products such as cholesterol and fecal bile salts and also may change the normal intestinal flora of the bowel. This process may serve as a cancer promoter by damaging the colonic mucosa and increasing the proliferational activity of the colonic epithelium.

Reduced dietary fiber may also serve as a promoter of the carcinogenic process by increasing the amount of contact time that the carcinogenic substance has with colonic mucosa, therefore increasing the potential for mutagenic changes in the bowel wall. Increased alcohol and caffeine intake has also been indicated to increase risk of large-bowel cancers.

Other dietary factors that serve as promoters of the carcinogenic process include genotoxic carcinogens such as charbroiled meats, fish, and fried foods. Dietary deficiencies of vitamins A, C, and E; selenium; and calcium have also been investigated and may result in future dietary recommendations. The American Cancer Society Updated Nutritional Guidelines (1999) mirror the 1992 U.S. Department of Agriculture (USDA) Food Guide Pyramid and the 1995 Dietary Guidelines for Americans. Additional recommendations can be found in Box 8–1.*

Genetic Factors

Genetic abnormalities and traits represent a new area of scientific technology that may help identify individuals at risk. Progressive genetic changes trigger a multistep process in which chromosomal and oncogenic changes occur and result in colorectal epithelium mutations forming malignant tumors in the colon.

Genetics plays a role in the predisposition to colorectal cancer. Persons with first-degree relatives who have colorectal cancer have a threefold risk of having the disease themselves. Polyposis syndromes such as Gardner's, Turcot's, and Peutz-Jeghers' are linked to increased risks for the development of colorectal cancers.

---

* References 9, 25, 30, 33, 36, 43, 45, 46.

* References 1, 11, 15, 21, 22, 33, 40, 46, 51–53.

168

BOX 8-1

Nutrition Guidelines of the American Cancer Society

Choose most of the foods you eat from plant sources.
  Eat five or more servings of fruits and vegetables each day.
  Eat other foods from plant sources, such as breads, cereals, grain products, rice, pasta, or beans several times each day.
Limit your intake of high-fat foods, particulary from animal sources.
  Choose foods low in fat.
  Limit consumption of meats, especially high-fat meats.
Be physically active. Achieve and maintain a healthy weight.
  Be at least moderately active for 30 minutes or more on most days of the week.
  Stay within your healthy weight range.
Limit consumption of alcoholic beverages, if you drink at all.

These autosomal dominant diseases are manifested by thousands of colonic adenomas that have a high malignant potential. Specific genes that are being evaluated include APL, HNPCC, Lynch I and II, and 1130K. Details of genetic relationships can be found in Chapter 2 of this text.

Other Predisposing Factors

Other predisposing factors include ulcerative colitis and Crohn's disease. These inflammatory bowel disorders are associated with dysplasia and associated malignant lesions. Potential for the malignant process is correlated to the disease's duration. In addition to inflammatory bowel disease, polyposis adenomas are the most common bowel polyps and account for 80% of all types of bowel polyps. These polyps increase their malignant potential as they grow larger and demonstrate cellular changes. This process takes 10 to 15 years from the time of diagnosis. Villous adenomas are another type of polyp that has been associated with increased malignancy and high fatality. These polyps produce excessive mucus and result in severe fluid and electrolyte disorders. Other relationships have been correlated with a history of breast, endometrial, and ovarian cancer. Aging, itself, is listed as a risk factor with over 90% of all patients diagnosed after the age of 50. The most recent area of investigation is examining the regular use of ASA products and nonsteroidal anti-inflammatory drugs (NSAIDs).*

---

* References 1, 33, 35-37, 45, 49, 50, 52.

PREVENTION, SCREENING, AND DETECTION

The American Cancer Society (ACS) recommends specific protocols for the screening and prevention of colorectal cancers. The ACS recommendations for colon cancer screening for an asymptomatic person include an annual digital rectal examination and an annual stool guaiac test for persons over age 50. Proctosigmoidoscopy should be done every 5 years. Table 8-1 shows complete ACS guidelines. Persons at high risk may need screening at an earlier age and more frequently than the general population.[12, 29, 39]

Because many tumors are found in the lower rectum, abdominal and rectal examinations should be performed at the time of a routine physical examination. Digital rectal examination (DRE) should be performed yearly to examine for polyps and cancers of the lower rectum (up to 7 cm) and the anal verge. This should also be done prior to scopy examination or before a barium enema.

The *fecal occult blood test (FOBT)* is an effective and inexpensive screening tool to examine for hidden blood. False-negative and false-positive results may occur for a variety of reasons. The primary cause may be inadequate instruction on sample collection, poor compliance with specific directions, and the fact that 50% of most polyps are not actively bleeding at the time of sample collection. Instructions should include various dietary, medication, and collection procedures.

All individuals should be on a meat-free, high-residue diet for 2 days before specimen collection. Red meats may contain nonhuman hemoglobin, which yields false-positive tests. Foods with peroxidase activity, such as tomatoes, turnips, beets, radishes, and cherries, should be eliminated because their consumption will yield a false-positive test. High-residue diets are recommended to encourage bleeding from small colonic lesions.

Medication ingestion may also yield false-negative or false-positive tests. Vitamin C and antacids produce

---

TABLE 8-1

Summary of American Cancer Society Recommendations for the Early Detection of Cancer in Asymptomatic People (2000)

Beginning at age 50, men and women should follow *one* of the examination schedules below:
  A fecal occult blood test every year and a flexible sigmoidoscopy every 5 years
  A colonoscopy every 10 years*
  A double-contrast barium enema every 5–10 years.*

A digital rectal exam should be done at the same time as sigmoidoscopy, colonoscopy, or double-contrast barium enema. People who are at moderate or high risk for colorectal cancer should talk with a doctor about a different testing schedule.

false-negative results even in the presence of active bleeding. Iron, aspirin, cimetidine, cytochromes, and halogens are known for false-positive results and should be avoided during the testing period. Diseases such as diverticulosis, hemorrhoids, and other gastrointestinal pathology have yielded false-positive tests because of an alternate bleeding source.

Sample collection also has a direct impact on test results. Diluted specimens obtained from toilet water may result in fecal blood loss from the sample or may be affected by the halogens, such as chlorine, that may be present in the water. Stool samples either too dry or wet may also alter results. The American College of Physicians recently made new recommendations that six samples should be collected, two from each of three separate bowel movements. Testing should be done within 7 days of sample collection and the sample should not be rehydrated. Sensitivity is thought to be no more than 25% to 50% depending on the bleeding. Newer fecal occult tests with a quiac base are now available. Hemoccult II, Hemocultsensa, and HemeSelect are immunochemical tests that demonstrate improved sensitivity. Access to FOBT collection is available in physician offices, clinics, and even grocery stores. Patients must be reminded to call for any positive test reading and that a false-positive result is possible if instructions are not followed completely.

A double-contrast barium enema should be performed every 5 to 10 years and compliment a colonoscopy examination. Barium enemas may yield false readings of up to 18% particularly with smaller lesions. The ACS recommends a colonscopy examination at least every 10 years as a secondary prevention screening. Although very accurate, colonoscopy does add additional patient preparation concerns and added cost. Table 8–1 summarizes the ACS guidelines for early detection. Patients with family histories or those who have undergone curative surgery will require strict guidelines.*

Sigmoidoscopy is also an appropriate method of screening for cancerous lesions of the colon and rectum. Approximately 50% to 65% of all colorectal cancers can be found within the range of this particular instrument (25 cm, or 10 inches). A flexible fiberoptic sigmoidoscope is available that can reach to the splenic flexure (60 cm, or 24 inches). This instrument provides for increased visibility and patient comfort and should be performed at least every 5 years.

CLASSIFICATION

The site of presentation is primarily the sigmoidorectal area. The majority (40–50%) of lesions occur in the

---

* References 9, 15, 25, 33, 43, 45, 50, 52, 53.

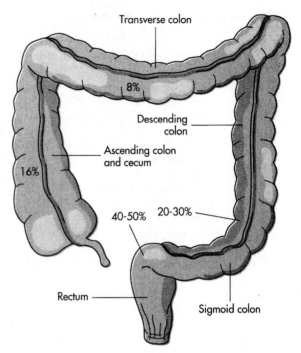

FIGURE 8–1 Incidence of cancer in various segments of the colon and rectum. (From Phipps WJ, Sands JK, Marek JF: *Medical surgical nursing: concepts and clinical practice,* St. Louis, Mosby, 1999.)

rectum, and 20% to 35% occur in the descending and sigmoid colon. Only 8% occur in the transverse colon and 16% in the cecum and ascending colon. A small percentage (4–8%) may occur as a second primary site[9, 25] (Fig. 8–1).

Most bowel cancers are *adenocarcinomas* and are moderately differentiated to well-differentiated cancers. Other forms of colorectal cancers consist of epithelioma, squamous cell carcinoma, sarcoma, lymphoma, leiomyosarcoma, and melanoma. Cancer of the anus occurs rarely, but recent research has shown an increase in men with a history of homosexual and bisexual activity or a history of anal condylomata acuminata. Other anal cancers include squamous cell, basal cell, and melanomas.[2]

CLINICAL FEATURES

General signs and symptoms exist for all colorectal cancers and may include a change in bowel habits, blood in the stool, abdominal pain, anorexia, flatulence, and indigestion. Later symptoms include loss of energy, weight loss, and a decline in general health. Symptoms may vary greatly according to size, location, tumor type, and the individual patient. Specific variances are seen between the right and left colon and the rectum. Patients with right-sided lesions do not display changes in bowel habits because of the liquid nature of the stool. Specific

CLINICAL FEATURES
Colorectal Cancer

General: Change in bowel habits, blood in stool, abdominal pain, anorexia, flatulence, indigestion

Late symptoms: Weight loss, fatigue, decline in general health

Right-sided lesions: Dull vague abdominal pain radiating to back, dark/mahogany-red blood in stool, weakness, anemia, malaise, indigestion, weight loss, liquid stool

Left-sided lesions: Change in bowel habits–cramps, gas pains, decrease in caliber of stool, bright-red bleeding, constipation, rectal pressure, incomplete evacuation of stool

Transverse colon: Palpable masses, obstruction, changes in bowel habits, bloody stools

Rectal: Changes in bowel habits, bright-red bleeding, tenesmus, severe pain in groin, labia, scrotum, legs, or penis

---

symptoms include a dull, vague abdominal pain radiating from abdomen to back. These tumors present as palpable masses in the right lower quadrant. Dark or mahogany-red blood may be present in the stool. Anemia leads to weakness and malaise, and indigestion and weight loss often occur.

In contrast, patients with left-sided lesions usually display a change in bowel habits because the area affected is the sigmoid colon and the rectum. Symptoms include cramps, gas pains, a decrease in the caliber of stool, bright-red bleeding, constipation, and a feeling of rectal pressure or incomplete evacuation of stool. Obstruction may occur and result in emergency surgery. Patients with transverse colon tumors have palpable masses, obstruction, a change in bowel habits, and bloody stools. Those with rectal cancers may display similar symptoms, such as changes in bowel habits, bright-red bleeding, tenesmus, and a late symptom of severe pain in the groin, labia, scrotum, legs, or penis. Unfortunately, colorectal cancer may be advanced before symptoms occur. Pain may only be the last symptom, and metastasis may be present before treatment is sought.

DIAGNOSIS

Persons at high risk for disease or who have symptoms and are guaiac positive require additional diagnostic testing (Box 8–2). A *barium enema* provides a clear picture of the large intestine and is useful for detecting smaller tumors. *Colonoscopy* may be performed at this time, especially if surgery is indicated. This examination provides increased visualization and the ability to biopsy

---

BOX 8-2
Diagnostic Work-up for Colorectal Cancer

Barium enema
Colonoscopy
Chest x-ray film
Liver scan
Bone scan
CBC, AST (SGOT), LDH, ALP, BUN*
Carcinoembryonic antigen (CEA)

* See text for abbreviations.

---

lesions. Potential metastatic lesions are evaluated using chest x-ray films and liver, bone, and other scans. Laboratory work includes a complete blood count (CBC), serum aspartate aminotransferase (AST, glutamic-oxaloacetic transaminase [SGOT]), lactate dehydrogenase (LDH), alkaline phosphatase (ALP), and blood urea nitrogen (BUN). A *carcinoembryonic antigen* (CEA) test may be used and a CA19-9 assay. This biologic marker is elevated in later stages of colorectal cancer and may have prognostic value at diagnosis or disease recurrence. Diagnosis is confirmed by tissue biopsy from the suspected site. Additional diagnostic evaluation includes a variety of procedures and varies with patients staging or suspected metastasis. New exams include Satumomb pentide that looks for extral heptatic abdominal metastasis and CEA scan used to detect hepatic metastasis.[6, 9, 10]

STAGING

The most widely used method for colorectal surgery is the *Duke's classification* or some modification of the original form, which was developed in 1932. The Duke's system classifies tumors into four major categories based on the degree and depth of tumor involvement and presence of lymph nodes. Subcategories were developed by Astler and Collier in 1954 in an attempt to delineate the importance of tumor wall penetration, as follows:

Duke's Classification

Stage A	Carcinoma limited to the mucosa
Stage B1	Carcinoma invades the muscle but is confined to the bowel wall
Stage B2	Carcinoma penetrates through the muscularis propria into the serosa and connective tissue
Stage B3	Same as B2 with adherence or invasion into adjacent organs, but with negative nodes
Stage C1	Lymph nodes positive for metastatic disease, but main tumor confined to bowel wall

TABLE 8–2
Comparison of Staging Systems

TMN System	Duke's System
Tis-N0-M0	
Tis: carcinoma in situ	
T1 or T2-N0-M0	A
T1: tumor invading submucosa	
T2: invading muscle layer	
T3 or T4-N0-M0	B
T3: tumor invades through muscle layer, into subserosa	
T4: tumor directly invades other organs or perforates visceral peritoneum	
Any T-N1, N2, or N3-M0	C
N1: one to three pericolic or perirectal lymph node metastases	
N2: four pericolic or perirectal lymph node metastases	
N3: any nodal metastasis along vascular trunk or apical node (1997 AJCC/UICC Staging Classification System has eliminated N3)	
Any T-any N-M1	D
M1: distant metastasis	

Data from Beahrs O and others: AJCC/UICC staging manual, ed 5, Philadelphia, Lippincott-Raven, 1998.

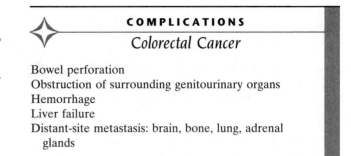

COMPLICATIONS
Colorectal Cancer

Bowel perforation
Obstruction of surrounding genitourinary organs
Hemorrhage
Liver failure
Distant-site metastasis: brain, bone, lung, adrenal glands

Stage C2   Lymph nodes positive for metastatic disease, and tumor completely penetrates bowel wall
Stage C3   Same as B3, with positive nodes
Stage D   Distant metastasis

The variances and minor modifications of various systems of colorectal staging resulted in the promotion of the *TNM system* by the Committee of the International Union Against Cancer (UICC).[3] Table 8–2 compares the Duke and TNM systems. Unlike other tumors, size is not a major factor. The depth of tumor penetration is the best indicator of prognosis.[19, 30, 46] Figure 8–2 shows growth of colon polyp to invasion.

METASTASIS

Most colorectal cancers spread by direct extension and penetration into layers of the bowel. Local invasion occurs to surrounding organs. Lymph node involvement and invasion into the vascular bed allow for disseminated disease. Lymphatic disease is present in 50% of all diagnosed cases. Nodal chains follow the pathway of the superior and mesenteric arteries. Colon cancer and cancer of the upper one half of the rectum spread by direct extension to the liver. Cancer of the lower half of the rectum spreads to portal veins and the inferior vena cava. Venous invasion permits distant metastasis, with the liver and lung as the most common sites. Additional sites include the brain, bone, and adrenal glands. Anal cancers spread directly into local muscles and to genitourinary organs. Metastatic spread at diagnosis significantly alters prognosis and treatment modalities. The most common metastatic sites are liver and lung.[19] The Complications box summarizes disease-related complications of colorectal cancer.

Liver Metastasis

Of all patients diagnosed with colorectal cancer, 25% will have liver metastasis at the time of their diagnosis. As many as 70% will display metastatic disease as the disease progresses. Methods to treat metastatic liver cancer include surgical resection, cryosurgery, regional infusion therapy, and vascular interruption with hepatic

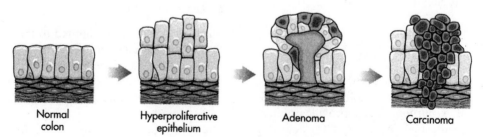

Normal colon   Hyperproliferative epithelium   Adenoma   Carcinoma

FIGURE 8–2   The progression to malignancy in bowel cancer. (From Phipps WJ, Sands JK, Marek JF: *Medical surgical nursing: concepts and clinical practice,* St Louis, Mosby, 1999.)

artery ligation. Each procedure has specific eligibility criteria based on the extensiveness of the metastatic disease. Risks and benefits vary. To date, no one specific treatment has been documented to be successful to manage liver metastasis.[7, 8, 13] (For specific instructions on the use of the Infusaid, Medtronic, and other pumps as treatment approaches, see Chapters 21 and 23.)

TREATMENT MODALITIES

Surgery

Colon resection with disease-free margins remains the surgical goal. Tumor and associated blood vessels are resected en bloc with the vascular and lymphatic structures to prevent seeding of malignant cells. A biopsy of the liver and regional lymph nodes is taken at the time of surgery to evaluate the extent of disease. Extensive procedures may be needed to attain the goal of reanastomosis and return to normal bowel function. Tumor size, tumor location, and additional metastases determine the type and the extent of surgery. Three major surgeries performed for colorectal cancer are *colon resection with reanastomosis, colostomy* (temporary or permanent), and *abdominal perineal resection* (Fig. 8–3). Table 8–3

outlines site-specific surgeries that may be done for various portions of the colon and rectum.

Localized tumors of the rectum can now be treated with a sphincter-sparing procedure using a reconstructed pouch. Anastomotic stapler devices have allowed greater ease of anostomosis in mid-rectal tumors and spared patients abdominoperineal resections. Radiolabeled monoclonal antibodies may be given intraoperatively to identify occult disease. Smaller tumors have been removed through colonoscope.[19, 23–25]

Each case must be evaluated individually to meet specific patient needs. Age, nutritional status, metastases, and such complications as perforation and obstruction may alter the surgical course. Additional surgical modalities may be required for palliation even when cure is not possible.[2, 4]

Chemotherapy

Chemotherapy alone has not been proved to be effective against colorectal cancer. Chemotherapy continues to be considered an adjunct to the initial surgical intervention. Various forms of combination drug therapy have been evaluated, with 5-fluorouracil (5-FU) including

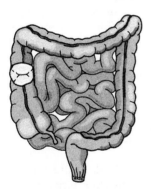

The ascending colostomy is done for right-sided tumors.

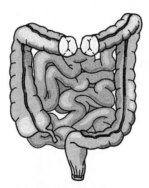

The transverse (double-barreled) colostomy is often used in such emergencies as intestinal obstruction or perforation because it can be created quickly. There are two stomas. The proximal one, closest to the small intestine, drains feces. The distal stoma drains mucus. Usually temporary.

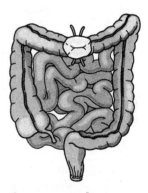

The transverse loop colostomy has two openings in the transverse colon, but one stoma. Usually temporary.

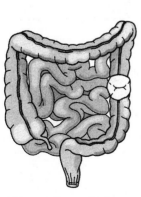

Descending colostomy

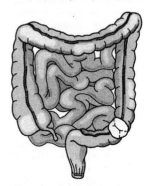

Sigmoid colostomy

FIGURE 8–3   Types of colostomies. (From Phipps WJ, Sands JK, Marek JF: *Medical surgical nursing: concepts and clinical practice*, St Louis, Mosby, 1999.)

TABLE 8-3

Major Surgeries for Colorectal Cancer

Location	Tumor Site	Procedure
Right colon	Cecum, ascending colon, proximal and midtransverse colon	Right colectomy or colostomy
Left colon	Splenic flexure and descending colon	Colectomy or colostomy
Sigmoid colon	Sigmoid portion of bowel	Sigmoid resection
Upper rectum	12 cm from anal verge	Anterior colon resection
Middle rectum	7–11 cm from anal verge	Pull-through procedure
Lower rectum	7 cm from anal verge	Abdominal perineal resection and colostomy

combinations of levamisole and leucovoran or both. A new agent Camptosar (irinotecan) has been used in various protocols for advanced colorectal cancer. Recent studies are underway to examine the effects of oxaliplatin (a neurotoxic platinum analogue) in combinations with Camptosar, 5-FU, and leucovoran. Table 8–4 shows the National Cancer Institute (NCI) current treatment guideline for cancer colorectal stages II, III, and IV.[28] Clinical trials are being evaluated for biologic therapy.[32, 43, 44] 5-FU continues to remain the drug of choice for treatment of colorectal cancer. Specific drug-related side effects can be found in Chapters 22 and 23.

Chemotherapy has also been used in attempts to prevent unresectable tumors confined to the liver from metastasizing. 5-FU has been administered by intra-arterial catheter into the hepatic artery, and floxuridine (FUDR), an analogue of 5-FU, has been administered by an implanted pump known as an Infusaid or Medtronic. The role of regional hepatic perfusion remains controversial in the treatment of metastatic disease.[5–8, 16, 26, 41]

Radiation Therapy

The role of radiation therapy in the management of colon tumors remain under investigation, but it is often used for patients with extensive microscopic tumor penetration, lymph node involvement, and direct tumor extension into the viscera or perineum. Various combination approaches have been attempted, including preoperative radiation, postoperative radiation, and a combination of both known as the "sandwich technique." *Preoperative* radiation therapy may damage malignant cells that could disseminate during surgery and may help shrink unresectable lesions. *Intraoperative* therapy is a modality that allows delivery of radiation to a large treatment area when the tumor is advanced, recurrent, or inoperable rectal cancer. Normal organs are moved from the pathway of radiation, and a large, single fraction beam is directed onto the tumor site. *Postoperative* radiation has proved effective in rectal cancer. Palliation may result from radiation treatment through reduction of tumor size, thereby relieving pain, bleeding, and pressure. New modalities using stereotactic radiation have been used to treat hepatic metastasis from colorectal cancer.[27, 42]

PROGNOSIS

Persons diagnosed with colorectal cancer must receive follow-up treatment after initial surgery, including peri-

TABLE 8-4

Treatment Recommendations for Stage II, III, and IV Colon Cancer

Stage	Recommended Treatment
II	Wide surgical resection and anastomosis
	Patients should be considered for participation in clinical trials of postsurgical adjuvant chemotherapy, radiation therapy, or biologic therapy.
III	Wide surgical resection and anastomosis. Adjuvant chemotherapy with 5-FU-containing regimens should be considered for patients who are not candidates for clinical trials.
	Eligible patients should be considered for entry into clinical trials evaluating postoperative treatments, including chemotherapy, radiation therapy, or biological therapy, alone or in combination.
IV/recurrent disease	Surgical resection/anastomosis or bypass of obstructing primary lesions in selected cases
	Surgical resection of isolated metastases
	Chemotherapy
	Clinical trials evaluating new drugs and biologic therapy
	Radiation therapy

From National Cancer Institute (PDQ). Colon cancer. 1999. Available at http://cancernet.nci.nih.gov/clinpdq/soa/Colon_Cancer_Physician.html.

odic physical examinations, colonoscopy, CEA levels, and traditional x-ray films as needed. Symptoms of weight loss and pain should be evaluated immediately. Disease recurrence may be observed locally or regionally in distant organs. Local recurrence at the original tumor site is a possibility and may cause obstruction and hemorrhage. Penetration beyond the bowel wall may result in fistula formation. Further surgery or combined adjunctive therapy may be indicated.

Spread to distant organs has a direct impact on the prognosis and the patient's ultimate survival. Survival time for persons with metastasis usually is less than 1 year. Age is an additional factor that affects the survival rate; persons under age 30 have a poorer prognosis, and patients over age 70 have a higher surgical morbidity rate. High CEA titers before surgery, the presence of obstruction at diagnosis, and poorly differentiated cancers also decrease the survival rate. Rectal tumors continue to be associated with poor prognosis, especially those located near the lower one third of the rectum. The overall survival rate of all stages is 40%. Survival rates continue to change as new treatment modalities and early detection methods are developed. Table 8–5 lists specific prognosis rates.

TABLE 8–5

Prognosis Rates for Colorectal Cancer

Duke's Classification	Survival Rate
A	80–90%
B	60%
C	25–45%
D	5%
Anal cancer	48–66%

CONCLUSION

Colorectal cancer provides an exciting challenge to the medical profession. Knowledge of the impact of dietary and environmental factors on colorectal statistics is a critical goal of research. Promotion of the ACS guidelines and large-scale, cost-effective screening may improve statistics and survival rates. Clinical trial research also provides hope for new treatment modalities for patients with disease recurrence. New surgical modalities offer reduced mortality and quality of life through reduced extensive operative procedures.

Nursing Management

SURGERY

Preoperative Teaching

Patient teaching and preoperative counseling are essential elements of nursing care for the patient preparing for colorectal surgery. Many patients will have already had several diagnostic and laboratory tests in an outpatient setting before they reach the hospital. Often they are aware of their diagnosis but may be in the stage of denial or disbelief. Patients and their families may be anxious or even angry at the diagnosis and will require additional attention and reinforcement of teaching preoperatively and postoperatively.

Teaching may begin with preparation of the colon for surgery. Most protocols involve a regimen of 2 or 3 days of liquid diets, a combination of laxatives and enemas, and the use of oral antibiotics to sterilize the bowel before surgery.[46] Antibiotics suppress both anaerobic and aerobic colonic organisms and reduce septic complications after surgery. Patients with bowel obstructions do not receive the usual bowel preparation.

Nursing Diagnoses

- *Knowledge deficit related to lack of experience in surgical routine and procedure*

- *Fear related to the diagnosis of cancer and outcomes of surgical procedure*
- *Knowledge deficit related to ostomy*

Outcome Goals

Patient will be able to:

- Verbalize understanding of surgical procedure and postoperative routine.
- Express fears and use effective coping mechanisms.
- Demonstrate care of ostomy, including stoma, peristomal skin, application of appliance, dietary concerns, and changes in life-style patterns.

Interventions

The nurse must provide support to an already anxious patient by explaining the rationale for the bowel preparation regimen. Close observation of the patient's tolerance of laxatives and enemas must be reported, including the side effects of nausea, vomiting, abdominal discomfort, and excessive diarrhea and the symptoms of electrolyte imbalance. Elderly and debilitated patients are at the greatest risk for discomfort and complications.

Preoperative Care

Preoperative teaching may begin at this time and should include a review of the patient's past experience with surgery. Basic teaching should include a review of the preoperative routine: preoperative medications, intravenous lines, recovery room procedures, and placement of a Foley catheter, nasogastric tube, and abdominal dressings. Postoperative exercises, such as coughing and deep breathing, wound splinting, and leg exercises, should be reviewed and practiced. Concerns about pain medication and diet restrictions may be discussed preoperatively. A basic review of anatomy is necessary for the person to understand the surgical procedure and colostomy placement.

Psychosocial issues and concerns must be addressed and support systems identified. A review of past coping mechanisms allows the individual to evaluate strengths and weaknesses. Ample time to discuss fears and concerns must be permitted to evaluate the dynamics of interpersonal relationships between patients and their support systems. Quality preoperative assessment allows for more effective intervention postoperatively.

If a colostomy is performed, a referral to an enterostomal therapist or other appropriate resource should be made as soon as possible. Preoperative teaching should review the type of surgery, a description of an ostomy, various pouching methods available, and marking of the stoma site. Marking the stoma site is important to eliminate the possibility of future skin problems and difficult pouch applications. One of the basic rules for stoma marking is that the stoma should be away from the waistline, folds, scars, or where the abdominal incision will be placed. The stoma should be placed so that the patient will be able to see and reach the pouch easily. The stoma site will be placed through the rectus abdominis muscle, which runs vertically through the abdomen. Approximately 3 inches (7.5 cm) of skin will be necessary to provide adequate pouch placement. Various positions should be attempted before marking the stoma. The stoma should be visualized in sitting, standing, and lying positions. The site is usually below the umbilicus and at the infraumbilical bulge. The stoma site is then marked with a dye such as methylene blue or gentian violet.[15] Marking the stoma validates the reality of the ostomy. Documentation of the patient's and family's reaction is important to meet future emotional needs.

Postoperative Care

Nursing Diagnoses

- *Pain related to incisional discomfort*
- *Infection, risk for, related to improper wound healing*
- *Bowel incontinence (or other elimination problem) related to loss of normal bowel function*
- *Skin integrity, impaired, related to abdominal incision and stoma drainage*

Outcome Goals

Patient will be able to:

- Verbalize level of comfort at pain-rating score of 0 to 3.
- Be free of signs and symptoms of infection, as demonstrated by adequate wound healing.
- Have adequate bowel function, as evidenced by evacuation of stool in 1 to 3 days.
- Maintain intact skin at incision and peristomal site.

Interventions

Care during the postoperative period focuses on meeting the patient's physical and metabolic needs. Observing the patient for initial complications includes assessment of vital signs and lung and bowel sounds. The incision is inspected for drainage or bleeding and approximation. The nasogastric tube and Foley catheter, if present, are monitored for the amount and color of drainage and patency. Accurate recording of intake and output is necessary to provide proper electrolyte balance. The stoma site is observed at each shift initially for color and size. A postoperative pouch usually covers the stoma, allowing for easy visibility. The stoma should appear pink and moist. Signs of necrosis and ischemia are present if the stoma appears blue or black or has a dusky appearance. This observation should be reported at once because this indicates stoma death. Drainage from the stoma should be scant and blood-tinged. A strict postoperative routine of coughing, deep-breathing exercises, early ambulation, and adequate pain control assists the patient toward early recovery and limits potential complications.

Despite good nursing care, postoperative complications may occur, including infection, paralytic ileus, pulmonary complications, anastomotic leak, urinary problems, stoma retraction, and prolapse.[46] Fevers may result from infection, respiratory difficulty, urinary infections, or thrombophlebitis. Elderly patients

---

COMPLICATIONS

Bowel Surgery

Infection (wound, urinary, lung)
Thrombophlebitis
Paralytic ileus
Pulmonary embolus
Hemorrhage
Anastomotic leaks

with preexisting medical illness such as diabetes and lung disease are at greatest risk.

Anastomotic leaks are more common in lower resections and often result in fistula formation. Skin care and adequate nutrition are essential components of proper wound healing. Paralytic ileus, a common complication after bowel surgery, results from the surgical manipulation of the bowels in surgery and can last up to 14 days or more. Increased abdominal girth, distention, nausea, and vomiting are classic signs of an ileus. Decompression of the bowel with a nasogastric tube, maintenance of the NPO (nothing by mouth) status, and increased activity usually result in a return to normal bowel function.

Postoperative wound infection is not usually a major concern because of prophylactic antibiotics and reduction of wound contamination with postoperative stoma pouching. Those patients with abdominoperineal resections are at greater risk for wound complications and infections. Sitz baths, dressing changes, and topical ointments assist in the healing process. Healing may be very slow, and meticulous skin care remains essential.

Postoperative Teaching

Nursing Diagnoses

- *Sexual dysfunction related to body function alteration and body changes*
- *Self-esteem disturbance related to altered body image*
- *Family processes, altered, related to diagnosis of cancer and ostomy placement*
- *Health maintenance, altered, related to knowledge deficit regarding diet modifications and ostomy care*

Outcome Goals

- Patient will express concerns related to sexual dysfunction and identify alternatives to cope with modification.
- Patient will verbalize concerns related to self-concept and express positive self-esteem.
- Patient and family will verbalize changes in family patterns and identify methods to incorporate new changes into life-style.
- Patient will verbalize understanding of dietary restrictions and ostomy care.

Interventions

Postoperative teaching addresses the patient's emotional and physical changes resulting from the ostomy and involves appropriate referral to resources as needed. Postoperative pouch application and stoma care should be a step-by-step process, moving from the simple to the complex components. Ostomy care includes pouch applications, emptying of the pouch, and use of skin products.

Pouch selection is based on the site of the stoma, manual dexterity, cost, and patient preference; all pouches should be well fitted and odor proof and should provide skin protection.[46] Special skin barriers may also be necessary, depending on the type of effluent discharged. Ileostomy drainage is particularly wet and contains enzymes that can cause skin irritation. Sigmoid colostomy effluent is solid but may also cause skin problems. Odor is managed with pouching, and ostomy deodorant sprays must be discussed. The enterostomal therapist is invaluable in selecting the appropriate product for the patient (see table below).

Colostomy irrigations may be an option for patients with a sigmoid colostomy. Patients should be told the

Ostomy Supplies*

Product	Use
Skin barriers	Paste, wafers, rings, or powders used to protect skin
Skin sealants	Plasticizing agents that produce a thin, protective film around skin
Skin cleaners	Foams, wipes, sprays, or liquids used to clean or remove residue from skin
Skin adhesives	Sprays or liquids used to increase adhesion of ostomy equipment
Pouches	Wafers cut to fit and presized: one piece or two piece, disposable or reusable
Belts and binders	Provide support and keep equipment in place
Convex inserts	Provide support and convexity
Pouch covers	Protect skin from moisture and provide concealment
Tail closures	Close end of pouches to prevent leakage
Tapes	Help pouches stay in place; prevent leakage; provide waterproofing
Stoma guide strips	Assist with centering pouches over stoma
Solvents	Assist with removal of residual tape or water residue
Stomocap	Cover for continent ostomy
Irrigation set and insertion cone	Used to irrigate colostomy
Faceplates	Used for retracted stomas

Patient should be referred to appropriate resources, including the enterostomal therapy nurse, American Cancer Society, and United Ostomy Association.

advantages of both systems, that irrigation control takes patience, and that a daily schedule can be established over time. Other types of ostomies cannot be regulated by irrigation because the effluent is constant and liquid. Figure 8–4 demonstrates various ostomy supplies.

The special dietary needs and restrictions of the ostomy patient are discussed, including adequate fluid intake and the avoidance of certain foods that may cause blockage, odor, or gas. A list of medications that are not absorbed in the intestine and may be expelled through the colostomy is also provided. Foods that contain seeds, nuts, or excessive bulk should be avoided because blockage is likely. Gas- and odor-producing foods are frequently the same foods that caused problems before surgery and usually are related to beans, cabbage, and brussels sprouts.

Trial and error and the use of commercial deodorant products assist with this problem. Discharge teaching includes specific problems that may be encountered, such as diarrhea or blockage. A dietary consultant can assist the patient in appropriate diet selection. A physician or enterostomal therapist should be notified if these problems arise. Stoma prolapse and stoma retraction also may occur if there is undue pressure on the stoma from an appliance or from edema or scar formation. Specific skin problems and use of products are discussed with the patient at this time. Discharge teaching may be an overwhelming task for a patient who is emotionally and physically drained from the events of surgery. Scheduling short visits with repetition is the most reliable method of teaching. Readiness to learn has the greatest impact on ostomy teaching.

Body image and sexuality concerns are discussed preoperatively and postoperatively. Signs of difficulty in dealing with the new ostomy may include failure to look at the stoma, making remarks about the stoma, or not permitting the significant other to assist with care of the appliance. Common concerns are fear of rejection, shame, a sense of disfigurement, and concerns of others' reactions. Continued feelings of low self-esteem lead to depression, withdrawal, and sexual dysfunction.[10, 34, 38] An ostomy visitor with a similar background may provide the additional support and encouragement needed at this time. Meeting a person who is able to work and continue with outside activities provides the patient with a positive outlook and encouragement.[14, 20]

Sexual counseling begins while the patient is in the hospital. A discussion about sexuality concerns ultimately includes the spouse or significant other. Suggestions to assist couples to deal with sexuality issues should begin with open communication and gradual introduction of sexual activity. Body image concerns may be dealt with by the use of pouch covers, nightgowns and shirts, or other methods to conceal the ostomy until the patient is comfortable with the issue. Altered sexual positions that are more comfortable and less traumatic on the stoma should also be discussed. Patients with abdominoperineal resections require referrals for further counseling, because 30% to 100% of all men with this surgery experience erec-

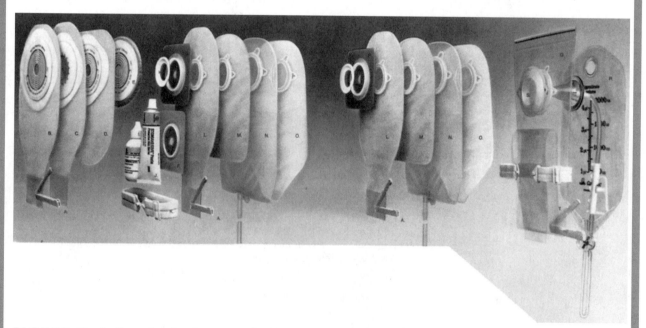

FIGURE 8–4 Examples of various types of colostomy equipment patients may use. (Courtesy of ConvaTec, Princeton, NJ.)

tile impotence. Damage to the parasympathetic nerve and loss of sensation have a severe impact on sexual performance. Referral to a urologist for a semirigid or inflatable penile implant is necessary if the patient finds he is unable to perform sexually and desires further medical intervention. Research on women with abdominoperineal resections is not conclusive, but reports include changes in sensation that alter the orgasmic process.[47]

Rehabilitation

Rehabilitation of the patient with colorectal cancer requires the combined efforts of several professionals. Physical, emotional, and spiritual concerns must be met to return the patient to the preoperative state of functioning. The ultimate goal of rehabilitation is to provide patients with the knowledge and support to reach their maximum capabilities within the limits of their condition. The United Ostomy Association and ACS can provide additional support and information for the patient and family. Additional referrals for counseling to deal with emotional and sexual concerns may also be necessary for long-term support. The availability of an enterostomal therapist and adequate access to ostomy supplies are additional supports for patients who have had ostomy surgery.

Radiation Therapy

Nursing Diagnoses

- *Skin integrity, impaired, risk for, related to effects of radiation treatment*
- *Diarrhea related to treatment side effects*
- *Fluid volume deficit, risk for, related to nausea and vomiting*
- *Health maintenance, altered, related to knowledge deficit regarding radiation side effects*

Outcome Goals

Patient will be able to:

- Maintain skin integrity without complications.
- Have normal bowel evacuation in 1 to 3 days.
- Control nausea and vomiting without evidence of fluid and electrolyte loss.
- Verbalize knowledge of side effects of radiation therapy.

Interventions

Patients receiving radiation therapy to the abdominal cavity require emotional and physical support throughout their treatment. Preradiation instruction reviews the frequency and length of treatments, skin markings and their care, and potential side effects and their management. Patients who have an ostomy may

---

COMPLICATIONS

Radiation Therapy

Skin irritation
Proctitis
Nausea/vomiting
Cystitis
Sexual dysfunction
Bone marrow suppression
Fatigue

---

need additional information about skin care to their stomas. Side effects experienced by patients receiving abdominal radiation include nausea, vomiting, diarrhea, cystitis, sexual dysfunction, bone marrow suppression, local skin reaction, and fatigue.[48]

Nausea and vomiting are of particular concern to patients receiving radiation therapy over the abdominal area. This is primarily related to the destruction of the epithelial lining of the bowel wall. The toxic waste production from cellular destruction produces increased stimuli to the nausea receptors in the medulla. Prolonged nausea and vomiting may produce weight loss and dehydration. Appropriate nursing measures include use of antiemetics 1 to 2 hours before radiation therapy and up to 12 hours after each treatment. Small, frequent meals are encouraged, with high protein and liquid supplements if needed. Weight, dietary intake, and hydration status should be monitored weekly. For patients with an ostomy, significant weight loss causes stoma shrinkage. Measurement of the stoma and pouch sizes may be needed.[15]

Diarrhea is another common symptom. It begins about 1 or 2 weeks after the start of radiation treatment and is caused by the rapid proliferation of the epithelial cells in the intestinal wall. Patients experiencing diarrhea should be instructed to eat low-residue, high-protein, high-carbohydrate diets. Fluids high in potassium are encouraged; milk products are discouraged. Antidiarrheal products are effective in controlling diarrhea. Patients are instructed to record the number and consistency of bowel movements. Rectal irritation from bowel movements or from radiation therapy to the rectum requires sitz baths, topical creams, and assessment by the radiologist and enterostomal therapist. Ostomy patients require increased pouch changes, assessment of peristomal skin, and use of a skin barrier to protect their skin. Severe excoriation of the peristomal skin requires a referral to the enterostomal therapist or the discontinuation of treatments until symptoms subside.

Abdominal radiation causes inflammation of the bladder, resulting in symptoms of cystitis, burning, back pain, hematuria, and foul-smelling urine. Instructions should be given on increasing fluid intake to 2 to 3 quarts of liquids per day and limiting caffeine products. Urine cultures, sensitivity specimens, and monitoring intake and output may be necessary.

Sexual dysfunction occurs for a variety of emotional and physical reasons. Changes in self-concept, decreased libido, impotence, fertility concerns, and vaginal lining changes may all occur as a result of radiation therapy. Instructions include alternative forms of sexual contact, use of a water-based lubricant, and appropriate referrals for severe sexual concerns and fertility issues.

Bone marrow suppression may also occur because of the proximity of the radiation dose to the treatment site and the pelvic bones. The significance of suppression depends on the length of treatment cycles, number of treatments, and total dose delivered. Patients are monitored for fatigue, infection, bleeding, and fever. Weekly laboratory studies should be obtained. Patient instructions include prudent handwashing to minimize the potential for infection.

Local skin reactions may occur at any time, resulting from the destruction of epithelial tissue. Reactions include itchy, dry skin, darkened areas near the radiation site, and mild excoriation. Patients are instructed to avoid excessive heat or cold and not to use creams or lotions near the treatment site. Only skin products applied by the radiologist should be used because an increased skin reaction occurs with nonprescribed creams.

Patients with ostomies experience increased radiation dermatitis near the peristomal skin site because of the direct exposure of mucous membrane to treatment field. Pouches are often removed before treatments and cause the patient increased concern about skin exposure. Assessment of the peristomal skin is done at this time. Careful skin cleansing and skin barriers assist with adequate protection. Severely excoriated areas require additional creams or powders near the stoma site. A referral to the enterostomal therapist should always be made if the skin condition worsens. Treatments are often delayed if symptoms progress.

Chemotherapy

Nursing Diagnoses

- *Knowledge deficit related to potential chemotherapy side effects*
- *Oral mucous membrane, altered, related to side effects of chemotherapy drugs*
- *Nutrition, altered: less than body requirements, related to nausea and vomiting*
- *Infection, risk for, related to altered immune status*

- *Injury, risk for, related to change in clotting factor*
- *Diarrhea related to chemotherapy side effects*
- *Self-esteem disturbance related to hair loss and body changes*

Outcome Goals

Patient will be able to:

- Verbalize knowledge of chemotherapy side effects.
- Maintain normal mucous membranes.
- Maintain body weight within 10% of pretherapy state.
- Be free of infection and have temperature within normal limits.
- Maintain normal platelet count.
- Maintain normal bowel evacuation pattern of 1 to 3 days.
- Verbalize changes in body image and methods to promote self-esteem.

Interventions

Patients receiving chemotherapy for colorectal cancer may be treated with a single or multidrug protocol as well as a combination of chemotherapy, radiation, and biotherapy. Side effects are usually dose, drug, and patient specific. General side effects include nausea, vomiting, diarrhea, and myelosuppression (see Chapters 23 and 24).

Nursing measures include adequate instructions on potential drug side effects. Diarrhea is of particular concern to the ostomy patient because skin breakdown may easily occur. Use of a protective barrier and additional paste or powder may be necessary. Recording the number and consistency of stools is of vital importance to assess hydration status. Small, frequent, high-protein meals rich in potassium are encouraged. Antidiarrheal agents may become necessary if bowel movements are too frequent.[15]

Constipation is treated with fluids, stool softeners, laxatives, and irrigations of the stoma if necessary. Mucositis is also found around the peristomal skin and the stoma itself. Bowel drainage from infused chemotherapy agents requires the use of protective skin barriers, careful pouch changes, and proper skin cleansing. Fungal infections near the stoma site may also result from prolonged myelosuppression. Antifungal powders near the peristomal skin assist in wound healing. Local trauma from low platelet counts may also be experienced near the stoma. Careful pouch removal is necessary to avoid trauma.[15]

Nausea and vomiting cause excessive weight loss that changes stoma size. This often requires a pouch change or size variance. Consultation for the appropriate pouch should be done before any significant changes.

Body image and self-esteem disturbances require emotional support to deal with the additional body changes of hair loss and ostomy formation. Support groups and counseling should be provided for these individuals.

Specialized treatment of metastatic liver cancer may be accomplished with an infusion pump. The Medtronics infusion pump allows patients increased freedom from hospitalization but requires extensive patient teaching concerning the pump's placement and management. Its placement is a surgical procedure; a disk-shaped pump is placed into a subcutaneous pocket, allowing access to the hepatic artery. The pump contains an access port, a chamber for the fluid to be infused, and a chamber filled with fluorocarbon. The vapor pressure of fluorocarbon at normal body temperature results in expansion of the pump and release of the chemotherapeutic drug (see Fig. 22–4).[3] Postoperative complications include development of a seroma, an accumulation of sterile fluid in the pump pocket. Seromas may require draining. Infections may also occur within the pocket site and may require surgical removal of the pump. Percutaneous access is used to fill the pump on a 2- to 4-week schedule. Each patient's schedule will vary. FUDR and a heparin solution are infused every 2 weeks. Between the doses of FUDR, a solution of normal saline and heparin is used to keep the pump open. Access to the pump for filling is done by a perfusion scan and injection of radioactive material to assist with proper placement.

Nursing Diagnosis

- *Knowledge deficit related to care of infusion pump and management of side effects from pump*

Outcome Goals

Patient will be able to:

- Explain correct use and care of infusion pump.
- Verbalize knowledge of the management of side effects from infusion pump placement and use.

Interventions

Specific teaching concerning the pump includes understanding its use and particular filling schedule. Side effects of FUDR must also be discussed and managed. Common side effects include nausea, vomiting, abdominal pain, diarrhea, fatigue, and chemical hepatitis. Symptoms are treated systemically except for hepatitis, which requires the removal of the drug from the pump. Patients must also be instructed to avoid blunt trauma to the pump site and to limit exposure to extremes of temperature and altitude, which may interfere with drug administration. The effect of intra-

---

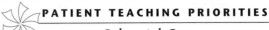

PATIENT TEACHING PRIORITIES

Colorectal Cancer

Surgery (Preoperative Care)

Turning, coughing, deep breathing
Wound splinting
Ambulation
Pain management
Pouch application
Bowel preparation
Postoperative complications

Chemotherapy

Drug name/regimen
Side effects
Complications
Follow-up schedule

Culture

Relationships
Communication
Values
Sexual concerns
Food habits
Health care beliefs
Teaching/learning process
Religious concerns
Body image
Pain
Death/dying beliefs

Surgery (Postoperative Care)

Ostomy and skin care
Pouch application
Diet modifications
Complications
Sexuality issues
Rehabilitation
Community support

Radiation

Treatment schedule
Side effects
Skin care
Dietary constraints

Community

Availability of enterostomal therapist services, hospital, clinics, ostomy supplier
Support groups
Home care agencies
Housing (privacy/bathroom facilities)
Acceptance of differences
Family resources (financial/emotional/physical availability)
Transportation resources
Rehabilitation resources
Community screening programs

arterial chemotherapy and its effectiveness in hepatic metastasis are still under evaluation.

Continued patient teaching is needed to support the patient with colorectal cancer through the postoperative course and through various treatment modalities. Patient teaching priorities and implications are summarized.

Geriatric Considerations

Special considerations should be given to the elderly population, who may demonstrate a lack of awareness of increased risk factors, signs and symptoms, and recommended screening for colorectal cancer. Awareness of the ACS guidelines and the availability of community screening programs are imperative to early diagnosis. Once a diagnosis is made and treatment indicated, the elderly patient may experience increased side effects from preexisting medical conditions and lack of physical stamina to tolerate aggressive therapy.

Postoperatively, elderly patients are at increased risk for pulmonary, circulatory, and bowel complications. Additional treatment modalities of radiation and chemotherapy impose further complications of fluid and electrolyte imbalance, infection, and skin concerns. Monitoring the immune and nutritional status of this population is essential.

Postoperative teaching of elderly patients may also require added time to allow for any vision and hearing

---

GERIATRIC CONSIDERATIONS
Colorectal Cancer

Education Needs

Awareness of screening recommendations
Knowledge of signs and symptoms
Understanding of risk factors
Treatment complications

Surgery

Pulmonary
Circulatory
Bowel

Chemotherapy and Radiation

Fluid and electrolyte imbalance
Infection
Skin impairment

Teaching Concerns

Vision/hearing impairment
Dexterity for pouch applications

Community Resources

Financial/home care referral

---

impairment as well as dexterity with pouch applications. Community resources and referrals should be made to assist with physical and financial support.[17, 18] The box summarizes geriatric considerations.

Chapter Questions

1. Considerations for patient teaching include all of the following *except:*
   a. Cultural variations
   b. Community resources
   c. Age differences
   d. Genetic variances
2. The primary location for presentation of colorectal cancer is the:
   a. Ascending colon
   b. Descending colon
   c. Rectum
   d. Transverse colon
3. Complications of abdominal radiation include:
   a. Cystitis
   b. Constipation
   c. Increased appetite
   d. Urinary retention
4. Risk factors for colorectal cancer include:
   a. High alcohol intake
   b. History of constipation

   c. Abnormal bowel habits
   d. Combination of factors, including diet, genetics, and predisposing factors such as bowel disorders
5. Late symptoms of colorectal cancer include:
   a. Anorexia
   b. Blood in the stool
   c. Change in bowel practices
   d. Weight loss
6. Appropriate immediate postoperative nursing diagnoses for a patient with colon cancer and a bowel resection include all of the following *except:*
   a. Sexual dysfunction
   b. Impaired skin integrity
   c. Pain
   d. Risk for infection
7. The American Cancer Society recommendations for colon cancer screening include:
   a. Digital rectal examination every year
   b. Persons at high risk to increase screening at an earlier age than the normal population
   c. Proctosigmoidoscopy every year for patients over age 50
   d. Colonoscopy examinations for every rectal bleeding episode

8. Treatment modalities for colon and metastatic liver cancer include all of the following *except:*
   a. Intra-arterial infusion of FUDR
   b. Local infusion of FUDR
   c. Radiation therapy, including IORT
   d. Complete surgical dissection
9. Reduced dietary fiber promotes carcinogenic changes by:
   a. Increases the contact time of carcinogenic substances within the colonic mucosa
   b. Promoting growth of polyps
   c. Promoting constipation concerns
   d. Reabsorbing fluids
10. Immediate postoperative home care teaching includes all of the following *except:*
   a. Dietary modifications
   b. Prevention, screening, and detection guidelines
   c. Potential complications: bleeding, infection,
   d. Self-care skin integrity interventions

BIBLIOGRAPHY

1. American Cancer Society: *Cancer facts and figures–2000,* Atlanta, The Society, 2000.
2. Arnell TD, Stamos MJ: Alternatives in therapy for low rectal cancer, *J Wound Ostomy Continence Nurs* 23(3): 150, 1996.
3. Beahrs O and others: *American Joint Commission on Cancer manual for staging of cancer,* ed 5, p. 83, Philadelphia, Lippincott-Raven, 1998.
4. Berger D, Roslyn J: Cancer surgery in the elderly, *Clin Geriatr Med* 13(1):119, 1997.
5. Berkery R, Cleri L, Skarin A: *Oncology pocketguide to chemotherapy,* ed 3, Baltimore, Mosby, 1997.
6. Berg D and others: *Disease management of colorectal cancer* (continuing education program) 6, pp. 1-66.
7. Bryson M: Caring for patients with liver cancer, *Nursing* 96(1):52, 1996.
8. Cancer Trials: *ACI will test new drugs for colorectal cancer throughout North America.* National Cancer Institute, 2000.
9. Cohen A, Minsky B, Schilsky R: Cancer of the colon: In DeVita V, Hellman S, Rosenburg S, editors: *Cancer: principles and practice of oncology,* ed 5, Philadelphia, Lippincott-Raven, 1997.
10. Cuhez A, Minsky B, Schilsky R: Cancer of the rectum. In DeVita V, Hellman S, Rosenburg S, editors: *Cancer: principles and practice of oncology,* ed 5, Philadelphia, Lippincott-Raven, 1997.
11. Clinton S, Giovannucci E: Chemoprevention, nutrition in the etiology and prevention of cancer. In Holland J and others, editors: *Cancer medicine,* Baltimore, Williams and Wilkins, 1997.
12. Declan-Fleming RY: Colorectal cancer screening and followup. *Surg Oncol* 7(3–4):125, 1999.
13. Doley J, Kemeny N: Metastatic cancer of the liver. In DeVita V, Hellman S, Rosenburg S, editors *Cancer: principles and practice of oncology,* ed 5, Philadelphia, Lippincott-Raven, 1997.
14. DeCosse J, Cennerazzo W: Quality of life management of patients with colorectal cancer, *CA Cancer J Clin* 47(4):198, 1997.
15. Desch C and others: Recommended colorectal cancer surveillance guidelines by the American Society of Clinical Oncology, *J Clin Oncol* 17:1312, 1999.
16. DeVita V: Principles of cancer management: chemotherapy. In DeVita V, Hellman S, Roseburg S, editors: *Cancer: principles and practice of oncology,* ed 5, Philadelphia, Lippincott-Raven, 1997.
17. Doenges M, Moorhouse M, Geissler A: *Nursing care plans,* ed 4, Philadelphia, Davis, 1997.
18. Exterman M: Assessment of the older cancer patient. Proceedings from ASCO 35th meeting, p 353, 1999.
19. Fong Y: Surgical therapy of hepatic colorectal metastasis, *CA J Clin* 49 (4), 231, 1999.
20. Freireich EJ: Regulatory issues. In DeVita V, Hellman S, Rosenburg S, editors: *Cancer: principles and practice of oncology,* ed 5, Philadelphia, Lippincott-Raven, 1997.
21. Greenwald P: Dietary carcinogens. In DeVita V, Hellman S, Rosenburg S, editors: *Cancer: principles and practice of oncology,* ed 5, Philadelphia, Lippincott-Raven, 1997.
22. Greenwald P: Dietary fiber. In DeVita V, Hellman S, Rosenburg S, editors: *Cancer: principles and practice of oncology,* ed 5, Philadelphia, Lippincott-Raven, 1997.
23. Greene F: Laparoscopic management of colorectal cancer, *CA J Clin* 49(4):221, 1999.
24. Guillem J, Paty P, Cohen A: Surgical treatment of colorectal cancer, *CA J Clin* 47(2):113, 1998.
25. Hoebler L: Colon and rectal cancer. In Groenwald SL and others, editors: *Cancer nursing principles and practice,* ed 4, Boston, Jones and Bartlett, 1997.
26. Karas B, Alpuche A: Refilling an implantable pump, *Nursing 95* 95(11):57, 1995.
27. Kelvin J: Gastrointestinal cancers. In Don K and others, editors: *Nursing care in radiation oncology,* ed 2, Philadelphia, Saunders, 1997.
28. MacDonald J: Adjuvant therapy of colon cancer, *CA J Clin* 49(4):202, 1999.
29. Markowitz A, Ninawer, S: Management of colorectal polyps, *CA J Clin* 47(2):93, 1998.
30. Marsh J: Carcinomas of the gastrointestinal tract. In Skeel R, Lachant N, editors: *Handbook of cancer chemotherapy,* ed 4, Boston, Little-Brown, 1995.
31. Monahan, F: *Medical-surgical nursing: foundations for clinical practice,* ed 2, Philadelphia, Saunders, 1998.
32. Morrison GB and others: Dihydropyrimidine dehydrogenase deficiency: a pharmocogentic defect causing severe adverse reactions to 5-fluorouracil based chemotherapy, *Oncol Nurs Forum* 24(1):83, 1997.
33. Pazdur, R, Royce M: *Myths and facts about colorectal cancer, what you need to know.* In Pazdur R, Coia R, Hoskins WJ, Wagman LD, editors: *Cancer management: a multidisciplinary approach* ed 3, Melville NY, PRR, 1999.
34. Phipps, N, Sands J, Marek J: *Medical surgical nursing concepts and clinical practice,* St. Louis, Mosby, 1999.
35. PDQ Database: *Anal cancer treatments—health professionals,* National Cancer Institute, 2000.
36. PDQ Database: *Colon cancer treatment—health professionals,* National Cancer Institute, 2000.

37. PDQ Database: *Q & A about screening, early detection and treatment for colorectal cancer,* National Cancer Institute, 2000.

38. PDQ Database: *Rectal cancer treatment,* National Cancer Institute, 2000.

39. PDQ Database: *Screening for colorectal cancer, screening/detection,* National Cancer Institute, 2000.

40. PDQ Database: *Selenium lowered incidence of lung, colorectal and prostate cancers,* National Cancer Institute, 2000.

41. Pharmacia & Upjohn, Inc: *A complete product profile, Camptosar® Irinotecan HCL Injection,* Kalamazoo, MI: Pharmacia Upjohn, 1997.

42. Riese N, Noll L: Chemical modifiers of radiation therapy. In Dow K and others, editors, *Nursing care in radiation oncology,* ed 2, Philadelphia, Saunders, 1997.

43. Rosenbaum E, Dollinger M: Colon and rectum. In Dollinger M, Rosenbaum E, Cable G, editors, *Everyone's guide to cancer therapy,* Kansas City, 1997, Andrews McMeek.

44. Rosenburg S: Principles of cancer management: biologic therapy. In DeVita V, Hellman S, Rosenburg S, editors: *Cancer: principles and practice of oncology,* ed 5, Philadelphia, Lippincott-Raven, 1997.

45. Rothenberg M: Colorectal cancer: a therapeutic update, *Semin Oncol* 2(5):1, 1998.

46. SGNA Core Curriculum Committee: *Gastroenterology nursing, a core curriculum,* St. Louis, Mosby, 1998.

47. Shank B, Cunningham J, Kelsen D: Cancer of the anal region. In DeVita V, Hellman S, Rosenburg S, editors: *Cancer: principles and practice of oncology,* Philadelphia, Lippincott-Raven, 1997.

48. Sitton E: Managing side effects of skin changes and fatigue. In Dow K and others, editors, *Nursing care in radiation oncology,* ed 2, Philadelphia, Saunders, 1997.

49. Strohl R: Nursing care of the client with cancer of the gastrointestinal tract. In Itano J, Taok O, editors, *Core curriculum for oncology nursing,* ed 3, Philadelphia, Saunders, 1992.

50. Warmkessel, JH: Caring for a patient with colon cancer, *Nursing* 27(4):34, 1997.

51. Willett WC: Goals for nutrition in the year 2000, *CA J Clin* 49 (6):331, 1999.

52. Willett WC: Cancer prevention: diet and RDR reduction. In DeVita V, Hellman S, Rosenburg S, editors: *Cancer: principles and practice of oncology,* ed 5, Philadelphia, Lippincott-Raven, 1997.

53. Winawer SJ and others: Prevention of colorectal cancer: guidelines based on new data, WHO Collaborative Center for the Prevention of Colorectal Cancer, *Bull WHO* 13:7, 1995.

Gastrointestinal Cancers

Betty Thomas Daniel

Gastrointestinal (GI) cancers accounted for 18.6% of the new cases of cancer diagnosed in the United States in 2000 and 23.5% of the cancer deaths in the same period. This represents a total of 226,600 new cases and 129,800 cancer deaths.[27] Progress has been made in treating some of the GI cancers, but others remain difficult to control. Symptoms of many of these cancers are vague and nonspecific until advanced disease develops, which makes treatment difficult and long-term survival rates low. However, prevention and early detection can reduce the impact of the disease and prolong survival.

Nurses have an important role to play in the prevention, early detection, diagnosis, and treatment of GI cancers. In some instances, prevention and early detection are not possible, but knowledge of the course of disease may improve the patient's quality of life.

Cancer of the Esophagus

EPIDEMIOLOGY

Cancer of the esophagus is a fairly uncommon cancer in the United States, but its incidence varies greatly throughout the world. It is considered endemic in the northern provinces of China, India, southeastern seaboard of South Africa, northern Iran, and along the northeast coast of the Caspian Sea. In northern China, esophageal cancer accounts for 20% of all deaths.[27, 59] In the United States the estimated number of new cases in 2000 was 12,300, and 12,100 of these patients will die of their disease.[27] The incidence of esophageal cancer increases sharply after the age of 40, and men have a significantly greater risk of developing the disease than women.[26, 75] Adenocarcinoma is more common in white men (ratio of 4:1), whereas squamous cell carcinoma is more common in African American men.[24, 45, 59]

ETIOLOGY AND RISK FACTORS

Although the etiology of esophageal cancer is not well defined, some identified risk factors are associated with chronic irritation of the esophagus.[24] In the United States and Western Europe, smoking and alcohol ingestion are the most prominent factors.[24, 26] In some Asian countries and South America, the consumption of hot tea and a hot beverage called *mate* have been identified as risk factors.[59] In Iran and China, silica fragments found in bread and millet are implicated.[26] Other factors that are implicated include a previous history of squamous cell carcinoma of the esophagus, oropharyngeal leukoplakia, tylosis palmaris, head and neck cancer, the presence of Barrett's esophagus, caustic injury, prior irradiation, esophageal achalasia, Plummer-Vinson syndrome, and a variety of nutritional deficiencies.[24, 59]

PREVENTION, SCREENING, AND DETECTION

Prevention of the disease focuses on counseling regarding alcohol and tobacco use and instructing patients with risk factors to report any problems with *dysphagia* (difficulty in swallowing) or *odynophagia* (pain on swallowing). These patients must be evaluated immediately so that any cancer present may be diagnosed as early as possible. Dietary instructions are also important. A diet of fresh citrus fruit, vegetables high in carotenoids, and milk and enriched flour as sources of riboflavin is recommended.[26] In areas where esophageal cancer is endemic, mass screening by brushing techniques is feasible, but in the United States the incidence of the disease does not justify this approach.[7] Instead, specific groups are targeted. Some experts recommend that selected persons with achalasia undergo periodic endoscopy with biopsies every 2 to 3 years. Persons with caustic ingestion should undergo esophagoscopy every 2 to 3 years beginning 15 to 20 years after ingestion. For affected members of tylosis families endoscopy is recommended every 2 to 3 years after age 30. Persons with documented Barrett's esophagus should undergo endoscopy with multiple biopsies every 1 to 2 years.[6]

CLASSIFICATION

Over the past two decades, the incidence of esophageal adenocarcinoma has risen in the United States and Eu-

Nursing Management

The nurse can assume a significant role in identifying persons at risk for esophageal cancer and in providing counseling on the signs and symptoms of esophageal cancer, life-style modifications to eliminate or reduce risk factors, and importance of annual health examinations by a health care professional. Because there are few or no early signs of esophageal cancer, other than vague GI symptoms of pressure, indigestion, or heartburn (pyrosis), nurses should be aware of persons who are chronic users of home remedies or over-the-counter medications for GI distress. Nurses should urge these persons to seek medical attention immediately.

Nursing Diagnosis

- *Knowledge deficit regarding prevention and early detection of esophageal cancer related to unfamiliar information*

Outcome Goals

Patient will be able to:

- Identify risk factors associated with development of esophageal cancer.
- Identify measures to minimize risks.
- Identify signs and symptoms to be reported to health care professionals related to early detection of esophageal cancer.

Interventions

- Assess for high-risk factors such as heavy alcohol and cigarette use or history of reflux esophagitis, hiatal hernia, or Barrett's esophagus.
- Provide instructions on healthy life-style behaviors:
    Have annual health examination by a health care professional.
    Stop use of cigarettes through a smoking cessation program.
    Eliminate or reduce consumption of alcoholic beverages.
    Eat balanced diet with adequate portions of recommended food groups.
- Provide instructions to report these signs and symptoms: persistent GI distress (regurgitation, reflux, heartburn, epigastric pain) requiring use of antacids, difficulty swallowing requiring changes in diet, or weight loss.

Many persons with esophageal cancer have had a significant weight loss just before they are diagnosed. They usually are experiencing dysphagia and have had to make some dietary adjustments. Depending on the severity of the dysphagia, they will need to change their oral intake and receive enteral feeding, or even total parenteral nutrition (TPN).

Nursing Diagnosis

- *Nutrition, altered: less than body requirements, related to dysphagia*

Outcome Goals

Patient will be able to:

- Identify signs and symptoms to report to health care professionals.
- Identify measures to obtain adequate nutrition.
- Demonstrate a stable nutritional status.

Interventions: *Mild Dysphagia*

- Assess patient for choking or regurgitation during and after meals.
- Obtain dietary consultation for calorie count and dietary modification as needed.
- Weigh patient every other day.
- Instruct patient to sit upright for meals and 30 to 60 minutes after meals. If in bed, raise head to at least 45-degree angle.
- Offer six to eight small feedings per day of high-protein, high-calorie liquefied foods and nutritional supplements.
- Avoid feedings within 2 hours of bedtime.
- Teach patient to use oral suction if he is anxious about aspiration.
- Provide oral and written instructions of measures to maintain stable nutritional status and prevent aspiration.

Interventions: *Severe Dysphagia (in Addition to Mild Dysphagia)*

- Monitor food and fluid intake daily.
- Weigh patient daily.
- Assess for fatigue, altered mental status, weight loss of 2 lb (1 kg) or more, and decreased serum albumin.
- Obtain dietary consultation for alternate routes of nutrition (enteral feedings via nasogastric or gastrostomy tubes, or TPN).
- Administer feedings per physician's orders.
- Instruct patient/caregiver to administer feedings.
- Instruct patient/caregiver to provide oral hygiene frequently.
- Instruct patient/caregiver about signs and symptoms to report to health care professionals.

rope, making it the most common subtype of esophageal cancer. Squamous cell carcinoma is the second most common subtype in the United States; however, it is first in other parts of the world.[7, 75] *Squamous cell carcinomas* arise from the surface epithelium and are found most often in the upper and middle portions of the esophagus. *Adenocarcinomas* most often occur in the lower portion of the esophagus and probably arise from the gastroesophageal junction. They are rarely found in the upper and middle esophagus. Other less common esophageal tumors include mucoepidermoid carcinoma, small-cell carcinoma, sarcoma, adenoid cystic carcinoma, and lymphoma.[7]

CLINICAL FEATURES

Dysphagia, weight loss, and odynophagia are the most common presenting symptoms of this disease. Dysphagia occurs in 95% of patients and is generally not noted until the esophageal lumen is narrowed to one half to one third of normal.[7, 59] Many patients complain of vague discomfort in swallowing for the past 3 to 6 months.[59, 71] Odynophagia is present in about 50% of patients.[58, 75] A weight loss of greater than 10% total body weight may occur before the patient seeks medical attention.[7] Because of this delay, most patients present with advanced disease. The symptoms of advanced disease usually result from the invasion or involvement of surrounding organs and structures.

DIAGNOSIS AND STAGING

All patients complaining of dysphagia should be tested by a plain chest x-ray and barium swallow.[58, 71, 75] Advanced infiltrative esophageal tumors have a characteristic irregular, ragged mucosal pattern with narrowing of the lumen. Endoscopy usually follows the barium

---

CLINICAL FEATURES

Advanced Carcinoma of Esophagus

Hematemesis
Melena
Coughing when swallowing (tracheoesophageal fistula)
Hemoptysis
Dysphonia (laryngeal paralysis)
Superior vena cava syndrome
Malignant pleural effusion
Malignant ascites
Bone pain
Hypercalcemia (paraneoplastic syndrome)

From DeVita V and others, editors: *Cancer: principles and practice of oncology,* ed 5, Philadelphia, Lippincott, 1997.

---

swallow and is required to confirm the presence of a malignant tumor. Biopsies and brushings can be obtained through the endoscope to confirm the histology of the lesion.[58, 71, 75] Endoscopic ultrasonography may be used to identify invasion of the tumor into the tissue layers to aid in staging of disease.[7, 71, 75] It is very accurate for diagnosing stage I and II lesions, but less accurate for stage III and IV lesions.[45] Computed tomography (CT) provides information about the distant metastasis. It is not useful in determining tumors that involve only the mucosa or submucosa, stage I and II lesions. However, the overall accuracy in detecting stage III and IV lesions is greater than 90%.[45]

In 1998, the American Joint Committee on Cancer (AJCC) changed the TNM staging system for esophageal cancer from a clinical one to a pathologic one (Table 9–1). This change was based on data that the depth of penetration of the tumor is a vital prognostic indicator. Both still have importance in the staging of esophageal cancer, particularly in patients managed with primary radiotherapy or chemoradiation, where there is no specimen to determine pathologic staging.[7, 42]

METASTASIS

Esophageal cancer can spread to almost any part of the body, but distant metastases are present in only 25% of the cases at initial presentation. However, they are almost always found during autopsy. Primary sites of metastasis include the lymph nodes (73%), lung (52%), liver (42%), adrenals (20%), bronchus (17%), and bone (14%).[67] Adenocarcinoma is also known to spread to the brain.[7] The presence of metastatic disease is indicative of a very poor prognosis. Survival with proven metastatic disease is less than 7 months.[67]

TREATMENT MODALITIES

The most effective approach to the treatment of esophageal cancer is a combined-modality therapy.[24] For the 40% to 60% of patients with localized disease, surgical resection is the primary treatment.[7, 58] For stage I disease, 5-year survival rates as high as 70% have been reported.[69] For those with more advanced localized disease, investigation has turned to preoperative chemotherapy, preoperative radiation, and preoperative chemoradiation.[58] Palliation is the primary goal for patients with advanced or metastatic disease, and surgery often provides the best long-term relief of dysphagia.[69]

Surgery

As with most solid tumors, surgery offers the best chance for a cure.[69] All patients without evidence of distant metastasis and who are clinically fit should un-

T A B L E 9 – 1
1983 and 1998 AJCC TNM Staging Systems for Esophageal Cancer

1983 Classification (Clinical)	1998 Classification (Pathologic)
PRIMARY TUMOR (T)	
Tis Carcinoma in situ	Noninvasive
T1 Tumor involves ≤ 5 cm of esophageal length, produces no obstruction, and has no circumferential involvement	Tumor invades lamina propria or submucosa
T2 Tumor involves > 5 cm of esophageal length, causes obstruction, or involves the circumference of the esophagus	Tumor invades muscularis propria
T3 Extraesophageal spread	Tumor invades adventitia
T4 NA	Tumor invades adjacent structures
REGIONAL LYMPH NODES (N)	
NX Regional nodes cannot be assessed	Same
N0 No nodal metastases	No regional nodal metastasis
N1 Unilateral, mobile, regional nodal metastases (if clinically evaluable)	Regional nodal metastasis
N2 Bilateral, mobile, regional nodal metastases (if clinically evaluable)	NA
N3 Fixed nodes	NA
DISTANT METASTASES (M)	
M0 No distant metastases	Same
M1 Distant metastases	Distant metastases (including cervical or celiac nodal metastases for tumors of the thoracic esophagus)

STAGE GROUPING						
Stage I	T1	N0 or NX	M0	T1	N0	M0
Stage II	T2	N0 or NX	M0			
Stage IIA				T2-3	N0	M0
Stage IIB				T1-2	N1	M0
Stage III	T3	Any N	M0	T3	N1	M0 or
				T4	Any N	M0
Stage IV	Any T	Any N	M1	Any T	Any N	M1

NA = Not applicable
From Bonin S, Coia L, Hoff P, Pazdur R, Paz I: Esophageal cancer. In Pazdur R, Coia L, Haskins W, Wagner L, editors: Cancer management: a multidisciplinary approach, ed 3, 1999. With permission of PRR, Inc., Melville, NY, 11747.

dergo surgery. If locally advanced disease or distant metastases are found during exploration, nonsurgical palliation should be performed due to the high mortality (as high as 20%) associated with surgical bypass.[69] The choice of surgical approach to an *esophagectomy* remains controversial.[7, 24, 75] In most cases, the stomach is used for the reconstruction, with the anastomosis performed in either the chest or the neck. If the patient has had a surgical procedure involving the stomach, or if the tumor extends so far as to require a total esophagectomy, the esophagus must be reconstructed using a portion of the small or large intestine.[71] Tumors in the distal esophagus involving the gastroesophageal junction are usually managed with a subtotal esophagectomy. The Ivor Lewis approach, with both thoracic and abdominal incisions, allows easy access to both the stomach and the thoracic esophagus. The transhiatal approach (Fig. 9–1) is used for tumors in the cervical or upper esophagus. These lesions require a total esopha-

gectomy because of the difficulty in achieving negative margins.[32, 69, 71]

With the increased popularity of endoscopic surgery during the 1990s, endoscopic esophagectomy procedures have been investigated. Esophagectomy continues to be associated with high mortality and prolonged morbidity; thus, the potential benefit of an endoscopic procedure was attractive. Because this is still a relatively new approach, few results have been reported. Factors being considered are the best approaches and the increased incidence of port-site metastases.[32]

Radiation Therapy

Radiation therapy is seldom used as a primary therapy because studies have shown that chemotherapy plus radiation therapy (chemoradiation) is superior to radiation alone.[29, 58] Neither preoperative nor postoperative radiation therapy offered any survival benefit over sur-

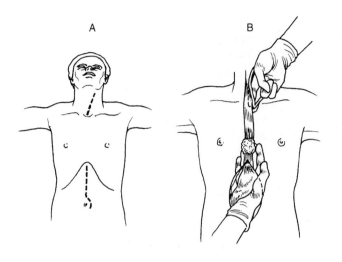

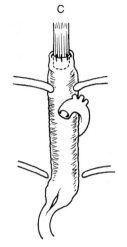

FIGURE 9–1 Transhiatal esophagectomy. A, The cervical and abdominal incisions. B, How manual dissection is used from both above and below. C, The stomach anastomosed to the esophagus in the neck. (From Jamieson G, Mathew G: Surgical management of esophageal cancer: the Western experience. In Daly J and others, editors: *Management of upper gastrointestinal cancer*, p. 187, Philadelphia, Saunders, 1999.)

gery alone. Patients offered radiation therapy alone are those with widespread metastasis, advanced and obstructing tumors, or a poor functional status that does not permit combined-modality therapy.[24] Unfortunately, this relief is short term. Dysphagia is relieved for up to 5 to 10 months for 60% to 80% patients.[24] Intraluminal brachytherapy has been also been explored for palliation in advanced tumors. The procedure allows high doses of radiation to be administered locally to a small volume of tissue.[7, 24, 45, 58, 67] Unfortunately, the additional toxicity compared to radiation alone, has limited its use.

Preoperative chemoradiation has been found to provide improved disease-free survival and a higher frequency of curative resections. Unfortunately, this has not translated into improved overall survival.[7] For patients with squamous cell carcinoma, primary chemoradiation has become the standard of treatment for locally confined disease.[7] Patients with adenocarcinoma are usually offered preoperative chemoradiation or primary chemoradiation with surgical salvage if needed.[7]

Chemotherapy

Studies using single-agent chemotherapy have shown some effectiveness in treating squamous cell carcinoma. However, studies regarding adenocarcinoma of the esophagus and cardia are limited; thus, it is unclear whether adenocarcinomas respond differently. Generally, the response to single-agent chemotherapy is brief and is associated with little palliative relief and no survival benefit.[24] Twelve agents have been identified with 15% or greater response rate. These include 5-fluorouracil, cisplatin, methotrexate, paclitaxel, mitomycin, vindesine, mitoguazone, vinorelbine, doxorubicin, and bleomycin.[24] Cisplatin-based chemotherapy is the most common combination used. Response rates of the combination protocols based on cisplatin are re-

ported as 25% to 50%.[75] The most common regimen used is 5-fluorouracil (5-FU) and cisplatin. Recently paclitaxel, 5-FU, and cisplatin have been used to treat patients with advanced esophageal cancer with an overall response rate of 44%.[7] High-dose cisplatin with etoposide has been used for patients with unresectable or metastatic esophageal adenocarinoma with a response rate of 27% to 65%. Another protocol for regionally advanced or metastatic esophageal carcinoma is 5-FU, recombinant interferon-α-2B, and cisplatin. Reported response rates are 27% to 65%.[67]

Preoperative (*neoadjuvant*) chemotherapy may provide the advantages of improving surgical outcome by reducing the tumor burden, eliminating micrometastatic disease, and allowing chemosensitivity evaluation of the agents given for possible use postoperatively.[24] Studies using neoadjuvant chemotherapy have been inconclusive; therefore, the use of preoperative chemotherapy remains under investigation. Adverse side effects depend on the agents used and may include nausea, vomiting, myelosuppression, nephrotoxicity, and peripheral neuropathy.

A number of studies have used concurrent neoadjuvant chemotherapy and radiation therapy. The purpose of preoperative radiation therapy is to control local recurrence while improving the resectability of the primary tumor. The purpose of chemotherapy is to eliminate metastatic disease. The high incidence of local recurrence and metastasis in patients with esophageal cancer provides the rationale for the increase in the number of clinical trials combining preoperative chemotherapy and radiation.[24] Researchers have learned that not only does thoracic radiation therapy control local recurrence, but a number of the chemotherapeutic agents used to treat esophageal cancer, such as 5-FU and cisplatin, act to potentiate the effect of radiation as well. However, the results of clinical trials are inconclu-

COMPLICATIONS

Esophageal Cancer Treatment[58]

After Esophageal Resection

Pneumonia
Pulmonary embolism
Gastric outlet obstruction
Hemorrhage
Atrial fibrillation
Anastomotic leak
Strictures
Laryngeal nerve palsy

Related to Radiation Therapy

Radiation pneumonitis
Pericarditis
Myocarditis
Spinal cord damage
Stricture
Fistula formation
Hemorrhage

---

sive and further studies are in progress using more aggressive regimens.[67]

The Complications box summarizes potential treatment-related complications of esophageal cancer.

PROGNOSIS

Although the prognosis for persons with esophageal cancer remains poor, the 5-year survival rate has increased in the past 30 years from 3% to 15%.[24, 75] Even with the improved treatment, 95% of patients diagnosed will die of their disease.[24, 75] Therefore, the majority of patients are in need of palliative care at diagnosis or shortly thereafter. The major problems experienced by patients with advanced disease include dysphagia and odynophagia, with resulting malnutrition.[24, 75] Radiation therapy has been used for palliation; however, the treatment cycle takes several weeks, and the response to therapy does not occur immediately.

Endoscopic palliation provides several alternatives with immediate relief. These include dilatation, esophageal prosthesis, laser ablation of obstructing lesions, photodynamic therapy (PDT), and endoluminal brachytherapy.[9, 75] The simplest approach is esophageal dilatation. Dilatation provides temporary relief and is often used as an adjunct for placement of an endoluminal stent for hospice patients.[75] Expandable endoluminal stents are easily placed endoscopically with fluoroscopic control. New designs of stents have decreased the complications of perforation, hemorrhage, and fistula formation. Laser therapy and PDT palliate by reducing the size of the obstructing tumor. Using an endoscope, a fiberoptic laser fiber is passed through the tumor causing vaporization of the tumor. A neodymium/yttrium-aluminum garnet laser is used for routine laser ablation. For PDT, patients are given a photosensitizer, then are treated with light delivered from an argon pump dye laser.[9, 75] These procedures usually allow the patient to continue oral feedings of liquids and possibly soft foods. If the patient develops anorexia or is unable to continue oral feedings, enteral feedings may be used. Percutaneous endoscopic gastrostomy is a low-risk method of placing a feeding tube. If necessary, a feeding tube may be placed under fluoroscopy, avoiding the need for a laparotomy and general anesthesia in severely ill patients. Total parenteral nutrition is usually not used in these patients if another route is possible. Chronic severe mediastinal and posterior chest pain is indicative of regional spread of cancer and is very incapacitating. If the patient is unable to take oral sustained-release analgesics, he may require a patient-controlled analgesia (PCA) pump for maximum comfort.

Cancer of the Stomach

Although cancer of the stomach has shown a significant decline in incidence, about 60% decrease from the 1930s to the 1970s, it remains one of the 10 most common causes of cancer deaths in the United States.[8, 27] The reason for the decline in incidence in some parts of the world but not in others remains an enigma. Although the United States reports an incidence of 10/100,000 population, Japan's incidence is 780/100,000.[53] It is postulated that the increased consumption of refrigerated foods rather than spiced, smoked, and pickled foods may be a factor.[1]

EPIDEMIOLOGY

In the United States an estimated 21,500 new cases of stomach cancer were diagnosed in 2000, and a total of 13,000 deaths were attributed to the disease.[27] Gastric cancer is more common in men than women; the ratio reported is 1.7:1, and is 1.5 times more common in African Americans than whites.[8] Two thirds of the patients with newly diagnosed gastric cancer are over 65 years of age, and 50% are older than 70.[27]

ETIOLOGY AND RISK FACTORS

Several nutritional, environmental, social, and medical factors have been associated with the development of cancer of the stomach (Table 9–2). Immigrant studies show that the second generation of families emigrating from countries of high incidence to low incidence have fewer cases of gastric cancer. This decrease has been

TABLE 9–2

Factors Associated with Increased Risk of Developing Stomach Cancer

NUTRITIONAL

Low fat or protein consumption
Salted meat or fish
High nitrate consumption
Low dietary vitamins A and C

ENVIRONMENTAL

Poor food preparation (smoked)
Lack of refrigeration
Poor drinking water (well water)
Occupation (rubber, coal workers)
Smoking

SOCIAL

Low social class

MEDICAL

Prior gastric surgery
Helicobacter pylori infection
Gastric atrophy and gastritis

From Alexander H, Kelsen D, Teppen J: Cancer and the stomach. In DeVita VT, Hellman S, Rosenberg SA editors: Cancer: principles and practice of oncology, ed 5, Philadelphia, Lippincott-Raven, 1997.

attributed to changes in dietary habits.[2, 39] Smoking is also associated with increased risk; however, data are inconclusive regarding use of alcohol.

Low socioeconomic status is also associated with increased incidence of gastric cancer. This is probably related to a number of social, occupational, and cultural factors. The lack of refrigeration of foods, diets including smoked or salted meats and fish, and the use of well water are all associated with high risk. Occupational risk factors have also been associated with higher incidence of stomach cancer. Metal workers, coal miners, rubber workers, and those exposed to dust from wood and asbestos have all been shown to have higher than normal incidence.[8, 53]

Familial occurrence of gastric cancer is rare, but a small increase in incidence has been noted in direct relatives of some people who have had gastric cancer. The most notable family with this disease is that of Napoleon Bonaparte.[2] It has been reported that diffuse gastric cancer is significantly more common in patients with blood group A and in relatives of patients with diffuse gastric cancer.

Pathologies and past medical history associated with the development of gastric cancer include gastric polyps, especially the villous adenoma; pernicious anemia; chronic reflux esophagitis; *Helicobacter pylori* infection; and gastric resection for benign disease. It is suggested that the presence of atrophic gastritis and achlorhydria

in persons with pernicious anemia may contribute to the development of gastric cancer.[2, 8, 39, 53]

PREVENTION, SCREENING, AND EARLY DETECTION

The key to prevention of cancer of the stomach lies in dietary intake. People of geographic areas and socioeconomic groups associated with the lowest incidence consume a diet different from those of highest incidence. Nutrition counseling to prevent gastric cancer should stress the importance of consuming a balanced diet high in fresh fruits and vegetables and moderate in amounts of animal protein and fats. Salted, smoked, and pickled foods should be consumed in low quantities.[39]

Screening and early detection programs have been very successful in Japan. Esophagogastroduodenoscopy (EGD) and upper GI series are the techniques used most. The diagnosis of early gastric cancer in Japan increased to over 65%.[38, 60]

In western countries, where the incidence of gastric cancer is low, widespread screening programs are not considered economically useful because of the low yield.[1, 8] It is important, however, to identify persons at high risk and follow them with annual endoscopic examinations. The high-risk group includes those with atrophic gastritis, pernicious anemia, intestinal metaplasia, gastric polyps, previous gastric surgery, or dysplasia.

CLASSIFICATION

Adenocarcinomas represent almost 95% of the malignant tumors of the stomach. Lymphoma, carcinoid, leiomyosarcoma, and squamous cell carcinoma comprise the remaining 5%.[2, 8, 53]

Several classification systems are used for stomach cancer. One developed by Borrmann, used exclusively in Japan, identifies five different types of stomach cancer: *type 1* includes polypoid or fungating cancers; *type 2* includes ulcerating lesions with elevated borders; *type 3* includes ulcerating lesions infiltrating the gastric wall; *type 4* includes diffusely infiltrating carcinomas (linitis plastica); and *type 5* includes unclassifiable cancers.[2] Broder's classification system is based on degree of histologic differentiation. Tumor cells are graded from 1 (*well differentiated*) to 4 (*anaplastic*).[2]

The most widely accepted system of classification was developed by Lauren in 1965.[2, 43] This system identifies two main groups of gastric cancers: diffuse gastric cancer (33%) and intestinal gastric cancer (53%). The remaining 14% are unclassified.[43] *Intestinal gastric cancers* are characterized by tubular or papillary glandular structures with varying degrees of differentiation. *Diffuse gastric cancers* are composed of poorly differentiated cells that infiltrate the gastric wall, and are associated with a very poor prognosis.[43]

Nursing Management

As with patients with cancer of the esophagus, patients with cancer of the stomach experience profound weight loss caused by the disease process and the treatment modalities, particularly radical subtotal or total gastrectomy. The preoperative patient assessment should include a nutritional evaluation encompassing a diet and weight loss history (especially the type and consistency of diet consumed), laboratory values (serum albumin, leukocyte count, total iron-binding capacity, ferritin, electrolytes), and calorie intake.

Nursing Diagnosis

- *Altered nutrition: less than body requirements, related to gastrectomy*

Outcome Goals

Patient will be able to:

- Explain rationale for altered nutrition and factors that contribute to malnutrition.
- Demonstrate measures to manage nutritional status.
- List signs and symptoms to report to the health care team.
- Demonstrate a stable nutritional status consistent with stage of disease.

Interventions

- Weigh patient daily.
- Take accurate intake and output readings every 24 hours.
- Monitor laboratory values, including electrolytes and leukocyte count.
- Provide patient/caregiver dietary instructions:
  Eat six small feedings per day.
  Limit fluids at mealtime, and drink fluids between meals.
  Progress slowly from liquid to soft diet.
  Choose high-protein and moderate-carbohydrate foods.
  Avoid greasy foods.
  Eat slowly.
- Provide instructions on signs and symptoms to report to health care team:
  Diarrhea
  Clay-colored stools
  Fatty stools
  Abdominal cramps
  Weakness
  Faintness
  Rapid heartbeat
- Provide instructions for diet if diarrhea occurs:
  Choose low-residue, bulk-forming foods (refined breads and cereals, pasta, rice, cheese, fish, chicken, bananas, applesauce, cooked vegetables).
  Avoid foods such as whole-grain breads or cereals, fresh fruits and vegetables, gas-forming foods, citrus fruits, and juices.
  Eat slowly.
  Notify health care team of need for antidiarrheal and/or antispasmodic agents.
- Provide instructions for diet if dumping syndrome occurs:
  Choose foods high in protein and fat and low in carbohydrates.
  Avoid concentrated sweets.
  Drink liquids between meals.
  Sit upright after meal for at least 60 minutes.
  Notify health care team if symptoms continue.
- Obtain dietary consult for assistance, evaluation, and diet planning.
- Administer enteral/parenteral feedings if ordered and provide instructions to patient/caregiver if necessary before discharge.

CLINICAL FEATURES

One of the most frustrating aspects of gastric cancer is that it has no early symptoms. Most patients present with locally advanced or metastatic disease.[2, 8] Symptoms are nonspecific and may have been present for several months. They include indigestion and epigastric discomfort (67%), nausea and vomiting (40%), hematemesis (15%), and anorexia (25%).[1, 2, 8, 62] Often the symptoms may reflect the location of the tumor. Dysphagia is associated with lesions in the cardia. Vomiting after meals is seen in obstructing tumors of the pyloric region of the stomach.[2, 39, 53]

DIAGNOSIS AND STAGING

Physical examination of the patient suspected of having gastric cancer is often normal. Abnormal findings usually reflect metastasis. Attention should be paid to whether the left supraclavicular node is enlarged (Virchow's node), or whether the left anterior axillary node is enlarged (Irish's node). A digital rectal examination should be performed to assess for the presence of a mass in the pouch of Douglas. Abdominal palpation may reveal evidence of Sister Joseph's nodules around the umbilicus. A pelvic examination should be performed to rule out metastasis to the ovary (Krukenberg tumor).[1] These abnormal findings are indicative of poor prognosis.

The two most useful diagnostic procedures for gastric cancer are the *esophagogastroduodenoscopy* (EGD) and the *double-contrast upper GI series*.[1, 2, 8, 39, 53] The latter is able to identify the site of the lesion and, with special compression techniques, detect depressions and elevations of the gastric mucosa.[1] However, an EGD has the advantage of being able to directly visualize the lesions and to obtain multiple biopsies.[8] The EGD is considered the most accurate procedure in diagnosing gastric cancer.[1, 2]

Once the initial diagnosis is made, a CT scan of the chest, abdomen, and pelvis is recommended to evaluate tumor extent, nodal involvement, and distant metastasis.[8] CT scans are not useful in determining depth of tumor penetration unless it penetrates outside the wall of the stomach, but they are very accurate in identifying distant metastasis and lymph node involvement. Endoscopic ultrasonography (EUS) has been found to be highly accurate in staging the depth of invasion of the primary tumor and assessing local lymph node involvement.[1, 53] Laparoscopy is more accurate in identifying liver and peritoneal metastasis.[43] Therefore, CT scans, EUS, and laparoscopy are critical in staging gastric cancer.[2, 8, 43]

Table 9–3 outlines the AJCC TNM criteria for classification and staging of cancer of the stomach.

METASTASIS

In addition to local extension to nearby organs and tissue, cancer of the stomach metastasizes most frequently to the liver (40%), lungs (40%), peritoneum, and bone marrow (10%). It is also known to spread more rarely to the brain, kidney, thyroid, ovary, local lymph nodes, and adrenal gland.[1]

TREATMENT MODALITIES

Surgery, chemotherapy, and radiation therapy are used to treat cancer of the stomach and have potential complications.[76]

Surgery

Surgery is the major treatment modality and is the only potentially curative treatment for cancer of the stomach.[2, 8, 39, 44] Preoperative staging is critical to identify patients who will best benefit from surgery.[60] Due to the advanced stages of disease on presentation, a decision must be made regarding the goal of surgery, curative or palliative. Generally, in the absence of metastatic disease, an aggressive surgical approach is justified.[53]

TABLE 9–3
TNM Clinical Classification System for Staging Gastric Carcinoma

PRIMARY TUMOR (T)

TX	Primary tumor cannot be assessed
T0	No evidence of primary tumor
Tis	Carcinoma in situ: intraepithelial tumor, without invasion of lamina propria
T1	Tumor invades lamina propria or submucosa
T2	Tumor invades muscularis propria or subserosa
T3	Tumor penetrates serosa (visceral peritoneum) without invasion of adjacent structures
T4	Tumor invades adjacent structures

REGIONAL LYMPH NODES (N)

NX	Regional lymph node(s) cannot be assessed
N0	No regional lymph node metastasis
N1	Metastasis in 1–6 regional lymph nodes
N2	Metastasis in 7–15 regional lymph nodes
N3	Metastasis in >15 regional lymph nodes

DISTANT METASTASIS (M)

MX	Presence of distant metastasis cannot be assessed
M0	No distant metastasis
M1	Distant metastasis

STAGE GROUPING

Stage 0	Tis	N0	M0
Stage IA	T1	N0	M0
Stage IB	T1	N1	M0
	T2	N0	M0
Stage II	T1	N2	M0
	T2	N1	M0
	T3	N0	M0
Stage IIIA	T2	N2	M0
	T3	N1	M0
	T4	N0	M0
Stage IIIB	T3	N2	M0
Stage IV	T4	N1	M0
	T1	N3	M0
	T2	N3	M0
	T3	N3	M0
	T4	N2	M0
	T4	N3	M0
	Any T	Any N	M1

From Meyers M: Gastric carcinoma: imaging, staging, and management. In Meyers M, editor: Neoplasms of the digestive tract: imaging, staging, and management, Philadelphia, Lippincott-Raven, 1998.

The operative procedure chosen depends on the anatomic location of the tumor and knowledge of the pattern of spread from that particular location.[53] For selection of procedure and reconstruction, the stomach may be divided into thirds (Fig. 9–2). The proximal third includes the gastroesophageal junction and the fundus; the middle third includes the fundus to midsection of the lesser curvature; and the distal third includes the remaining portion to the pylorus.[60] For tumors in the

COMPLICATIONS

Gastric Cancer Disease and Treatment[2]

DISEASE-RELATED COMPLICATIONS

Pain
Obstruction
Bleeding
Dysphagia

TREATMENT-RELATED COMPLICATIONS

Postoperative Complications[62]

Early	*Late*
Infection	Dumping syndrome
Hemorrhage	Reflux esophagitis
Acute pancreatitis	Chronic weight loss
Ileus, jaundice	Anemia
Anastomotic leak	Hypoproteinemia

Radiation Therapy Complications[2]

During Treatment	*Late*
Fatigue	Radiation nephritis
Nausea	Radiation hepatitis
Vomiting	Bleeding
Weight loss	Ulceration

Chemotherapy Complications

Myelosuppression	Alopecia
Oral mucositis	Extravasation
Nausea/vomiting	Fatigue
Diarrhea	Nephrotoxicity

proximal third, choice of surgical procedure remains controversial, but usually either a *radical subtotal gastrectomy* or a *total gastrectomy* is used. Tumors in the middle section usually require a total gastrectomy to obtain tumor-free margins. Tumors located in the distal third are usually treated with a radical subtotal gastrectomy.[8, 53, 60] After a subtotal gastrectomy, a gastroduodenostomy or gastrojejunostomy is used for the reconstruction.[8, 18] After a total gastrectomy, a Roux-en-Y esophagojejunostomy is performed for reconstruction.[8, 37]

Chemotherapy

Of all the gastrointestinal tract cancers, stomach cancer is the most responsive to chemotherapy, with the exception of islet cell cancers.[76] Chemotherapy is now being studied as adjuvant and neoadjuvant therapy for resect-

able tumors and for the treatment of advanced gastric cancer. Presently, there is no standard chemotherapy protocol because of the significant toxicity and the absence of evidence of improved survival.[39] Patients undergoing curative surgery, even those without nodal metastasis, have 5-year survival rates between 30% and 40%.[8] Therefore, treatment in addition to surgery is necessary for long-term survival. Drugs that have shown some activity against gastric cancer include 5-FU, tegafur, doxorubicin, epirubicin, mitomycin C, the nitrosoureas, cisplatin, trimetrexate, and methotrexate.[39, 44, 76] One of the older regimens that has been widely studied is FAM (5-FU, doxorubicin, mitomycin C). Reported response rate range from 30% to 40%, and median survival reported is 6 months to more than a year.[44] By substituting methotrexate for mitomycin C in combination with 5-FU and doxorubicin (FAMTX), researchers were able to show an improved response rate and median survival.[45] Other studies have been reported using 5-FU, and the nitrosourea methyl-CCNU, 5-FU, methyl-CCNU and doxorubicin, and 5-FU combined with BCNU.[2] The three different combination studies showed no significant difference in disease-free survival or overall survival.

In an effort to improve surgical outcomes and long-term survival, many studies have been directed toward preoperative (neoadjuvant) therapy. If there is a response to the neoadjuvant therapy, treatment can be continued postoperatively.[53] One such regimen is *EAP* (etoposide, doxorubicin [Adriamycin], cisplatin [Platinol]). Although this regimen is associated with significant dose-limiting myelosuppression, in some studies it has shown a significant improvement in survival.[2] Other regimens that have been investigated are *FAMTX* (5-FU, doxorubicin [Adriamycin], high-dose methotrexate, leucovorin rescue); 5-FU, leucovorin, and cisplatin; and 5-FU, leucovorin, and interferon-α.[2, 53]

Chemotherapy in the setting of advanced gastric cancer has also been investigated. The most widely used combinations are FAM and FAMTX.[8, 53, 76] For the elderly, particularly those with cardiac disease or impaired renal function, etoposide, leucovorin, and 5-FU (ELF) has been used.[66, 76] Other combinations include EAP, LV-FP (leucovorin, 5-FU, and cisplatin), MLP-F (methotrexate, 5-FU, cisplatin, and leucovorin), PMUE (cisplatin, mitomycin-C, UFT, and etoposide), and FLAME (5-FU, leucovorin, doxorubicin, methotrexate, and etoposide).[76] Unfortunately, the effect of chemotherapy on advanced gastric cancer has been disappointing.[53]

Because there is a high incidence of peritoneal recurrence of gastric cancer, intraperitoneal chemotherapy administration has been investigated.[53, 66, 76] The most recent investigation involved the use of hyperthermia and mitomycin C in the adjuvant setting. The intraperitoneal hyperthermic perfusion is considered safe and is

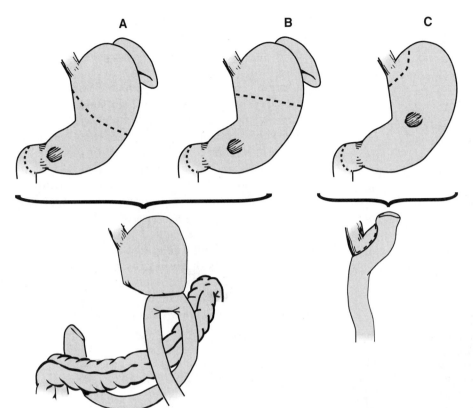

FIGURE 9–2 Gastric resection by thirds using location of tumor. (From Sarr M, McIlath D, Dalton R: Radical subtotal gastrectomy. In Donahue J, van Heerder J, Monson J: editors: *Atlas of surgical oncology,* Cambridge, MA, Blackwell Science, 1995.)

associated with no increase in postoperative complications.[53] The hyperthermic perfusion is usually administered during exploratory laparotomy after a primary resection in cases with either known carcinomatosis or with high risk of developing peritoneal disease.[2] The advantages of using intraperitoneal hyperthermic perfusion include the brief treatment (1–2 hours), effective method of administration to the peritoneal cavity, dose intensification without systemic toxicity, and the effectiveness of the synergy between hyperthermia and chemotherapy.[2] Intraperitoneal infusions of EAP after gastric resection in patients with peritoneal seeding has also been beneficial. Another innovation being investigated is the use of immunologic agents both alone and in combination with chemotherapy.[53]

Radiation Therapy

Radiation therapy may be used to control or eliminate recurrent or residual disease or for palliative treatment of bleeding, pain, or obstruction.[8, 76] Although radiation therapy has been used alone with some response, it is most often combined with chemotherapy. Using 5-FU as a radiosensitizing agent concomitantly with radiation has been shown to improve both survival and palliation.[44] *Intraoperative radiation therapy* (IORT) has been useful in the control of microscopic disease.[53, 76] The advantage of IORT is that radiosensitive normal tissue can be removed from the field. Combining IORT and postoperative radiation has been studied and may increase the long-term survival of patients with stage II, III, or IV disease.[44]

PROGNOSIS

The prognosis for patients with gastric cancer depends on the extent of the disease and on the treatment. The 5-year survival rate in the United States ranges from 5% to 15%.[1,2] Therefore, the prognosis for these patients remains poor. Most cases are diagnosed at an advanced stage, and even after surgery, disease is known to reoccur in 80% of patients.

Cancer of the Liver

Hepatocellular carcinoma (HCC) is relatively uncommon in the United States but is one of the most common malignancies in some parts of the world, especially in areas of China and sub-Saharan Africa.[11, 63] It is an aggressive tumor with an absence of early symptoms and a poor prognosis.[11] Left untreated, life expectancy is 3 to 6 months.[9]

EPIDEMIOLOGY

For reporting purposes in the United States, HCC is combined with biliary tract cancers (gallbladder carcinoma, cholangiocarcinoma, and periampullary carcinoma). Therefore, the incidence data are not completely reliable for primary liver cancers (HCC and hepatoma) alone. In the United States, the estimated number of new cases of liver and intrahepatic bile duct cancers in 2000 was 15,300, which resulted in 13,800 deaths.[27] Worldwide, HCC has an incidence of approximately 1,000,000 annually.[10, 46, 63] It is twice as common in men than women in the United States; however, this situation is quite different in Asia where the ratio is 4 to 7:1.[9] The incidence of HCC increases with age.[15] In the United States the peak age is 55 to 64 years, in Japan 50 to 59 years, in China 45 to 54 years, and in Africa 30 to 39 years.[27]

ETIOLOGY AND RISK FACTORS

Because of the widespread geographic variations in incidence, researchers have been particularly interested in studying the environmental factors implicated in the development of HCC. Box 9–1 summarizes the etiologic and risk factors known to be associated with primary liver cancers. Hepatitis B virus (HBV) and hepatitis C virus (HCV) infections are probably the most important cause worldwide. In China, approximately 90% of HCC patients had a history of HBV infection. In Japan, France, and Italy, HCV infections were associated with 60% to 80% of cases of HCC.[27, 30, 74]

Cirrhosis and alcohol consumption have been associated with the development of HCC. Cirrhosis associated with chronic HBV infection and hemachromatosis is a major risk factor in Asia and Africa. In the western world, however, alcoholic cirrhosis is more common and therefore may be a more important risk factor.[14] It is estimated that 15% of HCC cases in North American can be attributed to alcohol.[27, 30, 74]

Aflatoxins are produced by *Aspergillus flavus* and *A. parasiticus*. Aflatoxin B_1 (AFB_1) occurs when foods, especially peanuts and corn, are stored in warm, moist places. AFB_1 has the highest potency among the aflatoxins as a toxin and carcinogen. This is a widespread problem in humid regions of Africa and Asia, where HCC is most common.[14, 27, 30, 40, 55]

A number of chemical agents have been implicated in the development of primary liver cancer. Many of the improvements in living standards have been accompanied with the use of a wide variety of chemicals, many of which have been found to be toxic to the liver and have carcinogenic and mutagenic potential.[40] These include a variety of chemicals such as nitrites, hydrocarbons, solvents, chlorine, pesticides, primary metals, and polychlorinated biphenyls.[40] Thorotrast, a contrast medium used in the 1930s, emits high levels of radiation and is associated with a long half-life. It accumulates in the macrophages of the reticuloendothelial system, particularly the liver, and produces hepatic fibrosis, angiosarcoma, cholangiocarcinoma, and HCC.[40] The use of oral contraceptives and anabolic steroids has also been associated with HCC, but is uncommon.[22, 50, 63]

PREVENTION, SCREENING, AND DETECTION

Some of the strategies being used in endemic areas of the world to prevent liver cancer include changing the staple food from corn to rice in rural areas to avoid the ingestion of AFB_1. With advent of the vaccine against HBV, China is vaccinating newborns. Changing the source of drinking water to deep well water or tap water is another effort to avoid the exposure to chemicals.[30, 50] High-risk patients with chronic HBV or cirrhosis may be screened for the tumor marker α-fetoprotein (AFP). If the patients have 2 consecutive elevated AFP results, they are then screened by abdominal ultrasonography.[10, 30] The National Institutes of Health recommend screening for HCC in patients with chronic HBV infection, especially those with high risk (cirrhosis, men, nonwhites, and those with perinatally acquired infection), with AFP every 3 to 4 months and ultrasound every 4 to 6 months.[10] No recommendations were made for those with HCV infection or other causes of cirrhosis.

CLASSIFICATION

Hepatocellular carcinoma accounts for more than 90% of the adult primary cancers of the liver.[22] Three classifications have been identified: nodular, diffuse, and massive.[9, 33] The nodular type is composed of distinct solitary or multiple nodules of various sizes occurring in both lobes. The massive type forms a large discrete mass involving most or all of one lobe. The diffuse is most often associated with cirrhosis. Diffuse and massive types account for more than 90% of cases.[9]

BOX 9–1

Summary of Conditions Associated with Hepatocellular Carcinoma (HCC)[11]

Hepatitis B virus	Androgenic steroids
Alcoholism	Cirrhosis
Hepatitis C virus	Sex hormones
Aflatoxins	Occupational exposure to pesticides/insecticides
Hemochromatosis	Vinyl chloride

Nursing Management

The nursing care of the patient with primary liver cancer is very challenging. Because most patients with HCC are not candidates for liver resection, many will be treated by hepatic artery infusion therapy via an implanted infusion pump. The nurse's primary responsibility is educating the patient and family to manage this form of therapy.

Nursing Diagnosis

- *Knowledge deficit regarding management of hepatic artery infusion therapy related to lack of exposure*

Outcome Goals

Patient will be able to:

- State rationale for use of hepatic artery infusion.
- Demonstrate measures for care of implanted pump and management of side effects of chemotherapy.
- Identify signs and symptoms to report to health care team.

Interventions

- Assess patient's understanding of treatment, goals, patient's ability to manage care postoperatively, and availability of support from family and friends.
- Provide both verbal and written instructions regarding the implanted pump and chemotherapy:

  Purpose of pump and where catheter is placed anatomically in liver

  Management of pocket site: keep incision clean and dry until healed; resume usual activities when healed; avoid activities that may lead to blunt trauma to pump pocket or that may cause increased temperature, pressure, or altitude

  What to report to health care team: temperature greater than 101°F (38.3°C) for more than 24 hours, air travel, or change in residence requiring a change in altitude

  Side effects of chemotherapy drug(s) being infused and other medications

- Provide written list of phone numbers of health care team members and schedule of treatment cycles.

CLINICAL FEATURES

Patients with early HCC seldom have symptoms. Most patients present with advanced disease. The most common presenting symptoms of HCC are right upper quadrant abdominal pain and other vague symptoms such as fatigue, anorexia, weight loss, unexplained fever and jaundice.[9, 22, 30, 63] Pain is usually dull or aching, and often radiates up to the right shoulder.[22, 34] On physical examination hepatomegaly may be found in 50% to 90% of patients.[11] Other findings may include splenomegaly, ascites (30–60% of patients), and hepatic arterial bruits.[11, 63] The Clinical Features box lists signs and symptoms. HCC is also associated with several paraneoplastic syndromes that are important because they may be present before the local effects of the tumor and alert the health care professional to the presence of HCC.[9] The major paraneoplastic syndromes include hypoglycemia, hypercalcemia, erythrocytosis, carcinoid syndrome, and hypercholesterolemia. Less frequently sexual changes, porphyria cutanea tarda, hypertrophic osteoarthropathy, hypertension, and hyperthyroidism may be noted.[11, 34, 63, 68]

DIAGNOSIS AND STAGING

Diagnosis of liver cancer can be challenging. Patients presenting with a right upper quadrant abdominal mass should have a diagnostic work-up at once. The initial studies should include blood tests and diagnostic imaging.[28]

Blood tests should include AFP, des-γ-carboxy prothrombin (DCP), and hepatitis surface antigens. AFP is the principal tumor marker associated with HCC and

---

CLINICAL FEATURES

Hepatocellular Carcinoma (HCC)

Symptoms[65]

Abdominal pain
Abdominal mass
Weight loss
Anorexia/early satiety
Intermittent nausea/vomiting
Weakness, fatigue, malaise

Clinical Signs[11]

Hepatomegaly/splenomegaly
Jaundice
Abdominal bruits
Ascites
Paraneoplastic syndromes (hypoglycemia, erythrocytosis, hypercalcemia, hypercholesterolemia, dysfibrinogenemia, carcinoid syndrome, sexual changes, porphyria cutanea tarda)

is elevated in more than 85% of patients with the disease.[9] The normal range for AFP is 1 to 20 ng/mL, and elevations to greater than 400 ng/mL are almost always diagnostic for HCC.[9] However, AFP levels do correlate with the size of the primary tumor, extent of intrahepatic disease, or the presence of metastasis.[15] DCP is a fairly new marker that is tumor specific for HCC; however, it is less sensitive than AFP and is totally independent of AFP. Some patients may be found to be AFP negative, but may have increased DCP.[11, 15] DCP is elevated in 91% of patients with HCC, but may also be elevated in patients with vitamin K deficiency, chronic hepatitis, or cirrhosis.[11, 28]

Diagnostic imaging should specifically include an ultrasound and CT. The ultrasound is as sensitive and specific as CT and has the advantages of being relatively inexpensive and noninvasive.[9, 28, 61, 65] It is able to detect lesions less than 3 cm in size. Conventional CT is able to detect and demonstrate the extent of the liver tumors and is helpful in identifying any extrahepatic disease. For any tumor that appears to be resectable, CT with angiography is necessary to provide information regarding arterial and venous involvement. This study relies on uniform distribution of the contrast dye injected into the hepatic artery. Unfortunately, this is not always possible in the cirrhotic liver or if there is variant hepatic arterial anatomy present. CT with arterial portography (CTAP) provides the most accurate method of assessing hepatic lesions. This method involves injecting contrast into the superior mesenteric artery or the splenic artery, then delayed images are taken when contrast enters the portal system. CTAP is used to assess size of the primary tumor, the presence of intrahepatic spread of tumor, and the presence of portal or hepatic venous invasion by tumor.[11, 15] CTAP can determine metastases. Sensitivity of CTAP is reported as high as 97%.[15, 61, 65] Magnetic resonance imaging (MRI) with angiography is also used. It has demonstrated sensitivity and provides information relating to the anatomy of the tumor and major vessels.[63] A chest x-ray is usually obtained to determine presence of lung metastasis. CT scan of the brain or bone scans may be indicated if there is suspicion of metastasis to these areas.[61, 65]

A fine-needle aspiration or percutaneous needle biopsy is ultimately necessary to make a definitive diagnosis. Often this is performed under ultrasound guidance or fluoroscopy. Unfortunately, most HCCs are hypervascular, so there is a high risk of hemorrhage following this procedure. Also, patients may have ascites or a coagulopathy. Therefore, if the tumor appears resectable, a surgical approach is best for obtaining a tissue specimen. A preoperative liver biopsy should be used if the lesion is unresectable and histopathology is needed to determine appropriate alternative therapy.[61, 65]

BOX 9–2

TNM *Classification and Staging for Liver Cancer*

PRIMARY TUMOR (T)

T1: solitary tumor 2 cm or less, without vascular invasion

T2: solitary tumor 2 cm or less, with vascular invasion, or multiple tumors limited to one lobe, none more than 2 cm, without vascular invasion, or a solitary tumor more than 2 cm without vascular invasion

T3: solitary tumor more than 2 cm with vascular invasion, or multiple tumors limited to one lobe, none more than 2 cm, with vascular invasion, or multiple tumors limited to one lobe, any more than 2 cm, with or without vascular invasion

T4: multiple tumors in more than one lobe, or tumor(s) involve(s) a major branch of portal or hepatic vein(s)

LYMPH NODE (N)

N0: no regional lymph node metastasis
N1: regional lymph node metastasis

DISTANT METASTASIS (M)

M0: no distant metastasis
M1: distant metastasis

STAGE GROUPING

Stage I: T1-N0-M0
Stage II: T2-N0-M0
Stage III: T1-N1-M0 T2-N1-M0 T3-N0-M0 T3-N1-M0
Stage IVA: T4-any N-M0
Stage IVB: any T-any N-M1

In 1997, the AJCC adopted a staging system based on degree of liver involvement, extent of vascular invasion, nodal involvement, and the presence or absence of distant metastasis (TNM). Box 9–2 summarizes this system.

METASTASIS

The usual sites for HCC metastasis are the regional nodes, lung, bone, adrenal gland, and brain.[9, 61, 68]

TREATMENT MODALITIES

Surgery

Surgery is the only potentially curative treatment modality for patients with HCC. Unfortunately, only 10% to 30% of the patients meet the criteria for liver resection.[61]

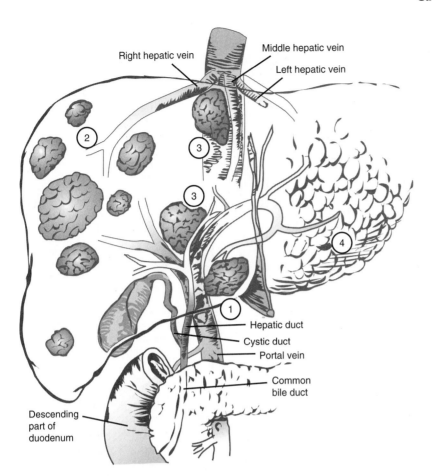

Right hepatic vein

Middle hepatic vein

Left hepatic vein

② ③ ③ ④ ①

Hepatic duct

Cystic duct

Portal vein

Common bile duct

Descending part of duodenum

FIGURE 9 – 3 Contraindications for hepatic resection for HCC. (From Curley SA: Surgical management of hepatocellular cancer. In Curley S, editor: *Liver cancer,* New York, Springer-Verlag, 1998.)

Findings that may contraindicate liver resection are found in Figure 9–3. Controversy regarding the feasibility of resection for patients with cirrhosis continues. It is critical to assess the functional hepatic reserve to make a decision regarding surgery for these patients.[15] A common test used to assess liver function uses chemicals that are normally rapidly acquired and metabolized by hepatocytes. Metabolism and clearance are decreased in cirrhotic livers. Indocyanine green (ICG) is given intravenously, and then blood samples are drawn at timed intervals to assess clearance from the plasma. A calcula-

tion is performed to arrive at percentage of clearance. Values between 15% and 20% indicate a lobectomy or two-segment resection will be tolerated. Values between 21% and 35% indicate a single segment or wedge resection will be tolerated. A value greater than 40% indicates that liver failure will probably occur even with a minimal resection.[15] Another method of determining candidates for resection is the Child-Turcotte classification of hepatic dysfunction (Table 9–4).

Hepatic resections used for HCC are based on anatomic segments of the liver (Figure 9–4). The type of

TABLE 9 – 4
Child-Turcotte Classification of Hepatic Dysfunction in Cirrhotic Patients

	Criteria by Class		
Parameter	A	B	C
Nutritional status	Excellent	Good	Poor
Ascites	None	Minimal, controlled	Moderate to severe
Encephalopathy	None	Minimal, controlled	Moderate to severe
Serum bilirubin	<2	2–3	>3
Serum albumin (g/dL)	>3.5	2.8–3.5	<2.8
Prothrombin time (% of control)	>70	40–70	<40

From Curley S: Surgical management of hepatocellular cancer. In Curley S, editor: Liver Cancer, New York, Springer-Verlag, 1998.

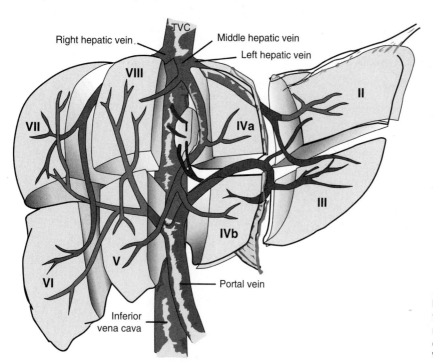

FIGURE 9 – 4 Segmental anatomy of the liver. (From Curley S: Surgical management of hepatocellular cancer. In Curley S, editor: *Liver cancer,* New York, Springer-Verlag, 1998.)

liver excision depends on the size, number, and locations of the lesions and the need for at least a 1-cm tumor-free margin.[52] Wedge resections are usually adequate for small lesions easily accessible. Tumors located in one or two different liver segments can be resected by removing the involved segments. Major liver resections involve the removal of at least three adjoining segments in their entirety: right lobectomy involves segments V, VI, VII, and VIII; left lobectomy involves segments II, III, and IV; right trisegmentectomy involves segments IV to VII; and a left lateral segmentectomy involves segments II and III.[52]

Total hepatectomy and orthotopic liver transplantation is an option for primary liver cancer patients with disease only in the liver, but who are not candidates for curative resections due to contraindications of tumor size, location, multicentricity, or poor hepatic functional reserve.[15] Because of high cancer recurrence rates and limited donor organs, it remains controversial.[14] Prognostic factors associated with recurrence include stage III or IV disease, tumor size greater than 5 cm, evidence of vascular invasion, absence of a pseudocapsule, and lymph node metastasis. Reported 5-year survival rates for patients after transplant are up to 35%.[9, 19]

Cryosurgery is a procedure used to treat multiple or bilobar unresectable primary and metastatic liver tumors. A probe is placed inside the tumor. Liquid nitrogen is circulated through the probe causing rapid freezing of the tumor cells. Each freezing takes 15 to 20 minutes, making it difficult to treat more than 3 or 4 tumors.[14] Cryosurgery has the advantage of being able to treat the tumor and a portion of the surrounding liver tissue. The disadvantage is that the patient is subjected to general anesthesia and a laparotomy.[35, 65]

Percutaneous ethanol injection (PEI) involves the direct injection of 95% ethanol into a tumor using ultrasound guidance.[9, 15] It has been used for patients with two to three lesions less than 4 cm each and for patients with cirrhosis who are ineligible for resection. The treatments are repeated once or twice a week for a total of six to eight treatments.[14] It is unclear whether this treatment has any effect on overall survival, but it does provide good palliation.[9, 31, 50, 51]

Chemotherapy

No systemically administered single chemotherapeutic agent or combination of agents has shown high activity against HCC.[9, 11, 14] Doxorubicin has been the most active, but the true response rate is substantially less than 20%. A number of combinations of agents have been studied, but none has been recognized as a standard therapy and none has demonstrated a survival advantage over any other.[9, 11, 72]

Because a large number of HCC patients have significant unresectable liver tumors without extrahepatic spread, regional chemotherapy has been investigated. *Regional chemotherapy* involves infusion of agents that are highly metabolized by the liver via the hepatic artery. Tumor cells derive more than 80% of their blood supply from the hepatic artery. However, normal hepatocytes derive their supply from the portal circulation. Thus, administering chemotherapy through the hepatic artery greatly increases the dose of drug delivered to the tumor but minimizes the effect on the hepatocytes and systemic toxicity.[14, 31, 41, 70, 72] *Intra-arterial chemotherapy* can be administered through temporary catheters placed into the axillary or femoral arteries. This method requires that the patient remain in bed for the duration of the infusion, which may be up to 5 days. Complications of this method include thrombosis of the hepatic and other intra-abdominal arteries, catheter displacement, sepsis, and hemorrhage. Drugs may also be administered via an *implantable pump,* which offers the advantages of allowing the patient to remain ambulatory and reducing catheter-related complications. The most common problems associated with the implantable pump have been gastroduodenal ulceration and inflammation.[25] The agents used most frequently for intra-arterial chemotherapy are floxuridine (FUDR) and 5-FU. Other drugs used in combination with FUDR and 5-FU include cisplatin, doxorubicin, mitomycin C, leucovorin, vinblastine, vincristine, and interleukin 2.[4, 14, 17]

Embolization and Chemoembolization

Embolization is the selective occlusion of hepatic vessels by injecting nondegradable particles, typically Gelfoam and Ivalon. Embolizations usually need to be repeated because of the formation of collateral circulation. *Chemoembolization* involves occlusion by particles into which chemotherapeutic agents have been adsorbed. Drugs used in this application include FUDR, doxorubicin, cisplatin, and mitomycin C, in different combinations.[5, 14, 35]

Radiation Therapy

Even though HCC is considered a radiosensitive tumor, the use of radiation therapy is restricted by the relative intolerance of the normal liver parenchyma. The whole liver will tolerate 30 Gy. Higher doses of radiation hepatitis increase the incidence of radiation hepatitis.[41, 56, 63] A cure or long-term remission of HCC requires significantly higher doses. To improve results, radiolabeled antibodies have been used with some success. The high concentration of ferritin in HCC has led to the use of antiferritin antibodies labeled with iodine-131; this technique allows tolerance of high doses. The dose-limiting toxicity is thrombocytopenia, because the bone marrow has a significant uptake of the antiferritin antibodies.[61] The Complications box summarizes typical treatment-related complications.

PROGNOSIS

With the increased knowledge regarding risk factors, diagnosis, and treatment of HCC, the overall prognosis remains grim. Early diagnosis in the United States is

---

✦ COMPLICATIONS
Hepatocellular Carcinoma (HCC)

Surgery Related[15]

Hemorrhage	Ascites
Coagulopathy	Infection/sepsis
Liver insufficiency/	Portal vein thrombosis
failure	Adult acute respiratory
Renal insufficiency/failure	distress syndrome
Pneumonia	Pleural effusion

Hepatic Artery Infusion Related[25]

Catheter occlusion, migration
Arterial thrombosis/aneurysm
Pump pocket hematoma/seroma
Drug toxicities: gastritis, nausea/vomiting/ulcer/diarrhea/sclerosing cholangitis
Chemical hepatitis
Localized infection
Pump malfunction
Biliary sclerosis

Hepatic Artery or Chemoembolization Related (1–3 days)[11]

Fever
Abdominal pain
Anorexia
Ascites
Cholecystitis

Radiation Therapy Related[11]

Nausea
Anorexia
Occasional vomiting
Fatigue

---

uncommon, and patients present with advanced disease. Patients who present with stage III or stage IV disease have a median survival of 4 months or less. Patients with regional lymph node involvement have a median survival of 7 months.[72]

Cancer of the Gallbladder

Gallbladder cancer is an uncommon malignancy, representing less than 2% of all cancers.[48] It is the fifth most common GI malignancy.[16] The overall 5-year survival rate for gallbladder cancer is less than 15%. In the early stages patients are usually asymptomatic. Once symptoms are present the disease is advanced.[9] The most common signs and symptoms are nonspecific and include right upper quadrant abdominal pain (75–97%), nausea and vomiting (40–64%), weight loss (37–77%), and jaundice (45%).[16] It is more common in women than men with a ratio of 3:1. It is more common in Hispanics, Southwestern Native Americans, Mexicans, and Alaskans. The median age of patients is 73 years. There is a correlation between gallbladder cancer and cholelithiasis or calcified gallbladders and typhoid carriers.[9]

The most common tumor type is *adenocarcinoma,* accounting for 85% of cases, and the remaining 15% are squamous cell or mixed tumors. The treatment of choice is *surgical resection.* However, only 80% of the patients are found to have resectable disease at the time of surgery.[16] A small number of patients are diagnosed during a cholecystectomy for chronic cholecystitis, when surgery alone is usually adequate. Patients with more extensive disease require more radical procedures.

The role of *radiation therapy* is controversial. Local recurrence is a common cause of death in patients who relapse after cholecystectomy. Thus adjuvant radiation therapy is often used.[16] Intraoperative radiation therapy also has been used to prevent local recurrence. The median survival for patients treated with intraoperative radiation therapy is less than 12 months.[16] Because there is little evidence that radiation therapy improves survival, this modality is more for palliation of biliary tract obstruction.

The role of *chemotherapy* has not been well defined, but it is offered to patients with metastatic or unresectable disease. The most common protocol used includes a combination of 5-FU, doxorubicin, and mitomycin (FAM).[9] Although patients who receive chemotherapy have slightly improved survival rates, more than 90% of patients with unresectable disease die within 1 year.[48] Due to the significant toxicity and limited benefit of combination therapy, it is recommended that patients be offered either clinical trials or 5-FU with or without leucovorin.[9]

Cancer of the Pancreas

Pancreatic cancer is the second most common GI cancer and the fifth leading cause of cancer death in the United States.[27, 64] Cancers of the pancreas fall into three different categories: those in the exocrine pancreas, those around the ampulla of Vater, and those in the islets of Langerhans. The pathologic and etiologic characteristics of the three types differ. The term *pancreatic cancer* usually refers to cancer of the exocrine pancreas.

EPIDEMIOLOGY

The estimated number of new cases of cancer of the pancreas reported in 2000 was 28,300, which resulted in 28,200 deaths. This represents 2% of the cancers diagnosed and 5% of the cancer deaths in the United States.[27] Over the past 10 years the incidence of cancer of the pancreas has been slowly but steadily increasing. The median age of patients with pancreatic cancer is about 70, with about two thirds of the new cases being persons over 65 years of age. The incidence is about 30% to 40% higher in the black population than in the white population; the black man is the person at highest risk worldwide.[9]

ETIOLOGY AND RISK FACTORS

Cigarette smoke is the most clearly identified carcinogen in pancreatic cancer. Cigarette smoke contains carcinogens, including nitrosamines, that have induced pancreatic cancer in laboratory animals.[9, 21, 64] Approximately 30% of pancreatic cancers are due to smoking.[21] Several dietary carcinogens have been implicated, generally a diet high in fats and cholesterol increase the risk.[21] There is conflicting information regarding caffeine and alcohol consumption.[9, 21] A history of chronic pancreatitis and diabetes mellitus may also be etiologic factors, but are also complications of the cancer.[64] The possibility of an autosomal dominant heredity pattern is being explored. As many as 3% to 5% of all pancreatic cancer may have an hereditary origin.[9, 21] The role of oncogenes is also being studied. Abnormalities in the expression of p53 tumor suppressor gene and K-*ras* oncogene have been found in over 50% of pancreatic cancer cases.[9]

PREVENTION, SCREENING, AND DETECTION

Because no specific risk factors have been conclusively identified for pancreatic cancer, it is impossible to determine how to prevent the disease. Avoiding cigarette smoke and eating a healthy balanced diet would probably reduce risk. Diets rich in vegetables, citrus fruits, fiber, and vitamin C have been associated with decreased rate for pancreatic cancer.[20, 21] No cost-effective test has been found that could be used to screen the asymptomatic population and identify patients for more invasive procedures. CA19-9, a serologic tumor marker for pancreatic cancer, may be useful for screening high-risk patients. Recent studies indicate that detection of K-*ras* in bile or pancreatic ductal secretions may be helpful in identifying early cancer of the pancreas.[20, 21] The most recently discovered tumor suppressor gene is DPC4 (deleted in pancreatic cancer). It may also be helpful in screening. However, these are still investigational.[20, 21]

CLASSIFICATION

Ninety-five percent of cancers involving the pancreas arise from the exocrine gland ductal system.[9] *Ductal*

Nursing Management

Patients who have had surgical intervention for pancreatic cancer have complex and challenging nursing needs. Preoperative assessment includes both psychological and physical parameters, including nutritional history, elimination problems, pain, jaundice, pruritus, fatigue or weakness, depression, or anxiety; laboratory values must be monitored for anemia and coagulation abnormalities. Postoperatively, nurses should be aware of the extent of the surgical resection and the reconstruction the patient has undergone to anticipate potential problems and plan for the care of the patient.

Nursing Diagnosis

- *Fluid volume deficit related to extensive abdominal surgery*

Outcome Goals

Patient will be able to:

- State rationale for potential and actual fluid loss.
- Demonstrate measures to correct or maintain adequate fluid volume.
- Maintain fluid volume evidenced by normal laboratory parameters.

Interventions: *Potential Fluid Loss*

- Check assessment parameters:
  Monitor fluid intake and output, and note fluid preferences.
  Examine mucous membranes for moistness and integrity.
  Monitor weight and vital signs.
  Monitor laboratory values: blood urea nitrogen (BUN), creatinine, electrolytes, serum osmolality, and hematocrit.
- Provide patient instructions:
  List signs and symptoms to report to health care team: thirst, dry skin and mucous membranes, fatigue, constipation, nausea/vomiting, diarrhea, or fever.
  Monitor appropriate fluid intake per day, as well as type and timing of fluid intake, to avoid possible problems such as dumping syndrome.
  Administer medications to minimize fluid loss.

Interventions: *Actual Fluid Loss*

- In addition to above assessment parameters, monitor type and amount of output (diarrhea, wound drainage, emesis), and weigh patient daily.
- Administer intravenous fluids per physician's orders.
- Offer small amount of fluids by mouth as appropriate.
- Administer replacement electrolytes per physician's orders.
- If tube feedings or TPN is ordered, administer and provide instructions to patient/caregiver as appropriate.
- When oral feedings are resumed, administer pancreatic enzymes per physician's orders, and provide instructions on same to the patient.

Nursing Diagnosis

- *Risk for injury related to unstable blood glucose levels*

Outcome Goals

Patient will be able to:

- State rationale for potential changes in blood sugar.
- Demonstrate self blood glucose monitoring, urine testing, and insulin injection.
- Identify signs and symptoms of hypoglycemia and hyperglycemia and measures to prevent/treat.

Interventions

- Assess patient for signs and symptoms of hypoglycemia and hyperglycemia; report to physician if occurs.
- Test urine for acetone every 4 to 6 hours or as ordered by physician.
- Monitor blood glucose levels every 6 hours, and administer sliding-scale insulin per physician's order.
- If patient is not receiving TPN, blood glucose may be monitored before each meal and bedtime with a dose of neutral protamine Hagedorn (NPH) insulin in the morning and/or evening and sliding-scale regular insulin before meals.
- Provide patient with written and verbal instructions regarding diabetic management.
- Evaluate for the need for home health referral.

adenocarcinoma accounts for 85% of all pancreatic cancers.[23] Other less common types include pancreatic acinar carcinoma and cystadenocarcinomas.[9] Two thirds of the carcinomas occur in the head, the rest in the body and tail of the pancreas.

CLINICAL FEATURES

The early signs and symptoms of pancreatic cancer are vague and nonspecific leading to a delay in diagnosis in most patients.[9, 21] The most common presenting symptoms of pancreatic cancer are pain, weight loss, and jaundice.[63, 64] The *pain* is generally described as dull, constant pain radiating to the middle or upper back. Severe pain is usually indicative of invasion of the celiac and mesenteric plexus and is a sign of locally advanced cancer.[21]

Anorexia and weight loss are also common. A typical patient has lost more than 10% of his body weight at diagnosis. The exact cause of the weight loss is unknown, but it may be related to malabsorption and decreased intake.[63, 64] *Jaundice,* occurring in 50% of patients, is due to extrahepatic bile obstruction. It is usually associated with less advanced disease than the other signs and symptoms.[21] Table 9–5 summarizes signs and symptoms of cancer of the head of the pancreas.[63–65]

DIAGNOSIS AND STAGING

Staging is critical to identify those 10% to 15% of patients who have potentially resectable disease at diagnosis.[48] If the tumor cannot be totally resected, surgery does not offer any survival advantage. Dynamic contrast-enhanced CT is the basis for determining treatment plans for patients with pancreatic cancer. The accuracy

of identifying lesions as small as 1 to 2 cm is approximately 95%.[9] If a mass is not seen on contrast-enhanced CT, patients undergo EUS and endoscopic retrograde cholangiopancreatography (ERCP).[21] If a mass is located, EUS is used to guide a fine-needle aspiration. The overall accuracy of EUS-guided fine-needle aspiration is 94%. Angiography and MRI have been surpassed by the accuracy of contrast-enhanced CT.[47]

There is no standardized clinical and pathologic staging system of pancreatic cancer existing in the United States. The AJCC has accepted a staging system for pancreatic cancer based on local, regional nodal, and distant metastatic involvement using the TNM system. Unfortunately, this system lends itself more to pathologic evaluation of resected specimens.[21, 47] Patients without surgery must rely on clinical staging from radiographic studies. Treatment and prognosis are based on whether the tumor is resectable, locally advanced, or metastatic, and the current TNM system does not correlate with this terminology. The advent of contrast-enhanced CT enables the clinician to accurately assess the tumor and its relationship to the celiac plexus and blood vessels. This knowledge makes it possible to make realistic treatment plans and avoid unnecessary surgical procedures. Table 9–6 depicts the current TNM classification system. Table 9–7 is a system for clinical staging that is proposed.[21]

METASTASIS

Of all cancers, pancreatic cancer is the tumor most likely to have metastasized by the time of diagnosis.[47] Metastasis occurs through the regional lymph nodes, to the liver, and to the peritoneum. Distant sites of metastasis include lung, adrenal glands, and ovary.[12]

TREATMENT MODALITIES

Even with the advances in treatment in recent years, pancreatic cancer continues to be the most difficult to treat of all GI cancers. Surgery, as a part of a multimodality approach, is only potentially curative. Unfortunately, early symptoms are vague and nonspecific and do not become severe until the cancer invades adjacent organs or metastasizes. Only 15% of patients meet the criteria for curative surgery.[12] Radiation therapy is used either preoperatively, to make locally advanced tumors resectable, or postoperatively, to eliminate residual disease in the tumor bed or lymphatics. Pancreatic cancer is very chemoresistant; however, new approaches are being investigated.[9]

Surgery

The majority of pancreatic cancers occur in the head of the pancreas. Patients who are amenable to curative

TABLE 9–5

Presenting Signs and Symptoms of Patients with Carcinoma of the Head of the Pancreas

Sign or Symptom	Percentage of Patients
Weight loss	90
Pain	75
Malnutrition	75
Jaundice	70
Anorexia	60
Pruritis	40
Courvoisier's sign	33
Diabetes mellitus	15
Ascites	5
Gastric outlet obstruction	5

From Spitz FR, Bouvet M, Fuhrman GM, Berger DH: Pancreatic adenocarcinoma. In Feig BW, Berger DH, Fuhrman GM, editors: The M. D. Anderson surgical oncology handbook, ed 2, Philadelphia, Lippincott Williams & Wilkins, 1999.

TABLE 9-6

TNM Clinical Classification System for Staging Pancreatic Cancer

PRIMARY TUMOR (T)

TX	Primary tumor cannot be assessed
T0	No evidence of primary tumor
T1	Tumor limited to the pancreas
	T1a Tumor ≤2 cm in greatest dimension
	T1b Tumor >2 cm in greatest dimension
T2	Tumor extends directly to duodenum, bile duct, or peripancreatic tissues
T3	Tumor extends directly to stomach, spleen, colon, or adjacent large blood vessels.

REGIONAL LYMPH NODES (N)

NX	Regional lymph nodes cannot be assessed
N0	No regional lymph node metastasis
N1	Regional lymph node metastasis
	pN1a Metastasis in a single regional lymph node
	pN1b Metastastis in multiple regional lymph nodes

DISTANT METASTASIS (M)

MX	Presence of distant metastasis cannot be assessed
M0	No distant metastasis
M1	Distant metastasis: hepatic metastasis, peritoneal seeding

STAGE GROUPINGS

Stage I	T1	N0	M0
	T2	N0	M0
Stage II	T3	N0	M0
Stage III	Any T	N1	M0
Stage IVA	T4	Any N	M0
Stage IVB	Any T	Any N	M1

From Meyers M: Overview: carcinoma of the pancreas: imaging, staging, and management. In Meyers M, editor: Neoplasms of the digestive tract: imaging, staging, and management, Philadelphia, Lippincott-Raven, 1998.

resection will undergo either a pancreaticoduodenectomy (Whipple procedure) or a total pancreatectomy. The pancreaticoduodenectomy involves the removal of the distal stomach, the gallbladder, the common bile duct, the head of the pancreas, the duodenum, and the upper jejunum.[12] Figure 9–5 illustrates reconstruction after the pancreaticoduodenectomy, which involves four steps. First, a pancreaticojejunostomy attaches the remaining pancreas to the small bowel. Second, as a part of the choledochojejunostomy, the jejunum is anastomosed to the common hepatic duct. Third, a standard gastrojejunostomy is then performed. This is followed by insertion of gastrostomy and feeding jejunostomy and closed-suction drains.[21, 63, 64] Routine placement of feeding tube allows nutritional support without the expense of intravenous hyperalimentation, and the patient can be discharged from the hospital on enteral feedings and instructions to advance diet as tolerated.

A *pylorus-preserving pancreaticoduodenectomy* is used for some benign diseases and for small periampullary lesions. By preserving the antral pyloric pump mechanism, the patient has improved long-term GI function and nutritional sequelae. The procedure decreases intestinal transit time, lessens diarrhea, normalizes glucose metabolism, and improves postoperative weight gain. The major disadvantage of the pylorus-preservation procedure is that it may compromise the tumor-free margin of tissue and prevent adequate removal of involved lymphatics.[54]

A *total pancreatectomy* is an extension of the pancreaticoduodenectomy and in addition involves removal of the body and tail of the pancreas and the spleen and a more extensive regional lymphadenectomy. Controversy continues over the advantages and disadvantages of the pancreaticoduodenectomy versus the total pancreatectomy. Some cite the multicentric nature of pancreatic cancer, the confidence of a total lymphadenectomy, and the avoidance of a pancreatic anastomosis as a rationale for routine total pancreatectomy. However, the documentation of multicentricity is less than 10%, which many believe does not justify the increased operative morbidity and life-long dependence on insulin. Also the incidence of anastomic leak is rare in centers that are experienced in the Whipple procedure.[9, 63, 64]

Palliation for cancer of the head of the pancreas is the objective of treatment more often than is cure. For most patients with unresectable disease, laparotomy for palliation is unnecessary. Advances in endoscopic, per-

TABLE 9–7

Clinical (Radiographic) Staging of Pancreatic Cancer

Stage	Clinical/Radiologic Criteria
I	Resectable (T1–3, selected T4*, NX, M0)
	No evidence of tumor extension to the celiac axis or SMA
	Patent SMPV confluence
	No extrapancreatic disease
II	Locally advanced (T4, NX–1, M0)
	Arterial encasement (celiac axis or SMA) or venous occlusion (SMPV)
	No extrapancreatic disease
III	Metastatic (T1–4, NX–1, M1)
	Metastatic disease (typically to liver, and peritoneum and occasionally to lung)

SMA, superior mesenteric artery, SMPV, superior mesentertic–portal vein.
* Resectable T4 tumors include those with isolated involvement of the superior mesenteric vein, portal vein, or hepatic artery without tumor extension to the celiac axis or SMA.
From Evans DE, Wolff RA, Abbruzzese JL: Cancer of the pancreas. In Pollock R, editor: Manual of clinical oncology, ed 7, New York, Wiley, 1999. Reprinted by permission of Wiley-Liss, Inc., a subsidiary of John Wiley & Sons, Inc.

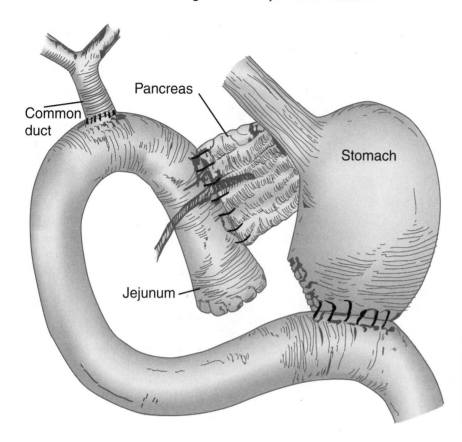

FIGURE 9–5 Reconstruction following conventional pancreaticoduodenectomy. (From Castillo CF, Warshaw AL: Cancer of the pancreas. In Rustgi AK, editor: *Gastrointestinal cancers: biology, diagnosis, and therapy*, p. 342. Philadelphia, Lippincott-Raven, 1995.)

cutaneous, and laparoscopic techniques allow stent placements, bypass procedures, and pain control.[20] Jaundice, gastric outlet obstruction, and pain are the problems most often relieved.[9] For the patient undergoing a surgical procedure that is found not to be a curative resection, palliative surgery is warranted to relieve symptoms and improve quality of life. A choledochojejunostomy or cholecystojejunostomy is used to bypass distal biliary obstruction. This is to relieve jaundice and pruritus and prevent ascending cholangitis. Duodenal obstruction is a late symptom of pancreatic cancer, but occurs in approximately 25% of patients. A gastrojejunostomy may be performed to prevent future bowel obstructions, and many believe this should be performed in all patients. Severe back pain experienced by many patients may be relieved with a chemoablation of the celiac plexus or by alcohol injection. Either may be performed intraoperatively or percutaneously.[9]

When surgery is not an option for the patient, obstructive jaundice may be relieved by either the endoscopic placement of a stent, which will provide internal drainage of bile, or the placement of percutaneous transhepatic catheter, which will provide either external or internal-external drainage. The percutaneous transhepatic catheter may be used to internalize the drainage via a stent. Complications of these procedures include cholangitis, hemorrhage, bile leak, and catheter obstruc-

tion. Laparoscopic cholecystojejunostomy is another alternative for biliary obstruction. It is usually used in patients with locally advanced nonmetastatic disease in whom endoscopic stenting has been unsuccessful.[21]

Chemotherapy

For unknown reasons, pancreatic cancer cells are relatively chemoresistant.[9, 64, 65] Both single and multiple chemotherapeutic agents have demonstrated less than 10% activity. Because patients with metastatic pancreatic cancer cannot be cured, the risks of chemotherapy must be carefully considered. Patients who are debilitated due to their disease should not be offered chemotherapy because it is unlikely to be of any benefit. Persons who strongly desire treatment who have good performance status may be offered clinical trials or standard chemotherapy.[9, 64, 65] Historically 5-FU has been the drug of choice for pancreatic cancer. In 1996, gemcitabine was approved by the Food and Drug Administration as first-line therapy for patients with locally advanced or metastatic disease and second-line therapy for patients previously treated with 5-FU.[3, 64] Gemcitabine has been shown to have a small but significant improvement in survival compared to 5-FU, but more importantly it has shown a greater clinical benefit by improvement in symptoms.[64, 65] Other combinations

---

COMPLICATIONS

Pancreatic Cancer Treatment

Hemorrhage
Fistula (intestinal, pancreatic, or biliary)
Cardiopulmonary problems
Gastric retention
Intra-abdominal sepsis
Late complications (jaundice, gastrointestinal ulcer-
ation, diabetes mellitus, dumping syndrome)

Data from reference 12.

---

now in use that show improved responses include strep-tozotocin, mitomycin C, and 5-FU (SMF); 5-FU, doxo-rubicin (Adriamycin), and mitomycin C (FAM); and FAM with the addition of streptozotocin.[64, 65] Studies are also in progress investigating the usefulness of monoclonal antibodies and hormonal therapies in treating pancreatic cancer; however, these show little improvement in response rates. Gene therapy is also being researched. The approaches being used include replacement of tumor suppressor genes and to inhibit the ras protein function.[9]

Radiation Therapy

The use of radiation therapy in treating cancer of the pancreas has been limited by the proximity of the pancreas to dose-limiting structures such as the kidneys, bowel, liver, and spinal cord. However, with the development of new scanning techniques and modern treatment planning software, external beam radiation therapy (EBRT) is now being used to improve local disease control and long-term survival.[57]

Radiation therapy with concomitant chemotherapy (5-FU) has shown survival benefit in patients with locally advanced pancreatic cancer.[21] Currently chemoradiation is used preoperatively (neoadjuvant) or postoperatively (adjuvant), and for palliation. Electron beam intraoperative radiation therapy combined with EBRT shows improved survival. Intraoperative radiation therapy has the advantage of being able to deliver tumor-specific high-dose radiation therapy while avoiding adjacent normal tissue.[57] Another promising study is the use of paclitaxel or gemcitabine weekly during 2 weeks of neoadjuvant radiation therapy, followed by surgery with intraoperative radiation therapy, then more systemic therapy.[21] The Complications box summarizes treatment-related complications.

PROGNOSIS

The prognosis for persons with cancer of the pancreas is relatively poor. The reported 5-year survival rate for pancreatic cancer is 1% to 4%.[20, 64] This figure has increased only slightly from that reported in the early 1960s. Improved surgical techniques and supportive care have not led to improved survival. The 5-year survival rate in patients who have had a pancreatoduodenectomy is 15% to 20%, with a median survival of 15 to 24 months.[20] Patients with locally advanced nonmetastatic disease have a median survival of 6 to 10 months. Those with metastatic disease survive only 3 to 6 months.[20]

Cancer of the Small Intestines

Neoplasms of the small intestines are rare. They comprise only 1% of GI malignancies.[6] The estimated number of new cases for 2000 was 4700, which resulted in 1200 deaths.[27] The four primary types of neoplasms found in the small intestines include adenocarcinoma (42%), carcinoid (29%), lymphoma (18%), and leiomyosarcoma (11%).[6, 49] Risk factors that have been associated with small-bowel cancers include familial adenomatous polyposis, Crohn's disease, celiac disease, urinary-ileo anatomosis, ileostomy, nodular lymphoid hyperplasia, and immunodeficiency diseases.[6] Symptoms of cancer of the small intestine are vague and not localizing, occurring late in the disease course.[36] Due to the vague symptoms and the rarity of this malignancy, there is usually a delay of months before a diagnosis is made. By the time the patient presents, symptoms are those of advanced disease and include pain (32–86%), perforation (10%), bleeding (20–53%), and weight loss (32–67%).[13, 36] Treatment depends on the histologic type of tumor and location.[13] Most commonly the approach to curative treatment is surgery. Adenocarcinoma of the duodenum is approached with a pancreaticoduodenctomy. Tumors in the lower portion require a segmental duodenectomy and primary anastomosis. Five-year survival varies widely from 0% to 60%, because lymph node metastases are frequent.[14] Early carcinoid tumors are managed with wide resection because they are usually multiple and found throughout the bowel. Carcinoid often spreads to the liver before diagnosis and the patient presents with symptoms of carcinoid syndrome, flushing of head and neck, and watery secretory diarrhea.[13, 48] Treatment includes resection of liver metastasis, medical management with octreotide, and sometimes hepatic arterial embolization.[48] Lymphomas and sarcomas are treated with surgical resection and adjuvant chemotherapy. Radiation therapy has been used as adjuvant therapy; however, it is considered to be high risk with long-term side effects and is not often used.[13]

GERIATRIC CONSIDERATIONS
Gastrointestinal Cancers

Factors Related to Cancer Prevention and Early Detection

Encourage low-fat, high-fiber diet within ethnic, social, and economic limitations.

Encourage smoking cessation and avoidance of exposure to other health hazards (e.g., sun, chemicals, petroleum products).

Be suspicious of symptoms such as malaise, fatigue, anorexia, weight loss, and altered bowel habits as possible indicators of cancer and not automatically attributed to nonmalignant illnesses associated with aging.

Factors Related to Modalities of Therapy

Alterations in hepatic and renal function may necessitate adjustment of dosage and schedule of chemotherapy protocols.

Decreased bone marrow cellularity may place patient at risk for prolonged myelosuppression chemotherapy with toxic effects on bone marrow.

Decreased nutritional intake may be exacerbated because of nausea and taste changes associated with many chemotherapeutic agents typically used for GI malignancies.

Fatigue may be increasing problem after courses of therapy, requiring additional assistance with activities of daily living.

Comorbid disease (e.g., obesity, poor nutritional status, lung and cardiovascular disease, altered immune function) places the older adult at greater risk for surgical morbidity and mortality.

Teaching should be tailored to take into account older adult's life experiences and cognitive and physical impairments (e.g., reading comprehension, decreased vision and hearing, altered tactile sense, misconceptions regarding cancer and cancer treatment, past experience with cancer and family members).

Modified from Boyle DM and others: Oncology nursing society position paper on cancer and aging: the mandate for oncology nursing. *Oncol Nurs Forum* 19:913, 1992.

PATIENT TEACHING PRIORITIES
Gastrointestinal Cancers

Prevention and Early Detection

Risk factors
Dietary habits
Avoidance of cigarette smoking
Moderate or no alcohol consumption
Signs and symptoms to report to health care professional (e.g., dysphagia, odynophagia, chronic indigestion, jaundice, weight loss not associated with dieting, change in bowel habits)
Annual physical examination and cancer checkup

Diagnostic Procedures

Purpose of procedure
Preparation needed by patient
Procedure description
Postprocedural care by patient

Treatment Modalities

Surgery—preoperative instructions include operative experience and immediate postoperative period; discharge instructions include self-care needs and any further treatment plans
Chemotherapy—name of agent, possible side effects and measures to control, route of administration, dose, schedule, and any directions needed for self-administration
Radiation therapy—description of procedure and schedule and duration of treatment, skin care measures, and management of any side effects

Supportive Care

Community resources (e.g., home health care agencies, inpatient and outpatient hospice care)
Use of any medical equipment in the home
Referrals necessary for psychosocial support for patient and caregiver
Referrals for financial assistance if needed

Nursing care guidelines for patients with GI cancer follow the practices recommended for the patient's particular therapy. Refer to Chapter 32 for interventions related to death and dying.

CONCLUSION

Gastrointestinal cancers remain a nursing practice challenge. The overall prognosis ranges from 5% to 15%. Progress has been made in treatment modalities. However, prevention, early detection, and the seeking of health care early when initial symptoms occur can reduce the impact and prolong patient survival.

Chapter Questions

1. You are providing teaching for an esophageal cancer patient who will be receiving radiation therapy. What is one of the complications you will want to include?
   a. Right upper quadrant abdominal pain
   b. Chills and sweating

c. Mouth pain

d. Esophageal stricture

2. In interviewing a patient, the nurse learns that the patient is a chronic user of antacids for indigestion and epigastric pain. He is 62 years old and has come to the clinic because his wife is concerned that the symptoms are not relieved by the antacids as well as they had been. What advice should the nurse give them?

a. Referral to a gastroenterologist for further work-up of symptoms

b. Change to a bland diet

c. Change to a different antacid

d. Eating six to eight small meals a day

3. A close association exists between which of these risk factors and gastric cancer?

a. Epstein-Barr virus

b. *Helicobacter pylori* infection

c. Hepatitis B infection

d. Human immunodeficiency virus

4. The treatment of choice for cancer of the pancreas is:

a. Autologous stem cell transfusion

b. External beam radiation therapy

c. Intra-arterial chemotherapy

d. Multimodality therapy including surgery, chemotherapy, and radiation therapy

5. Which of the following statements is *true?*

a. In the United States, more than 90% of all primary liver cancers are hepatocellular carcinomas.

b. The most common type of esophageal cancer is squamous cell carcinoma.

c. Leiomyosarcomas account for up to 50% of the gastric malignancies.

d. The most common cancers in the pancreas are endocrine in origin.

6. Which of the following is the second most common GI malignancy in the United States?

a. Esophageal

b. Gastric

c. Liver

d. Pancreatic

7. If you were counseling a client regarding risk factors for gastric cancer, which of the following would you include?

a. Avoid use of tobacco and alcohol.

b. Avoid diets high smoked, salted, and pickled foods.

c. Avoid exposure to pesticides and herbicides.

d. Avoid tobacco, and drink alcohol and coffee in moderation only.

8. Your patient has been recently diagnosed with hepatocellular carcinoma and is a good candidate for liver resection. He tells you he read about a person who had a liver transplant, and he wonders if he might be able to have one. How would you respond?

a. Liver transplants are not an option for persons with cancer.

b. Liver transplants are an option for select patients with cancer, but because of high recurrence rates and because donors are scarce they are still controversial.

c. Liver transplants are standard treatment for primary liver cancer.

d. The use of liver transplants is indicated only for patients who have poor hepatic functional reserve.

9. The occurrence of cancer of the small intestines is associated with:

a. Crohn's disease

b. Hepatitis C

c. Pernicious anemia

d. Tylosis palmera

10. How would you describe cancer of the gallbladder?

a. Rare form of GI malignancy with a poor prognosis

b. Uncommon cancer that has one of the better prognoses in relation to other GI cancers

c. Slow-growing cancer that affects middle-aged adults

d. Form of cancer that does not require any treatment until it becomes symptomatic

BIBLIOGRAPHY

1. Albert C: Clinical aspects of gastric cancer. In Rustgi KA, editor: *Gastrointestinal cancers: biology, diagnosis, and therapy,* Philadelphia, Lippincott-Raven, 1995.

2. Alexander HR, Kelsen DG, Tepper JC: Cancer of the stomach. In DeVita VT Jr, Hellman S, Rosenberg SA, editors: *Cancer: principles and practice of oncology,* ed 5, Philadelphia, Lippincott-Raven, 1997.

3. Barton-Burke M: Gemcitabine: a pharmacologic and clinical overview, *Cancer Nurs* 22:176, 1999.

4. Bergsland EK, Warren RS: Antiangiogenic agents in the treatment of liver tumors. In Clavien P-A, editor: *Malignant liver tumors: current and emerging therapies,* Malden, MA, Blackwell Science, 1999.

5. Bleiberg H, Gerard B: Current and new systemic treatment of hepatobiliary tumors. In Clavien P-A, editor: *Malignant liver tumors: current and emerging therapies,* Malden, MA, Blackwell Science, 1999.

6. Bond JH: Screening, detection, and early diagnosis of gastrointestinal cancer. In Wanebo HJ, editor: *Surgery for gastrointestinal cancer: a multidisciplinary approach,* Philadelphia, Lippincott-Raven, 1997.

7. Bonin SR and others: Esophageal cancer. In Pazdur R, Coia R, Hoskins WJ, Wagman LD, editors: *Cancer management: a multidisciplinary approach,* ed 3, Melville, NY, PRR, 1999.

8. Bonin SR and others: Gastric cancer. In Pazdur R, Coia R, Hoskins WJ, Wagman LD, editors: *Cancer management: a multidisciplinary approach* ed 3, Melville, NY, PRR, 1999.

9. Brower ST and others: Pancreatic cancer, hepatobiliary cancer, and neuroendocrine cancers of the GI tract. In Pazdur R, Coia R, Hoskins WJ, Wagman LD, editors: *Cancer management: a multidisciplinary approach* ed 3, Melville, NY, PRR, 1999.

10. Brown RS, Scharschmidt BF: Liver cancer. In Kramer BS, Gohagen JK, Prorok PC, editors: *Cancer screening: theory and practice,* New York, Marcel Dekker, 1999.

11. Carr BI, Flickinger JC, Lotze MT: Hepatobiliary cancer. In DeVita VT Jr, Hellman S, Rosenberg SA, editors: *Cancer: principles and practice of oncology,* ed 5, Philadelphia, Lippincott-Raven, 1997.

12. Castillo CF, Warshaw AL: Laparoscopic staging with selected resection in pancreatic cancer. In Wanebo JH, editor: *Surgery for gastrointestinal cancer: a multidisciplinary approach,* Philadelphia, Lippincott-Raven, 1997.

13. Coit DG: Cancer of the small intestine. In DeVita VT Jr, Hellman S, Rosenberg SA, editors: *Cancer: principles and practice of oncology,* ed 5, Philadelphia, Lippincott-Raven, 1997.

14. Curley SA, Jones DV: Management of hepatocellular carcinoma. In Meyers MA, editor: *Neoplasms of the digestive tract: imaging, staging, and management,* Philadelphia, Lippincott-Raven, 1998.

15. Curley SA: Surgical management of hepatocellular carcinoma. In Curley SA, editor: *Liver cancer,* New York, Springer-Verlag, 1998.

16. Curley SA: Diagnosis and treatment of primary gallbladder cancer. In Curley SA, editor: *Liver cancer,* New York, Springer-Verlag, 1998.

17. Cusak JC Jr: Induction of apoptosis in liver tumors. In Clavien P-A, editor: *Malignant liver tumors: current and emerging therapies,* Malden, MA, Blackwell Science, 1999.

18. Dalton RR, Sarr MG, McIlrath DC: Radical subtotal gastrectomy. In Donohue JH, van Heerden JA, Monson JRT, editors: *Atlas of surgical oncology,* Cambridge, MA, Blackwell Science, 1995.

19. Dodd GD III, Halff GAQ, Rhim H: Thermal ablation of liver tumors by radiofrequency, microwave, and laser therapy. In Clavien P-A, editor: *Malignant liver tumors: current and emerging therapies,* Malden, MA, Blackwell Science, 1999.

20. Evans DE, Abbruzzese JL, Rich TA: Cancer of the pancreas. In DeVita VT Jr, Hellman S, Rosenberg SA, editors: *Cancer: principles and practice of oncology,* ed 5, Philadelphia, Lippincott-Raven, 1997.

21. Evans DE, Wolff RA, Abbruzzese JL: Cancer of the pancreas. In Pollock RE, editor: *Manual of clinical oncology,* ed 7, New York, Wiley-Liss, 1999.

22. Falkson G, Falkson CI, Garbers LM: Hepatocellular carcinoma. In Benson AB, editor: *Gastrointestinal oncology,* Boston, Kluwer Academic Publishers, 1998.

23. Farley DR, Sarr MG: Management of the apparent periampullary malignancy: preoperative evaluation and operative treatment. In Wanebo JH, editor: *Surgery for gastrointestinal cancer: a multidisciplinary approach,* Philadelphia, Lippincott-Raven, 1997.

24. Flood WA, Forastiere AA: Esophageal cancer. In Benson AB, editor: *Gastrointestinal oncology,* Boston, Kluwer Academic Publishers, 1998.

25. Gallagher JT, Vauthey J-N: Selective continuous intra-arterial chemotherapy for liver tumors. In Clavien P-A, editor: *Malignant liver tumors: current and emerging therapies,* Malden, MA, Blackwell Science, 1999.

26. Garland CF, Garland, FC, Gorham ED: Etiology, epidemiology, and potential prevention of gastrointestinal cancer. In Wanebo JH. editor: *Surgery for gastrointestinal cancer: a multidisciplinary approach,* Philadelphia, Lippincott-Raven, 1997.

27. Greenlee RT, Murray T, Bolden S, Wingo PA: Cancer statistics, 2000. *CA Cancer J Clin* 50:7, 2000.

28. Helton, WS: Diagnostic and therapeutic approaches to the patient with liver malignancy. In Clavien P-A, editor: *Malignant liver tumors: current and emerging therapies,* Malden, MA, Blackwell Science, 1999.

29. Hennessy TPJ: Combined modality therapy: esophageal adenocarcinoma. In Daly JM, Hennessy TPJ, Reynolds JV, editors: *Management of upper gastrointestinal cancer,* London, Saunders, 1999.

30. Heyneman LE, Nelson RC: Pathology of primary and secondary liver tumors. In Clavien P-A, editor: *Malignant liver tumors: current and emerging therapies,* Malden, MA, Blackwell Science, 1999.

31. Izzo F and others: Alternative treatment approaches to early stage or unresectable hepatocellular carcinoma confined to the liver. In Curley SA, editor: *Liver cancer,* New York, Springer-Verlag, 1998.

32. Jamieson GG, Mathew G: Surgical management of esophageal cancer: the western experience. In Daly JM, Hennessy TPJ, Reynolds JV, editors: *Management of upper gastrointestinal cancer,* London, Saunders, 1999.

33. Jaskiewicz K: Pathology of hepatocellular carcinoma. In Rustgi KA, editor: *Gastrointestinal cancers: biology, diagnosis, and therapy,* Philadelphia, Lippincott-Raven, 1995.

34. Johnson PJ: Presentation and approach to diagnosis. In Leong AS-Y, Liew C-T, Lau JWY, Johnson PJ, editors: *Hepatocellular carcinomas: contemporary diagnosis, investigation and management,* London, Arnold Publishers, 1999.

35. Johnson PJ: Future prospects. In Leong AS-Y, Liew C-T, Lau JWY, Johnson PJ, editors: *Hepatocellular carcinomas: contemporary diagnosis, investigation and management,* London, Arnold Publishers, 1999.

36. Kane RA, Kruskal JB, Eustace S: Imaging strategies for the diagnosis, staging, and follow-up of gastrointestinal malignancies. In Wanebo JH, editor: *Surgery for gastrointestinal cancer: a multidisciplinary approach,* Philadelphia, Lippincott-Raven, 1997.

37. Karpeh MS, Shiu M, Brennan MF: Total gastrectomy. In Donohue JH, van Heerden JA, Monson JRT, editors: *Atlas of surgical oncology,* Cambridge, MA, Blackwell Science, 1995.

38. Kennedy BJ: Gastric cancer staging and natural history. In Wanebo JH, editor: *Surgery for gastrointestinal cancer: a multidisciplinary approach,* Philadelphia, Lippincott-Raven, 1997.

39. Kim J-P: Cancer of the stomach. In Pollock RE, editor: *Manual of clinical oncology,* ed 7, New York, Wiley-Liss, 1999.

40. Leong AS-Y: Epidemiology, risk factors, etiology, premalignant lesions and carcinogenesis. In Leong AS-Y, Liew C-T, Lau JWY, Johnson PJ, editors: *Hepatocellular carcinomas: contemporary diagnosis, investigation and management,* London, Arnold Publishers, 1999.

41. Leung TWT: Non-surgical management. In Leong AS-Y, Liew C-T, Lau JWY, Johnson PJ, editors: *Hepatocellular carcinomas: contemporary diagnosis, investigation and management,* London, Arnold Publishers, 1999.

42. Levine MS: Diagnosis of esophageal carcinoma by barium studies. In Meyers MA, editor: *Neoplasms of the digestive tract: imaging, staging, and management,* Philadelphia, Lippincott-Raven, 1998.

43. Lewandrowski KB, Compton CC: The pathology of gastric cancer and conditions predisposing to gastric cancer. In Rustgi KA, editor: *Gastrointestinal cancers: biology, diagnosis, and therapy,* Philadelphia, Lippincott-Raven, 1995.

44. Mansfield PF: Management of gastric carcinoma. In Meyers MA, editor: *Neoplasms of the digestive tract: imaging, staging, and management,* Philadelphia, Lippincott-Raven, 1998.

45. Meyers MA: Carcinoma of the esophagus: imaging, staging, and management. In Meyers MA, editor: *Neoplasms of the digestive tract: imaging, staging, and management,* Philadelphia, Lippincott-Raven, 1998.

46. Meyers MA: Hepatocellular carcinoma: imaging, staging, and management. In Meyers MA, editor: *Neoplasms of the digestive tract: imaging, staging, and management,* Philadelphia, Lippincott-Raven, 1998.

47. Meyers MA: Carcinoma of the pancreas: imaging, staging, and management. In Meyers MA, editor: *Neoplasms of the digestive tract: imaging, staging, and management,* Philadelphia, Lippincott-Raven, 1998.

48. Meyers MA: Carcinoma of the gallbladder: imaging, staging, and management. In Meyers MA, editor: *Neoplasms of the digestive tract: imaging, staging, and management,* Philadelphia, Lippincott-Raven, 1998.

49. Meyers MA: Small bowel malignancies: imaging, staging, and management. In Meyers MA, editor: *Neoplasms of the digestive tract: imaging, staging, and management,* Philadelphia, Lippincott-Raven, 1998.

50. Morse MA, Clavien P-A, Lyerly HK: Overview: immunologic, genetic, apoptotic, and neovascular therapies for liver tumors. In Clavien P-A, editor: *Malignant liver tumors: current and emerging therapies,* Malden, MA, Blackwell Science, 1999.

51. Morse MA, Clary B: Pro-drug converting gene therapy for liver tumors. In Clavien P-A, editor: *Malignant liver tumors: current and emerging therapies,* Malden, MA, Blackwell Science, 1999.

52. Nordlinger B, Arla E: Hepatocarcinoma: results with resection (western experience). Morse MA, Clavien P-A, Lyerly HK: Overview: immunologic, genetic, apoptotic, and neovascular therapies for liver tumors. In Clavien P-A, editor: *Malignant liver tumors: current and emerging therapies,* Malden, MA, Blackwell Science, 1999.

53. Pearlstone DB, Staley CA: Gastric carcinoma. In Feig BW, Berger DH, Furhman GM, editors: *The M. D. Anderson surgical oncology handbook,* Philadelphia, Lippincott Williams & Wilkins, 1999.

54. Pisters PWT, Lee JE, Evans DE: Standard forms of pancreatic resection. In Reber HA, editor: *Pancreatic cancer: pathogenesis, diagnosis, and treatment,* Totowa, NJ, Humana Press, 1998.

55. Porte RJ, Clavien P-A: Epidemiology and natural history of liver tumors. In Clavien P-A, editor: *Malignant liver tumors: current and emerging therapies,* Malden, MA, Blackwell Science, 1999.

56. Rich TA: Radiation therapy for pancreatic cancer. In Reber HA, editor: *Pancreatic cancer: pathogenesis, diagnosis, and treatment,* Totowa, NJ, Humana Press, 1998.

57. Robertson JM, Lawrence TS: Radiation therapy for liver tumors. In Clavien P-A, editor: *Malignant liver tumors: current and emerging therapies,* Malden, MA, Blackwell Science, 1999.

58. Roth JA and others: Cancer of the esophagus. In DeVita VT Jr, Hellman S, Rosenberg SA, editors: *Cancer: principles and practice of oncology,* ed 5, Philadelphia, Lippincott-Raven, 1997.

59. Schmitt CM, Brazer SR: Clinical aspects of esophageal cancer. In Rustgi KA, editor: *Gastrointestinal cancers: biology, diagnosis, and therapy,* Philadelphia, Lippincott-Raven, 1995.

60. Schwarz RE, Karpeh MS, Brennan MF: Surgical management of gastric cancer: the western experience. In Daly JM, Hennessy TPJ, Reynolds JV, editors: *Management of upper gastrointestinal cancer,* London, Saunders, 1999.

61. Selzner M, Clavien P-A: Resection of liver tumors: special emphasis on neoadjuvant and adjuvant therapy. In Clavien P-A, editor: *Malignant liver tumors: current and emerging therapies,* Malden, MA, Blackwell Science, 1999.

62. Siewert JR, Sendler A, Bottcher K: Early gastric cancer. In Daly JM, Hennessy TPJ, Reynolds JV, editors: *Management of upper gastrointestinal cancer,* London, Saunders, 1999.

63. Spitz FR, Bouvet M, Yahanda AM: Hepatobiliary cancers. In Feig BW, Berger DH, Furhman GM, editors: *The M. D. Anderson surgical oncology handbook,* Philadelphia, Lippincott Williams & Wilkins, 1999.

64. Spitz FR and others: Pancreatic adenocarcinoma. In Feig BW, Berger DH, Furhman GM, editors: *The M. D. Anderson surgical oncology handbook,* Philadelphia, Lippincott Williams & Wilkins, 1999.

65. Strauss RM: Hepatocellular carcinoma: clinical diagnostic and therapeutic aspects. In Rustgi KA, editor: *Gastrointestinal cancers: biology, diagnosis, and therapy,* Philadelphia, Lippincott-Raven, 1995.

66. Stucky-Marshall L: New agents in gastrointestinal malignancies: part 2: gemcitabine in clinical practice, *Cancer Nursing* 22:290.

67. Swisher SG, Mansfield PF: Management of esophageal carcinoma. In Meyers MA, editor: *Neoplasms of the digestive tract: imaging, staging, and management,* Philadelphia, Lippincott-Raven, 1998.

68. Tang Z-Y: Liver cancer. In Pollock RE, editor: *Manual of clinical oncology,* ed 7, New York, Wiley-Liss, 1999.

69. Tempero MA, Vaziri IA, Rasmussen B: Upper gastrointestinal cancer. In Kirkwood JM, Lotze MT, Yasko JM, editors: *Current cancer therapeutics,* ed 3, Philadelphia, Churchill Livingstone, 1998.

70. Tempero M: Chemotherapy for pancreatic cancer. In Reber HA, editor: *Pancreatic cancer: pathogenesis, diagnosis, and treatment,* Totowa, NJ, Humana Press, 1998.

71. Vaporciyan AA, Swisher SG: Esophageal cancer. In Feig BW, Berger DH, Furhman GM, editors: *The M. D. Anderson surgical oncology handbook,* Philadelphia, Lippincott Williams & Wilkins, 1999.

72. Venook AP, Warren RS: Regional chemotherapy for hepatic neoplasms. In Wanebo JH, editor: *Surgery for gastrointestinal cancer: a multidisciplinary approach,* Philadelphia, Lippincott-Raven, 1997.

73. Wanebo JH: Treatment of gallbladder cancer. In Wanebo JH, editor: *Surgery for gastrointestinal cancer: a multidisciplinary approach,* Philadelphia, Lippincott-Raven, 1997.

74. Washington K: Pathology of primary and secondary liver tumors. In Clavien P-A, editor: *Malignant liver tumors: current and emerging therapies,* Malden, MA, Blackwell Science, 1999.

75. Wood DE, Vallieres E, Pellegrini CA: Esophageal cancer. In Pollock RE, editor: *Manual of clinical oncology,* ed 7, New York, Wiley-Liss, 1999.

76. Woodward TA, Levin B: Cancer of the stomach: chemotherapy and radiation therapy. In Rustgi KA, editor: *Gastrointestinal cancers: biology, diagnosis, and therapy,* Philadelphia, Lippincott-Raven, 1995.

Genitourinary Cancers

Maureen E. O'Rourke

Genitourinary (GU) malignancies include cancers of the urinary and genital organs in men and urinary organs in women. Taken as a group, the incidence of GU malignancies in the year 2000 is projected to be 275,100 new cases, and these GU malignancies are expected to account for 57,200 deaths in the United States alone.[56] Refinements and increased sophistication in both diagnostic approaches and treatment modalities continue to result in improved patient outcomes both in terms of increased survival and enhanced quality of life.

This chapter reviews the diagnosis and management of common GU malignancies, including those involving the prostate, testis, bladder, kidney, and penis, with special emphasis on issues related to prevention, detection, current management, and quality of life concerns.

Prostate Cancer

EPIDEMIOLOGY

Prostate cancer is the most frequently diagnosed malignancy and the second leading cause of male cancer death in the United States.[56] The median age at diagnosis is 72 years, with the incidence rate steadily increasing with each decade after age 50. For African American men the incidence rate is approximately 1.5 times that of white men, and the death rate is slightly more than twice as great among African Americans. Hispanic men are affected at about half the rate of African Americans. The global distribution of prostate cancer reveals predominance in the United States and Canada, the British Isles, and among Northern European countries, such as Norway, Sweden, and the Netherlands. Eastern Europe and Asia have the lowest incidence rates.[56] Mortality rates are lowest in the former Soviet Union countries and Japan, and highest in North America, Western Europe, and the British Isles. The highest mortality rates documented over the period of 1994 to1997 were in Trinidad/Tobago (35.5/100,00 men).[56]

ETIOLOGY AND RISK FACTORS

The exact etiology of prostate cancer is unknown, although it appears to result from interplay between endogenous hormones and environmental influences. As in the case of all malignancies, it is postulated that the normal cells of the prostate are subjected to some initiating event and then later to a single or series of promoting events leading to the development of progression and metastasis.

The majority of prostate cancers are adenocarcinomas and occur mainly in the peripheral zone of the gland (70%), with the other 30% being distributed between the transitional zone and the central zones.[116] Transitional zone carcinomas tend to be less aggressive in nature.[25] No single factor has been identified to account for carcinogenesis. Histologic presence of the disease appears to be similar worldwide, whereas clinically significant disease has substantial geographic variation. Current scientific thinking suggests that prostate cancer results from a combination of environmental factors as well as personal risk factors.[69]

Age

Prostate cancer is associated with the aging process. More than 75% of cases diagnosed are among men over the age of 65. After age 50, both incidence and mortality rates increase at nearly exponential rates. Diagnosis before the age of 50 years is associated with decreased relative survival.[16] The biologic explanation for the link between increased age and such drastic increases in incidence remains unclear. Histologic tumors have been documented in 70% to 90% of men over the age of 80 at autopsy.[131] Within the United States, male life spans have extended and one theory proposes that this extension has allowed histologic disease the opportunity to progress and become clinically significant.

Racial and Ethnic Factors

Within the United States, the risk of developing prostate cancer among white men over the period of 1990 to 1996 was 147.3/100,000 (age adjusted), whereas the incidence for African American men over that same time period was 229.9/100,000. Mortality rates reflect a similar pattern, with 23.7/100,000 white men dying of the disease as compared to 54.8/100,000 population among African Americans.[56] This racial differential extends beyond incidence and mortality rates. Fourteen percent of African American men have distant metastasis at the time of diagnosis versus only 8% among white men.[16] Research findings support the theory that prostate cancer behaves more aggressively biologically among African American men. Moul and colleagues reported that among men treated with curative intent via radical prostatectomy, being African American was a poor prognostic factor for disease recurrence.[102] African American men, especially those over age 65, present with higher Gleason scores.[102, 116, 129] Younger African American men appear to fare poorly as well, having a worse prognosis stage for stage. Access to health care alone does not adequately explain the variance, because at least one study conducted by the U.S. Department of Defense documented high rates of risk, higher stages at diagnosis, and higher rates of progression among African American men despite equal access to military health care.[107]

Differences in testosterone levels between white and African American men may account for some of the prognostic variation. Total testosterone and free testosterone levels have been noted to be 15% and 13%, respectively, higher among healthy African American men of college age. African American men have also been demonstrated to have higher prostate-specific antigen (PSA) levels and PSA densities as compared to other racial groups.[1] Additionally, African American men have been noted to have positive surgical margins (58%) more frequently than white men (40%).[120]

Other racial variations have been noted. Although incidence and mortality rates among Asian/Pacific Islanders, Native Americans, and Hispanic Americans remain significantly lower than both whites and African Americans,[56] a trend toward increasing incidence and mortality has been noted among Native Americans. Over the period of 1969 to 1994, prostate cancer has become the leading cause of male cancer mortality among Native Americans.[52]

Dietary Factors

Strong correlations have been noted between high levels of dietary fat and prostate cancer.[173] Diets high in fat content may increase the relative risk of developing prostate cancer by a factor of 1.6 to 1.9.[16] Epidemiologic research and migrant studies have associated a high-fat diet with prostate cancer, but how dietary fat is related to prostate cancer is unclear. The effect of dietary fat may be mediated through endogenous hormones. A low-fat, high-fiber diet has been shown to affect male sex hormone metabolism by lowering both circulating testosterone and estradiol levels. Testosterone is necessary for normal prostate epithelium to grow. Early prostate cancer has been shown to be estrogen dependent. The absence of prostate cancer in androgen-deficient men and the reduction of prostate cancer in experimental animals by prolonged administration of male sex hormones suggest that altered hormone metabolism may play a role in the progression of prostate cancer.

Relationships between other dietary nutrients and prostate cancer development have been described. Although vitamin A intake from animal sources may be tied to increased risk, intake from plant sources may be associated with decreased risk.[54, 65, 128, 143] Lycopene, a potent carotenoid antioxidant found in high concentrations in tomatoes, may be associated with decreased risk.[53] Studies have also identified vitamins D and E and selenium intake as potential mediating factors. No conclusive evidence exists at this time, however.[54]

Vasectomy

The literature is replete with research findings examining the relationship between vasectomy and prostate cancer risk. Although numerous studies have documented a slight increase in relative risk (1.85),[53] other studies have failed to demonstrate similar findings. If this risk truly exists, it is small and may be tied in with the fact that men who obtain vasectomies demonstrate health-seeking behaviors and are more likely to be screened for and thus diagnosed with prostate cancer. Results from the largest study ever conducted on this issue demonstrated that when confounding variables such as race, age, and family history of prostate cancer were considered, no significant differences were noted in the prevalence of prostate cancer among men who had and had not undergone vasectomies.[146]

Genetics and Family History

Men with first-degree relatives having prostate cancer are estimated to have a 2.1- to 2.8-fold greater risk of developing prostate cancer than men of the general population.[148] Having both an affected first- and second-degree relative increases risk up to 6-fold.[16] Some research has suggested that men who have a family history of breast cancer are also at increased risk. BRCA1 and BRCA2 gene mutations are suspect. HPC1 has been identified as a major prostate cancer susceptibility locus, accounting for 33% of cases of hereditary prostate cancer.[16]

Other Relevant Risk Factors

Conflicting data exist on the relationship of benign prostatic hyperplasia (BPH) and the development of prostate cancer. It is possible that BPH does not predispose men to the development of malignancy, but it may expose men to more frequent screening and thus a higher chance of being diagnosed.

No occupational exposures have been firmly linked with prostate cancer. Cadmium exposure among welders and electroplate workers may weakly increase risk. The mechanism of action is unknown but believed to be related to cadmium's zinc antagonist properties. Zinc is critical for numerous metabolic pathways.[16]

Infection has been proposed as a possible risk factor, but research has failed to demonstrate a clear association. Despite a century of theorizing, sexual behavior and fertility fail to demonstrate a clear relationship with the development of prostate cancer.[117]

ANATOMY

The prostate gland is a small, firm, walnut-sized, organ weighing about 20 g. The gland is shaped like an inverted pyramid. The superior surface, referred to as the *base*, lies at the neck of the urinary bladder; the inferior apex rests on the urogenital diaphragm (Fig. 10–1). The portion of the urethra passing centrally from the superior base to the inferior apex is referred to as the prostatic urethra. Dense, fibrous tissue surrounds the gland. The ejaculatory ducts penetrate the gland posteriorly and superiorly. There are no true lobar divisions in the gland. Visualizing the prostate gland as having a central area or zone, a submucosal or transitional zone, and a horseshoe-shaped peripheral area may help with understanding disease distribution and the area accessible to digital rectal examination (DRE). Palpable areas in-

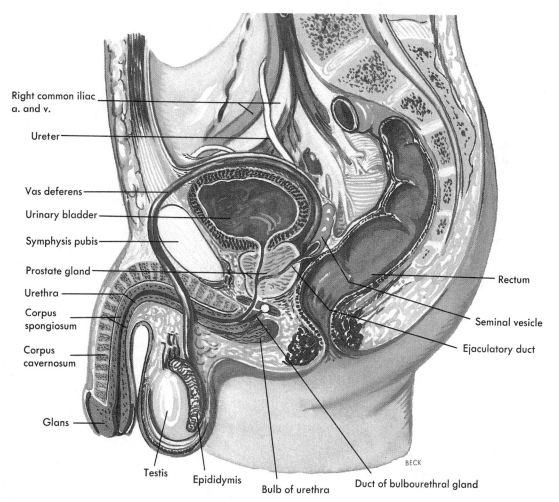

FIGURE 10–1 Male pelvic organs. (From Thibodeau G, Patton K: *Anthony's textbook of anatomy and physiology*, ed 16, St. Louis, Mosby, 1999.)

clude posterior or posterolateral region of the peripheral zone with a median furrow, which is felt as a shallow midline depression, and the two superiorly positioned seminal vesicles are identifiable landmarks on rectal palpation. The prostate serves as a sex accessory gland, with the seminal vesicles contributing viscous secretions to semen.

PREVENTION, SCREENING, AND DETECTION

Substantial controversy surrounds the issues of prostate cancer screening and early detection, and published guidelines by the leading health care authorities reflect a lack of consensus. The most recently updated guidelines published by the American Cancer Society (ACS) recommend that both PSA testing and DRE should be offered annually, beginning at age 50, to men who have at least a 10-year life expectancy and to younger men who are at high risk. High-risk men are identified as those of African American descent and men with a family history of prostate cancer. The ACS further recommends that men should be given specific information regarding the potential risks and benefits of screening. The ACS bases their recommendation on data supporting screening as a means of detecting tumors at a more favorable stage; however, they note that reductions in mortality from prostate cancer cannot directly be attributed to screening. An abnormal PSA is defined as a value of 4.0 ng/mL or higher.[166]

The American Urological Association, the American College of Radiology, and the Prostate Cancer Education Council all recommend screening for prostate cancer.[66] Other agencies such as the United States Preventive Health Services, the Canadian Task Force on Periodic Examination, the National Cancer Institute, and the American College of Physicians have not endorsed routine screening for prostate cancer.[4, 162] Controversy stems in part from concerns over the diagnosis of potentially clinically insignificant tumors and the lack of randomized trials demonstrating the efficacy of treatment in reducing morbidity and mortality as compared to conservative expectant management alone.

SCREENING AND DIAGNOSTIC TOOLS

PSA

PSA remains the single best test for early diagnosis. PSA is a serine protease produced by malignant cells in the prostate as well as normal and hyperplastic prostate cells. An elevated PSA is not diagnostic of prostate cancer. Any disruption of normal prostate epithelial cell architecture allows PSA to diffuse into the tissue and ultimately into the circulation. Elevated levels are seen following DRE (though thought to be clinically insig-

nificant), in men with BPH and prostatitis, following transrectal ultrasonography, and in those with urinary retention.

Efforts to enhance the specificity of PSA have included examining PSA density, velocity, and the development of age-specific PSA reference ranges. PSA density represents the quotient of serum PSA divided by one half of the prostatic volume. PSA density was thought to be important based on observations that serum PSA values could normalize based on calculations of the volume of the prostate, known to be larger in cases of BPH. Theoretically, this data could result in fewer unnecessary prostate biopsies. PSA density testing has lost favor in recent years because of concerns regarding the significant costs associated with subjecting men to transrectal ultrasound with each PSA reading.[15]

PSA velocity refers to the examination of serial PSA readings over time. Some researchers have noted that velocity is useful in stratifying men with carcinoma versus those without if three consecutive readings are taken over a 2-year time period.[23] Velocity appeared to be most relevant in men with PSA values greater than 4.0 ng/mL. Others have questioned the value of PSA velocity based on findings that PSA values vary from day to day, implying that short intervals between testing may allow normal biologic variations to mask significant PSA changes that may be indicative of carcinoma.[14, 15]

Though a number of researchers have proposed age-specific PSA reference ranges, the predictive value of the 4.0 ng/mL cutoff has withstood the test of time. At present, there is a lack of consensus in the scientific community regarding the application of age-specific reference ranges.[14, 15]

Another area under study is the investigation of PSA molecular forms and examination of the ratio of free-to-total PSA. In several studies, free PSA has been found to be lower among men with carcinoma.[27, 87] A significant hurdle to be overcome before free-to-total ratios gain clinical acceptance is the wide variability among the available commercial assays.

DRE and Other Tests

A DRE should be performed by a skilled professional health care practitioner. The examination is brief, taking only seconds. The examiner inserts the well-lubricated gloved index finger approximately 2 to 3 cm (about 1 inch) into the anal orifice and gently presses against the lower wall of the rectum, systematically palpating the accessible surface of the prostate gland. This examination is facilitated when the subject is leaning forward with arms resting on the examination table, toes pointed inward, and the knees slightly flexed. Alternative positions include side-lying in fetal position or kneeling face down on the examination table.[167] Any change in size, consistency, or contour detected in the gland may represent an inflammatory process, infarction, or calculus, in addition to tumor. A disadvantage to this screening procedure, however, is that only the lateral and posterior areas of the gland can be palpated, precluding estimation of tumor volume and extent.

Transrectal ultrasound (TRUS) is used to determine whether the disease is confined to the gland itself and to guide the needle biopsy process. The use of high-frequency transducers has enabled the visualization of internal prostatic anatomy, an opportunity previously available only to pathologists studying radical prostatectomy or autopsy specimens. TRUS shows most prostatic lesions, both malignant and benign, as hypoechoic. Magnetic resonance imaging (MRI), with its ability to illustrate glandular subtleties and determine capsular penetration and seminal vesicle involvement, may be helpful in the staging of prostate cancer.[136] Use of an endorectal coil has been demonstrated to enhance MRI sensitivity and specificity in the diagnosis of capsular penetration and seminal vesicle invasion.[94]

Computed tomography (CT) continues to be used for evaluation of nodes, tissue, and organs and to estimate prostatic size. CT provides poor visualization of the prostate and its surrounding structures, yields wide variation in interpretation of findings, and does not provide information necessary to differentiate between inflammation and malignancy.[91] Spiral or helical CT using thin multiplanar sections may overcome some of these shortcomings.[30] Radioimmunoscintigraphy is currently under study as a new methodology for the identification of lymph node metastasis. Radionucleotide scanning continues to be a primary modality for detecting or confirming metastatic bone involvement.

Bone scans, though highly sensitive, are relatively nonspecific and findings must be correlated with plain radiographs. Bone scans are predominantly recommended for patients with PSA levels of 20 ng/mL or greater to rule out bony metastasis.

Biopsy

When a suspicious area is identified in the prostate, or when a PSA level is significantly elevated, a biopsy is indicated. Prostatic needle biopsy for a core of tissue is accomplished with good yield and low morbidity by transrectal approach. This approach has been demonstrated to be superior to either blind biopsy or the transperineal approach.[42] Biopsy is performed on an outpatient basis. An 18-gauge spring-loaded needle is used to obtain multiple specimens. Refinements in the design of biopsy needles have decreased the risk of cancer seeding and implantation. There is no special prebiopsy patient preparation. The patient is placed in the lithotomy position and local anesthesia is administered. An ultrasound probe is inserted into the rectum to guide needle placement. Patients may experience discomfort as well as a sensation of fullness or pressure. After the procedure, a urine specimen is examined for the presence of hematuria.[69]

Discharge instructions include teaching about the normal postprocedure findings. Hematuria with small clots may occur for 24 hours. Patients may experience ecchymosis at the biopsy site and are instructed to avoid strenuous activity for 24 hours. Patients also should be instructed to contact the physician if they develop any signs of infection such as fever, chills, or dysuria.[70]

CLINICAL PREVENTION TRIALS

The Southwest Oncology Group (SWOG) along with the Eastern Cooperative Oncology Group (ECOG) and the Cancer and Leukemia Group B are currently conducting an intergroup prostate cancer prevention trial. The study is sponsored by the National Cancer Institute and is a double-blind placebo-controlled trial. Eighteen hundred men have been randomized to receive either finasteride (5 mg/d) or a placebo for a period of 7 years. Men aged 55 and older with normal prostates and PSA levels of 3 or less were eligible.[22, 44]

The theoretical basis for this study revolves around hormonal manipulation. Androgens are required for the growth and development of prostatic tissue. Lutenizing hormone-releasing hormone (LHRH) is produced by the pituitary and stimulates the release of lutenizing hormone (LH) and follicle-stimulating hormone (FSH). LH in turn stimulates Leydig cells within the testicles to produce testosterone. In the prostate gland, testosterone is converted by the enzyme 5α-reductase to dihydrotestosterone (DHT). It is DHT that binds to androgenic receptors and is primarily responsible for cell growth. Finasteride is a testosterone analogue, which acts as an inhibitor of 5α-reductase. After all enrollees have been in the study for 7 years, each man will undergo a prostate biopsy. The two groups will then be compared.[22, 44]

Other chemopreventive approaches have focussed on examination of vitamin A modulators, nonsteroidal anti-inflammatory agents, and antiangiogenesis agents.

CLASSIFICATION

Ninety-five percent of prostate cancers are *adenocarcinomas*. Ductal carcinomas, including transitional and squamous cell carcinomas, endometrioid carcinomas, and sarcomas, account for the remainder. The classically used Gleason system ascertains a degree of glandular differentiation and tumor growth pattern in relation to prostate stroma. A score is assigned both to the predominant pattern of differentiation, ranging from well-

TABLE 10-1
Prostate Cancer Staging Systems

Whitmore-Jewett	Description	AJCC
A	Incidental finding of carcinoma on examination of prostate tissue after prostatectomy or transurethral resection	T1
A_1	Histologically well- or moderately well-differentiated tumor or tumor consisting of <5% of resected specimen	T1a
A_2	Histologically poorly differentiated or anaplastic tumor or tumor consisting of >5% of resected specimen	T1b
B	Clinically palpable tumor confined to prostate	T2
B_1	Focal ≤1.5 cm	T2a
B_2	Diffuse >1.5 cm ≥2 foci T2b	T2b
C	Extension beyond prostate capsule to seminal vesicles or contiguous tissue	T3
D	Metastatic tumor	N-M
D_1	Regional nodal involvement	M1 to M3
D_2	Metastasis to any of the following: Bone, lymph nodes above aortic bifurcation, other organs	M

formed to undifferentiated tumors, and to any secondary pattern of differentiation observed microscopically. Histologic grading is based on the most undifferentiated portion or on the predominant pattern observed. Scores range from 2 to 10 and have been shown to be predictive of associated lymph node metastases. In general, degree of tumor differentiation and abnormality of histologic growth pattern directly correlate with likelihood of metastases and with death.[104, 105] Prognosis is worse in patients with pelvic lymph node involvement. Ductal-acinar dysplasia, identified by nuclear and cytoplasmic abnormalities, is now characterized as prostatic intraepithelial neoplasia (PIN). PIN is considered a premalignant lesion and demonstrates cellular changes indicative of cellular alterations in regulation and differentiation. PIN has been further classified as high or low grade, with low grade having low correlation with the development of subsequent carcinoma.[61]

DIAGNOSIS, STAGING, AND CLINICAL FEATURES

The first clinical staging system was introduced by Whitmore and Jewett.[71] The American Urologic System consists of stages A, B, C, and D, that have been translated into tumor-node-metastasis (TNM) categories by the American Joint Commission on Cancer (AJCC) and the Committee of the International Union Against Cancer.[5, 12, 71] Table 10–1 outlines the TNM classification for prostate cancer. Stage A, or T1, disease is asymptomatic, suspected on DRE, and found incidentally on pathologic examination of resected prostate tissue for management of prostatic hypertrophy. Stage A is further subdivided into A_1, or T1a, which is a pathologically graded, well-differentiated tumor or tumor foci repre-

senting 5% or less of resected tissue; and A_2, or T1b, which is a moderately or poorly differentiated tumor involving greater than 5% of the resection. Stage B, or T2, disease is a palpable tumor confined to the prostate. B_1, or T2a, disease is a focal lesion 1.5 cm or less in diameter; B_2, or T2b, is diffuse disease greater than 1.5 cm in diameter or two or more tumor foci at a time. Stage B_1, or T2, prostate cancer may also be asymptomatic. Clinically determined involvement of seminal vesicles or adjacent structures is staged as C, or T3, disease. At this stage, local irritative symptoms include painful urination, frequency, and hematuria. Obstructive symptoms may also be present, ranging from hesitancy and interrupted urinary stream, to full urinary obstruction. Stage D, or N-M, represents metastatic disease with D_1, or M, indicative of tumor metastatic to bone, other organs, or nodes above the aortic bifurcation.[99]

Symptoms associated with advanced disease may include painful urination; urinary frequency; hematuria; bone, back, or joint pain; weight loss; and fatigue. Prostate cancer spreads by direct extension to the seminal vesicles and contiguous structures, bladder, membranous urethra, and pelvic sidewalls. The rectum is essen-

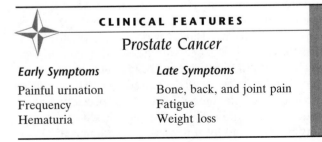

CLINICAL FEATURES

Prostate Cancer

Early Symptoms	*Late Symptoms*
Painful urination	Bone, back, and joint pain
Frequency	Fatigue
Hematuria	Weight loss

tially spared because it is offered a degree of protection by Denonvilliers' fascia. Lymphatic spread to pelvic nodes or hematogeneous deposition to bone is frequently encountered.[69]

BIOLOGIC MARKERS

Laboratory quantification of PSA provides a marker for monitoring response to therapy. PSA, a serine protease produced by normal and neoplastic ductal epithelium, serves to lyse the seminal coagulum. First purified from normal prostate tissue in 1979, PSA has since been found in seminal fluids, in BHP tissue, and in malignant tissue.[14, 15] Monoclonal and polyclonal antibodies that react with PSA have been developed to provide more precise laboratory determination of the level of PSA present. The ability of PSA to predict localized disease reliably continues to be evaluated (see prior discussion). Although PSA is prostate specific, it is not prostate cancer specific. PSA is also used as the primary measure of treatment success. Rising PSA levels after treatment are generally viewed as biologic failure, but it remains unclear whether such biologic treatment failures translate into clinical treatment failures.

TREATMENT MODALITIES

Prostate cancer has been shrouded by a cloak of uncertainty, extending from issues surrounding the value and efficacy of screening and early detection, to uncertainty regarding which, if any, treatment option is superior. There is no consensus within the scientific community regarding optimal treatment for early stage disease at this point. Within the confines of Western medicine, three basic options are offered for the management of early stage prostate cancer: radical prostatectomy, radiation therapy (either external beam or brachytherapy), or "expectant management," sometimes referred to as "watchful waiting." Cryotherapy is currently under investigation. Selection of treatment is based on projected survival, as well as patient and physician preferences. A substantial body of literature exists examining patient preferences for prostate cancer treatment and more recently describing the actual decision-making process as experienced by men and their spouses in the face of a prostate cancer.[35, 36, 108, 109, 111] Multiple treatment decision models have been published for physician use, including specific practice guidelines established by the National Comprehensive Cancer Network (NCCN).[98] The key factors for consideration within each model include the patient's age and projected survival, coexisting medical problems, stage of disease, and other tumor factors such as grade and the Gleason score, and consideration of the expected side effects associated with each treatment modality. The meaning of the can-

cer experience and the patient's personal or vicarious experiences and opinions of each treatment option are fundamental issues to be considered.[108]

Treatment options can be summarized as follows[156]:

Stage I disease: Options generally include careful observation without further treatment for most patients, more definitive treatment for younger men in otherwise good health

Stage II disease: Options include radical prostatectomy, external bean or interstitial implant radiotherapy, watchful waiting

Stage III disease: Options include external beam radiotherapy with or without hormonal manipulation, hormonal manipulation alone, radical prostatectomy in limited cases. Watchful waiting is an additional option for older men and or those men who are asymptomatic with coexisting medical conditions.

Stage IV disease: Hormonal therapy, orchiectomy, external beam radiotherapy, palliative pain management with radioisotopes or external beam radiation therapy, watchful waiting, chemotherapy for hormone-refractory disease.

Surgery

Surgery in the form of radical prostatectomy has historically been the primary therapy for localized prostate cancer. The procedure, first described by Young in 1905,[174] has undergone numerous refinements, the most notable being the nerve-sparing retropubic approach introduced by Walsh.[168, 169]

The retropubic approach remains the dominant surgical technique because it provides access to regional lymph nodes in the pelvis and affords nerve-sparing potential, improving postoperative potency. Regional lymph node sampling permits assessment of the presence or absence of tumor in adjacent nodes. If tumor is present in nodes, radical prostatectomy may be deferred and patients may be treated with a more palliative as opposed to curative intent.

Stages A, B_1, B_2, T_1, and T_2 lesions may be treated surgically by radical prostatectomy.[98, 156] Surgery is usually reserved for patients in good health who are younger than 70 years, who have no evidence of metastatic disease, and who desire this option.[175]

Immediate postoperative nursing care includes maintaining catheter patency, prevention of urinary tract infections, and the administration of analgesia for pain management. Teaching includes discussion of catheter maintenance following discharge (may be in place for several weeks postoperatively), early initiation of Kegel exercises to strengthen pelvic floor muscles, progressive ambulating, and avoidance of vigorous activity until cleared by the physician. Nurses should assess patients' knowledge regarding potential incontinence following catheter removal and provide anticipatory teaching regarding the use of incontinence management aids. Nursing research has demonstrated that patients have an incomplete understanding of the potential adverse effects of prostate cancer treatment, and that the management of incontinence is a more pressing symptom management priority in the immediate postoperative period than impotence.[110]

Postoperative complications include incontinence, impotence, urethral stricture, and general complications associated with anesthesia and surgery itself. Morbidity and mortality increase considerably with advanced age. Reports of incontinence following radical prostatectomy are variable, owing to the lack of precise definitions of incontinence and inconsistent measurement intervals for assessment. Among patients with radical prostatectomy the reported incidence of postoperative incontinence ranges from 3%[45] to 69%.[8] Another source cites a range of 2% to 87%.[26] Low estimates should be interpreted with caution, because these are usually reflective of study samples including large numbers of younger men. After a 12-month period, little additional recovery of continence is expected.[26] Researchers have reported that patients over the age of 70 have incontinence rates double those of younger cohorts.[155] Incontinence is very common immediately after catheter removal in the postoperative period, with approximately 56% of men in one large series (n = 180) requiring the use of absorbent pads. In that same series, 11 patients ultimately required artificial sphincters to regain continence. The literature consistently reveals more difficulties with urinary control following radical prostatectomy as compared with external beam radiotherapy. In terms of quality of life, urinary incontinence has been found to have a significant positive association with tension, fatigue, and depression, and a significant negative association with vigor and social well-being.[84]

Impotence is another significant threat to quality of life following radical prostatectomy. Despite nerve-sparing techniques, reports of potency are highly variable in the medical literature. Talcott and colleagues reported that 79% of the men in their sample who had undergone bilateral nerve-sparing prostatectomy had inadequate erections for vaginal penetration.[155] Jonler and associates reported that only 9% of their patients had full erections and 39% partial erections,[74] figures corroborated by Fowler.[48] Experienced surgeons report preserved potency in the range of 40% to 70%.[24, 121]

Pharmacologic erection or surgical implantation of a penile prosthesis may manage disease-related or treatment-related impotence. Additionally patients may try vacuum assist devices to obtain adequate erections for vaginal penetration. New pharmacologic options include the use of prostaglandin urethral suppositories and the use of oral sildenafil citrate (Viagra). Results and patient satisfaction have been variable, but sildenafil citrate has had some benefit in improving erectile dysfunction among men following radical prostatectomy or radiotherapy for prostate cancer treatment.[78, 176] Erectile dysfunction is often multifactorial, and the influence of other preexisting medical conditions, the status of preprostate cancer therapy potency, and the effects of life stress, alcohol, and tobacco use, as well as prescription and nonprescription medications must be considered in counseling men regarding this distressing side effect. Potential disease-related and treatment-related complications are summarized in the Complications box.

Radiation Therapy

The delivery of radiotherapy may take several forms: traditional external beam delivery, three-dimensional conformal radiotherapy, or brachytherapy. External beam therapy continues to be the most widely applied technique. In the case of prostate cancer it is applied in the treatment of stages I to III disease, and in stage IV disease for palliative purposes. Patients with stage I or II disease who have positive surgical margins or pathologic findings of seminal vesicle involvement experience local relapse rates of 20% to 50% and may benefit from postoperative radiotherapy beginning 6 to 12 weeks postoperatively.[6, 165]

External beam radiotherapy can result in long-term remissions paralleling those achieved with radical pros-

---

COMPLICATIONS

Prostate Cancer

DISEASE-RELATED COMPLICATIONS

Infection
Painful urination
Urinary frequency
Hematuria
Impotence

TREATMENT-RELATED COMPLICATIONS

Treatment Modalities	*Treatment Complications*
Surgery (prostatectomy)	Impotence
	Incontinence, other urinary symptoms
Radiation (external, internal)	Incontinence, other urinary symptoms
	Impotence
	Altered bowel functioning

tatectomy. Candidates for definitive (versus palliative) therapy include men with stage I, II, or III disease that is clinically confined to the prostate or surrounding tissues. Additionally, candidates should have negative bone scans. Because patients treated with external beam radiotherapy lack the benefit of surgical staging, it must be appreciated that they may be clinically understaged, which may affect their treatment success rates.[156]

External beam radiation therapy is delivered daily over a 7-week period. The radiation field includes the prostate and seminal vesicles, with a margin to allow for patient motion. Field sizes depend on patient anatomy.

External beam radiation can also be delivered conformally. The goal of this technique is to concentrate high radiation doses to the tumor while sparing critical adjacent structures (bladder and rectum). Tumor doses may exceed 65 Gy, and higher doses are used for more advanced disease. Three-dimensional conformal radiation therapy (3D-CRT) uses CT scanning to create a three-dimensional reconstruction of the prostate and surrounding structures. Standard simulation procedures are used in conjunction with three-dimensional reconstructions to facilitate treatment planning. Immobilization casts are used to maintain patient positioning during treatment administration.[165]

The risk of treatment-related side effects is influenced by the dose to normal tissue and volume of tissue treated. Radiotherapy-related side effects are categorized as acute and late toxicities. Acute toxicity, occurring within 90 days of treatment, is usually reversible and occurs within rapidly dividing cells. Late reactions occur in more slowly dividing cells and may be permanent. The onset of late effects is variable, occurring anytime after the 90-day period, even months to years after the completion of therapy. (See Chapter 22 for more information regarding general side effects and nursing management of radiation therapy.)

With the exception of generalized fatigue, side effects are site specific and occur only within the treatment field. Symptoms relating to bladder toxicity include cystitis, urethral stricture, urinary frequency, dysuria, and nocturia. Griffiths and Neal[57] cite the overall incidence of urinary incontinence after external beam radiotherapy as 3% to 7%; however, others offer slightly higher rates. Patients with a history of prior transurethral resection of the prostate (TURP) have higher rates of incontinence.[80] Tenesmus, diarrhea, and mucosal bleeding may result from gastrointestinal mucosal irritation. Onset is usually within the second to third week of therapy, corresponding to a dose rate between 15 and 30 Gy.[165] Prompt intervention is indicated to prevent dehydration and electrolyte imbalance. Pharmacologic management of these symptoms is achieved with the use of antispasmodics and antidiarrheal agents including kaolin, pectin,

loperamide, atropine, diphenoxylate hydrochloride, and opium preparations such as paregoric.[165]

Patients should be instructed to follow a low-residue diet and to maintain adequate fluid intake. Proctitis may be treated with sitz baths and topical applications of hydrocortisone. Patients should be instructed to maintain adequate elimination patterns and to monitor for signs and symptoms of urinary or rectal irritation. Treated areas should not be exposed to sunlight because local skin reactions have been reported. Skin assessment is critical.

Erectile functioning is affected by radiation therapy. Impotence is often multifactorial and the contributions of such factors as cardiovascular disease, diabetes, tobacco and alcohol use, and prescription and nonprescription medications must be considered. Patients who are potent prior to external beam therapy tend to remain potent, in contrast to those with poor initial function. Disruptions in potency are caused by radiation damage to the small blood vessels and nerves responsible for erection. The effects of radiation on erectile function may be delayed.

Forty percent of the active marrow is within the pelvic bones, predisposing patients receiving large-field radiation to myelosuppression. Older patients and those with bony metastasis are at increased risk. The incidence of myelosuppression as a dose-limiting toxicity, however, appears to be low.[88]

A third treatment delivery option for radiotherapy is interstitial implantation, also known as brachytherapy. Patients having organ-confined disease and a life expectancy of more than 5 years are considered eligible candidates. Results have been favorable for patients with localized disease, with 65% 10-year survival reported in at least one major study.[122]

Brachytherapy may be performed as a solo treatment modality or before or after external beam radiation therapy. Implants may be permanent or temporary, using palladium-103, iridium-192, and iodine-125 sources. Placement is guided by CT enhancement and TRUS. The procedure is performed on an outpatient basis using spinal or general anesthesia. Needles are placed transperineally through a template guide. Radioactive seeds are loaded through the needles directly into the prostate. The needles are withdrawn after all seeds are placed. Following implantation, a cystourethroscopy may be performed to assess for bleeding or to retrieve errant seeds. A Foley catheter may be placed to monitor output for volume and quality. When the urine is free of clots, 200 mL sterile water is injected into the bladder and then the catheter is removed. The patient is monitored to ascertain that he can void spontaneously.[165]

Nursing care of patients following prostatic brachytherapy includes teaching regarding the management of side effects. Mild dysuria, frequency, and mild pain may occur. Patients should report any obstructive symptoms. Patients are encouraged to maintain a high level of fluid intake and to complete the full course of prophylactic antibiotic therapy as prescribed. Rarely patients require an indwelling catheter or intermittent self-catheterization if edema causes severe obstructive symptoms. Symptoms generally subside within 3 to 4 months. Hematuria caused by the trauma of needle insertion is common and resolves within 72 hours. Patients may resume sexual intercourse within 2 weeks, but should wear a condom for 2 months to protect their partner from possible seed expulsion.[165]

Patient education should include information regarding radiation safety. Urine straining is no longer a general recommendation. Patients are instructed to observe urine for lost seeds. However, they are no longer instructed to attempt to retrieve the seeds; rather they should allow the seeds to be flushed into the sewer system. Body secretions including urine and feces may be flushed as usual.[2, 165] (See Chapter 22 for more detailed information on brachytherapy treatment delivery and radiation safety protocols.)

Radiation also plays a role in palliation for prostate cancer. External beam irradiation to selected sites may provide significant pain relief. Strontium-89, a systemic radioisotope, targets specific sites of metastatic disease when administered intravenously.[119, 126] Response rates of 70% to 80% have been reported.[126]

Hormonal Therapy

Hormonal manipulation is the mainstay of treatment for advanced prostate cancer and is accomplished either surgically or medically. The scientific basis for hormonal manipulation is predicated on an understanding of normal prostate growth and function (reviewed previously). Prostatic epithelial cells depend on DHT for growth and differentiation. A schematic representation of the hypothalamic-pituitary-gonadal axis that regulates the physiologic balance of circulating testosterone is shown in Figure 10–2. The goal of hormonal manipulation is to stop the growth of androgen-dependent prostate cancer cells and to induce apoptosis or cell death. The loss of androgenic stimulation to prostatic cancer cells results in cellular death within 24 hours.[93]

Removal of the testes, the source of 95% of the major circulating androgen testosterone, through bilateral orchiectomy, is a cost-effective intervention that interrupts the gonadal portion of the axis. Although the surgical procedure is associated with minimal risk, choice of this option as opposed to medical castration is a personal one. Orchiectomy is irreversible and the side effects are associated with significant morbidity.

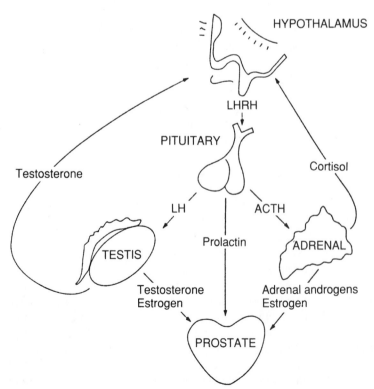

FIGURE 10–2 Hypothalamic-pituitary-testicularadrenal axis. LHRH, luteinizing hormone-releasing hormone; LH, luteinizing hormone; ACTH, adrenocorticotropic hormone. (Modified from Crawford ED: Combined androgen blockade, *Urology* 34[suppl]:24, 1989, with permission from Elsevier Science.)

Medical castration was initially accomplished by the administration of exogenous estrogens such as diethyl stilbestrol (DES), but it is now more commonly accomplished by the administration of LHRH agonists. LH, normally is released from the anterior pituitary in response to the pulsatile release of LHRH, which is synthesized in the hypothalamus. The presence of LH results in the testicular secretion of a physiologic level of testosterone with corresponding spermatogenesis (production of spermatozoa). Medically induced continuous LHRH stimulation, however, results in desensitization of the pituitary gland and inhibits LH production.[19] Within the first 5 to 8 days of treatment, there is an initial increase in testosterone levels resulting from increased LH production induced by the LHRH agonist. This initial rise corresponds with a disease flare and may exacerbate bone pain or result in obstructive urinary symptoms. This flare may be avoided by the administration of an antiandrogen such as finasteride to block testosterone at the receptor level. Laboratory monitoring is necessary to ensure that castration levels of testosterone have been achieved (<20 mg/dL). If these levels are not achieved, the addition of an antiandrogen is necessary.[98] Although the cost of LHRH agonists is covered by Medicare, self-administration is not covered. Longer-acting depot formulations are now available and offer some cost savings.[152]

Peripheral tissue and adrenal androgens account for the remaining 5% of circulating testosterone. Antiandrogens, such as flutamide, bicalutamide, and nilutamide, are nonsteroidal compounds that bind to androgen receptors but do not have hormonal activity themselves. These drugs are taken orally. Pure antiandrogens do not alter the level of circulating male hormone but rather block the hormone from reaching the target tissue, the prostate gland.[19] Testosterone levels are maintained within normal range and thus potency is not affected by the administration of these agents. Pure antiandrogens are associated with a range of side effects including breast tenderness, gynecomastia, hot flashes, and generalized weakness and energy loss. Liver dysfunction has also been reported. Antiandrogen therapy is not covered by Medicare.[152]

Steroidal antiandrogens inhibit LH secretion from the pituitary and block androgens at the receptor level. Because testosterone levels are affected by this mechanism, these agents are associated with decreased libido and erectile dysfunction. The most commonly prescribed steroidal antiandrogen in the United States is megesterol acetate.

Nursing care of patients receiving hormonal therapy includes teaching potential side effects and self-care activities to ameliorate these. Bothersome side effects include hot flashes, fatigue, impotence, and osteoporosis. Additionally, patients may experience weight gain and appetite changes. Therapeutic interventions to control hot flashes are limited. Administration of megesterol acetate,[86] clonidine,[17] and medroxyprogesterone (Depo-Provera)[18] have been recommended. Management of impotence may be mechanical or pharmacologic. Sildenafil, alprostadil urethral suppositories, and alprostadil penile injections are among the pharmacologic options. External vacuum devices and implanted penile prostheses are other options. Bisphosphonates may be beneficial in maintaining bone density among men treated with hormonal manipulation and at high risk for the development of osteoporosis.

Expectant Management or Watchful Waiting

One option for the management of prostate disease is that of expectant management, surveillance, or watchful waiting. This conservative management strategy involves no local therapy on diagnosis, with initiation of treatment only when the patient becomes symptomatic from either locally advanced disease or metastatic disease. Again, selection of this option is largely based on patient preference, but it is generally reserved for patients with low-grade disease who are older than 70 years of age, with a life expectancy of less than 10 years. The rationale for expectant management is based on the observation that the incidence rates for prostate cancer far exceed the death rates. More men die "with" the disease than "of" the disease. Proponents of this approach argue that there is significant evidence that aggressive therapy has not improved overall prostate cancer survival but has significantly diminished quality of life.[112] Frequently cited supporting literature includes European and Scandinavian studies by Adolfsson,[3] and Johansson[73] reporting low death rates among men selecting this option. The National Cancer Institute and the Veterans Affairs Cooperative Studies Group have undertaken a large-scale, randomized trial comparing radical prostatectomy with expectant management for the treatment of clinically localized prostate cancer (Prostate Intervention Versus Observation Trial [PIVOT]). Launched in 1995, the study is ongoing. It is hoped that data from this trial and simultaneous European studies will provide clear scientific evidence as to the value of aggressive treatment versus a strategy of observation only.

Cryotherapy

Although initially introduced in the 1960s as a treatment option for prostate cancer, cryotherapy was abandoned due to the high rate of complications experienced. In recent years, there has been a renewed interest in this treatment modality resulting from technique refinements. This therapy involves the direct application of ice to the prostate gland via percutaneously inserted cryogenic probes. Probe placement is guided by ultrasound, and continuous temperature monitoring is conducted throughout the procedure. Reported complications include urethral sloughing, urinary incontinence, bladder neck contracture, and impotence.[172] Wong,[172] and Saliken[132] have reported high rates of urinary complications, whereas Badalament[7] reported lower rates and high levels of patients satisfaction. Wong[172] reported 90% negative follow-up biopsies in one group with mean PSA levels of 0.3 ng/mL at 30 months. Saliken reported negative follow-up biopsies at 6 months in 68 of 69 patients, and undetectable PSA levels at that same interval.[132] Although cryoablation appears to be an emerging therapy for prostate cancer, data must be complied regarding side effects, both immediate and delayed. The long-term efficacy of cryotherapy as compared to radical prostatectomy or radiotherapy has not yet been established.

Chemotherapy

The development of recurrent or progressive disease following curative intent therapy remains a formidable challenge in the area of prostate cancer management. An additional challenge is the case of the development of hormone-refractory disease. Although further treatment options are available, the main focus of care is supportive. Management of distressing symptoms and their impact on quality of life poses the greatest nursing challenge. Identified physiologic problems include fatigue, anemia, appetite disturbances, obstruction (both urinary and bowel), spinal cord compression, and pain. Specific side effects related to treatment modalities also require attention. Pain management is a major focus of nursing care.[43]

In the case of advanced disease, selection of further treatment depends on multiple factors, including prior treatment, site of recurrence, comorbid conditions, and individual patient considerations. Prolonged disease control is often possible with hormone therapy, with median cancer-specific survival of 6 years after local failure.[164] Chemotherapy has limited value in the treatment of patients with refractory disease after hormonal therapy. Recent updates report results of trials using estramustine and etoposide, cytoxan, DES and prednisone, and single-agent DES. The regimens were generally well tolerated and produced measurable declines in PSA values. Other regimens include vinblastine and estramustine, mitoxantone in combination with prednisone, and combinations including doxorubicin.[76] Docetaxel (Taxotere) is also under study presently.[106] There has been renewed interest in the use of ketoconazole as a second-line hormonal agent in combination with hydrocortisone.[144]

Emerging Therapies

Current efforts are being directed to develop novel strategies for the treatment of prostate cancer. A variety of methods aimed at augmenting immune response are currently under investigation. Phase I and II clinical trials are in progress investigating the use of cytokine adjuvant therapy, cytokine gene-transduced vaccines, DNA peptide vaccines, and dendritic cell-based vaccines.[159] Additionally, gene therapy aimed at affecting alterations in genes p53, p21, PML, BRCA1, Rb, c-myc, Bcl-2, and TGF-β is under investigation.[114] A recent focus of research has been the insertion of "suicide genes" into prostate cancer tumor cells.

Special Nursing Considerations— Erectile Dysfunction

Erectile dysfunction and impotence are distressing adverse effects affecting men and their partners following therapy for prostate cancer. A variety of diagnostic tests are used to evaluate the extent and nature of erectile dysfunction.

The *nocturnal penile tumescence test* allows assessment of penile tumescence and the degree of rigidity the patient experiences. A device called a RigiScan with a strain gauge at the base of the penis tip has the ability to record tumescence and rigidity during erections. If normal tumescence and rigidity are demonstrated during sleep, vascular impotence is less likely. Doppler pulse waveform analysis initially was used to evaluate penile arterial vasculature. This procedure has now been replaced with high-resolution ultrasonography and pulsed Doppler spectrum analysis. This test evaluates the function of the arterial system during vasodilator-induced secretions (penile injections). High-resolution imaging and identification of the arteries can be done, and the whole penis can be scanned to assess the internal corporeal tissue. The inner diameter of the cavernous arteries and blood flow velocity are assessed before and after injection of a vasodilator. The ultrasound and pulsed Doppler evaluations are done in a flaccid state. The patient then assumes a supine position, a rubber band is placed on the base of the penis, and a vasodilator is injected into the corpora cavernosa. Arterial dilation and flow are evaluated, as well as cavernosa venous emptying capacity. Baseline organic erectile functioning results from failure to initiate (neurogenic), failure to fill (arteriogenic), or failure to store.

Options for treatment of erectile dysfunction can involve *pharmacotherapeutic agents* such as intracavernous prostaglandin injections, urethral prostaglandin suppositories, oral agents such as sildenafil (Viagra), penile implants, or external devices including vacuum

Nursing Management

Nurses and physicians are in a pivotal position to promote compliance with screening recommendations, especially among African American men and men with a family history of prostate cancer who are identified to be at high risk. Men should be fully informed about PSA testing and the implications of the results. A multidisciplinary approach will facilitate informed treatment decisions and the management of disease-related sequelae such as incontinence, impotence, and pain. This approach enhances psychosocial adjustment related to sexuality.

GERIATRIC CONSIDERATIONS

Because approximately 87% of prostate cancer patients are 65 years of age or older, special attention to the unique concerns of this population is appropriate. With the transition to older adulthood and accommodation to the gradual shift in family responsibilities, retirement, and declining economic opportunities, the aging adult is challenged to achieve ego integrity. Along with the acceptance of age-related limitations, the senior adult is adjusting to physiologic aging, retirement, reduced income, and deaths of relatives, friends, and conceivably spouse while maintaining a safe and solvent environment, often in a relocation setting. The older person is often concerned about finances, loss of independence, and placing a burden on family or society. Frequently the senior adult approaches the health care system and care providers from a docile perspective and may not aggressively pursue or report symptoms, resulting in delay of diagnosis or lack of symptom resolution. The older adult with Medicare has acute care coverage but may not have comprehensive coverage for preventive or supportive care, including oral and subcutaneous medications. Transportation to and from appointments may be a factor impeding treatment.

Intellectual function is usually maintained in older adulthood, although short-term memory may gradually decline, underscoring the need for offering information repetitively using a variety of communication techniques. Special attention to establishing a framework for open communication and identifying components of the individual's dilemma, such as reimbursement, are suggested for facilitating compliance and rehabilitation for the older adult. And finally, the older adult may accommodate the symptoms, interpreting them as related to age rather than disease, and delay in seeking prudent medical intervention.

---

pump mechanisms. External devices are generally recommended for individuals who are receiving anticoagulant therapy or who have blood dyscrasias. Choices are highly individualistic and determined by cost, ease of use, comfort, and partner preferences. Compared with inflatable protheses, *semirigid devices* are not as expensive, are easier to implant, and have lower long-term mechanical failure rates. Men who have penile fibrosis as a result of other diseases or infection may not be candidates for implants. Table 10–2 outlines the differ-

TABLE 10 – 2
Semirigid Penile Prostheses

Type	Advantages	Disadvantages
Simple	Least expensive	Difficulty with outward erectile appearance
Hinged	Has softer zone for positioning for micturition No dressing Fewer sizes necessary	Cost, postoperative complications
Malleable	Central metal core so penis can be bent down and up for coitus, Best rigidity	Cost, postoperative complications
Positionable	Central cable that runs through a series of polyfone segments Superior cosmetic results	Cost, postoperative complications
Mechanically activated	Only nonhydraulic device available	Most expensive

ent types of implants available. Common complications related to implant procedures include perforations during dilation of the corpora, erosion, infection, or mechanical complications related to the implant.

Assessment of the patient's baseline erection functioning before treatment including other potential contributory factors can assist the clinician in planning a sexual rehabilitation program. Erectile function may return spontaneously up to 2 years after a radical prostatectomy. Support and appropriate management of the impotent patient are essential to maintaining the patient's sexual quality of life during this period.

Testicular Cancer

EPIDEMIOLOGY

Testicular cancer is a relatively uncommon disease, with an estimated 6900 new cases diagnosed per year within the United States. Three hundred deaths are anticipated in 2000 from this malignancy.[56] Testicular cancer represents the most common malignancy in men aged 15 to 35 and the second most common malignancy from ages 35 to 39. Occurring during the prime of life for most patients, testicular cancer has a major emotional impact. Testicular tumors occur more often in white men than African American men in the United States, and as in the case of other malignancies, survival rates differ by race with African American men having only an 88% chance of 5-year survival as compared to white men having a 96% chance.[56] The disease represents one of the most curable solid tumors and serves as a paradigm for the multimodal treatment of solid malignancies. Dramatic increases in survival are a result of a combination of effective diagnostic techniques, improvement in tumor markers, effective multidrug chemotherapeutic regimens, and modification of surgical techniques.

Germ cell tumors (GCTs) of the testes represent the most common solid tumor among men between the ages of 20 and 35, and occur with three modal peaks: infancy, age 25 to 40, and again at approximately age 60. Geographic incidence varies, with the highest incidence being reported in Scandinavia, Switzerland, Germany, and New Zealand. The lowest incidence is reported in Africa and Asia.[10] The rising incidence of GCTs worldwide has been a source of increasing concern. Incidence rates have doubled worldwide over the past 40 years.[10] A recently published report indicated a significant rise among active duty members of the United States Armed Forces. Incidence rates increased from 8.62/100,000 men in 1988 to 15.38/100,000 men in 1996.[158]

ETIOLOGY AND RISK FACTORS

The etiology of testicular cancer is unknown, but certain conditions are associated with an increased incidence of this malignancy. Specifically, testicular tumors are more likely to occur in an atrophic testis or a cryptorchid (undescended) testis. The relative risk of testicular cancer in patients with cryptorchidism is thought to be 5 times the normal expected risk. Family history of testicular cancer is associated with 3 to 12 times the average risk, history of a prior germ cell testicular tumor is associated with 23 to 27 times greater risk, and certain intersex syndromes are associated with greater than 100 times the average risk.[161]

Despite case studies suggesting a link between DES use during pregnancy and the development of GCTs, no conclusive evidence exists to support this as a risk factor. Organ transplant patients experience a 20 to 50 times greater risk of developing testicular cancer than the general male.[84] Many sources have noted that a history of trauma to the testes often precedes diagnosis, yet this also has not been supported by research findings to support a causal association. Epidemiologic studies have failed to support viral infection as a cause,[10] although testicular tumors are a common malignancy related to acquired immunodeficiency syndrome (AIDS).

PREVENTION, SCREENING, AND DETECTION

Prevention of testicular cancer is not a reasonable expectation because etiologic factors are unknown. However, early detection is accomplished best by testicular self-examination (TSE). Although the U.S. Preventive Services Task Force states that there is insufficient evidence to support routine screening or TSE among asymptomatic men, the ACS recommends TSE for all men beginning at puberty. TSE is facilitated by the heat of a warm bath or shower. Each testicle is examined with both hands. The index and middle fingers are placed on one side of the testicle. The thumbs are placed on the other side. A gentle rolling motion allows for complete palpation of each testicle (Fig. 10–3). One testicle may be larger than the other. Any lump, new finding, or worrisome area needs to be reported. The normal testis is homogeneous in consistency, freely movable, and separable from the epididymis.

The classic presentation of a testicular tumor is a small-sized painless mass ranging from several millimeters to centimeters. Patients may present with diffuse pain, swelling, or hardness of the testes.[10, 11] A trial of antibiotic therapy is sometimes prescribed on initial presentation if no discrete mass is noted. The health care provider should palpate the testes and surrounding structures for a scrotal mass, examine the breasts for ynecomastia, transilluminate intrascrotal lesions, and

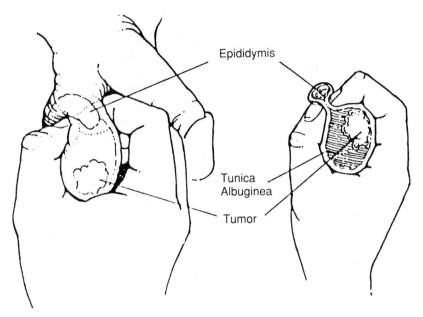

Labels: Epididymis, Tunica Albuginea, Tumor

FIGURE 10-3 Testicular self-examination (TSE). Care is taken with digital separation of testis from posterior elements, including epididymis and cord, for thorough palpation of intrascrotal contents. (Modified from Donohue JP: The testis. In Paulson DF, editor: *Genitourinary surgery,* New York, Churchill Livingstone, 1984.)

perform abdominal examination for a palpable mass, as well as evaluate the supraclavicular region, axillae, and inguinal area for adenopathy. Proper examination of a scrotal mass, including separation of the anterior testis within the tunica albuginea from the posterior adnexal elements, including the epididymis and cord, must be performed so that the intrascrotal contents may be palpated (see Fig. 10–3). The tunica albuginea functions as a natural barrier to expansive local growth. Ultrasound may reveal one or more hypoechoic areas or diffuse abnormalities with microcalcifications.[10] The clinical features associated with testicular cancer are outlined in the Clinical Features box.

Once a palpable nodule exists within the testicle, local involvement or metastases may occur via either the lymphatic (in an orderly manner) or the hematogenous route. Lymphatic metastasis generally tends to follow the spermatic vessels to primary landing sites in the retroperitoneum. Involvement of the epididymis or spermatic cord may lead to pelvic and inguinal lymph node metastases. Common sites of distant metastases include the lungs, bone, or liver and may occur as a direct tumor invasion.[79]

Lymphatic metastasis is common to all forms of germinal testicular tumors. Distant metastases occur most frequently to the pulmonary region. Subsequent spread may occur in the liver, viscera, brain, or bone. Bony metastases are encountered late in the course of the disease. Central nervous system metastases may occur.[145]

Posteroanterior and lateral chest x-ray films provide an initial assessment of the lung parenchyma and mediastinal structures. Chest CT may be ordered to detect pulmonary metastases. Abdominal and pelvic CT scans remain the most common imaging modality for evaluation of the retroperitoneum. CT remains favored over ultrasound and MRI at present due to cost and length of scanning times, and its use has led to near abandonment of lymphangiography. The ability to detect disease in lymph nodes of normal size remains a limitation.[50]

CLASSIFICATION

Cancer of the testes includes a sizeable group of diverse tumors in terms of morphology and clinical behavior. General tumor categories include GCTs (seminomas, embryonal cancers, teratomas, choriocarcinomas and yolk sac tumors), sex cord-stromal or gonadal stromal tumors, mixed germ and stromal cell tumors, adnexal and paratesticular tumors, and other malignancies such

CLINICAL FEATURES

Testicular Cancer

Classic Presentation

Nontender, enlarged testis

History

Trauma
Mumps, orchitis
Episodic testicular pain or heaviness

Symptoms

Abdominal aching
Low back pain
Gynecomastia
Breast tenderness

as mesothelioma and lymphoma. Additionally, the testes may be the site of metastatic disease.[10, 11] Approximately 95% of all testicular tumors are GCTs originating in the primordial germ cells essential for spermatogenesis, and of these more than 90% are cured. Testicular cancer is broadly divided into two groups: a pure form or a mixture of cell types. Most clinicians distinguish primarily between seminoma and nonseminoma. When both seminoma and nonseminoma are present, management is based on the nonseminoma.[103] α-Fetoprotein (AFP) and human chorionic gonadotropin (HCG) are serum tumor markers of critical importance in the diagnosis and prognosis of testicular cancer. Nonseminomas are associated with elevated HCG or AFP or both, whereas seminomas are associated with elevated serum HCG alone.[11] Elevations in lactic dehydrogenase (LDH) correlate with large-volume disease in GCTs.[50]

CLINICAL STAGING

If an intratesticular mass is identified on ultrasound or by physical examination, further evaluation is needed. The diagnostic work-up includes history and physical, urinalysis and culture/sensitivity, AFP and HCG levels, chemistry profile, and chest radiograph.[103] Radical inguinal orchiectomy follows, but patients should be counseled to attempt sperm banking before this procedure. Both clinical examination and radical orchiectomy are required for clinical staging. Staging is accomplished using the TNM system, although alternative systems such as Royal Marsden Hospital Staging Classification, and the Indiana University Staging System for Disseminated Disease are also used.

The extent of the primary tumor (T) is classified after radical orchiectomy. In testicular cancer, the most important aspect in the pathology is whether there has been invasion of the cord, epididymis, tunica albuginea, rete testis, scrotum, lymphatic system, or blood vessels.[103] An inguinal incision rather than a trans-scrotal incision is made to approach the mass. Violation of the scrotal lymphatic vessels and open biopsy are avoided to prevent lymphatic spread.[40] Trans-scrotal biopsy is contraindicated during the diagnostic evaluation because of the risk of local tumor dissemination.[83]

TREATMENT MODALITIES

Seminoma Therapy

Seminomas account for 47% of GCTs of the testis[124] and most present as clinically localized disease confined to the testis.[63] Pure seminomas exhibit dramatic radiosensitivity. Removal of the affected testicle, or radical inguinal orchiectomy, is the initial treatment for all stages of seminomas. This procedure is performed on an outpatient basis.

Following orchiectomy, stage I seminomas are treated with radiation to the retroperitoneal and ipsilateral (same side) lymph nodes.[103] The contralateral testis is shielded from the radiation beam. Prophylactic radiation to the mediastinal area is not recommended because relapse at this site is rare.[55] Surveillance has been suggested as an alternative to radiation for stage I seminoma; however, between 15% and 20% of surveillance patients relapse within 12 months.[103]

Combination chemotherapy with a cisplatin, etoposide, and bleomycin regimen is effective in treating bulky tumors. Platinum-based chemotherapy is the treatment of choice for stage II disease, advanced supradiaphragmatic adenopathy, or widespread metastatic disease.[100] Approximately 90% of patients with advanced disease will achieve cure with platinum-based chemotherapy regimens.[97, 100] Nursing considerations are directed at decreasing the treatment-induced symptomatology in the management of seminoma. After orchiectomy, measures are taken to promote comfort and to minimize postoperative morbidity. Discussions regarding concerns about body image and sexuality should be encouraged. Reassurance is needed that potency is not permanently impaired. Radiotherapy to the retroperitoneal area is generally well tolerated. Nausea and vomiting, diarrhea, myelosuppression, and azoospermia may occur as a result of the radiation or chemotherapy. Aggressive treatment with antiemetic therapy is necessary. Patients should be instructed to increase fluid intake and begin a low-residue diet that is high in protein and carbohydrates. Foods or beverages that increase GI motility should be eliminated. Measures should be taken to prevent infection and bleeding from chemotherapy-induced myelosuppression. A brief review of fertility issues follows.

Nonseminoma Therapy

The majority of nonseminomas have more than one cell type. The cell type is important for deciding chemotherapy and risk of metastases.

The cure rate for stage I disease approaches 95%. The two basic treatment options after radial inguinal orchiectomy are observation or nerve-sparing retroperitoneal lymph node dissection (RPLND).[103] Close follow-up is critical. Twenty to thirty percent of patients have disease relapse, but respond well to chemotherapy with etoposide/cisplatin, or bleomycin/etoposide/cisplatin. If RPLND reveals no nodal involvement, no adjuvant chemotherapy is administered; however, if nodes are positive, adjuvant chemotherapy is indicated for a patient who may not be willing or able to maintain close follow-up.[103] Nerve-sparing *retroperitoneal lymphadenectomy* (RPL) preserving ejaculatory ability can be performed.[47] Stage II nonseminoma is also highly curable, with success rates greater than 95%. Radical inguinal orchiectomy (avoiding scrotal violation), followed by RPLND with or without fertility-preserving technique, along with follow-up, remains a standard of care.[81] Patients with persistent tumor marker elevations following RPLND are treated with two cycles of adjuvant chemotherapy. Relapse-free survival is nearly 100%.[81, 101]

The cure rate for stage III nonseminoma with standard chemotherapy is about 70%. Patients who are not cured with standard chemotherapy usually have large, bulky disease. In advanced disease, the most common sanctuary sites are the contralateral testis and the central nervous system.[130] Patients with brain metastases are treated with chemotherapy and simultaneous whole brain irradiation and consideration of surgical excision.

Patients who do not have a complete response to first-line therapy or who have a relapse following complete response are treated with salvage therapy regimens containing cisplatin, ifosfamide, and vinblastine. Nearly 50% of these patients will achieve a complete response. Standard treatment consists of four cycles.[103]

Specific Nursing Considerations

Patients being treated for testicular cancer face unique threats to their body image and sexuality. Promoting an honest open atmosphere to enhance communication is critical. Inclusion of the patient's sexual partner in discussions should be a priority. Specific complications associated with treatment modalities are discussed in the Complications box. Fertility issues must be addressed with regard to both surgery and radiation. Inguinal orchiectomy does not affect sexual functioning or fertility. Radiotherapy with its propensity for fatigue may affect libido, but does not affect potency. Radiotherapy does, however, impair spermatogenesis. RLND is known to result in retrograde ejaculation with resultant infertility. Nerve-sparing techniques preserve anterograde ejaculation in 90% of cases.[137] Additional considerations include site specific side effects related to radiotherapy, and toxicities associated with chemotherapeutic agents, including synergistic responses.

Fertility

Testicular cancer is predominantly a disease of young men, many of whom have not yet established a family. It is estimated that between 40% and 60% of patients are hypofertile at diagnosis. Orchiectomy renders improvement, however, with 75% fertility following surgery. The mechanisms by which fertility is recovered remain unclear, but it is postulated that hormonal production (β-HCG or estrogen) by the tumor and the production of antisperm antibodies ceases.[58] Surgical treatment (after orchiectomy) appears to have little ef-

COMPLICATIONS
Testicular Cancer Disease and Treatment

Potential organ system, body image, and reproductive capacity complications associated with testicular cancer and treatment are serious and significant. Compliance is paramount to achievement of optimal success in the management of testicular tumors. With cure a likely expectation, the individual with a testicular tumor, his support network, and his clinicians are encouraged to maintain an outcome-focused approach while encouraging compliance with prescribed therapeutic regimens.

Treatment Modality	Treatment Complications
Orchiectomy Unilateral	May cause poor semen quality, body image concerns
Bilateral	Sterility, infertility
Retroperitoneal lymph node dissection (RPLND)	Body image concern, spermatogenesis deficiency
Chemotherapy	Body image concern
	Bone marrow suppression
	Organ function impairment: renal, neurologic, otologic, pulmonary
	Alopecia
	Fatigue
	Spermatogenesis impairment
Radiation therapy	Body image concern
	Spermatogenesis impairment
	Skin integrity compromise
	Fatigue

fect on spermatogenesis but may impair ejaculation. Infradiaphragmatic radiation is a common treatment used for stage I seminoma after orchiectomy, leading to concerns regarding radiation effects on the contralateral testicle. Although this testicle is shielded, studies have revealed that it received an unintended scatter dose of 78 cGy. Semen analysis revealed reductions to oligospermic levels between 1 and 4 months, and that most men were azoospermic 2.5 to 7.5 months after radiation. Semen recovery was noted for the majority of men within 7.5 to 20 months.[62] Seventy-six percent of men in one study successfully achieved paternity following infradiaphragmatic radiation with gonadal shielding, and the mean interval from orchiectomy to paternity was 4 years.[46] (See Chapter 33 for a more complete discussion of the impact of cancer on sexuality.)

Chemotherapeutic agents are especially toxic to the differentiating spermatogonia within the testes, and alkylating agents are considered to be the most toxic to the testes.[160] Both the endocrine and exocrine compo-

Nursing Management

The psychological and physical experiences of the diagnosis and treatment of testicular cancer are severe. Yet, with the remarkable success associated with aggressive treatment, the promotion of compliance with prescribed therapeutic regimens is of paramount importance. A multidisciplinary approach is necessary. Promoting an atmosphere of trust and openness is a nursing priority. Diligent attention to symptom management and quality of life issues will promote compliance with treatment.

nents of the testes are affected by chemotherapy, and the toxic effects depend on baseline testes function, the dose and duration of chemotherapy, and the age and health of the patient overall. Paternity is compromised by chemotherapy. Hansen and colleagues reported that among 22 men treated with cisplatin-based chemotherapy for testicular cancer, only 30% of those attempting conception were successful.[64] Examination of sex chromosomes after chemotherapy with mitroxantrone (Novantrone), vincristine, vinblastine, and prednisone revealed a fivefold increase in abnormalities on sperm chromosomes 8, X, and Y.[125] The clinical significance of these abnormalities is unknown, but the findings suggest that sperm banking during chemotherapy may be ill advised. Additionally, patients should be counseled to use contraceptives during chemotherapy and for a period of 3 months after its completion.[160]

At present, the most effective means to preserve fertility in patients undergoing treatment for testicular cancer is cryopreservation of sperm prior to the initiation of treatment. All specimens that demonstrate motile or viable sperm should be considered for preservation. Recent technologic advances such as in vitro fertilization (IVF) and sperm micromanipulation have made pregnancy possible even with the poorest quality sperm. Sperm recovery is independent of the time it has been cryopreserved.[160]

Treatment options exist for men who do not recover antegrade ejaculation following RPLND. Administration of sympathomimetic agents such as imipramine hydrochloride and pseudoephedrine hydrochloride several days before ejaculation have been used with varying degrees of success. Additionally new techniques allowing sperm aspiration from the vas deferens and epididymis enable anejaculatory men to achieve fertility with assistive technology such as IVF. Emerging treatments aimed at preserving fertility in testes exposed to radiation or chemotherapy include the application of a variety of hormonal regimens designed to protect spermatogenesis.[160]

Penile Cancer

EPIDEMIOLOGY

Penile carcinoma accounts for 0.3% to 0.6% of all malignancies among men in the United States, with approximately 1 to 2 cases occurring per 100,000 men each year.[133] The estimated number of new cases of penile cancer, combined with other male genital organ malignancies (but excluding testes and prostate) is 1100 for the year 2000, with an expected 300 deaths.[56] Incidence rates are higher in Asia, Africa, and South America.[118]

ETIOLOGY AND RISK FACTORS

Penile cancer is generally associated with older age, with most cases being diagnosed in men in the sixth or seventh decade of life. Cases have been reported in younger men and in children. The etiology is unknown, although several risk factors have been identified.[134] Nearly 100% of affected men are uncircumcised. A growing body of evidence links human papillomavirus (HPV), specifically HPV type 16, with the disease. Cases associated with HPV occur at a younger age.[70] Men who have been exposed to ultraviolet radiation for psoriasis treatment are also at increased risk for the development of penile cancer.[153] Phimosis and poor hygiene are commonly associated with this disorder.[118]

CLASSIFICATION

Several staging systems are currently in use: the TNM system and the Jackson system. The Jackson system involves four stages:

Stage I: tumors limited to glans and/or prepuce
Stage II: tumors invading shaft
Stage III: tumors with operable metastatic nodes
Stage IV: tumors invading adjacent structures or with inoperable nodes or distant metastases

Lesions may be further classified as precancerous, cancer in situ, or squamous cell carcinoma.

Precancerous Lesions. Condyloma acuminata are soft papillomatous growths of viral origin, known for their ability to destroy adjacent tissue. These lesions are locally highly aggressive but do not metastasize. These lesions present as leukoplakia and appear as scaly patches or plaques on the penis or urethral meatus. They may precede or coexist with carcinoma.[118]

Carcinoma in Situ. Carcinoma in situ (CIS) of the penis appears as an erythroplasia in the form of a red velvety plaque on the glans or the prepuce. The lesions may be solitary or multiple. When the plaque evolves to ulceration, it may signal the development of a carcinoma. One example is Bowen's disease.[118]

Kaposi's Sarcoma. Chun and colleagues cite 37 cases of Kaposi's sarcoma involving the glans penis in the medical literature.[28] The presentation and management of Kaposi's are discussed in Chapter 13.

Squamous Cell Carcinoma. Squamous cell carcinoma accounts for 95% of all penile cancers.[21] The growth patterns of these lesions may be superficial or vertical, with vertical being the more aggressive. Squamous cell carcinomas of the penis are usually moderately to well differentiated.

PRESENTATION AND DIAGNOSIS

Patients generally present for evaluation of an ulcerated nodule or nonhealing ulcer. Swelling or discharge from the prepuce may also precede diagnosis. Rarely, patients present with inguinal adenopathy. Diagnostic evaluation includes inspection and palpation of the penis. More than 50% of patients delay seeking evaluation for at least 6 months after the onset of their first symptoms. Lesions must be differentiated from those of sexually transmitted infectious diseases.[118] Diagnosis is established by biopsy.

Diagnostic evaluation includes urethroscopy and cavernosography with contrast media. Ultrasound examination and MRI are also used to view adjacent structures. Lymph nodes are assessed by direct palpation, with fine-needle aspiration performed on suspicious nodes. Bipedal lymphangiography and CT scanning have been unable to detect regional lymph node invasion that escapes physical examination.[68] Sentinel node biopsy is under investigation; however, there have been reports of inguinal metastases following sentinel node biopsy.[115]

Metastasis generally occurs throughout the lymphatic channels by lymphatic embolization. Pelvic lymph node metastasis occurs only in the presence of inguinal node involvement. Depth of tumor invasion and tumor grade are directly related to nodal metastases.[95] The tumors may invade the penile urethra. If death occurs, it is caused by local complications such as hemorrhage from ulcerated metastases or infection. Death secondary to systemic complications of widely disseminated disease is extremely rare.[118]

TREATMENT

Treatment of penile carcinoma is controversial. Survival depends primarily on nodal metastases, yet there is a lack of consensus on the optimal management of regional lymph nodes. Radical inguinal or ileoinguinal

lymphadenectomy can cure 40% to 50% of patients with positive nodes, but approximately half of the patients with clinically enlarged nodes have no metastases in actuality.[34, 118] The standard treatment for T1 to T4 lesions is partial amputation. For those tumors limited entirely to the foreskin, circumcision is sufficient treatment. In the case of partial penectomy, a 2-cm margin is necessary to prevent local metastases.[133] Partial penectomies leave a stump of less than 3 cm, resulting in problems such as spraying during micturition. When penile lesions are located at the base, a total penectomy with creation of a perineal urethrostomy is the treatment of choice. One of the most common and life-threatening complications of penectomy (partial or total) is hemorrhage. Technique refinements reported by Samm and Steiner may minimize this complication.[133] More conservative surgical approaches focusing on tumor excision while maintaining organ form and function are receiving attention in the literature[34, 134] along with multimodality therapy including laser hyperthermia, chemotherapy, and radiation.[138]

Laser surgery is routinely performed for superficial lesions, precancerous lesions, and CIS. The carbon dioxide laser is preferred over the YAG laser. The procedure is performed under local anesthesia. Circumcision is also recommended.[118]

Radiotherapy offers a conservative approach for T1N1 tumors less than 4 cm in diameter. Both external beam and brachytherapy are used. Circumcision is performed before brachytherapy. Complications following radiotherapy are common. Acute reactions include edema, mucositis, and local infections. Circumcision, diligent hygiene, and antibiotic therapy may minimize these complications. Later complications include telangiectasia and discoloration and superficial necrosis in up to 40% of cases. Urethral meatus stenosis is the most frequent late complication, occurring in up to 30% of cases.[51] Treatment of urethral meatal stenosis involves dilation or surgical repair. Deep fibrosis is dose and volume dependent, generally confined to those patients with tumors greater than 4 cm. Necrosis is the most serious complication related to radiotherapy. It occurs following biopsy in previously irradiated areas. Necrosis is volume and dose dependent and is more frequent among patients treated with brachytherapy versus external beam therapy.[38] Necrotic lesions generally heal poorly and require amputation in up to 50% of cases.[118]

Squamous cell penile tumors do respond to chemotherapy. Bleomycin, methotrexate, and cisplatin are among the most commonly used agents, in combination with radiotherapy or laser surgery as an option to partial or total penectomy.[60, 118] Toxicity from these agents remains a problem.

The focus of treatment for advanced disease is palliation. Combination therapy is the most effective treatment at present for advanced disease.[118] Responses are of short duration.

Long-term survival of patients with penile cancer is directly related to nodal status. Five-year disease-free survival approaches 85% among those with negative nodes as compared to 56% among those with unilateral nodal metastases only.[154]

Bladder Cancer

EPIDEMIOLOGY

Bladder carcinoma is the most common malignant tumor of the urinary tract, with approximately 53,200 new cases and 12,200 deaths anticipated in the United States in the year 2000.[56] Incidence rates are high in African counties, most especially in Egypt, where schistosomiasis is endemic. Incidence rates within the United States have continued to increase; however, trends in 5-year disease-free survival indicate modest but steady improvement in survival for both whites and African Americans. African Americans continue to lag behind in the area of survival with 62% 5-year relative cancer survival as compared to 82% among whites.[56] Improvements in survival can be attributed to a stage migration to more localized disease and to treatment.[32] There is a marked male predominance. Within the United States 38,300 new cases will be diagnosed among men as compared to 14,900 new cases among women.[56] Bladder cancers are rarely diagnosed before the age of 40, the median age of diagnosis being 65 years.[135]

ETIOLOGY AND RISK FACTORS

The first reports linking chemical carcinogenic exposure to bladder cancer date back to 1895 when Rehn reported three cases of bladder cancer among workers in a German dye factory. Since then, numerous investigations have demonstrated a relationship between bladder cancer and exposure to aromatic amines. Specific compounds that have been identified include 2-naphthylamine, 4-aminobiophenyl, benzidine, chlornaphazine, and 4-chloro-o-toludine.[31, 149] These chemicals are used in textile, rubber and cable, paint, and printing industries. Occupational exposures are believed to account for 25% of the cases among whites and 10% of cases among nonwhites in the United States.[163] Cigarette smoking is considered the most significant risk factor, contributing to more than 50% of cases. The mechanism by which damage occurs is thought to be related to changes in the uroepithelium, and cellular changes are dose and duration sensitive. Some occupations are associated with higher than average risk, including aluminum workers, motor vehicle operators,

drycleaners, chemical workers, pesticide applicators, miners, chimney sweeps, and cooks.[59, 139, 140, 149, 151, 157]

A high consumption of fried meats and fats has been associated with increased risk. Increased consumption of vitamin A may be protective.[150] A combination of vitamins A, B_6, E, and zinc has been suggested to be highly protective.[75] The risk posed by artificial sweeteners and coffee remains a controversial topic. Exposure to certain drugs such as phenacetin and cyclophosphamide is associated with increased risk.[82, 141] Infection with *Shistosoma haemotobium* is associated with increased risk of both transitional and squamous cell bladder carcinoma.[141] Recurrent urinary tract infections have been associated with increased risk of squamous cell carcinoma, especially among paraplegics with indwelling Foley catheters and recurrent bladder calculi.[77] Genetic changes are well documented in bladder cancer. The loss of the long arm of chromosome 9 appears in all grades, and alterations in p53 have been noted.[113]

CLASSIFICATION—TERMINOLOGY UPDATE

There has been a recent concerted effort by the World Health Organization (WHO) and the International Society of Urologic Pathology (ISUP) to standardize classification and grading terminology in an effort to foster worldwide communication and comparison. They have recommended that the term "transitional cell" be replaced with "urothelial" or "urothelium"; thus, the current terminology is "urothelial carcinoma."[13] They further recommend that the term "superficial" also be abandoned. Although these are the current recommendations, the use of these terms has not yet become fully accepted. Tumors are now classified as flat or papillary neoplasms. The two staging systems currently in use are the Jewett-Strong system,[72] which was later modified by Marshall,[92] and the AJCC system.[5] Box 10-1 presents the revised terminology for bladder neoplasms.

Urothelial carcinoma (formerly called transitional cell carcinoma) is the most common carcinoma of the bladder in the United States, accounting for 90% of cases. The remainder of bladder cancers are squamous cell carcinoma (5%) and adenocarcinoma (<1%). The most significant prognostic indicators include the depth of invasion at presentation, multifocality, history of prior uroepithelial lesions, tumor size, and tumor grade.[123] Pathologic grade based on cell atypia, nuclear abnormalities, and number of mitotic features is of great prognostic importance.

CLINICAL FEATURES

The most common presenting sign of bladder cancer is gross hematuria. This hematuria is often described as "painless," and bladder irritability (urgency, dysuria, or

---

BOX 1 0 – 1

Revised Terminology—Bladder Neoplasms

PAPILLARY UROTHELIAL NEOPLASMS OF THE BLADDER

New Terminology	*Old Terminology*
Papilloma	Papilloma
Papillary neoplasia of low malignant potential	Grade 1 carcinoma
Low-grade carcinoma	Grade 2 carcinoma
High-grade carcinoma	Grade 3 carcinoma

FLAT UROEPITHELIAL NEOPLASMS OF THE BLADDER

Reactive atypia
Atypia of uncertain clinical significance
Dysplasia
Carcinoma In situ

Adapted from Bostwick DG and others: Diagnosis and grading of bladder cancer and associated lesions, *Urol Clin North Am* 26:493, 1999.

---

frequency) is likely to be present. Intermittent bleeding is characteristic and may lead to delayed diagnosis as either the patient or physician may postpone further investigation if the urine clears. Because urinary tract infections (UTIs) are often seen, patients with cancer of the bladder are treated with antibiotics for what is thought to be hemorrhagic cystitis, a common phenomenon in women. The presence of unexplained gross or microscopic hematuria should always be evaluated. Obstructive symptoms are associated with large tumor burden or metastases. Tumor pushing on the urethral orifice may cause urinary hesitancy or decrease in stream force. Patients may experience flank pain caused by hydronephrosis if ureteral obstruction occurs. Back pain, rectal pain, or suprapubic pain may suggest metastatic disease.

DIAGNOSIS

Physical examination generally reveals no suggestive signs of bladder cancer, although rarely a mass may be detected on rectal examination. The diagnostic steps indicated in a patient with hematuria include urinalysis, intravenous pyelogram (IVP; also referred to as an excretory urogram), cystoscopy, and urine cytology. IVP allows for visualization of the upper tracts to help exclude a nonvesical source of hematuria and to determine if there is any evidence of obstruction or a persistent bladder-filling defect.

Cystoscopy is used to verify the presence of a bladder tumor and to characterize its gross appearance and as a means of obtaining a biopsy specimen. Areas of erythema may represent CIS. Cystoscopy with multiple random bladder biopsies is performed with the patient under local anesthesia using an intraurethral topical anesthetic with or without intravenous sedation. Associated procedures, such as transurethral resection, bimanual examination, or retrograde studies of the upper tracts, are more readily performed with the patient sedated. A bimanual pelvic examination helps to determine the presence of a palpable or fixed mass. In addition to tissue biopsies, cells may be captured from bladder mucosa through bladder washings or voided urine, because malignant cells from urinary epithelial surfaces exhibit characteristic morphologic changes.

Flow cytometry, a technique that allows examination of the DNA content of cells within the urine, is useful for providing information for staging and grading purposes. Flow cytometry can be performed on bladder wash specimens, urine specimens, and biopsy specimens. High grade and aneuploidy (large amounts of DNA per cell) are associated with poor prognosis.

A wide array of tumor markers have been identified, including blood group antigens, tumor-associated and proliferating antigens, oncogenes, peptide growth factors, and factors promoting and inhibiting angiogenesis. Additionally cellular adhesion molecules and cell cycle regulatory proteins have recently been identified.[147] These biomarkers may prove to be critical prognostic

CLINICAL FEATURES

Bladder Cancer

Classic Presentation

Hematuria
　Solitary
　Recurrent
Infection
　Absent
　Present

History

Exogenous exposure
　Present
　Absent
Tobacco habit
　Present
　Absent

Symptoms

Vesical irritability
　Frequency
　Spasms
　Pain

indicators, suggesting not only the predicted clinical course of the disease, but response to treatment as well.

If the tumor is invasive additional studies may be indicated, including abdominal and pelvic CT scans, chest x-ray films, and bone scans if metastases are suspected. Urine cytology may be of screening value in industrial settings and can be used to detect lesions at an early stage of follow-up. DNA flow cytometry of urine may be used as a diagnostic and screening mechanism in high-risk patients. Clinical staging, even with CT or MRI, often underestimates the extent of tumor.

TREATMENT

The management of bladder cancer is based on multiple factors. Recurrence and progression depend on the initial anatomic and histologic classification, the depth of invasion at presentation, multifocality, history of prior uroepithelial lesions, tumor size, and tumor grade.[123] The patient's age and general stage of health, functional status, self-care abilities and personal preferences, and presence of associated GU problems (e.g., UTI, ureteral obstruction, and compromised renal function) factor into the treatment decision. Treatment planning is based on the depth and degree to which the cancer has penetrated into the bladder wall. Before treatment it is essential to determine if the tumor has seeded downward from the renal pelvis or has originated as a ureteral primary tumor. Metastasis occurs by lymphatic and hematogeneous routes and usually spreads to the lymph nodes, liver, lung, and bones.

The bladder is also a common site for contiguous spread from malignant lesions of neighboring viscera, most notably the uterine cervix and prostate. The bladder may be invaded by carcinoma of the sigmoid colon, rectum, or uterine body. Secondary tumors can promote urinary irritative symptoms or obstruction. The Complications box outlines treatment-specific complications of bladder cancer.

Noninvasive Tumors

Historically, most patients with noninvasive stage I bladder cancer have been managed with transurethral resection (TUR) and fulguration with or without intravesical therapy. Treatment of multiple papillary uroepithelial (transitional) cell lesions with TUR depends on the tumor's location and size. Most surgeons begin removing lesions at the dome of the bladder. With this method, if bleeding occurs, it drains to the bladder base, not obscuring the surgeon's vision. Tumors that cannot be removed by standard TUR require cystectomy. Following resection, an indwelling catheter may be left in place. The catheter may be connected to gravity drainage or a continuous irrigation system. The catheter is left in place for 2 to 3 days or until the urine is clear. It is

---

◆ **COMPLICATIONS**

Bladder Cancer Treatment

Treatment Modality	Treatment Complications
Intravesical therapy	Body image concerns
	Myelosuppression
	Irritative symptoms
Radical cystectomy	Body image concerns
	Loss of body function
	Sexuality/sensuality disturbance
Systemic chemotherapy	Body image concerns
	Bone marrow suppression
	Organ function impairment: renal, cardiac, neurologic
	Alopecia
	Fatigue

---

important to monitor the patient for any signs of clot retention and urinary outlet obstruction. Patients should be informed that they may experience some bleeding on urination as the postoperative site heals.

Chemotherapeutic or immunotherapeutic agents may be instilled directly into the bladder postoperatively. Intravesical chemotherapy is believed to offer an advantage over systemic chemotherapy because it allows active agents to come into direct contact with the uroepithelium. Additionally this mode of delivery reduces the occurrence of systemic toxicity, although this varies depending on the agents selected.[32] The goal of intravesical therapy is to prevent tumor recurrence or progression after TUR of the primary lesion and to treat possible residual tumor after resection. The most common indication is prophylactic use because 50% to 70% of patients will have recurrence when treated with TUR.[41] Intravesical therapy usually begins within 10 to 14 days after resection. Patient preparation involves restricting fluids in an attempt to limit urine output and to facilitate retention of chemotherapy or immunotherapy for the requisite 2 hours. A urinalysis is performed before the procedure; infection is a contraindication. A Foley catheter is inserted. Topical lidocaine may be applied to the urethra to minimize discomfort. The prescribed agents are slowly instilled into the catheter by gravity. The catheter is clamped to retain the therapeutic agents, and patients are repositioned every 30 minutes to allow maximal bladder tissue exposure. Following catheter removal, patients may be discharged and instructed to increase fluid intake to flush residual medication from the bladder and minimize irritation. Patients receiving Bacille Calmette-Guérin (BCG) must remain at the treatment center until they have voided to ensure proper disposal of contaminated urine. Patients are instructed that burning, frequency, and urgency are expected side effects. These may be managed with topical anesthetics and nonsteroidal anti-inflammatory agents. Blood in the urine or any signs of infection should be reported to the health care provider immediately.[49] A number of drugs are used for intravesical therapy. Examples of agents in current use include thiotepa, doxorubicin, mitomycin C, epirubicin, ethoglucid, and mitoxantrone.[41] BCG is considered one of the most effective therapies; however, treatment and maintenance schedules and optimal dose have not been established.[33] Two drug combinations are also used. Interleukin-12 (IL-12), either alone or in combination with radiotherapy, has been used and phase I clinical trials are now in progress. There is a lack of scientific evidence to suggest the superiority of any one drug. IL-12 is also being used in gene therapy models in vivo.[29]

Patients are followed postoperatively with periodic cystoscopies and bladder washings for cytology, usually every 3 months for the first year and at 6-month intervals for the next 2 years. If cystoscopies and cytologies are negative, the patient then undergoes cystoscopy annually. Electrocautery or electorfulguration may be performed on patients who have been previously diagnosed with appropriate biopsies and experience recurrent lesions. This procedure is used on small lesions 2 to 3 mm in size or when lesions are located near the bladder neck and are not accessible to resection. The major problem with fulguration is that it destroys cellular morphology and does not provide adequate information on the depth of invasion.

Laser treatment and photodynamic therapy may be used for patients with recurrent localized disease. The YAG lasers have been most widely used. Results are comparable to those achieved by electrocautery, with tumor recurrence rates of up to 18% at 1 year.[67, 90] The procedure is bloodless and requires only local anesthesia. The disadvantage is the cost and availability of the equipment. Photodynamic therapy with intravenous porfimer sodium (Photofrin) is used as a sensitizer 2 to 3 days before ultraviolet illumination of the whole bladder. The procedure is performed in the operating room under general or spinal anesthesia. Nursing care involves patient teaching and management of side effects. Patients experience irritative bladder symptoms that generally peak on the second day after treatment. Symptoms can be relieved with antispasmodic agents and topical anesthetics. Sun exposure can result in severe sunburn. Patients should be instructed to avoid sunlight exposure for 8 weeks after treatment. Current use of this therapy is mainly confined to patients who are refractory to conventional intravesical therapy.[170]

Invasive Tumors

The standard treatment for tumors invading the muscle is surgical removal of the bladder by radical cystectomy. If distant disease is detected on MRI, CT, or bone scan, systemic treatment is required. In the absence of distant disease, an exploratory laparotomy with pelvic node dissection is performed. The cystectomy will generally not be performed if nodal involvement within the pelvis is detected. For men, the procedure involves a cystoprostatectomy. Women undergo both cystectomy and hysterectomy. Urinary diversions are created in the form of ileal conduits or by directing urine flow into an internal urinary reservoir with drainage to the abdominal wall or to the urethra.[135]

The *ileal conduit* is constructed from a small piece of bowel. The ureters are anchored into the ileal conduit, which protrudes through the skin as a bud stoma in the right lower quadrant for application of an external ileostomy drainage device (Fig. 10–4). *Continent diversion* has been used successfully in selected male and female populations. In a Kock pouch procedure a midportion of isolated ileum is folded and opened onto itself, creating a continent pouch with a nipple-valve stoma.[142] The stoma is generally below the undergarment line. A small gauze pad may cover the stoma, which provides access for intermittent catheterization by the individual approximately every 6 hours.

Preoperative consultation and education with an enterostomal therapist (ET) are essential to treatment and rehabilitation. Pretreatment management of the ileal stoma site should be done jointly with the surgeon and the ET while the patient is in the supine, sitting, and standing positions. Optimal stomal placement is crucial for postoperative management. The standard of care for urinary diversion focuses on patient adjustment to body image and quality of life. The surgeon positions the ileostomy location below the belt line and close to the pubis for concealment, because these patients do not wear external appliances. If cosmetic concealment is not a significant concern to the patient, placement higher on the abdominal wall may make intermittent catheterization easier. The criteria for urinary diversions are outlined in Box 10–2.

Bladder-sparing options include aggressive endoscopic resection alone or resection followed by chemotherapy or radiation. The decision to spare the bladder is based on the location, depth and size of the lesion, and the status of the noninvolved uroepithelium.[135] Radiation delivered after surgery or with chemotherapy may intensify the effects and delay tissue healing. Therefore, treatment is withheld for 4 to 6 weeks postoperatively.

Early reactions to radiation usually occur during the first 3 or 4 weeks of therapy and tend to resolve within

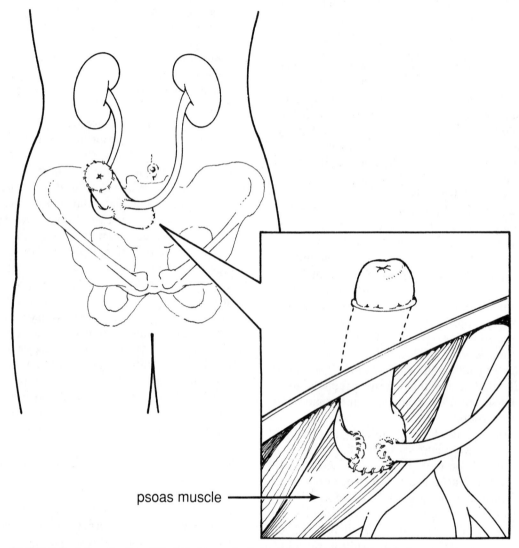

FIGURE 10–4 Completed ileal loop. Ileal conduit has been anchored to psoas muscle, and ureters lie without tension or angulation. A protruding bud stoma has been created. (Modified from Richie JP: Techniques of ureterointestinal anastomoses and conduit construction. In Crawford ED, Borden TA, editors: *Genitourinary cancer surgery*, Philadelphia, Lea & Febiger, 1982.)

BOX 10-2

Criteria for Continent Urinary Diversions

1. The reservoir substitute for the lower tract should collect and store urine under low pressure.
2. The diversion must prevent reflux into the upper urinary tracts.
3. The diversion should not cause recurrent infections from stasis or reflux.
4. The diversion should not cause fluid and electrolyte or acid–base imbalances.
5. Malabsorption nutritional disorders should be minimized.
6. Continence should be maintained so that patients can control emptying of the reservoir at socially acceptable and convenient intervals.

4 weeks of completion. Urinary frequency, urgency, and dysuria may occur as bladder capacity is reduced. Hematuria may result from mucosal inflammation. Patients occasionally require a respite from treatment as symptoms intensify or as skin integrity becomes compromised. Pharmacologic treatments provide relief and are used to prevent infection. Antispasmodics or parasympathetic blockers provide relief of symptoms and promote analgesia. Patients are instructed to empty the bladder frequently and increase intake of fluids, such as water and cranberry juice. Caffeine, alcohol, tobacco, and spices tend to irritate the bladder mucosa and should be avoided.

Late effects of radiation occur 1 year or more after treatment. Internal fibrosis, telangiectasia, chronic urinary frequency, and permanent diminished bladder capacity may occur. Combined modalities of surgery and radiotherapy may lead to fistula formation, although the occurrence is rare. Development of a fistula after treatment may indicate tumor recurrence.

Neither chemotherapy nor radiotherapy alone are standard options for invasive bladder cancer. Treatment with concurrent chemotherapy and radiotherapy has been associated with improved rates of local control compared with radiotherapy alone. Multiple trials are in progress to evaluate the role of chemotherapy administered before cystectomy, after cystectomy, or in conjunction with radiotherapy to improve local disease, prevent distant metastases, or preserve the bladder. Chemotherapy regimens in current usage include CAP (cyclophosphamide, Adriamycin, cisplatin); MVAC (methotrexate, vinblastine, doxorubicin [Adriamycin], cisplatin); and MVEC (methotrexate, vinblastine, epirubicin, cisplatin).[135]

Stage III disease carries a high risk for extramural tumor and lymph node involvement. Preoperative radiotherapy followed by radical cystectomy has been widely used for stage III cancer. Because the frequency of distant metastases is becoming apparent with improved surgical techniques, systemic preoperative or postoperative chemotherapy is now being evaluated in clinical trials. To date, improved rates of local control have been achieved using a combination of cisplatin and external beam radiotherapy.

Currently, only a small percentage of patients with advanced stage IV bladder cancer can be cured. The prognosis of patients with T4 tumors is generally poor with either radical cystectomy or radiotherapy. The focus of care for many stage IV patients should be on symptom management and supportive care. Urinary diversion may be indicated not only for palliation of symptoms related to bladder tumors, bleeding, and pain, but also for preservation of renal function in patients who are candidates for chemotherapy. Because of the overall poor results with drug treatment, patients with meta-

Nursing Management

Reduction of risk factors associated with development and promotion of bladder neoplasms is necessary. Nurses must continue their efforts promoting smoking cessation.

Approximately 80% of bladder cancers are superficial when first diagnosed. These superficial presentations have a demonstrated pattern of recurrence. Patients should be encouraged to view the disease as a chronic process requiring a life-time pattern of serial cystoscopies, cytology, surgical resection for pathologic evaluation of suspicious lesions, and intravesical chemotherapy as indicated. Postponement of potentially curative therapy (i.e., radical cystectomy) in the event of bladder cancer locally confined to the muscularis may render salvage therapy useless. The development of measures to promote patient compliance to established regimens of surveillance in superficial bladder cancer for early detection and initiation of effective therapy with recurrences is suggested as an area for nursing research. This need is underscored by the high mortality rate associated with bladder cancer.

static disease should be provided with the opportunity to participate in clinical research trials.

Renal Cell Cancer

EPIDEMIOLOGY

Approximately 3% of all tumors diagnosed in the United States each year are tumors of the kidney. Thirty-one thousand new cases are expected within the year 2000, and renal cancer is expected to cause 11,900 deaths during that same period. The ratio of men to women is 1.5:1.[56] It is estimated that renal cell carcinoma is increasing worldwide at a rate of approximately 2% yearly.[9] In adults, most cases occur in persons aged 50 to 60 years, but cases have been reported in children as young as 6 months.[85]

ETIOLOGY AND RISK FACTORS

The etiology of renal cancer is unknown. Associated abnormalities include deviations involving chromosome 3, p53, and the VHL gene.[20] A wide variety of environmental, genetic, cellular, and hormonal factors have been examined, including obesity, dietary fat intake, tobacco use, phenacetin, and occupational exposures to asbestos and petroleum. Numerous epidemiologic studies suggest that tobacco may play a significant role. An increase in renal cell carcinoma has been observed among persons with autosomal dominant polycystic kidney disease and tuberous sclerosis.[96, 171] Up to 35% of patients with von Hippel-Lindau disease develop renal cell carcinoma.[85]

CLASSIFICATION AND STAGING

Two staging systems are applied to renal cell carcinoma, the Robson Modification of the Flocks/Kadefsky Staging System[127] and the AJCC TNM system.[5] The staging system for renal cell cancer is based on the degree of tumor spread beyond the kidney. Blood vessel involvement may not always be a poor prognostic indicator. The TNM system defined by the AJCC can be abbreviated into a tumor stage grouping as follows: T1, tumor confined to the kidney and capsule; T2, tumor larger than 2.5 cm and limited to the kidney; T3, tumor extending into major veins or exhibiting perinephric invasion; and T4, tumor invading beyond Gerota's fascia.

CLINICAL FEATURES

Renal cell carcinomas arise from the proximal convoluted tubule epithelium and are adenocarcinomas. Renal cell carcinomas are historically characterized by a mixture of clear, granular, or spindle-like sarcomatoid cells arranged in solid, cystic, tubular, or papillary patterns. More than 95% of parenchymal tumors are adenocarcinomas and are referred to as hypernephroma, *renal cell carcinoma, clear cell cancer,* or Grawitz tumor. Squamous cell carcinoma and nephroblastoma are also identified.[37] Wilms' tumor occurs in children. Renal carcinomas locally invade the capsule, are highly angioinvasive and often spread to the renal vein and vena cava, and result in widespread hematogeneous and lymphatic metastases. The most common sites for nonlymphatic metastases are lung, bone, liver, and brain. Renal cell carcinoma can metastasize to unusual sites, such as the testes and skin. Renal cell carcinomas have been reported to regress spontaneously.

DIAGNOSIS

The classic triad of hematuria, palpable flank mass, and costovertebral pain is associated with advanced tumors and occurs in only 10% to 20% of patients.[20] Analgesics generally relieve the pain. Pain unresponsive to additional treatments may indicate invasion of adjacent muscle and nerve routes. Early stage renal cell cancer is usually "silent" and is coincidentally detected when the patient is undergoing work-up for a non–cancer-related procedure such as cardiac angiography or gallbladder ultrasound. There appears to be high variability in symptom presentation. Up to 88% of patients with the disease have hypochromic anemia as a result of hemolysis or hematuria.[85] Renal cell carcinomas are known to secrete hormones, including parathyroid hormone and erythropoietin, resulting in hypercalcemia and erythrocytosis. Hypertension is typically encountered and may be mediated by tumor secretion of renin.

Nursing Management

With the identification of certain etiologic factors, lifestyle or environmental modification to decrease the risk of developing kidney cancer is a reasonable goal. Specifically, encouraging cessation or moderation of tobacco use, promoting advoidance of developing a tobacco habit in youth, and stressing dietary modification to decrease or limit high-fat content are positive steps in decreasing cancer risk. Minimizing occupational or life-style exposure to petrochemicals is also suggested.

CLINICAL FEATURES

Renal Cell Cancer

Pain
Hematuria
   Intermittent
   Uncontrolled
Anemia
Fever
Fatigue

Unfortunately, approximately one third of patients have metastases at diagnosis. The most common metastatic sites are the lungs (75%), soft tissues (36%), bones (20%), and the liver (18%).[89]

Box 10–3 details paraneoplastic syndromes associated with renal cancer.

The differential diagnosis includes a variety of conditions including benign inflammatory processes such as abscess and pyelonephritis; additionally, hematomas, cystic masses, and hydronephrosis must be considered. CT, MRI, ultrasound, arteriography, and excretory urography are used in the diagnostic process. Venacavo-grams provide information regarding tumor involvement of the vena cava.[20] MRI is replacing this modality. Bone scans are not routinely performed unless the patient specifically complains of bone pain or an elevation of serum alkaline phosphatase is noted.[101] CT-guided fine-needle biopsy is the current diagnostic standard.

TREATMENT MODALITIES

State-of-the-art treatment using surgery cures more than half the patients with early stage renal cell cancer. Poor prognosis is associated with stage IV disease as a result of the tumor's lack of sensitivity to existing chemotherapy and radiotherapy. Patients with advanced disease should be considered for clinical experimental protocols.

Surgery

For more than two decades, *radical nephrectomy* has proved to be an efficient treatment modality for localized renal carcinomas. Surgical resection is the standard curative therapy for stage I or II renal cell carcinoma. Resection may be simple or radical. In a radical nephrectomy the kidney, perinephric fat, Gerota capsule, and regional nodes are removed, as well as the adjacent adrenal gland. Nephron-sparing surgery is indicated in cases when a radical nephrectomy would render a patient functionally anephric requiring dialysis such as in the case of patients with only a single kidney or bilateral renal carcinoma.[101]

Nephrectomy remains the standard of care for patients with stage III renal disease. The focus of care for patients with stage IV disease is palliation. Following radical nephrectomy 20% to 30% of patients with localized tumors will experience relapse. Median time to relapse is 1 to 2 years. Attempts to delay relapse have included adjuvant radiotherapy or systemic therapy including α-interferon. As yet there has been no demonstrated benefit from the addition of these treatment modalities[101] other than symptom control among patients with advanced disease.[20] Renal cell carcinoma is largely refractory to chemotherapy. Clinical trials using circadian-based floxuridine (FUDR) infusions have yielded limited success.[39] Clinical trials continue to investigate the use of cytokine therapy consisting of α-interferon and IL-2. Gene therapy is also under investigation and may provide new options in the future.

PROGNOSIS

Unfortunately, the prognosis for any patient with treated renal cell cancer who has relapsing, recurring, or progressing disease, regardless of stage or cell type, is poor. Survival is equated with early diagnosis of incident carcinoma. Local recurrence occurs infrequently, and

---

BOX 10–3

Syndromes Associated with Renal Carcinomas

SYNDROMES

Hypercalcemia
Nonmetastatic hepatopathy
Hypertension
Erythrocytosis
Pyrexia
Galactorrhea
Cushing's syndrome
Gynecomastia
Serum glucose abnormalities

SEROLOGIC FACTORS AND OTHER SYNDROMES

Prostaglandins
Alkaline phosphatase
Neuromyopathy
Amyloidosis
Coagulation factors
Iron metabolism
α-Fetoprotein
Vasculitis
Fibroblast growth factor

From Sufrin G and others: Paraneoplastic and serologic syndromes of renal adenocarcinoma, *Semin Urol* 7(3):159, 1989.

failure is related to metastatic disease through nodal or hematogeneous spread.

CONCLUSION

Genitourinary malignancies represent a broad array of carcinomas. Although prostate cancer represents the most frequently diagnosed male malignancy, penile cancers represent less than 1% of all male malignancies. Despite the variability in incidence and prognosis, each of the GU malignancies represents a significant threat to mortality and quality of life. The uniqueness of this group of malignancies lies in intense threat to body image and sexuality. Although it is encouraging to note the major treatment advances over the past decade, and the emerging treatment options, it is more encouraging still to note the increased emphasis on quality of life. Nurses are challenged to retain and refine their focus on quality of life, especially in the face of increasingly aggressive multimodality therapy.

Acknowledgments. The contributor would like to acknowledge the authors of this chapter in previous editions: Marilyn Davis and Jeanne Parzuchowski.

Nursing Management

The following focus points include the diagnostic phase, initiation and completion of therapy, evaluation of response to therapy, introduction of a new treatment modality, discovery of metastatic or recurrent disease, and finally the exhaustion of all viable treatment options. Nursing interventions are predicated on continuous acknowledgment of the individuality of each patient, maintenance of a patient-centered focus rather than a disease-centered approach, and awareness of predictable points in the cancer continuum that may precipitate or exacerbate stress.

The selected nursing diagnoses include anxiety, health-seeking behaviors, altered urinary elimination, and altered sexuality patterns. Interventions follow each diagnostic grouping as a guide for creation of evaluative and therapeutic nursing strategies. The Teaching Priorities box lists teaching priorities for prevention, early detection, and risk modification tactics.

Nursing Diagnosis

- *Anxiety related to:*
    GU cancer incidence and mortality rates
    Screening (digital rectal examination [DRE], testicular self-examination [TSE], physical examination)
    Diagnostic procedures: biopsies for histologic and cytologic review
    Staging extent of disease: imaging modalities
    Localized disease: surgery, radiation therapy, laser therapy, bladder instillation of chemotherapy and biologic response modifier (BRM) therapy
    Locally, regionally advanced, or metastatic disease: radical surgery, radiation therapy, chemotherapy, BRM therapy, hormonal therapy
    Continuing care: encounters with health care professionals and systems, outcome or response to therapy, finances
    Supportive care: pain control, maintenance of independence, nutrition, mobility, quality of life issues

Outcome Goal

Patient will be able to:

- Demonstrate decreased anxiety and be knowledgeable of planned treatment.

Interventions

- Review purpose of surgery, radiation therapy, che-

PATIENT TEACHING PRIORITIES

Genitourinary Cancers

Prevention

Avoid or limit exposure to exogenous carcinogens.
Discourage development of tobacco habits.
Maintain low-fat diet.

Early Detection

Encourage early investigation of GU findings, such as mass, pain, hematuria, and altered urinary patterns.
American Cancer Society (ACS) screening guidelines
Perform monthly TSE.
Annual DRE (men 40 years and older)
Annual prostate-specific antigen (PSA) test (men 50 years and older).

Risk Modification

Encourage cessation or moderation of tobacco habits.
Avoid obesity.
Limit exposure to petrochemicals.

motherapy, hormonal therapy, and BRM therapy treatments and rationale for treatment.
- Explain common terms and procedures, provide written literature, and show actual equipment.
- Familiarize patient with terminology, equipment, simulation, dosimetry port films, linear accelerator, and implants.
- Discuss potential sequelae of radiation, surgery, and chemotherapy, such as alteration in skin integrity and change in elimination patterns.
- Explain role of various medical personnel with whom patient will interact.
- Allow time for discussions, write down key words or expressions, and provide diagrams or models reviewing anatomic and physiologic functions for clarification.
- Encourage patient to write down questions as they arise, and discuss concerns about cancer and the treatment as a strategy for eliciting individual concerns.
- Elicit degree of comprehension and comfort using a technique for recall of information previously presented.

Nursing Diagnosis

- *Health-seeking behaviors related to:*
  Prevention or risk reduction in development of GU cancers, specifically bladder and kidney cancer
  Promotion of early detection:
  Monthly TSE
  Annual DRE for men 40 years and older
  Annual PSA testing

Outcome Goals

Patient will be able to:

- Effectively communicate feelings, demonstrate ability to perform self-care, and seek assistance as necessary.
- State name, type, and description of treatment, reason for therapy, expected outcomes and potential side effects, and professionals involved.

Interventions

- Encourage cessation or moderation of tobacco habits.
- Discourage development of tobacco habits.
- Promote low-fat diet.
- Avoid or minimize exposure to exogenous chemicals or agents known to be associated with initiation or promotion of malignancies.

- Encourage early investigation of any GU findings, including a mass, pain, hematuria, or alteration of urinary patterns.
- Provide current and accurate information on diagnostic and therapeutic modalities.
- Encourage positive outlook with a view of the positive statistics on disease remission or disease stabilization.

Nursing Diagnosis

- *Elimination, altered, related to:*
  Decreased bladder capacity secondary to partial cystectomy, instillation of intravesical agents, radiation
  Urinary diversion: radical cystectomy with ileal conduit or continence techniques
  Obstruction: cancerous tissue growth or edematous or fibrous tissue reaction to therapy
  Retention: possible chronic or intermittent catheterization after prostatectomy or drug therapy (e.g., antihistamines, epidural analgesics)
  Incontinence from urethral instrumentation or after prostatectomy
  Increased gastrointestinal motility secondary to radiation therapy

Outcome Goals

Patient will be able to:

- Monitor changes in patterns of elimination and report to health care provider.
- Adhere to diet as recommended.
- Report rectal bleeding, diarrhea, tenesmus, abdominal discomfort, urinary frequency, nocturia, urinary urgency, dysuria, hematuria, or lower back pain.
- Communicate feelings about body image changes.

Interventions

- Promote acceptance of change in body image secondary to disease or treatment process.
- Provide information and ensure continuing care for the individual with a urinary diversion.
- Provide resource and referral information for patients on a bladder catheterization program and those experiencing any degree of incontinence.
- Instruct patient about signs and symptoms of cystitis and avoidance of foods that irritate the bladder lining.
- Assess and document ongoing patterns of bowel elimination.
- Teach patient signs and symptoms of proctitis.
- Instruct on use of topic anesthetic agents.
- Teach Kegel exercises.

- Monitor weight and nutritional status weekly, and observe for evidence of fluid volume depletion. Provide patient with low-residue, high-protein, and high-carbohydrate diet.

Nursing Diagnosis

- *Sexuality patterns, altered, related to:*
    Pathophysiologic changes associated with cancer or treatment
    Surgery: unilateral or bilateral orchiectomy, transurethral resection, modified or extensive node dissection, interruption of neural pathways essential for potency preservation
    Radiation therapy: interstitial prostatic implants or external beam therapy
    Hormonal manipulation
    Chemotherapy
    BRM therapy
- *Self-image and self-esteem disturbances related to:*
    Diagnosis
    Loss of body part or function
    Potential loss of autonomy and independence
    Financial concerns
    Temporary or permanent role changes
    Decreased libido

Males

- *Potential for fertility impairment related to: disease, chemotherapy, radiation therapy, surgical interventions*
- *Potential for impotence: hormonal, systemic, or surgical ablative therapy; arteriosclerotic changes promoted by radiation therapy; cavernous nerve removal (radical prostatectomy)*
- *Dry orgasms after removal of prostate and seminal vesicles*

Females

- *Inadequate vaginal lubrication and infertility secondary to surgical procedure*
- *Radical cystectomy with removal of ovaries, fallopian tubes, uterus, cervix, and anterior portion of vagina*

Interventions

- Assess patterns of sexuality expression before diagnosis as a guide to predicting or planning for similar pattern of maintenance or attainment during and after treatment.
- Use technique of permission-granting general discussion regarding disease and treatment followed by specific individual questions.
- Review anticipated physiologic impact of disease and treatment on libido and potency.
- Consider general themes associated with age, gender, disease, and treatment modalities while focusing on the person's perception of cancer and potential impact on life-style.
- Maintain an awareness of personal biases and values, and allow for possibility of nontraditional partner or expressions of sexuality.
- Encourage enhancement of satisfaction and pleasure from everyday encounters.
- Review options for management of impotence, including injectable drugs (prostaglandins, papaverine), oral drugs (sildenafil citrate), urethral suppositories, vascular reconstruction, surgery, vacuum devices, and surgically implanted semirigid or inflatable penile prostheses.
- Ensure that patient/partner can identify aspects of sexuality and sexual function that may be threatened by the surgical procedure (e.g., prostatectomy, cystectomy, ileal conduit).
- State factors that influence sexual identity, and identify behaviors that facilitate acceptance of surgery.
- Maintain satisfying social and sexual role concept.
- Verbalize importance of seeking professional assistance if normal life-style, socialization, or sexual function is impaired.
- Provide patient/partner with factual information; give assurance that it is okay to share feelings and concerns; assist with coping and adjustment to illness.
- Provide information about use of lubricant products.

Chapter Questions

1. Which of the following is *not* a risk factor for the development of prostate cancer?
   a. Race
   b. Vasectomy
   c. Age
   d. High-fat diet
2. The quotient of serum PSA divided by one half the prostatic volume is referred to as:
   a. PSA velocity
   b. Free-to-total PSA ratio

c. PSA density

d. Age-referenced PSA

3. The site of action of luprolide (Lupron) is:

a. Pituitary-hypothalamic axis

b. Adrenal gland

c. Testes

d. Liver

4. Which biomarker or biomarkers are useful for the diagnosis and follow-up of seminomas?

a. CEA

b. AFP

c. HCG

d. AFP and HCG

5. In counseling a patient regarding sperm banking and fertility issues prior to treatment for testicular cancer, you advise the patient that:

a. All patients are eligible for sperm banking if ejaculatory function is intact.

b. Patients are ineligible for sperm banking if they test positively for sexually transmitted disease.

c. No contraception is necessary during chemotherapy treatment because all sperm will be destroyed.

d. Sperm recovery after chemotherapy is unlikely.

6. The classic symptom triad associated with renal cell carcinoma is:

a. Pain, hematuria, palpable flank mass

b. Pain, hematuria, weight loss

c. Pain, hematuria, urinary frequency

d. Pain, hematuria, fever

7. Standard treatment for invasive bladder tumors is:

a. Chemotherapy

b. Radiotherapy

c. Cystectomy

d. Partial cystectomy

8. In counseling a patient who is considering treatment options for early stage prostate cancer you include which of the following pieces of information:

a. Impotence is not a significant risk due to the widespread availability of nerve-sparing surgery.

b. Some degree of postoperative incontinence is nearly universal.

c. Radiotherapy is associated with a higher incidence of bowel dysfunction than surgery.

d. Impotence is more common among men treated with radiotherapy.

9. Current treatment options for erectile dysfunction include all of the following *except*:

a. Oral medication

b. Urethral prostaglandin suppositories

c. Surgical creation of an artificial sphincter

d. Vacuum devices

10. Which of the following is *not* a risk factor for the development of bladder cancer?

a. High intake of vitamin A

b. Tobacco

c. Schistosomiasis

d. Aniline dyes

BIBLIOGRAPHY

1. Abdalla I, Ray P, Vijayakumar S: Race and serum prostate-specific antigen levels: current status and future directions, *Semin Urol Oncol* 16:207, 1998.

2. Abel LJ and others: Nursing management of patients receiving brachytherapy for early stage prostate cancer, *Clin J Oncol Nurs* 3(1):7, 1999.

3. Adolfsson J: Deferred treatment for clinically localized prostate cancer, *Eur J Surg Oncol* 21:333, 1995.

4. American College of Physicians: Clinical Guideline: Part III. Screening for prostate cancer, *Ann Intern Med* 126:480, 1997.

5. American Joint Committee on Cancer: *AJCC cancer staging manual* ed 5, Philadelphia, Lippincott-Raven, 1997.

6. Ancher MS, Prosnitz LR: Multivariate analysis of factors predicting local relapse after radical prostaectomy—possible indications for postoperative radiotherapy, *Int J Radiat Biol Phy* 21:941, 1991.

7. Baldalament RA and others: Patient-reported complications of cryoablation therapy for prostate cancer, *Urology* 54:295, 1999.

8. Bates TS and others: Prevalence and impact of incontinence and impotence following total prostatectomy assessed anonymously by the ICS-Male questionnaire, *Eur Oncol* 33:165, 1998.

9. Boring CC and others: Cancer statistics: 1993, *CA Cancer J Clin* 43:7, 1993.

10. Bosl GJ and others: Cancer of the testes. In DeVita VT, Hellman S, Rosenberg S, editors: *Cancer: principles and practice of oncology* ed 5, Philadelphia, Lippincott-Raven, 1997.

11. Bosl GJ, Motzer RJ: Testicular germ cell cancer, *N Engl J Med* 337:242, 1997.

12. Bostwick DG and others: Staging of prostate cancer, *Semin Surg Oncol* 10(1):60, 1994.

13. Bostwick DG and others: Diagnosis and grading of bladder cancer and associated lesions, *Urol Clin North Am* 26:493, 1999.

14. Brawer MK: Prostate-specific antigen: current status, *CA Cancer J Clin* 49:264, 1999.

15. Brawer MK: Prostate-specific antigen, *Semin Surg Oncol* 18:3, 2000.

16. Brawley OW and others: The epidemiology of prostate cancer. Part II: risk factors, *Semin Urolog Oncol* 16:193, 1998.

17. Bressler LR and others: Use of clonidine to treat hot flashes secondary to leuprolide or goserelin, *Ann Pharmacother* 27:182, 1993.

18. Brosman SA: Depo-Provera as a treatment for hot flashes in men on androgen ablation therapy, Proceedings of the 90th Annual Meeting of the American Urological Association, Abstract #87. *J Urol* 153(4):448A, 1995.

19. Brufsky A, Kantoff PW: Hormonal therapy for prostate cancer. In Ernstoff MS, Heaney JA, Peschel RE, editors:

Urologic cancer Cambridge, MA, Blackwell Science, 1997.

20. Bukowski RM, Novick AC: Clinical practice guidelines: renal cell carcinoma, *Cleve Clin J Med* 64(suppl 1):SI, 1997.

21. Burgers JK and others: Penile cancer: clinical presentation, diagnosis, and staging, *Urol Clin North Am* 19(2): 247, 1992.

22. CancerNet, National Cancer Institute: Prostate cancer prevention trial recruitment of 18,000 men completed, *http://www.graylab.ac.uk/cancerner/600047.html.* Last update 1/1/97; accessed 3/2/00.

23. Carter HB and others: Prostate-specific antigen variability in men without prostate cancer: effect of sampling interval on prostate-specific antigen velocity, *Urology* 45:591, 1995.

24. Catalona WJ, Basler JW: Return of erections and urinary continence following nerve-sparing radical retropubic prostatectomy, *J Urol* 150:905, 1993.

25. Catalona WJ, Smith DS: Cancer recurrence and survival rates after anatomic radical retropubic prostatectomy for prostate cancer: Intermediate-term results, *J Urol* 160(6):2428, 1998.

26. Cespedes RD and others: Collagen injection for post-prostatectomy incontinence, *Urology* 54:597–602, 1999.

27. Christensson A and others: Serum prostate-specific antigen complexed to alpha 1-antichymotrypsin as an indicator of prostate cancer, *J Urol* 150:100, 1993.

28. Chun YS and others: A case of Kaposi's sarcoma of the penis showing a good response to high-energy pulsed carbon dioxide laser therapy, *J Dermatol* 26(4):240, 1999.

29. Clinton SK and others: Interleukin-12: opportunities for the treatment of bladder cancer, *Urol Clin North Am* 27:147, 2000.

30. Coakley FV, Hircak H: Radiologic anatomy of the prostate gland: a clinical approach, *Radiol Clin North Am* 38(1):15, 2000.

31. Cohen SM, Johnsson SL: Epidemiology and etiology of bladder cancer, *Urol Clin North Am* 19:421, 1992.

32. Crawford ED: Diagnosis and treatment of superficial bladder cancer: an update, *Semin Urol Oncol* 14(1) (suppl 1):1, 1996.

33. Dalbagni G, Herr HW: Current use and questions concerning intravesical bladder cancer group for superficial bladder cancer, *Urol Clin North Am* 27:137, 2000.

34. Davis JW and others: Conservative surgical therapy for penile and urethral carcinoma, *Urology* 53:386, 1999.

35. Davison BJ and others: Information on decision making preferences of older men with prostate cancer, *Oncol Nurs Forum* 22:1401, 1995.

36. Degner LF, Sloan JA: Decision making during serious illness: What role do patients really want to play? *J Clin Epidemiol* 45:941, 1992.

37. DeKernion JB, Berry D: The diagnosis and treatment of renal cell carcinoma, *Cancer,* 45(7 suppl):1947, 1980.

38. Delannes M and others: Iridium-192 interstitial therapy for squamous cell carcinoma of the penis, *Int J Radiat Oncol Biol Phys* 24:479, 1992.

39. Dexus FH and others: Circadian infusion of floxuridine in patients with metastatic renal cell carcinoma, *J Urol* 146:709, 1991.

40. Donohue JP and others: The role of the retroperitoneal lymphadenectomy in clinical stage B testis cancer: The Indiana University experience (1965–1989), *J Urol* 153(1):85, 1995.

41. Duque JLF, Loughlin KR: An overview of the treatment of superficial bladder cancer: Intravesical chemotherapy, *Urol Clin North Am* 27:125, 2000.

42. Eskew L and others: Systematic 5 region prostate biopsy is superior to sextant method for diagnosing carcinoma of the prostate, *J Urol* 157:199, 1997.

43. Esper P, Redman BG: Supportive care, pain management, and quality of life in advanced prostate cancer, *Urol Clin North Am* 26(2):475, 1999.

44. Feigl P and others: Design of the prostate cancer prevention trial (PCPT), *Control Clin Trials* 16:150, 1995.

45. Feneley MR and others: A review of radical prostatectomy from three centers in the UK. Clinical presentation and outcome: *Br J Urol* 78:911, 1997.

46. Fossa SD and others: Long term morbidity after infradiaphragmatic radiotherapy in young men with testicular cancer, *Cancer* 64:404, 1989.

47. Foster RS and others: The fertility of patients with clinical stage I testis cancer managed by nerve-sparing retroperitoneal lymph node dissection, *J Urol* 152(4):1139, 1994.

48. Fowler FJ Jr and others: Patient-reported complications and follow-up treatment after radical prostatectomy—the National Medicare experience: 1988–1990 (updated June 1993), *Urology* 42(6):622, 1993.

49. Games J: Nursing implications in the management of superficial bladder cancer, *Semin Urol Oncol* 14(1) (suppl 1):36, 1996.

50. Gatti JM, Stephenson RA: Staging of testis cancer, *Urol Clin North Am* 25:397, 1998.

51. Gerbaulet A, Lambin P: Radiotherapy of cancer of the penis. Indications, advantages, pitfalls, *Urol Clin North Am* 19:325, 1992.

52. Gilliland FD, Key CR: Prostate cancer in American Indians, New Mexico, 1969–1994, *J Urol* 159:893, 1998.

53. Giovannucci E and others: A prospective cohort study of vasectomy and prostate cancer in US, *JAMA* 269: 873, 1993.

54. Giovannucci E and others: Intake of caretenoids and retinol in relation to risk of prostate cancer, *J Natl Cancer Inst* 87:1767, 1995.

55. Gospodarowicz M and others: Early stage and advanced seminoma: role of radiation therapy, surgery, and chemotherapy, *Semin Oncol* 25:160, 1998.

56. Greenlee RT and others: Cancer statistics 2000, *CA Cancer J Clin* 50(1):7, 2000.

57. Griffiths TRL, Neal DE: Localized prostate cancer: early intervention or expectant therapy? *J R Soc Med* 90:665, 1997.

58. Grtiz ER and others: Long term effects of testicular cancer on sexual functioning in married couples, *Cancer* 64:1560, 1989.

59. Gustavasson P and others: Excess of cancer among Swedish chimney sweeps, *Br J Intern Med* 745:777, 1988.

60. Haas GP and others: Cisplatin, methotrexate and bleomycin for the treatment of carcinoma of the penis: a Southwest Oncology Group study, *J Urol* 161:1823, 1999.

61. Haggman MJ and others: The relationship between prostatic intraepithelial neoplasia and prostate cancer: Critical issues, *J Urol* 158:12, 1997.

62. Hahn EW, Feingold SM, Simpson L, et al: Recovery from azoospermia induced by low-dose radiation in seminoma patients, *Cancer* 50:337, 1982.

63. Hanks G and others: Seminoma of the testes: long-term beneficial and deleterious effects, *Int J Radiat Oncol Biol Phys* 24(5):913, 1992.

64. Hansen SW and others: Long-term fertility and Leydig cell function in patients treated for germ cell cancer with cisplatin, vinblastine, and bleomycin versus surveillance, *J Clin Oncol* 8:1696, 1990.

65. Heshmat MY and others: Nutrition and prostate cancer: a case control study, *Prostate* 6:7, 1985.

66. Hoffman RM and others: Prostate-specific antigen testing practices and outcomes, *J Gen Intern Med* 13:106, 1998.

67. Holzbeierlin JM, Smith JA: Surgical management of non-invasive bladder cancer (stages Ta/T1/CIS), *Urol Clin North Am* 27:15, 2000.

68. Horenhaus S and others: Squamous cell carcinoma of the penis: accuracy of tumour nodes and metastasis classification system, and the role of lymphangiography, computed tomography scan and fine needle aspiration, *J Urol* 146:1279, 1991.

69. Horrell CJ: Assessment and diagnosis. In Held-Warmkessel J, editor: *Contemporary issues in prostate cancer: a nursing perspective* Sudbury, MA, Jones & Bartlett, 2000.

70. Iwasawa AK and others: Detection of human papilloma virus deoxyribonucleic acid in penile carcinoma by polymerase chain reaction and in situ hybridization, *J Urol* 149:59, 1993.

71. Jewett HJ: The present status of radical prostatectomy for stages A and B prostatic cancer, *Urol Clin North Am* 2(1):105, 1975.

72. Jewett HJ, Strong GH: Infiltrating carcinoma of the bladder: relation of depth of penetration of the bladder wall to incidence of local extension and metastases, *J Urol* 55:366, 1946.

73. Johansson JE and others: Fifteen year survival in prostate cancer: results and identification of high-risk patient population, *JAMA* 277:467, 1997.

74. Jonler M and others: Sequelae of radial prostatectomy, *Br J Urol* 74:352, 1994.

75. Kamat AM, Lamm DL: Chemoprevention of urological cancer, *J Urol* 161:1748, 1999.

76. Kamradt JM and others: Oral chemotherapy for hormone-refractory prostate cancer, *Urol Clin North Am* 26(2):419, 1999.

77. Kantor AF and others. Epidemiologic characteristics of squamous cell carcinoma and adenocarcinoma of the bladder, *Cancer Res* 48:3853, 1988.

78. Kedia S and others: Treatment of erectile dysfunction with sildenafil citrate (Viagra) after radiation therapy for prostate cancer, *Urology* 54:308, 1999.

79. Klepp O and others: Prognostic factors in clinical state I nonseminomatous germ cell tumors of the testis: multivariate analysis of a prospective multicenter study, *J Clin Oncol* 8(3):509, 1990.

80. Lee WR and others: Urinary incontinence following external-beam radiotherapy for clinically localized prostate cancer, *Urology* 48:95, 1996.

81. Leibovitch I and others: The clinical implications of procedural deviations during orchiectomy for nonseminomatous germ testes cancer, *J Urol* 151a(93):939, 1995.

82. Levine, LA, Richie JP: Urologic complications of cyclophosphamide, *J Urol* 141:1063, 1989.

83. Liebovitch I and others: Malignant testicular neoplasms in immunosuppressed patients, *J Urol* 155:1938, 1996.

84. Lim AJ and others: Quality of life: radical prostatectomy versus radiation therapy for prostate cancer, *J Urol* 154:1420, 1995.

85. Linehan WM and others: Cancer of the kidney and ureter. In DeVita VT, Hellman S, Rosenberg S, editors, *Cancer: principles and practice of oncology,* ed 5, Philadelphia, Lippincott-Raven, 1997.

86. Loprinzi CL and others: Megesterol acetate for the prevention of hot flashes, *N Engl J Med* 331:347, 1994.

87. Luderer AA and others: Measurement of the proportion of free-to-total prostate-specific antigen improves diagnostic performance of prostate-specific antigen in the diagnostic gray zone of total prostate-specific antigen, *Urology* 46:187, 1995.

88. Maher KE: Male genitourinary cancers. In Dow KH, Bucholtz JD, Iwamoto R and others, editors: *Nursing care in radiation oncology,* ed 2, Philadelphia: Saunders, 1997.

89. Maldazys JD, Dekernion JB: Prognostic factors in metastatic renal carcinoma, *J Urol* 136:376, 1986.

90. Malloy TR and others: Superficial transitional cell carcinoma of the bladder treated with an Nd:YAG laser, *J Urol* 131:151, 1984.

91. Manyak MJ: Clinical applications of radioimmunoscintigraphy with prostate-specific antibodies for prostate cancer, *Cancer Control* 5:493, 1998.

92. Marshall VF: The relation of preoperative estimate to the pathologic demonstration of the extent of vesical neoplasms, *J Urol* 68:714, 1952.

93. Martikainen P and others: Programmed death of nonproliferating androgen-independent prostate cancer cells, *Cancer Res* 51:4693, 1991.

94. Masi A and others: Magnetic resonance with an endorectal coil and fast spin echo sequence in the staging of prostate carcinoma. The correlation with histopathological data, *Radiol Med* 94:496, 1997.

95. McDougal WS: Carcinoma of the penis: Improved survival by regional lymphadenectomy based on histological grade and depth of invasion of primary lesion, *J Urol* 154:1364, 1995.

96. McLaughlin JK and others: A population based case control study of renal cell carcinoma, *J Natl Cancer Inst* 72:275, 1984.

97. Mencel PJ and others: Advanced seminoma: treatment results, survival, and prognostic factors in 142 patients. *J Clin Oncol* 12:120, 1994.

98. Millikan R, Logothetis C: Update of the NCCN guidelines for the treatment of prostate cancer, *Oncology* 11(11A):180, 1997.

99. Montie JE: Staging of prostate cancer: current TNM classification and future prospects for prognostic factors, *Cancer* 75(7)(suppl):1814, 1995.

100. Motzer RJ and others: Etoposide and cisplatin adjuvant therapy for patients with pathologic stage II germ cell tumors, *Clinical Papers and Current Comments: Highlights of Genitourinary Cancer Research* 2:455, 1998.

101. Motzer RJ and others: NCCN practice guidelines for kidney cancer, *Oncology* (Huntington) 12(11A):398, 1998.

102. Moul JW and others: Black race is an adverse prognostic factor for prostate cancer recurrence following radical prostatectomy in an equal access health care setting, *J Urol* 155:1667, 1996.

103. National Comprehensive Cancer Network: NCCN practice guidelines for testicular cancer, *Oncology* (Huntington) 12(11A):417, 1998.

104. Oesterling JE and others: Correlation of clinical stage, serum prostatic acid phosphatase and preoperative Gleason grade with final pathological stage in 275 patients with clinically localized adenocarcinoma of the prostate, *J Urol* 138(1):92, 1987.

105. Oesterling JE: The use of prostate-specific antigen in staging patients with newly diagnosed prostate cancer, *JAMA* 269(1):57, 1993.

106. Oh WK, Kantoff PW: Docetaxel (Taxotere)-based chemotherapy for hormone-refractory locally advanced prostate cancer, *Semin Oncol* 26(5)(suppl 17):49, 1999.

107. Optenberg SA and others: Race, treatment and long-term survival from prostate cancer in an equal access medical delivery system, *JAMA* 274:1599, 1995.

108. O'Rourke ME: *Prostate cancer treatment selection: the family decision process.* Doctoral dissertation, University of North Carolina Chapel Hill, 1997.

109. O'Rourke ME: Narrowing the options: the process of deciding on prostate cancer treatment, *Cancer Invest* 17:349, 1999.

110. O'Rourke ME: Urinary incontinence as a factor in prostate cancer treatment selection. *J Wound, Ostomy, Continence Nurs* 27(3):146, 2000.

111. O'Rourke ME, Germino BB: Prostate cancer treatment selection: a focus group exploration, *Oncol Nurs Forum* 25:97, 1998.

112. O'Rourke ME, Griffin AS: Expectant management: the art and science of watchful waiting. In Held-Warmkessel J, editor: *Contemporary issues in prostate cancer: a nursing perspective,* Sudbury, MA, Jones & Bartlett, 2000.

113. Ozen H: Bladder cancer, *Curr Opin Oncol* 10:273, 1998.

114. Palapattu GS and others: Gene therapy for prostate cancer: new perspectives on an old problem, *Urol Clin North Am* 26(2):353, 1999.

115. Pettaway CA and others: Sentinel node dissection for penile carcinoma: The M. D. Anderson Cancer Center experience, *J Urol* 154:1999, 1995.

116. Pienta KJ and others: Effects of age and race on the survival of men with prostate cancer in the metropolitan Detroit tricounty area: 1973 to 1987, *Urology* 150:797, 1993.

117. Pienta KJ and others: Prostate cancer. In Pazdur R, Coia LR, Hoskins WJ, editors: *Cancer management: a multidisciplinary approach: medical, surgical, and radiation oncology,* Melville, New York, PRR, 1999.

118. Pizzocaro G and others: Up-to-date management of carcinoma of the penis, *Eur Oncol* 32:5, 1997.

119. Porter AT and others: Results of a randomized phase-III trial to evaluate the efficacy of strontium-89 adjuvant to local external beam irradiation in the management of endocrine resistant metastatic prostate cancer, *Int J Radiat Oncol Biol Phys* 25:805, 1993.

120. Powell IJ and others: The predictive value of race as a clinical prognostic factor among patients with clinically localized prostate cancer: a multivariate analysis of positive surgical margins, *Urology* 49:726, 1997.

121. Quinlan DM and others: Sexual functioning following radical prostatectomy: Influence of preservation of neurovascular bundles, *Br J Urol* 74:352, 1994.

122. Ragde H and others: Ten-year disease free survival after transperineal sonography-guided iodine-125 brachytherapy with or without 45-gray external beam irradiation in the treatment of patients with clinically localized, low to high Gleason grade prostate carcinoma, *Cancer* 83:989, 1998.

123. Reuter VE: Bladder: risk and prognostic factors—a pathologist's perspective, *Urol Clin North Am* 26:481, 1999.

124. Richie J: Detection and treatment of testicular cancer, *CA Cancer J Clin* 34:151, 1993.

125. Robbins WA and others: Chemotherapy induces transient sex chromosomal and autosomal aneuploidy in human sperm, *Nat Gen* 16:74, 1997.

126. Robinson RG: Strontium-89: precursor targeted therapy for pain relief of blastic metastatic disease, *Cancer* 72(11, suppl):3433, 1993.

127. Robson CJ and others: The results of radical nephrectomy for renal cell carcinoma, *J Urol* 101:297, 1969.

128. Rose DP and others: International comparisons of mortality rates for cancer of the breast, ovary, prostate, and colon, and per capita food consumption, *Cancer* 58:2363, 1986.

129. Ross R and others: Serum testosterone levels in healthy young black and white men, *J Natl Cancer Inst* 76:45, 1986.

130. Roth B and others: Neoplasms of the testes. In Holland J, Frei E, Bast R and others, editors: *Cancer Medicine,* vol 2, ed 3, Philadelphia, Lea & Febiger, 1993.

131. Sakr WA and others: The frequency of carcinoma and intraepithelial neoplasia of the prostate in young males, *J Urol* 150:379, 1993.

132. Saliken C and others: Outcome and safety of US-guided percutaneous cryotherapy for localized prostate cancer, *J Vasc Intervent Radiol* 10:199, 1999.

133. Samm BJ, Steiner MS: Penectomy: a new technique to reduce blood loss, *Urology* 53:393, 1999.

134. Schelhammer PF: Penile cancer. In Krane SJ, Sisky MB, & Fizpatrick JM, editors: *Clinical Urology,* Philadelphia, Lippincott, 1994.

135. Scher H and others: NCCN urothelial cancer practice guidelines, *Oncology* (Huntington) 12(7A):225, 1998.

136. Schiebler ML and others: Current role of MR imaging in the staging of adenocarcinoma of the prostate, *Radiology* 189(2):339, 1993.

137. Sheinfeld J, Herr H: Role of surgery in the management of germ-cell tumors, *Semin Oncol* 25:203, 1998.

138. Shirahama T and others: A new treatment for penile conservation in penile carcinoma: a preliminary study of combined laser hyperthermia, radiation and chemotherapy, *Br J Urol* 82(5):687, 1998.

139. Silverman DT and others: Occupational risks of bladder cancer in the United States. I: white men, *J Natl Cancer Inst* 81:1472, 1989.

140. Silverman DT and others: Motor exhaust-related occupations and bladder cancer, *Cancer Res* 46:2113, 1986.

141. Silverman DT and others: Epidemiology of bladder cancer, *Hematol Oncol Clin North Am* 6:1, 1992.

142. Skinner DG and others: Clinical experience with the Kock continent ileal reservoir for urinary diversion, *J Urol* 132(6):1101, 1984.

143. Slattery ML and others: Food consumption trends between adolescent and adult years and subsequent risk of prostate cancer, *Am J Clin Nur* 52:752, 1990.

144. Small EJ and others: Simultaneous antiandrogen withdrawal and treatment with ketoconazole and hydrocortisone in patients with advanced prostate cancer, *Cancer* 80:1755, 1997.

145. Spears WT and others: Brain metastases and testicular tumors: long-term survival, *Int J Radiat Oncol Biol Phys* 22(1):17, 1992.

146. Stanford J and others: Vasectomy and risk of prostate cancer, *Cancer Epidemiol Biomarkers Prev* 8:881, 1999.

147. Stein JP and others: Prognostic markers in bladder cancer: a contemporary review of the literature, *J Urol* 160:645, 1998.

148. Steinberg GS and others: Family history and the risk of prostate cancer, *Prostate* 17:337, 1990.

149. Steineck GS and others: Urothelial cancer and some industry-related chemicals: an evaluation of the epidemiologic evidence, *Am J Med* 17:371, 1990.

150. Steineck GS and others: Vitamin A supplements, fried foods, fat, and urothelial cancer: a case efferent study in Stockholm in 1985–1987, *Int J Cancer* 45:1006, 1990.

151. Steineck G and others: Industry-related urothelial carcinogens: Application of a job-exposure matrix to census data, *Am J Ind Med* 16:209, 1989.

152. Stempkowski L: Hormonal therapy. In Held-Warmkessel J, editor: *Contemporary issues in prostate cancer: a nursing perspective,* Sudbury, MA, Jones & Bartlett, 2000.

153. Stern RS and Members of the Photochemotherapy Follow-up Study: Genital tumors among men with psoriasis exposed to ultraviolet radiation, *N Engl J Med* 332:1093, 1990.

154. Srivinas V and others: Penile cancer: relation of extent of nodal metastases to survival, *J Urol* 137:880, 1987.

155. Talcott JA and others: Patient-reported impotence and incontinence after nerve-sparing radical prostatectomy, *J Natl Cancer Inst* 89:1117, 1997.

156. Tester W, Brouch MD: Treatment decision making. In Held-Warmkessel J, editor: *Contemporary issues in pros-tate cancer: a nursing perspective,* Sudbury, MA, Jones & Bartlett, 2000.

157. Theriault G and others: Bladder cancer in the aluminum industry, *Lancet* 1:947, 1988.

158. Thompson IM and others: Increased incidence of testicular cancer in active duty members of the Department of Defense, *Urology* 53:806, 1999.

159. Tjoa BA, Murphy GP: Progress in active immunotherapy of prostate cancer, *Semin Surg Oncol* 18:80, 2000.

160. Turek PJ and others: Fertility issues and their management in men with testes cancer, *Urol Clin North Am* 25(3):517, 1998.

161. Ulbright TM: Testis risk and prognostic factors, *Urol Clin North Am* 26:611, 1999.

162. United States Preventive Health Services Task Force: *Guide to clinical preventive services,* ed 2, Baltimore, MD, Williams & Wilkins, 1996.

163. Vineis P and others: Effects of timing and type of tobacco in cigarette-induced bladder cancer, *Cancer Res* 48:1849, 1988.

164. Vogelzang NJ and others: Goserelin versus orchiectomy in the treatment of advanced prostate cancer: final results of a randomized trial, *Urology* 46(2):220, 1995.

165. Volpe HM: Radiation therapy. In Held-Warmkessel J, editor: *Contemporary issues in prostate cancer: a nursing perspective,* Sudbury, MA, Jones & Bartlett, 2000.

166. von Eschenbach A and others: American Cancer Society Guidelines for the early detection of prostate cancer, *Cancer* 80(9):180, 1997.

167. Waldman AR: Screening and early detection. In Held-Warmkessel J, editor: *Contemporary issues in prostate cancer: a nursing perspective,* Sudbury, MA, Jones & Bartlett, 2000.

168. Walsh PC, Doker PJ: Impotence following radical prostatectomy: insight into etiology and prevention, *J Urol* 128:492, 1982.

169. Walsh PC, Lepor H: The role of radical prostatectomy in the management of prostate cancer, *Cancer* 60(3 suppl):526, 1987

170. Walther MM: The role of photodynamic therapy in the treatment of recurrent superficial bladder cancer, *Urol Clin North Am* 27:163, 2000.

171. Washeka R, Hanna M: Malignant renal cell tumors in tuberous sclerosis, *Urology* 37:340, 1991.

172. Wong WS and others: Cryosurgery as a treatment for prostate cancer: results and complications, *Cancer* 79:963, 1997.

173. Woutersen RA, Appel MJ: Dietary fat and carcinogenesis, *Mutat Res* 443(1-2):11, 1999.

174. Young HH: The early diagnosis and radical cure of carcinoma of the prostate: being a study of 40 cases and a presentation of a radical operation which was carried out in 4 cases, *Bull Johns Hopkins Hosp* 16:315, 1905.

175. Zincke H and others: Radical prostatectomy for clinically localized prostate cancer: long-term results of 1,143 patients from a single institution, *J Clin Oncol* 12:2254, 1994.

176. Zippe CG and others: Sildenafil citrate (Viagra) after radical retropubic prostatectomy: pro, *Urology* 54: 583, 1999.

Gynecologic Cancers

Shirley E. Otto

The American Cancer Society (ACS) estimates that 77,500 women were diagnosed with a malignancy of the genital tract in 2000. Although dramatic improvements in the prevention, diagnosis, and treatment of women with gynecologic cancers have occurred during the past decade, an estimated 26,500 women will die from gynecologic malignancies in 2000.[32]

This chapter reviews the epidemiology, etiology, risk factors, routes and sites of metastasis, and treatment strategies for gynecologic cancer. The nurse's role in the education of the public about preventive health behaviors, self-examination skills, and recommended screening activities is discussed. In addition, critical elements of nursing care for the patient diagnosed with specific gynecologic cancers are described.

Cervical Cancer

EPIDEMIOLOGY

Although the incidence rates of invasive cervical cancer have steadily declined since the 1940s, the ACS estimates that 12,800 women were diagnosed with the disease in 2000. Patterns of occurrence have been described based on age and socioeconomic status. Invasive cervical cancer occurs most often among women between ages 35 and 50 years. Recent trends indicate an increasing incidence of cervical cancer in younger women. In the United States differences are noted between ethnic groups, with a twofold difference between the African American and white populations. Approximately 80% of cervical cancer occurs in developing countries. Urban populations frequently show higher rates than rural populations. The incidence is lower for the Japanese populations but is higher in Hispanics and American Indians. Worldwide, cancer of the cervix is the *second most common cancer* (breast is number one) among women, but remains the *most common cause of cancer mortality*.[16, 25, 53]

Cervical cancer develops primarily at the *squamocolumnar junction,* the area on the cervix where squamous cells that line the vagina and cover the outer portion of the cervix and where columnar cells that line the endocervical canal meet. The squamocolumnar junction occurs on the outer portion of the cervix (*exocervix*) in younger women. As women age, changes in the vaginal pH trigger a process of squamous metaplasia in which the squamous cells begin to cover the columnar cells, resulting in an area called the *transformation zone.* Over time, the squamocolumnar junction moves from the exocervix into the endocervical canal.[24, 25]

Invasive cervical cancer is usually preceded by a 10- to 20-year history of preinvasive cellular changes ranging from mild dysplasia to carcinoma in situ (CIS) (Fig. 11–1). If untreated, a small proportion of women with mild dysplasia will eventually develop invasive cancer. Since the advent of cytologic screening in the 1940s, the incidence has been decreasing; however, there has been a steady increase in the incidence of preinvasive disease of the cervix. Even with the widespread use of the Papanicolaou (Pap) smear for early detection of preinvasive and invasive cervical disease, an estimated 4600 woman will die of cervical cancer in 2000.[24, 25, 32]

ETIOLOGY AND RISK FACTORS

The etiology of cervical cancer is unknown. Data have suggested a strong association between sexual history and practices and the incidence of cervical cancer. In addition, diet and life-style have been identified as cofactors for development of the disease. Cofactors associated with an increased risk include decreased levels of vitamins A and C and folic acid in the diet, tobacco use, alcohol abuse, immunosuppression, and oral contraceptive use. The role of genital hygiene also is being explored as a possible cofactor in the development of cervical cancer.[12, 16, 17]

Sexual practices associated with an increased risk for cervical cancer include onset of sexual intercourse

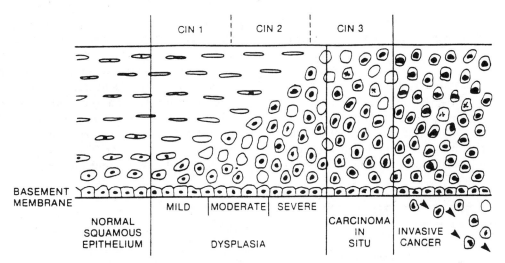

FIGURE 11–1 Progression of cervical intraepithelial neoplasia (CIN). (From Jones HW, Wentz AC, Burnett LS: *Novak's textbook of gynecology,* ed 11, Baltimore, Williams & Wilkins, 1988.)

before 18 years of age and multiple sexual partners. Increasingly, data have indicated that the number of sexual partners of the male partner(s) has a significant role in the development of cervical cancer. A history of infection with sexually transmitted viruses, such as herpes simplex virus type 2 (HSV-2) and the human papillomavirus (HPV, specifically types HPV-16 and HPV-18), initial pregnancy before 18 years of age, and multiple pregnancies place an individual woman at increased risk for cervical intraepithelial neoplasia (CIN) and invasive cervical cancers. Women infected with human immunodeficiency virus (HIV) are at increased risk for cervical squamous intraepithelial lesions, a precursor to invasive cervical cancer.[16, 24–26, 53, 63]

In the late 1960s an increase in the incidence of clear cell adenocarcinoma of the cervix was noted in women younger than 30 years. On review of medical histories for these women, a commonality was noted. Most of the women had been exposed in utero to *diethylstilbestrol* (DES), a synthetic estrogen given to women with high-risk pregnancies. Although the use of DES during pregnancy was discontinued in the early 1960s, a study of the incidence of cervical and vaginal carcinomas among women exposed to DES continues.[17, 24, 25]

PREVENTION, SCREENING, AND DETECTION

Prevention

Prevention is the key strategy for eradication of cervical cancer. Based on available knowledge about factors that place women at high risk for cervical cancer, the nurse can develop cervical cancer prevention programs for the public. Programs for teenagers may include strategies such as avoidance of penile-vaginal intercourse and

use of barrier contraceptives to prevent pregnancy and sexually transmitted diseases (STDs). For women of all ages, limitation of the number of sexual partners and use of barrier contraceptives, such as condoms and diaphragms, are recommended to reduce the risk of cervical cancer. Dietary modifications that may reduce the risk of cervical cancer include increased ingestion of foods high in vitamins A and C and folic acid. In addition, strategies to prevent initiation or to encourage discontinuation of tobacco and alcohol use could be included. Discussion regarding appropriate use of oral contraceptives should also be considered. Because invasive cervical cancer is preceded by a preinvasive stage in most patients, the ACS guidelines for screening should be taught as a cancer prevention strategy.[8, 12, 39, 53, 97]

The target population for teaching prevention of cervical cancer is teenagers. Points to be stressed include an overview of normal physiologic changes that occur on the cervix during puberty and adolescence, the importance of using barrier contraception, and initiation of routine Pap smears and pelvic examinations whenever the teenager becomes sexually active. Emphasis on the ability to diagnose preinvasive lesions of the cervix and on the effectiveness of conservative treatment in eradicating preinvasive disease may lessen the fear of cancer and enhance compliance.[8, 24, 25]

Screening

The primary screening test for cervical cancer is the *Papanicolaou smear.* Screening for cervical cancer with the Pap smear with a pelvic examination has resulted in a 50% decrease in mortality rate from cervical cancer. The specimen is obtained by collecting a sample of cells from the squamocolumnar junction with a cotton swab, wooden spatula, or a cytobrush. The lowest false-negative rate and the highest predictability are achieved by sampling cells from the exocervix and the endocervical canal. A *pelvic examination* is also recommended to evaluate the shape and consistency of the cervix and adjacent tissues.[25, 53, 80, 97]

The ACS recommendations for screening of asymptomatic women for cervical cancer include an annual Pap smear and pelvic examination for all women who are or have been sexually active or who are 18 years of age. After three or more normal, consecutive, annual Pap smears, the Pap smear and pelvic examination can be performed less frequently at the physician's discretion. Although debate continues about the cost effectiveness of the Pap smear for women older than 65 years, data indicate that the incidence of invasive cervical cancer increases with age in general and particularly among older, lower socioeconomic women who have never had a Pap smear. Therefore, women should not be denied the opportunity to have a Pap smear and

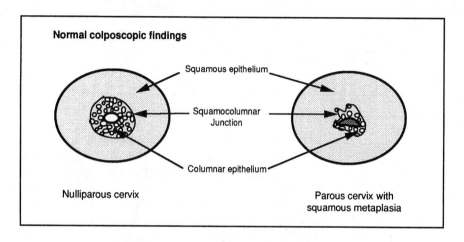

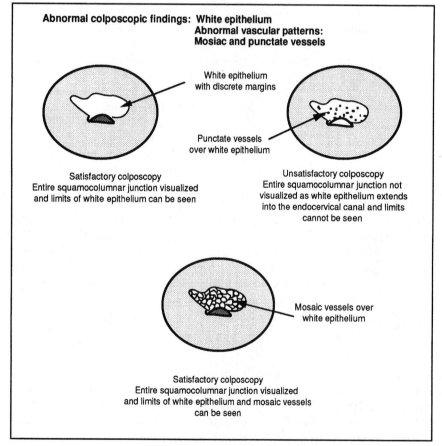

FIGURE 11-2 Graphic representation of cervical findings using the colposcope.

pelvic examination based on age alone. Recent changes in Medicare coverage allow for a Pap smear every 3 years.[8, 12, 25, 53, 61, 80]

Detection

A thorough history and physical examination are used to detect cervical cancer in symptomatic women. A clinical examination is performed to visualize the cervix, obtain a Pap smear, conduct a colposcopic examination, and palpate the cervix and adjacent tissues. The majority of invasive cervical carcinomas may be visualized on inspection. Cervical carcinoma presents in two primary patterns. The most common presentation is an *exophytic lesion.* These lesions occur primarily on the portion of the cervix, resemble polyps, spread superficially across the cervix, and bleed easily. *Endophytic lesions* invade toward the endocervical canal. These tumors often go undetected as they expand within the endocervical canal and form a barrel-shaped lesion.[16, 24, 25, 42]

A colposcopic examination may be performed in women with significant symptoms or grossly suspicious lesions on the cervix. The *colposcope* is a binocular optical device used to magnify and illuminate the cervical tissues. After application of a 3% to 5% acetic acid solution, the clinician evaluates the transformation zone and the squamocolumnar junction, if visible, for abnormalities in color and contour of tissues and vascular patterns (Fig. 11–2). The clinician obtains a colposcopically directed biopsy from the most abnormal areas for evaluation.[24, 25]

The rectovaginal, bimanual examination allows the clinician to evaluate the size, contour, and consistency of the cervix, corpus, ovaries, and vaginal and rectal tissues. Gross extension of the tumor to adjacent structures such as the rectum, vagina, and paracervical tissues also can be evaluated. Additionally patients with abnormal cytology should undergo endocervical curettage at the time of the colposcopic examination.[17, 25, 61]

CLASSIFICATION

Cervical carcinomas are classified histologically by the tissue of origin. Historically, more than 80% of cervical cancers are *squamous cell carcinomas.* Squamous cell carcinomas have been divided further into *keratinizing, nonkeratinizing,* and *small cell* types based on histologic descriptors. *Adenocarcinomas* and *adenosquamous carcinomas* account for an increasingly greater proportion of cervical cancers (11–16%), particularly in women under 35 years of age. The increase in cervical cancers with adenomatous features is important because of the poorer prognosis associated with the disease.[24, 25]

CLINICAL FEATURES

The most common presenting symptom of women with cervical cancer is *abnormal vaginal bleeding,* which may present as a decrease in the interval between the menstrual periods, an increase in the length or amount of menstrual flow, intermenstrual, and/or postmenopausal bleeding. The woman also may describe episodes of "contact" bleeding after intercourse or douching. Less often the woman may complain of a persistent, thin, watery, blood-tinged, odoriferous vaginal discharge. Symptoms of more advanced disease include urinary complaints such as difficulty starting the stream of urine, urinary urgency, hematuria, or pain with urination. Advanced disease resulting in pressure or invasion of the rectum may result in constipation, rectal tenesmus, rectal bleeding, and malodorous, serosanguinous, or yellowish, vaginal discharge. Involvement of regional lymph nodes may result in edema of the lower extremities. Weight loss, pain of the lower back, groin, and lower extremities also may be present with advanced disease.[24, 25, 53] Please see the Clinical Features and Complications boxes.

CLINICAL FEATURES
Gynecologic Cancers

Cervical: abnormal vaginal bleeding—increase in the amount, frequency, and/or length; postcoital, irregular, or postmenopausal bleeding; urinary urgency; discharge; dysuria; hematuria *late stage disease*—malodorous serosanguinous, yellowish vaginal discharge, weight loss

Endometrial: *abnormal* bleeding—may be prolonged, irregular, or excessive; pain in the hypogastric, pelvis, and/or lumbosacral area, rapidly enlarging nonpregnant uterus.

Ovarian: dyspepsia, indigestion, anorexia, or early satiety; urinary frequency; constipation; full or heavy sensation in the pelvis or with increasing abdominal girth—*usually most of these symptoms represent presence of advanced disease.*

Vulvar: pain, pruritus, bleeding, discharge, dysuria, presence of lump or mass in vulvar area

Vaginal: *Painless* vaginal bleeding—postcoital, perimenopausal or postmenopausal; foul-smelling vaginal discharge; dyspareunia

Fallopian: vaginal bleeding; intermittent, colicky, dull, aching pain; profuse, watery vaginal discharge

Gestational trophoblastic disease: first-trimester vaginal bleeding, hyperemesis, and uterine size inconsistent with estimated gestational age, abnormal ultrasound appearance of the intrauterine contents.

COMPLICATIONS
Gynecologic Cancers

Disease Related

Sexual dysfunction
Infertility
Sterility
Alteration in bowel and bladder function
Loss of pregnancy
Changes in self-concept

Treatment Related

Infertility
Sterility (temporary/permanent)
Fistula formation
Infection
Bleeding
Wound dehiscence
Vaginal fibrosis/stenosis
Ureteral obstruction
Myelosuppression
Alopecia
Alteration in bowel and bladder function
Termination of pregnancy
Altered sexual function

DIAGNOSIS AND STAGING

Diagnosis and staging form the basis of treatment for cervical carcinomas. A tissue biopsy is required for the diagnosis of cervical cancer. The exocervix and the endocervical canal are easily accessible to punch biopsy and curettage, respectively. Because the treatment of preinvasive cervical disease is more conservative, the tissue biopsy is needed to rule out or confirm the presence of invasive cancer. If an adequate tissue sampling for making the determination is not obtained, a more extensive tissue sampling with conization of the cervix is required (Fig. 11–3). Pathologic confirmation of preinvasive or invasive disease is mandatory before initiation of treatment.[24, 25]

Staging for cervical cancer is done clinically. Data obtained from the clinical examination (inspection, palpation, colposcopy), radiographic examinations (chest, kidneys, sigmoid colon and rectum, skeleton, intravenous pyelography), barium enema, cystoscopy or proctoscopy, and pathologic evaluation of biopsy and curettage materials are used to determine the extent of disease and ultimately plan treatment. Protein markers for detection of cervical cancer recurrence and *vaccines* for *prevention* of cervical cancer are under investigation. Table 11–1 presents staging systems for cervical cancer that have been developed by the American Joint Committee on Cancer (AJCC) and the International Federation of Gynecology and Obstetrics (FIGO).[16, 25, 55]

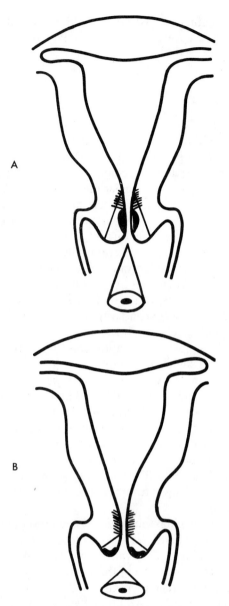

FIGURE 11–3 Cone biopsy for endocervical and exocervical disease. (a) Endocervical disease: increased depth of cone biopsy to remove all abnormal areas. (b) Exocervical disease: increased width of cone biopsy to remove all abnormal areas. (From DiSaia PJ, Creasman WT: *Clinical gynecologic oncology,* ed 4, St. Louis, Mosby, 1997.)

METASTASIS

Cervical carcinomas are slow-growing tumors that invade by direct extension to adjacent tissues of the uterus, vagina, rectum, bladder, and parametrial tissues. Lymphatic invasion also occurs in regional and distant lymphatic channels. Cervical cancer rarely spreads hemato-

TABLE 11–1
Staging Classification for Cervical Cancer

		Primary Tumor (T)
TNM	**FIGO**	**Definition**
TX		Primary tumor cannot be assessed
T0		No evidence of primary tumor
Tis	0	Carcinoma in situ
T1	I	Cervical carcinoma confined to uterus (extension to corpus should be disregarded)
T1a	Ia	Preclinical invasive carcinoma, diagnosed by microscopy only
T1a1	Ia1	Minimal microscopic stromal invasion
T1a2	Ia2	Tumor with invasive component 5 mm or less in depth taken from base of epithelium and 7 mm or less in horizontal spread
T1b	Ib	Tumor larger than T1a2
T2	II	Cervical carcinoma invades beyond uterus but not to pelvic wall or to lower third of vagina
T2a	IIa	Without parametrial invasion
T2b	IIb	With parametrial invasion
T3	III	Cervical carcinoma extends to pelvic wall and/or involves lower third of vagina and/or causes hydronephrosis or nonfunctioning kidney
T3a	IIIa	Tumor involves lower third of vagina, no extension to pelvic wall
T3b	IIIb	Tumor extends to pelvic wall and/or causes hydronephrosis or nonfunctioning kidney
T4	IVa	Tumor invades mucosa of bladder or rectum and/or extends beyond true pelvis
M1	IVb	Distant metastasis

Regional Lymph Nodes (N)

Regional lymph nodes include paracervical, parametrial, hypogastric (obturator), common, internal and external iliac, presacral, and sacral

TMN	**Definition**
NX	Regional lymph nodes cannot be assessed
N0	No regional lymph node metastasis
N1	Regional lymph node metastasis

Distant Metastasis (M)

TMN	**FIGO**	**Definition**
MX		Presence of distant metastasis cannot be assessed
M0		No distant metastasis
M1	IVb	Distant metastasis

Stage Grouping

Stage 0:	Tis-N0-M0
Stage IA:	T1a-N0-M0
Stage IB:	T1b-N0-M0
Stage IIA:	T2a-N0-M0
Stage IIB:	T2b-N0-M0
Stage IIIA:	T3a-N0-M0
Stage IIIB:	T1-N1-M0
	T2-N1-M0
	T3a-N1-M0
	T3b-any N-M0
Stage IVA:	T4-any N-M0
Stage IVB:	any T-any N-M1

From American Joint Committee on Cancer: Manual for staging cancer, *ed 5, Philadelphia, Lippincott-Raven, 1997.*

logically; however, metastatic disease can occur in the lungs or liver.

TREATMENT MODALITIES

The treatment of preinvasive cervical disease is based on the extent of disease (Fig. 11–4). Women with preinvasive disease may be treated conservatively with *cryosurgery, electrocautery,* or *carbon dioxide laser ablation.* Each of these techniques allows destruction of superficially abnormal cells with cold, heat, or light energy, respectively. Of the three methods, the laser ablation allows for more control of the pattern and depth of tissue destruction.[17, 24, 25]

A *cold-knife conization* or *loop electrosurgical excision procedure* (LEEP) of the cervix may be used as treatment. With either procedure, the entire transformation zone and squamocolumnar junction is removed (see Fig. 11–3). Conization of the cervix often is recommended as treatment for women who desire to maintain fertility. However, many physicians recommend hysterectomy after completion of childbearing. For women with preinvasive disease who do not desire to maintain fertility or who are high risk for noncompliance with follow-up examinations, hysterectomy may be considered as definitive treatment.[17, 24, 25, 45]

Localized cervical carcinoma (stages I–IIA) may be treated with surgery alone, radiation therapy alone, or a combination of both. Comparable survival rates have been demonstrated among the three treatment plans. The choice of treatment is based on extent of disease and the patient's general health status, desire to maintain

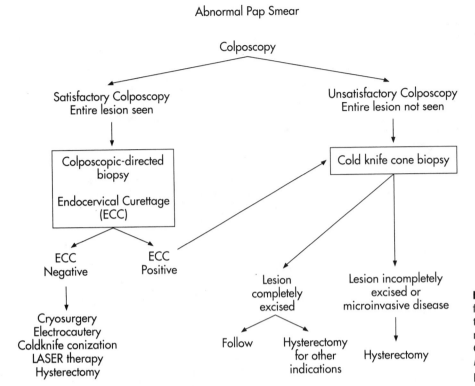

Abnormal Pap Smear

FIGURE 11–4 Decision tree for management of cervical intraepithelial neoplasia (CIN). (From Flannery M: Reproductive cancers. In Clark JC, McGee RF, editors: *Core curriculum for oncology nursing*, Philadelphia, Saunders, 1992.)

childbearing function, and indication of intent to comply with follow-up recommendations. Ideally the treatment decision should be made jointly by the woman, the gynecologic oncologist, and the radiation therapist after review of the risks and benefits of treatment alternatives.[24, 25]

Surgical treatment of women with invasive cervical cancer most often includes a *radical hysterectomy* with *bilateral pelvic lymphadenectomy*. Advantages of a radical approach to treatment include the gathering of additional pathologic information about the spread of the disease to local and regional lymph nodes and the need for adjuvant radiation therapy and maintenance of ovarian function. Disadvantages of radical surgical treatment include potential alteration in bowel and bladder function, risks of intraoperative and postoperative complications, and the loss of childbearing function. For a select number of women with stage IA disease who desire to maintain fertility, conization of the cervix may be used as definitive treatment.[24, 25]

Radiation with external beam (*teletherapy*) and internal or interstitial beam (*brachytherapy*) offers women with early stage disease equally effective treatment. Advantages of radiation are that the treatment can be given on an outpatient basis, intraoperative and postoperative complications are avoided, and treatment time is shortened. Disadvantages include long-term effects of radiation on normal tissues, such as radiation enteritis, blad-

der damage, fistula formation, vaginal stenosis, and ureteral obstruction.[48, 51]

Advanced cervical carcinoma (stages IIB–IV) is treated primarily with radiation therapy alone, although recent clinical trials include antineoplastic agents, radiosensitizing agents, hyperbaric oxygen, and hyperthermia administered in conjunction with radiation. Coordination between the medical oncologist and the radiation oncologist is mandatory to maximize therapeutic benefit while carefully monitoring immediate and long-term consequences of combined therapy.[25, 51]

The incidence of persistent or recurrent cervical cancer is approximately 35%. Women with advanced disease at diagnosis are in the highest-risk group. Recent data from randomized clinical trials has shown that the addition of concurrent cisplatin-based chemotherapy to radiation prolongs survival and a 30% to 50% reduction in disease recurrence risk with the concurrent cisplatin-based chemoradiation. For locally recurrent or persistent disease, treatment options include pelvic exenteration, radiation therapy to previously nonradiated areas, and antineoplastic therapy.[17, 25]

Pelvic exenteration is considered for curative treatment of women with recurrent disease if no evidence of extrapelvic disease, tumor fixed to the pelvic wall, or ureteral obstruction from the tumor is present preoperatively. The procedure consists of removal of the uterus, cervix, vagina, rectum, bladder, urethra, and lateral supporting tissues and carries significant morbidity. In women whose disease has not spread to the bladder or rectum, variations on the procedure may be performed: a posterior pelvic exenteration or anterior pelvic exenteration, respectively (Fig. 11–5). Patients must be monitored carefully after the surgery for potential complications of the procedure, such as infection, bleeding, wound dehiscence, and fistula formation. In addition, the patient is faced with learning new self-care skills (ostomy care), evaluating components of self-image and body image, and learning new sexual expression behaviors and attitudes.[25, 99]

Radiation therapy for disease recurrence consists mainly of external therapy and occasionally with interstitial implants and has a 25% survival rate. Women with a central recurrence who have not received prior radiation therapy to the area are candidates for this form of treatment[66] (see Chapter 22).

Antineoplastic agents, as single agents (cisplatin, paclitaxel, gemcitabine, carboplatin, ifosfamide, 5-

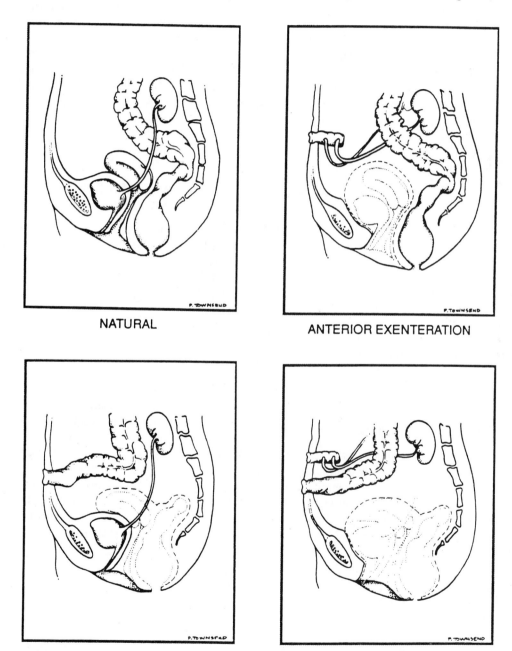

NATURAL

ANTERIOR EXENTERATION

POSTERIOR EXENTERATION

TOTAL EXENTERATION

FIGURE 11–5   Pelvic exenteration for treatment of cervical cancer. (From DeStefano MS, Bertin-Matson K: Gynecologic cancers. In McCorkle R and others, editors: *Cancer nursing: a comprehensive textbook,* ed 2, Philadelphia, Saunders, 1997.)

fluorouracil (5-FU), doxorubicin, methotrexate, vinblastine, vinorelbine, and bleomycin) or in combination, have been used to treat women with recurrent cervical cancer; however, responses to combination chemotherapy versus single-agent cisplatin have shown a limited overall survival. Currently there are a number of ongoing trials of neoadjuvant administration of chemotherapy prior to surgical or radiation therapy. Information from these studies compared to historical controls suggest there is an increased complete response rate, a decrease in the incidence of positive pelvic lymph nodes, and an increase in 2- to 3-year disease-free survival, especially in stage I and II disease. Combination regimens for neoadjuvant chemotherapy appear to provide better response rates versus single agents. Based on the evidence, it is likely that concurrent chemotherapy with radiation therapy will become a new standard of care for patients with bulky and advanced cervical cancer.[13, 24, 25, 83]

Previous issues regarding combination radiation therapy and chemotherapy include the following[17, 24]:

1. Previous radiation therapy to the pelvis may result in fibrosis of the bone marrow and a decreased tolerance of the chemotherapy agents' hematologic effects.
2. Decreased vascularization of recurrent tumors may limit the chemotherapy agents' ability to reach the target tissues.
3. Fibrosis from previous radiation therapy can also damage and obstruct the ureters.
4. The combination of ureteral obstruction and nephrotoxicity of many antineoplastic agents may result in the kidneys being unable to clear the drug metabolites from the body.

TREATMENT DURING PREGNANCY

As the incidence of preinvasive and invasive cancer is increasing in younger women of childbearing age, the issue of treatment for the woman who is pregnant has become more common. Careful discussion among the woman, partner, gynecologic oncologist, and obstetrician about potential risks of the disease, evaluation procedures, and treatment is recommended at each step of the evaluation and treatment process. Pregnant women with an abnormal Pap smear are evaluated with colposcopy and biopsies. If the squamocolumnar junction can be visualized entirely with colposcopy and if directed biopsies are sufficient to rule out the presence of invasive cancer, the clinician can follow the woman to term with interval Pap smears and colposcopy examinations. Appropriate treatment is deferred until after delivery. If, however, the limits of the colposcopically abnormal area are not visualized or if biopsies cannot rule out

invasive cancer, a conization of the cervix is recommended. Profuse bleeding and spontaneous abortion of the fetus are potential complications of the procedure.[17, 24, 25, 45]

Invasive cancer of the cervix occurs in 0.2% to 4% of pregnancies. Women with stage IA disease usually can be followed with Pap smears, colposcopy, and biopsies to term. In the presence of invasive cancer, immediate treatment is recommended. For women at less than 24 weeks' gestation, the pregnancy is terminated. Radical hysterectomy or radiation therapy can be used as primary treatment. Treatment of women between 24 and 28 weeks' gestation is more complicated. The risk of delaying treatment to allow for fetal development must be weighed carefully against the risk of progressive disease. After 28 weeks' gestation, the fetus is considered viable and is delivered by cesarean section to decrease the risk of maternal bleeding and spread of the disease. Radical hysterectomy is performed for definitive treatment after delivery.[24, 25]

FOLLOW-UP AFTER CERVICAL CANCER TREATMENT

After treatment for cervical cancer, all patients are examined on a scheduled frequency. Follow-up with cervical cytology, colposcopy, and pelvic examination at 3-month intervals for the first year; every 3 to 4 months during the second year; every 6 months for the next 3 years; and then annually beginning 5 years after treatment is recommended for early detection of recurrent invasive cervical cancer.[25]

PROGNOSIS

Clinical stage of the disease at the time of diagnosis is the most important determinant of survival, regardless of the treatment modality. Survival for cervical carcinoma is strongly associated with depth of tumor invasion into the underlying tissue stroma. The incidence of lymph node metastasis correlates with the size of the primary tumor, depth of stromal invasion, tumor grade, and patient age. Correlation of depth of stromal invasion with pelvic node metastasis is:

<1 mm invasion: extremely rare metastasis
1.0–3.0 mm invasion: <1% metastasis
3.1–5.0 mm invasion: approximately 4% pelvic nodal metastasis

The overall 5-year survival rate for patients diagnosed with CIS approaches 100%; negative nodes 85% to 90%; tumor emboli only in one pelvic node 82.5%; unilateral pelvic nodes positive 59% to 70%; bilateral pelvic nodes positive 22% to 40%; and common iliac nodes positive 25%.[25]

Endometrial Cancer

EPIDEMIOLOGY

Endometrial cancer has been the most common gynecologic malignancy among women in the United States since 1972. Worldwide the highest incidence occurs in North America, Europe, and South America. African American women in the United States have a *lower incidence* rate but a *higher mortality* rate than white women. An estimated 36,100 women will be diagnosed with endometrial cancer in 2000. The average age at diagnosis is 58 years.[14, 18, 53]

ETIOLOGY AND RISK FACTORS

Although the etiology of endometrial cancer is unknown, unopposed endogenous and exogenous *estrogen* are the major risk etiologic risk factors associated with the development of endometrial cancer. When ovarian production or progesterone during ovulation does not balance endogenous estrogen, regular sloughing of the endometrial lining does not occur (menses). A build-up of estrogen in the endometrial lining may lead to hyperplasia and cancer. With advancing age the amount of estrogen produced by the body decreases. However, researchers have suggested that as estrogen production is lowered, the body increases the production of estrogen precursors. These estrogen precursors are known to have carcinogenic potential and may play a role in the development of *adenomatous hyperplasia,* a premalignant condition.[7, 12, 18, 53]

Women who have Stein-Leventhal syndrome or who have an intact uterus and are receiving hormone replacement therapy with estrogen alone, as opposed to estrogen and progesterone combination therapy, are at higher risk of developing endometrial cancer. Risk factors for cancer of the endometrium include advancing age, early onset of menstruation, late menopause, and concurrent conditions. Women who have a history of postmenopausal bleeding, have never been pregnant, and have a late menopause are at higher risk for cancer of the endometrium. Concurrent conditions, such as obesity (21–50 lb = 3 times risk, > 50 lb = 10 times risk), diabetes, hypertension, endometrial hyperplasia, use of tamoxifen, or previous history of breast, colon, or ovarian cancer, also increase the risk for endometrial cancer.[14, 17, 32, 53]

PREVENTION, SCREENING, AND DETECTION

Prevention

As knowledge of the etiology of endometrial cancer evolves, the primary focus of prevention is targeted toward high-risk women. Maintenance of ideal body weight is recommended to avoid obesity and to decrease the risk of hypertension and diabetes. Treatment of premalignant changes of the endometrium such as endometrial hyperplasia with progesterone is suggested as a prevention strategy. To control the symptoms of menopause in women with an intact uterus, the addition of cyclic progesterone to the estrogen replacement regimen is recommended to reduce the risk of development of endometrial cancer. Pregnancy also serves as a protective factor because menses is halted for a short time, thereby decreasing the amount of circulating estrogens.[14, 53]

Screening

No reliable, valid, and cost-effective tests are recommended for periodic screening of asymptomatic women for endometrial cancer. Because the majority of endometrial cancers are stage I and the outcome for these patients is relatively favorable, mass screening is usually not cost effective and does not affect the survival outcome. However, the ACS recommends that asymptomatic, high-risk women have an endometrial tissue sampling done at menopause.

Detection

A complete history, physical examination, and diagnostic evaluation guide the detection of endometrial cancer in symptomatic women. The history includes a review of risk factors and the presence of clinical signs and symptoms for endometrial cancer. The physical examination includes evaluation of the size, consistency, and shape of the uterus, which are determined by palpation on the rectovaginal, bimanual examination. The depth of the uterine cavity is determined by inserting a uterine sound. An endometrial biopsy is obtained for histologic confirmation of the disease. A dilation and curettage (D&C) is considered the standard and should be performed whenever the endometrial biopsy is insufficient for diagnosis or contains atypical cells not diagnostic for carcinoma.[1, 8, 14]

CLASSIFICATION

The primary types of endometrial cancer are adenocarcinoma, sarcomas, mucinous carcinoma, serous carcinoma, clear cell carcinoma, and epidermoid carcinoma. More than 95% are endometrial *adenocarcinomas* and less than 5% are sarcomas. These exophytic or polypoid lesions tend to invade the uterine muscle. Variants of adenocarcinoma include *adenocanthoma* (contains benign squamous elements) and *adenosquamous carcinoma* (contains malignant squamous elements). The aggressive nature of these lesions results in a higher incidence of invasion of the myometrium and lymph nodes, distant metastases, and a lower survival rate compared with adenocarcinomas. Mixed mullerian tumors, sarcomas, clear cell carcinomas, and epidermoid carcinomas are rare and are associated with higher incidences of local and distant metastases and lower survival rates than adenocarcinomas.[14, 53]

CLINICAL FEATURES

The most common presenting symptom in women with endometrial cancer is prolonged, excessive, or irregular *premenopausal or postmenopausal bleeding.* Additional symptoms may include a yellow, watery vaginal discharge, *pyometria* (accumulation of pus in the uterus), *hematometria* (accumulation of blood in the uterus), or pain in the hypogastric or lumbosacral areas or the pelvis. Women with advanced disease may present with intestinal obstruction, ascites, jaundice, respiratory distress, or hemorrhage. On physical examination, the uterus may be enlarged or have an irregular contour. In advanced stages, extension of tumor into the vagina, bladder, or bowel may be palpated on bimanual, rectovaginal examination. Enlarged inguinal lymph nodes also may be palpated.[14, 17, 53] See Clinical Features for Gynecologic Cancers box.

DIAGNOSIS AND STAGING

The diagnostic evaluation includes physical examination, vaginal probe ultrasonography, color flow Doppler studies, tissue sampling, with laboratory and radiographic studies to determine the histologic type, degree of differentiation, and extent of disease. Ideally the gynecologic oncologist and radiation oncologist collaborate on the physical examination and a thorough evaluation of potential sites of metastatic disease: cervix, vagina, tissues surrounding the urethral meatus, parametria, and regional lymph nodes. Cervical biopsies, endocervical curettage, endometrial biopsy, or a fractional D&C are done to rule out the presence of a cervical malignancy and to obtain a tissue sample for diagnosis. Cervical biopsies and endocervical curettage are collected first to minimize the risk of contamination of the cervical specimen with endometrial tissue that may be dislodged by the uterine sound or dilator. Although obtaining the necessary specimens can be uncomfortable for the patient, the diagnostic evaluation usually can be performed in the outpatient setting.[4, 14, 76]

Laboratory studies routinely include a complete blood count (CBC), CA-125 levels, blood chemistry profile (SMA), and liver and renal chemistries. Additional radiographic studies to determine the presence of metastatic disease may include a chest x-ray film, magnetic

resonance imaging (MRI), and computed tomography (CT). If involvement of the bladder or rectum is suspected, intravenous pyelography (IVP), barium enema, cystoscopy, and proctosigmoidoscopy may be done.[14, 53]

Surgical staging is performed with a minimum of an exploratory laparotomy, total hysterectomy, bilateral salpingo-oophorectomy, and cytology. Staging is based on the depth of myometrial invasion, degree of cellular differentiation, spread to lymph nodes, and the extent of cervical involvement and metastatic disease.[14, 24, 76] Figure 11–6 presents the schema for staging cancer of the endometrium.

METASTASIS

Most endometrial cancers originate in the fundus of the uterus and spread by direct extension to the entire endometrium, through the layers of the uterine wall (myometrium and serosa), or through the endocervical canal to the cervix. The disease may also spread outside the uterus to the structures of the parametria and abdominal cavity, such as the ovaries, fallopian tubes, vagina, bladder, rectum, omentum, or bowel. Lymphatic metastases occur primarily to the pelvic and para-aortic lymph nodes. The endometrium is highly vascular; therefore hematogeneous spread, particularly with sarcomas, is common. Lung, liver, bones, and brain metastases may occur.[14, 24]

TREATMENT MODALITIES

Development of a plan for treatment of endometrial cancer is a collaborative effort between the gynecologic oncologist and radiation oncologist. Factors that influence the treatment plan selected include the type of tumor, degree of differentiation, stage of disease, and the woman's general health status.[14, 24, 58]

Surgery

Surgical resection provides the best chance for cure and guides the potential need for adjuvant therapy. Controversy exists regarding the extent of surgical staging, in particular the necessity and rationale for removing or sampling the draining lymphatics. An emerging practice in the United States is to perform more aggressive lymph node dissections. Because abnormal bleeding brings most women to the health care system with early stage disease, localized treatment is typically chosen. Usually a *total abdominal hysterectomy* and *bilateral salpingo-oophorectomy* (TAH-BSO) is the most common primary treatment for women with early stage disease. More extensive surgery, radical abdominal hysterectomy and bilateral pelvic lymphadenectomy, has been used for treatment, but surgical risks are higher and

Data Form for Cancer Staging

Patient identification

Name _____

Address _____

Hospital or clinic number _____

Age _____ Sex _____ Race _____

Institution identification

Hospital or clinic _____

Address _____

Oncology Record

Anatomic site of cancer _____

Histologic type _____

Grade (G) _____

Date of classification _____

Chronology of classification

[ ] Clinical (use all data prior to first treatment)

[ ] Pathologic (if definitively resected specimen available)

Clin	Path	TNM category	FIGO* stage	DEFINITIONS Primary Tumor (T)
[ ]	[ ]	TX		Primary tumor cannot be assessed
[ ]	[ ]	T0		No evidence of primary tumor
[ ]	[ ]	Tis		Carcinoma in situ
[ ]	[ ]	T1	I	Tumor confined to corpus uteri
[ ]	[ ]	T1a	IA	Tumor limited to endometrium
[ ]	[ ]	T1b	IB	Tumor invades up to or less than one half of the myometrium
[ ]	[ ]	T1c	IC	Tumor invades to more than one half of the myometrium
[ ]	[ ]	T2	II	Tumor invades cervic but does not extend beyond uterus
[ ]	[ ]	T2a	IIA	Endocervical glandular involvement only
[ ]	[ ]	T2b	IIB	Cervical stromal invasion
[ ]	[ ]	T3 &/or N1	III	Local and/or regional spread as specified in T3a, b, N1 and FIGO IIIA, B, and C below
[ ]	[ ]	T3a	IIIA	Tumor involves serosa and/or adnexae (direct extension or metastasis) and/or cancer cells in ascites or peritoneal washings
[ ]	[ ]	T3b	IIIB	Vaginal involvement (direct extension or metastasis)
[ ]	[ ]	N1	IIIC	Metastasis to the pelvic and /or paraaortic lymph nodes
[ ]	[ ]	T4†	IVA	Tumor invades bladder mucosa and/or bowel mucosa
[ ]	[ ]	M1	IVB	Distant metastasis. (*Excluding* metastasis to vagina, pelvic serosa or adnexae. *Including* metastasis to intraabdominal lymph nodes other than paraaortic, and/or inguinal lymph nodes.)
		Lymph Node (N)		
[ ]	[ ]	NX		Regional lymph nodes cannot be assessed
[ ]	[ ]	N0		No regional lymph node metastasis
[ ]	[ ]	N1		Regional lymph node metastasis
		Distant Metastasis (M)		
[ ]	[ ]	MX		Presence of distant metastasis cannot be assessed
[ ]	[ ]	M0		No distant metastasis
[ ]	[ ]	M1	IVB	Distant metastasis

Clin	Path	Stage Grouping AJCC/UICC				FIGO
[ ]	[ ]	0	Tis	N0	M0	
[ ]	[ ]	IA	T1a	N0	M0	Stage IA
		IB	T1b	N0	M0	Stage IB
		IC	T1c	N0	M0	Stage IC
[ ]	[ ]	IIA	T2a	N0	M0	Stage IIA
		IIB	T2b	N0	M0	Stage IIB
		IIIA	T3a	N0	M0	Stage IIIA
[ ]	[ ]	IIIB	T3b	N0	M0	Stage IIIB
[ ]	[ ]	IIIC	T1	N1	M0	Stage IIIC
			T2	N1	M0	
			T3a	N1	M0	
			T3b	N1	M0	
[ ]	[ ]	IVA	T4	any N	M0	Stage IVA
[ ]	[ ]	IVB	any T	any N	M1	Stage IVB

Staged by _____ M.D.

_____ Registrar

Date _____

FIGURE 11–6 Corpus uteri (endometrium)—data form for cancer staging. (From American Joint Committee on Cancer: *Manual for staging cancer,* ed 5, Philadelphia, Lippincott-Raven, 1997.)

no significant improvement in survival rates has been reported. Vaginal hysterectomy with laparoscopic surgical staging may be an alternative for selected patients, but further studies are needed to determine which group of women are best suited for this approach.[14, 24, 43, 59, 76]

Radiation Therapy

Selected patients may benefit from radiation therapy, which may be given either preoperatively or postoperatively. Radiation therapy may consist of intracavity brachytherapy, vaginal cuff irradiation, and external beam. The specific type of therapy is modified according to the patient's needs and disease status. Survival rates for women treated with radiation therapy alone, even with early stage disease, are not as high as those observed when surgery alone is used as the primary treatment. In women with bulky disease, poorly differentiated tumors, or greater depth of myometrial invasion, preoperative or postoperative radiation therapy may be recommended. Advantages of preoperative and postoperative radiation therapy are detailed in the literature.[14, 24, 34, 98] (See also Chapter 22.)

Hormonal Therapy

Endometrial cancer is a hormone-dependent tumor. Increased levels of progesterone and estrogen receptors have been identified in more well-differentiated tumors. Therefore clinicians are using estrogen and progesterone receptor analyses as one factor to determine those women who may benefit from hormone manipulation either as an adjuvant therapy or as treatment for recurrent disease. Depo-Provera, Provera, Delalutin, and Megace are the most common progestational agents currently used for women who are estrogen and progesterone receptor positive. Response rates with hormonal manipulation range from 30% to 70%, with the highest response rate occurring in women with well-differentiated tumors.[14, 24]

---

* *FIGO:* Federation Internationale de Gynecologie et d'Obstetrique

† *Note:* The presence of bullous edema is not sufficient evidence to classify a tumor T4.

Chemotherapy

Antineoplastic agents are reserved for women who have estrogen/progesterone-negative tumors, who have failed hormone therapy, or who have disseminated disease. However, antineoplastic agents, used either as single agents or in combination, have resulted in no significant improvement in survival rates from endometrial cancer. Agents typically used include cisplatin, docetaxel, doxorubicin, hexamethylmelamine, vincristine, carboplatin, and ifosfamide. Evaluation of the effectiveness of combined hormonal and antineoplastic agents in women with endometrial cancer is ongoing.[14, 24, 67, 79]

PROGNOSIS

Properly staged patients with a stage IA, grade I cancer have an excellent prognosis and need only surgery since the 5-year survival is 99%. These patients are followed by physical examination including pelvic examination every 3 months for 2 years; then every 6 months for 3 years, then yearly. Relative 5-year survival rates associated with a diagnosis of endometrial cancer have improved significantly between 1960–1962 and 1990–1992. The 5-year survival rate for women diagnosed with early stage endometrial cancer is 85%; if diagnosed at a regional stage 49% to 70%; and with distant metastasis, 19%. The overall 5-year survival for all stages combined is 77.5%.[14, 24]

Ovarian Cancer

EPIDEMIOLOGY

The 23,100 new cases of ovarian cancer account for approximately 30% of all gynecologic cancers diagnosed in the United States in 2000. The lifetime likelihood that a woman will develop ovarian cancer is estimated to be 1 in 55, with a higher frequency associated with certain familial syndromes. Ovarian cancer is more common in women over age 60, but often occurs in women with a family history before or during their early forties. Ovarian cancer causes more deaths (14,000 deaths and equals more than all other gynecologic diseases combined [12,500] for the year 2000) and accounts for 6% of all cancer deaths among women. The highest incidence of ovarian cancer is reported in highly industrialized countries. The disease occurs less frequently in women from Asia and Latin America.[32, 53, 77, 95]

ETIOLOGY AND RISK FACTORS

The etiology of ovarian cancer is unknown. However, age, genetics, history of other cancers, and menstrual history have been associated with an increased incidence of the disease. Most ovarian cancers are diagnosed in the 50- to 59-year-old age group. Families with a history of ovarian cancer across multiple generations have been identified but are uncommon. A familial or personal history of other cancers, including breast, colon, and uterine, increases the risk of ovarian cancer. The incidence of ovarian cancer is greater among women who are single, nulliparous, and infertile; the incidence is lower among women who use oral contraceptives. Researchers are currently evaluating the role of uninterrupted ovulation in the pathogenesis of ovarian cancer.[30, 53, 77, 95]

PREVENTION, SCREENING, AND DETECTION

Prevention and Screening

Because the etiology of ovarian cancer remains a mystery, no recommendations exist for prevention of the disease. Women in higher-risk categories, as described previously, are encouraged to seek routine gynecologic care, including an annual pelvic examination. Palpation of a normal-size ovary in postmenopausal women is cause for a further diagnostic evaluation. However, the overall yield of one case of ovarian cancer in 10,000 pelvic examinations is low. Furthermore, the occurrence of widely disseminated metastatic disease in women with palpable disease is high, and survival rates in this group are low.[8, 12, 77, 95]

The cost effectiveness with the use of tumor markers and vaginal ultrasound to screen high-risk women for ovarian cancer has been studied. Researchers have noted variable specificity and sensitivity outcomes with tumor markers, such as α-fetoprotein (AFP) for rare endodermal sinus tumors, carcinoembryonic antigen (CEA), and CA-125 for epithelial ovarian tumors. Serial CA-125 levels have been used to monitor selected high-risk women with a strong familial history of ovarian cancer. A third method of screening women at high risk for ovarian cancer has been serial vaginal ultrasounds. Because of the variability in results, none of the tests is recommended for screening asymptomatic populations. Consequently many women continue to be diagnosed with ovarian cancer after the disease has spread throughout the abdominal cavity, lymphatic channels, and vascular system.[53, 77, 95]

Within the past decade there is increasing interest in using family history to identify patients at high risk for ovarian cancer. Certain hereditary syndromes have been described, which include hereditary breast-ovarian cancer syndromes associated with changes at chromosome 17q (BRAC1) and chromosome 13q (BRAC2) and hereditary nonpolyposis colon cancer syndromes (see Chapter 2). These familial ovarian cancers typically appear at a younger age than sporadic ovarian cancer.

Options regarding prevention of ovarian cancer in the high-risk patients, prophylactic oophorectomy or tubal ligation, remain controversial. Other factors that offer some degree of protection include oral contraceptives, pregnancy, and breast-feeding. Following a low-fat, high-fiber diet also may help.[24, 38, 53, 77, 82, 95]

Detection

Most women with early stage ovarian cancer are asymptomatic. Therefore the clinician must maintain an index of suspicion for ovarian cancer. A careful personal and family history is important to identify women at high risk for the disease. Attention to generalized, vague complaints among women during their middle-age years often will alert the clinician to the possibility of ovarian cancer. Finally, a pelvic examination and palpation of an adnexal mass or a postmenopausal ovary raise suspicion for ovarian cancer.[95]

CLASSIFICATION

Ovarian carcinomas are classified as epithelial, sex cord-stromal, or germ cell tumors. *Epithelial tumors,* most frequently found in women 40 to 65 years of age, account for 90% of all ovarian malignancies diagnosed in the United States. *Sex cord-stromal tumors* occur much less frequently (5%) than the epithelial tumors. These tumors often are associated with femininizing or masculinizing effects. Women with sex cord-stromal tumors have a better prognosis than women with epithelial malignancies. *Germ cell tumors* account for about 5% of all ovarian malignancies. These tumors, particularly dysgerminoma, endodermal sinus tumors, and embryonal carcinoma, occur most frequently in younger women. Because most ovarian malignancies are epithelial tumors, the remainder of this section focuses on this specific ovarian neoplasm.[53, 77, 95]

CLINICAL FEATURES

Vague gastrointestinal symptoms such as dyspepsia, indigestion, anorexia, and early satiety may be some of the first symptoms of ovarian cancer. Pressure of the tumor on the rectum and bladder may result in symptoms of urinary frequency, constipation, or pelvic pressure and discomfort. Progressive disease is marked by an increase in abdominal girth, pain, shortness of breath, intestinal or ureteral obstruction, and muscle wasting.[53, 77, 95] (See Clinical Features box.)

DIAGNOSIS AND STAGING

Diagnosis and staging (Table 11–2) of women with ovarian cancer are achieved by tissue sampling and inspec-

tion of the abdominal cavity at the time of exploratory laparotomy. The initial approach and exploration of the abdomen are well defined and methodical to allow careful evaluation of the extent of disease and to remove (debulk) as much of the tumor burden as possible. Before surgical exploration, however, a series of laboratory and radiographic tests is recommended. A CBC, biochemical profile, and CA-125 level are obtained. In addition, a chest x-ray film, cystoscopy, proctoscopy, IVP, barium enema, CT, MRI, or ultrasound may be ordered. The stage of ovarian cancer at diagnosis is an important indicator of prognosis.[20, 21, 77, 95]

METASTASIS

Ovarian carcinoma spreads by direct extension to adjacent pelvic organs such as the opposite ovary, uterus, fallopian tubes, bladder, rectum, and peritoneum, seeding of the peritoneal cavity, and lymphatic and vascular channels (Fig. 11–7). Spread occurs primarily by shedding of malignant cells that float within and form micrometastases throughout the peritoneal cavity. Common sites of metastatic disease include the omentum and surfaces of the bowel, uterus, bladder, and peritoneum. Free-floating malignant cells are washed beneath the diaphragm and removed through lymphatic channels located in the diaphragm. This pattern of flow of peritoneal fluid accounts for the high incidence of metastatic ovarian disease found on the undersurfaces of the diaphragm.[77, 95]

Lymphatic invasion can occur in the pelvic, para-aortic, and aortic nodes even in early stage disease. Partial or complete obstruction of lymphatic channels in the diaphragm result in the accumulation of malignant ascitic fluid. Although rare, metastasis can occur through vascular invasion to distant sites. The most common sites of hematogenous spread include the liver, lung, and pleura.[40, 77, 95]

TREATMENT MODALITIES

Treatment of ovarian cancer is based on surgical staging of the disease, malignant potential of the tumor, and the bulk of remaining disease. Surgery, radiation therapy, chemotherapy, or autologous peripheral blood stem cell transplantation are used in varied combination regimens.[11, 91, 95]

Surgery

Volume of residual disease is related both to response to chemotherapy and to survival. The standard of care with disease confined to the abdominal cavity is to resect as much disease as possible at the initial onset of treatment. Surgery has a major role in the diagnosis, primary

TABLE 11-2
Staging Classification for Ovarian Cancer

Primary Tumor (T)		
TNM	**FIGO**	**Definition**
TX		Primary tumor cannot be assessed
T0		No evidence of primary tumor
T1	I	Tumor limited to ovaries
T1a	Ia	Tumor limited to one ovary; capsule intact, no tumor on ovarian surface
T1b	Ib	Tumor limited to both ovaries; capsules intact, no tumor on ovarian surface
T1c	Ic	Tumor limited to one or both ovaries with any of the following: capsule ruptured, tumor on ovarian surface, malignant cells in ascites, peritoneal washing
T2	II	Tumor involves one or both ovaries with pelvic extension
T2a	IIa	Extension and/or implants on uterus and/or tube(s)
T2b	IIb	Extension to other pelvic tissues
T2c	IIc	Pelvic extension (2a or 2b) with malignant cells in ascites or peritoneal washing
T3 and/or N1	III	Tumor involves one or both ovaries with microscopically confirmed peritoneal metastasis outside pelvis and/or regional lymph node metastasis
T3a	IIIa	Microscopic peritoneal metastasis beyond pelvis
T3b	IIIb	Macroscopic peritoneal metastasis beyond pelvis 2 cm or less in greatest dimension
T3c and/ or N1	IIIc	Peritoneal metastasis beyond pelvis more than 2 cm in greatest dimension and/or regional lymph node metastasis
M1	IV	Distant metastasis (excludes peritoneal metastasis)

Regional Lymph Nodes (N)

Regional lymph nodes include hypogastric (obturator), common iliac, external iliac, internal iliac, lateral sacral, para-aortic, and inguinal

TMN	Definition
NX	Regional lymph nodes cannot be assessed
N0	No regional lymph node metastasis
N1	Regional lymph node metastasis

Distant Metastasis (M)

TMN	FIGO	Definition
MX		Presence of distant metastasis cannot be assessed
M0		No distant metastasis
M1	IV	Distant metastasis (excludes peritoneal metastasis)

Stage Grouping

Stage IA:	T1a-N0-M0
Stage IB:	T1b-N0-M0
Stage IC:	T1c-N0-M0
Stage IIA:	T2a-N0-M0
Stage IIB:	T2b-N0-M0
Stage IIC:	T2c-N0-M0
Stage IIIA:	T3a-N0-M0
Stage IIIB:	T3b-N0-M0
Stage IIIC:	T3c-N0-M0
	any T-N1-M0
Stage IV:	any T-any N-M1

Data from American Joint Committee on Cancer: Manual for staging cancer, *ed 5, Philadelphia, Lippincott-Raven, 1997.*

treatment, evaluation of response to therapy, and palliative care for women with ovarian cancer (Box 11-1). In addition to the exploratory laparotomy required for staging, surgery is used as primary treatment for women with borderline and malignant tumors of the ovary. For younger women with tumors of borderline malignant potential, conservative treatment with unilateral oophorectomy may be considered definitive treatment. However, in women beyond childbearing years, every attempt is made to remove the uterus, cervix, fallopian tubes, and ovaries if the disease is considered surgically resectable. Beyond a TAH-BSO, surgical resection of the bulk of remaining tumor is attempted. Resection of the bladder, colon, or omentum may be indicated. The extent of the debulking procedure is based on evaluation of potential risks of more extensive resection and potential benefits in terms of survival and quality of life.[46, 50, 77, 95]

The use of surgical exploration (second-look procedure) to evaluate the response to primary therapy for ovarian cancer is controversial. Advocates of second-look procedures indicate that the procedure allows for

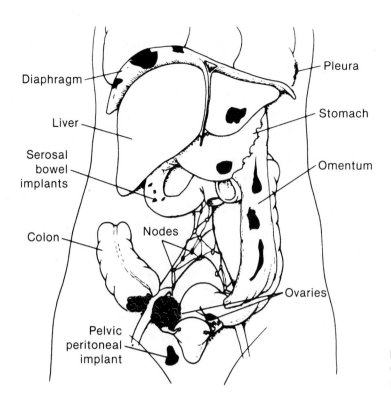

FIGURE 11-7 Patterns of metastasis for ovarian cancer. (From DiSaia PJ, Creasman WT: *Clinical gynecologic oncology,* ed 4, St. Louis, Mosby, 1997).

direct inspection of the abdominal cavity, sampling of ascitic fluid, and sampling of abdominal tissues at risk for persistent microscopic disease. If persistent disease is found, the surgeon is able to debulk the tumor burden before retreatment. If no disease is documented, therapy is usually discontinued and the woman enters a clinical follow-up scheme. Opponents of the second-look procedure argue that the procedure requires hospitalization, a major abdominal surgery, and disruption of the patient's normal activities.[46, 50, 77, 95]

Surgery has also been used in providing palliative care to women with advanced ovarian cancer. Bowel resection and bowel or urinary diversion may be done to relieve obstructive symptoms in selected patients. The relative risks and benefits of such procedures are weighed carefully before surgical intervention.[17]

Radiation Therapy

Teletherapy to the pelvis and abdomen and the instillation of radioactive isotopes in the peritoneal cavity have been used in the treatment of women with early stages (I and II) of ovarian cancer. Although adequate doses of radiation can be delivered to the pelvis and abdomen to eradicate the disease, the tolerance of normal tissues within the treatment field to the tumoricidal doses is limited. To overcome this barrier, shielding techniques for vital organs such as the kidneys and liver, multifield techniques and various fractionation techniques have been used to limit damage to normal tissues and organs.[46, 95]

The extent of residual disease and the differentiation of the tumor determine the response to radiation therapy. Women with well-differentiated tumors that are less than 2 cm in size have the best response rates. Radioactive isotopes (e.g., ^{32}P) have been used to treat residual disease in the peritoneal cavity. Women, who have limited residual disease, less than 2 cm, are the most likely candidates for ^{32}P therapy. Disadvantages of the treatment include potential inability of the entire peritoneal cavity to be exposed to the isotope because of adhesions or location and the occurrence of small-bowel obstruction or stenosis.[46, 95]

Chemotherapy and Peripheral Blood Stem Cell Transplantation

For women with high-risk, early stage, epithelial ovarian tumors and for women with disseminated disease, antineoplastic therapy has resulted in improved survival outcomes. Historically, alkylating agents have been used most often as either single agents or in combination regimens for treatment of women with ovarian cancer. Current therapies include cisplatin-based chemotherapy at conventional doses without paclitaxel; paclitaxel plus cisplatin at conventional doses; and high-dose chemotherapy with peripheral blood stem cell transplantation (PBSCT). Early results from high-dose chemotherapy with PBSCT indicate that it has a high response rate; however, there is no indication that it leads to prolonged survival. Clinical trials with new combinations of paclitaxel/carboplatin with oral etoposide, gemcitabine, epir-

---

BOX 11-1

Steps in Surgically Staging Ovarian Cancer

Step 1. If ascites is present, remove as much as possible for cytology. If no ascites is present, obtain cell washings from the pelvis, both abdominal gutters, and both subdiaphragmatic areas.

Step 2. Determine whether the mass is malignant; if malignant, perform appropriate pelvic procedure (total abdominal hysterectomy and bilateral salpingo-oophorectomy unless patient desires further childbearing and there is no evidence of spread beyond the ovary).

Step 3. Carefully examine pelvic peritoneum; if lesions are present, remove as much as possible and biopsy any lesion that cannot be removed. If no lesions are seen, sample at a minimum the peritoneum of lateral pelvic sidewalls, bladder, rectosigmoid, and cul-de-sac.

Step 4. Examine the paracolic gutters, and remove any lesions seen. If no lesions are seen, obtain a 1 × 3-cm strip of peritoneum on either side.

Step 5. Examine the omentum, and remove any that contains visible tumor (including the supracolic omentum if involved by tumor). If no lesions are seen, remove the infracolic omentum.

Step 6. Examine and palpate both diaphragms and surface of the spleen and liver. If lesions are present, remove as much as possible; biopsy if they cannot be removed. If no lesions are seen, a 1 × 2-cm strip of peritoneum should be carefully excised from the right hemidiaphragm. (NOTE: Only peritoneum is needed, and care should be taken not to create a pneumothorax.)

Step 7. Beginning at either the rectum or cecum, carefully inspect the entire large colon and remove and biopsy any suspicious lesion of the intestine or mesentery.*

Step 8. Beginning at either the ileocecal valve or ligament of Treitz, carefully inspect the entire small bowel and mesentery and remove or biopsy any lesions.*

Step 9. If, after all the above procedures, no gross disease larger than 1 or 2 cm is left, the pelvic and para-aortic lymph nodes should be sampled.

* If resection of intestine is necessary to cytoreduce the tumor optimally or to relieve obstruction, this should be performed.

From Hoskins WJ, Perez CA, Young RC: Cancer of the ovary. In DeVita VT Jr, Hellman S, Rosenberg SA, editors: *Cancer: principles and practice of oncology*, ed 5, Philadelphia, Lippincott-Raven, 1997.

---

ubicin, topotecan, liposomal doxorubicin, and/or hexamethylmelamine have recently begun.* (See Chapters 23 and 25.)

Because metastasis in ovarian cancer occurs primarily through exfoliation of malignant cells within the peritoneal cavity, researchers have explored the use of antineoplastic agents intraperitoneally to treat the disease. For individuals with no residual disease but who are at high risk for recurrence, intraperitoneal chemotherapy (cisplatin or paclitaxel) has been used as adjuvant therapy. In women with minimal residual disease, the intraperitoneal route of administration has been used to provide high concentrations of antineoplastic drug(s) to disease within the peritoneal cavity while limiting the concentrations of the agent(s) in the circulation and thus limiting systemic toxic effects. Prospective randomized trials in previously untreated patients are in progress. Until the completion of these trials high-dose chemotherapy with PBSCT and intraperitoneal chemotherapy should be considered investigational.[9, 74, 75, 81]

PROGNOSIS

Prognostic factors for ovarian cancer include: (1) age—older patients have poorer survival; (2) grade—poorly differentiated lesions are associated with poorer survival; (3) histology type—clear cell and mucinous types are associated with poorer survival; (4) stage—more extensive disease produces a poorer survival; (5) volume of disease—patients with stage III disease with a larger volume of residual disease leads to a poorer survival. Five-year survival rates according to the stage are stage I, 95%; stage II, 65%; stage III, 20%; and stage IV, 5%.[77, 95]

Vulvar Cancer

EPIDEMIOLOGY

Vulvar carcinoma accounts for approximately 3400 cases in the United States for the year 2000. Although the incidence of invasive vulvar cancer is small, the incidence rates of *vulvar intraepithelial neoplasia* (VIN) and CIS are increasing. VIN occurs most often in women in their forties, CIS in women in their fifties, and invasive disease in women in their sixties. No ethnic or geographic variations have been noted in the incidence rates. The most frequent sites for vulvar carcinoma include the labia majora, labia minora, clitoris, and perineum. Approximately 800 patients will die from vulvar cancer in 2000.[25, 32]

---

* References 27, 62, 64, 70, 74, 87, 96.

ETIOLOGY AND RISK FACTORS

The etiology of vulvar carcinoma is unknown. However, several factors have been associated with an increased incidence of the disease. These include concurrent diseases such as hypertension, diabetes mellitus, cardiovascular disease, obesity, cervical cancer, early menopause, nulliparity, and chronic vulvar irritation. Syphilis and lymphogranuloma inguinale have been associated with invasive vulvar cancer, but no specific cause-and-effect relationships have been established. Additionally there may be an association of vulvar cancer with HPV.[12, 53, 63]

PREVENTION, SCREENING, AND DETECTION

Prevention and Screening

No specific measures are recommended for the prevention of vulvar cancer. In recent years, emphasis has been placed on teaching women vulvar self-examination as a strategy for screening in asymptomatic women.[12]

Detection

Many women with vulvar cancer are asymptomatic. Therefore a thorough history and physical examination are required to identify women with existing risk factors and to inspect and palpate vulvar tissue for abnormalities. Physical examination of the vulva, groins, and pelvis is mandatory.[25] (See Geriatric Considerations box.)

GERIATRIC CONSIDERATIONS

Gynecologic Cancers

Vulvar and vaginal cancer disease onset occurs most often in the late fifth, sixth, to the seventh decade of life.

Patients should be taught the need for annual health examinations, including bimanual pelvic examination with a thorough inspection and palpation of the perineal, vulvar and vaginal areas.

Other chronic diseases (e.g., hypertension, diabetes, arthritis) may exacerbate with the onset or progression of the disease and the side effects of the multiple therapies.

Age-related modifications may require a reduction in drug regimens and other therapies.

Elderly women may live alone and have limited financial, social, and health care resources. Nurses should assess needs and intervention strategies and consult with multiple referral systems (e.g., American Cancer Society, Social Services, Meals On Wheels, Home Health Agencies).[15, 21, 22, 28, 85, 88]

CLASSIFICATION

Invasive cancers of the vulva are classified as squamous cell, basal cell, adenocarcinoma, and malignant melanoma. Ninety percent of all malignancies of the vulva are squamous cell carcinomas.

CLINICAL FEATURES

The most common presentation of invasive vulvar cancer is in the postmenopausal woman with a vulvar lump or mass, pain, or pruritus of several months' duration. Vulvar tissues may be reddened, white, warty, or abnormally pigmented. Vulvar bleeding, discharge, and dysuria may be present.[25, 53] (See Clinical Features box.)

DIAGNOSIS AND STAGING

Diagnosis of vulvar cancer is made by a wedge biopsy, which includes some surrounding skin and underlying dermis and connective tissue. A thorough examination of abnormality areas is noted via inspection, palpation, and colposcopic examination. Once a diagnosis of invasive disease is made, the woman undergoes a metastatic work-up that may consist of cystoscopy, proctoscopy, barium enema, IVP, lymphangiography, CT, and MRI. Sentinel node biopsy as a surgical staging method (see Chapter 7 for a complete description of this procedure) is being explored. Staging for vulvar carcinoma is done clinically.[25, 50, 92] Figure 11–8 presents the classification system for staging.

METASTASIS

Direct extension occurs to adjacent structures including the vagina, perineum, clitoris, and anus. Lymphatic embolization to regional lymph nodes may occur early in the disease. At clinical diagnosis, approximately 10% of superficially invasive vulvar cancer have undergone lymph node metastasis. Carcinomas of the vulva follow a predictable, slow pattern of spread by direct extension to these adjacent tissues and by lymphatic spread to inguinal and pelvic lymph nodes. The frequency of lymph node metastasis to the inguinofemoral nodes is related to the size of the lesion and depth of stromal invasion. Hematogenous spread rarely occurs. The frequency of groin lymph node metastasis in relation to lesion size in vulvar carcinoma is: lesion size less than 1 cm/5% metastasis; 1 to 2 cm/16% metastasis; 2 to 4 cm/33% metastasis; and greater than 4 cm/53% metastasis.[25, 69]

TREATMENT MODALITIES

Treatment of women with vulvar cancer is based on the size and extent of the lesion, depth of stromal invasion,

Data Form for Cancer Staging

Patient identification
Name _____
Address _____
Hospital or clinic number _____
Age _____ Sex _____ Race _____

Institution identification
Hospital or clinic _____
Address _____
Oncology Record
Anatomic site of cancer _____
Histologic type _____

Grade (G) _____
Date of classification _____
Chronology of classification
[ ] Clinical (use all data prior to first treatment)
[ ] Pathologic (if definitively resected specimen available)

Clin	Path		
		DEFINITIONS	
		Primary Tumor (T)	
[ ]	[ ]	TX	Primary tumor cannot be assessed
[ ]	[ ]	T0	No evidence of primary tumor
[ ]	[ ]	Tis	Preinvasive carcinoma (carcinoma *in situ*)
[ ]	[ ]	T1	Tumor confined to the vulva or to the vulva and perineum, 2 cm or less in greatest dimension
[ ]	[ ]	T2	Tumor confined to the vulva or to the vulva and perineum, more than 2 cm in greatest dimension
[ ]	[ ]	T3	Tumor involves any of the following: lower urethra, vagina, or anus
[ ]	[ ]	T4	Tumor involves any of the following: bladder mucosa, upper part of urethral mucosa, rectal mucosa or tumor fixed to the bone
		Lymph Node (N)	
		Regional lymph nodes are the femoral and inguinal nodes	
[ ]	[ ]	NX	Regional lymph nodes cannot be assessed
[ ]	[ ]	N0	No regional lymph node metastasis
[ ]	[ ]	N1	Unilateral regional lymph node metastasis
[ ]	[ ]	N2	Bilateral regional lymph node metastasis
		Distant Metastasis (M)	
[ ]	[ ]	MX	Presence of distant metastasis cannot be assessed
[ ]	[ ]	M0	No distant metastasis
[ ]	[ ]	M1	Distant metastasis (Pelvic lymph node metastasis is M1)

Clin	Path	**Stage Grouping** AJCC/IUCC				
[ ]	[ ]	0	Tis	N0	M0	
[ ]	[ ]	I	T1	N0	M0	I
[ ]	[ ]	II	T2	N0	M0	II
[ ]	[ ]	III	T1	N1	M0	III
			T2	N1	M0	
			T3	N0	M0	
			T3	N1	M0	
[ ]	[ ]	IVA	T1	N2	M0	IVA
			T2	N2	M0	
			T3	N2	M0	
			T4	any N	M0	
[ ]	[ ]	IVB	any T	any N	M1	IVB

Staged by _____ M.D.
_____ Registrar
Date _____

FIGURE 11–8 Vulva—data form for cancer staging. (From American Joint Committee on Cancer: *Manual for staging cancer,* ed 5, Philadelphia, Lippincott-Raven, 1997.)

and evidence of metastatic disease. The clinician also considers functional and cosmetic results when planning treatment. For women with preinvasive disease, VIN, or CIS, in a limited area, a conservative approach with topical 5-FU, cryotherapy, laser therapy, wide local excision, skinning vulvectomy, or simple vulvectomy can be used for primary treatment. With each treatment the chance for control of disease with minimal disruption of function or cosmesis in carefully selected women is good. Women undergoing conservative treatment must be followed at 3- to 6-month intervals.[25, 52, 69, 92, 93]

In women with invasive disease less than 2 cm in diameter, less than 5 mm of invasion, and negative inguinal lymph nodes on frozen section, wide local excision alone may be done. If the inguinal lymph nodes are positive, a radical vulvectomy with complete, bilateral groin dissection is done. The trend over the past 15 years has been toward less radical surgery for early stage

vulvar cancer in an attempt to decrease the significant physical and psychological morbidity associated with en bloc dissection. Sentinel node dissection combined with pathologic ultrastaging is being investigated. This method appears to be highly sensitive for detecting subclinical micrometastases in the regional lymphatics area. This technique potentially provides a more accurate assessment with less surgical morbidity than conventional inguinofemoral lymphadenectomy. For women who are not candidates for surgical intervention, radiation therapy for early stage disease has been used successfully.*

Historically, clinicians have used a surgical approach to the treatment of vulvar carcinoma, although the risks of wound breakdown, lymphedema, and sexual dysfunc-

_____

* References 10, 22, 28, 35, 69, 92, 93.

tion were high. Radiation therapy was not used because of the high incidence of short-term side effects (moist desquamation, maceration) on the skin over the vulvar, perineal, and groin areas. Given the advanced age of women usually diagnosed with the disease, concurrent health problems that increase surgical risks, and improved techniques of delivering high doses of radiation therapy while sparing the skin, clinicians again are evaluating the role of radiation therapy in the treatment of women with vulvar cancer. The treatment plan for women with locally advanced disease can consist of a combination of surgery, radical surgery (vulvectomy, anterior exenteration, and posterior exenteration), and preoperative or postoperative radiation therapy. For women with distant metastasis, a combination of radiation therapy to control central disease and chemotherapy for systemic disease is typically used as palliative treatment.[22, 25, 50, 68, 93]

Chemotherapy has been used to treat limited numbers of women with vulvar cancer. The use of chemotherapy and radiation therapy to shrink large tumors to allow better surgical resection continues to be evaluated but has demonstrated excellent results to date. Agents used in these protocols include 5-FU, cisplatin, methotrexate, cyclophosphamide, bleomycin, mitomycin C, via single-agent administration or combination therapy.[25]

PROGNOSIS

Survival of patients with vulvar cancer is associated with the stage of disease at diagnosis and more specifically the status of pelvic lymph nodes. Five-year survival for patients with vulvar cancer treated with a curative intent includes stages I, 92%; stage II, 80%; stage III, 53.5%; stage IV, 14.6%; and overall. 70.3%. The overall 5-year survival rate of patients with positive lymph nodes is 50% and overall survival rate for patients treated with palliation is 47%.[25]

Vaginal Cancer

EPIDEMIOLOGY

Carcinoma of the vagina accounts for approximately 2100 cases in 2000. The disease, preinvasive and invasive, occurs primarily in the fifth and sixth decades of life, respectively. Incidence rates have been declining with the use of screening cytology for cervical disease and development of more rigid diagnostic criteria for vagina carcinoma. However, 600 deaths related to vaginal cancer were estimated for 2000.[19, 32]

ETIOLOGY AND RISK FACTORS

The etiology of vaginal cancer is unknown. However, prior radiation to a field including the vagina, DES exposure in utero, and increasing age place a woman at higher risk for the disease. Some speculation exists regarding the role of HPV in vaginal carcinoma.[19, 53]

PREVENTION, SCREENING, AND DETECTION

Prevention and Screening

No recommendations for the prevention and screening of women for vaginal cancers exist. However, a thorough physical examination including inspection and palpation of the vaginal tissues, cervical cytology, and bimanual examination should be done routinely as part of a gynecologic examination for women who are sexually active or 18 years of age or older.[8, 12, 25]

Detection

Many women with vaginal carcinoma are asymptomatic. Detection of preinvasive and invasive lesions is accomplished by thorough inspection of the vaginal tissues, colposcopic examination, and palpation of the tissues along the length of the vaginal wall. Preinvasive lesions of the vagina may only be visualized by colposcopic examination that reveals areas of whitened tissues or atypical vascular patterns. Lesions occur most often on the posterior wall and the upper third of the vagina.[8, 12, 25]

CLASSIFICATION

Most carcinomas of the vagina are squamous cell cancers (93–97%). Other cell types include clear cell carcinomas associated with exposure to DES in utero, malignant melanomas, and sarcomas.

CLINICAL FEATURES

Most patients present with postcoital, perimenopausal, or postmenopausal painless bleeding. Patients may also present with symptoms related to the location of the tumor, such as urinary frequency, and discomfort from anterior tumors and constipation or tenesmus from posterior tumors.[25, 31, 53] (See Clinical Features box.)

DIAGNOSIS AND STAGING

The diagnosis of vaginal carcinoma may be made using colposcopy in the setting of an abnormal Pap smear. Definitive diagnosis of preinvasive and invasive carcinoma of the vagina is made by tissue biopsy of a gross or colposcopically detected lesion. An examination under anesthesia with appropriate biopsies may be necessary if the patient is elderly or has significant vaginal stenosis to preclude an adequate office examination. Staging is done clinically based on inspection of the vagina and palpation of pelvic structures on rectovaginal, bimanual examination. The clinician notes special attention to the location and size of the primary lesion. Metastatic disease is assessed by review of findings from laboratory and radiographic studies, including biochemical profile, chest x-ray film, IVP, barium enema, cystoscopy, and proctoscopy. MRI, CT scans, and lymphangiography may be used to rule out metastatic disease. Table 11–3 presents staging system for carcinoma of the vagina.[25, 31, 54, 61]

METASTASIS

Squamous cell carcinoma of the vagina spreads primarily by direct extension to adjacent tissues, including the urethra, bladder, rectum, parametria, and pelvic sidewall. In addition, spread can occur through extensive lymphatic channels surrounding the vagina and can extend to the rectal, pelvic, para-aortic, and femoral lymph nodes. Hematogenous dissemination to other organs includes lungs, liver, bone, and supraclavicular lymph nodes. This process is usually a late manifestation of this disease.[25]

TREATMENT MODALITIES

Treatment of vaginal neoplasia must be individualized based on tumor location, size, and clinical stage. The close proximity of other organs such as bladder, urethra, and rectum limits the doses of radiation given and restricts the surgical margins that can be obtained without performing an extensive resection. Additionally, psychosexual issues and attempts to maintain a functional vagina are an integral part of the treatment planning. For women with premalignant lesions of the vagina, local excision, carbon dioxide laser, or topical chemotherapy (5-FU) may be used for primary treatment. Partial or total vaginectomy may be done for treatment of women with multifocal disease involving more than a single portion or the full length of the vagina. Radiation therapy for treatment of preinvasive vaginal neoplasia is reserved for women who are poor surgical candidates.[31, 54]

Surgery

Surgery is recommended as treatment for women with early stage disease (stage I and II). This treatment has consisted of radical hysterectomy, vaginectomy with formation of a split thickness of skin graft neovagina, and lymphadenectomy or local excision followed by local irradiation to the tumor bed. Based on the tumor location, size, extent of the lesion, depth of invasion, and evidence of metastasis a total hysterectomy, radical hysterectomy, partial vaginectomy and pelvic lymphadenectomy, or in very selected cases anterior or posterior

TABLE 11–3
Staging Classification for Vaginal Cancer

Primary Tumor (T)		
TNM	FIGO	Definition
TX		Primary tumor cannot be assessed
T0		No evidence of primary tumor
Tis	0	Carcinoma in situ
T1	I	Tumor confined to vagina
T2	II	Tumor invades paravaginal tissues but not to pelvic wall
T3	III	Tumor extends to pelvic wall
T4	IVa	Tumor invades mucosa of bladder or rectum and/or extends beyond true pelvis
M1	IVb	Distant metastasis

Regional Lymph Nodes (N)	
TMN	Definition
NX	Regional lymph nodes cannot be assessed
N0	No regional lymph node metastasis
Upper two thirds of vagina:	
N1	Pelvic lymph node metastasis
Lower one third of vagina:	
N1	Unilateral inguinal lymph node metastasis
N2	Bilateral inguinal lymph node metastasis

Distant Metastasis (M)		
TNM	FIGO	Definition
MX		Presence of distant metastasis cannot be assessed
M0		No distant metastasis
M1	IVb	Distant metastasis

Stage Grouping	
Stage 0:	Tis-N0-M0
Stage I:	T1-N0-M0
Stage II:	T2-N0-M0
Stage III:	T1-N1-M0
	T2-N1-M0
	T3-N0, N1-M0
Stage IVA:	T1-N2-M0
	T2-N2-M0
	T3-N2-M0
	T4-any N-M0
Stage IVB:	any T-any N-M1

Data from *American Joint Committee on Cancer: Manual for staging cancer, ed 5, Philadelphia, Lippincott-Raven, 1997.*

exenteration (see Fig. 11–5) may be recommended. Surgery may also be recommended for women who have locally recurrent disease after primary treatment with radiation therapy.[25, 31, 54]

Radiation Therapy

Because of the proximity of the bladder and rectum as well as the potential for local and regional lymph node metastasis, radiation therapy alone or in combination with surgery is recommended as treatment for women with stage II and higher carcinoma of the vagina. Various combinations of teletherapy as well as interstitial and intracavity therapy are the treatments of choice for selected patients, for example, stage I with a greater than 2 cm lesion; patients with stage II to IV require initial external beam therapy to shrink the size of the primary tumor.[25] (See also Chapter 22.)

Chemotherapy

The results of chemotherapy in treating women with advanced or recurrent vaginal carcinomas, including clear cell and melanoma, have been disappointing. Cisplatin, irinotecan, 5-FU, vincristine, cyclophosphamide, and doxorubicin, actinomycin D have been used as single agents and in combined protocols with radiation therapy. More promising results have occurred with chemotherapy used to treat women with vaginal sarcomas and endodermal sinus tract tumors.[25, 31]

PROGNOSIS

A marked improvement in the survival rates in patients with vaginal cancer has occurred in the past three decades. Survival at 5 years after diagnosis of primary vaginal cancer includes stage I, 65% to 81%; stage II, 50% to 66%; stage III, 15% to 39%; and stage IV, 0% to 25%. Overall survival rates combined for all stages range from 42% to 56%. The decrease in survival rate compared to cervical or vulva cancer may reflect that a higher portion of vaginal tumors are at an advanced stage at the time of diagnosis and more difficult to treat because of close proximity to other organs.[10, 25]

Fallopian Tube Cancer

EPIDEMIOLOGY

Cancer of the fallopian tubes accounts for only 0.1% of all cancers of the female reproductive system. Approximately 300 cases are reported annually in the United States. This cancer occurs in the fifth or sixth decade of life with ages ranging from 14 years to 88 years with a mean age of 56.7 years. Two thirds of the patients are postmenopausal and present with a pelvic mass, and nulliparity was found in approximately one third of the cases.[95]

ETIOLOGY AND RISK FACTORS

The etiology of cancer of the fallopian tubes is unknown. Researchers have hypothesized that chronic inflammation of the tubes and tubal tuberculosis may contribute to the development of the disease. However, because the number of cases of fallopian tube cancer is so small, meaningful data with respect to etiology and risk factors are limited.[17, 95]

PREVENTION, SCREENING, AND DETECTION

Prevention and Screening

Currently, no recommendations are made specifically for the prevention and screening of women for cancer of the fallopian tubes. However, as the pelvic examination is done for screening for other gynecologic malignancies, the clinician must always be alert to the possibility of a pelvic mass being cancer of the fallopian tube. The presence of persistent positive cervical cytology in a woman without evidence of cervical, endometrial, or vaginal cancers should alert the clinician to possible cancer of the fallopian tube.[17, 95]

Detection

Clinical examination is done to detect the presence of ascites and a pelvic mass. On clinical examination a pelvic mass is palpable in more than two thirds of women with fallopian tube cancer. Because fallopian tube carcinoma is rare and symptoms and clinical findings are similar to those in ovarian carcinoma, the diagnosis is rarely made before surgery.

CLASSIFICATION

Adenocarcinoma is the most common histologic type of cancer of the fallopian tube. Sarcomas, mixed mesodermal tumors, lymphomas, hydatidiform moles, and choriocarcinoma have also been reported. Because the number of cases of carcinoma of the fallopian tube is so small, the clinical significance of both histology and grade of the tumor is unknown.[95]

CLINICAL FEATURES

The postmenopausal woman may present with symptoms of vaginal bleeding; intermittent, colicky, dull, aching pain; and profuse, watery, serosanguineous vaginal discharge. If the tumor is large, pressure or a sense of heaviness on the bladder or rectum may be reported.

In women with metastatic disease, ascites may be present and the woman may complain of abdominal fullness and pressure.[17, 95] (See Clinical Features box.)

DIAGNOSIS AND STAGING

Diagnosis of fallopian tube carcinoma is made at the time of surgery for definitive treatment of a pelvic mass. Because the disease has a pattern of spread similar to that of ovarian cancer, a similar surgical approach is recommended. Although many clinicians use the FIGO system for ovarian cancer, no official staging system for cancer of the fallopian tube exists.[95]

METASTASIS

Carcinoma of the fallopian tube metastasizes primarily by direct extension to adjacent tissues and organs, seeding of the abdominal cavity, and lymphatic spread to local and regional nodes. The pattern of metastasis is thought to be related to the site of the primary lesion. For women with lesions in the proximal portion of the tube, metastasis is more likely to occur in the myometrium and endometrium. For women with lesions in the lateral position of the tube, metastasis is more likely to occur to the ovaries and aortic nodes.[95]

TREATMENT MODALITIES

Surgery is the cornerstone of the initial treatment and usually follows the practice for epithelial ovarian cancer. Usually a TAH-BSO and omentectomy is performed followed by removing as much tumor as possible with collection of ascitic or peritoneal fluid, sampling of pelvic and para-aortic lymph nodes, and a careful evaluation of the extent of the disease. For women with residual disease, treatment with interperitoneal radioactive isotopes (^{32}P or ^{198}Au), pelvic or abdominal teletherapy, or systemic single-agent or combination chemotherapy with cyclophosphamide, doxorubicin, progestins, cisplatin, or chlorambucil is recommended.[95]

PROGNOSIS

The prognosis for patients with cancer of the fallopian tube is similar to that of patients with ovarian cancer and is related to the stage of disease in general and specifically to the depth of penetration of the tubal wall. The survival rate for all stages has been reported as 40%, with the rate as high as 88% in patients with stage I disease. Survival data are not as reliable for fallopian tube cancer as for other gynecologic malignancies because the number of cases is low and treatment varies considerably across published reports.[95]

Gestational Trophoblastic Disease

EPIDEMIOLOGY

Gestational trophoblastic disease (GTD) consists of several disorders that arise from placental trophoblastic tissue after abnormal fertilization. These include hydatidiform mole, choriocarcinoma, chorioadenoma, and placental site trophoblastic tumor. Although the disease accounts for only 1% of all cancers of the female reproductive system in the United States, clinical studies report an incidence of 0.5 to 1.08/1000 pregnancies. Population studies in Japan report an incidence of 2.5/1000 pregnancies compared to a Chinese incidence of 0.78/1000 pregnancies. Large differences in incident racial groups have not been confirmed.[6, 86]

ETIOLOGY AND RISK FACTORS

As previously stated GTD includes a variety of tumors that originate in the trophoblastic layer of the chorionic villae during pregnancy. The tumors may range from benign hydatidiform moles to locally invasive moles to choriocarcinomas. A woman who has had a hydatidiform mole has an approximately 1000-fold higher chance of developing choriocarcinoma than one who has a live birth.[6, 86]

PREVENTION, SCREENING, AND DETECTION

Prevention and Screening

No recommendations for prevention or screening of asymptomatic women for GTD are available.

Detection

The detection of GTD is based on careful review of findings on history, clinical examination, and laboratory studies. Disparities such as uterine size inconsistent with estimated gestational age, abnormal ultrasound appearance of the intrauterine contents, and abnormal human chorionic gonadotropin (HCG) levels are keys to the early detection of GTD.

CLASSIFICATION

Gestational trophoblastic disease is classified morphologically as either hydatidiform moles, invasive moles, or choriocarcinoma. Invasive moles and choriocarcinoma have a higher incidence of metastasis to surrounding tissues and thus carry a poor prognosis. Tables 11–4 and 11–5 list the classification and prognostic scoring for GTD.[6, 94]

TABLE 11-4

Classification of Gestational Trophoblastic Disease (GTD)

I. Nonmetastatic disease: no evidence of disease outside uterus
II. Metastatic disease: any disease outside uterus
  A. Good prognosis metastatic disease
    1. Short duration (last pregnancy < 4 months)
    2. Low pretreatment HCG titer (< 100,000 IU/24 h or < 40,000 mIU/mL)
    3. No metastasis to brain or liver
    4. No significant prior chemotherapy
  B. Poor prognosis metastatic disease
    1. Long duration (last pregnancy > 4 months)
    2. High pretreatment HCG titer (> 100,000 IU/24 h or > 40,000 mIU/mL)
    3. Brain or liver metastasis
    4. Significant prior chemotherapy
    5. Term pregnancy

From DiSaia PJ, Creasman WT: Clinical gynecologic oncology, ed 4, St. Louis, Mosby, 1997.

CLINICAL FEATURES

The most common symptom of GTD is vaginal bleeding, particularly during the first trimester. A history of hyperemesis may be reported. Clinical examination reveals an enlargement of the uterus in excess of the estimated length of gestation with an abnormal ultrasound appearance of the intrauterine contents and absent fetal heart sounds; fetal parts cannot be palpated. Finally, elevations of the HCG titers that exceed those found during the course of a normal pregnancy and postpartum period should alert the clinician to the possibility of the disease.[6, 49, 86] (See Clinical Features box.)

DIAGNOSIS AND STAGING

Diagnosis of GTD is confirmed by tissue examination from expulsion of grapelike villi, vaginal bleeding, or evacuation of tissues from the uterus. Clinical examination of the uterus, pelvis, and vagina before and during surgery for evidence of metastasis is recommended. Evaluation of the patient via CT scans of the pelvis, abdomen, and chest, with laboratory and radiographic studies to rule out the presence of metastatic disease in the lungs, brain, and liver, are necessary.[6, 49, 86]

METASTASIS

Metastasis from GTD occurs primarily by local extension to surrounding tissues of the pelvis or through hematogenous spread. The most common sites of distant metastasis include the lungs, brain, and liver.[6]

TREATMENT MODALITIES

With increasingly effective chemotherapy the role of surgery has diminished in overall significance. Aggressive multimodality therapy results in cure rates for 80% to 90% of patients with high-risk disease.[6, 49, 57, 86]

Surgery

The cornerstone of therapy for *placental site* trophoblastic tumors is surgery. Hysterectomy as primary therapy for hydatidiform mole is acceptable for women who have completed childbearing. Patients with low-risk metastatic disease who have limited extrauterine disease are also candidates for hysterectomy in conjunction with chemotherapy. Hysterectomy is generally not as useful

TABLE 11-5

World Health Organization: Prognostic Scoring for Gestational Trophoblastic Disease

Prognostic Factors	Score			
	0	1	2	4
Age	< 39	> 39		
Antecedent pregnancy	Hydatidiform mole	Abortion	Term	
Months from last pregnancy	4	4–6	7–12	12
HCG (IU/L)	10	10- 10	10- 10	10
ABO (female × male)		O × A	B	
		A × O	AB	
Largest tumor (cm)		3–5	5	
Site metastasis		Spleen	GI	Brain
		Kidney	Liver	
Number of metastases		1–4	4–8	8
Prior chemotherapy			Single drug	2 or more drugs
< 4: low risk	5–7: middle risk	> 8: High risk		

From DiSaia PJ, Creasman WT: Clinical gynecologic oncology, ed 4, St. Louis, Mosby, 1997.

in management of high-risk metastatic disease; however, surgical resection of chemoresistant metastatic lesions has a definite role in the treatment of high-risk patients with a poor prognosis.[6, 86] Chemotherapy regimens are often combined with the surgical management of this disease. Emergency laparoscopy or laparotomy may be required for hemorrhage, necrosis, and perforation from a metastatic site in the bowel.[6, 57, 86]

Chemotherapy

Patients with nonmetastatic disease and low-risk metastatic disease are treated with single-agent chemotherapy using methotrexate or actinomycin D. The usual schedule and dose (e.g., methotrexate 0.4 mg/kg IM; actinomycin D 9–13 μg/kg IV) includes a 5-day regimen or a weekly treatment schedule for each of these drugs. Following the serum HCG values at weekly interval monitors the therapy response. Varied chemotherapy drug dosing, route, and infusion time protocols use combinations of etoposide, methotrexate, actinomycin D, ifosfamide, bleomycin, cisplatin, vincristine, cyclophosphamide, and folinic acid are indicated for women middle and high-risk disease, choriocarcinoma, or persistent invasive hydatidiform mole.[3, 5, 6, 44, 57, 86]

Radiation Therapy

Radiation therapy also has a role in the treatment of women with metastatic disease. Women with metastasis to the brain or elevated levels of HCG in the spinal fluid receive whole brain radiation. Corticosteroids are administered concomitantly to minimize cerebral edema. Metastatic lesions to the liver may be treated with radiation therapy.

Response to Therapy

The cure rate of GTD exceeds 90%. Measurement of serial β-HCG values provides a reliable means to determine response to therapy and to detect recurrent disease in cases of molar pregnancy and gestational trophoblastic neoplasia. After evacuation of hydatidiform moles and chemotherapy, β-HCG levels are monitored weekly. For approximately 80% of women diagnosed, the levels return to normal and no additional treatment is needed. For women with metastatic disease, β-HCG levels are evaluated before each course of treatment. Once the β-HCG levels have returned to normal and have remained within normal levels for 3 weeks, monitoring at monthly intervals is begun and continued for 1 year. Current recommendations include measures to prevent pregnancy during the 1-year follow-up period.[6, 47, 86]

PROGNOSIS

Prognosis for patients with GTD is reported based on the percentage of patients who achieve remission with treatment. For patients with nonmetastatic disease, remission (HCG levels within normal range for 3 consecutive weeks) rates with single-agent chemotherapy range from 90% to 100%. Remission rates for patients with metastatic disease are related to the site(s) of metastasis. With combined chemotherapy and radiation therapy, patients with metastatic disease to the lungs or vagina had higher remission rates (74%) than those with metastatic disease at other sites.[2, 6, 47]

CONCLUSION

The specialty of gynecologic oncology has experienced some of the most impressive successes in the use of screening, early diagnosis, and treatment techniques to modify the natural history and incidence of selected gynecologic cancers. These successes have resulted in a significant decrease in mortality. Throughout the phases of care, prevention, screening, diagnosis, treatment, and rehabilitation, nurses have a critical role in improving the quantity and quality of survival. Challenges remain, but the rewards are seen in the daily lives of the many survivors of gynecologic cancers. Patients are often faced with adjusting to significant structural, functional, and cosmetic changes as a result of the disease and treatment. The nurse assumes a key role in addressing rehabilitation concerns. In collaboration with others on the health care team, identification of rehabilitation needs for both the woman and her significant others and referral to appropriate rehabilitation personnel and services may be necessary. The nurse also has an important role in the long-term evaluation of the success of rehabilitative efforts.

Nursing Management

Women at risk or with a diagnosis of gynecologic malignancy present a range of challenges to the nurse. Prevention, screening, and early detection activities are nursing interventions that have the potential to improve both survival and quality of survival for these women.

Counseling on healthy life-style choices that can reduce cancer risks; teaching and valuing the importance of routine gynecologic surveillance and care, including self-examination skills, Pap smear, and bimanual pelvic examination; and educating women about the early signs and symptoms of gynecologic cancers are critical elements of the role the nurse plays in prevention and early detection. The Patients Teaching Priorities box presents specific content for a teaching plan for women at risk for selected gynecologic malignancies.[36, 38, 60, 66]

Throughout the diagnostic phase the nurse becomes an advocate and resource for the woman and her significant others. The nurse is responsible for instruction on the rationale for, procedures involved in, and sensations experienced during diagnostic tests and pretest and posttest care. The nurse also assumes a role in listening to concerns that the woman and her significant others may have about the requirements and results of the diagnostic evaluation.

During the treatment phase the nurse assists the woman in meeting the physical and psychosocial demands imposed by the disease and treatment. In collaboration with the patient, significant others, physician, social worker, physical, respiratory, and occupational therapists, nutritionist, and chaplain, the nurse develops and coordinates implementation of a plan of care designed to provide a safe environment, minimize the incidence of complications from disease and treatment, monitor for signs and symptoms of complications of the disease and treatment, promote independence in self-care, include significant others in the plan of care, and promote coping strategies that foster self-worth and a positive self-concept. Elements common to the nursing care of patients receiving surgery, radiation therapy, chemotherapy, biotherapy, and bone marrow transplantation are included in Chapters 21, 22, 23, 24, and 25, respectively.*

Women facing gynecologic cancers have the potential to experience many common responses to the disease and treatment. Structural changes in anatomy resulting from surgery and radiation therapy for gynecologic cancers may result in altered sexuality patterns.[10, 22, 23, 33]

Aggressive treatment and progressive disease place the patient at risk for complications. Common complications associated with progressive disease include altered bowel elimination related to obstruction; fluid volume excess: ascites related to intra-abdominal metastasis; and fluid volume excess: lymphedema related to blocked lymphatic channels. Nursing care for patients experiencing these problems focuses on maintaining safety, comfort, and mobility.[90]

Aggressive treatment for gynecologic cancers carries increased risks of complications. Because the bladder and bowel lie in proximity to the female reproductive system, altered bowel and urinary elimination related to treatment may result. Problems experienced include decreased sensation to defecate or void, enteritis, cystitis, and fistula formation. Radical surgery and radiation therapy, particularly involving the vulva, may result in impaired skin integrity.[89]

Women with gynecologic cancers are often faced with adjusting to significant structural, functional, and cosmetic changes as a result of the disease and treatment. The nurse assumes a key role in addressing rehabilitation concerns, which may range from care of ostomies resulting from pelvic exenteration, sexual

---

 PATIENT TEACHING PRIORITIES

Gynecologic Cancers

Patient teaching reflects cultural sensitivity, age-appropriate considerations, and use of multiple reinforcers: written, audio, visual, and verbal. Teaching includes content that represents the identified needs of patients across the care continuum, including:

Prevention, screening, and detection practices for all the gynecologic cancers

Disease symptomatology (cervical, endometrial, ovarian, vaginal, vulvar, fallopian cancers; gestational trophoblastic disease)

Treatment modalities with pertinent side effects and purpose, rationale, and potential schedule

Monitoring of blood counts

Wound management

Bowel and bladder elimination

Self-care management

Signs of infection (fever, chills, erythema, bleeding, drainage with odor)

Sexual dysfunction issues (infertility, sterility, libido, intercourse)

---

*References 10, 22, 23, 28, 66, 73, 88.

counseling (see Chapter 33), health maintenance issues, and psychological concerns (see Chapter 32). In collaboration with others on the health care team, identification of rehabilitation needs for both the woman and her significant others and referral to appropriate rehabilitation services and agencies may be necessary. Potential agencies include the American Cancer Society, United Ostomy Association, National Coalition for Cancer Survivorship (see Chapter 28).*

Women can be encouraged to participate in support programs or groups such as Can-Surmount. The nurse also plays an important continuous role in long-term evaluation of the success of rehabilitative efforts (see Chapter 28).

Nursing Diagnosis

- *Knowledge deficit related to prevention and early detection of gynecologic malignancies*

CERVIX

Assessments

- Assess baseline knowledge of personal risk factors for cervical cancer.
- Identify personal risk factors for cervical cancer: age at onset of sexual activity, number of sexual partners, sexual history of partners, number of pregnancies, exposure to herpes simplex virus (HSV-2), history of sexually transmitted diseases (STDs), history of cervical dysplasia, method of contraception, genital hygiene measures, and history of alcohol or tobacco abuse.[23, 53, 66, 88]
- Identify any concerns the woman may have related to personal risks for cervical cancer.

Outcome Goal

Patient will be able to:

- Describe personal risk factors for cervical malignancies.

Interventions

- Teach advantages of barrier contraception use.
- Teach methods to discontinue smoking: "cold turkey," nicotine patch or gum, I Quit, and hypnosis.
- Educate woman about the benefits and schedule of routine Pap smears and pelvic examinations.
- Review signs and symptoms of cervical cancer: abnormal menstrual, intramenstrual, or postcoital bleeding; vaginal discharge; and pain.

- Provide age-appropriate and culturally sensitive written materials about cervical cancer.
- Provide a list of community resources for information and services available to women at risk or with a diagnosis of cervical cancer.

VULVA

Assessments

- Assess knowledge of personal risk factors for vulvar cancer.
- Identify personal risk factors for vulvar cancer: age; chronic vulvar irritation; concurrent diseases such as hypertension, diabetes, cardiovascular disease, and obesity; and history of cervical cancer.
- Identify any concerns the woman may have related to personal risks for vulvar cancer.

Outcome Goal

Patient will be able to:

- Participate in life-style choices that modify the risk of vulvar malignancies: sexual risk factors (HPV-16, HSV-2, multiple sex partners), smoking, chronic vulvar disease.

Interventions

- Teach steps of vulvar self-examination: inspection and palpation.
- Encourage woman to report significant changes in the texture, color, or sensations of the vulva to a physician: a lump, pruritus, bleeding, or discharge.
- Educate women about the benefits of an annual health examination, including evaluation of the vulva and groins.
- Provide age-appropriate and culturally sensitive written materials on vulvar cancer.
- Provide a list of community resources for information and services available to women at risk or with a diagnosis of vulvar cancer.[21, 23, 28, 38, 66, 88]

ENDOMETRIUM

Assessments

- Assess baseline knowledge of personal risk factors for endometrial cancer.
- Identify personal risk factors for endometrial cancer: young age at onset of menstruation; menopause after 52 years of age; nulliparity; obesity; history of Stein-Leventhal syndrome, diabetes, or hypertension; family history of breast, colon, or endometrial cancer; and use of unopposed estrogens; reproductive factors: low fertility index, nulli-

---

*References 10, 22, 28, 37, 41, 72, 85, 90.

parity, late menopause, anovulation, and polycystic ovarian disease.
- Identify concerns that the woman may have related to personal risks for endometrial cancer.

Outcome Goal

Patient will be able to:

- Demonstrate compliance with recommended screening behaviors to detect endometrial malignancies in asymptomatic women.

Interventions

- Discuss life-style choices that can reduce endometrial cancer risks: maintenance of ideal body weight and reduction of fat intake to 30% of total caloric intake.
- Describe health promotion activities to screen for endometrial cancer: annual Pap smear and bimanual pelvic examination and endometrial biopsy in women at high risk for endometrial cancer. Use of combination estrogen and progesterone for hormone replacement therapy (HRT).
- Review signs and symptoms of endometrial cancer: prolonged, excessive, or intramenstrual bleeding in premenopausal women; postmenopausal spotting or bleeding; or yellow, watery, vaginal discharge.
- Provide age-appropriate and culturally sensitive written materials about endometrial cancer.
- Provide a list of community resources for information and services available to women at risk or with a diagnosis of endometrial cancer.*

OVARY

Assessments

- Assess baseline knowledge of personal risk factors for ovarian cancer.
- Identify personal risk factors for ovarian cancer: history of infertility, nulliparity, and personal or family history of breast, ovarian, colon, or uterine cancer. Reproductive (nulliparity, early menarche, late menopause, infertility, hormonal therapy). Genetic factors (BRAC-1, BRAC-2, p53).
- Identify concerns that women may have related to personal risks for ovarian cancer.

Outcome Goal

Patient will be able to:

- Report signs and symptoms of ovarian malignancies to a member of the health care team.

*References 23, 28, 36, 53, 66, 73, 88.

Interventions

- Discuss life-style choices that can reduce ovarian cancer risks: use of oral contraceptives, serial CA-125 levels, vaginal ultrasounds for high-risk women, potential prophylactic oophorectomy.
- Describe health promotion activities to screen for ovarian cancer: annual bimanual pelvic examination.
- Review signs and symptoms of ovarian cancer: dyspepsia, indigestion, loss of appetite, early satiety, pelvic pressure or discomfort, urinary frequency, increasing abdominal girth, and weight loss.
- Provide age-appropriate and culturally sensitive written materials about ovarian cancer.
- Provide a list of community resources for information and services available to women at risk or with a diagnosis of ovarian cancer.[53, 73, 77, 78, 88, 90]

Nursing Diagnosis

- *Sexuality patterns, altered, related to impact of structural, functional, and psychological changes associated with treatment for gynecologic cancers*

Assessments

- Assess woman's and significant other's perception of patient as a sexual being.
- Evaluate factors that contribute to woman's self-concept and expression of sexuality.
- Identify perceived threats to sexuality imposed by disease and treatment.
- Assess factors that may facilitate or hinder adaptation to the structural, functional, and psychological changes resulting from treatment.

Outcome Goals

Patient will be able to:

- Identify potential threats to sexual expression of patient and partner resulting from diagnosis and treatment of gynecologic cancers.
- Discuss effects of surgery, radiation therapy, chemotherapy, biologic therapy, and stem cell or bone marrow transplantation on sexuality.
- Participate in self-care activities to minimize impact of disease and treatment for gynecologic cancers on sexuality and patterns of sexual behavior.
- Report nonacceptable changes in sexual expression and behaviors related to disease and treatment to member of health care team.

Interventions

- Review normal anatomy and physiology of the reproductive system with woman and significant other.
- Describe strategies recommended for minimizing effects of treatment that can influence sexuality patterns.
- Discuss the potential structural, functional, or psychological effects of treatment: surgery, radiation therapy, and chemotherapy.

Interventions: *Surgery*

- Inform woman that only a small portion of vagina is resected as a component of either a simple or radical hysterectomy. Edges of vagina are sutured to form a closed tube. Vagina has ability to stretch during intercourse.
- Discuss that removal of ovaries results in lack of estrogen. Vaginal tissues may become dry and lose elasticity. Oral estrogen replacement therapy or vaginal estrogen creams may be ordered by physician unless contraindicated by presence of a hormone-dependent tumor (e.g., endometrial or breast cancer).[23, 28, 29, 37, 60]

Interventions: *Radiation Therapy*

- Inform woman that radiation also can affect vaginal tissues, making them thinner, drier, and less elastic over time. If woman is not sexually active, vaginal stenosis may occur after radiation therapy.
- Teach use of vaginal dilators to prevent vaginal stenosis:
  Lubricate dilator with water-based lubricant or estrogen cream.
  Insert dilator gradually to full length of vagina.
  Leave dilator inserted in vagina for 10 minutes each day.
  Remove and wash dilator thoroughly with soap and water.[66, 78]

Interventions: *Chemotherapy*

- Inform woman that common side effects of chemotherapy, including hair loss, stomatitis, nausea, vomiting, and fatigue, can influence both perceptions of body image and self-concept and desire for sexual intimacy (see Chapter 33).
  Encourage open discussions about perceptions of body image and self-concept with health care team and significant others.
  Encourage patient to assume an active role in decision making about care.
  Recognize incremental achievements in progress toward patient outcome goals.

Recommend participation in American Cancer Society's Look Good, Feel Better program.[65, 73, 78, 85]
- Encourage open discussions with patient and partner about potential effects of treatment on sexuality patterns.
- Teach patient and partner strategies to reexplore pleasurable experiences during intimacy.
- Suggest increasing the length of time for foreplay to allow for adequate vaginal lubrication.
- Suggest use of vaginal water-based lubricant or vaginal estrogen cream.
- Describe sexual positions that provide woman with more control over depth of penetration.
- Discuss benefits of engaging in sexual behaviors that require minimal energy (hugging, kissing, closeness) and that are initiated when well rested.[21, 22, 28]
- Recommend a schedule for resuming sexual activity.
- Review signs and symptoms of altered sexuality patterns to be reported to the health care team: feelings of decreased self-worth, negative feelings about body image or self-concept, and any changes in expression of sexuality that are not satisfying or pleasurable to self or partner.
- Evaluate impact of disease, treatment, and effectiveness of suggestions in maintaining a satisfactory sexuality pattern.
- Refer for sexual counseling if problems persist.

Nursing Diagnosis

- *Fluid volume excess: ascites related to intra-abdominal metastasis*

Assessments

- Assess weight and abdominal girth daily.
- Assess condition of skin over abdomen, buttocks, bony prominences, and back for changes in color, temperature, or texture.
- Evaluate effect of ascites on level of comfort, mobility, respiratory effort, and activities of daily living (ADL).

Outcome Goals

Patient will be able to:

- Report effects of ascites on ADL and comfort to member of health care team.
- Participate in strategies to minimize untoward effects of ascites.
- List signs and symptoms that require immediate medical intervention.

Interventions

- Position patient with head elevated 30 to 90 degrees to allow for maximum respiratory expansion with minimal effort.
- Monitor intake and output ratio each day.
- Assist patient with ADL as needed.
- Encourage wearing loose clothing around the trunk and abdomen: larger-size bra, bikini-cut panties, and pantyhose made for pregnant women.
- Encourage compliance with low-salt diet.
- Monitor for signs and symptoms of respiratory or gastrointestinal distress that require medical intervention: marked shortness of breath, protracted nausea or vomiting, and acute changes in pattern of pain.
- Provide supportive care as physician performs palliative paracentesis:

  Instruct patient in terms of what will be involved in procedure, what sensations may be experienced during and after procedure, and elements of postprocedural care.

  Position patient in comfortable position.

  Administer any premedications ordered for anxiety.

  Measure amount of ascitic fluid removed and prepare specimen for laboratory as ordered.

  Monitor subjective (pain, relief of shortness of breath) and objective responses (blood pressure, pulse, respirations) of patient to procedure.

  Observe site after procedure for continued drainage, discharge, redness, pain, or warmth.[20, 38, 56, 85, 88, 90]

Nursing Diagnosis

- *Fluid volume excess: lymphedema related to blocked lymphatic channels*

Assessments

- Assess for predisposing factors that could contribute to occurrence of lymphedema of lower extremities: concurrent cardiac, renal, or liver disease; previous lymphadenectomy or radiation therapy of pelvic nodes; and diet.
- Assess pattern of lymphedema: onset, location, and aggravating and alleviating factors.
- Evaluate impact of lymphedema on life-style, comfort, skin integrity, and ADL.
- Evaluate serial measurements, presence on peripheral pulses, and range of motion of affected extremities.

Outcome Goals

Patient will be able to:

- List personal risk factors for lymphedema.

- Describe pattern of lymphedema to member of health care team.
- Discuss impact of lymphedema on ADL and comfort.
- Participate in strategies to minimize risk of complications of lymphedema.
- Report significant changes in lymphedema to member of health care team.

Interventions

- Protect affected extremity: wear loose, protective clothing and avoid restrictive jewelry, irritants, and temperature extremes.[72]
- Avoid invasive procedures to affected extremity.
- Elevate extremity as much as possible.
- Monitor for and report changes in color, temperature, intactness of skin over the affected extremity, and quality of peripheral pulses to physician.[72]
- Consult physical therapy to evaluate use of compression equipment and to develop program of exercise to maintain range of motion in extremity.

Nursing Diagnosis

- *Bowel elimination, altered (e.g., bowel incontinence; diarrhea; constipation), related to disease or treatment for gynecologic cancers*

Assessments

- Assess characteristics of stool: amount, consistency, odor, and color.
- Assess bowel elimination patterns: frequency, presence of constipation, diarrhea, pain with defecation, or incontinence.
- Identify factors that contribute to bowel elimination patterns: dietary intake, fluid intake, activity level, and medication history.[37]

Outcome Goals

Patient will be able to:

- Discuss personal risk factors for changes in bowel or bladder elimination.
- Perform self-care activities related to management of altered bowel or bladder elimination.
- Participate in activities to minimize risk of complications of altered bowel or bladder elimination.
- List community resources available related to management of changes in bowel or bladder elimination.
- List signs and symptoms of complications of altered bowel and bladder elimination that require immediate professional intervention.

Intervention

- Discuss changes that may occur in bowel elimination patterns after surgery or radiation therapy: adhesions with bowel obstruction, decreased sensation of need to defecate, radiation enteritis, and rectovaginal fistula.

Interventions: Surgery

- Discuss that women treated with hysterectomy or radical hysterectomy will note decreased bowel function postoperatively because of manipulation of bowel during surgery. Bowel is kept at rest postoperatively by avoiding oral fluid and food intake until bowel sounds return. Flatulence is common and may be uncomfortable. Attention to pattern of bowel elimination is necessary in first weeks after surgery to minimize risk of constipation associated with use of pain medication, changes in fluid and food intake, and inactivity.
    - Ensure that woman institutes bowel regimen as ordered by physician before surgery to cleanse bowel of stool.
    - Encourage strategies to stimulate bowel function: walking, heating pads, and bowel stimulants.
    - Monitor bowel sounds every 8 hours.
    - Instruct patient to notify team of presence of flatulence or passage of stool.[29, 37, 88]
- Discuss that for women undergoing a total or posterior pelvic exenteration, a bowel diversion will be constructed.
    - Instruct patient in skills to evaluate condition of stoma, application of collection devices, care of peristomal skin, and irrigation techniques.
    - Teach critical changes in character of stool, condition of stoma or peristomal skin, or functioning of diversion to report to health care team.[22, 23]

Interventions: Radiation Therapy

- Inform woman that the most common immediate side effect of radiation therapy to bowel is diarrhea.
    - Observe for signs and symptoms of dehydration.
    - Assess condition of the perianal and perineal skin.
    - Teach women elements of good perineal hygiene after each bowel movement: cleanse the area with water, pat area dry thoroughly, and apply barrier cream as needed to maintain skin integrity.
    - Instruct in dietary changes to increase bulk of stool: avoid fresh fruits and vegetables.
    - Administer antidiarrheals as ordered by physician.

- Discuss that long-term effects of radiation therapy on bowel include radiation enteritis and rectovaginal fistula formation.
    - Place bowel at rest.
    - Instruct in dietary changes to increase bulk of stool: avoid fresh fruits and vegetables.
    - Administer antidiarrheals as ordered by physician.
    - Administer anti-inflammatory agents to decrease inflammation in bowel.
    - Teach significant changes to be reported to health care team: blood in stool, marked increase in the volume of diarrhea, symptoms of dehydration, and passage of stool from vagina.

Interventions: Progressive Disease

- Inform woman that bowel obstruction is a common symptom of progressive disease.
    - Monitor for signs of bowel obstruction: colicky, cramping, lower abdominal pain; alternating diarrhea and constipation; abdominal distention; vomiting; and hyperactive, high-pitched bowel sounds above obstruction and absent bowel sounds below obstruction.
    - Prepare patient for nasogastric tube as ordered by physician.
    - Report significant changes in character of symptoms that indicate need for immediate medical attention: increase in severity of pain, decrease in abdominal girth, rebound tenderness, and acute absence of bowel sounds.

Nursing Diagnosis

- *Urinary elimination, altered, related to disease or treatment for gynecologic cancers*

Assessments

- Assess urinary elimination patterns before initiation of treatment: frequency, nocturia, and incontinence.
- Identify factors that contribute to urinary elimination patterns: volume and timing of fluid intake, concurrent diseases such as diabetes, and medications.

Intervention

- Discuss changes that may occur as a result of surgery or radiation therapy: decreased sensation to void, incomplete emptying of bladder, cystitis, and vesicovaginal fistula formation.

Interventions: Surgery

- Inform woman that after hysterectomy or radical hysterectomy, innervation to bladder may be damaged. Decreased sensation of need to void and incontinence are common effects. A suprapubic catheter is usually placed after surgery. Bladder retraining occurs with catheter in place until residual urines of less than 50 mL are achieved after voiding.

Encourage to drink as much fluid as possible.

Limit fluid intake after 7 PM.

Establish regular schedule for voiding.

- Discuss that for women undergoing a total or anterior pelvic exenteration, a urinary diversion will be constructed.

Teach skills to evaluate condition of stoma, application of collection devices, and care of peristomal skin.

Discuss critical changes in character of urine, condition of stoma or peristomal skin, and functioning of diversion to report to health care team.

Interventions: *Radiation Therapy*

- Inform woman that the primary short-term effect of radiation on bladder tissues is radiation cystitis. Frequency, dysuria, and bleeding are common symptoms.

Encourage a daily fluid intake of 3000 mL.

Consult physician to order medications to minimize discomfort.

Reassure patient that symptoms will improve with time.

- Discuss that the primary long-term effect of radiation therapy is weakening of tissues between vagina and bladder and formation of a fistula. Depending on size of fistula, urine may leak or flow through vagina. Approaches to treatment range from catheter placement to surgical repair.

Institute care strategies to keep patient dry: pouching, indwelling catheter, and protective clothing.

Teach perineal care measures: rinse perineum thoroughly with warm water after each voiding, pat area dry, and apply skin barrier as ordered.

Monitor condition of perineal skin daily.

- Review signs and symptoms of alteration in urinary elimination to report to health care team: frequency, pain, changes in the amount or character of the urine, inability to void, and passage of urine through vagina.[28, 66, 78]

Nursing Diagnosis

- *Skin integrity, impaired, related to surgery or radiation therapy for treatment of vulvar cancer*

Assessments

- Assess skin over vulva, perineum, gluteal folds, and groin areas before initiation of treatment.

- Evaluate for factors that predispose woman to impaired skin integrity: presence of diabetes, obesity, and age.
- Assess steps in routine perineal hygiene measures.
- Evaluate perceived and actual ability (skill and range of motion) of patient to provide self-care during treatment.

Outcome Goals

Patient will be able to:

- Discuss personal risk factors for impaired skin integrity.
- Perform self-care activities to minimize risk of impaired skin integrity.
- List signs and symptoms of complications of impaired skin integrity that require immediate professional intervention.[37, 72, 78, 89]

Interventions

- Discuss potential structural and functional effects of treatment of vulvar cancer with surgery (wound breakdown) and radiation therapy (erythema, dry to moist desquamation).
- Develop a plan of care to minimize risks of side effects of treatment.

Interventions: *Surgery*

- Discuss that wounds from a radical vulvectomy are difficult to heal, particularly if preoperative radiation therapy has been given. Key elements of wound care for these patients are keeping wound clean and dry.

Irrigate surgical wounds with half-strength hydrogen peroxide.

Pack wounds with gauze.

Dry perineum with a hair dryer on coolest setting.

Use bed cradles and positioning to increase circulation of air to wound.

Interventions: *Radiation Therapy*

- Discuss that tissues of vulva, perineum, and groin areas are extremely radiosensitive. Erythema often occurs early in course of therapy and is associated with edema, warmth, and tenderness of tissues. Moist desquamation occurs later in course of treatment and is accompanied by marked redness of tissues, serous drainage, and pain. Radiation is usually stopped until changes subside.

Suggest comfort measures such as wearing loose cotton panties or no panties, avoiding pantyhose, using cool compresses to the perineum, and taking pain medications as ordered by physician.

Recommend measures to keep tissues clean and dry.

Discourage use of any topical agents other than those recommended by radiation oncologist.

- Review signs and symptoms of infection and skin breakdown that should be reported to health care team: redness, increased pain, purulent drainage, foul-smelling discharge, fever, swelling, and ulceration.

Nursing Diagnosis

- *Health maintenance, altered, related to lack of endogenous estrogen in presence of estrogen/progesterone-dependent malignancy*

Assessments

- Assess life-style factors that contribute to health maintenance: diet, activity, and stress reduction techniques.
- Assess woman's perception of physical and psychological changes experienced attributed to lack of estrogen.
- Evaluate extent to which changes have a negative impact on quality of life.
- Evaluate personal and family history for presence of osteoporosis, cardiac disease, and psychiatric problems.

Outcome Goals

Patient will be able to:

- Discuss relative risks and benefits of estrogen replacement.

- Participate in alternative strategies to minimize postmenopausal symptoms and decrease risks of osteoporosis and heart disease.

Interventions

- Discuss rationale for avoiding estrogen replacement therapy in presence of estrogen/progesterone-dependent cancer.
- Describe potential risks to health maintenance from lack of estrogen: increased risks of osteoporosis, cardiovascular disease, psychiatric disease, and vasomotor changes.
- Instruct in strategies to maintain bone integrity: diet rich in calcium-containing foods, calcium supplements, regular exercise program, modifications in home environment to decrease risk of falls, and periodic evaluation of bone density in high-risk women.
- Teach strategies to minimize risk of cardiovascular disease: low-fat diet, regular exercise program, and periodic evaluation of serum cholesterol and triglyceride levels.
- Discuss alternative methods to minimize postmenopausal symptoms: diet, exercise, and medications such as Bellergal-S.
- Suggest use of water-based lubricants for vaginal dryness.
- Encourage expression of psychological responses to disease and treatment. If depressive symptoms persist or if woman has suicidal ideations, refer to psychologist or psychiatrist for medical management.[20, 56, 88, 90]

Chapter Questions

1. Worldwide cervical cancer statistics reflect the following incidence and mortality rates:
   a. Most common cancer, most common cause of cancer death, among women
   b. Second most common cancer, second most common cause of cancer death, among women
   c. Most common cancer, third most common cause of death, among women
   d. Second most common cancer, most common cause of cancer death, among women
2. In counseling women about cancer prevention, which of the following behaviors would be most

important to include reducing the incidence of cervical cancer?
   a. Obtain a Pap smear at least every 5 years after three consecutive annual Pap smears.
   b. Include foods high in fiber in the diet.
   c. Use a barrier form of contraception.
   d. Abstain from alcohol consumption.
3. Endometrial cancer is the most common gynecologic cancer for women the United States; incidence and mortality rates for African American and white women are reflected by:
   a. African American have a higher incidence rate but lower mortality rate than white women.
   b. African American have a higher incidence rate and a higher mortality rate than white women.

c. African American have a lower incidence rate and a lower mortality rate than white women.

d. African American have a lower incidence rate but a higher mortality rate than white women.

4. The most common presenting clinical symptoms for endometrial cancer include:

a. Abnormal vaginal bleeding, increase in amount and frequency, dysuria

b. Prolonged, excessive, irregular, premenopausal or postmenopausal bleeding

c. Painless, postcoital bleeding, full or heavy sensation in pelvis

d. Pruritus, dysuria, dyspepsia, abnormal vaginal bleeding

5. Survival of patients with vulvar cancer is associated with the stage of the disease at diagnosis and the status of the pelvic lymph nodes; survival rates are reflected as follows:

a. Stage I, 92%; stage II, 80%; stage III, 53.5%; stage IV, 14.6%; and overall 70.3%

b. Stage I, 85%; stage II, 70%; stage III, 59%; stage IV, 22%; and overall 60%

c. Stage I, 99%; stage II, 85%; stage III, 49%; stage IV, 19%; and overall 77.5%

d. Stage I, 95%; stage II, 65%; stage III, 20%; stage IV, 5%; and overall 40%

6. Surgery and chemotherapy are major treatments used for gestational trophoblastic disease; what reliable test(s) is used most frequently in diagnosing and monitoring the response to treatment?

a. β-HCG levels, CT scans

b. β-HCG levels, ultrasound

c. Serial 125 levels, ultrasound

d. α-Fetoprotein levels, MRI

7. The nursing intervention most helpful to a patient with ascites secondary to intra-abdominal metastatic ovarian carcinoma is:

a. Dry perineum with a hair dryer on coolest setting.

b. Suggest water-based lubricants for vaginal dryness.

c. Position patient with head of the bed elevated 30 to 90 degrees.

d. Suggest wearing restrictive clothing to manage edema.

8. A 28-year-old woman who had a radical hysterectomy 7 days ago is returning to the office with a suprapubic catheter in place, for follow-up care. The assessment most important for the nurse to determine if the catheter can be removed is:

a. Presence of urinary incontinence

b. Ratio of oral intake to urinary output

c. Total urinary output over 24 hours

d. Volume of postvoiding residuals

9. Options regarding prevention of ovarian cancer in the high-risk patient include:

a. Prophylactic hysterectomy, tubal ligation, cyclic progesterone and estrogen replacement

b. Prophylactic oophorectomy, tubal ligation, oral contraceptives

c. Prophylactic oophorectomy, prophylactic hysterectomy, oral contraceptives

d. Prophylactic oophorectomy, tubal ligation, cyclic progesterone and estrogen replacement

10. The treatment for vaginal cancer must be individualized based on the following criteria:

a. Tumor location, size of tumor, clinical stage, psychosexual issues

b. Type of tumor, degree of differentiation, stage of disease, general health status

c. Size and extent of the lesion, depth of stromal invasion, evidence of metastatic disease

d. Surgical staging, malignant potential of the disease, bulk of remaining disease

BIBLIOGRAPHY

1. Abramovich D and others: Serum CA-125 as a marker of disease activity in uterine papillary serous carcinoma, *J Cancer Res Clin Oncol* 125(12):697, 1999.

2. Amr MR: Return of fertility after successful chemotherapy treatment of gestational trophoblastic tumors, *Int J Fertil Womens Med* 44(3):146, 1999.

3. Aoki Y and others: Failure of high-dose chemotherapy with peripheral blood stem cell support for refractory placental site trophoblastic tumor, *Gynecol Obstet Invest* 47(3):214, 1999.

4. Ayhan A and others: Endometrial adenocarcinoma in pregnancy, *Gynecol Oncol* 75(2):298, 1999.

5. Bae SN, Kim SJ: Telomerase activity in complete hydatidiform mole, *Am J Obstet Gynecol* 180(2 Part II):328, 1999.

6. Baker VV: Gestational trophoblastic disease. In Abeloff MD, Armitage JO, Lichter AS, Niederhuber JE, editors: *Clinical oncology*, ed 2, New York, Churchill Livingstone, 1999.

7. Beard CM and others: Endometrial cancer in Olmsted County, MN, trends in incidence, risk factors and survival, *Ann Epidemiol* 10(2):97, 2000.

8. Beavers T: Evidence-based cancer screening, *Highlights Oncol Pract* 16(4):91, 1999.

9. Bertelsen K, Grenman S, Rustin GJ: How long should first-line chemotherapy continue? *Ann Oncol* 10(Suppl 1):17, 1999.

10. Bezjak A: Quality of life in women with cancer. In Kavanagh JJ, Singletary SE, Einhorn N, DePetrillo AD, editors: *Cancer in women*, Malden, MA, Blackwell Science, 1998.

11. Biffi R, Martinelli G, G, Pozzi S, Cinieri S, Cocorocchio E, Peccatori F, Ferrucci PF, Pistorio R, Andreoni B: Totally implantable central venous access ports for high-dose chemotherapy administration and autologous stem cell transplantation: analysis of overall and septic complications

in 68 cases using a single type of device, *Bone Marrow Transplant* 24(1):89, 1999.

12. Boyle P, Maisonneuve P: Cancer prevention in women; clues from epidemiology. In Kavanagh JJ, Singletary SE, Einhorn N, DePetrillo AD, editors: *Cancer in women,* Malden, MA, Blackwell Science, 1998.

13. Burnett AF and others: A phase II study of gemcitibine and cisplatin in patients with advanced, persistent, or recurrent squamous cell carcinoma of the cervix, *Gynceol Oncol* 76(1):63, 2000.

14. Byers LJ, Fowler JM, Twiggs LB: Uterus. In Abeloff MD, Armitage JO, Lichter AS, Niederhuber JE, editors: *Clinical oncology,* ed 2, New York, Churchill Livingstone, 1999.

15. Camp-Sorrell D: Surviving the cancer, surviving the treatment: acute cardiac and pulmonary toxicity, *Oncol Nurs Forum* 26(6):983, 1999.

16. Canavan TP, Doshi NR: Cervical cancer, *Am Fam Physician* 61(5):1369, 2000.

17. Clark JC: Gynecological cancers. In Otto SE, editor: *Oncology nursing,* ed 3, St. Louis, Mosby, 1997.

18. Creasman WT: HRT and women who have had breast or endometrial cancer, *J Epidemiol Biostat* 4(3):217, 1999.

19. Creasman WT, Phillips JL, Menck HR: The National Cancer Data Base report on cancer of the vagina, *Cancer* 83(5):1033, 1998.

20. Dahlin CM: Care and compassion in conveying bad news, *Clin J Oncol Nurs* 3(2):73, 1999.

21. Damaron BI: *Nurse-physician-patient communication: the vital triangle,* Medical Education Resources, Inc., Wyeth Genetics Institute, 2000.

22. De Petrillo AD, Thompson LJ: Sexual rehabilitation in gynecology oncology. In Kavanagh JJ, Singletary SE, Einhorn N, DePetrillo AD, editors: *Cancer in women,* Malden, MA, Blackwell Science, 1998.

23. De Stefano MS, Bertin-Matson K: Gynecologic cancers. In McCorkle R, Grant M, Frank-Stromborg M, Baird SB, editors: *Cancer nursing: a comprehensive textbook,* ed 2, Philadelphia, Saunders, 1996.

24. DiSaia PJ, Creasman WT: *Clinical gynecologic oncology,* ed 4, St. Louis, Mosby, 1997.

25. Elkas JC, Farias-Eisner R, Berek JS: Cervix, vulva, and vagina. In Abeloff MD, Armitage JO, Lichter AS, Niederhuber JE, editors: *Clinical oncology,* ed 2, New York, Churchill Livingstone, 1999.

26. Ellerbrock TV and others: Incidence of cervical squamous intraepithelial lesions in HIV-infected women, *JAMA* 283(8):1031, 2000.

27. Ferrucci PF and others: Evaluation of acute toxicities associated with autologous peripheral blood progenitor cell reinfusion in patients undergoing high-dose chemotherapy, *Bone Marrow Transplant* 25(2):173, 2000.

28. Flannery M: Nursing care of the client with genital cancer. In Itano JK, Taoka KN, editors: *Core curriculum for oncology nursing,* ed 3, Philadelphia, Saunders, 1998.

29. Froiland KG: Complex wound care: use of negative pressure therapy for wound healing in an ovarian cancer patient, *Nursing interventions in oncology* 12:8, 2000. Associates in Medical Marketing, Newtown, PA.

30. Frank T: Hereditary breast and ovarian cancer, *Genetic susceptibility to breast and ovarian cancer,* Myriad Genetic Laboratories, Inc., UT, 2000.

31. Goodman A: Primary vaginal cancer, *Surg Oncol Clin N Am* 7(2):347, 1998.

32. Greenlee RT and others: Cancer statistics 2000, *CA Cancer J Clin* 50:7, 2000.

33. Groenwald SL and others: *Cancer nursing: principles and practice,* ed 5, Boston, Jones & Bartlett, 2000.

34. Greven KM: Tailoring radiation to the extent of disease for uterine-confined endometrial cancer, *Semin Radiat Oncol* 10(1):29, 2000.

35. Hacker NF: Radical resection of vulvar malignancies: a paradigm shift in surgical approaches, *Curr Opin Obstet Gyncol* 11(1):61, 1999.

36. Haas BK: Focus on health promotion: self-efficacy in oncology nursing research and practice, *Oncol Nurs Forum* 27(1):89, 2000.

37. Haisfield-Wolfe ME, Rund C: A nursing protocol for the management of perineal-rectal skin alterations, *Clin J Oncol Nurs* 4(1):15, 2000.

38. Harris KA: The informational needs of patients with cancer and their families, *Cancer Pract* 6(1):39, 1998.

39. Haverkos K, Roher M, Pickworth W: The cause of invasive cervical cancer could be multifactional, *Biomed Pharmacother* 54(1):54, 2000.

40. Haylock PJ: Cancer metastasis: an update, *Semin Oncol Nurs* 14(3):172, 1998.

41. Highfield MEF: Providing spiritual care to patients with cancer, *Clin J Oncol Nurs* 4(3):115, 2000.

42. Holmquist ND: Revisiting the effect of the Pap test on cervical cancer, *Am J Public Health* 90(4):620, 2000.

43. Holub Z and others: Laparoscopic surgery in obese women with endometrial cancer, *J Am Assoc Gynecol Laparosc* 7(1):83, 2000.

44. Homesley HD: Single-agent therapy for nonmetastatic and low-risk gestational trophoblastic disease, *J Reprod Med* 43(1):69, 1998.

45. Hulka JF, Reich H: *Textbook of laparoscopy,* ed 3, Philadelphia, Saunders, 1998.

46. Kapp KS and others: The prognostic significance of peritoneal seeding and size of postsurgical residual in patients with stage III epithelial ovarian cancer treated with surgery, chemotherapy, and high-dose radiotherapy, *Gynecol Oncol* 74(3):400, 1999.

47. Kim JH and others: Subsequent reproductive experience after treatment for gestational trophoblastic disease, *Gynecol Oncol* 71(1):108, 1998.

48. Koh WJ, Panwala K, Greer B: Adjuvant therapy for high-risk, early stage cervical cancer, *Semin Radiat Oncol* 10(1):51, 2000.

49. Kohorn EI, McCarthy SM, Taylor KJ: Normostatic gestational trophoblastic neoplasia. Role of ultrasonography and magnetic resonance imaging, *J Reprod Med* 43(1):14, 1998.

50. Koops HS and others: Sentinel node biopsy as a surgical staging method for solid cancers, *Radiother Oncol* 51(1):1, 1999.

51. Lanciano R: Optimizing radiation parameters for cervical cancer, *Semin Radiat Oncol* 10(1):36, 2000.

52. Lavie O and others: Thrombocytosis in women with vulvar carcinoma, *Gynecol Oncol* 71(1):82, 1999.

53. Lee CO: Gynecologic cancers: part I—risk factors, *Clin J Oncol Nurs* 4(2):67, 2000.

54. Lee YS: Early experience with laparoscopic pelvic lymphadenectomy in women with gynecologic malignancy, *J Am Assoc Gynecol Laparosc* 6(1):59, 1999.

55. Liang CC, Tseng CJ, Soong YK: The usefulness of cystoscopy in the staging of cervical cancer, *Gynecol Oncol* 76(2):200, 2000.

56. Looney M: Death, dying, and grief in the face of cancer. In Burke CC, editor: *Psychosocial dimensions of oncology nursing care,* Pittsburgh, Oncology Nursing Press, 1998.

57. Lurain JR: Management of high-risk gestational trophoblastic disease, *J Reprod Med* 43(1):44, 1998.

58. Maggino T and others: An analysis of approaches to the management of endometrial cancer in North America: a CTF study, *Gynecol Oncol* 68(3):274, 1998.

59. Mariani A and others: Potential therapeutic role of para-aortic lymphadenectomy in node-positive endometrial cancer, *Gynecol Oncol* 76(3):348, 2000.

60. Mayer D: Cancer patient empowerment, *Oncol Nurs Updates* 6(4):1, 1999.

61. McIntosh DG: Pap smear screening after hysterectomy, *Compr Ther* 24(1):14, 1998.

62. Meden H, Marx D, Roegglen T, Schauer A, Kuhn W: Overexpression of the oncogene c-erbB-2 (HER2/neu) and response to chemotherapy in patients with ovarian cancer, *Int J Gynecol Pathol* 17(1):61, 1998.

63. Melbye M, Frisch M: The role of human papillomaviruses in anogenital cancers, *Semin Cancer Biol* 8(4):307, 1998.

64. Messori A and others: Treatments for newly diagnosed advanced ovarian cancer: analysis of survival data and cost-effectiveness evaluation, *Anticancer Drugs* 9(6):491, 1998.

65. Miller SE: Stomatitis and esophagitis. In Yasko JM, editor: *Nursing management of symptoms associated with chemotherapy,* Bala Cynwyd, PA, Pharmacia & Upjohn, Meniscus Health Care Communications, 1998.

66. Mitchell S: Gynecologic cancer. In Dow KH, Bucholtz JD, Iwamoto RR, Fieler VK, Hilderley L, editors: *Nursing care in radiation oncology,* ed 2, Philadelphia, Saunders, 1999.

67. Moore DH and others: Dactinomycin in the treatment of recurrent or persistent endometrial carcinoma: a phase II study of the Gynecologic Oncology Group, *Gynecol Oncol* 75(3):473, 1999.

68. Moore DH and others: Preoperative chemoradiation for advanced vulvar cancer: a phase II study of the Gynecologic Oncology Group, *Int J Radiat Oncol Biol Phys* 42(1):79, 1998.

69. Morgan MA, Mikuta JJ: Surgical management of vulvar cancer, *Semin Surg Oncol* 17(3):168, 1999.

70. Nieto Y, Shpall EJ: Autologous stem-cell transplanatation for solid tumors in adults, *Hematol Oncol Clin North Am* 13(5):939, 1999.

71. North American Nursing Diagnosis Association: *Nursing diagnosis: definitions and classification,* Philadelphia, The Association, 1999.

72. Olson K, Tkachuk L, Hanson J: Preventing pressure sores in oncology patients, *Clin Nurs Res* 7(2):207, 1998.

73. Oncology Nursing Society: *Cancer chemotherapy guidelines and recommendations for practice,* Pittsburgh, Oncology Nursing Press Inc., 1999.

74. Ozols RF: Paclitaxel plus carboplatin in the treatment of ovarian cancer, *Semin Oncol* 26(1 Suppl 2):84, 1999.

75. Ozols RF and others: Intraperitoneal treatment and dose-intense therapy in ovarian cancer, *Ann Oncol* 10(Suppl 1):59, 1999.

76. Petereit DG: Complete surgical staging in endometrial cancer provides prognostic information only, *Semin Radiat Oncol* 10(1):8, 2000.

77. Piver MS, Eltabbakh G: *Myths and facts about ovarian cancer, What you need to know,* ed 2, Melville, NY, PRR, 2000.

78. Poulson J: Symptom management and supportive care in women with advanced cancer. In Kavanagh JJ, Singletary SE, Einhorn N, DePetrillo AD, editors: *Cancer in women,* Malden, MA, Blackwell Science, 1998.

79. Pustilnik T, Burke TW: Adjuvant chemotherapy for high-risk endometrial cancer, *Semin Radiat Oncol* 10(1):23, 2000.

80. Rex D: Should we colonoscope women with gynecological cancer? *Am J Gastroenterol* 95(3):812, 2000.

81. Rieger PT: *Clinical handbook of biotherapy,* Boston, Jones and Bartlett, 1999.

82. Rieger PT: Management of cancer in the next millennium: DNA holds the key, *Highlights Oncol Pract* 16(4):110, 1999.

83. Rose PG and others: Paclitaxel and cisplatin as first-line therapy in recurrent or advanced squamous cell carcinoma of the cervix: a gynecologic oncology group study, *J Clin Oncol* 17(9):2676, 1999.

84. Ross AA: Minimal residual disease in solid tumor malignancies: a review, *J Hematother* 7(1):9, 1998.

85. Rust DM: Anorexia and cachexia. In Yasko JM, editor: *Nursing management of symptoms associated with chemotherapy,* Bala Cynwyd, PA, Pharmacia Upjohn, Meniscus Health Care Communication, 1998.

86. Rustin GJS, Begent RHJ: Gestational trophoblastic disease. In Kavanagh JJ, Singletary SE, Einhorn N, DePetrillo AD, editors: *Cancer in women,* Malden, MA, Blackwell Science, 1998.

87. Schilder RJ, Shea TC: Multiple cycles of high-dose chemotherapy for ovarian cancer, *Semin Oncol* 25(3):349, 1998.

88. Sivesind DM, Rohaly-Davis JA: Coping with cancer: patient issues. In Burke CC, editor: *Psychosocial dimensions of oncology nursing care,* Pittsburgh, Oncology Nursing Press, Inc., 1998.

89. Smith DB: Urinary continence issues in oncology, *Clin J Oncol Nurs* 3(4):161, 1999.

90. Socci M: Palliative nursing in advanced cancer care, *Nurs Interventions Oncol,* 12:19, Newtown, PA, Associates in Medical Marketing, 2000.

91. Sugimoto A, Thomas G: Early-stage ovarian carcinoma. In Kavanagh JJ, Singletary SE, Einhorn N, DePetrillo AD, editors: *Cancer in women,* Malden, MA, Blackwell Science, 1998.

92. Terada KY, Shimizu DM, Wong JH: Sentinel node dissection and ultrastaging in squamous cell cancer of the vulva, *Gynecol Oncol* 76(1):40, 2000.

93. Tewari K and others: Interstitial brachytherapy in the treatment of advanced and recurrent vulvar cancer, *Am J Obstet Gynecol* 181(1):91, 1999.

94. Tham KF, Ratnam SS: The classification of gestational trophoblastic disease: a critical review, *Int J Gynecol Obstet* 60(Suppl 1):S39, 1998.

95. Thigpen JT: Ovaries and fallopian tubes. In Abeloff MD, Armitage JO, Lichter AS, Niederhuber JE, editors: *Clinical oncology,* ed 2, New York, Churchill Livingstone, 1999.

96. Wandt H and others: Sequential cycles of high-dose chemotherapy with dose escalation of carboplatin with or without paclitaxel supported by G-CSF mobilized peripheral blood progenitor cells: a phase I/II study in advanced ovarian cancer, *Bone Marrow Transplant* 23(8):763, 1999.

97. Wee CC and others: Screening for cervical and breast cancer: is obesity an unrecognized barrier to preventive care? *Ann Intern Med* 132(9):697, 2000.

98. Wolfson AH: The role of radiotherapy for high-risk endometrial cancer, *Semin Radiat Oncol* 10(1):15, 2000.

99. Zanetta G and others: Unusual recurrence of cervical adenosquamous carcinoma after conservative surgery, *Gynecol Oncol* 76(3):409, 2000.

Head and Neck Cancers

Andrea Sampson Haggood

Andrea Sampson Haggood

Although not among the five leading causes of death from cancer in the United States, the significance of head and neck cancers lies in what they represent to the patient, family, and professional as an acutely visible and disabling threat to future function and well-being. It is one's face, even more so than one's voice, spoken words, emotions (verbalized and withheld), or mannerisms (involuntary and intentional), that presents each individual to the world. Left untreated, cancers in this area can result in disabilities, which may be grossly offensive to the individual, and lead to fatalities. Even if treated, patients and their significant others will have to face the potential for disfigurement, physiologic dysfunction, sensory loss, changes in body image, altered social interaction, altered sexuality, spiritual distress, and cancer-related death.

Providing care and education for these patients and their significant others can present a significant challenge for the nurse. However, nurses are uniquely skilled and positioned to support and guide the patient and family through their adjustment to illness, treatment, and rehabilitation, ultimately affecting future quality of life. Given the intricacies involved in patient care and disease management for the person with head and neck cancer, nursing care is presented in great detail in this chapter. Nursing care guidelines are included throughout for surgery, cosmesis, radiation therapy, chemotherapy, rehabilitation, and self-care management.

EPIDEMIOLOGY AND ETIOLOGY

In the United States, it is estimated that carcinomas of the head and neck account for approximately 4% to 5% of all new malignancies, and approximately 63,900 new head and neck malignancies and 14,000 deaths (including 18,400 new thyroid cancers and 1200 thyroid cancer-related deaths) will occur in 2000.[21, 34, 71, 137] The worldwide incidence consists of more than 500,000 cases of head and neck neoplasms.[130, 137, 150, 157] In other parts of the world (e.g., India), where oral cancers account for as many as 50% of all malignancies, head and neck cancer is much more prevalent.[100] Over 90% of head and neck cancers are of *squamous cell* histology.[21, 28, 80, 101] Other cell types include various salivary gland tumors (e.g., adenocarcinoma, adenoid cystic tumor, mucoepidermoid cancer), thyroid tumors, verrucous carcinomas, lymphoepitheliomas, and rare lymphomas and soft tissue sarcomas.[17, 80, 124, 137]

The most common site of head and neck cancer is the oral cavity (48%), followed by the larynx (25%), and then the oropharynx (10%).[80] At diagnosis, more than 60% of patients present with locally advanced (stages III and IV) disease.[21, 136] Although an increasing number of patients have been seen in their third and fourth decade of life, especially with oral cavity malignancies,[136, 137] the incidence of head and neck malignancies increases markedly after age 50,[21, 34] with more than 50% occurring in persons over age 65.[124] There continues to be a higher incidence of head and neck cancers among men, except for thyroid cancers, which have a higher incidence in women. The year 2000 projected male/female incidence ratio in the United States is 2.5 : 1[34] in contrast to the 4 to 5 : 1 male/female ratio in the 5 to 10 years prior to 1995.[9, 119, 136] This trend toward increasing numbers of women with head and neck cancer is attributed to the increasing consumption of tobacco and alcohol by women.[21] Excluding thyroid cancer, which has an overall survival rate of 95%,[34] 5-year survival rates for all head and neck cancers approach 50% with stage I and II ranging from 40% to 95%, and stage III and IV ranging from 0% to 50%. Five-year survival rates vary by stage and site: oral cavity, 40% to 70%; oropharynx, 35% to 50%; larynx, 50% to 80%; nasopharynx 26%; and nose and sinuses 15% to 40%.[80] One third of all patients with head and neck cancer will ultimately die as a consequence of their disease.[156] In the last 20 to 30 years, there has been no statistically significant change in survival rates among whites or African Americans.[34, 80, 156] African Americans, in general, have higher incidence rates and lower survival rates than whites, and they tend to be diagnosed at a later stage of disease.[34, 100] In one study the most important explanatory factor for ethnic differences in oral and pharyngeal cancer incidence was alcohol consumption. After controlling for smoking, heavy drinking (more than 30 drinks per week) resulted in a 9-fold increase risk of oral and pharyngeal cancers among whites, in contrast to a 17-fold increase in African Americans.[133] The American Cancer Society (ACS) suggests that survival differences can largely be attributed to the more advanced stage of disease at diagnosis among African Americans.[9] The aerodigestive tract serves as a conduit for air, fluid, and food; therefore, the body is constantly exposed to a broad range of potential carcinogenic agents. Life-style choices and occupational exposures have been studied and correlate positively to head and neck cancer. Although extensive evidence exists regarding risk of tobacco and alcohol consumption and the associated development of head and neck cancer, the degree of risk associated with other etiologic factors is not as well documented. Table 12–1 summarizes various etiologic factors implicated in the

TABLE   12 – 1
Etiology of Head and Neck Cancer: Specific Sites

Site	Carcinogens/Occupations	Other Factors
Skin	Inorganic arsenics in drugs, water, or occupational environment Ultraviolet rays of sun, ionizing radiation Polycyclic aromatic hydrocarbons, coke ovens, gas workers Chloroprene (neoprene) in synthetic rubber	Burns Riboflavin deficiency Syphilis: lip
Nose and sinuses	Wood dust (furniture industry) Shoe industry (leather manufacturing) Textile workers Radiochemical (Thorotrast) Radium dial painters and chemists (osteogenic sarcomas) Mustard gas Nickel refining Isoprophyl oil BCME: bis(chloromethyl)ether—alkylating agent (produces esthesioneuroepithelioma in animals)	?Chronic sinusitis ?Cigarette smoke
Nasopharynx	Nitrosamines (N-nitrosodimethylamine)	Epstein-Barr virus Genetics: Chinese from Kwantung province 25 times more susceptible Vitamin C deficiency Salted fish
Oral cavity	Cigarettes, reverse smoking Ethyl alcohol Snuff, chewing tobacco, betel nut Textile industries Coke ovens Leather manufacturing	Syphilis: tongue Nutrition: vitamin B (riboflavin) deficiencies
Hypopharynx-larynx	Cigarettes Asbestos (ship builders) Mustard gas Polycyclic aromatic hydrocarbons (coke ovens) Ethyl alcohol Wood exposure	Nutrition: riboflavin deficiency
Esophagus	Ethyl alcohol Cigarettes	Nutrition: riboflavin, nitrosamines Race and nationality: Eskimos, Iranians, blacks
Thyroid	Radiation exposure	Iodine deficiencies Genetics
Salivary glands	Radiation	Genetics: Eskimos

Modified from Jesse TC: Etiology of head and neck cancer. In Suen JW, Myers EN, editors: Cancer of head and neck, New York, Churchill Livingstone, 1981.

incidence of head and neck cancer. Under investigation are various host-specific factors that affect ones susceptibility to cancer.[151] Studies are being conducted regarding genetic polymorphisms, which affect one's ability to activate or detoxify carcinogens in tobacco and repair DNA damage. There are also studies of specific genotypes and phenotypes, which render one mutagen sensitive.[15, 132, 157] Further investigation is clearly indicated, particularly in areas such as molecular genetics, where much of the research is fragmented and preliminary.[22]

PREVENTION, SCREENING, AND DETECTION

The primary risk factor for developing cancer of the oral cavity, pharynx, and larynx is *tobacco use* (smoked and smokeless).[21, 130, 133] It acts as an initiator, promoter, and cocarcinogen, having a linear dose-effect response on the tissues with which it has contact, with smokers having a relative risk 6 to 25 times that of nonsmokers.[133] The level of risk depends on the type of tobacco, daily amount consumed, the duration of the habit, the types of tobacco, the manner in which it is used, and depth of inhalation.[133, 150] "Tar" (polycyclic aromatic hydrocarbons) is the primary source of tumorigenic activity in tobacco smoke. Benzo(a)pyrene, vinyl chloride, polonium-210, nickel, and cadmium are some other carcinogenic agents identified in tobacco smoke.[33, 133] The primary constituent responsible for oral cancers is thought to be N^1-nitrosonor nicotine, which has tumor-promoting properties in animals and is present in cigarette smoke condensate, chewing tobacco, and snuff. Relative risk decreases significantly with each year of smoking cessation, but the risk for head and neck neoplasia never returns to that of a nonsmoker.[130]

In combination with *alcohol,* tobacco has been associated with 80% to more than 95% of squamous cell cancers of the head and neck.[136, 137] The risk factors alcohol and tobacco have a maximum effect in the oral cavity and oropharynx in the horseshoe-shaped area that includes the anterior floor of the mouth, the ventrolateral tongue, and the lingual aspect of the retromolar trigone (where saliva pools), as well as the soft palate.[133] Some studies suggest that alcohol, which is both a solvent and an irritant, has an independent carcinogenic action on the oral cavity, pharynx, and larynx, in addition to its synergistic effects with tobacco, when consumed in large amounts.[133, 137] Marijuana smoke, which contains a higher concentration of "tar" than tobacco smoke, has been implicated in the development of head and neck cancer.[27, 31, 150] Precancerous lesions (erythroplakia more so than leukoplakia) are associated with cancers of the oral cavity, alveolar ridge, gums, and floor of the mouth in people who have dipped or chewed tobacco.[96, 118, 145]

Up to 15% of malignancies of the aerodigestive tract may have viral etiologies.[131] The *Epstein-Barr virus* (EBV) related to nasopharyngeal cancer is the virus best described as a risk factor for head and neck cancer. Now mounting evidence exists that the human papillomaviruses (HPVs) and herpes simplex virus type 1 (HSV-1) may be involved in the development of cancers in the aerodigestive tract.[33, 92, 130] Cancers of the thyroid have been found to occur more frequently in persons who received small doses of radiation therapy[20] previously for acne, chronic tonsillitis, enlarged thymus, or middle ear disease. Nutritional deficiencies (e.g., Plummer-Vinson syndrome), poor oral hygiene, mechanical irritation, occupational exposures, and immunosuppression have also been linked with cancer development in specific sites within the aerodigestive tract.

Risk for second primary tumors in patients with head and neck cancer ranges from 10% to 40%; they may be *synchronous* primaries (simultaneous lesions or those presenting within 6 months of initial diagnosis) or *metachronous* second primaries (appearing 6 months or more after initial diagnosis).[21, 37, 91, 130, 145] Second and sometimes third primaries, usually occurring in the lung, head, and neck region and esophagus, are explained by the phenomenon of diffuse mucosal atypia called "field cancerization."[130] This is the process by which the mucosal surfaces of the upper aerodigestive tract and the surrounding tissues have undergone changes (initiation, promotion, and proliferation) in response to repeated exposure to carcinogenic insult.[33, 147] Genetic alterations resulting in the inactivation of oncogenes, inactivation or mutation of tumor-suppressor genes, and amplification of growth factors and their receptors have been linked with the development of head and neck neoplasms.[130] Because these malignancies occur in a small percentage of patients who neither smoke nor drink, they may have a genetic predisposition to developing head and neck cancer.[137, 165]

CLASSIFICATION

Carcinomas arising in the head and neck region are classified according to *anatomic regions* rather than cell type. These regions include the (1) oral cavity, (2) oropharynx, (3) nasal cavity, (4) nasopharynx, (5) paranasal sinuses, (6) hypopharynx, (7) larynx, (8) salivary glands, and (9) thyroid gland. Each of these regions is subdivided into specific sites (Fig. 12–1 and Table 12–2). The tumor characteristics of each area, therapeutic management, and prognosis may differ depending on the disease's natural history, the sites of metastases, and the disease's biologic behavior.[43, 63]

DIAGNOSIS

Optimal treatment and patient survival require accurate identification of the primary tumor, local/regional

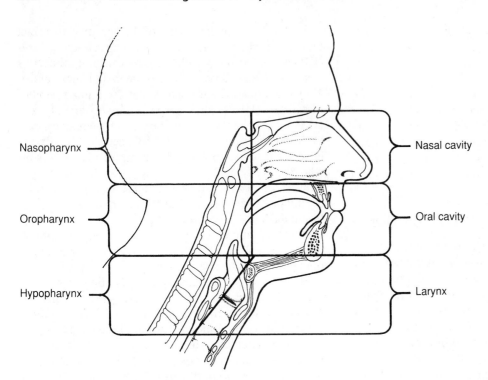

Nasopharynx

Oropharynx

Hypopharynx

Nasal cavity

Oral cavity

Larynx

FIGURE 12–1 Region of head and neck.

spread and invasiveness, distant metastasis, and synchronous second primaries. All patients should undergo a thorough head and neck examination with the use of a mirror or a fiberoptic nasopharyngolaryngoscope. Radiologic examinations should be completed before obtaining a biopsy. A biopsy can alter the mucosa and bone detail and can cause the radiologist to misinterpret the film. Direct triple endoscopy or *panendoscopy* (laryngoscopy, bronchoscopy, and selectively used nasopharyngoscopy) with multiple biopsies performed under general anesthesia is the definitive diagnostic and staging procedure.[101, 130, 136] Fine-needle aspiration (FNA) of a suspicious cervical node is performed if no obvious primary is identified. Because open biopsy may jeopardize curative therapy, it is a last resort if panendoscopy and FNA fail to identify a primary site or histopathology.[130] An essential element in head and neck staging is the physician's documentation, including a precise diagram and written description of the extent of disease, to provide all consulting disciplines with accurate data.

STAGING

Head and neck tumors are classified by the American Joint Committee for Cancer (AJCC) Staging and End Results Reporting (Table 12–3). Patient information that affects clinical staging of head and neck tumors is listed in Box 12–1. Head and neck *T classifications* are a general indication of the extent of the primary tumor. These T classifications can be subclassified according to

how the tumor affects other anatomic sites. Tumors of the oral cavity and lip are classified primarily by the T stage of the lesion. Cancer staging of tumors of the pharynx (nasopharynx, oropharynx, hypopharynx), larynx, and paranasal sinuses is determined by the extent of the primary tumor, depth of tumor invasion, and the number of sites involved. The depth of invasion can significantly affect normal function and mobility of involved and neighboring structures, such as in the hypopharyngeal/laryngeal region, where the tumor may invade bone or affect cranial nerves (e.g., nasopharyngeal cancer). The *N classifications* indicate location (unilateral or bilateral), number, and size of cervical lymph node metastasis and are uniform for all sites. *M classifications,* which indicate distant spread of disease, are determined by clinical and radiographic findings.[58, 137] Using the concept of the greater the T size, the greater the stage, increased extension or invasion results in a higher stage; increased stage of disease is directly related to a poorer prognosis. Staging of head and neck disease ranges from stage I to IV varying by the primary site, according to the extent of the tumor, number and location of the lymph nodes, and the presence or absence of distant metastasis.[58]

PRETREATMENT EVALUATION

Rationale for Treatment Options

The therapeutic measures available for the management of head and neck cancer include surgery, radiation ther-

TABLE 12–2
Major Subdivisions of Aerodigestive Tract

Site	Function	Anatomic Relationship	Clinical Features
Oral cavity	Maintain oral competency for swallowing, articulation	Sensory motor innervation of tongue is bilateral; central chamber of salivary system; sensory innervation mediated by lingual nerve (V); motor innervation to muscles by hypoglossal nerve (XII) Lymphatic drainage to submaxillary and upper cervical lymph nodes and retropharyngeal lymph nodes	Early symptoms: painless "white spot," persistent ulcerations, difficulty with denture fit, difficulty swallowing, blood-tinged sputum
Oropharynx	Mouth and pharynx perform together in alimentary functions of swallowing, emesis, and respiratory functions of crying, speaking, coughing, and yawning	Boundaries include soft palate, tonsils, tonsillar fossa, and base of tongue; glossopharyngeal nerve (IX) mediates motor and sensory innervation to pharynx and posterior one third of tongue; soft palate and pharynx innervated by vagus nerve (X) Lymphatic drainage to jugulodigastric (tonsillar) node and retropharyngeal lymph nodes	Irregular ulcerations of mucosal surfaces, painless growth, dysphagia, pain on swallowing, otalgia, persistent sore throat Late symptoms: speech difficulties, palatal resultant incompetence with nasal regurgitation, dysphagia with or without aspiration, trismus
Nasal cavity	Conditions affecting inspired air before entrance: olfaction humidification, temperature control, cleansing, antibacterial and antiviral protection	First cranial nerve (olfactory) innervates mucous membranes to mediate sense of smell Drainage into submandibular nodes	Similar to chronic sinusitis
Nasopharynx	Anatomic boundary that lies behind nasal cavities and above soft palate	Open space situated just below base of skull behind nasal cavity; inferior wall bordered by soft palate, pharyngeal orifice of eustachian tube, abducens nerve (VI), oculomotor nerve (III), trochlear nerve (IV), and optic nerve (II) Behind eustachian tube lies internal carotid artery, internal jugular vein, and glossopharyngeal (IX), vagus (X), spinal accessory (X), and hypoglossal (XII) nerves Lymph node chain that drains these areas: posterior cervical triangles, supraclavicular nodes, and jugular chain	Persistent poorly localized frontal headaches; temporal, parietal, and orificial pain; decreased hearing, tinnitus; multiple nerve palsies, sensory losses Blood in postnasal drip very significant Profuse epistaxis an infrequent presenting symptom
Paranasal sinuses	Air-filled cavities within bones of skull lined by mucous membranes that drain into nasal cavities	Four pair of maxillary, ethmoid, and frontal sphenoid tumors drain into submaxillary, retropharyngeal, and jugular lymph nodes	Chronic sinusitis, bump on hard palate, swelling, numbness and/or pain of cheek, swelling gums, toothache, increased lacrimation, visual changes: diplopia exophthalmos Persistent unilateral rhinorrhea: epistaxis *Table continued on following page*

TABLE 12-2

Major Subdivisions of Aerodigestive Tract *Continued*

Site	Function	Anatomic Relationship	Clinical Features
Hypopharynx	Anatomic boundary extending from tip of epiglottis to lower border of cricoid cartilage	Lower subdivision of oropharynx, also called laryngopharynx, divided into pyriform sinuses and posterior cricoid area; posterior and lateral pharyngeal walls	Painless, enlarged cervical lymph nodes; odynophagia accompanied with progressive dysphagia and rapid weight loss
	Structures important for swallowing and airway protection	Pharyngeal constrictions innervated by glossopharyngeal (IX) and vagus (X) nerves	Otalgia on same side of tumor Hoarseness, dysphagia
		Lymphatic drainage: primary along internal jugular vein and retropharyngeal and paratracheal nodes	
Larynx	Serves for speech production, maintenance of airway, and airway protection	Located directly below hypopharynx; sensory innervation supplied from internal laryngeal branch of superior laryngeal nerve of vagus and recurrent laryngeal nerve	Persistent hoarseness; change in quality, pitch, voice; pain; hemoptysis; dysphagia; cough; aspiration
		Divided into three anatomic sites: (1) supraglottic, (2) glottic, and (3) subglottic	
		Lymph drainage to anterior jugular nodes	
Salivary glands	Production of saliva	Divided into major glands: paired parotid, submandibular, sublingual, and minor salivary glands	Painless, rapidly growing mass with or without associated nerve paralysis
		Lymphatic drainage usually to deep jugular or intraglandular or paraglandular lymph nodes; innervation of this area includes mandibular branch of seventh cranial, lingual, and hypoglossal (XII) nerves	
Thyroid gland	Endocrine gland	Highly vascular gland located in anterior and lower part of neck; composed of small central part, isthmus, and two lobes; isthmus covers second, third, and fourth tracheal rings; thyroid related medially to esophagus and recurrent laryngeal nerve and laterally to carotid sheath, containing carotid artery; internal jugular vein and vagus nerve	Neck pain, tightness or fullness in neck, hoarseness, dysphagia, dyspnea
		Lymphatic drainage of thyroid gland mainly through lymphatic vessels that accompany arterial blood supply	

apy, and chemotherapy. Treatment modalities may be used alone or in combination. Surgery or radiation therapy is used as standard treatment for patients with very early limited or advanced resectable head and neck cancers. The ultimate goal of all head and neck therapy is patient survival and quality of life. Treatments may be given in an attempt to achieve cure, control, or palliation. If the goal is cure, treatment focuses on local con-

TABLE 12-3
Staging for Head and Neck Cancer

CANCER OF THE LIP, ORAL CAVITY, OROPHARYNX, HYPOPHARYNX, AND LARYNX			
Stage 0	Tis	N0	M0
Stage I	T1	N0	M0
Stage II	T2	N0	M0
Stage III	T3	N0	M0
	T1	N1	M0
	T2	N1	M0
	T3	N1	M0
Stage IVA	T4	N0	M0
	T4	N1	M0
	Any T	N2	M0
Stage IVB	Any T	N3	M0
Stage IVC	Any T	Any N	M1

CANCER OF THE NASOPHARYNX			
Stage 0	Tis	N0	M0
Stage I	T1	N0	M0
Stage IIA	T2a	N0	M0
Stage IIB	T1	N1	M0
	T2	N1	M0
	T2a	N1	M0
	T2b	N0	M0
	T2b	N1	M0
Stage III	T1	N2	M0
	T2a	N2	M0
	T2b	N2	M0
	T3	N0	M0
	T3	N1	M0
	T3	N2	M0

Stage IVA	T4	N0	M0
	T4	N1	M0
	T4	N2	M0
Stage IVB	Any T	N3	M0
Stage IVC	Any T	Any N	M1

CANCER OF THE PARANASAL SINUSES			
Stage 0	Tis	N0	M0
Stage I	T1	N0	M0
Stage II	T2	N0	M0
Stage III	T3	N0	M0
	T1	N1	M0
	T2	N1	M0
	T3	N1	M0
Stage IVA	T4	N0	M0
	T4	N1	M0
Stage IVB	Any T	N2	M0
	Any T	N3	M0
Stage IVC	Any T	Any N	M1

CANCER OF THE SALIVARY GLAND			
Stage I	T1	N0	M0
	T2	N0	M0
Stage II	T3	N0	M0
Stage III	T1	N1	M0
	T2	N1	M0
Stage IV	T4	N0	M0
	T3	N1	M0
	T4	N1	M0
	Any T	N2	M0
	Any T	N3	M0
	Any T	Any N	M1

Used with the permission of the American Joint Committee on Cancer (AJCC®), Chicago, Illinois. The original source for this material is the AJCC® Cancer Staging Handbook, 5th edition (1998) published by Lippincott-Raven Publishers, Philadelphia, Pennsylvania.

BOX 12-1

Patient Information Needed for Staging Head and Neck Tumors

Facts About Tumor

Exact location
Histologic type
Estimated degree of local invasion
Local behavior (e.g., exophytic or invasive)
Cytologic grade
Involvement of other structures

Local Lymph Node Involvement

Location of all suspicious nodes (unilateral/bilateral)
Size
Firmness
Presence of extracapsular spread

Distant Metastasis

Organ system involved
Degree of tumor replacement

Presence or Absence of Second Cancer

---

trol of the disease and prolonged relapse-free survival. When cure is no longer possible, palliation and control of symptoms become the focus of therapy. Table 12-4 outlines the advantages and disadvantages of the three therapeutic measures, which are briefly discussed next.

Surgery. Surgery is as effective as radiation in eliminating limited cancers of the head and neck region. Surgery may be done effectively without functional and cosmetic loss in small early cancers, which are easily accessible. Surgical failures are usually related to the surgeon's inability to remove the tumor en bloc. A disadvantage of surgery is the potential for structural, functional, or cosmetic loss.[98, 110]

Radiation Therapy. Radiation therapy can control the disease in situ, avoids surgical sacrifice of anatomic parts, and preserves functions of speech, swallowing, smell, and cosmesis. Despite acute and long-term sequelae, radiation is classified as the best "tissue- and organ-sparing" treatment available. Radiation therapy has excellent cure rates for patients with limited disease (T1-N0-M0 and T2-N0-M0).[21, 40, 152] Failed radiation therapy in head and neck cancers differs from failed surgery or chemo-

TABLE 12–4
Advantages and Disadvantages of Treatments for Head and Neck Cancers

Modality	Advantages	Disadvantages
Surgery	Ability to remove central-resistant hypoxic tumor cells Immediate reconstruction Provides most accurate estimate of disease extent No carcinogenic effect No biologic resistance by tumor	Potential for structural, functional, or cosmetic loss Only provides local/regional treatment May leave behind viable malignant tissue Must sacrifice some healthy tissue to excise malignancy effectively
Radiation therapy	Curative if disease is small and localized Acute side effects generally disappear after treatment Limited residual deformity or functional loss (in most patients) Focused delivery of tumoricidal dose	Time consuming Not effective as single treatment for large tumors Potential long-term sequelae: soft tissue damage May have carcinogenic effects Some tumors radioresistant
Chemotherapy/biologic therapy	Potential chemopreventive systemic treatment for killing lymphatic and hematogenous metastasis Minimal residual deformity or loss of function	Limiting factors: normal tissue tolerance and tumor responsiveness

therapy. Cancer cells that are hypoxic are insensitive to radiation and do not respond well to treatment. Local failure also can occur when occult malignant cells outside the irradiated field are present, when distant metastases through lymphatic and hematogenous spread are present at treatment, or when tissue and organ tolerance to radiation is less than that of the tumor.

Chemotherapy. Chemotherapy is being used in the treatment of patients with advanced or recurrent disease. The curative role of chemotherapy is still undergoing evaluation; however, its adjuvant or palliative roles in the treatment of this disease have been recognized. Normal epithelial tissues depend on certain substances to maintain their integrity and to promote cellular renewal. The role of chemotherapy is now being evaluated for its preventive potential in premalignant lesions (e.g., leukoplakia or erythroplasia of the oral cavity). Vitamin A and its natural analogues, retinoids, are necessary for the normal development and differentiation of epithelial tissues.[75, 90] (See Chapters 23 and 24 for discussions of drug side effects, specific chemotherapy and biotherapy agents, and treatment combinations.)

Combined Research. The ultimate goal of clinical head and neck research is to provide optimal therapies for each patient. Historically, treatment recommendations may have been based on limited experience and knowledge. The Southwest Oncology Group, Radiation Oncology Group, Veterans Administration Head and Neck Study Group, and other intergroup study groups have attempted to answer questions about the natural history and treatment of head and neck cancers as well as patient rehabilitation. These diversified groups are evaluating

new therapies, including drugs, surgical techniques, radiation delivery systems, and biologic approaches. The strength of the cooperative group studies is that larger populations are evaluable, which can support statistically significant findings. These findings will direct the diagnosis and treatment of patients with head and neck cancer.*

Factors Affecting Treatment Decisions

Treatment decisions are always affected by factors related to the tumor, patient, and the health care provider. In choosing a treatment option, especially in head and neck cancer, the treatment team must put in perspective what is to be achieved. Clearly, survival is important and easily measured, but the quality of life during that survival is even more important.[1, 17, 30, 31, 55] The choice of treatment modalities depends on many factors: (1) tumor site and size, (2) extent of lesion and disease, (3) histology and aggressiveness, (4) need for reconstruction, (5) previous treatment, (6) patient's physical and emotional condition, (7) availability of health care providers and resources to provide comprehensive treatment and rehabilitation programs, and (8) quality of life. *Quality of life* is especially relevant because symptoms and side effects of the disease and treatment can significantly affect patients' adjustment to illness. Quality of life issues emphasize the impact of these symptoms on the patient's physical function, physiologic and emotional status, social function and well-being, and financial status, in contrast to the standard performance

---

* References 4–8, 61, 65, 83, 84, 141, 142.

scales currently used (e.g., Karnofsky and Zubrod).[1, 31] Because the potential for disease recurrence still remains high, quality of life is of significant value when making treatment decisions.

Tumor-Related Factors. Appropriate therapy requires an accurate assessment of the tumor. The size and extent of the primary tumor are equally as important as type and site in determining the treatment. A guide to size and extent of primary head and neck tumors may be found in the AJCC *Cancer Staging Manual.*[58] In general, smaller cancers without metastases (T1 or T2-N0) do not require multimodality treatment. For larger primary tumors (T3 or T4), combined modalities offer a greater chance for quality survival. Patients with regional metastasis classified as N1 or with extension into soft tissues of the neck have benefited from the addition of radiation, which has been shown to prevent recurrence within the neck. Primary lesions that present with regional metastases or distant disease may be best approached by combination therapy incorporating surgery, radiation, and systemic or regional chemotherapy.[28, 160]

Patient-Related Factors. Patient-related factors that affect treatment decisions include general health, previous therapy, dental health, social habits, motivation, economic resources, individual needs, and cultural beliefs and values. Many patients have other health conditions (e.g., chronic lung, cardiovascular, hepatic, or renal disease) that limit the clinician's ability to perform surgery or give maximum doses of chemotherapy. The patient brings a unique set of psychosocial experiences to the treatment milieu. An evaluation of the psychosocial status of the patient and significant others may be more important and more difficult to obtain than an evaluation of the patient's physical status.* Many patients with head and neck cancer are chemical (alcohol/tobacco) abusers and may have associated personality disorders. An evaluation of the patient's smoking and drinking habits is essential in forming the treatment plan. History of previous psychiatric difficulties (e.g., clinical depression) can be a "red flag" indicating those at risk for ineffective coping during or after treatment.[152] The nurse must assess the patient for orientation to current medical status, appropriateness of responses to questions and health care directions, and interactions with family or significant others. The choice of therapy is often influenced by the patient's or family member's misconceptions and knowledge of myths related to cancer and the health care system, based on previous health-related experiences. With the initial assessment, the nurse should attempt to determine how motivated the patient is to comply with the demands of illness and treatment and to survive. Insight into motivation may be gained by obtaining infor-

mation related to previous ability to work and work habits; life-style; economic status; social networks; perceived resources; health-seeking behaviors and history; culturally related attitudes, values, and beliefs that affect the patient's perception of health and illness; compliance with treatment regimens; and self-care practices.[14, 35, 48, 103, 120, 140] Finally, the nurse must remember that treatment cannot be administered if patients choose not to have therapy. The treatment team has the responsibility to educate patients who elect to take their "chances" about the natural course of their disease and the ultimate outcome. Regardless of the patient's decision, physical support and symptom control should be offered and continued. Offering educational materials and activating support systems early within the course of disease provide the patient with opportunities for control and self-care and facilitate the nurse–patient relationship.[114, 135]

Health Care Resources. Treatment of head and neck cancers is influenced not only by the availability of specialists, facilities, equipment, resources, and health care reimbursement, but also by the patient's ability to gain access to that care. The skills and experience of the head and neck surgeon, radiotherapist, and medical oncologist vary in each treatment center. Patients receiving treatment in centers that participate in clinical research trials are afforded opportunities to participate in treatment protocols otherwise unavailable. Patients ideally should receive treatment where a comprehensive rehabilitation team is readily available, including dentists, maxillofacial prosthodontists, speech pathologists, nurse specialists, social workers, physical and occupational therapists, and clinical dietitians. If these opportunities are limited, it may be efficacious for the physician to refer the patient to centers that provide such services.

Treatment and Rehabilitative Planning

Treatment and rehabilitative planning are dictated by the anatomic location and the extent of the primary tumor. Before initiation of treatment, the patient should be evaluated by an interdisciplinary team.[137] Pretreatment assessment by the interdisciplinary groups can accomplish several goals: establish the diagnosis, stage the disease, plan treatment, and integrate prescriptive rehabilitative programs.[35, 48, 87, 88, 109] Nursing assessment in the pretreatment phase identifies any potential or actual nursing diagnoses that can minimize complications of therapy and promote adjustment of the patient, family, and significant others to the illness, treatment, and rehabilitation.[93, 124, 143, 144]

Psychosocial Assessment. In general, patients with head and neck cancer and their families respond to the diagnosis of cancer with shock, anxiety, fear, denial, and grief.[14, 55, 57, 93, 140] The patient is faced with a potential threat to body image and self-esteem. The patient may experience

---

* References 30, 57, 64, 103, 120, 143, 144.

severe and permanent facial disfigurement and functional loss that closely resemble those experienced by the burn patient.[11] The face and neck left uncovered by clothing are subject to the full view of others. Physical disfigurement or functional loss may pose a threat to the patient's coping, sexuality, and socialization patterns.[4,29,140] Patients may feel stigmatized and may become socially isolated. Depression related to the prognosis, altered body image, and decreased self-esteem can become a major impediment to the rehabilitative process.[72] If surgery is planned, the patient may fear undergoing anesthesia or dying during the surgical procedure.

Potential altered body image or a patient's perception of distortion in body image often plays a significant role in the ability to cope with the illness and the treatment plan.[17, 26, 29, 30, 55, 115] A person's body image is a picture or concept of the physical and emotional self, which is incorporated into the person's psychologic construct. Many head and neck cancer patients initially refuse surgery in an attempt to preserve or maintain the concepts of self and function.[57] Body image, self-esteem, and sexuality can be threatened by the results of the surgical procedure. The patient who faces loss of cosmesis, structure, or function (e.g., laryngectomy, tongue or jaw/neck dissection) experiences a major adjustment in body image and may have problems coping. The degree of disfigurement and the patient's perceptions associated with the surgery may intensify the emotional response. The nurse must remember that patients diagnosed with early stage disease may not face the same issues as those with advanced or recurrent disease. A nursing diagnosis of potential altered patterns of sexuality can be related to changes in appearance, fear of the partner, change in oral and respiratory function, alcohol abuse, or nonacceptance of surgery. Salient questions that should be incorporated into a psychosocial nursing assessment and suggested interventions are listed later in this chapter. These nursing interventions support both patient and family and assist the patient to cope with and adjust to illness.*

Pulmonary Assessment and Health History. Patients with head and neck cancer may have other significant medical problems. The physician will evaluate the patient for a history of cardiopulmonary disease, diabetes, bleeding disorders, and renal disease. Careful review and documentation of preexisting medical disorders, along with routine paraclinical data, blood chemistries, cardiography, and chest x-ray films, should be evaluated. Disorders such as hypertension, end-stage cardiopulmonary disease, uncontrolled or labile diabetes, or bleeding disorders may preclude or significantly modify surgical interventions. Prognostic signs associated with cardiac disease that carry a high surgical risk for the patient

include (1) history of poor exercise tolerance, (2) increasing angina, (3) chronic diabetes, (4) uncontrolled or acute congestive heart failure, (5) severe uncontrolled hypertension, (6) dysrhythmias, (7) acute electrocardiograph changes indicating injury or ischemia, and (8) myocardial infarction within 6 months of surgery. Patients with respiratory insufficiency or a significant smoking history should undergo a respiratory evaluation. Patients with respiratory insufficiency or chronic obstructive lung disease cannot adequately meet the body's oxygenation needs during stress. The nurse or respiratory therapist[21] can implement an aggressive pulmonary hygiene and rehabilitation program. To circumvent complications of atelectasis or aspiration pneumonia, the patient should be instructed on proper posture, lung expansion techniques, and breathing exercises.

Nicotine ingestion is clearly a source that contributes to poor wound healing and loss of reconstructive flaps. Some patients are more sensitive to the peripheral vasoconstrictive and ischemic effects of nicotine than others, and the harmful microcirculatory effects of nicotine may persist weeks after cessation of smoking. When cessation of smoking is critical to the survival of the flap, as with a free island flap, the physician may order preoperative urine nicotine levels. Treatment decisions may be significantly influenced by the patient's ability to quit smoking.[25, 51, 66, 83, 164] A lengthy discussion of smoking cessation programs is not within the scope of this text, but programs such as Fresh Start (American Cancer Society) and In Control (American Lung Association) are among the available resources. A thorough nursing assessment also should include documentation of the use of drugs or chemicals.

Alcoholism is common in this patient population; thus a large percentage of these patients will also have associated medical and psychological problems related to acute and chronic abuse (e.g., chronic liver disease, peripheral neuropathies, damaged central nervous system [CNS]). Liver function tests and standard coagulation screening tests, including platelet count, partial thromboplastin time, and prothrombin time, should be evaluated. If chronic alcohol abuse is suspected, the nurse should monitor the patient for clinical problems and signs and symptoms related to withdrawal. The alcohol withdrawal syndrome, which includes symptoms ranging from mild tremulousness to delirium tremens, represents the body's defense reaction to withdrawal of the CNS depressant. Anxiety, tremulousness, increased visual imagery, and tachycardia are compensatory mechanisms that are no longer depressed by alcohol. Manifestations of symptoms may be quite variable from time of cessation of alcohol. Agitation, increased anxiety, and mild tremulousness usually occur within the first 24 to 36 hours. Seizures related to withdrawal most frequently occur within 24 to 48 hours. Tremulousness

---

*References 11, 64, 84, 88, 93, 95, 103, 107, 116, 140.

and agitation often precede delirium tremens. In some patients, severe manifestations may be delayed for 3 to 5 days after cessation of drinking. The medical management of alcohol withdrawal syndrome should include (1) maintaining patient hydration, (2) providing adequate calories, (3) administering vitamin supplementation, (4) suppressing CNS hyperactivity with sedation, and (5) monitoring for electrolyte imbalance, metabolic imbalance, and acidosis.[149]

Nutritional Assessment. Sixty percent of patients with head and neck cancer will present with malnutrition.[49, 80] Each of the three major treatment modalities used singly or in combination may affect the patient's nutritional status. Limited caloric intake for extended periods can deplete protein stores.[12, 54, 68, 124] Before, during, and after treatment weight loss is common among these patients. Therefore, a pretreatment nutritional assessment should be completed.[12, 16, 24, 29, 32] A recent loss of 10% or more of actual body weight, unrelated to dieting or other concurrent medical conditions (e.g., diabetes, infection, alcoholism), is a critical indicator for continued nursing assessment and implementation of a nutritional plan.[18, 67, 139, 146]

The aim of nutritional support in head and neck cancer patients is twofold: to rebuild or maintain protein and to maintain fat stores. Reduced nutritional intake places the patient at risk for a physiologic state of negative nitrogen balance with a resultant loss of protein stores. A reduction in total plasma protein and protein stores places the patient at risk for blood volume loss and hypotension, decreased immune competence, and poor wound healing.[49] If the patient is unable to maintain adequate nutrition, the physician may prescribe oral high-calorie, high-protein supplemental feedings. Most physicians choose the oral or enteral route if the patient has a functional gastrointestinal tract. Patients may require placement of a nasogastric, gastrostomy, or jejunostomy feeding tube.[21, 59] Jejunostomy tubes are placed when the patient is at high risk for aspiration. The nurse may need to prepare the patient psychologically and educationally if placement of a feeding tube is required. The psychologic and social impact of not being able to eat normally can be devastating to the patient and can result in ineffective coping or social isolation. Nursing education and interventions directed at assisting the patient to cope with these physical changes could help the patient circumvent feelings of not being "normal" or of being "socially unacceptable." Patients should be afforded the opportunity to continue experiencing all sensory input (e.g., smell, sight) and maintaining normal socialization patterns and life-style. The nurse and clinical dietitian may encourage the patient and family to puree normal high-calorie, high-protein meals in the blender before administration. Prepackaged supplements are also available if normal food preparation and blenderized meals are not a practical option. (See Chapter 29 for a complete review of nursing diagnoses, assessment, interventions, and care plans related to nutrition.)

Communication and Cognitive Motor Skills. A thorough nursing assessment of the patient's reading, comprehension, and communication skills should be accomplished before the initiation of the definitive therapy. Education should be tailored to the patient's specific need and educational level. If patients have limited reading or writing skills, education may need to be accomplished by using simple explanations, pictures, or videos. Explanations without medical jargon facilitate effective communication. Alternative forms of communication will need to be established with the patient before undergoing definitive surgical procedures such as laryngectomy, glossectomy, or palatal resection. Also, a thorough hearing, speech, and visual examination should be accomplished in patients undergoing these procedures. Deficits in any of these functional areas need to be identified before surgery to facilitate appropriate rehabilitation. Table 12–5 outlines functional losses related to the four types of laryngectomies. Pretreatment consultation with a speech and language pathologist facilitates communication among the patient, family, and nurse; establishes a trusting relationship among professional, patient, and family; and decreases anxiety. Meeting members of the rehabilitation team before treatment serves as a nonverbal statement to the patient that wellness and rehabilitation are the primary treatment foci. If a trained speech and language pathologist schedules the patient for a laryngectomy, a presurgical visit (with a specialty in rehabilitation of the patient with head and neck disease) before hospital admission may allay the patient's fears and anxieties.

Dental Assessment

Dental care is important before, during, and after head and neck cancer treatment.[21, 74, 92, 113, 137] Assessing the dental history gives the nurse insight into the patient's knowledge, beliefs, and resources toward preventive care, as well as susceptibility to dental disease. Oral pathology may be present if the patient has not been evaluated or treated by a dentist. An accurate dental history is critical to prevention of oral complications during therapy. The following questions should be incorporated into a nursing dental history:

1. When was the patient's last dental visit, and what type of procedures were done?
2. How often does the patient see a dentist?
3. Does the patient have a relevant history of:
   a. Sore swollen gums, drainage, or boils?
   b. Toothaches or teeth sensitive to hot, cold, or chewing?
   c. Loose teeth?

TABLE 12-5

Functional Loss Associated with Laryngectomy

Procedure	Structures Removed	Structures Remaining	Functions
TOTAL LARYNGECTOMY			
Loss of laryngeal sphincter mechanism may lead to aspiration. Swallowing mechanism must be intact so that when food lands on vocal cords, patient coughs to remove it and swallows instantly.	Hyoid bone Entire larynx Epiglottis, false/true cords Cricoid cartilage Two/three rings of trachea	Tongue Pharyngeal walls Lower trachea	Loss of voice (resulting from tracheal laryngectomy) Normal swallowing
PARTIAL SUPRAGLOTTIC/HORIZONTAL LARYNGECTOMY			
During supraglottic laryngectomy, muscles that elevate larynx are transected, thereby limiting elevation of larynx. This, along with loss of supraglottic structures, further downgrades swallowing. Because cough is necessary to clear larynx, patient's pulmonary functions must be adequate.	Hyoid bone Epiglottis False cords	True cords Cricoid cartilage Trachea	Normal voice Increased risk for aspiration Normal airway
HEMIVERTICAL LARYNGECTOMY			
Interferes very little with swallowing. Removal of arytenoid cartilage may cause aspiration in a small percentage of patients. Free or pedicled muscle or submucosal cartilage grafts may prevent aspiration. If surgical resection extends to base of tongue, swallowing may be affected related to inability to move bolus. Aspiration may occur.	One true cord, one false cord Arytenoid cartilage One-half thyroid cartilage	Epiglottis One true cord, one false cord Cricoid	Hoarse but serviceable voice Normal airway Normal swallowing
PARTIAL LARYNGECTOMY/LARYNGOFISSURE			
Procedure may affect predominantly deglutition and phonation.	One vocal cord	All other structures	Hoarse but serviceable voice Normal airway Normal swallowing

4. Does the patient have loose, poorly fitting dentures or recurring problems with denture sores?
5. Does the patient have bad breath odor?
6. What kind of toothpaste or dental floss does the patient use?

Oral assessment by the dentist, hygienist, or nurse can facilitate identification of oral disease. The hard and soft oral tissue should be systematically and thoroughly examined. Equipment needed for an oral examination includes good light source, gloves, tongue blade, and unsterile 2 × 2-gauze square. Labial mucosa, vestibule, anterior dentition, and gingiva can be examined by retracting the lips. Buccal mucosa, vestibule, posterior dentition, and gingiva can be examined by retracting the cheeks. Dorsum and lateral surfaces of the tongue can be inspected by grasping the tip of the tongue using a 2 × 2 gauze. Wrapping tongue to palate allows for examination of the floor of the mouth and lingual frenulum. By tilting the patient's head back, with chin up and mouth wide open, the hard palate, maxillary dentition,

and gingival can be inspected. All patients with dentures should have them evaluated for proper fit. Instability and excessive movement of the dentures can potentially cause irritation and may become a source of infection. The nurse should pay particular attention to all denture-bearing surfaces: floor of mouth, hard and soft palate, and lateral borders of the tongue. Demonstrated gingival recession, hypertrophy or decayed teeth, denture sores, or exposed roots should be documented, and the dentist should be consulted.

An individual dental treatment plan that reflects the patient's present and future dental needs should be developed. All corrective procedures should be completed before initiation of any treatment. The dentist or hygienist will take a full-mouth x-ray film (panorex), scale the teeth, and evaluate the roots. A pretreatment panorex identifies the presence of teeth in edentulate patients when radiation to this area is planned. Teeth should be extracted and restored, dental plaque and calculus removed, and periodontal disease corrected before initiation of treatment. If advanced periodontal disease exists on the teeth, it is best to extract the teeth in the involved area. Periodontal disease and poor oral care are major sources of infection during treatment. All these procedures should be completed 10 to 14 days before the initiation of therapy. This waiting period allows for adequate healing of extraction sites. The nurse should enlist the patient's active participation in this dental care and oral hygiene. Patient education should include (1) oral hygiene instructions emphasizing the importance of cessation of use of tobacco and alcohol products; (2) fluoride application and oral hygiene instructions taught initially and on an individual basis or as outlined on the radiation care plan; (3) nutritional counseling, especially limiting sucrose intake; and (4) avoiding commercially available mouthwashes that contain alcohol. The type of floss is not as important as compliance. The mechanical action of vertically moving the floss against the tooth disrupts bacterial colonization. Daily fluoride application should be encouraged as part of a preventive dental and oral care regimen. Fluoride is an anticarious agent with antibacterial properties that promotes remineralization of the enamel. Three types of fluoride are available for use: acidulated phosphate fluoride, neutral sodium fluoride, and stannous fluoride.[74] The fluoride of choice, as with oral rinses and toothpastes, should be nonirritating to the mucosa, readily available, and convenient. Patients undergoing radiation therapy with teeth included in the treatment field should have custom fluoride carrier trays, which will need to be prescribed by the dentist. These fluoride-filled trays are placed over dry teeth for at least 5 minutes to obtain a therapeutic effect (Fig. 12–2). The patient should spit out the excess fluoride after removing the tray, but should not rinse, eat, or drink for 30 minutes after application. When patients are experiencing epi-

TABLE 12–6
Fluoride Sources

Type	Method of Application
Sodium fluoride	Carrier technique
Stannous fluoride	Mixed with water and brushed on
Acidulated phosphate fluoride	Brushed on

sodes of severe mucositis or xerostomia, they may need to convert to a brush-on technique if placement of carrier trays is painful. Regardless of the fluoride delivery method used, fluoride must be used daily and continuously when patients undergo radiation.

Most dentists will recommend a neutral sodium or stannous fluoride gel. It is important for the nurse to understand the differences in fluoride preparations and application techniques (Table 12–6). All patients with dentures should be instructed to keep the dentures and denture-soaking containers clean. Ideally, soaking containers should be disposable and the cleaning solution (any commercial brand) should be discarded and replaced daily.[46] Common soaking solutions that have been found to inhibit microbial growth include chlorhexidine gluconate (Stuart Pharmaceuticals, Wilmington, DE), Chloroseptic (Norwich Eaton Pharmaceuticals, Norwich, NY), or Efferdent (Warner-Lambert Company, Morris Plains, NJ). Chlorhexidine oral rinse is used as an anticarious agent. *Streptococcus mutans,* a component of caries-producing dental plaque, has proved to be sensitive to chlorhexidine rinse solutions.[46, 159] Mouth rinses with 0.1% or 0.2% aqueous solution of chlorhexidine used twice a day have proved effective in inhibiting plaque formation. In addition to a meticulous oral care program, the nurse should educate the patient about the importance of a balanced diet that emphasizes limiting sucrose intake. Sugarless gum and mints are acceptable and should be encouraged.

In patients who have required mandibular reconstruction, osseointegrated dental implants are now a safe option 6 months after surgery. Implants are generally placed in nonirradiated patients because of the increased risk of infection secondary to the radiation-induced compromised blood supply. With the advent of hyperbaric oxygen therapy, implants are now being placed in irradiated patients.[101, 166]

TREATMENT MODALITIES

Marked improvements in the treatment of head and neck cancer have been made in the 1990s compared with therapies offered in the 1960s. New surgical techniques, radiotherapeutic approaches, and chemotherapy are now used earlier in patient management. However,

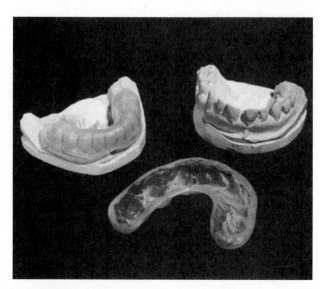

FIGURE 12–2 Oral cavity molds used to prepare individual carrier fluoride trays.

overall cure rates are still only 50%[34] and relapses occur in 40% to 80% of individuals who are diagnosed with advanced disease, depending on the status of the surgical margin.[160] Unfortunately, the incidence of local/regional failures is as high as 60%, with systemic metastases developing in more than 10% of this patient population. The sites of occurrence for second primary tumors vary from 10% in the larynx to 40% in the oropharynx, with the remainder in the esophagus, lung, and bladder. The second tumors usually prove to be the cause of death.

Surgery

The primary goal of surgery for head and neck cancer is removal of the primary disease and all metastatic lymph nodes in hope of controlling local disease and preventing recurrent disease. A secondary goal is to preserve structure and function as much as possible without compromising the treatment.[44, 101] A final goal is to maximize the cosmetic and functional outcome.*

Surgery plays a major role in the diagnosis and staging of head and neck tumors. Surgical approaches to the treatment of these tumors depend greatly on the site and size of the primary lesion, the presence of cervical lymph nodes, and whether the patient has distant metastases.[21, 137] Although surgical management of benign lesions usually involves local excision, malignant lesions require wide resections with or without regional lymphadenectomy and reconstruction at the time of definitive procedure. When cure is no longer within the scope of treatment, the physician can offer palliative surgical options (e.g., tracheostomy, gastrostomy, jejunostomy placement, venous access, implantable ports).

Presurgical Assessment. Preoperative patient assessment, medical evaluation, and health team communication focused on rehabilitation can minimize postoperative complications and help the patient to cope with illness. Additional time spent in preoperative education and planning may actually decrease postoperative complications, decrease the period of inpatient convalescence, and improve the overall quality of postoperative survival. Guidelines for preoperative and postoperative nursing care are presented later in this section.

A presurgical nutritional evaluation is essential because patients with head and neck cancer often experience weight loss and interference with food and fluid intake. A reduction in nutritional intake, protein stores, and total plasma volume places the patient at risk for blood loss and hypotension. The nurse should monitor the patient for clinical signs and symptoms of hypovolemia, such as persistent tachycardia, dizziness, or syncope. The physician may order a volume replacement with red blood cells, albumin, or normal saline. The most efficient tissue oxygenation in microcirculation takes place in normal persons with a hemoglobin level greater than 10 g and a hematocrit level greater than 30%.* The nurse should be aware that if volume depletion has occurred rapidly, a false increase in the hemoglobin and hematocrit levels might be present for a short time. Preoperatively, the nurse should initiate a dietary consultation. It may be necessary to give the patient oral supplements, enteral feedings by tube, or short-term parenteral therapies before surgery. Follow-up nutritional support should be evaluated on an ongoing basis by the nurse, dietitian, physician, and patient.

During the preoperative phase the nurse needs to assess the patient's cognitive skills, motor skills, and ability to communicate. Any potential sensory deficits (e.g., vision, hearing, fine motor writing skills) could affect the patient's ability to participate in the postoperative rehabilitative process.

Surgical Procedures. Cosmesis, body image, and function can be affected significantly by the type of primary and reconstructive procedures.† In addition to the primary surgery, the patient may require a lymph node dissection. The head and neck have about 300 lymph nodes, about 30% of the total lymph nodes in the body. Approximately 75 nodes are present on each side of the neck, most of which are in the deep jugular and spinal accessory chains (Fig. 12–3).

The nodes most frequently involved in metastatic carcinoma are those in the deep jugular chain, which extends from the base of the skull to the clavicle. The decision to perform a neck dissection is based on the presence of lymph nodes or, in a clinically negative neck, based on the probability of metastasis.[76, 104, 105, 119, 129, 138] Table 12–7 lists the types of radical neck procedures, structures removed, and advantages and disadvantages of each procedure. *Modified neck dissection* is a term used to describe several different procedures that are modified from the classic, complete, or radical neck dissections.

Patients who have had a radical or modified procedure may benefit from a preoperative physical therapy evaluation. Functional parameters that are evaluated include head rotation and arm and shoulder mobility (Fig. 12–4). When the spinal accessory nerve has been sacrificed, the head and shoulder range of mobility is significantly affected and the patient faces the potential for permanent disability and chronic pain.[47, 101, 102, 129, 134, 138]

Reconstruction. The primary goal of most head and neck surgery before 1981 was to remove the cancer,

Text continued on page 303

---

*References 26, 36, 38, 56, 70, 76, 85, 94, 101, 112, 164.

---

* References 16, 24, 50, 54, 66, 67, 83, 126.

† References 3, 13, 45, 79, 101, 102, 129, 131, 138, 145.

Nursing Management

HEAD AND NECK SURGERY

Nursing Diagnoses

- *Knowledge deficit related to surgery, preoperative/postoperative procedures*
- *Altered health maintenance related to new postoperative self-care behaviors*
- *Anxiety related to the surgical experience and unpredictable outcome*

Interventions: *Preoperative*

- Review purpose of surgery and rationale (e.g., temporary versus permanent tracheostomy).
- Explain common terms and procedures, provide written literature (show videos), and show actual equipment. Patient will need to be familiar with terminology/equipment.
- Discuss potential sequelae of surgery:
    Change in body appearance
    Change in body function (e.g., breathing, speaking, swallowing, coughing, mobility)
- Explain roles of various medical and nursing personnel and purpose of visits:
    Medicine
    Respiratory therapy
    Nursing/clinical nurse specialist/nurse practitioner
    Home care coordinator
- Determine means of nonverbal communication to be used in the postoperative period (as appropriate).
- Instruct and have patient give verbal return demonstration on all self-care (e.g., coughing, deep breathing, ambulation).
- Document (in nursing notes):
    Patient's level of understanding
    Patient's ability to perform self-care behavior
    Patient education materials given

Outcome Goals: *Preoperative*

Patient will be able to:

- Demonstrate decreased anxiety.
- Demonstrate knowledge about planned surgical procedure.
- Effectively communicate feelings.
- Demonstrate ability to perform self-care, and seek assistance as necessary.
- Name surgery and describe it.
- State reason for surgery, physical changes, and expected outcomes.

- State expectations of intraoperative care and professionals involved.
- State immediate postoperative care, and perform self-care behaviors.
- State patient is less anxious when questioned.
- Describe nonverbal means of communication for use in postoperative period (as appropriate).

Interventions: *Postoperative*

- Instruct patient on self-care behaviors:
    Provide patient education materials and community resources.
    Teach patient to report symptoms of discomfort.
    Teach patient the importance of ambulation, coughing, deep breathing, and rehabilitation.
- Document:
    Patient's response to surgery, functional level, self-care level, and ability to perform procedures
    Patient's level of understanding
    Patient's ability to perform self-care
    Patient education materials given
- Discharge patient with written instructions
- Specific self-care behaviors (e.g., tracheostomy/laryngectomy care exercise, wound management, oral/dental hygiene, signs and symptoms to report to physician)
- Tips for tracheostomy care:
    When performing tracheostomy care at home, patient may use clean technique.
    Keep peristomal area clean and dry to protect it from erosive secretions and prevent infections. From 3 to 5 mL of sterile or disinfected (e.g., quart of water boiled for 15 minutes with a teaspoon of salt added) saline may be instilled in tracheostomy to lavage and irritate trachea and bronchi, thereby stimulating a cough to clear tenacious secretions.
    Wear stoma cover/bib to protect stoma, filter out dust and other airborne particles, warm the air entering the trachea, and help retain some of expired humidity.
    Avoid extremes of temperatures; exposure to dust, gas fumes, and aerosolized vapors; and submersion of stoma under water.
- Emergency procedures (list of appropriate nursing/medical personnel to contact in case of emergency)
- Medic-Alert wallet card and necklace/bracelet should be carried/worn at all times to indicate that person is a neck breather.
- Home care referral

Outcome Goals/Rationale: *Postoperative*

Patient will be able to:

- Demonstrate decreased anxiety.
- Demonstrate knowledge about postoperative care and rehabilitation.
- Effectively communicate feelings.
- Demonstrate ability to perform self-care.
- Demonstrate realistic expectations for assistance needed for postoperative care.
- Identify community resources to assist with disease management and adjustment to illness
- State emergency procedures and names of personnel to contact. NOTE: These instructions ensure a safe homebound environment even if patient demonstrates independence in hospital setting. It is not unusual for patient to become overwhelmed with information and experience difficulty processing it on discharge.

Nursing Diagnoses

- *Ineffective breathing pattern related to diversional methods (tracheostomy, laryngectomy)*
- *Ineffective airway clearance related to tracheal edema, secretions*
- *Risk for injury related to hematoma formation between flap and underlying tissue*
- *Altered tissue perfusion related to arterial erosion rupture around/at surgical site*
- *Impaired skin integrity related to surgery flap reconstruction, flap failure*
- *Impaired swallowing related to superior laryngeal nerve injury, loss or weakness of tongue*
- *Impaired verbal communication related to airway diversion or loss/weakness of tongue*

Potential Clinical/Collaborative Problems

- Respiratory distress
- Hypoxia, airway obstruction, tracheal edema, aspiration
- Hemorrhage
- Hematoma
- Arterial rupture
- Failure of flap survival
- Nerve damage

Interventions: *Postoperative*

- Monitor signs and symptoms of respiratory distress:
  Restlessness, agitation, confusion
  Complaint of air hunger, inability to breathe
  Diminished or absent air exchange in breath sounds over tracheostomy, laryngectomy tube
  Use of accessory muscle retractions of soft tissues around airway
- Monitor signs and symptoms of hemorrhage:
  Continuous oozing of blood or bleeding around surgical site, drains, tracheostomy, laryngectomy, unrelated to manipulation of auctioning, reconstruction
  Presence of unusual edema around wound, stoma, reconstructive site, drainage tubes
- Monitor signs and symptoms of hematoma:
  Check drains for patency.
  Notify physician immediately if presence of air, serum, or milky fluids.
  Normal, excessive, absent. Air indicates dead space; milky drainage may indicate fistula formation with thoracic duct. Leakage can lead to severe fluid/electrolyte loss.
- Monitor signs and symptoms of infection:
  Vital signs
  Drainage/odor
  Intake/output
- Monitor wound and surrounding tissue for signs and symptoms of arterial erosion/rupture:
  Evidence of arterial erosion
  Color (red, pallor, black)
  Vascularity (evidence of bleeding and/or bruising, pulsations, arterial exposure)
  Temperature changes (warm, cool, unilateral)
  Edema (presence or absence)
  Turgor (taut, mobile)
- Monitor signs and symptoms of thoracic duct leakage:
  Milky white drainage often mixed with serous fluid in drainage tubes
- Monitor signs and symptoms of fluid and electrolyte imbalance.
- Monitor signs and symptoms of nerve injury:
  Superior laryngeal nerve dysphagia
  Recurrent laryngeal nerve
  Lingual nerve
  Hypoglossal nerve
  Glossopharyngeal nerve
  Facial nerve
  Phrenic nerve
  Spinal accessory nerve
- Monitor signs and symptoms of flap reconstructive failure:
  Monitor wound, flap, surrounding tissue every 2 hours for 72 hours, then every 4 hours.
  Color (redness, pallor, cyanosis), tension, kinking, pressure, hematoma
  Vascularity (presence or absence of blanching)
  Temperature (warm, cool, unilateral)
  Edema (presence or absence)

Turgor (taut, mobile, shiny, wrinkled)

Odor (not malodorous)

"Red flap": flap appears bright red and when tested for capillary filling feels tense or thick on digital palpation. This occurs when blood flow is excessive. A red flap occurs when there is partial venous obstruction.

"White flap": one that has limited or no blood supply; related to tension, constriction, pressure, or occlusion; can stop blood flow. With dearterialization, flap has no capillary refill, is cool to touch, and becomes white.

"Blue flap": occurs when input of blood exceeds output. This imbalance occurs when arterial pressure remains the same and venous pressure increases (e.g., hematoma) or with constriction of vascular pedicle related to patient lying on flap, with a tight pressure dressing, or with formation of a clot at venous anastomotic site.

- Monitor signs and symptoms of infection:

  Tenderness

  Thickness (inspect level of tissue repair, presence or absence of tumor)

  Moisture (dry; drainage–amount, color, odor; fistula formation)

- Monitor pressure—external pressure of flap.

Postoperative nursing care should focus on preventing and minimizing complications. Immediate postoperative care focuses on maintaining and monitoring the airway. Patient's head should be elevated to reduce edema. Nurse should make sure that drains are kept functional and clear to avoid accumulations of fluid under surgical site or reconstructed flap. Intake and output must be monitored to avoid overhydration or underhydration. If patient has a nasogastric tube, first postoperative day patient is kept NPO, and tube is placed on suction to avoid gastric contents, air, vomiting, or aspiration from occurring. Feedings usually are initiated on second or third postoperative day. Early ambulation is encouraged, and upper aerodigestive system may require frequent, gentle suction to prevent atelectasis, infection, and aspiration. If patient has undergone a mandible/tongue or palatal or larynx resection, nurse must provide patient with paper or magic slate or picture board to facilitate communication. Speech rehabilitation should be started as soon as patient's surgical condition is stable. Whether or not patient is to receive any additional therapy, he or she should be monitored for local or regional recurrence or new disease. Nurse should instruct patient on the importance of maintaining all scheduled appointments; most physicians will follow patient monthly for the first year. During this period,

patient should be prepared to undergo additional tests to evaluate her response to treatment or identify any recurrences or new disease (e.g., chest x-ray film, blood chemistries).

It is generally recommended that patient be seen every month for the first year, every 2 months for the second year, every 3 months for the third year, every 6 months for the fourth and fifth year, and every 6 to 12 months thereafter. Early detection of local or regional recurrences or a new primary lesion provides patient with the best opportunity for cure or control of disease.

Outcome Goals/Rationale: *Postoperative*

- If tracheostomy is not placed during surgical procedure, tissue swelling (tracheal edema) may occur during the first 24 hours; patient should be observed for airway obstruction. Intrinsic laryngeal edema or hematoma and increased anxiety or apprehension can increase potential for obstruction. Elevating patient's head to facilitate lymphatic arterial flow reduces edema.

- Continuous oozing of blood after first 24 hours postoperatively is not normal; may require surgical intervention for control.

- Surgical incision should be assessed carefully the first 24 hours for bleeding drainage and patency of drainage tubes. Serious complications can lead to skin flap wound breakdown. If suction apparatus and tubes are not functioning, skin flaps may not adhere, and necrosis may occur.

- If drain suction becomes plugged, malfunctions, or has excessive oozing or bleeding, vascular link-up occurs and fluid collects; sets site for compromised circulation and infection.

- Drains prevent development of dead space. Continuous bloody drainage may indicate formation of hematoma or fistula formation.

- Hematoma formation is prevented by placement of suction catheter draining superiorly and anteriorly or placement of flap to recipient site, eliminating dead space. Fluid or air collects between flap and underlying tissue. Gravity permits venous drainage through flap.

- Meticulous wound care as ordered by physician should be provided.

- Careful monitoring of intake and output avoids overhydration or underhydration.

- Exposure of adventitial layer of artery to atmosphere facilitates drying and destroys blood supply of layers. Once artery is exposed to the air, destruction of wall occurs in approximately 6 to 10 days.

- Contributing factors to arterial erosion include poor wound healing, exposure of artery at surgery, tumor growth invasion, previous radiation, fistula formation, or infection.

- Raising head of patient's bed facilitates venous drainage; raising it 30 to 45 degrees promotes lymphatic venous drainage.
- Major lymphatic leak from thoracic duct represents loss of fluid and protein and may require surgical closure or protein replacement.
- Branch of vagus that innervates base of tongue may cause swallowing impairment.
- Responsible for adduction/abduction of vocal cords.
- Bilateral pareses require immediate tracheostomy.
- Numbness on ipsilateral tongue can occur if severed.
- If severed, unilateral tongue paralysis results, which causes impairment of speech and mastication; innervates the genioglossus muscle and is responsible for tongue movement.
- Innervates posterior two thirds of tongue. Damage can result in altered taste sensation on ipsilateral side and difficulty in swallowing.
- Result of trauma, especially in the area of parotid, may result in droop or asymmetry of musculature around the mouth (drooping periostosis).
- If severed, paralysis of diaphragm can result.
- Innervates trapezius muscle, which stabilizes and supports shoulder; allows lateral abduction of arm.
- Often affected in neck dissections. Injury results in painful shoulder, droopy atrophy of trapezius muscle, and immobility of head and shoulder.
- Major surgery can create deficits that may not be approximated and closed by direct suture. Skin flaps with or without muscle provide tissue and bulk protection to vital structures (e.g., carotid artery). Purpose is to maintain vascular integrity. Maximum redness should occur first 8 to 12 hours and decrease after 2 to 3 days. If arterial or venous supply is hindered, flap may necrose or slough. Flap and recipient sites should survive if no unusual kinking, pressure, hematoma, or infection occurs. Tension compromises blood supply; kinking causes decreased blood supply to distal portion of flap and compromises venous outflow, resulting in increased capillary permeability and occlusion of lymphatics and arterioles. Pressure compromises blood supply. Position patient to permit gradual flow of lymph and blood. Elevate head of bed 30 to 45 degrees.
- Normal tissue and flaps are warm to the touch and recover color slowly after tested for blanching. Flaps have fine wrinkles, an indication of minimal edema.
- Abnormal findings (shiny, taut, reddish) indicate circulatory embarrassment and venous congestion.

After testing for blanching, flap recovers color quickly.

- Foul purulent drainage is seen.
- Room temperatures that are extreme cold can be a contributing factor to flap loss; maintain room temperature.
- Flap necrosis can lead to formation of fistula, septicemia, arterial rupture, and prolonged hospitalization.
- External pressure on muscle flap compromises circulation, facilitates venous congestion, and leads to decreased permeability and occlusion of lymphatics.

Nursing Diagnoses

- *Body image disturbance related to head/neck cancer surgery*
- *Sexual dysfunction related to altered self-esteem and change in appearance*
- *Self-esteem disturbance related to anatomic changes, role disturbance, disruption of life-style, uncertain future, altered sexuality patterns, body image changes*

Interventions: *Preoperative*

- Review purpose of interview: obtaining information and a sexual history early in a relationship with a patient validates to patient/partner that sexuality is an important part of health and rehabilitation and therefore it is appropriate for concerns to be discussed.
- Progress from less sensitive questions. Ask patient/partner if they have any questions at conclusion of history.
- Include following components of preoperative nursing assessment in interview:
  Specific sexual needs of patient/partner
  Sexual history (provide privacy, assure confidentiality)
  Coping style and adjustment to previous illness or surgery
  Attitudes about sex
  Patient's attitudes about altered body image and perception of sexuality
  Effects of illness on partner/patient. Does patient's present or postoperative physical condition limit partner's ability for sexual expression?
  Demonstration of nurse's acceptance; facilitation of patient's comfort and adjustment to illness and surgery
  Determination of involvement of partner in providing actual physical care and whether or not partner is fatigued

Assessment of whether partner feels guilty about initiating or making sexual demands

Patient's/partner's reactions to impending physical change

Existence of pain, fatigue, depression, limited mobility that would affect normal expressions of sexuality

Interference by illness on patient's roles. Has being ill interfered with (mother, father, wife, husband, etc.)?

Impact of surgery on patient's self-perception

Effect of illness/disability on patient's sexual function

Outcome Goals: *Preoperative*

Patient/partner will be able to:

- Identify aspects of sexuality/sexual function that may be threatened by surgical procedure (e.g., tracheostomy; laryngectomy; tongue, jaw/neck dissection/reconstruction).
- State factors that influence sexual identity.
- Identify behaviors that facilitate acceptance of surgery.

- Maintain satisfying social and sexual/role concept.
- Verbalize importance of seeking professional assistance if normal life-style, socialization, or sexual function is impaired.

Interventions: *Postoperative*

- Assess that patient/partner wants to know about surgical procedure and changes in function that may be related to surgical procedure.
- Assess patient's attitude about altered body image and perception of sexuality.
- Do pain, fatigue, and limited mobility affect normal expressions of sexuality?
- What is patient's/partner's reaction to altered body image?

Outcome Goals: *Postoperative*

Patient/partner will be able to:

- Provide factual information.
- Give assurance that it is acceptable to share feelings and concerns.
- Assist with coping/adjustments to illness.

replace the anatomic structure, and restore cosmesis. With the advent of muscle, musculocutaneous, and free tissue transfer, more attention is dedicated to restoration of functional losses and rehabilitation. Surgeon and communication scientists are coordinating efforts to identify and improve reconstructions of the oral cavity that focus on swallowing and speech function. Video fluoroscopic studies are done to evaluate the patient's communicative ability, tongue strength, and range of motion. When done preoperatively and postoperatively, these studies can help measure the patient's progress in rehabilitation. Patient education is essential to a patient's adjustment to illness, empowerment, and rehabilitation when considering reconstructive surgery.[97–99]

The goals of reconstructive surgery are better accepted if the patient understands the reasons for considering various surgical options, such as flap versus graft or secondary wound healing. Patients must understand that no restorative surgery can return them to complete normalcy and that function and imperfection in contour are an expected outcome. When immediate reconstruction is performed, it is important and reasonable to anticipate possible need for revisions or future procedures. Surgical removal of head and neck tumors can result in functional and socially unacceptable cosmetic deformities. Many patients undergo immediate reconstruction. Patients may be faced with more than one surgical procedure for reconstruction, including autoge-

nous tissue and all-aplastic material.* Normal physiology is best achieved when the surgeon uses autogenous tissue. Soft-tissue defects can be closed by direct approximation (suturing), free skin grafts, pediculed tissue (using local, regional, or distant flaps), or free flaps transferred by microvascular anastomoses. Skeletal tissue is best provided by living vascularized bone grafts or flaps.[38, 125, 155, 158, 164] Nonvascularized bone grafts or all-aplastic material can be used for bone replacement.[38, 128, 129, 136–138] Small defects can usually be covered by primary closure.

Moderate-sized defects may require skin grafting or local skin flaps (Figs. 12–5 and 12–6). Table 12–8 outlines factors that affect the surgeon's choice of flap. Several types of flaps are available for reconstruction: (1) tongue flaps are used to cover internal mucosal defects such as floor of mouth, pharyngeal wall, or cheek; (2) skin flaps consist of skin, the subcutaneous tissues, and the fascia of the underlying muscle; and (3) myocutaneous flaps incorporate an island of desired skin and underlying subcutaneous tissue, and fascia is severed from all surrounding tissues (Fig. 12–7). A full thickness of underlying muscle is lifted with its blood supply. When reconstruction is not technically feasible, the patient may require fitting with a prosthesis (e.g., exter-

---

* References 36, 38, 45, 70, 76, 79, 94, 102, 129, 131, 134, 137, 138.

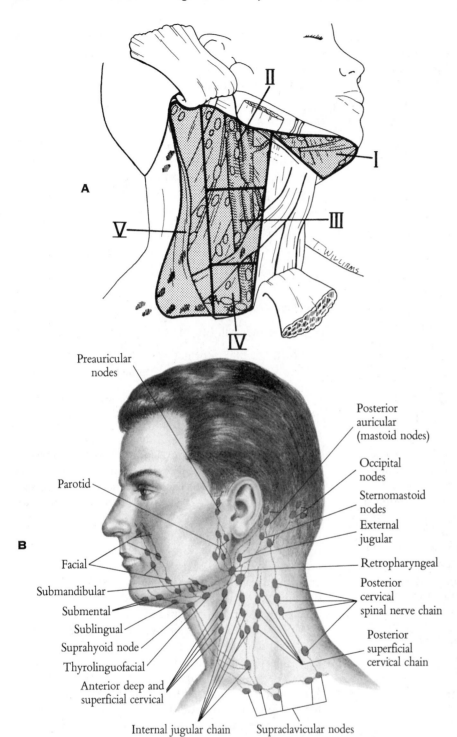

Preauricular
nodes

Posterior
auricular
(mastoid nodes)

Occipital
nodes

Sternomastoid
nodes

External
jugular

Parotid

Retropharyngeal

Facial

Posterior
cervical
spinal nerve chain

Submandibular

Submental

Sublingual

Posterior
superficial
cervical chain

Suprahyoid node

Thyrolinguofacial

Anterior deep and
superficial cervical

Internal jugular chain   Supraclavicular nodes

FIGURE 12-3   A, Schematic of lymph node regions of neck. **B,** Lymphatic drainage system of head and neck. (A from Cummings CW and others, editors: *Otolaryngology—head and neck surgery,* ed 3, St Louis, Mosby, 1999; B from Seidel HM and others: *Mosby's guide to physical examination,* ed 3, St Louis, Mosby, 1995.)

nally for a total ear or nose, internally for a palate). Preoperative consultation with a maxillofacial prosthodontist is necessary. This preoperative consultation allows the patient and professional to evaluate all options for reconstruction. The surgeon and prosthodontist must work collaboratively. Appropriate planning for surgical resection and reconstruction allows for

the anchoring and stabilization of a prosthesis (Fig. 12–8).

Radiation Therapy

Radiation therapy for head and neck tumors can be divided into three treatment categories: curative, pallia-

TABLE 12–7
Radical Neck Procedures

Procedure	Structures Removed	Advantages	Disadvantages
Comprehensive (classic) neck dissection: bilateral or unilateral			
Radical neck dissection	En bloc removal of nodal regions I to VI and all lymph node-bearing tissues on one side of neck, superficial and deep fascia, sternocleidomastoid muscle, omohyoid muscle, submandibular gland, tail of parotid gland, internal and external jugular veins, connective tissue of carotid sheath, transverse cervical vessels, spinal accessory nerve, greater auricular nerve, cutaneous branches of the cervical plexus; excision may also include external carotid artery, portion of digastric muscle, branches of vagus nerve, and hypoglossal nerve	Low probability of leaving nodal disease behind	Trapezius muscle dysfunction with shoulder drop, resulting in pain and limitation in motion Mild to moderate neck deformity If bilateral procedure is performed, cerebral edema may persist Painful neuromas may occur Loss of carotid artery
Modified radical neck dissection	Unilateral removal of nodal regions I to V with preservation of spinal accessory nerve, internal jugular, and/or sternocleidomastoid muscle	Low incidence of shoulder drop and shoulder disability Carotid artery not sacrificed Cosmetic deformity not as severe as with comprehensive neck dissection If cervical plexus preserved, decreased incidence of sensory deficit and painful neuromas	Possible omission of occult positive nodes Increased risk of hematoma under sternocleidomastoid muscle Increased risk of surgeon cutting into positive nodes and seeding neck Increased difficulty in performing secondary procedure and if disease recurs
Type I	Spinal accessory nerve preserved		
Type II	Spinal accessory nerve and internal jugular preserved		
Type III (functional or Bocca) neck dissection	Spinal accessory nerve, internal jugular, and sternocleidomastoid preserved		
Selective neck dissection	Spinal accessory, internal jugular, and sternocleidomastoid muscles preserved	Same as for modified neck dissection, plus improved lymphatic drainage because selected lymph node groups retained	Increased possibility of cutting into or omitting occult positive nodes
Lateral neck dissection	En bloc removed of nodal regions II, III, and IV		
Anterolateral neck dissection	Supraomohyoid neck dissection: en bloc removal of nodal regions II, III, and IV Expanded supraomohyoid neck dissection: en bloc removal of nodal regions I, II, III, and IV		
Posterolateral neck dissection	Removal of suboccipital and retroauricular lymph node groups and nodal regions II, III, IV, and V		

Table continued on following page

TABLE 12–7
Radical Neck Procedures *Continued*

Procedure	Structures Removed	Advantages	Disadvantages
Extended neck dissection	Any neck dissection extended to include lymph node groups not usually removed or structures not routinely removed (e.g., carotid artery, levator scapular muscle)	Lower probability of leaving occult disease behind	Increased risk of cerebrovascular accident (stroke) if carotid is resected Increased risk of shoulder dysfunction if levator scapular muscle excised

Data from Robbins KT: Neck dissection. In Cummings CW and others, editors: Otolaryngology—head and neck surgery, ed 3, St. Louis, Mosby, 1999.

tive, or adjunctive to surgery or chemotherapy.[61, 77, 78, 81, 82, 86] Treatment planning is based on the nature, size, location, and growth of the tumor; volume of disease; organs to be spared; and purpose of treatment. Radiation energies of 1 million volts or greater and radioactive isotopes are usually the primary sources of treatment in head and neck cancers. These are termed *megavoltage radiation sources,* and they possess some very important physical advantages in the treatment of head and neck cancers, such as skin-sparing effects, increase in depth of dose, formation of a sharp beam (which minimizes unnecessary damage to adjacent tissues and organs), and a bone-sparing effect related to decreased absorption by soft tissue and bone.[60, 78, 162]

The inherent properties of head and neck tumors determine their responsiveness to radiation therapy. These tumors can be exophytic, infiltrative, or ulcerative. Exophytic small tumors tend to be homogenous and well-vascularized, thus are very responsive to radiation therapy.[78] Infiltrative and ulcerative tumors tend to be more extensive than is clinically apparent and frequently have a large hypoxic compartment, thus they are more radioresistant.[78]

Radiation as a primary treatment to the head and neck is usually delivered with a "shrinking field" technique. With conventional fractionation, the initial dose of 45 to 50 Gy is administered to the region encompassing the tumor and the clinically affected/potentially af-

The following exercises have been developed to increase the movement and strength in your neck, arms, and shoulders.

Neck Range of Motion
1. Bring chin to chest in a relaxed way and then let it fall gently backwards so a stretch on the neck muscles is felt.
2. Slowly turn head as far as possible to one side as if attempting to look over that shoulder. Do the same to the other side.
3. Bend the head toward the shoulder on the unaffected side. A stretching will be felt on the operated side.

Shoulder Mobility
1. Standing with shoulders relaxed and head facing forward, let arm on the affected side hang freely. Make circles with the shoulder by moving it:
   a) forward
   b) upward
   c) backward
   d) downward
2. With a wand or cane in front of body and shoulders and arms relaxed, raise wand as high as possible keeping elbows extended. After you are able to raise it directly overhead, slowly lower it behind the neck. Raise wand overhead and return it to starting position.
3. Stand facing a wall with your feet a few inches from it. Slide the hand on your affected side up the wall as far as possible, using the wall for support. Perform the same exercise with your affected side facing the wall. Repeat the motion of sliding your hand up the wall but do not turn your body when doing this exercise.

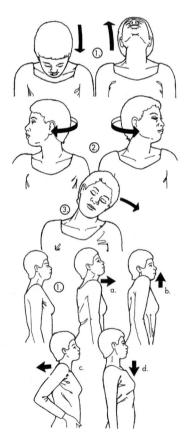

FIGURE 12–4 Exercises after neck dissection. (From Sigler BA, Schuring LT: *Ear, nose, and throat disorders,* St Louis, Mosby, 1993.)

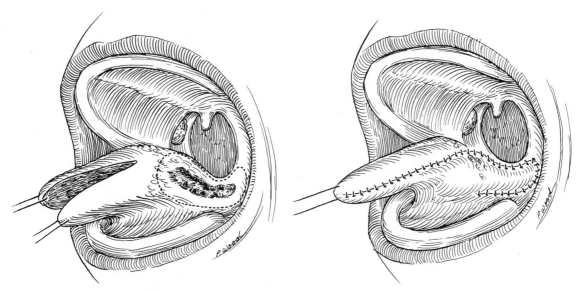

FIGURE 12–5 Tongue flap used for reconstruction of lateral oropharynx. (From Genden EM, Thawley SE, O'Leary MJ: Malignant neoplasms of the oropharynx. In Cummings CW and others, editors: *Otolaryngology—head and neck surgery,* ed 3, St Louis, Mosby, 1999.)

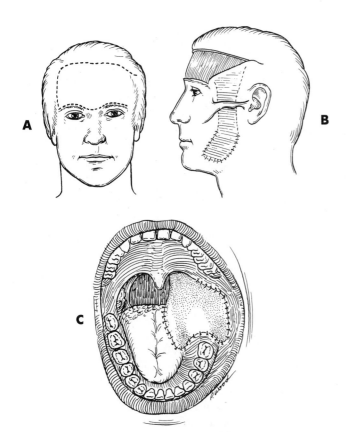

FIGURE 12–6 A, Forehead flap based on superficial temporal artery and portions of occipital artery. **B,** Rotation of forehead flap medial to zygomatic arch for reconstruction of oropharynx. Flap is pulled interiorly to fill resected area. **C,** Completion of forehead flap reconstruction. (From Genden EM, Thawley SE, O'Leary MJ: Malignant neoplasms of the oropharynx. In Cummings CW and others, editors: *Otolaryngology—head and neck surgery,* ed 3, St Louis, Mosby, 1999.)

fected nodes for 4.5 to 5 weeks. The fields are then reduced to cover the tumor and a small margin, and a "boost" of therapy is given to complete the 7 to 7.5 weeks of therapy at a dose between 60 and 70 Gy.[78, 121] With massive tumors there is often a third reduction at 60 to 65 Gy and therapy may continue for up to 8 weeks. Care must be taken to limit the radiation exposure of the spinal cord to 45 Gy to avoid radiation myelitis.[78, 121]

In the past 10 years, altered fractionation schemes have been tried for inoperable tumors of the oral cavity, which poorly tolerate higher doses of radiation. Hyperfractionation is administered twice a day, 1.2 Gy per fraction, for a total of 76 to 80 Gy. Accelerated hyperfractionation is administered two fractions per day, spaced 4 hours apart, with a 2-week break at 38.4 Gy, for up to 67 Gy in 6 weeks. This is an area that is still under investigation.[121, 153]

In treatment of head and neck cancers, radiotherapy may be given preoperatively to prevent marginal recurrences and to control subclinical disease at the primary site or in the nodes. It is also used to convert technically inoperable tumors to operable ones. The combination of preoperative irradiation and surgery is successful in decreasing both local and regional recurrence.* However, the major disadvantages of preoperative radiation are: (1) the normal tissue reaction to radiation may obscure the surgeon's ability to determine the exact extent of the tumor margin; (2) the risk for postoperative complications are higher; and (3) the dose that can be safely delivered preoperatively is less than the dose that can be delivered postoperatively, thus may be less than

---

*References 4–7, 10, 60, 78, 122, 136.

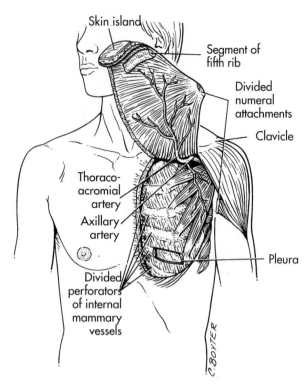

FIGURE 12–7 Diagrammatic representation of myocutaneous flap procedure. (From Mathes S, Nahai F: *Clinical applications for muscle and musculocutaneous flaps,* St Louis, Mosby, 1982.)

that necessary to control gross disease and it is difficult to add a meaningful dose postoperatively.[28, 78] Preoperative radiation is usually given for 1 month, followed by a 1-month rest period, which allows time for the acute tissue reaction to subside but stays within a time frame when radioactive cell kill is still occurring.[163]

Postoperative radiation therapy may also be given to treat residual disease at the surgical margins and subclinical disease in the lymph nodes or may be implanted in the wound. Radiation treatments are usually given about 3 or 4 weeks (preferably no more than 6 weeks) after surgery to allow wound healing. Treatment usually lasts 6 to 8 weeks.[78, 145, 148]

In addition to external beam radiation, *radioactive isotopes* and *intracavitary implants* are sources of radia-

TABLE 12–8
Factors That Affect Surgeon's Choice of Flaps

Tissue Considerations	Physician Considerations
Size of arc	Will the flap cover the defect?
Vascular supply	Will the flap survive?
Accessibility	How close to defect is the new tissue?
Donor site	Functional loss and contour of donor site
Sensation	Maintain nerve supply

tion that may be applied closely to tumors by hollow containers loaded with radioactive sources. These techniques are beneficial when treating tumors of the antrum, sinuses, and nasal cavity. These interstitial or intracavitary implants can be used for the treatment of the tongue, tonsils, nasopharynx, oral cavity, and metastatic neck nodes.[121, 123, 146] Interstitial irradiation is often used in the management of early, localized T1 lesions of the nasal vestibule with no detectable lymph nodes. Larger and more infiltrating (T2) squamous cell carcinomas are treated by implants alone or with external beam radiation. This technique is termed *brachytherapy.* The advantage of brachytherapy is that it permits the delivery of irradiation at a high volume over a short period while delivering a relatively low dose to surrounding tissues.[21, 78, 106, 121] Interest in protocols that examine "organ preservation" have been developed in the area of advanced laryngeal cancers.

Pretreatment Assessment. Immobilization devices (e.g., head straps, bite blocks, light cast molds), portal planning films and simulation, and dosimetry port films all must be prepared before initiation of radiation treatment. Pretreatment medical work-ups, including physical examinations, radiographs with or without contrast, computed tomography (CT), magnetic resonance imaging (MRI), nutritional evaluation, and paraclinical laboratory studies, should be completed before initiation of treatment. If anemia, weight loss, or electrolyte imbalance exists, every medical effort should be made to correct imbalances, because anemic patients do not tolerate radiation therapy well and tumors do not respond as well. Once the type and amount of radiotherapy are determined, the nurse, including the following questions, should complete a pretreatment psychosocial assessment:

How does the patient interpret his current physical status?

Is there a previous history of effective versus ineffective individual family coping and powerlessness?

What is the patient's knowledge deficit related to radiation therapy, pretreatment planning, and actual treatment delivery?

Does the patient demonstrate any cognitive or learning disabilities, such as illiteracy, sensory limitations, and vision, speech, hearing, or motor disabilities?

Patient education is developed based on information obtained in the initial nursing assessment. Simple, nontechnical, concise explanations should be used rather than medical terminology. Pretreatment patient education should include the rationale for why radiation therapy was chosen over other treatments, actual length of treatment session, duration of treatment, and oral, nutritional, and skin care. This education will eliminate

An opening (fistula) has been created between the tracheostoma (windpipe) and esophagus (food passage) in order to place a speech valve (prosthesis). Temporarily, a red rubber catheter will stent the fistula open. Once healing has taken place, a speech prosthesis will replace the catheter.

If the Prosthesis Comes Out

1. Insert a red rubber catheter (10, 12, 14 Fr) into fistula approximately 6-8 inches.
2. Tie a knot in the external end of the catheter to prevent passage of stomach contents.
3. Tape external end of catheter to skin of chest.
4. If catheter cannot be inserted, contact your physician or speech therapist immediately. This may indicate closure of the fistula.

Replacing the Prosthesis

1. Remove prosthesis.
2. Cleanse neck and stoma.

3. Using inserter that is supplied with prosthesis, reinsert clean prosthesis into fistula.
4. Tape in place.
5. Clean prosthesis with hydrogen peroxide and water. Rinse well.
6. The voice prosthesis will last from 2 weeks to several months between changes. The length of time a prosthesis remains in place is dependent upon you. If food or fluid leaks around the prosthesis, it should be changed. If leakage continues, contact your speech therapist for a new size or length of prosthesis.

To Use the Prosthesis

1. Cover your stoma with your thumb. This will allow air from your lungs to pass through the opening of the prosthesis into the esophagus. The walls of your throat and the structures in your mouth will form the words for speech.

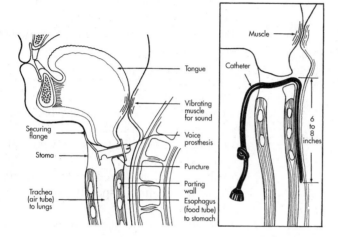

FIGURE 12–8 Care of tracheoesophageal puncture. (From Sigler BA, Schuring LT: *Ear, nose, and throat disorders,* St Louis, Mosby, 1993.)

the myths and misconceptions that the patient and family may experience related to radiation therapy and its side effects.

Although radiation therapy holds some distinct advantages over other treatment modalities, the patient remains at risk for acute and chronic side effects. Acute complications include mucositis and oral ulcerations with resultant pain or discomfort, superficial infections, dermatitis, and hypogeusia. Chronic side effects may include chronic xerostomia, radiation caries, soft-tissue necrosis, osteoradionecrosis, and trismus.* The type and extent of complications vary depending on the dose, type, fractionation, duration of radiation, and the volume of tissue radiated. Therefore, it is important to consider these factors before counseling patients regarding self-care behaviors. Most complications can be prevented or minimized with collaborative efforts of the patient, family, physician, nurse, dentist, dental hygienist, physical therapist, speech therapist, and dietitian, thus enhancing the patient's overall quality of life.†

Complications

Mucositis. Radiation-induced mucositis is a frequently occurring acute problem. Radiation impairs mitosis nonspecifically. Mucositis, ulceration, and inflammation of the mucous membranes are expected and often painful side effects of high-dose radiotherapy to the head and neck. Mucosal erythema usually begins within 2 to 3 weeks of the initiation of therapy. The normal mucosa thins from direct killing of parietal replicating cells. The rate of mucosal breakdown and ulceration is directly related to the timing and total dosage of radiotherapy. The daily dosage of radiotherapy will determine the degree of erythema, mucositis, or xerostomia. During this time the radiation destroys the basal cell layer at a rate faster than proliferation of new cells. Mucosal ulcerations result spontaneously or can be caused by minor trauma from dentures, abrasive foods, or teeth. The ulcerations vary in site and severity, generally occurring along the buccal and labial mucosa, adjacent to teeth. Preradiation patient teaching on oral care can circumvent ulcerations related to trauma. All these changes can compromise the natural epithelial barrier that protects the oral cavity from pathogenic bacteria and fungus. Preexisting periodontal disease exacerbates the ulcerations. Mucositis can develop

---

*References 10, 20, 21, 53, 78, 108, 111, 113, 145, 146, 154.

†References 1, 16, 17, 21, 30, 48, 64, 73, 100, 108, 124, 143, 145, 146.

Nursing Management

HEAD AND NECK RADIATION THERAPY

Nursing Diagnoses

- *Knowledge deficit regarding radiation therapy to head and neck*
- *Altered oral mucous membrane related to radiation therapy to head and neck (mucositis, xerostomia, caries)*
- *Altered nutrition: less than body requirements related to oral pain, difficulty swallowing (dysphagia), difficulty chewing, xerostomia-imposed fluid restrictions, change in tolerance to temperatures of food (cold, hot), change in tolerance to acidic or highly seasoned food, change in taste (hypogeusia), poorly fitted dentures or inability to wear dentures (see the table below)*
- *Acute pain related to mucositis, xerostomia, difficulty chewing, swallowing*
- *Chronic pain related to radiation caries, or osteoradionecrosis*
- *Risk for injury related to oral hygiene*
- *Altered dentition related to radiation therapy associated osteoradionecrosis*
- *Risk for impaired skin integrity related to radiation therapy*

Interventions

- Review purpose of radiation therapy and rationale for treatment.

Supraglottic Swallow

Action	Effect
Take deep breath	To aerate lungs
Perform Valsalva maneuver (bear down)	To approximate vocal cords
Place food in mouth and swallow	Some food will enter airway and remain on top of closed vocal cords
Cough	To remove food from top of vocal cords
Swallow	To swallow food removed from top of vocal cords
Breathe	Restoring breathing before cough-swallow sequence would result in aspiration of food collected by vocal cords

From Sigler BA, Shuring LT: Ear, nose, and throat disorders, St Louis, Mosby, 1993.

- Explain common terms and procedures, provide written literature, and show actual equipment (e.g., light cast molds, bite blocks). Patient will need to be familiar with terminology and equipment (e.g., simulation/dosimetry port films, cobalt/linear accelerator implants).
- Discuss potential sequelae of radiation:
  Change in body appearance (e.g., skin)
  Change in body function (e.g., mucositis, xerostomia, swallowing)
  Potential for infection
  Potential for radiation caries
  Potential for soft tissue and osteoradionecrosis
  Nutritional stomatitis and taste loss
  Trismus
- Explain roles of various medical, nursing personnel, technicians, dosimetrists, and purpose of visits.
- Instruct and have patient give verbal/return demonstration on all self-care:
  Oral hygiene (for dentulous and edentulous patients)
- Provide instructions for edentulous patients:
  Brush teeth often, especially after eating and at bedtime.
  Use soft, nylon toothbrush with even bristles.
  Place bristles at an angle to where your gums and teeth meet.
  Use short back-and-forth strokes to clean front, back, and all chewing surfaces of teeth and tongue.
  Tongue can harbor bacterial plaque and should be gently brushed.
  Use toothpaste that contains fluoride.
  Use dental floss at least once a day to clean sides of teeth where toothbrush does not reach.
  Ease the floss between teeth so that it is close to the tooth as you guide it up and down. Do not snap floss between teeth because it may damage your gums.
  Oral hygiene. Cleanse inside of mouth gently with moist clean gauze or toothette. Massage gums gently with finger.
  Clean dentures or partials every day with denture brush and denture cleaner (e.g., soap and water or baking soda and water).
  Change dental soaking cup and brush frequently, every 2 weeks.
  Store dentures in container of water to keep shape when not in mouth.
  Remove dentures several hours daily as prescribed by dentist.

- Instruct dentulous and edentulous patients to rinse mouth often. Rinse mouth several times daily. This helps relieve dryness and promotes comfort, cleansing, and healing. Mix solution (1 tsp table salt, 1 tsp baking soda, and 1 qt warm water), swish in mouth, and expectorate.
    Instruct dentulous patient on fluoride application and daily application of topical fluoride.
    Instruct on rationale/application of daily fluoride application after brushing, flossing, and rinsing.
    Instruct patient not to eat or drink anything for 30 minutes after application.
- Instruct patient to report to physician/nurse/dentist clinical problems early related to:
    Xerostomia
    Loss of taste
    Inability to maintain nutritional intake
    Inability to maintain hydration
    Infection
- Instruct patient on stomatitis/taste loss, nutritional maintenance, and foods to be avoided.
    Consult dietitian.
    Encourage patient to substitute aroma of foods for taste to stimulate appetite; eat frequent smaller meals; avoid extreme temperatures.
    Apply soothing ointments to lips for dryness/cracking.
    Moisten foods with sauces, gravies, creams, and other liquids.
    Eat pureed food.
    Chew sugarless gum.
    Take vitamin B complex if prescribed.
    Restrict all sucrose intake (i.e., candies, cakes, pastries).

Outcome Goals/Rationale

Patient will be able to:

- Demonstrate decreased anxiety and be knowledgeable of planned radiation therapy.
- Effectively communicate feelings, demonstrate ability to do self-care, and seek assistance as necessary.
- State name, type, length of treatment, and description of radiation.
- State reason for radiation therapy, expected outcome, and potential side effects.
- Patient will state expectations of radiation treatment and professionals involved.
- Oral care instructions should be determined by the patient's physician, radiation oncologist, and dentist.
- Patient will state expectations and reasons for all oral care.

- Patients at risk for infection and radiation caries must adhere to a strict oral hygiene program coupled with dental visits. Patients who remain at risk for radiation caries should assume an active role in this prevention.
- Patient will brush teeth at least four times daily, particularly after meals and at bedtime.
- Patient will use Bass technique of brushing, in which toothbrush bristles are adapted to teeth and gingiva at 45-degree angle and vibrated in short back strokes. This method is effective in cleaning gingival sulcus.
- Toothpaste is not necessary to remove plaque from teeth. Fluorinated paste is recommended if used.
- Patient will use dental floss to cleanse the interproximal tooth surfaces inaccessible to toothbrush.
- Edentulous patients with or without prostheses will cleanse soft tissues of oral cavity gently to stimulate circulation.
- Patient will frequently change denture storage container and brush to decrease potential for infection/colonization of bacteria.
- Patient will remove dentures from oral cavity to allow oral tissues to rest.
- Frequent oral irrigations with alkaline lavage will help buffer acidity of oral cavity and promote cleansing lubrication of oral mucosa. Variations or other rinses may be recommended by physician and dentist.
- Patient will state self-care behaviors and will perform application.
- Patient will obtain a fluoride prescription and fluoride carrier tray from dentist.
- Five-minute application daily decreases radiation caries and dental sensitivity.
- Fluoride is available in gel, rinses, and tablets. A 11.23% neutral sodium gel applied in custom carrier is most often used.
- Edentulous patients do not require fluoride application.
- Patient will state expectations and rationale for regular dental visits and early reporting of symptoms.
- Patient will state reason for maintaining nutritional intake and self-care behaviors.

Patient will be able to:

- Maintain weight/hydration.
- State reason for nutritional maintenance.
- State expected outcome and rationale for avoiding:
    All forms of tobacco
    All forms of alcohol, including mouthwashes
    Having teeth pulled after radiation therapy
- Damage to microvilli and outer surface taste cells of tongue and their innervating nerve fibers decreases ability to taste. Taste loss, xerostomia, sore-

ness, dryness, difficulty chewing, swallowing, and sucrose restrictions can result in weight loss and nutrition deficiency.

- Taste acuity will return following therapy. Vitamin B complex therapy is effective for patients who experience angular cheilosis and lingual manifestation related to malnutrition. Angular cheilosis may also be caused by a loss of vertical dimension between mandible and maxilla.
- Sucrose intake for dentulous patients has little nutritional value and promotes radiation caries.

Potential Collaborative/Clinical Problems

- Mucositis
- Xerostomia
- Radiation caries
- Soft tissue necrosis and osteoradionecrosis

During course of radiation therapy and at follow-up visits:

Interventions: *Mucositis*

- Monitor signs and symptoms of mucositis:
    Oral pain
    Burning
    Discomfort
    Difficulty chewing/swallowing/speaking
    Sensitivity to temperature extremes/highly seasoned foods
    Unable to tolerate wearing dentures

Outcome Goal/Rationale

Mucosal erythema is usually expected within 2 to 3 weeks after initiation of treatment. Radiation destroys basal cell layer, thereby thinning mucosa. Ulcerations can occur spontaneously or as a result of trauma from brushing, dentures, food, or teeth. Swallowing can become difficult if pharyngeal mucosa is involved.

Medical Interventions

- Have patient take systemic analgesic as prescribed.
- Apply viscous lidocaine to produce topical anesthesia. NOTE: Viscous lidocaine application may adversely affect patient's taste sensation. Patients may be unable to detect temperature extremes and inadvertently bite themselves.

Nursing Interventions

- Maintain patient comfort:
    Use moist gauze, toothette, or water rinse to cleanse teeth and mouth if toothbrush causes discomfort.
    Temporarily suspend fluoride application if discomfort occurs.

Avoid alcohol or mouthwashes containing alcohol (alcohol dries and irritates mucous membranes).
Suggest methods to assist patient with cessation of alcohol and tobacco consumption.
Avoid coarse, spicy, acidic foods and extreme temperatures. Consult with dietitian.
Maintain soft bland or liquid diet.
Remove dentures or prosthesis that rests within radiation field (exception: mealtime, if tolerated).

Interventions: *Xerostomia*

- Monitor signs and symptoms of xerostomia:
    Dry mouth
    Burning sensation
    Difficulty swallowing
    Difficulty speaking
    Decreased ability to tolerate wearing a prosthetic appliance

Outcome Goals/Rationale

Radiation to the major and minor salivary glands results in a significant decrease in salivary secretions and changes in pH, viscosity, volume, and inorganic constituents of saliva. Alterations in quality and quantity of saliva inhibit saliva to cleanse, lubricate, and buffer the oral cavity, predisposing patient to caries and periodontal disease. Salivary flow decreases, and saliva is thick, viscous, and stringy. Saliva contains microbial compounds important in mechanical removal of pathogens from mouth.

Medical Intervention

- Refer patient to physician/dentist.

Nursing Interventions

- Encourage use of prescribed synthetic salivas to lubricate mouth and buffer oral microflora.
- Carry out frequent oral irrigations as prescribed.
- Have patient drink water and sugar-free beverages throughout day as prescribed.
- Puree foods or use food processor.
- Moisten foods with gravies and sauces.
- Have patient use humidifier at home.
- Encourage use of sugarless gum and candy and ice chips.
- Have dentist instruct on wearing dentures.

Interventions: *Radiation Caries*

- Monitor signs and symptoms of radiation caries:
    Tooth sensitivity
    Pain
    Destruction of teeth

Outcome Goals/Rationale

Xerostomia and associated changes in salivary flow related to radiation can create environment for a highly acidic and cariogenic oral microflora. Total output of salivary production results in reduction of caries-protective electrolytes and immunoproteins. Reduced consumption of high-detergent foods (coarse, roughage) that cleanse teeth also contributes to caries formation. Carious lesions can occur up to 3 months after radiation therapy, appear on the cervical margin of teeth, and progress to complete destruction of the crown. Patients are at risk for caries for their entire lives.

Medical Intervention

- Refer patient to physician/dentist:
  Maintenance of oral hygiene program
  Frequent alkaline lavage
  Restriction of sucrose intake

Nursing Intervention

- Reinforce all prescriptions.

Interventions: Tissue Necrosis

- Monitor signs and symptoms of tissue necrosis and osteoradionecrosis:
  Throbbing pain
  Bleeding
  Suppuration
  Fetid odor in breath
  Difficulty eating

Outcome Goal/Rationale

Soft-tissue necrosis is the progressive enlarging of mucosal ulcers that become necrotic and may develop in radiated soft tissue as a result of radiation-induced fibrosis and impaired blood supply. Osteoradionecrosis is a progressive condition as a result of radiation on the osteocytes, regional blood supply, and bone marrow. Bony exposure, infection, and necrosis can occur, resulting in bone sequestration and fracture. Osteoradionecrosis is common in the mandible, usually results from trauma, and usually occurs within a year of treatment. This process can progress to pathologic fracture, infection of surrounding soft tissues, and oral-cutaneous fistula formation.

Interventions: Infection

- Monitor signs and symptoms of infection:

Complaints of pain, burning, tenderness
Bleeding (gingiva)
Tooth mobility
Elevated temperature

Outcome Goal/Rationale

Infection can occur during or after radiation. Oral infections are most common (e.g., candidiasis [thrush], periodontal disease [pyorrhea]). Periodontal disease is manifested by hyperemic and edematous gingiva.

Medical Interventions

- Use topical nystatin mouth rinses daily.
- Ensure frequent physician/dental visits.
- Administer antibiotics if indicated.

Nursing Interventions

- Maintain meticulous oral hygiene.
- Carry out oral irrigations.
- Provide for consistent monitoring of oral cavity.
- Monitor vital signs, specifically temperature.

Interventions: Trismus

- Monitor signs and symptoms of trismus:
  Impaired ability to open mouth widely
  Impaired ability to chew
  Impaired ability to speak

Outcome Goal/Rationale

Muscles of mastication undergo fibrosis related to radiation. This may indicate disease recurrence and occurs 3 to 6 months after completion of therapy. Fibrosis of the muscles of mastication and temporomandibular joint, although uncommon, may result in trismus.

Medical Intervention

- Use prosthetic appliances and elastics prepared by dentist/prosthodontist.

Nursing Interventions

- Refer patient to physician/dentist.
- Instruct patient to exercise masticatory muscles before, during, and after treatment: opening and closing mouth 20 times in row three times a day.
- Maintain meticulous oral hygiene.

and persist to a degree that radiation treatments may be temporarily discontinued.

Pain. Pain related to oral mucositis, if not managed properly, can have a profound negative effect on hydration, nutrition, and sleep. Pain or discomfort related to

mucositis should not automatically limit the patient from maintaining adequate hydration and nutrition or from practicing oral hygiene procedures. Adequate pain control can be achieved by prescribing topical anesthetics alone or in conjunction with nonnarcotic and narcotic analgesics. In addition, an early nursing consultation with a dietitian is one of the simplest ways to circumvent complications. The dietitian can make recommendations for alternative food preparation and supplements.

Infection. Oral mucositis with ulcerations puts the patient at risk for developing oral infections.[40, 146] Oral infections seen in patients undergoing radiation may be bacterial, fungal, or viral in origin. One of the most common acute infections seen in patients is *candidiasis,* or *moniliasis,* resulting from radiation-induced changes of the normal oral flora. The nurse should monitor the patient for the classic white patches that scrape off, leaving burning tissue.

For *fungal infections,* the physician may prescribe topical and systemic antifungal agents. Antifungal agents are usually mixed with sucrose to make the drug more palatable. To prevent caries formation, a non–sucrose-containing, antifungal agent should be used. A patient who wears a dental prosthesis or uses fluoride carrier trays must be instructed that these are to be removed from the oral cavity and immersed in an antifungal agent for 8 hours to avoid reintroduction of fungal organisms into the oral cavity. Toothbrushes and denture-soaking containers should be changed frequently.

The nurse performs a weekly routine oral examination to detect new lesions early in their development, noting carefully size, shape, location, and appearance. Cultures or smears of new lesions may be ordered by the physician to document and facilitate treatment of any superimposed infection.

Palliative treatment of mucositis related to radiation includes oral rinses and application of topical anesthetics. Sodium bicarbonate oral rinse (1 tsp baking soda in 32 oz water or normal saline) should be used at least six times a day. Topical anesthetics can be used, progressing from the least potent and toxic to the more potent and toxic.

Dermatitis. Dermatitis, an acute condition characterized by a sunburned appearance, results from radiation inhibiting mitosis of epithelial cells. The patient may experience significant pain or discomfort and become reluctant to perform any self-care. Treatment of this condition is discussed in detail in Chapter 31.

Xerostomia. Xerostomia (dry mouth) occurs when radiation therapy causes sclerosis of the acini of the salivary gland. Saliva regulates the pH in the oral cavity, which controls bacterial flora, and lubricates and cleanses the teeth. When the amount of saliva and consistency (thick) are changed, generalized oral disease can occur, creating an environment conducive to caries formation. The oral pH becomes more acidic when salivary flow decreases and allows a major caries-forming organism, *Streptococcus,* to grow. Salivary flow can be accurately measured before and after radiation therapy by having the patient undergo *sialometric testing.* This allows the clinician to measure the patient's ability to produce saliva when stimulated, either by total stimulation or stimulation of paired major salivary glands.

Radiation therapy also affects taste bud function. Alteration in taste (*dysgeusia*) and decreased taste (*hypogeusesthesia*) can occur. The degree of taste alteration and impairment depends on the site and dose of radiation. Taste sensations are decreased because food must be in solution to be tasted. Taste buds, as with other normal cells, will regenerate after completion of radiation if adequate nutrition is maintained. Most patients experience a degree of return of function within 4 to 12 months, but some patients may have permanent taste alterations. Most patients undergoing radiation therapy state that the taste sensation of sweetness lasts the longest. This is related to the fact that normally more taste buds are devoted to the detection of sweet tastes than sour or salty tastes. The nurse must remember that with this alteration in taste sensation, the patient may naturally increase sugar intake to obtain the same level of sweetness. Alternative sources for sugar should be identified to prevent radiation caries.

Palliation of xerostomia, hypogeusia, and impaired swallowing can be achieved by adequate hydration of the oral cavity with nonsucrose liquids. Most salivary substitutes consist of sodium carboxymethyl cellulose combined with fluoride and other agents. In 1992, a multi-institution, randomized, double-blind study demonstrated that pilocarpine has a direct treatment benefit for hyposalivation in patients after radiation therapy. Pilocarpine is a cholinergic, parasympathomimetic agent that acts as an agonist on the muscarinic receptors. When given orally, it stimulates salivary flow.*

If the patient prefers not to carry a thermos of water or some other liquid to sip on frequently, several artificial saliva products are commercially available, such as Moi-Stir (Kingswood Laboratory, Carmel, IN), Orex (Young Dental, Maryland Heights, MD), Sahvart (Westport Pharmaceuticals, Westport, CT), and Xerolube (Scherer Laboratories, Dallas, TX). In addition, the patient should be instructed to moisten the lips with lanolin or cocoa butter. Rinses or creams containing synthetic steroids (e.g., Kenalog) should be avoided because they have the potential to facilitate fungal growth in preexisting conditions conducive to fungus. Patients may stimulate unaffected salivary glands by sucking or chewing on sucrose-free sour candies or gum. A dietary consultation will aid the patient in learning additional food preparation techniques to facilitate chewing and swallowing (e.g., addition of sauces and gravies to dry foods, stimulation of taste sensations by the aroma of warm foods).[12, 29, 32, 50, 108]

---

* References 21, 29, 89, 108, 127, 143, 166.

Radiation Caries. Radiation caries can result from radiation-induced xerostomia, poor oral hygiene, and high sucrose intake. These lesions form within 2 to 3 months compared with several months in the normal patient. Classically, radiation caries occur in areas of the tooth that are normally self-cleaning, such as the incisional edges of the anterior teeth, near the gum line, and the cuspids. The preventive treatment regimen for radiation caries should include five key segments: pretreatment evaluation, periodontal care, oral hygiene instructions, daily fluoride application, and limited sucrose intake.[61, 108] Once radiation caries form, teeth are at a high risk for fractures, and actual extractions are not recommended.

Osteoradionecrosis. Osteoradionecrosis (infection into the bone) is by far the most devastating of all the chronic sequelae of radiation to the head and neck. Despite improved technology of shielding and treatment delivery, patients remain at risk for this long-term side effect.[10, 20, 53, 166]

Radiation causes hypoxic, hypocellular hypovascularization, resulting in tissue breakdown, cellular breakdown, cellular death, and collagen lysis that exceeds synthesis. Rather than a primary infection of irradiated bone, this has been described as a complex metabolic and tissue hemostatic deficiency created by radiation-induced cellular injury and replication. This injury weakens the bone and tissue, decreasing the ability to respond to injury, and produces favorable conditions for trauma and infection to occur. The mandible, with its single-source blood supply, has a higher incidence of osteoradionecrosis than the maxilla, which has a broad-based blood supply.[20, 53, 113]

Monitoring the patient for osteoradionecrosis is extremely important. Nurses play a significant role in prevention of this phenomenon. Patient education, postradiation follow-up appointments, and the importance of regular examinations should be presented as *essential* and *nonoptional*. At these visits the nurse should perform a thorough oral examination, documenting the presence or absence of chronic oral ulcerations, defective teeth, caries, defective restorations, or poorly fitting dentures. If any of these are identified, the patient should be immediately referred to the dentist for an examination. Follow-up visits should include concurrent medical and dental evaluations. Although prevention is the best approach to managing this potential clinical problem, local irrigations, high-dose extended antibiotics, and surgical procedures to remove dead bone tissue may be indicated.

Trismus. Patients who receive radiation that directly affects the muscles of mastication or the temporomandibular joint (TMJ) may develop trismus. Trismus may occur during therapy or may become problematic up until 6 months after completion of radiotherapy. Patient education about mouth-opening exercises is extremely important. A simple exercise of opening the mouth as widely as possible 20 times, three to four times a day, should minimize muscle fibrosis and loss of mobility. If trismus is noted, the degree of opening must be recorded and monitored at the patient's regular follow-up appointments. The dentist or maxillofacial prosthodontist may prescribe special appliances similar to those prescribed by an orthodontist, such as wedges, or appliances with screws, springs, or elastic for the patient to wear. Most physicians use all possible conservative measures to treat this side effect, leaving surgical interventions as a last approach. Any surgical procedure on devitalized tissue and bone may result in poor healing and infection.

Chronic Side Effects. Chronic side effects of radiation include anorexia, dysgeusia, and generalized lethargy.[21] Ideally, every patient undergoing radiation for head and neck cancer should be seen by a nurse and registered dietitian before, during, and after radiation. Nutritional evaluation and support should be provided for at least 6 months after completion of radiation. Weight loss or potential for weight loss should be anticipated during radiation therapy. Weight loss will continue after radiation, being maximal at 3 months and remaining virtually unchanged for 6 months after treatment.[16, 19, 24, 32, 59]

Health care education for patients undergoing radiation therapy should include the following:

Importance of returning for all appointments
Maintaining individualized oral hygiene program—brushing, flossing, fluoride, and ongoing dental assessment
Nutrition, weight maintenance, and monitoring weight gain
Maintaining or returning to normal life-styles, work, recreation, family, and social life

A comprehensive nursing care plan and guidelines for monitoring for potential collaborative and clinical problems are given in the Nursing Management feature on radiation therapy.

Chemotherapy

The role of chemotherapy in the treatment of head and neck cancer has changed since more single active agents and combinations have been discovered.[6, 7, 28, 137] In the past, systemic chemotherapy was used as a palliative treatment or for patients who had persistent, recurrent disease or disseminated metastases after standard therapy (surgery/radiation).[2, 28, 51, 53, 61, 137] A brief discussion of agents under evaluation for the treatment of head and neck cancers is included in this chapter. Individual agents, classification, metabolism, toxicity, and indications are discussed in Chapter 23.

Medical oncologists are using chemotherapy in conjunction with standard therapy, surgery, and radiation. Clinical trials designed to answer questions related to efficacy, timing, and sequencing of treatment are ongoing in national cooperative and intergroup studies.* Chemotherapy sequencing and timing may be given in four ways and are listed in Box 12–2.

These sequences and combinations seek to answer the following questions related to treating head and neck cancer:

What is the best combination to use?
When should chemotherapy be included in the treatment plan?
When and in what sequence should chemotherapy be used (e.g., preoperatively, before radiation, or in conjunction with radiation)?
Is there a benefit of using chemotherapy as part of multimodality therapy?
Does giving chemotherapy first delay or lessen the need for extensive radiation or surgery?
Does chemotherapy have an effect on disease-free survival, overall survival, and quality of life?
What is the incidence of chronic or delayed side effects?
Does chemotherapy cause a change in patterns of recurrence?

The physician monitors the patient's response to chemotherapy by clinical and physical examination, by x-ray films, and by validating absence of tumor by having the surgeon obtain multiple biopsies. Nurses are responsible for educating and monitoring the patient for clinical problems related to the chemotherapy, such as adjustment to illness, knowledge deficits, potential for effective individual/family coping, altered comforts, and potential for infection.

Chemotherapeutic drugs that have demonstrated significant activity in head and neck cancer include doxorubicin, methotrexate, bleomycin, cyclosphophamide, cisplatin, carboplatin, and 5-fluorouracil (5-FU, vinblastine and vincristine). These first-line agents are currently being used singly or in combinations for the treatment of head and neck cancer. If the patient fails to respond clinically, the physician may prescribe second-line therapies such as paclitaxel and gemcitabine; paclitaxel with cisplatin and 5-FU; paclitaxel with ifosfamide, docetaxel-based therapy.[21, 90, 142] Other new chemotherapeutics are the topoisomerase I inhibitor, topotecan, and the topoisomerase II inhibitor amonafide.[62] Studies are also being performed with oral chemotherapeutics, including teglafur/uracil with IV cisplatinum or carboplatinum, eniluracil with IV 5-FU, and hydroxyurea in combination with radiation therapy and IV 5-FU.[21, 23] Investigations are ongoing with cytoprotective agents such as amifostine (WR-2721), leucovorin, and MESNA.[5–8, 62, 84] Regional and interarterial chemotherapy is also under study. Organ preservation has been a phenomenal outcome of combined therapy with radiation and chemotherapy, but in general, chemotherapy has produced little or no difference in survivorship.[62] The new chemotherapeutics have shown no significant improvement in response, except possibly the taxanes.[62] Consequently, there is increasing interest in trials with biological therapies and gene therapy.[62] Other trials with head and neck therapy involve the administration of retinoids, carotenoids, and vitamin E as chemoprevention therapy.[118]

The nurse and patient need to monitor for transient, acute, subacute, and chronic side effects related to these agents. One of the most important aspects of nursing care is educating and reinforcing to the patient the importance of maintaining scheduled appointments. Response to therapy and early detection of toxicities or new lesions can be determined only if the patient keeps the appointment. Patients may be tempted to delay or skip a treatment until they "get stronger," "feel better," "gain weight," or "conduct personal business." Early detection of side effects related to chemotherapy can facilitate patient comfort and safety. Documentation of toxicities and side effects is critical because subsequent therapies are determined and calculated by the patient's tolerance to treatment.

Pretreatment Assessment. The general clinical status of the head and neck cancer patient is one of the best predictors of the patient's ability to tolerate chemotherapy, respond well to it, and survive. A pretreatment assessment of the patient's clinical status must be thoroughly evaluated and should include age; nutritional status; disease staging (TNM); documentation of other disease processes (e.g., cardiac, pulmonary, tuberculosis); function and reserve of lung, liver, kidney, bone marrow; and prior therapies (e.g., chemotherapy, radia-

---

BOX 12–2

Chemotherapy Sequencing and Timing

Induction chemotherapy: used before standard treatment; also called neoadjuvant, prostandard, or prestandard therapy
Concurrent chemotherapy: used as total treatment or postoperatively in patients with resectable tumors
Sandwich chemotherapy: used after surgery or before radiotherapy
Maintenance chemotherapy: used after standard therapies

---

* References 4–8, 21, 28, 39, 51, 52, 81, 82, 86, 137.

tion, surgery). The treatment of squamous cell carcinoma of the head and neck has reached the stage where chemotherapy may be potentially curative. Successful development of chemotherapeutic regimens that are curative for patients with advanced stages of disease hold the potential for effectively treating many with earlier stage disease.

Use of MRI, positron emission tomography (PET), and flow cytometry holds the potential to identify head and neck tumors or cellular characteristics that may direct the course of therapy. The use of flow cytometry to detect and measure tumor parameters has doubled over the past four decades. This technique involves passing a beam of light through a head and neck cancer cell. In theory, any part of the cell that can be caused to fluoresce by interruption of a beam of light when it passes through all the DNA/RNA structures can be measured and studied. These techniques have proved efficacious in hematologic malignancies and may be able to identify tumor characteristics that could predict how head and neck tumors would respond to chemotherapy, radiotherapy, or surgery.[41, 42, 117]

The patient's overall performance status is consistently associated with prognostic outcome, including determining the response to systemic chemotherapy and survival. The better the patient's performance status, the greater the patient's ability to tolerate therapy and the greater the likelihood that she will respond and survive longer.

Al-Sarraf and coworkers[4] identified and reported two groups of prognostic factors that play an important role in determining the overall survival of the patient with recurrent or systemic disease (Box 12-3).

As many as 30% of patients who are unwilling to alter their life-styles, particularly those who continue to smoke and drink, experience the occurrence of second cancers.

A complete nursing biopsychosocial evaluation should be included in the pretreatment evaluation. Emphasis should be placed on determining the patient's level of education, educational needs, literacy, and ability to learn and comprehend. Toxic effects related to chemotherapy could be life-threatening in patients who are unable to understand and monitor for these side effects.

BOX 12-3

Prognostic Factors in Recurrent and Systemic Head and Neck Cancer

Good Prognostic Factors

Good performance status
Minimal disease
Local recurrence only
No bony erosion
Good response to induction (adjuvant) chemotherapy
Good response to previous chemotherapy
Long disease-free interval
First-line chemotherapy
Good organ function
Complete response to chemotherapy

Poor Prognostic Factors

Poor performance status
Bulky disease
Systemic/visceral disease
Bone metastasis and/or hypercalcemia (and local bone invasion)
Lymphangitis spread (skin)
Failure of radiotherapy (persistent disease)
Failure of induction (adjuvant) chemotherapy
Patients receiving first-line chemotherapy for recurrent and/or systemic cancer
Organ impairment
Less than complete response to chemotherapy

Modified from Al-Sarraf M: Head and neck cancer: chemotherapy concepts, *Semin Oncol* 15(1):70, 1988.

REHABILITATION

As treatment protocols increase, more patients are being diagnosed with secondary primary lesions or distant metastasis. The patient who has been treated for head and neck cancer is at significant risk for recurrent disease at the primary site or the neck.[21, 119, 137] The patient should also be monitored for a metachronous primary in the head and neck area, lung, or esophagus. Ongoing assessment and evaluation of response to treatment are essential for early diagnosis of disease and validation of health. Routine follow-up of patients should include a thorough examination of the head and neck with indirect laryngoscopy: once a month for the first year, every 2 months during the second year, and every 3 months the third year, every 6 months the fourth and fifth year, and every 6 months to 1 year after treatment. Patients with new symptoms of significant weight loss, dysphagia, chronic soreness, or persistent hoarseness should have an endoscopic examination with biopsy when tumor is not visible by examination. Nurses share the responsibility to educate patients and reinforce the importance of maintaining scheduled appointments. Careful and meticulous follow-up is a significant link to long-term survival in this patient group. Nurses should emphasize the importance of maintaining a healthy life-style. The patient should be educated on the importance of cessation of alcohol and tobacco, notifying physician of early symptoms, and keeping appointments.

RECURRENT DISEASE

Treatment options of recurrent disease are limited. The clinical management and treatment of recurrent disease depend on accurate specific site and staging of the disease. Recurrent head and neck cancer is, by definition, a failure to the standard definitive local therapy. Approximately 40% of these patients will have recurrence overall, 20% locoregionally, 10% with distant metastasis, and another 10% with both local and distant disease. Many of these patients relapse within 6 to 24 months after treatment and have a median survival of 6 months from initial diagnosis to recurrence. In the past, re-irradiation of recurrent tumors in the head and neck was performed with extreme caution. In select patient populations, re-irradiation has been combined with surgery or chemotherapy in attempts to control the disease.[8, 122] Managing the psychosocial consequences of cancer recurrence provides nursing with a unique opportunity to implement interventions that can fulfill the emotional and spiritual needs of both patient and family.[29, 95, 146]

In addition to recurrent disease, the physician is often challenged with other common clinical problems, which may significantly limit treatment options. The physician must identify the treatment regimen that holds the highest therapeutic value and lowest risk/benefit ratio.[160] Diseases related to life-styles, chronic obstructive pulmonary disease, and liver or renal disease substantially affect the physician's ability to deliver adequate therapeutic doses of chemotherapy such as cisplatin, bleomycin, or methotrexate. Age-related diseases, such as underlying cardiac problems, hypertension, and diabetes, can limit tolerance to chemotherapy.

Common tumor-related factors can affect the timing and choice of such treatment as 5-FU and cisplatin. Malnutrition secondary to tumor or alcohol use can have a major negative influence on treatment. Meningeal carcinomatoses and cranial nerve involvement may occur when the patient's tumor involves the base of the skull. These patients may require lumbar punctures and placement of an Ommaya reservoir for intrathecal instillation of methotrexate. Hypercalcemia related to bone or tumor involvement will require aggressive hydration and furosemide treatment before chemotherapy can be administered. Infection related to local wound cellulitis or recurring aspiration pneumonia may result in sepsis, requiring antibiotic therapy and delaying the administration of chemotherapy. In addition, bleeding from the carotid or small vessels can produce a significant obstacle. Chemotherapies that cause nausea and vomiting can precipitate bleeding. Many patients may require surgical intervention for fulguration, or occasional embolization of the artery to control bleeding.[69]

Choice of treatment for recurrent head and neck cancer is also significantly influenced by the patient's

COMPLICATIONS

Head and Neck Cancer Treatment

Surgery

Potential for structural, functional, or cosmetic loss, such as changes in body appearance and function (breathing, speaking, swallowing, coughing, mobility)
Respiratory distress; hypoxia, airway obstruction, tracheal edema, aspiration; hemorrhage; hematoma; arterial rupture; failure of flap survival; nerve damage

Radiation Therapy

Mucositis	Xerostomia
Pain	Radiation caries
Infection	Osteoradionecrosis
Dermatitis	Fungal infections
Trismus	Dysgeusia

Chemotherapy

Mucositis	Dehydration
Infection	Electrolyte imbalance
Immunosuppression	Nausea and vomiting
Weight loss	Diarrhea

General Considerations

Patients with head and neck cancers receiving multi-modality therapy may experience severe and permanent facial disfigurement and functional loss that resembles what is experienced by the burn patient.

PATIENT TEACHING PRIORITIES

Head and Neck Cancers

Rationale for pretreatment evaluation:

Psychosocial assessment—potential changes in body image (structural, functional, and cosmetic changes)
Cardiopulmonary assessment and health history
Nutritional assessment; communication/cognitive motor skills; dental assessment

Rationale for treatment:

Surgery: review purpose, rationale, and potential sequelae; explain common terms and procedures; discuss preoperative and postoperative nursing interventions.
Radiation therapy: review purpose, rationale, and potential side effects of the therapy; explain the procedures, purpose of positioning the body, and scheduling of the radiation therapy treatments.
Chemotherapy: review purpose, rationale, and potential side effects of the therapy; discuss chemotherapy treatment schedule and need for weekly blood tests to monitor the side effects of drugs.
Rehabilitation: initiate referrals to social worker, speech pathologist, physical therapist, occupational therapist, clinical dietitian, and nurse specialist.

GERIATRIC CONSIDERATIONS

Head and Neck Cancers

Age-related losses such as vision, hearing, communication, fine motor skills (writing), and swallowing/eating functions will be further compromised by effects of surgery/radiation therapy and/or chemotherapy.

Nutritional and dental assessment with appropriate interventions will need to be adapted to age-related changes (diet history—likes/dislikes; dentures and/or lack of because of age or finances).

Pretreatment evaluation: psychosocial, cardiopulmonary, and health history factors will require age-related adjustments and appropriate interventions.

Treatment-related factors: surgery, radiation therapy, chemotherapy, and rehabilitation will require age-related adjustments and appropriate interventions. Patients with chronic diseases such as hypertension, cardiopulmonary insufficiency, diabetes, chronic obstructive pulmonary disease, arthritis, and chronic renal disease will require medical treatment adjustments.

Surgery: potential exists for longer recovery and rehabilitation period.

Radiation therapy: treatment schedule may require adjustment for recovery of side effects; fatigue/immunosuppression, weight loss, stomatitis, and infection.

Chemotherapy: drug dosage, frequency of infusion, and monitoring of blood count will require adjustment (drug toxicities may increase related to previously mentioned chronic diseases). Transportation, financial and family resources, and home care responsibilities will require assessment and intervention based on the deficits and/or availability.

---

previous exposure to radiotherapy or chemotherapy and ability to tolerate further bone marrow suppressive treatments.[84, 86]

The complications, patient teaching priorities, and geriatric considerations for these patients are presented in the respective boxes.

CONCLUSION

Cancers of the head and neck are estimated to be the most prevalent cancers in the world.[33] Whereas the physician's goals are improving treatment and patient survival, the nurse is challenged with assisting the patient to adjustments related to the disease, treatment, and rehabilitation. The most important nursing challenge, however, is in the areas of early detection, prevention, patient education, and quality of life.[30, 31, 48, 64, 80] The incidence of head and neck cancers will never significantly decrease until patient use of the most common cocarcinogen (tobacco) ceases. Herein lies a challenge to all health care professionals.

Nursing Management

Individualized nursing care plans addressing lack of knowledge related to chemotherapy and monitoring for potential side effects related to chemotherapy should be established. Family or significant others should always be incorporated into the teaching and care plan because they can assist in monitoring the patient's response to treatment and adjustment to illness.

Routine home care nursing referral for patients receiving chemotherapy is recommended after the initial treatment and for those persons who continue to demonstrate knowledge deficits related to chemotherapy. The home care nurses can monitor for side effects of chemotherapy, reinforce patient teaching, validate the patient's ability to perform self-care, and monitor for adequate hydration and nutrition.

DENTAL EVALUATION

The goal of dental therapy for patients undergoing chemotherapy is the same as with radiation therapy and surgery: to reduce potential infections and morbidity and avoid unnecessary delays of chemotherapeutic treatments. Chemotherapeutic agents such as 5-FU, methotrexate, or bleomycin, alone or in combination with radiation therapy, affect tissues with high turnover rates, such as the oral mucosa. Mucosal tissues, in general, are subject to chronic physical trauma and infection. As discussed previously, when the patient experiences decreased host resistance, changes in normal bacteria—viral and fungal flora—have the potential to become pathogens and infect the patient.

Once chemotherapy has been initiated, the focus of dental therapy should be directed at maintaining oral hygiene and decreasing the potential for infection. Guidelines for oral hygiene and dental care are similar to those for the patient undergoing radiotherapy.

NUTRITIONAL ASSESSMENT

Common nutritional problems experienced by these patients relate not only to the treatment modality, but also to altered physiologic function related to tumor involvement. A pretreatment nursing nutritional assessment is important to identify any anticipated problems related to the patient's ability to maintain weight and hydration. The nutritional assessment should include a careful dietary history (including previous alcohol exposure) and daily intake, weight loss, and patient completion of a 3-day dietary recall. These data enable the health care professional and patient to develop a reasonable pretreatment nutritional plan. The nutritional plan ideally should be implemented before initiation of chemotherapy and monitored closely throughout the entire course of treatment. Having the patient complete the 3-day recall provides the nurse and clinical dietitian with an excellent tool for patient education. Patient education booklets such as *Eating Hints* and other dietary materials are available free from the National Institutes of Health and American Cancer Society.

Fluctuations of 2 to 3 lb between monthly visits is acceptable, but any rapid weight loss unrelated to infection or chemotherapy side effects may require the physician to place the patient on short-term or long-term enteral or parenteral nutrition. Patients with head and neck cancer undergoing combinations of chemotherapy that incorporate platinum or platinum derivatives should be monitored for signs and symptoms of dehydration and fluid and electrolyte imbalances. These agents are extremely nephrotoxic, and a key nursing intervention to circumvent toxicity is to maintain hydration and have the patient maintain a strict intake and output record. Likewise, patients should be provided with written guidelines for the monitoring of their hydration and should know when to notify the nurse or physician if they are unable to maintain hydration. Patients should be provided information on alternative sources of fluid, such as ice cream, gelatin, popsicles, and milkshakes. Symptom control (e.g., nausea and vomiting) and prescriptive therapies will depend on the chemotherapeutic agent given and the patient's response to treatment.

Chapter Questions

1. Squamous cell carcinoma accounts for what percentage of head and neck cancers?
   a. < 10%
   b. 30%
   c. 60%
   d. > 90%
2. The most common site of head and neck cancer is:
   a. Hypopharynx
   b. Pharynx
   c. Oropharynx
   d. Oral cavity
3. All of the following are risk factors for head and neck cancer *except:*
   a. Alcohol abuse
   b. Tobacco use
   c. Vitamin A supplementation
   d. Virus (EBV)
4. The head and neck area contains approximately 300 lymph nodes, and ___% of total lymph nodes in the body:
   a. 10%
   b. 30%
   c. 50%
   d. 60%
5. Postoperative clinical features that indicate respiratory distress include:
   a. Agitation, air hunger, confusion, diminished or absent air exchange
   b. Agitation, air hunger, fatigue, diminished air exchange
   c. Agitation, air hunger, temperature change, increased air exchange
   d. Agitation, air hunger, pain, increased air exchange
6. Treatment and rehabilitative interdisciplinary pretreatment evaluations include the following assessment(s):
   a. Communication/cognitive motor skills, dental, nutritional, hepatic, and psychosocial
   b. Communication/cognitive motor skills, dental, nutritional, pulmonary, and psychosocial
   c. Communication/cognitive motor skills, dental, nutritional, renal, and psychosocial
   d. Communication/cognitive motor skills, dental, nutritional, endocrine, and psychosocial
7. The most common side effects of radiation therapy treatment for head and neck cancers include:
   a. Mucositis, pain, bleeding, infection

b. Mucositis, pain, bleeding, xerostomia
c. Mucositis, pain, infection, xerostomia
d. Mucositis, pain, bleeding, anorexia

8. Which of the following observations/characteristics might indicate flap failure following a radical neck dissection and reconstructive surgery?
a. Fine wrinkles
b. Warm to the touch
c. Blanching present
d. Shiny appearance

9. Radiation therapy mucositis may be aggravated by:
a. Alkaline lavage
b. Alcohol consumption
c. Saline rinses
d. Soft diet

10. Functional loss associated with a total laryngectomy includes:
a. Loss of voice, normal swallowing
b. Hoarse voice, normal swallowing
c. Loss of voice, increased risk for aspiration
d. Hoarse voice, increased risk for aspiration

BIBLIOGRAPHY

1. Aaronson NK, Beckman J: *The quality of life for cancer patients,* New York, Raven, 1987.
2. Al-Kourainy K and others: Excellent response to cisplatinum based chemotherapy in patients with recurrent or previously untreated advanced nasopharyngeal carcinoma, *Am J Clin Oncol* 11:427, 1988.
3. Allison GR, Rappaport I, Salibian AH: Adaptive mechanisms of speech and swallowing after combined jaw and tongue reconstruction in long-term survivors, *Am Surg* 154:419, 1987.
4. Al-Sarraf M: Head and neck cancer: chemotherapy concepts, *Semin Oncol* 15(1):70, 1988.
5. Al-Sarraf M and others: Current progress in head and neck cancer: The Wayne State Experience. In Jacobs JR and others, editors: *Head and neck cancer: scientific perspectives in management and strategies for cure,* New York, Elsevier, 1987.
6. Al-Sarraf M and others: Concurrent radiotherapy and chemotherapy with cisplatin inoperable squamous cell carcinoma of the head and neck: RTOG study, *Cancer* 54:259, 1987.
7. Al-Sarraf M and others: Combined modality therapy (CMT) in patients with head and neck cancer (HN-CA): timing of chemotherapy (CT). In Salton JT, editor: *Radiation Therapy Oncology Group (RTOG) 6 study: adjunct therapy of cancer,* Philadelphia, Saunders, 1990.
8. Al-Sarraf M and others: Chemoradiotherapy versus radiotherapy in patients with advanced nasopharyngeal cancer: Phase III Randomized Intergroup Study 0099. *J Clin Oncol* 16:1310, 1998.
9. American Cancer Society: *Cancer facts and figures—2000,* Atlanta, The Society, 1996.
10. Amour RJ and others: Postoperative irradiation for squamous cell carcinoma of the head and neck: an analysis of treatment results and complications, *Int J Radiat Oncol Biol Phys* 16:25, 1989.
11. Anderson BL: Sexual functioning morbidity among cancer survivors, *Cancer* 55(7):1835, 1985.
12. Anderson L, Ward D: Nutrition. In Otto SE, editor: *Oncology nursing,* ed 3, St Louis, Mosby, 1997.
13. Baker SR, editor: *Microsurgical reconstruction of the head and neck,* New York, Churchill Livingstone, 1989.
14. Barsevick AM, Much J, Sweeney C: Psychosocial response to cancer. In Groenwald SL and others, editors: *Cancer nursing principles and practices,* ed 4, Boston, Jones and Bartlett, 1997.
15. Barstch H and others: Gene polymorphism of CYP genes, alone or in combination as a risk modifier of tobacco-related cancers, *Cancer Epidemiol Biomarkers Prevent Am* 9:3, 2000.
16. Basset MR, Dobie RA: Patterns of nutritional deficiency in head and neck cancer, *Otolaryngol Head Neck Surg* 91:119, 1983.
17. Belcher AE: Nursing aspects of quality of life enhancement in cancer patients, *Oncology* 4(5):197, 1990.
18. Berendt, MC: Alterations in nutrition. In Itano JK, Taoko KN, editors: *Core curriculum for oncology nursing practice,* ed 3, Philadelphia, Saunders, 1998.
19. Beumer J, Curtis TA, Morrish RB: Radiation complications in edentulous patients, *J Prosthet Dent* 36:193, 1976.
20. Beumer J and others: Osteonecrosis: predisposing factors and outcomes of therapy, *Head Neck Surg* 6:819, 1984.
21. Bildstein CY, Blendowski CB: Head and neck malignancies. In Groenwald SL and others, editors: *Cancer nursing: principles and practices,* ed 3, Boston, Jones and Bartlett, 1997.
22. Brachman DG: Molecular biology of head and neck cancer, *Semin Oncol* 21:320, 1994.
23. Brockstein BE, Vokes EE: Oral chemotherapy in head and neck cancer, *Drugs* 1999, 58(Suppl.):91, 1999.
24. Brookes GBH: Nutritional status: a prognostic indicator in head and neck cancer, *Otolaryngol Head Neck Surg.* 93:69, 1985.
25. Brown M: Wound healing. In Cummings CW and others, editors: *Otolaryngology–head and neck surgery,* ed 3, St. Louis, Mosby, 1998.
26. Buchbinder D and others: Functional mandibular reconstruction of patients with oral cancer, *Oral Surg Oral Med Pathol* 68(4):499, 1989.
27. Caplan GA, Brigham BA: Marijuana smoking and carcinoma of the tongue: is there an association? *Cancer* 6:1005, 1990.
28. Carew JF, Shah JP: Advances in multimodality therapy for laryngeal cancers, *CA-A Cancer J Clin* 48:211, 1998.
29. Carper E, McGuire M, Boland N: Head and neck cancer nursing. In Harrison LB, Sessions RB, Hong WK, editors: *Head and neck nursing: a multidisciplinary approach,* Philadelphia, Lippincott-Raven, 1999.
30. Cassileth BR and others: The satisfaction and psychosocial status of patients during treatment of cancer, *J Psychosoc Oncol* 7(4):47, 1989.
31. Cella DF: Quality of life as an outcome of cancer treatment. In Groenwald SL and others, editors: *Cancer nurs-*

ing: principles and practices, ed 4, Boston, Jones and Bartlett, 1997.

32. Chencharick JD, Mossman KL: Nutritional consequences of radiotherapy of the head and neck cancer, *Cancer* 51:811, 1983.

33. Clayman GL, Lippman SM, Laramore GE, Hong WK: Head and neck cancer. In Holland JF and others, editors: *Cancer Medicine,* ed 4, Baltimore, Williams & Wilkins, 1997.

34. Collins SL and others: Head and neck. In Abeloff MD and others, editors: *Clinical oncology,* New York, Churchill Livingston, 1995.

35. Conti J: Cancer rehabilitation: why can't we get out of first gear? *J Rehabil* 56(4):19, 1990.

36. Cook TA and others: Cervical rotation flaps for midface resurfacing, *Arch Otolaryngol Head Neck Surg* 117:77, 1991.

37. Cooper JS and others: Second malignancies in patients who have head and neck cancers: incidence, effect on survival and implications for chemoprevention based on the RTOG experience, *Int J Radiat Oncol Biol Phys* 17:449, 1989.

38. Cordeiro PG: General principles of reconstructive therapy for head and neck cancer. In Harrison LB, Sessions RB, Hong WK, editors: *Head and neck cancer: a multidisciplinary approach,* Philadelphia, Lippincott-Raven, 1999.

39. Corry J and others: Radiation with concurrent late chemotherapy intensification ('chemo boost') for locally advanced head and neck cancer, *Radiother Oncol J Eur SocTher Radiol Oncol* 54:123, 2000.

40. Crane L: Infections in patients with head and neck cancer. In Jacobs JR and others, editors: *Head and neck cancer: scientific perspectives in management and strategies for cure,* New York, Elsevier, 1987.

41. Crissman JD: Prognostic value of histopathologic parameters in squamous cell carcinoma of the oropharynx, *Cancer* 54:2995, 1984.

42. Crissman JD and others: Histopathologic diagnosis of early cancer, *Head Neck Cancer* 1:134, 1985.

43. Cummings CW, Frederickson JM, Harker LA, Krause CJ, Schuller DE, Richardson MA, editors: *Otolaryngology—head and neck surgery,* ed 3, St. Louis, Mosby, 1999.

44. David DJ and others: Mandibular reconstruction with vascularized crest: a 10 year experience, *Plast Reconstr Surg* 82:792, 1988.

45. Demirkan F and others: Oromandibular reconstruction using a third free flap in sequence in recurrent carcinoma, *Br J Plast Surg* 52:429, 1999.

46. Depalo LG, Minah GE: Isolation of pathogenic microorganisms for dentures and denture soaking containers of the myelosuppressed cancer patients, *J Prosthet Dent* 49:20, 1983.

47. DeSanto L, Beahrs OH: The modified and radical neck dissection for squamous cell carcinoma of the upper aerodigestive system. In Jacobs JR and others, editors: *Head and neck cancer: scientific and clinical perspectives in management and strategies for cure,* New York, Elsevier, 1987.

48. Dudas S, Carlson CE: Cancer rehabilitation, *Oncol Nurs Forum* 15:183, 1988.

49. Dudrick SJ, Brown W, Biggs CL: Nutritional management of patients with head and neck tumors. In Thawley SE and others, editors: *Comprehensive management of head and neck tumors,* Philadelphia, Saunders, 1999.

50. Elias EG, McCaslin DL: Nutrition in the patient with compromised oral function. In Peterson DE and others, editors: *Head and neck management of the cancer patient,* Boston, Martinus Nijhoff, 1986.

51. Ensley JF and others: The correlation of specific variables of tumor differentiation with response rate of survival in patients with advanced head and neck cancer treated with induction chemotherapy, *Cancer* 63:1487, 1989.

52. Ensley JF and others: Improved responses to radiation and concurrent cisplatin (CACP) in patients with advanced head and neck cancer (SCCHN) that fail induction chemotherapy. In *Proceedings of the Sixth International Conference on Adjuvant Therapy of Cancer,* March 1990, Tucson, AZ.

53. Epstein JB and others: Osteonecrosis: study of relationship of dental extractions in patients receiving radiotherapy, *Head Neck Surg* 10:48, 1987.

54. Fearon KCH and others: Influence of whole body protein turnover rate on resting energy expenditure in patients with cancer, *Cancer Res* 48:2590, 1988.

55. Ferrans C: Quality of life: conceptual issues, *Semin Oncol Nurs* 6:248, 1990.

56. Fisher J, Jackson T: Microvascular surgery as an adjunct to craniomaxillofacial reconstruction, *Br J Plast Surg* 42:146, 1989.

57. Fisher S: The psychosexual effects of cancer and cancer treatment, *Oncol Nurs Forum* 10(2):6367, 1983.

58. Fleming ID and others: *American Joint Commission on Cancer manual for staging of cancer,* ed 5, Philadelphia, Lippincott-Raven, 1997.

59. Foltz AT: Nutritional disturbances. In Groenwald SL and others, editors: *Cancer nursing: principles and practices,* ed 4, Boston, Jones and Bartlett, 1997.

60. Fowler JF: Rationales for high linear energy transfer radiotherapy. In Steel GG, Adams GS, Peckman, editors: *The biological basis of radiotherapy,* New York, Elsevier, 1983.

61. Fu KK and others: Combined radiotherapy and chemotherapy with bleomycin and methotrexate in advanced inoperable head and neck cancer: update of a Northern California oncology group randomized trial, *J Clin Oncol* 5:1410, 1987.

62. Ganly I, Kaye SB: Recurrent squamous-cell carcinoma of the head and neck: overview of current therapy and future prospects, *Ann Oncol* 11:11, 2000.

63. Genden EM, Thawley SE, O'Leary MJ: *Malignant neoplasms of the oropharynx.* In Cummings CW, Frederickson JM, Harker LA, Krause CJ, Schuller DE, Richardson MA, editors: *Otolaryngology head and neck surgery,* ed 3, St. Louis, Mosby, 1999.

64. Germino B, O'Rourke ME: Cancer and the family. In McCorkle R, Grant M, Frank-Stromborg M, Baird SB, editors: *Cancer nursing: a comprehensive textbook,* ed 2, Philadelphia, Saunders, 1996.

65. Goepfert H: Squamous cell carcinomas of the head and neck: past progress and future promise, *CA Cancer J Clin* 48:195, 1998.
66. Goltrup F and others: The dynamic properties of tissue oxygenation in healing flaps, *Surgery* 95:527, 1984.
67. Goodwin WJ, Torres J: The value of the prognostic nutritional index in the management of patients with advanced carcinoma of the neck, *Head Neck Surg* 6:932, 1984.
68. Gotay C: Research in cancer rehabilitation. In McGarvey C, editor: *Physical therapy for the cancer patient,* New York, Churchill Livingstone, 1990.
69. Gralla RJ and others: The management of chemotherapy-induced nausea and vomiting, *Med Clin North Am* 71:289, 1987.
70. Grayden JE: Factors that predict patients' functioning following treatment for cancer, *Int J Nurs Stud* 25(2):117, 1988.
71. Greenlee RT and others: Cancer statistics 2000, *CA Cancer J Clin* 50:7, 2000.
72. Grimm PM: Coping with psychosocial issues. In Itano JK, Taoko RN, editors: *Core curriculum for oncology nursing,* ed 3, Philadelphia, Saunders, 1998.
73. Guillamondequi OM, Larson DL: The lateral trapezium musculocutaneous flap: its use in head and neck reconstruction, *Plast Reconstr Surg* 67:143, 1981.
74. Harriot JC and others: Dental preservation in patients irradiated for head and neck tumors: a 10 year experience with topical fluoride and a randomized trial between two fluoridation methods, *Radiother Oncol* 1:72, 1983.
75. Harris L, Smith S: Chemotherapy in head and neck cancer, *Semin Oncol Nurs* 5(3):174, 1989.
76. Hidlago D: Aesthetic improvements in free flap mandible reconstruction, *Plast Reconstr Surg* 88(4):574, 1991.
77. Housset M and others: A perspective study of three treatment techniques for T1-T2 base of tongue lesions: surgery plus post op radiation, external radiation plus interstitial implantation and external irradiation alone, *Int J Radiat Oncol Biol Phys* 13:511, 1987.
78. Hussey DH, Wen B: Principles of radiation oncology. In Bailey BJ and others, editors: *Head and neck surgery—otolaryngology,* ed 2, Philadelphia, Lippincott-Raven, 1998.
79. Inigo F: Frontotemporal fasciocutaneous island flap for the facial aesthetic subunit reconstruction, *J Craniofac Surg* 10:320, 1999.
80. Iwamoto RR: Nursing care of the client with head and neck cancer. In Itano JK, Taoko RN, editors: *Core curriculum for oncology nursing,* ed 3, Philadelphia, Saunders, 1998.
81. Jacobs JR and others: Cisplatin and 5-fluorouracil infusion therapy before definitive treatments in advanced head and neck carcinoma: an RTOG study, *Arch Otolaryngol* 113:193, 1987.
82. Jacobs JR and others: Chemotherapy following definitive surgery for advanced squamous cell carcinoma of the head and neck: a Radiation Therapy Oncology Group Study, *Am J Clin Oncol* 12:85, 1989.
83. Jobsis FF, Boyd JB, Barwick WJ: Metabolic consequences of ischemia and hypoxia. In Serafin D, Buncke EU, editors: *Microsurgical composite tissue transplantation,* St. Louis, Mosby, 1974.
84. Kish J and others: Clinical results in recurrent head and neck carcinoma. In Jacobs JR and others, editors: *Head and neck cancer: scientific and clinical perspectives in management and strategies for cure,* New York, Elsevier, 1987.
85. Komisar A: The functional result of mandibular reconstruction, *Laryngoscope* 100:364, 1990.
86. Kramer S and others: Combined radiation therapy and surgery in the management of advanced head and neck cancers: final report of Study 7303 of the Radiation Therapy Oncology Group, *Head Neck Surg* 1:19, 1987.
87. Kudsk EG, Hoffman GS: Rehabilitation of the cancer patient, *Prim Care* 14:381, 1987.
88. Lamb M: Alterations in sexuality and sexual functioning. In Baird SB, McCorkle R, Grant M, editors: *Cancer nursing: a comprehensive textbook,* Philadelphia, Saunders, 1991.
89. Leveque FG and others: A multicenter, randomized, double-blind, placebo-controlled, dose-titrated study of oral pilocarpine for treatment of radiation-induced xerostomia in head and neck cancer patient, *J Clin Oncol* 11(6):1124, 1993.
90. Liggett WH, Forastiere AA: *Chemotherapy for head and neck cancer.* In Cummings CW, Frederickson JM, Harker LA, Krause CJ, Schuller DE, Richardson MA, editors: *Otolaryngology head and neck surgery,* ed 3, St. Louis, Mosby, 1999.
91. Licciardello JT, Spitz MR, Hong WK: Multiple primary cancer of the head and neck: second cancer of the head and neck, esophagus and lung, *Int J Radiat Oncol Biol Phys* 17:467, 1989.
92. Little W, Falace DA: *Dental management of the medically compromised patient,* St. Louis, Mosby, 1980.
93. Loescher LJ and others: Physiologic and psychological implications of surviving adult cancer (2 parts), *Ann Intern Med* 111:411, 1989.
94. Lukash FN, Sachs SA: Functional mandibular reconstruction: prevention of the oral invalid, *Plast Reconstr Surg* 84:227, 1989.
95. Mahon SM: Managing the psychosocial consequences of cancer recurrence: implications for nurses, *Oncol Nurs Forum* 16:39, 1989.
96. Mashberg A, Samit A: Early diagnosis of asymptomatic oral and oropharyngeal squamous cancers, *CA Cancer J Clin* 46:328, 1995.
97. Mathes S, Nahai F: *Clinical applications for muscle and musculocutaneous flaps,* St. Louis, Mosby, 1982.
98. Maxwell MB: Principles of treatment planning. In Groenwald SL and others, editors: *Cancer nursing: principles and practices,* ed 4, Boston, Jones and Bartlett, 1997.
99. McConnel FMS, Teichgraeber JF, Adler RK: A comparison of three methods of oral reconstruction, *Arch Otolaryngol Head Neck Surg* 113:496, 1987.
100. McCorkle R and others: *Cancer nursing: a comprehensive textbook,* ed 2, Philadelphia, Saunders, 1996.

101. McGuire M: Current trends in management of head and neck cancer, *Dev Supportive Cancer Care* 3:30, 1999.

102. McGuirt WF Sr: Differential diagnosis of neck masses. In Cummings CW, Frederickson JM, Harker LA, Krause CJ, Schuller DE, Richardson MA, editors: *Otolaryngology head and neck surgery,* ed 3, St. Louis, Mosby, 1999.

103. McPhetride L: Nursing history: one means to personalize care, *Am J Nurs* 68:68, 1968.

104. Medina JE, Houck JR, O'Malley BB: Management of cervical lymph nodes in squamous cell cancer of the head and neck. In Harrison LB, Sessions RB, Hong WK, editors: *Head and neck cancer: a multidisciplinary approach,* Philadelphia, Lippincott-Raven, 1999.

105. Mendenhall W and others: Is elective neck treatment indicated for T2 squamous cell carcinoma of the glottic larynx? *Radiat Ther Oncol* 14:199, 1989.

106. Mendenhall W and others: The role of radiation therapy in laryngeal cancer, *CA Cancer J Clin* 40(3):150, 1990.

107. Metcalf MC, Fischman SH: Factors affecting sexuality of patients with head and neck cancer, *Oncol Nurs Forum* 12(2):21, 1985.

108. Miaskowski C, Buchsel P, editors: *Oncology nursing, assessment and clinical care,* St. Louis, Mosby, 1999.

109. Miller SD, Levine DR: Rehabilitation of speech, voice, and swallowing function after treatment of head and neck cancer. In Harrison RB, Sessions RB, Hong WK, editors: *Head and neck cancer: a multidisciplinary approach,* Philadelphia, Lippincott-Raven, 1999.

110. Million R, Cassisi RR, editors: *Management of head and neck cancer: a multidisciplinary approach,* Philadelphia, Lippincott, 1994.

111. Morrish RB and others: Osteonecrosis in patients irradiated for head and neck carcinoma, *Cancer* 47:1980, 1981.

112. Muldooney JB and others: Oral cavity reconstruction using the free arm radial flap, *Arch Otolaryngol Head Neck Surg* 13:1219, 1987.

113. Murray CG, Daly TE, Zimmerman SO: The relationship between dental disease and radiation necrosis of the mandible, *Oral Surg* 49:99, 1980.

114. Myers EN, Suen JY: *Cancer of the head and neck,* Philadelphia, Saunders, 1996.

115. NANDA. Nursing diagnosis definitions and classifications, 1999–2000, Philadelphia, NANDA, 1999.

116. Nishimoto PW: Sexuality. In Itano JK, Taoko RN, editors: *Core curriculum for oncology nursing,* ed 3, Philadelphia, Saunders, 1998.

117. O'Malley BB, Yeung H: General principles of head and neck radiology. In Harrison LB, Sessions RB, Hong KB, editors: *Head and neck cancer: a multidisciplinary approach,* Philadelphia, Lippincott-Raven, 1999.

118. Papadimitrakopoulou VA, Shin DM, Hong WK: Chemo prevention of head and neck cancer. In Harrison LB, Sessions RB, Hong WK, editors: *Head and neck cancer: a multidisciplinary approach,* Philadelphia, Lippincott-Raven, 1999.

119. Parker RG, Enstrom JE: Second primary cancers of the head and neck following treatment of initial primary head and neck cancer, *Int J Radiat Oncol Biol Phys* 14:561, 1988.

120. Pasacreta J, McCorkle R: Psychosocial aspects of cancer. In McCorkle R and others: *Cancer nursing, a comprehensive textbook,* ed 2, Philadelphia, Saunders, 1996.

121. Perez CA, Brady LW, editors: *Principles and practice of radiation oncology,* ed 3, Philadelphia, Lippincott-Raven, 1999.

122. Pomp J, Levendag PC, Putten WLJ: Reirradiation of recurrent tumors in the head and neck, *Am J Clin Oncol* 11:543, 1988.

123. Puthawala AA and others: Limited external beam and interstitial iridium-192 irradiation in the treatment of carcinoma of the base of tongue: a 10 year experience, *Int J Radiat Oncol Biol Phys* 14:839, 1988.

124. Reese JL: Head and neck cancers. In McCorkle R, Grant M, Frank-Stromberg M, Baird SB, editors: *Cancer nursing: a comprehensive textbook,* ed 2, Philadelphia, Saunders, 1996.

125. Reuther JF, Steinau H, Wagner R: Reconstruction of larger defects in the oropharynx with revascularized intestinal grafts: an experimental clinical report, *Plast Reconstr Surg* 73:345, 1984.

126. Reynolds JV and others: Arginine, protein calorie malnutrition and cancer, *J Surg Res* 45:513, 1988.

127. Rieke JW and others: Oral pilocarpine for radiation-induced xerostomia: integrated efficacy and safety results from two prospective randomized clinical trials, *Int J Radiat Oncol Biol Phys* 31(3):661, 1995.

128. Rirken M and others: Rectus abdominis free flap in head and neck reconstruction, *Arch Otolaryngol Head Neck Surg* 117:857, 1991.

129. Robbins KT: Neck dissection. In Cummings CW, Frederickson JM, Harker LA, Krause CJ, Schuller DE, Richardson MA, editors: *Otolaryngology head and neck surgery,* ed 3, St. Louis, Mosby, 1999.

130. Rodriguez-Monge EJ, Shin DM, Lippman SM: Head and neck cancer. In Padzur R, editor: *Medical oncology: a comprehensive review,* Huntington, NY, PRR, 1995.

131. Sangers JR and others: Tongue reconstruction with a combined brachioradialis-radial forearm flap, *J Reconstruct Microsurg* 16:7, 2000.

132. Saunders JA: The genetic basis of head and neck carcinoma, *Am J Surg* 174:459, 1997.

133. Schleper JR: Prevention, detection, and diagnosis of head and neck cancer, *Semin Oncol Nurs* 5(3):139, 1989.

134. Schusterman MA and others: Use of the A0 plate for immediate mandibular reconstruction in cancer patients, *Plast Reconstr Surg* 88(4):588, 1991.

135. Seidel HM and others: *Mosby's guide to physical examination,* ed 3, St. Louis, Mosby, 1995.

136. Shah JP, Lydiatt W: Treatment of cancer of the head and neck, *CA Cancer J Clin* 45(6):352, 1995.

137. Shaha AR, Strong EW: Cancer of the head and neck. In Murphy GP, Lawrence W, Lenhard RE, editors: *American Cancer Society textbook of clinical oncology,* ed 2, Atlanta, American Cancer Society, 1995.

138. Sharma PK, Schuller DE, Baker SR: *Malignant neoplasms of the oral cavity.* In Cummings CW, Frederickson

JM, Harker LA, Krause CJ, Schuller DE, Richardson MA, editors: *Otolaryngology head and neck surgery*, ed 3, St. Louis, Mosby, 1999.

139. Sheldon JM, Shike M: Nutritional management of patients with head and neck cancer. In Harrison LB, Sessions RB, Hong WK, editors: *Head and neck cancer: a multidisciplinary approach*, Philadelphia, Lippincott-Raven, 1999.

140. Shell JA: Body image disturbance. In Carroll Johnson RM, Gorman LM, Bush NJ, editors: *Psychosocial nursing care along the cancer continuum*, Pittsburgh, Oncology Nursing Press Inc., 1998.

141. Shin DM: Paclitaxel (Taxol)/Ifosfamide–based chemotherapy in patients with recurrent or metastatic squamous cell carcinoma of the head and neck, *Semin Oncol* 27(Suppl):36, 2000.

142. Shin DM, Lippman SM, Hong WK: Chemoprevention of head and neck tumors. In Thawley SE and others, editors: *Comprehensive management of head and neck tumors*, ed 2, Philadelphia, Saunders, 1999.

143. Sigler BA: Nursing care for head and neck tumor patients. In Thrawley SE, Panye WR, editors: *Comprehensive management of head and neck tumors*, ed 2, Philadelphia, Saunders, 1999.

144. Sigler BA: Nursing care of the head and neck cancer patient, *Oncology* 2:49, 1988.

145. Sigler BA, Schuring LT: *Ear, nose, and throat disorders*, St. Louis, Mosby, 1993.

146. Sigler BA, Edwards A: Nursing care. In Myers EN, Suen JY, editors: *Cancer of the head and neck*, ed 3, Philadelphia, Saunders, 1996.

147. Slaughter DL, Southwick HW, Smejkal W: "Field cancerization" in oral stratified squamous epithelium: clinical implications of multicentric origin, *Cancer* 6:963, 1953.

148. Slotman GJ, Doolittle CH III, Glicksman AS: Preoperative combination chemotherapy and radiation therapy plus radical surgery in advanced head and neck cancer: 5-year results with impressive complete response rates and high survival. *Cancer* 69:2736, 1992.

149. Smeltzer SC, Bare BG, editors: *Brunner & Suddarth's medical-surgical nursing*, ed 9, Philadelphia, Lippincott Williams & Wilkins, 2000.

150. Spitz MR: Epidemiology and risk factors for head and neck cancer, *Semin Oncol* 21(3):281, 1994.

151. Spitz MR, Trizna Z: Molecular epidemiology and genetic predisposition for head and neck cancer. In Harrison LB, Sessions RB, Hong WK, editors: *Head and neck cancer, a multidisciplinary approach,* Philadelphia, Lippincott-Raven, 1999.

152. Stoll BA: *Coping with cancer stress,* Dordrecht, Martinus Nijhoff, 1986.

153. Strohl RA: Radiation therapy for head and neck cancers, *Semin Oncol Nurs* 5(3):166, 1989.

154. Sweeney PJ and others: Radiation therapy in head and neck cancer: indications and limitation, *Semin Oncol* 21(3):296, 1994.

155. Taylor I and others: Free vascularized bone graft: plastic and reconstruction of patients with oral cancer, *Oral Surg Oral Med Pathol* 68(4):499, 1992.

156. Tecknos TN, Coniglio JU, Netterville JL: Guidelines to patient management. In Bailey BJ: *Head and neck surgery—otolaryngology,* Philadelphia, Lippincott-Raven, 1998.

157. Thawley SE and others, editors: *Comprehensive management of head and neck tumors,* ed 2, Philadelphia, Saunders, 1999.

158. Tiwari RM: Masseter crossover flap reconstruction of oral-oropharyngeal defects. In Wolf T, Carey TE, editors: *Head and neck oncology research: Proceedings of the 2nd International Head and Neck Oncology Research Conference,* Arlington, VA, Kugler, September 1987.

159. Tonenelli PM, Hume WR, Kenny EB: Chlorhexidine: a review of the literature, *J West Soc Periodont* 31:5, 1983.

160. Vikram B: Adjuvant therapy in head and neck cancer, *CA-A Cancer J Clin* 48:199, 1998.

161. Wang CC, Blitzer PH, Siuit HD: Twice-day radiation therapy for cancer of the head and neck, *Cancer* 55:2100, 1985.

162. Wang CC and others: Treatment with preoperative irradiation and surgery of squamous cell carcinoma of the head and neck, *Cancer* 64:3233, 1989.

163. Weichselbaum R, Beckett MA: The maximum recovery potential of human tumor cells may predict clinical outcome in radiotherapy, *Int J Radiat Oncol Biol Phys* 13:709, 1987.

164. Weiland AJ: Vascularized bone grafts: reconstructive surgery. In Green DP, editor: *Operative hand surgery,* New York, Churchill Livingstone, 1988.

165. Wenig BM: General principles of head and neck pathology. In Harrison LB, Sessions RB, Hong WK, editors: *Head and neck cancer, a multidisciplinary approach,* Philadelphia, Lippincott-Raven, 1999.

166. Zlotlow IM: Dental oncology and maxillofacial prosthetics. In Harrison LB, Sessions RB, Hong WK, editors: *Head and neck cancer, a multidisciplinary approach,* Philadelphia, Lippincott-Raven, 1999.

Human Immunodeficiency Virus (HIV) and Related Cancers

Cynthia F. Brogdon

On June 5, 1981, the first cases of an illness later defined as *acquired immunodeficiency syndrome* (AIDS) were reported by California health care providers to the Centers for Disease Control and Prevention (CDC).[4] This first cluster of five Los Angeles men presented with unusual opportunistic infections and were thought to represent a geographically localized epidemic of an unknown infectious disease. Just 4 years later, in 1985, 14,049 cases of AIDS were reported in the United States. Later that same year, the *human immunodeficiency virus* (HIV) was identified as the causative agent of AIDS; more than 7000 Americans had already died of the disease.[4]

We are now well into the second decade of this epidemic, and HIV continues to infect 16,000 persons each day across the globe.[18] Although scientific and clinical progress has been made and new treatments and comprehensive models of care developed, HIV disease remains an incurable illness spreading rapidly throughout the United States and the world.

Nurses have a pivotal role in treatment and prevention of this disease. Patient education about risk behaviors and risk reduction techniques will help prevent new infections and will undoubtedly save countless lives. Appropriate, compassionate nursing care for those already infected may extend survival and will improve the quality of life for those afflicted with HIV disease.

Human Immunodeficiency Virus

EPIDEMIOLOGY

Infection with HIV has occurred in approximately 600,000 to 900,000 Americans and progressed to AIDS in more than 700,000. This epidemic has killed over 400,000 Americans, and the numbers increase daily.[3] Throughout the world, more than 12 million people are infected with HIV, and almost 2 million have progressed to an AIDS diagnosis. It is estimated that more than 1 million people have died of AIDS worldwide. Although changes in risk behaviors have slowed the spread of HIV infection in some areas of the United States, HIV transmission has accelerated in others. More than 40,000 new infections are expected this year in the United States alone.[3] In 1991, the World Health Organization (WHO) estimated 40 million infections worldwide by the year 2000. Although difficult to track, especially in third world countries with limited health care and virtually no surveillance, the CDC now estimates 42 million people have been infected with HIV since the onset of the pandemic.[7]

Throughout the epidemic the numbers of those infected have steadily increased each year. Early in the U.S. epidemic, more than 80% of those infected were homosexual men. Currently, approximately 60% of new infections occur in this population. Those persons now at greatest risk for acquiring HIV infection in the United States include heterosexual women and their children and intravenous drug users (IDUs). Women now represent 30% of new U.S. cases and IDUs almost 25%. HIV infection continues to affect racial minorities disproportionately: of the new HIV infections among men, it is believed that 50% occur among African American men and African American women represent 64% of all new infections among women each year.[3]

Worldwide, HIV continues to ravage heterosexual men, women, and their children. New infections in Asia have increased dramatically in the past 2 years, and areas of Africa have infection rates as high as 35% to 50% among the general population.

ETIOLOGY AND RISK FACTORS

Since the first description of AIDS in 1981, an extraordinary scientific adventure has ensued. In just over a decade, remarkable advancements have occurred in our understanding of the disease and its causative agent, HIV. The origin of HIV is still largely unknown, although evidence appears to support the hypothesis of an African origin. The first reports of an AIDS-like illness date back to the early 1960s in central Africa. HIV in humans probably has an animal origin, most likely nonhuman primates.

HIV is a human retrovirus and belongs to the lentivirus subfamily. Currently, five human retroviruses have been identified: human T-cell lymphotrophic virus type 1 (HTLV-1), HTLV-2, HTLV-5, HIV-1, and HIV-2. HTLV-2 has not been conclusively associated with human disease. HTLV-1 and HTLV-5 have been associated with human T-cell leukemia and lymphoma, conditions characterized by proliferation of CD4$^+$ (T4) helper cells. HIV-1 and HIV-2 both cause depletion of CD4 cells, resulting in loss of cellular immunity, as characterized by AIDS. HIV-1 is the predominant cause of AIDS in the United States, accounting for more than 95% of AIDS cases. HIV-2 seems to be limited to geographic distribution and is most prevalent in West Africa.[6]

The life cycle of HIV is similar to that of the other retroviruses. Mature virions interact with specific host receptors and then use the host cell for viral replication. HIV interacts with the CD4 glycoprotein, which occurs on the membrane of specific cells, primarily the CD4$^+$ (T4) helper lymphocytes. These specific white blood cells contain the CD4 glycoprotein on their membranes, allowing the virus to fuse. The viral core is subsequently injected into the cell cytoplasm, where the viral RNA genome is translated into DNA by a retroviral enzyme called *reverse transcriptase.* Infection and subsequent viral replication eventually deplete the host's CD4 cells, resulting in a dramatic loss of the protective immune response against invading microorganisms.

The routes for transmission of HIV are well documented: (1) intimate sexual contact; (2) parenteral exposure to blood, blood-containing body fluids, and blood products; and (3) mother-to-child contact during the perinatal period. Although HIV has been identified in a variety of body fluids, those consistently shown to be infectious are blood, semen, and vaginal secretions. Transmission has also been associated with breast milk, although this appears to occur infrequently. HIV is transmitted directly from person to person by sexual contact; from direct inoculation with contaminated blood products, needles, or syringes; and from an infected mother to her newborn. HIV is not transmitted by casual contact, including sneezing, coughing, or spitting; handshakes; toilet seats, bathtubs, showers, or swimming pools; or utensils, dishes, or linens used by an infected person. HIV disease is a blood-borne, sexually transmitted disease. Although certain sexual practices may be associated with higher risks for infection than others, any practice that exposes one to infected blood, semen, or vaginal secretions carries the potential for viral transmission.[5]

The natural history of HIV infection is associated with an unpredictable course of disease progression. Most patients undergo a prolonged period of clinically silent infection, often lasting more than 10 years.[12] Although the virus is consistently detectable throughout this time, patients typically have only subtle immunologic alterations. Once the patient becomes symptomatic, however, decreases in the number of CD4 helper cells can be detected and viral replication increases. In the well-studied "San Francisco Cohort" of men enrolled to follow hepatitis B, 69% had developed AIDS at a median follow-up time of 14 years and only 8% still had a CD4 lymphocyte count of greater than 500 cells/mm^3.[11]

It is postulated that several potential cofactors may be associated with HIV disease progression. These cofactors, which may be of a viral, host, or environmental nature, are thought to directly influence the replication of HIV or the severity of its pathogenic effects. Viral cofactors that may influence the progression of the disease include herpes simplex virus (HSV), cytomegalovirus (CMV), and Epstein-Barr virus (EBV). Host cofactors may include a variety of cytokines and intracellular mediators. Environmental cofactors may include repeated exposure to HIV, which may induce hyperactivation of the immune system, resulting in an expansion of the pool of HIV-replicating cells. As viral replication increases, depleting the body of CD4 helper lymphocytes, the body's defense mechanisms are progressively weakened. Infections that were once disarmed by the healthy immune system are eventually able to cause serious and potentially life-threatening disease. These *opportunistic infections* (OIs) include a variety of organisms, such as viruses (HSV, EBV, CMV), protozoa (*Pneumocystis carinii, Toxoplasma*), *Mycobacterium* (*tuberculosis* and *avium* [*avium-intracellulare*] complex), and fungi (*Histoplasma, Cryptococcus*). In addition to the various OIs, the profound immune dysfunction also allows the development of several neoplasms, including non-Hodgkin's lymphoma, Kaposi's sarcoma, and cervical carcinomas.

PREVENTION, SCREENING, AND DETECTION

Because HIV disease is blood borne and sexually transmitted, prevention efforts must be directed toward ways to avoid exposure to contaminated blood and body fluids. With less than 3% of AIDS cases attributed to exposure to contaminated blood products, the greatest exposure risk is through sexual contact. AIDS prevention efforts must therefore focus on ways to reduce sexual transmission.

Historically, it has been difficult to talk about sexuality in the American culture. It has been a subject laden with moral judgments and an area seldom addressed in the U.S. health care system. Nurses are in an excellent position to discuss sexuality with patients. Typically, it is the nurse who has an intimate rapport with the patient, talking about sensitive subjects and related health concerns. It is usually the nurse with whom the patient feels most at ease and the nurse who is most accessible to patients. The nurse has a major role in the education of individuals and groups in the prevention of HIV disease.

Prevention efforts must include accurate, reliable, and clear information about risk factors for HIV disease and ways to decrease these risks. Prevention education programs must include the topics of practicing safer sexual techniques and using clean drug paraphernalia, as well as public health measures such as blood product screening and perinatal counseling. Prevention efforts must focus on behaviors that put patients at risk for infection.

Safe Sex Counseling

Any exchange of blood, semen, or vaginal secretions can potentially put an individual at risk for HIV disease. Common sexual practices that are therefore risky behaviors include vaginal or anal penetration without a condom and possibly oral sexual practices. Use of barrier products such as latex condoms while engaging in these behaviors greatly reduces the likelihood of exposure to potentially infectious blood, semen, or vaginal secretions. In addition, education about condom use should include the use of prelubricated condoms. Nonoxynol 9, a frequently used spermicidal lubricant, may also have some antiviral properties. Use of condoms prelubricated with nonoxynol 9 may therefore further increase the protection afforded by condoms. Use of additional water-based lubricants should also be encouraged. Petroleum-based lubricant use should be discouraged because these agents may cause latex breakdown. Prevention education must also include risk reduction techniques such as minimizing the number of sexual partners and engaging in a mutually monogamous sexual relationship. In addition, sexual practices that do not put the individual at risk for potentially infectious fluids should be discussed. Mutual masturbation, massage, and body rubbing are safe sexual practices with no exchange of body fluids.

Intravenous Risk Reduction

The use of contaminated needles for subcutaneous, intramuscular, or intravenous injection represents a serious risk for HIV infection. Prevention education must include ways to clean needles and other paraphernalia used to inject drugs. Educational efforts may include information about substance abuse counseling and programs, but use of a bleach solution to disinfect needles and paraphernalia must also be discussed.

Perinatal Transmission

Women who are infected with HIV may pass the virus on to their newborns via three potential routes: during gestation, during delivery, and through breastfeeding. Although the exact mechanism of perinatal transmission is unknown, the current estimate of risk to the newborn from an infected mother is approximately 30% in the United States. A groundbreaking study of mother-to-infant transmission was completed in 1994. This study revealed the risk of mother-to-infant transmission could be reduced by more than 67% if women were treated with AZT during the pregnancy and newborns were then treated postpartum. In this study, only 18.3% of treated mothers had infants who were infected with HIV. Based on this study, the U.S. Public Health Service now recommends that HIV-positive pregnant women be advised of these results and be offered AZT.[3]

Public Health Measures

Prevention programs must also educate the public about the measures that are currently in place to screen and protect the blood supply from contamination. Currently, each unit of donated blood is tested for HIV infection and several other blood-borne infections such as hepatitis. Because HIV screening of blood products has been conducted since 1985 in the United States, only recipients of transfusions before this time are at significant risk for infection via the blood supply.

Screening

The HIV antibody testing plays an essential role in prevention and treatment of this disease process. The most common form of screening for HIV disease is the use of the antibody test with the *enzyme-linked immunosorbent assay* (ELISA) technique and the *Western blot* technique. The ELISA test uses spectrophotometry to detect serum antibody reactions to specific HIV viral proteins. The ELISA is highly sensitive and specific with sensitivity of 98.4% to 99.6%. A positive ELISA test must be confirmed by the Western blot technique.

Both the ELISA and the Western blot techniques depend on antibody formation. Approximately 90% of the population will form antibodies in response to HIV exposure within 6 weeks to 3 months after exposure. A negative antibody test may occur in the "window phase" between the dates of actual exposure leading to infection and development of detectable serum antibodies.

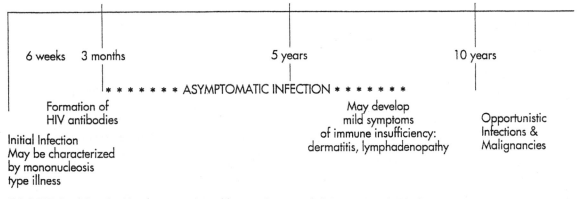

FIGURE 13–1   Usual progression of human immunodeficiency virus (HIV) disease in the United States.

Although approximately 90% of the population will form antibodies in response to HIV exposure within 6 weeks to 3 months after exposure, this period may be as long as 6 months.[8]

Because newborn infants maintain maternal antibodies for as long as 18 months, antibody testing is unreliable until the infant is 18 months of age. A newer test, the *polymerase chain reaction* (PCR), is now available. The PCR does not rely on antibody formation; instead, genetic subunits of the virus are identified, confirming infection.

Maintaining patient confidentiality is essential in HIV testing. Every measure possible should be taken to ensure that privacy is guaranteed. Unauthorized disclosure, stigmatization, and discrimination against HIV-positive individuals continue to occur with unfortunate regularity.

CLINICAL FEATURES

It has been estimated that one million Americans are infected with HIV; approximately one half are unaware they carry the virus that causes AIDS. Although some (fewer than 50%) of those infected will develop a viral syndrome resembling mononucleosis or influenza within a few days or weeks of infection, most are unaware the symptoms are related to the initial infection with HIV. Acute infection is followed by a period of asymptomatic HIV infection. In these early stages of HIV disease, there are no symptoms of infection. Infected persons may remain asymptomatic for several years, with half remaining asymptomatic for 10 years or longer.[11]

As HIV depletes the body of sufficient numbers of T4 helper cells, subtle symptoms of immunodeficiency may emerge. Patients may develop persistent generalized lymphadenopathy or minor dermatologic manifestations such as seborrhea. During this time a slow, persistent destruction of the immune system occurs with a gradual decline in the number of CD4 cells.

With continued destruction of the immune system, OIs and malignancies begin to develop and cause clinical symptoms. Clinical findings that appear to predict rapid progression to end-stage HIV disease (otherwise known as AIDS) include unexplained weight loss greater than 10% of usual body weight and persistent fever, diarrhea, or night sweats of longer than a 2-week duration.

Figure 13–1 provides an explanation of the usual progression of HIV disease in the United States. Table 13–1 lists specific clinical features of various OIs.

DIAGNOSIS AND STAGING

The spectrum of HIV infection ranges from asymptomatic infection to potentially life-threatening OI. In the past many clinicians used an informal staging system that put patients into one of three categories: (1) HIV positive, (2) AIDS-related complex (ARC), and (3) AIDS. In this staging system, "HIV positive" referred to patients who were completely asymptomatic but HIV positive. Those patients classified as "ARC" exhibited constitutional symptoms, including persistent generalized lymphadenopathy, persistent fevers, involuntary weight loss, or diarrhea. Any patient who had experienced an OI was classified as "AIDS."

Today, clinicians have become much more sophisticated about the stages of HIV disease and realize that it is a chronic, progressive illness characterized by four distinct categories. Although end-stage HIV disease is usually referred to as AIDS, most clinicians also use the staging system recommended by the CDC. The CDC Classification System for HIV Infection in Adults is currently the most widely used staging system (Table 13–2).

Perhaps the single most important advance in HIV care, viral load testing, now allows the clinician to more accurately stage the patient with HIV disease based on the measurable status of the immune system. Viral load studies measure the level of plasma HIV-1 RNA, which

Opportunistic Infections (OIs)

Opportunistic Infections	Clinical Features
BACTERIAL INFECTIONS	
Mycobacterium avium-intracellulare	General: persistent fever, night sweats, fatigue, weight loss, abdominal pain, weakness, lymphadenopathy, hepatosplenomegaly
FUNGAL INFECTIONS	
Candidiasis	Oral: white patches on tongue or buccal mucosa
	Vaginal: vulvar pruritus, vaginal discharge
Cryptococcosis	Meningitis: headache, fever, progressive malaise, altered mental status, seizures
	Pneumonia: fever, shortness of breath, cough
Histoplasmosis	Fever, weight loss, shortness of breath, lymphadenopathy
PROTOZOAL INFECTIONS	
Cryptosporidiosis	Diarrhea, abdominal cramping, nausea, vomiting, fatigue, weight loss, dehydration
Pneumocystis carinii	Pneumonia: fever, nonproductive cough, shortness of breath, weight loss, night sweats, fatigue
Toxoplasmosis	Encephalitis: altered mental status, seizures, fever, coma
VIRAL INFECTIONS	
Cytomegalovirus	Retinitis: unilateral visual deficit or change
	Gastrointestinal: dysphagia, wasting, nausea, fever, diarrhea
Herpes simplex	Painful blisters or ulcers

is proportional to the rate of viral replication and CD4 lymphocyte destruction. The significance of viral load testing was established in the Multicenter AIDS Cohort Study where HIV-1 RNA of greater than 100,000 copies/mL was associated with a 10-fold greater risk of progression to AIDS. In fact, viral load testing was the single most important predictor of HIV progression.[11]

Viral load testing is now used to determine appropriate treatment of infected individuals; Table 13–3 illustrates the use of viral load testing as a treatment guideline.

METASTASIS

HIV disease is a chronic, systemic infection. The infection itself primarily infects a specific group of lymphocytes (the CD4 lymphocytes) but also has the potential

for direct infection of the monocytes and macrophages and possibly muscle and nerve cells. In addition, many patients experience HIV infection directly affecting the central nervous system (CNS). As the disease progresses, almost every organ system is affected by one or more of the OIs that occur secondarily to the profound immunodeficiency that results from the original HIV infection. Most patients experience illness affecting the skin and mucous membranes, respiratory tract, gastrointestinal (GI) tract, and CNS.

TREATMENT MODALITIES

Chemotherapy

Several treatment options are now available to slow the progression of the illness, but currently no cure exists for HIV disease. However, the associated OIs that occur as a result of HIV infection can be treated and, in some patients, prevented.

In general, patients with HIV infection may remain relatively free of clinical symptoms for several years. Because of the variability of the disease progression, immune system surveillance on a regular basis is an important component of HIV treatment. It is recommended that patients with HIV disease obtain a physical examination and laboratory evaluation every 3 to 6 months. Currently the CD4 count and viral load testing are the most important indicators in tracking progressive deterioration of immune system function in HIV-infected individuals. If the CD4 cell count falls below 500 cells/mm^3, initiation of antiretroviral therapy is indicated: (1) regardless of the CD4 count or viral load in symptomatic patients, (2) when CD4 counts are below 500 cells/mm^3 or viral load is less than 20,000 copies/mL, and (3) at the discretion of the clinician in asymptomatic patients with CD4 counts of greater than 500 cells/mm^3 and viral loads of less than 20,000 copies/mL (Table 13–4). Zidovudine (Retrovir, AZT) was the first drug approved to treat HIV infection and is still often used. AZT is most often used now, however, as a component of combination therapy or as a single agent in pregnant HIV-positive women. Three other similar drugs are available: Videx (didanosine, ddI), HIVID (zalcitabine, ddC), and stavudine (d4T). All three of these antiretrovirals belong to a class of drugs known as the *nucleoside analogues* and work to slow the rate of viral replication. These drugs are not cures for HIV infection.

In early 1996 a new class of antiretroviral drugs became available (see Table 13–4). These new drugs, members of a class known as the *protease inhibitors*, have a different mechanism of action than the previously available *reverse transcriptase inhibitors* (AZT, ddI, ddC, d4T). The protease inhibitors include ritonavir and saquinavir and represent a significant breakthrough in

CDC Classification System for HIV Infections in Adults

Stage	Classification	Description
I	Acute infection	Occurs at time of initial HIV infection and may last from days to weeks; characterized by mononucleosis-like or influenza-like syndrome, with approximately 50% of patients reporting or recalling symptoms
II	Asymptomatic infection	Occurs after stage I and may last for several years
III	Persistent generalized lymphadenopathy (PGL)	Characterized by palpable lymph node enlargement of ≥1 cm at two or more extrainguinal sites, persisting for longer than 3 months
IV	Other diseases	PGL not prerequisite Subgroup A: constitutional disease—fever persisting for > 1 month, involuntary weight loss > 10% of usual body weight, diarrhea persisting for > 1 month Subgroup B: neurologic disease—dementia, myelopathy, peripheral neuropathy Subgroup C: secondary infectious diseases—specific infectious diseases identified by CDC; typically referred to as *opportunistic infections* Subgroup D: secondary cancers—includes Kaposi's sarcoma, non-Hodgkin's lymphoma, primary lymphoma of brain Subgroup E: other conditions—includes other conditions specified by CDC (e.g., chronic lymphoid interstitial pneumonitis)

the management of HIV disease. For the first time, patients have the option of using combination therapy with two drugs (e.g., AZT and ritonavir), both of which have different side effects and toxicities. As in the treatment of malignancies and other infectious diseases, the most successful therapy involves the use of multiple drugs that have different mechanisms of action and different side effects.

Several other drugs are available to treat specific OIs that occur as the immune system is depleted. Various degrees of success have been achieved with these regimens in treating the OI. In some patients, prophylaxis for recurrent or even primary OIs may be effective.

Pneumocystis carinii infection is the most common OI occurring in HIV-infected patients. This protozoan is a ubiquitous organism acquired by most persons during childhood. Most often in HIV infection, *P. carinii* causes pneumonia. Until recently, *P. carinii* pneumonia (PCP) was an almost universally life-threatening OI in patients with HIV disease. Although it remains the most common OI, occurring in as many as 85% of HIV patients, the mortality rate from PCP has been greatly reduced since the use of intravenous trimethoprim-sulfamethoxazole or pentamidine therapy. Oral trimethoprim-sulfamethoxazole has now been shown to be highly effective in preventing recurrence of PCP as well. In addition, initiation of oral PCP prophylaxis in patients known to be at high risk for PCP infection has reduced the primary occurrence rate.

Biotherapy

Anemia, leukopenia, and thrombocytopenia are part of the natural history of HIV disease. These cytopenias can result from marrow failure or cell-destructive processes. Drugs used to treat HIV disease and associated infections or malignancies can also cause them. Several HIV drug therapies have been shown to be myelotoxic. Many drugs used to treat OIs as well as Retrovir (AZT) may have to be interrupted in certain patients secondary to myelotoxicity. Use of colony-stimulating factors (CSFs) such as granulocyte and granulocyte-monocyte CSFs (G-CSFs and GM-CSFs) has proved useful in decreasing myelotoxicity and often allows successful completion of therapy.

Erythropoietin (EPO) can be used for treatment of Retrovir-induced marrow suppression. Although this therapy has not been successful in all patients, a significant number have required fewer transfusions and have

Viral Load in HIV Positive Patients Treatment Recommendations

Viral Load and Clinical Factors	Recommendations
Any viral load with OI	Treat with combination antiretrovirals
CD4 count < 350–500 cells/mm³ or viral load > 20,000 copies/mL	Treat with combination antiretrovirals
Asymptomatic disease with CD4 > 500 cells/mm³ and viral load < 20,000 copies/mL	Treat or observe
If viral load does not decrease by at least 0.5 log after 6 weeks	Change antiretroviral regimen

TABLE 13-4
Antiretroviral Drugs for HIV Disease

Category/Specific Drugs	Side Effects
NUCLEOSIDE REVERSE TRANSCRIPTASE INHIBITORS (NRTIs)	
Zidovudine (azidothymidine, AZT, ZDV, Retrovir)	Bone marrow suppression, GI upset, headache, myopathy
Didanosine (dideoxyinosine, ddl, Videx)	Peripheral neuropathy, pancreatitis, diarrhea, hepatitis, Lactic acidosis/hepatic steatosis
Zalcitabine (dideoxycytidine, ddC, HIVID)	Peripheral neuropathy, pancreatitis, oral ulcers, lactic acidosis/hepatic steatosis
Stavudine (d4T, Zerit)	Peripheral neuropathy, lactic acidosis/hepatic steatosis
Lamivudine (3TC, Epivir)	Lactic acidosis/hepatic steatosis
Abacavir (ABC, Ziagen)	Hypersensitivity
Adefovir (Preveon)	Nausea, Fanconi-like syndrome
NON-NUCLEOSIDE REVERSE TRANSCRIPTASE INHIBITORS (NNRTIs)	
Nevirapine (Virammune)	Skin rash, erythema multiforme
Delaviridine (Rescriptor)	Rash, erythema multiforme
Efavirenz (Sustiva)	Dizziness, skin rash, confusion, encephalopathy
PROTEASE INHIBITORS	
Indinavir (Crixivan)	Nephrolithiasis, nausea, diarrhea, lipodystrophy, hyperlipidemia, diabetes*
Saquinavir (Fortovase)	Nausea, diarrhea, lipodystrophy, hyperlipidemia, diabetes*
Ritonavir (Norvir)	Nausea, emesis, taste alterations, diarrhea, lipodystrophy, hyperlipidemia, hepatitis, diabetes*
Nelfinavir (Viracept)	Nausea, diarrhea, flatulence, lipodystrophy, hyperlipidemia, diabetes*
Amprenavir (Agenerase)	Nausea, headache, skin rash, lipodystrophy, hyperlipidemia, diabetes*

* *The relationship between this agent and diabetes has not been fully established.*[10, 11, 21]

been able to continue antiviral, antiinfective, or antineoplastic therapy while receiving EPO.[14]

Future Therapies

In the early years of the AIDS epidemic, there was steadfast hope that a vaccination could be developed to stop the spread of this deadly virus. Many researchers across the United States have conducted countless trials of various vaccines, but none has yet proved to be successful. The rapid rate of mutation of HIV has made it difficult for scientists to match this with a vaccine that would stimulate appropriate antibody responses. Although vaccine research is continuing, most researchers believe that a vaccine for the general population will likely not be available for many years.[3] Vaccine research historically has focused on the prevention of infection. Much current vaccine research, however, is evaluating administration of a vaccine to patients who are already HIV infected. Through the use of an inactivated virus vaccine, researchers hope to spur the body's production of an antibody specific for fighting HIV as well as the production of CD4 cells. By stimulating the immune system's response to HIV, researchers hope that the vaccine might be able to halt or even reverse the spread of the virus in newly infected individuals.

An increasing number of researchers now believe that *gene therapy* represents the only hope of cure for HIV disease. Gene therapy involves the insertion of a gene into a human cell. The new gene would direct the natural, antiviral human cell response. Theoretically the new gene would program the human cell to destroy HIV. Although research is now only in the early stages in this new arena, the therapy appears promising.

HIV has potential disease-related and treatment-related complications as listed in the Complications box.

PROGNOSIS

Although HIV disease appears to be a universally fatal illness, a small number of patients ($< 5\%$) appear to be long-term nonprogressors. These individuals are clearly infected with HIV but do not progress in the usual pattern of immunosuppression. The usual time to progression of profound immunodeficiency varies widely among patients. In countries such as the United States where more information and treatment options have become available, HIV disease has become a more manageable, chronic illness. The nurse plays a primary role in educational efforts to prevent this disease and provide compassionate and appropriate care to those already infected.

COMPLICATIONS

HIV *Disease and Treatment*

Disease-Related Complications

Profound immunosuppression

Development of various opportunistic infections/malignancies

Constitutional symptoms: fever, night sweats, weight loss

Persistent generalized lymphadenopathy

Financial loss, including employment, health insurance, housing

Societal stigmatization and discrimination

Treatment-Related Complications

Anemia, neutropenia, thrombocytopenia

Fatigue

Nausea, vomiting, weight loss

HIV-*Related Cancers*

The HIV epidemic has been characterized not only by the occurrence of opportunistic infections, but also by the development of specific cancers. It is well established that profound immune suppression is associated with an increased risk of developing a malignant disease. Generally, these tumors occur at an earlier age and behave more aggressively. As the patient's immune system function declines, the risk of malignancy increases. Viral infections are etiologically linked to approximately 20% of all malignancies worldwide and the risk of the development of a malignancy associated with a viral etiology appears to increase in immune-compromised individuals.[1] People with AIDS are at an increased risk of Kaposi's sarcoma (KS), non-Hodgkin's lymphoma (NHL), and Hodgkin's disease. All of these cancers have been associated with specific human herpesvirus (HHV) infections: KS with HHV-8, NHL and Hodgkin's disease with EBV, a closely related HHV.

Kaposi's sarcoma and NHL are the primary types of cancer associated with HIV infection. There are also reports of other cancers occurring at a higher than expected rate in HIV patients: childhood leiomyosarcoma, lung cancer, anorectal cancer, malignant testicular tumors, basal cell carcinoma, squamous cell carcinoma, and even malignant melanoma.[1,2]

Since the addition of new therapies for HIV disease, particularly the introduction of protease inhibitors into combination therapy regimens, there has been a substantial decline in morbidity and mortality. As the immune suppression of HIV disease is more optimally managed, we expect to see an associated decline in the incidence of malignant disease. It appears that KS has decreased in incidence by approximately 35%. The incidence of NHL appears to be declining as well, although this trend is less clear. Some centers have reported a continuing increase in the numbers of patients with NHL, some have found little change in the numbers of NHL patients, and others have identified reductions in the number of first admissions for NHL as high as 63%.[10,17,21] These data are difficult to interpret for several reasons: (1) Researchers have used various end-points to measure trends (i.e., number of first admissions, measurement of an HIV-associated malignancy as a presenting illness, etc.), (2) The use of protease inhibitors and combination regimens, often referred to as HAART or highly active antiretroviral therapy, is a relatively recent occurrence (primarily since 1997), and it may be too soon to see the effect of these therapies on the incidence rates of malignant diseases, (3) There is no clear association of reduction in incidence and a single antiretroviral regimen.

Kaposi's Sarcoma

AIDS was first reported to the CDC in 1981 as a combined epidemic of PCP and KS. After thorough investigation, clinicians and researchers discovered PCP and KS were diseases that occurred as a result of the profound immune suppression caused by HIV. KS remains the most common neoplasm in HIV-infected patients. Although some progress has been made in understanding this malignant process, much remains to be understood.

EPIDEMIOLOGY

Prior to the advent of the HIV epidemic, KS was a rare type of tumor and was categorized by three characteristic forms: (1) classical (occurring primarily in elderly men of Mediterranean descent), (2) African (an endemic form described in the 1950s in central Africa), and (3) iatrogenic (occurring in patients with chronic immune suppression, primarily those after transplant). After the discovery of KS in HIV patients, a fourth category was added: AIDS-related KS. In HIV-positive individuals, the incidence of KS is 75,000-fold greater than in the HIV-negative population. Histologically, this vascular neoplasm is indistinguishable in these various forms. KS is characterized by a proliferation in the dermis of aberrant vascular structures, lined by spindle-shaped cells.

The incidence of KS in HIV-positive patients has gradually declined since the epidemic was first discovered in the United States. From 1981 to 1982, KS accounted for more than 75% of the AIDS-defining illnesses. The current incidence of KS in HIV-positive patients in the United States is thought to be less than 15%.

ETIOLOGY AND RISK FACTORS

KS is a tumor of vascular origin, presents as a multifocal neoplasm, and is capable of arising simultaneously at multiple sites. In addition to HIV disease, other immunodeficient states, such as iatrogenically induced immunosuppression, as seen in renal transplant patients, have also been the setting for KS. However, immunodeficiency may not be a prerequisite for the development of KS. The host's genetic makeup may be a factor contributing to the development of KS in AIDS patients. An increased frequency of major histocompatibility antigens DR-5 and DR-2 has been reported in some studies of HIV-associated KS. The absence of the HIV genome in the KS tumor lends further support to an indirect role for HIV in AIDS-KS.

Among the HIV-positive population, homosexual and bisexual men are at the highest risk for KS. Although the pathogenesis of KS in HIV patients is not fully understood, it is likely a complex interaction involving immunosuppression, dysregulated cytokine production, and infection by HHV8, a sexually transmitted herpes virus. Although all types of patients with AIDS have been found to have KS (heterosexual, homosexual, IDU), the incidence is greatest in homosexual HIV-positive men.

PREVENTION, SCREENING, AND DETECTION

Because AIDS-KS is likely a result of a sexually transmitted disease (HHV8), prevention must include education about risky sexual behaviors. As with prevention of HIV disease, prevention of KS must involve barrier protection such as condoms and avoidance of potentially infectious body fluids, including blood, semen, and vaginal secretions. Because HIV-infected patients are at significant risk for AIDS-KS, all HIV patients should be screened routinely for potential signs and symptoms of KS. Such screening requires visual inspection of all body surfaces, including oral mucosa. Because no laboratory test exists for KS, patients must be educated to report any suspicious lesions immediately to their health care providers.

CLASSIFICATION

Before the advent of the HIV epidemic, KS was seen as an indolent, cutaneous vascular tumor in elderly men, particularly of Jewish or Mediterranean descent. This classic or endemic form of KS is rarely life-threatening. Multifocal, widespread lesions at the onset of the illness usually characterize AIDS-KS (also called epidemic

KS). AIDS-KS has a wide range of virulence in patients with HIV disease, ranging from limited stable involvement to fulminant disease with rapid, continuous development of new lesions. AIDS-KS is usually classified based on the site of the lesions.

A single lesion or multiple pigmented lesions characterize mucocutaneous KS. These are generally nonblanchable macules or papules, which may progress to nodules. Subcutaneous nodular lesions may vary in size from several millimeters to several centimeters in diameter. Although these lesions may appear on any cutaneous surface, the upper trunk, head, neck and feet are the most common sites. Mucocutaneous lesions tend to enlarge and coalesce, sometimes forming extensive plaques. As cutaneous lesions progress, lymphatic obstruction may develop, producing edema. Lymphadenopathic KS primarily affects the peripheral lymph nodes. Oral KS lesions can produce bleeding, tooth displacement, and pain.

Visceral involvement in epidemic KS may occur as the disease progresses or a visceral surface may be the presenting site. Visceral KS most often affects the lungs and GI tract. GI involvement is often asymptomatic except for oropharyngeal lesions. Pulmonary involvement in epidemic KS may occur in as many as 50% of patients.[18, 19]

CLINICAL FEATURES

Multifocal, widespread lesions at the onset of illness characterize AIDS-KS. These lesions may involve the skin, oral mucosa, lymph nodes, or visceral organs, including the lung, liver, spleen, and GI tract. Most patients have skin lesions that appear as flat or raised plaques ranging in size from a few millimeters to several centimeters. Colors range from blue-purple to red-brown. Although lymph node involvement occurs frequently, it is often difficult to distinguish from HIV-associated lymphadenopathy. Visceral involvement is extremely common as the disease progresses.[18, 19] GI involvement may be asymptomatic, although advanced disease may result in blood loss, diarrhea, and weight loss. Pulmonary involvement, although uncommon, may result in radiographic abnormalities and symptoms of cough, dyspnea, and fever. Although lesions from KS have been observed at autopsy in all organs, including the brain, pancreas, heart, and major vessels, these lesions remain generally asymptomatic.

DIAGNOSIS AND STAGING

AIDS-KS is generally diagnosed by examining biopsies of skin or mucous membrane lesions. Although AIDS-KS has often been diagnosed without biopsy, the visual appearance may be similar to several other dermatologic presentations, including fungal infection, lymphoma, dermatofibroma, and bacillary epithelioid angiomatosis (cat-scratch disease). Biopsy with histologic examination reveals a background of spindle-shaped cells with irregular proliferation of vascular spaces. Endothelial cells often appear large and malignant. AIDS-KS involving the lungs or GI tract is usually diagnosed by endoscopic examination. Although radiologic studies may be helpful in the evaluation of intestinal KS, lesions may be missed. Endoscopic examination may reveal violaceous macules or nodules. Although biopsy may be attempted on these lesions, it is often difficult to obtain an adequate specimen for biopsy. Computed tomography (CT) scan may be helpful in the identification of hepatic and splenic lesions. The appearance of multiple low attenuation enhancing lesions are characteristic on CT scan. Although pulmonary involvement in AIDS-KS is common, most patients remain asymptomatic until the disease is advanced. Chest radiographs may reveal perihilar linear infiltrates or nodular opacities. KS-related pleural effusions are a common finding on chest x-ray. Bronchoscopy is the preferred diagnostic procedure, although bronchoscopic biopsies are diagnostic in few cases. Gallium scans may be helpful in excluding lymphoma or infection.[18, 19]

Several staging systems have been proposed for AIDS-KS, but none has achieved universal acceptance. The Oncology Committee of the National Institute of Allergy and Infectious Diseases (NIAID) has developed a proposal for staging criteria using a description of the tumor's extent, the status of the patient's immune system, and presence or absence of other HIV-related disease manifestations (Table 13–5).

METASTASIS

Despite the overall progressive course of AIDS-KS, there may be a wide range of disease progression. A rapid course with short survival is seen in patients with opportunistic infections, systemic symptoms, and low CD4 counts. This rapid course is typically associated with aggressive, disseminated disease involving the lungs and visceral organs. In patients with no history of OIs or systemic symptoms and in those with CD4 counts greater than 200 cells/mm^3, the disease may be limited to cutaneous lesions and relatively slow progression.

TREATMENT MODALITIES

Curative therapy for AIDS-KS does not exist. AIDS-KS, however, is rarely life-threatening. Most patients with AIDS-KS ultimately die of OIs related to the profound immunodeficiency produced by HIV infection. Treatment of AIDS-KS is therefore usually instituted

TABLE 13–5
Staging Classification for AIDS-KS

Stage	Definition
TUMOR (T)	
T-0	Confined to skin and/or lymph nodes
	Minimal oral KS
T-1	Tumor-associated edema or ulceration
	Extensive oral KS
	Gastrointestinal KS
	Other visceral KS
IMMUNE SYSTEM (I)	
I-0	T4 helper cells $\geq$ 200/mm^3
I-1	T4 helper cells $\leq$ 200/mm^3
SYSTEMIC ILLNESS (S)	
S-0	No history of opportunistic infection or thrush
	No constitutional symptoms
	Karnofsky performance score $\geq$ 70
S-1	History of opportunistic infection and/or thrush
	Constitutional symptoms
	Karnofsky performance < 70
	Other related HIV illness

to relieve symptoms and to eliminate or reduce cosmetically unacceptable lesions.

In patients who have minimal cutaneous disease, several treatment options exist. Observation alone is a possibility, because the lesions themselves are not usually painful and typically cause no morbidity or mortality. Patients, however, may choose one of the local modalities to reduce unacceptable cosmetic appearance. Local modalities include surgical excision, cryotherapy, and radiation therapy and intralesional injection.

Generally, KS is very responsive to *radiation therapy,* and good palliation can usually be obtained. Excellent responses can be obtained in treatment of cutaneous KS using whole body electron beam therapy, fractionated focal x-ray therapy, or single-dose treatments. Radiation therapy is particularly useful when a prompt local response is desired. Electron beam therapy is highly effective in cutaneous KS although relapse is common. Although the optimal dose of radiation is controversial, 20 to 40 Gy is the most common range used. It is important to note, however, that patients with AIDS-KS seem to be unusually sensitive to radiation in specific areas, including the oral cavity, pharynx, and feet.[15, 18]

Intralesional injections with vincristine, vinblastine, or α-interferon have been effective in the management of isolated lesions, although relapse is common, typically within 4 to 6 months. β- Human chorionic gonadotropin (β-HCG) has also been used as an intralesional agent.

Patients with more rapidly progressive disease may benefit from *chemotherapy.* Chemotherapy is most appropriate for patients who have relatively limited disease and for those with relatively intact immune function. Single-agent chemotherapy can produce cosmetic and symptomatic improvement with little toxicity or significant immune impairment. Overall, single-agent chemotherapy may control disease in approximately 30% to 50% of patients, although responses are usually partial and of limited duration. Single-agent chemotherapy regimens may employ vinblastine, bleomycin, VP-16, or doxorubicin. Interferon may also be used as a single-agent systemic agent. Interferon offers unique mechanisms of action, including antiviral, immune modulator, and antiangiogenic activities. Although initial responses may not be seen with interferon for as long as 8 weeks, there is a relatively long duration of action and response rates may exceed 40% in patients with limited HIV disease. Single-agent regimens of paclitaxel at 150 to 175 mg/m^2 have demonstrated substantial activity against advanced KS. Liposomal encapsulated doxorubicin has also shown good response, generally in the range of 70% to 90%. Due to the excellent response rates, along with diminished toxicity, use of liposomal encapsulated doxorubicin as single-agent therapy has generally become the initial treatment of choice for rapidly progressive disseminated KS.

Combination chemotherapy has also been used successfully in the treatment of AIDS-KS. Although there is no standard regimen of choice in combination chemotherapy, the use of multiple agent regimens had produced response rates of as high as 80%, with complete responses in 30% of patients. Combination therapy is generally preferred for patients with widespread KS, which results in functional impairment secondary to edema, pain, or disfigurement. Visceral KS may also be managed with combination chemotherapy. Combination regimens may include vinblastine and vincristine; vinblastine and bleomycin; doxorubicin, bleomycin, and vinblastine; doxorubicin, bleomycin, and vincristine; or vinblastine, vincristine, and methotrexate. The combination regimen of ABV (doxorubicin, bleomycin, and vincristine/vinblastine) is the most frequently used combination regimen.[18]

Myelotoxicity and *neurotoxicity* have been the major adverse effects. However, the availability of hematopoietic growth factors (G-CSF, GM-CSF) may alleviate the myelotoxicity in a number of patients. With less myelotoxicity and improved disease response, a survival advantage may be obtained in the future.

AIDS-KS has potential disease-related and treatment-related complications.

COMPLICATIONS
AIDS-KS *Disease and Treatment*

Potential Disease-Related Complications

Disfigurement related to skin lesions
Airway obstruction related to pulmonary lesions
Nausea, vomiting, diarrhea related to gastrointestinal lesions

Potential Treatment-Related Complications

Radiation
  Skin: erythema, dry/wet desquamation
  Abdomen: gastritis, nausea, vomiting
  General: fatigue
Chemotherapy
  Neutropenia
  Increased risk of opportunistic infection (OI)
  Nausea, vomiting
  Alopecia
Interferon therapy
  Flulike syndrome
  Weight loss
  Rash
  Neutropenia and resultant increased risk of OI

PROGNOSIS

Despite significant progress in the treatment options available for patients with AIDS-KS, this unfortunately has not translated into an improvement in overall survival. Because optimal therapy of all stages is still in an early phase of development, patients are encouraged to enter into clinical trials whenever possible. Although curative therapy for AIDS-KS does not yet exist, KS is rarely life-threatening. Most patients with AIDS-KS ultimately die of OIs that develop as a result of the profound immunodeficiency that develops secondary to HIV infection.

Non-Hodgkin's Lymphoma

Non-Hodgkin's lymphomas (NHLs) are a diverse group of lymphoid malignancies. Intermediate-grade and high-grade NHLs occur at an increased frequency in HIV-infected persons. Additionally, these lymphomas demonstrate distinct biologic properties in this subgroup of patients. Although HAART has led to marked decreases in the incidence of most AIDS-associated opportunistic infections and malignancies, trends in HIV-associated lymphomas have been less clear. HIV-related NHL appears to be decreasing in frequency as immune deficiency is improved, but still represents 27% of all new cases of lymphoma.[18]

EPIDEMIOLOGY

The epidemiology data indicate a disproportionate number of cases among HIV-infected patients, with rates 191 times higher than the general population.[13] The median age of diagnosis in HIV-related NHL ranges from 26 to 40 years; the median age among HIV-negative patients is 56. Clearly, immunosuppression as a result of HIV infection is a risk factor in the development of NHL. Over 85% of NHL cases in HIV-positive patients are of intermediate- and high-grade B-cell tumors; the remaining lymphomas include T-cell malignancies such as lymphoblastic lymphoma, cutaneous T-cell lymphoma and peripheral T-cell lymphoma. AIDS-associated B-cell NHL (AIDS-NHL) occurs in 3% to 10% of all persons with HIV infection. Approximately 80% are systemic lymphomas, whereas 20% are present as primary CNS tumors. AIDS-NHL occurs at similar frequencies among all HIV-positive groups with two notable exceptions: AIDS-NHL occurs at twice the frequency in whites compared to African Americans and at twice the frequency in men than women.[9]

ETIOLOGY AND RISK FACTORS

The etiology of lymphoid neoplasia in the setting of HIV infection remains unclear. Lack of similarity in the molecular characteristics of these tumors suggests that several different mechanisms may be responsible for the development of lymphoma in HIV-infected individuals. Pathogenesis of many of these lymphomas has been linked to latent infection of B lymphocytes with the *Epstein-Barr virus* (EBV). EBV does seem to be present in approximately 50% of the tumors with monoclonal origins, but not in those of polyclonal origin. Other viral infections may also play a role in the etiology of AIDS-NHL. KSHV8, the human herpes virus generally associated with KS, has been isolated in a rare form of lymphoma known as body cavity lymphoma, which generally occurs in the pleura, pericardium, and peritoneum.

Hyperstimulation of B cells also appears to play a role in the development of AIDS-NHL. Hyperstimulation of B cells in HIV patients may result from depression of T-cell regulation, intrinsic B-cell defects, or alterations in regulatory cytokines. Chronic stimulation of B cells may result in spontaneous proliferation and transformation of the B-cell line.

Immunodeficiency also appears to play a critical role in the development of AIDS-NHL, particularly among the EBV-associated tumors. Systemic lymphomas, however, may be less closely linked to profound immune deficiency than other forms. Although HAART is relatively new, recent reviews of trends in malignant diseases since the introduction of HAART reveals significant reductions in the incidence of KS (55%), the incidence of AIDS-NHL dropped by considerably less (only 37%). These data may indicate the partial immune reconstitution seen with HAART therapy may simply be insufficient to prevent the occurrence of AIDS-NHL. It should be noted, however, that primary CNS lymphomas do seem to be closely related to profound immune deficiency, and occur at a median CD4 count of less than 50 cells/mL.[9]

Genetic factors also play a role in the development of AIDS-NHL. Activation of the *c-myc* cellular oncogene occurs in over half of the EBV-associated AIDS-NHLs. Additionally, translocations and point mutations are also seen in certain forms of NHL, including the t(8:14) translocation in AIDS-related Burkitt's lymphoma.

PREVENTION, SCREENING, AND DETECTION

Currently, there is no known way to prevent or screen for NHL. Clinicians should be suspicious of a NHL diagnosis in any HIV-infected patient who presents with a history of a lump or other mass. Laboratory studies are difficult to evaluate in this patient population. A complete blood count is usually normal, although anemia may be present and lymphopenia can occur in as many as 50% of patients. Erythrocyte sedimentation rate and lactic acid dehydrogenase may be elevated, although these elevations may also be attributable to HIV diseases or OI.

CLASSIFICATION

NHLs in HIV-infected patients are classified similarly to those occurring in noninfected patients. Rappaport introduced a classification system for the various histologic types of NHL in the late 1950s. This classification system has been formalized and is now commonly referred to as the *Working Formulation*.

In the Working Formulation classification scheme, the HIV-associated NHLs are generally placed in the intermediate-grade and high-grade categories. Most cases of HIV-related NHL consist of high-grade NHL with B phenotype. The most represented histologies are Burkitt's lymphomas, immunoblastic lymphomas, and the otherwise nonspecified "undifferentiated" lymphomas. Diffuse large cell lymphoma (DLCL), particularly of the high-grade immunoblastic type (IBL), is the most frequently diagnosed HIV-related NHL.

With the use of the more recent REAL (Revised European and American Lymphoma) classification system, the most common subtypes (approximately 50%) would include the diffuse large B-cell lymphomas (previously IBLs and DLCLs). Approximately 40% of AIDS-NHLs are identified as small noncleaved cell lymphomas, also known as Burkitt's or high-grade B cell, Burkitt-like, in the REAL system. The remaining 10% of AIDS-NHL cannot be classified.[18]

CLINICAL FEATURES

Patients presenting with HIV-associated NHL are a heterogeneous group. The most common symptom of NHL is painless lymphadenopathy that may involve the abdominal nodes. Systemic AIDS-NHL is often widespread at presentation, with extranodal involvement. One third of patients with NHL have had preceding persistent generalized lymphadenopathy (PGL). Patients may present with systemic "B" symptoms such as fever, chills, and weight loss, although these symptoms may be difficult to differentiate from those associated with HIV infection and related OIs. Because extranodal sites such as the GI tract, bone marrow, spleen, and liver may be affected, patients may have symptoms of vague abdominal discomfort, back pain, GI complaints, or ascites. Other unusual sites of disease may include the anus, rectum, heart, adrenal glands, mouth, muscle, and soft tissues.

DIAGNOSIS AND STAGING

The findings of lymphadenopathy, splenomegaly, or hepatomegaly suggest lymphoma, but NHL may also present as an abdominal mass or as a discrete lesion of the lung or CNS. A complete physical examination is essential. In addition, routine tests, including a complete blood count and chemistries, should be obtained. Abnormal liver function tests may suggest involvement of the hepatic system, and liver biopsy may be indicated. Bone marrow involvement is common in HIV-associated NHL, and bone marrow aspiration and biopsy should be performed early in the diagnostic workup. Chest x-ray evaluation may reveal mediastinal, hilar, or parenchymal involvement, and more sophisticated nuclear medicine studies such as the CT scan and magnetic resonance imaging (MRI) can be used to scan the liver and spleen. Gallium-67 scans and other tests, including a GI series or endoscopy, may also be helpful. Patients with neurologic symptoms should have brain MRI or CT scans and cerebrospinal fluid evaluation to rule out the presence of leptomeningeal lymphoma.

Final diagnosis is based on morphologic evaluation of fixed, paraffin-embedded haematoxylin/eosin-stained tissue. The clinical value of the staging laparotomy has yet to be demonstrated, and bone marrow evaluation may provide adequate information.

Although its prognostic significance is unknown, the Ann Arbor Staging Classification is used to categorize the extent of disease, as follows:

Stage I   Involvement of a single lymph node region or of a single extralymphatic organ or site

Stage II   Involvement of two or more lymph node regions on the same side of the diaphragm

Stage III   Involvement of lymph node regions on both sides of the diaphragm

Stage IV   Disseminated involvement of one or more extralymphatic organs or tissues

Prognostic features may be helpful in the staging process as well. Those features indicating a poorer prognosis include: poor performance status, CD4 count below 200, presence of extranodal disease, presence of bone marrow involvement, and the presence of EBV sequences in tumors.

METASTASIS

Few patients present with stage I disease or II. In fact, most patients present with stage IV disease, which is further complicated by frequent involvement of the bone marrow and the CNS. In addition, the immunodeficiency and possible history of previous OIs may potentiate the aggressive course of the disease. Widely disseminated disease is diagnosed at the initial presentation in more than two thirds of patients. Also common to this population is the occurrence of unusual sites of lymphomatous disease, including the myocardium, adrenals, ear lobes, maxillae, gallbladder, orbit, and rectum.[18]

TREATMENT MODALITIES

Treatment of patients with HIV-related NHL is often complicated by their underlying immunodeficiency. As a group, these patients generally do not respond well to treatment. Those patients more likely to tolerate intensive therapy and to do relatively well are those without a prior history of profound immunodeficiency or OIs. Unfortunately, many patients have significant immunodeficiency at presentation. In addition, most patients have advanced stage IV disease of a high-grade type with possible involvement of the bone marrow and/ or CNS. The neutropenia frequently seen in this patient population secondary to the HIV infection further complicates the use of conventional multiagent chemotherapy regimens.

Recent approaches to treatment have focused on variations in the dosing of the standard chemotherapeutic agents. Hematopoietic growth factors have also been used to alleviate the myeloid toxicity associated with chemotherapy. These trials have demonstrated that hematologic toxicity can be reduced by using reduced dosages of chemotherapy and by using myeloid growth factors with standard doses. It is still unclear, however, which of these treatment approaches will be associated with improved response and survival.[18]

In general, standard chemotherapy doses should be given to patients with CD4 counts greater than 200 cells/mm³. Growth factor support is also recommended in this population. For patients with more compromised immune function (with CD4 cell counts < 200), reduced-dosage chemotherapy regimens are advised because these patients are less likely to tolerate cytotoxic therapy. The most frequently used regimen is that of mBACOD, which includes methotrexate, bleomycin, doxorubicin, cyclophosphamide, vincristine, dexamethasone, and folinic acid, and CHOP, which includes cyclophosphamide, doxorubicin, vincristine, and prednisone. For patients who are profoundly ill with significantly compromised immune status, the option of only palliative therapy should be considered.

A small number of patients have been treated with high-dose chemotherapy followed by allogeneic or syngeneic bone marrow transplantation. Clinical trials to evaluate the merit of this therapy are currently in progress.

Leptomeningeal lymphoma is generally treated with radiotherapy and biweekly intraventricular infusions of cytosine arabinoside, methotrexate, and hydrocortisone through an Ommaya reservoir. Therapy is continued until no lymphoma cells are detected in the cerebrospinal fluid. Use of CNS prophylaxis in patients who present with systemic lymphoma, but not CNS involvement, is controversial.

Immunotherapy regimens have also been used in this patient population in an effort to stimulate the endogenous immune response to the lymphoma. Interleukin-2 (IL-2) has been used, with small numbers reporting complete responses (2 of 12 patients). Adoptive immunotherapy is also being studied. In this approach, the patient's T lymphocytes are removed and expanded ex vivo. The cells are then treated with a variety of biologic agents to improve their cytotoxicity against the lymphoma prior to their return to the patient. Although the numbers of patients in these studies are small and the trials are ongoing, these immunomodulatory approaches may prove beneficial in the treatment of this disease.[18]

Non-Hodgkin's lymphoma has potential disease-related and treatment-related complications.

PROGNOSIS

The prognosis for patients with HIV-associated NHL is poor. Median survival for patients with peripheral NHL treated with a variety of standard chemotherapeutic regimens ranges from 4 to 7 months in patients with fewer than 100 CD4 cells. For those with CNS involvement, the prognosis is even poorer, with median survival

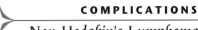

COMPLICATIONS
Non-Hodgkin's Lymphoma (NHL) Disease and Treatment

Disease-Related Complications

Pain secondary to lymphadenopathy and associated dysfunction

Mental status changes secondary to central nervous system involvement

Abdominal pain secondary to hepatic, splenic, or gastrointestinal involvement

Fatigue secondary to constitutional symptoms of fever, chills, and weight loss

Treatment-Related Complications

Infection related to myelotoxicity of chemotherapy

Fatigue related to myelotoxicity of chemotherapy

Altered nutrition secondary to emetigenic potential of chemotherapy, mucositis, stomatitis

Pain related to mucositis associated with chemotherapy

Pain and self-care deficit secondary to peripheral neuropathy related to chemotherapy

Altered respiratory function related to chemotherapy

of approximately 2.5 months. Treatment for these patients, however, has a significant impact on survival, because the anticipated survival for untreated patients would be on the order of weeks.

Patients with CD4 counts greater than 100 have a median survival of 24 months. These patients are more likely to tolerate intensive therapy, because they present without prior history of OI and with higher performance status.

Other HIV-Related Malignancies

In addition to the more common HIV-related malignancies such as KS and NHL, a variety of other malignancies are also becoming evident. Unfortunately, it is becoming apparent that as patients live longer with HIV disease, more malignancies may become clinically significant.

PRIMARY CNS LYMPHOMA

Primary CNS lymphoma (PCNSL) is of B-cell origin in the majority of reported cases. It is not simply a manifestation of systemic NHL, but instead is a discrete entity. HIV-infected individuals demonstrate an increased frequency of primary CNS lymphoma, and it is now estimated that its incidence represents 10% to 20% of all cases of AIDS-NHL. The frequency in HIV-infected individuals is 1000 times higher than in the general population.

It is difficult to diagnose CNS lymphoma in the setting of HIV disease because the differential diagnoses include a variety of OIs involving the CNS. Presenting signs and symptoms may include confusion, lethargy, memory loss, hemiparesis or dysphasia, seizures, or headaches. Peripheral adenopathy is usually absent.

Computed tomography brain scanning is usually non-specific for CNS lymphoma, and lumbar puncture is rarely diagnostic. Open brain biopsy is technically required to confirm the diagnosis. Approximately 90% of patients with PCNSL exhibit B symptoms, including fever, night sweats, and weight loss of 10% or more, and have CD4 counts below 50 cells/mm^3. PCNSLs are usually high-grade large-cell lymphomas, and virtually all contain EBV virus, suggesting a strong association between PCNSL and EBV.

The current treatment approach includes combination radiation therapy and corticosteroids. Typical course involves the administration of 4000 to 5000 rads over 3 weeks. Response rates vary widely, from 17% to 60%. The prognosis for these individuals remains poor, with long-term survival of only a few months.[18]

CERVICAL CANCER

The gynecologic problems associated with HIV infection include a variety of sexually transmitted diseases, pelvic inflammatory disease, genital ulcers, vaginal candidiasis, and cervical intraepithelial neoplasia (CIN), which can be a precursor to cervical cancer. The most common neoplasia of the cervix, squamous cell neoplasia, has been linked to early age of first sexual intercourse, multiple sexual partners, and infection with the human papillomavirus (HPV). HPV is also thought to be the causative agent for most condylomata acuminata (genital warts).

Genital warts in HIV-infected women may exist as multiple small lesions or as unusually large and profuse lesions. External warts often extend to adjacent, moist epithelium, including the vagina, cervix, urethra, and rectum. Cervical dysplasia, the premalignant changes noted on Papanicolaou (Pap) smear screening, can result from HPV infection and can progress to cervical cancer. Cervical dysplasia occurs at an unusually high rate in HIV-infected women, at 5 to 10 times the expected rate. Cervical cancer caused by HPV is potentially fatal and is the most serious gynecologic disease for HIV-infected women. In addition, cervical dysplasia and cancer may be more aggressive and persistent among HIV-positive women than among uninfected women.[18, 19]

The presence and severity of CIN correlates with both absolute number and function of CD4 cells. Women with more profound immunodeficiency are more likely to have high-grade lesions than asymptomatic HIV-positive women. Lymph node involvement is common, although greatly enlarged nodes may also result from HIV disease. Women with HIV disease also have higher recurrence and death rates with shorter intervals to recurrence.

The best way to screen for cervical dysplasia and cervical cancer is controversial. Pap smears may yield a high rate of false-negative results when compared to colposcopic evaluation, so colposcopic examination should be considered for HIV-positive women, particularly those who are found to be HPV positive.

Although observation of low-grade dysplastic lesions may be adequate in HIV-negative women, observation is not sufficient in the HIV-positive population. For patients with early disease, studies are evaluating the use of topical 5-fluorouracil and oral isotretinoin. Because CIN is more common in HIV-infected women and progresses at a more rapid rate to high-grade dysplasia, effective management of cervical carcinoma in HIV-positive women is contingent on early detection. CIN in HIV-positive women does not respond well to standard therapy and response rates appear to be related to CD4 counts. Recurrence rates as high as 61% have been reported after electrosurgical excision.

Wide excision of stage I cervical cancers by simple or radical hysterectomy appears to be equivalent to radiation therapy in HIV-negative patients. Although similar results may be seen in the HIV-positive population, this is not currently validated by clinical trials. Radical hysterectomy and pelvic lymphadenectomy may be performed safely for HIV-positive patients with later stage lesions. Later stage lesions are usually treated by radiation therapy. In patients with advanced or systemic disease, chemotherapy may be used along with radiation therapy, although careful monitoring of hematologic toxicities must be performed. Drugs that are relatively sparing of the bone marrow, such as cisplatin, bleomycin, and vincristine, may be used.[18]

ANAL CARCINOMA

Anal carcinoma in HIV-infected men is similar to cervical carcinoma in HIV-infected women. Increasing numbers of men with concurrent HIV and HPV infection are now showing signs of intra-anal cytologic abnormalities. More than 50% of patients with abnormal anal cytology have been shown to have HPV DNA on specimen. The prevalence of these abnormalities seems to increase with time in serial follow-up.[20]

Anal intraepithelial neoplasia (AIN), as with CIN, can develop into a malignant process. Because there is no widespread screening program for anal disease, it has been difficult to assess the true incidence of AIN in HIV-infected men. Data generated through cancer and AIDS registries, however, has estimated the risk of anal carcinoma in homosexual HIV-positive men at 80 times greater than the general population. Approximately 15% of symptomatic HIV-positive men, however, have been shown to have AIN, and this number increases to about 30% over longitudinal follow-up. The risk appears to increase with advancing immunosuppression.[16, 17] Because anal cancer may take several years to develop from AIN, it seems likely that the rate of anal cancer will continue to increase as immunosuppressed individuals live longer.

Patients with anal carcinoma have a much higher incidence of venereal warts compared with patients with carcinoma of the colon or rectum. What role HIV plays in the pathogenesis of this malignancy has yet to be defined. HIV may promote the development of HPV-related malignancies or may allow a broadened expression of the latent HPV.

Early stages of anal cancer and AIN usually are not associated with any symptoms. Some individuals may notice rapid growth of an external anal lesion or may develop new onset of anal pruritus or a change in bowel habits. In advanced disease, anal cancer may be associated with weight loss, pelvic pain, and even obstruction of the anal canal.

The natural history of AIN is currently under study. It is not yet known what percentage of those with AIN will go on to develop anal cancer if left untreated. It seems likely, however, that treatment of AIN will prevent the development of anal cancer. It therefore seems reasonable to perform an anal Pap test and anoscopy on any HIV-positive patient with new-onset signs or symptoms related to anal carcinoma and on those who have a history of venereal warts. Although the optimal forms of treatment have not yet been identified, fulguration or cryotherapy of anal lesions through the use of a proctoscope or sigmoidoscope seems reasonable. If the lesion has progressed to anal carcinoma, chemotherapy and possibly radiation therapy may be considered.

OTHER MALIGNANCIES

The development of malignancy in HIV-positive patients is a complex process, which involves a variety of interactions between the immune system and multiple infectious agents, including HIV, EBV, HHV8, and HPV. It is not surprising to find an increased incidence of various cancers in this patient population. Although the most prevalent malignancies are KS and NHL, several other malignancies may occur at higher rates in this population of patients when compared to those who are not HIV positive.

Although only a few cases of *malignant melanoma* have been reported in HIV-positive patients, this incidence may increase as survival is extended in this population. The incidence of malignant melanoma in renal transplant patients, a group with iatrogenic immunosuppression, is reported to be approximately four times that of the general population. Because this is probably related to immunosuppression, the same increase may occur in the HIV-infected population. The possibility of an increased incidence of *hepatocellular carcinoma* also seems likely in HIV-infected patients who are concurrently infected with chronic hepatitis B. Other malignancies, which have been reported in HIV-positive patients, include testicular cancer, basal cell carcinoma, lung cancer, squamous cell carcinoma, and Hodgkin's disease.

CONCLUSION

HIV disease has quickly become an overwhelming epidemic, claiming the lives of hundreds of thousands of people throughout the world and threatening to defeat the current health care delivery systems. It is a sexually transmitted, blood-borne viral infection that destroys the host's immune system, resulting in life-threatening opportunistic infections and a variety of malignant processes. Throughout the world, more than 12 million people have been infected with HIV. More than 40,000 new infections are expected this year in the United States alone. Worldwide, HIV continues to ravage men, women, and children. As the number of infected individuals continues to grow and as scientific advances are made with this disease, extending the life span of those infected, health care systems will be burdened even more with the ever-increasing load of patients requiring comprehensive, extended care. Caring for the patient with HIV disease is a complex issue given the life-threatening nature of the disease, the relative youth of the affected population, and the sociopolitical issues surrounding the epidemic (see Patient Teaching Priorities box). Nurses have played critical roles in defining the need for comprehensive, compassionate care of patients with HIV disease.

PATIENT TEACHING PRIORITIES

HIV *and Related Cancers*

Risk reduction techniques: minimize the number of sexual partners and engage in a mutually monogamous sexual relationship.

Safe sex counseling: any exchange of blood, semen, or vaginal secretions can potentially put an individual at risk for HIV disease.

Intravenous risk reduction: use of contaminated needles for any injection represents a serious risk for HIV infection.

Signs and symptoms of infectious process: these include fever, chills, shortness of breath, cough, pain, diarrhea, nausea, vomiting, skin breakdown, weight loss, and a sense of mental confusion.

Self-help care strategies: know where and when to seek medical, psychosocial, and financial assistance.

Nursing Management

The nursing management of the patient with HIV disease is complex and demanding. Because the disease has such an unpredictable course, the nurse must be prepared to provide appropriate care to those with early asymptomatic disease, to those who have acute opportunistic infections (OIs), to those battling AIDS-related malignancies, and to those in the terminal stages of their illness (see Complications: HIV Disease and Treatment box).

Nursing Diagnosis

- *Infection, risk for related to disease process, with viral destruction of T4 helper cells; neutropenia related to medication, treatment, or infection; knowledge deficit regarding infection control precautions; or impaired skin integrity*

Assessments

Patients with HIV infection are at risk for developing infections at any stage of the disease because of a number of factors. A variety of signs and symptoms may alert the nurse to an impending or current infection: neutropenia; decreased T4 helper count; fever, chills; impaired skin integrity with or without draining wounds; shortness of breath, cough; mental status change; and nausea, vomiting, or diarrhea.

Outcome Goals

- Patient will remain free of infection.
- Infections will be identified early and treatment initiated quickly.

Interventions

- Carefully monitor vital signs and laboratory results for signs of possible infection.
- Institute a low-microbial diet for patients with an absolute neutrophil count less than 500 cells/cm^3. Patients should receive only pasteurized dairy products and no fresh fruits or vegetables.
- Perform appropriate physical assessment, including careful examination of skin integrity and respiratory and gastrointestinal status.
- Perform appropriate mental status examinations.
- Maintain asepsis when caring for patient, including appropriate handwashing and limiting infectious visitors.
- Educate patient in protective strategies, such as handwashing, diet precautions (e.g., thorough cooking of meat products), pet care precautions, and avoidance of rectal thermometers and suppositories.

Nursing Diagnosis

- *Coping, ineffective individual*

Patients with HIV disease face a chronic, life-threatening illness. In addition, they face stigmatization and often overwhelming discrimination. Ineffective coping may be related to anxiety secondary to having a life-threatening illness, multiple losses secondary to the illness and resultant debilitation, changes in life-style secondary to HIV infection, or changes in self-concept.

Assessments

- Ineffective coping occurs when the individual is unable to manage stressors successfully secondary to lack of personal or external resources.[9] Ineffective coping may be evidenced by:
    Behavioral changes, including sudden mood swings, social withdrawal, anger, depression, anxiety
    Decreased self-esteem
    Inability to solve problems

Outcome Goals

Patient will be able to:

- Devise new coping strategies and enhance current strategies.
- Express feelings and maintain relationships.

Interventions

- Establish a therapeutic nursing relationship using empathy, acceptance, and support.
- Facilitate expression of patient's feelings.
- Assist patient in identification of past and current coping strategies and effective and ineffective skills.
- Identify resources available to patient, including family members, friends, clergy, and support groups.
- Use multidisciplinary resources, including social services, clergy, and psychiatry.

Nursing Diagnosis

- *Knowledge deficit related to disease and treatment*

Patients with HIV disease often have an overwhelming amount of information to assimilate regarding their illness and treatment. Knowledge deficits may be related to disease process, various treatment modalities, infection control, or protective mechanisms.

Assessments

Patients exhibit knowledge deficits in a variety of ways. Signs and symptoms that may alert the nurse to potential and actual deficits include new HIV diagnosis, institution of new treatment, inability to perform procedures correctly (e.g., failure to wash hands), failure to maintain infection control mechanisms (e.g., not using condoms during sexual contact), or repeated infections.

Outcome Goals

Patient will be able to:

- Verbalize correct knowledge of illness and treatments.
- Practice appropriate infection control precautions for protection of self and others.

Interventions

- Assess patient's knowledge and learning patterns.
- Provide a variety of educational resources, including videos, printed materials, and one-on-one instruction.
- Provide baseline education to patient regarding illness trajectory, infection control, protective mechanisms, laboratory evaluation, and medication administration.
- Explain all procedures and treatments to patient.
- Encourage patient and family to ask questions.

Nursing Diagnosis

- *Body image disturbance related to cutaneous lesions*

Assessments

A person's self-concept results from thoughts and feelings related to his identity, self-esteem, role performance, and body image.[9] Changes in physical appearance often accompany AIDS-KS and place the patient at risk for disturbance in body image and self-concept. Indications of this disturbance include social withdrawal or isolation, statements of low self-worth, and depression.

Outcome Goals

Patient will be able to:

- Have an improved self-concept.
- Identify and implement strategies for coping with physical disturbance of lesions.
- Maintain social and intimate relationships.
- Verbalize statements reflecting self-worth.

Interventions

- Establish a therapeutic nursing relationship based on acceptance and encouraging open sharing of feelings.
- Identify sources of threats to body image and self-concept.
- Educate patient in use of self-affirmation techniques.
- Facilitate incorporation of past adaptive coping behaviors.
- Involve family and significant others in support of patient.
- Use multidisciplinary group such as dermatology, psychology, social work, and support groups.
- Educate patient in techniques to reduce visibility of lesions.

Nursing Diagnosis

- *Skin integrity, impaired*

Impairment of skin integrity may be related to KS lesions, poor nutritional status secondary to chemotherapy/radiation treatment, or radiation therapy.

Assessments

- Signs and symptoms of actual or impaired skin integrity include erythema, scaling, or broken skin resulting from:
  Draining wounds
  Radiation therapy
  Limited activity patterns

Outcome Goals

- Patient will remain free of skin breakdown and associated infection.
- Breaks in skin integrity will heal.

Interventions

- Assess skin surfaces at least every 8 hours for erythema, breakdown, excessive moisture, or other changes.
- Keep skin clean and dry; provide skin care at least every 4 hours.
- Provide appropriate beds, mattresses, or other appliances for pressure relief.
- Maintain adequate hydration and nutrition.
- Use multidisciplinary team, including dermatology, skin care, and specialty nurse.

Nursing Diagnosis

- *Knowledge deficit related to Kaposi's sarcoma (KS) disease and treatment*

Assessments

Signs and symptoms that may alert the nurse to potential and actual knowledge deficits include new KS diagnosis, institution of new treatment, failure to report new suspicious lesions, and altered coping skills.

Outcome Goals

Patient will be able to:

- Verbalize correct knowledge of illness and treatments.
- Report suspicious lesions.
- Exhibit adequate coping skills.

Interventions

- Assess patient knowledge and learning patterns.
- Provide a variety of educational resources, including videos, printed materials, and one-on-one instruction.
- Explain all procedures and treatments to patient.
- Encourage patient and family to ask questions.

Nursing Diagnosis

- *Nutrition, altered: less than body requirements related to anorexia secondary to chemotherapy or chronic infection; nausea, vomiting, or diarrhea secondary to OI or treatment; impaired swallowing related to mucositis secondary to infection or treatment; or knowledge deficit*

Assessments

Patients with HIV infection in general are at risk for the development of malnutrition. The nutrition of these patients is further compromised when treatments for non-Hodgkin's lymphoma (NHL) are instituted. In addition, these treatment modalities may further compromise the immune status, resulting in GI opportunistic infections, which may further deplete the nutritional status. Signs and symptoms of altered nutritional status include weight loss; anorexia, nausea, and vomiting; dehydration; and mucositis.

Outcome Goal

Patient will be able to:

- Achieve or maintain body weight.

Interventions

- Monitor weight at least weekly with daily recording of intake and output.
- Assess for signs and symptoms of malnutrition, such as weight loss, weakness, fatigue, and decreased intake.
- Monitor laboratory data, such as serum protein, albumin, and electrolyte levels.
- Minimize anorexia, nausea, and vomiting by administering antiemetics; offering small, frequent meals at cool or room temperature; and avoiding spicy foods.
- Assist with good oral hygiene.
- Consult dietitian.
- Educate patient in nutritional needs and ways to reduce nausea, anorexia, and pain.

Chapter Questions

1. Which of the following represents a significant risk factor for transmission of HIV infection?
   a. Intimate kissing
   b. Sharing food or beverages with a person with AIDS
   c. Use of barrier products such as latex condoms
   d. Unprotected sexual intercourse
2. How long does it take after infection for an HIV test to become positive in the average adult?
   a. 24 hours
   b. 72 hours
   c. 2 weeks
   d. 6 to 12 weeks
3. How soon does the average patient develop opportunistic infections after initial infection?
   a. 10 years
   b. 5 years
   c. 2 years
   d. 1 year
4. The cell most frequently infected and destroyed by HIV is:
   a. CD4 suppressor T cell
   b. CD8 suppressor T cell
   c. CD4 helper T cell
   d. CD8 helper T cell
5. The best example of combination antiretroviral therapy for HIV disease is:
   a. AZT + ddI + ddC + biotherapy drugs
   b. ddC + ddI + adriamycin + biotherapy drugs
   c. Protease inhibitor + nucleoside analogues + adriamycin
   d. AZT + ddI + protease inhibitor + biotherapy drugs
6. The most important diagnostic test for a person with AIDS includes:
   a. ELISA
   b. Polymerase chain reaction

c. Viral load studies

d. Western blot

7. An AIDS-related malignancy characterized by multifocal, widespread lesions of the skin and oral mucosa is most likely:

a. Cervical cancer

b. Hodgkin's disease

c. Kaposi's sarcoma

d. Non-Hodgkin's lymphoma

8. *Pneumocyctitis carnii* is the most common opportunistic infection, occurring in ___% of HIV-infected patients.

a. 100%

b. 85%

c. 75%

d. 65%

9. The most current U.S. population distribution of *NEW* HIV-infected individuals include:

a. Homosexual men 80%; women 10%; intravenous drug users 15%

b. Homosexual men 60%; women 30%; intravenous drug users 25%

c. Homosexual men 55%; women 20%; intravenous drug users 35%

d. Homosexual men 70%; women 30%; intravenous drug users 15%

10. AIDS-related cervical cancer is most likely related to:

a. Human papillomavirus

b. Concurrent herpes simplex infection

c. Epstein-Barr virus

d. *Toxoplasma* infection

BIBLIOGRAPHY

1. Blattner, WA: Human retroviruses: their role in cancer, *Proc Assoc Am Physicians* 111(6):563, 1999.

2. Brockmeyer N, Barthel, B: Clinical manifestations and therapies of AIDS associated tumors, *Eur J Med Res* 3(3):127, 1998.

3. Centers for Disease Control and Prevention: A glance at the HIV epidemic, *MMWR* 48(8):1, 1999.

4. Centers for Disease Control and Prevention: First 500,000 AIDS cases—United States, 1995, *MMWR* 44(46):840, 1995.

5. Centers for Disease Control and Prevention: HIV and its transmission, *MMWR* 48(8):61, 1999.

6. Centers for Disease Control and Prevention: Human immunodeficiency virus type 2, *MMWR* 47(9):8, 1998.

7. Centers for Disease Control and Prevention: CDC's international activities support global HIV prevention efforts, *MMWR* 48(4):1, 1999.

8. Gee G: *AIDS: concepts in nursing practice,* Baltimore, Williams & Wilkins, 1988.

9. Grulich AE: AIDS associated non-hodgkin's lymphoma in the era of highly active antiretroviral therapy. *J Acquir Immune Defic Syndr* 21(Suppl):S27, 1999.

10. Jacobson LP and others: Impact of potent antiretroviral therapy on the incidence of Kaposi's sarcoma and non-Hodgkin's lymphomas among HIV-1 infected individuals. Multicenter AIDS Cohort Study: *J Acquir Immune Defic Syndr* 21(Suppl 1):S34, 1999.

11. Johnson SC, Gerber JG: Advances in HIV/AIDS therapy, *Adv Intern Med* 45:1, 2000.

12. Lusso P, Gallo R: Pathogenesis of AIDS, *J Pharmaceut Pharmacol* 44(suppl 1):160, 1992.

13. Maiman M: Cervical cancer as an AIDS defining illness. *Obstet Gynecol* 89(1):76, 1997.

14. McPhedran P: Using hematopoietic hormones in HIV disease, *AIDS Clin Care* 4(6):43, 1992.

15. Northfelt D: AIDS-associated Kaposi's sarcoma, *AIDS File* 6(1):1, 1992.

16. Palefsky J: Anal cancer among HIV-positive men, *AIDS File* 6(1):9, 1992.

17. Rabkin CS and others: Kaposi's sarcoma and non-Hodgkin's lymphoma incidence trends in AIDS Clinical Trial Group study participants: *J Acquir Immune Defic Syndr* 21(Suppl 1):S31, 1999.

18. Smith C: AIDS related malignancies, *Ann Med* 30(4):323, 2000.

19. Thompson D: Invincible AIDS, *Time,* August 3, 1992, p 30.

20. Silvestris N: AIDS related Kaposi's sarcoma: principal pathogenic mechanisms, *J Exp Clin Cancer Res* 18(3):311, 1999.

21. Sparano JA and others: Effect of highly active antiretroviral therapy on the incidence of HIV associated malignancies at an urban medical center: *J Acquir Immune Defic Syndr* 21(Suppl 1):S18, 1999.

Leukemia

Rosanne Eble Ososki

The leukemias are a complex collection of diseases that were first described in 1845 by Virchow. He described a condition in which the relationship between red and colorless corpuscles was the reverse of normal. He coined the term *weisses blut,* or "white blood."[72]

The two major classifications of leukemia are *acute* and *chronic.* These two types of leukemia are similar in that they are the products of dysfunctional bone marrow, but they differ dramatically in disease presentation, treatment, and prognosis. The cell line of origin can characterize acute and chronic leukemia as *myeloid* or *lymphoid.*

An understanding of any leukemia must begin with knowledge of normal bone marrow function, which is described in the first section of this chapter. This chapter is divided into three major sections: acute leukemias, chronic leukemias, and nursing management of the patient with leukemia. Hairy-cell leukemia and myelodysplastic syndromes are also discussed.

Much of the scientific knowledge of adult leukemia is derived from the studies done on pediatric leukemia. Although pediatric leukemia is referred to in this chapter, especially in the section on acute lymphoblastic leukemia, the focus of this chapter is the adult patient with leukemia.

PATHOPHYSIOLOGY

Leukemia is a malignant hematologic disorder characterized by a proliferation of abnormal white blood cells (WBCs) that infiltrate the bone marrow, peripheral blood, and other organs. Leukemia may present as an acute or chronic disease process.

Elements of the blood are formed in the bone marrow, vertebrae, clavicle, scapula, sternum, ribs, skull, proximal ends of long bones, and pelvis in children. In adults, most of the blood cells are produced in the pelvis, sternum, and vertebrae. The body can be imagined to have three pools of blood cells (Fig. 14–1). The first

pool of cells are the *pluripotent stem cells* of the bone marrow, the most primitive form of blood cell from which all blood cells originate. The stem cell pool is responsible for the generation of new cells to meet the body's requirements throughout the person's lifetime. The pluripotent stem cell can proliferate and differentiate. The decision to proliferate or differentiate is based on the body's current needs. With every stem cell division, one daughter cell remains in the stem cell pool, so the lifetime pool of stem cells is never depleted. An injury to the stem cell pool, such as a lethal dose of radiation, prevents the production of blood cells and results in marrow aplasia. The stem cell pool cannot be assessed by a routine bone marrow examination. Studies of the stem cell population are called *colony-forming assays* and are performed by in vitro culturing. In the bone marrow, blood cells mature within a framework of supportive cells and blood vessels that supply nutrition and growth factors for proliferation and differentiation.[14, 42] Proliferation of stem cells is mediated by specific *colony-stimulating factors* (CSFs) acting on progenitor cells to give rise to granulocytes, erythrocytes, macrophages, and megakaryocytes.[6]

The second pool of cells is *precursor cells* for red blood cells (RBCs), platelets, granulocytes, and lymphocytes. A stem cell becomes committed to a certain blood cell line when it leaves the stem cell pool. In the second pool the cells differentiate and mature. Figure 14–1 illustrates the steps of cell differentiation and maturation. In the second pool, cells at the blast phase of development cannot function as mature blood cells, but they can undergo mitosis. At this stage of development the *blast cells* (the least differentiated cells with commitment as to their bloodline) may be responsive to specific CSFs. Each cell divides multiple times at the early stages shown. As the cells divide, they differentiate, enabling them to carry out only specific functions, and they lose their proliferative response to CSFs. In the myeloid series, cells lose their proliferative ability after the my-

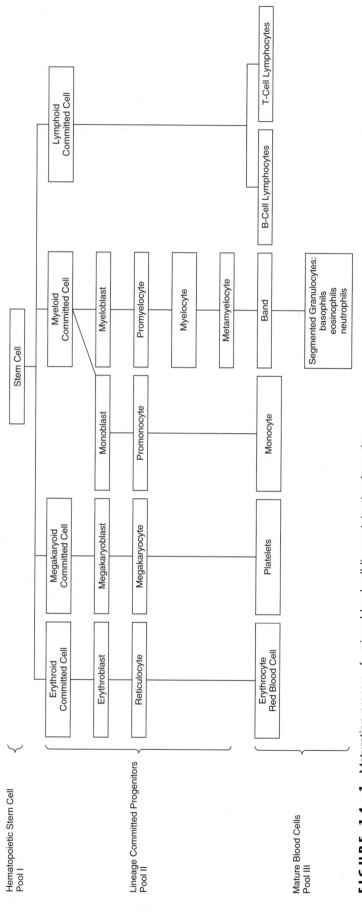

FIGURE 14 – 1 Maturation process of various blood cell lines originating from the stem cell.

Hematopoietic Stem Cell
Pool I

Lineage Committed Progenitors
Pool II

Mature Blood Cells
Pool III

Stem Cell

Erythroid Committed Cell

Megakaryoid Committed Cell

Myeloid Committed Cell

Lymphoid Committed Cell

Erythroblast

Megakaryoblast

Monoblast

Myeloblast

Reticulocyte

Megakaryocyte

Promonocyte

Promyelocyte

Myelocyte

Metamyelocyte

Erythrocyte Red Blood Cell

Platelets

Monocyte

Band

Segmented Granulocytes: basophils eosinophils neutrophils

B-Cell Lymphocytes

T-Cell Lymphocytes

elocytic stages.[14, 42] The process by which stem cells undergo self-renewal or commitment to differentiate is not known.

When the precursor cells of the second pool are mature, they are released into the *peripheral circulation,* the third pool. Each mature blood cell performs a specific function (RBCs—oxygen transport; granulocytes—phagocytosis; platelets—clotting). The mature circulating cells cannot undergo mitosis and must be replaced at the end of their life span (RBCs—120 days; granulocytes—6 to 8 hours; platelets—8 to 10 days). Mature blood cells are released from the bone marrow in response to the body's need.

In leukemia the control factors regulating the orderly differentiation and maturation of the blood cells are absent. This lack of regulatory control results in the arrest of the maturation process of a specific cell line. The involved immature cell form proliferates and accumulates in the bone marrow, resulting in crowding of the normal marrow cells. This marrow crowding impairs the production and function of normal cell lines; ultimately, leukemic cells, which are released into the circulating blood, replace the marrow. The leukemic cells may also invade body organs. In chronic lymphocytic leukemia, cell death is not regulated and the cells accumulate.

The specific type of leukemia depends on which stem cell line is affected (myeloid or lymphoid) and the point of maturation at which growth is arrested. Acute leukemias result from arrest of immature blood cells; chronic leukemias involve more mature blood cells and are due to failure of cells to die in chronic lymphocytic leukemia (CLL). In chronic myeloid leukemia (CML), the progenitor cells undergo more frequent mitosis than normal. Leukemic cells actually generate more slowly than normal WBCs, but the mechanisms controlling cellular division are errant, allowing more cells to be capable of division at any point in time.

Acute Leukemias

Acute leukemia is a severe and aggressive disease characterized by rapid onset and a rapidly terminal course if untreated. There are two types of acute leukemia: *lymphocytic* or *lymphoblastic* (ALL) and *myeloid* or *myelogenous* (AML).

In acute leukemia, the leukemic or blast cells function abnormally and accumulate in the peripheral blood, bone marrow, reticuloendothelial system (RES), and possibly the central nervous system (CNS). The overproduction of leukemic cells in the bone marrow impairs normal hematopoiesis, resulting in anemia, granulocytopenia, and thrombocytopenia.

Acute Lymphocytic (Lymphoblastic) Leukemia

EPIDEMIOLOGY AND ETIOLOGY

The exact etiology of ALL is unknown. High-dose radiation, chemicals, drugs, viruses, and genetic abnormalities have been implicated in the etiology of this disease.[130] A causal relationship between the human T-cell leukemia virus types I (HTLV-I) and T-cell leukemias and lymphoma is suspected but not proved.[2]

An estimated 30,800 new cases of leukemia will occur in 2000, divided equally between acute and chronic leukemias. Adults are diagnosed more frequently than are children (28,200 versus 2600). ALL will have approximately 3200 new cases with 1800 of them children.[2] ALL is the least common of the four major leukemia categories—AML, ALL, CML, and CLL.[5] In adults the most common are acute myelocytic (approximately 9700) and chronic lymphocytic (approximately 8100).[2] Whites are more frequently affected than African Americans. Twenty percent of acute leukemias in adults are ALL.[114]

Acute lymphocytic leukemia has a bimodal distribution. The initial peak in children occurs at less than 5 years of age. The second peak occurs after age 60, remaining stable from ages 20 to 60.[78]

CLINICAL FEATURES

The most common presenting complaints are a result of anemia, neutropenia, and thrombocytopenia caused by a rapidly expanding leukemic cell population. Symptoms are malaise, fatigue, bony pain, bleeding, bruising, and fever. Pain, especially in children, results from increased blasts in the bone marrow. CNS involvement is present in 10% of patients.[32, 112] Most CNS manifestations involve meningeal infiltrates resulting in increased intracranial pressure and cranial nerve palsies, most frequently involving cranial nerves III, IV, VI, and VIII. Parenchymal involvement of the brain is rare in leukemia, as is testicular involvement at diagnosis. Enlargement of the testes may be unilateral or bilateral. Lymphadenopathy is present in almost 80% of patients. The spleen or liver or both are also involved in 70% to 75% of patients.[32]

DIAGNOSIS

The diagnosis of acute leukemia is often indicated by the peripheral blood smear; however, a bone marrow evaluation is essential to finalize the diagnosis and provide specimens for further histochemical staining, immunophenotyping, and cytogenetics. The differentiation between AML and ALL based on cell morphology alone is inaccurate.[33]

The WBC count is greater than 10,000/mm³ in 50% to 60% of patients at diagnosis and greater than 100,000/mm³ in 10%. Another 30% to 40% of patients have WBC counts less than 10,000/mm³.[33] Leukemic cells may be seen in the blood. Despite high WBC counts, absolute neutrophil counts are low. Anemia is almost universal; two thirds of patients present with a platelet count less than 50,000/mm³.[32] The bone marrow aspirate is used to obtain the *differential* count, which quantitates the percentage of each of the hematologic components in the marrow. Lymphoblasts comprise at least 30% of the marrow cells in ALL.

Smears of the bone marrow aspirate are specially stained to define the specific subtype of ALL. A portion of the bone marrow aspirate is heparinized for cytogenetic analysis. These studies may reveal certain patterns of gene translocations or rearrangements that are prognostically significant.

A core biopsy of the bone is obtained during the bone marrow procedure. This specimen is used to determine the marrow cellularity. *Cellularity* refers to the ratio of hematopoietic tissue to adipose tissue in the marrow. The amount of blood-forming, or *red*, marrow decreases with the aging process and is replaced by fat, or *yellow*, marrow. Normocellular marrow for an adult is 30% to 40% cellularity. Young adults and children have bone marrow that is much more cellular. Older adults have more fat in their marrow. These age-related changes are reflected in defining marrow cellularity: *normocellular* marrow has normal proportions of the hematopoietic cells and adipose cells; *hypocellular* marrow has a reduced number of hematopoietic cells and an increase in adipose elements; and *hypercellular* marrow has an increased number of hematopoietic cells and a decreased amount of adipose tissue.[71] A bone marrow report for a newly diagnosed ALL patient is usually hypercellular with increased lymphoblasts (e.g., cellularity = 90%; lymphoblasts = 80%).

Infiltration of the cerebrospinal fluid (CSF) by leukemic cells is seen in 5% of children and fewer than 10% of adults.[32, 118] The CSF specimen is centrifuged and stained to determine the presence of leukemic cells. A low glucose level or a high protein level may indicate either leukemic infiltration or an infectious process. Platelet transfusions may be required before the procedure in patients with thrombocytopenia to decrease the potential risk of bleeding. Patients with high numbers of circulating blast cells may have their CSF specimens contaminated with circulating blast cells. This may lead to an inaccurate diagnosis of CNS involvement.

Table 14–1 presents the physical findings, laboratory values, bone marrow, and CSF results in ALL and AML.

CLASSIFICATION

Classification of leukemias at diagnosis is necessary to determine prognosis and select therapy. The ALLs are a heterogeneous group of disorders with subgroups that have distinct clinical and prognostic features.[33] The *French-American-British (FAB) classification system,* developed in 1976, is based on cellular morphology and immunophenotypic features and is universally accepted.[40] Cytogenetic analysis further defines the specific clonal abnormalities found in acute leukemia. Information about the role of molecular genetic techniques and the relationship of retroviruses and oncogenes is increasing knowledge about the nature of acute leukemia.

The three FAB classes of ALL are L₁, L₂, and L₃.[100] The L₁ classification is most common in childhood leukemias, representing 80% of children but only 30% of adults. Morphologically the leukemia cells are small, homogeneous, and nongranular with scanty cytoplasm. The common adult form of ALL is the L₂ classification in 65% to 70% of cases.[79] Microscopically these blasts appear larger and are heterogeneous. The L₃ classification is very rare and resembles Burkitt's lymphoma in about 2% to 7% of patients.[80] Morphologically the L₃ blasts are large and homogeneous with moderately abundant cytoplasm.

Lymphoblastic leukemias originate in either B-cell or T-cell progenitors at various stages of differentiation and proliferation. Assessing the reactivity of leukemic cells to several monoclonal antibodies specific for different cell types establishes their expression, or *immunophenotype*. These are also called *cell surface marker studies*. Different antigens are expressed as the cell matures, which aids in identification[31] (Table 14–2).

About 75% of adult cases are of B-cell lineage. Most express the *common ALL antigen,* or CALLA (CD10). They are divided into early pre–B-cell, pre–B-cell, and B-cell ALL. Approximately 25% of ALL cases are of T-cell lineage, either pre-T cell or T cell.[31] About 25% of adult ALL coexpress myeloid antigens; these patients do worse.

PROGNOSIS

Approximately 80% to 90% of adults treated for ALL will achieve complete remission (CR), and 30% to 40% will be cured.[97] In children, 90% will achieve CR, and 60% to 85% will be cured.[35]

The different response rates between adults and children are caused by differences in disease biology. Adults with ALL generally have poor prognostic indicators, and therefore their response is different from that seen in children.[55]

TABLE 14-1

Physical Findings and Laboratory Results in ALL and AML Patients

	Acute Lymphocytic Leukemia	Acute Myelogenous Leukemia
PHYSICAL EXAMINATION		
Fever	Often present	May be present
Infection	Frequently present	30% have serious infections
Bleeding	Mild in 30%	30% have significant bleeding or petechiae
		75% have intracutaneous bleeding
Adenopathy	Present in 80%	Rare
Splenomegaly/+ or hepatomegaly	Frequently present	Occurs in 25%
Gingival hypertrophy	Rare	Present with monocytic element
Neurologic findings	Headaches, visual disturbances	Rare
LABORATORY VALUES		
White blood cell count (WBC)	50–60% WBC > 10,000	30% decreased
	30–40% WBC < 100,000/mm^3	30% normal
	10% WBC > 100,000/mm^3	30% increased
	Often neutropenic	WBC > 50,000/mm^3 in 25%
	Most have blasts	10% have no blasts
Platelets	< 50,000/mm^3 in 60%	< 20,000/mm^3 common
Uric acid	Increased	Increased in 50%
Lactate dehydrogenase (LDH)	Increased	Typically increased
Bone marrow		
Cellularity	Hypercellular	Hypercellular
Blasts	30% or greater	30% or greater
Erythroid elements	Decreased	Increased
Morphology	Normal	Bizarre granulation of mature granulocytes
Cerebrospinal fluid		
Cytology: infiltration with leukemic cells at presentation	Children: 5%	< 5% occurrence: greater risk in M$_4$ and M$_5$
	Adult: < 10%	greater risk with WBC > 100,000

TABLE 14-2

Immunologic, Morphologic, and Cytogenetic Features of ALL

Immunophenotype	Incidence % Children	Incidence % Adults	Effect on Prognosis	FAB Morphology	Common Cytogenetic Abnormalities	Other Presenting Features
Early pre-B cell CALLA positive	2/3	< 2/3	Favorable	L$_1$: 90% L$_2$: 10%	t(12;21)	CALLA negative Poor prognosis
Pre-B cell	20	15–25	Moderately favorable	L$_1$: 90% L$_2$: 10%	t(1;19)	
B cell	1–2	1–2	Favorable with high-dose chemotherapy	L$_1$: 10% L$_2$: 15% L$_3$: 75%	t(8;14) t(8;22) t(2;8)	High rate of CNS involvement ↑ uric acid, ↑ LDH Hepatosplenomegaly Lymphadenopathy
Pre-T cell T cell	10–15	10–15	Favorable with high-dose chemotherapy	L$_1$: 95% L$_2$: 5%	t(1;14) t(11;14) del (9p)	Mediastinal mass in 50–60% High rate of CNS involvement

Adapted from Kinney MC, Lukens JN: Classification and differentiation of the acute leukemias. In Lee GR and others, editors: Wintrobe's clinical hematology, Philadelphia, Williams & Wilkins, 1999:2209; and Whitlock JA, Gaynon PS: Acute lymphocytic leukemia. In Lee GR and others, editors: Wintrobe's clinical hematology, Philadelphia, Williams & Wilkins, 1999:2241.

FAB, French-American-British classification system; CALLA, common ALL antigen; CNS, central nervous system; LDH, lactate dehydrogenase.

The most important prognostic factors for remission duration are cytogenetic abnormalities, time to achieve CR, initial WBC count, age, and immunologic subtype.[100]

Age

Infants younger than age 1 year and children older than age 10 years have a worse prognosis than do those between 1 and 9 years old. Adults have a worse outcome than children; adults older than 60 have the worst prognosis.[32] Older adults have more adverse biologic features plus other coexisting medical conditions contributing to a poorer prognosis.[97]

White Blood Cell Count

A high initial WBC count is a poor prognostic indicator and has an adverse effect on remission duration.[62, 114] A National Cancer Institute (NCI) workshop has suggested a WBC greater than $50,000/mm^3$ as a poor risk for children.[32] Adults with a WBC count greater than $30,000/mm^3$ also have a poor prognosis.[100]

Time to Response

Prognostic models by Hoelzer, Kantarjian, and Gaynor all list time to CR that is longer than 4 weeks as a high-risk factor.[32, 79]

Cytogenetics

Cytogenetic characteristics are one of the most important prognostic factors for ALL. Abnormalities can be related to the number of chromosomes or structural characteristics. In children, *ploidy (increased number of chromosomes)* is the most important prognostic factor; those with more than 50 chromosomes have the best prognosis.[32] Structural cytogenetic abnormalities are thought to either generate a novel gene (an oncogene) whose protein product acts on the host cell to induce malignancy or it may cause a loss or inactivation of genes whose proteins normally suppress cancer (a tumor suppressor gene). These structural abnormalities take the form of point mutation, gene amplification, gene deletion, or chromosomal translocation.[5, 142]

The most common structural abnormality in adults is the *Philadelphia chromosome* (Ph). In this translocation, a portion of chromosome 9 and 22 exchange places: t(9;22). This leads to a poorer prognosis. Other karyotypes that signal poorer prognosis are t(11;19), t(4;11), and t(1;19). A favorable cytogenetic abnormality is t(10;14).[40, 114]

Immunophenotype

The CALLA-positive early pre–B-cell ALL and T-cell ALL have the most prolonged remission duration. CALLA-negative, early pre–B-cell ALL and pre–T-cell ALL have lower 5-year response rates. B-cell ALL is now expected to do better when high-dose chemotherapies are used.[100]

Other Risk Factors

Leukemia of the CNS is a high-risk factor.[32] Splenomegaly, hepatomegaly, thrombocytopenia, high lactate dehydrogenase (LDH), and weight loss have been shown to indicate a worse prognosis in single studies and require confirmation.[80, 114]

Table 14–3 lists the factors affecting prognosis in ALL.

TREATMENT MODALITIES

The treatment goal in ALL is to achieve a cure. Standard treatment regimens for this disease consist of two parts: induction therapy and postremission therapy. Prophylactic treatment to prevent CNS disease is incorporated into both parts of treatment.

The purpose of induction therapy is to induce CR. A bone marrow aspirate and biopsy containing less than 5% lymphoblasts and the return of normal hematopoiesis document a CR. The elimination of extramedullary disease is needed. Postremission therapy is administered over 2 to 3 years after CR to eradicate completely any remaining clinically undetectable leukemia cells that may potentially cause disease relapse. High-dose therapy over a shorter time period may also be used.

Induction Therapy

The primary chemotherapeutic agents used to induce remission are (1) vincristine, (2) a corticosteroid (usually prednisone), and (3) anthracycline (doxorubicin, daunorubicin).[32, 40, 97] Remission rates range from 70% to 85%, with a low mortality rate resulting from induction. Some induction regimens use additional drugs (L-asparaginase, cyclophosphamide, methotrexate, 6-mercaptopurine [6-MP], cytarabine [ARA-C]), but these do not appear to increase response rates.[31, 32] An exception appears to be mature B-cell ALL, which may respond to the use of high-dose cyclophosphamide, alternating with high doses of methotrexate and ARA-C.[155]

Central Nervous System Treatment

The CNS may serve as a "sanctuary" site for leukemia cells. Leukemic involvement in the CSF at the time of

TABLE 14-3
Prognostic Indicators for ALL

Factor	Good	Poor
FAB	L_1, L_2	L_3
Immunophenotype	T cell	Null cell
	B cell	Early pre-B ALL, CALLA negative
	Early pre-B ALL, CALLA positive	
Age	< 30 y	> 60 y
Gender	Female	Male
WBC at diagnosis	< 30,000/mm^3	> 30,000/mm^3
CR	< 4 wk	> 4 wk
Cytogenetics	Normal karyotype	Cytogenetic abnormalities: t(4;11), t(1;19), t(9;22), t(8;14)
	Chromosome 14 changes	
CNS involvement	No	Yes
Mediastinal mass	Yes	No

FAB, French-American-British classification system; CALLA, common ALL antigen; WBC, white blood cell count; CR, complete remission; CNS, central nervous system.

diagnosis is seen in 5% of children and fewer than 10% of adults.[32, 118] However, if the CNS is not treated, as many as 50% to 75% of adults will develop CNS involvement.[32] CNS prophylaxis is a critical component of postremission therapy for leukemia-free survival. Cranial irradiation plus intrathecal chemotherapy with methotrexate or ARA-C was the standard for children with ALL. This often resulted in neuropsychological deficits and endocrine dysfunction. Newer treatments include intrathecal ARA-C or methotrexate (or both) without cranial irradiation and high-dose systemic chemotherapy with CNS penetration (e.g., high-dose methotrexate or ARA-C). The latter treatment is also used in adults.[40, 97, 121]

Patients who have CNS leukemia should be treated more aggressively. This includes intraventricular chemotherapy and cranial irradiation. An Ommaya reservoir may be inserted. The advantages of drug administration through an Ommaya include ease of access to CSF and higher and more predictable levels of the drug in ventricular CSF than when administered by lumbar puncture.[31, 32]

Postremission Therapy

Without some form of postremission therapy, ALL will almost certainly recur. The optimal form of this therapy remains controversial, but the two most widely used types of therapy are consolidation/intensification and maintenance.

Consolidation/Intensification Therapy. The role of consolidation/intensification in children has improved prognosis in those with high-risk features.[121] The role in adults is less clear. Consolidation or intensification is early treatment with chemotherapy after obtaining CR with combinations of drugs of comparable intensity given in repeated courses over several months. This appears to provide an advantage for T-cell and B-cell ALL without the need for maintenance.[100] Neither the optimal drugs nor the optimal durations of treatment are known.

Maintenance Therapy. Maintenance therapy is lower-dose treatment given continuously for 2 to 3 years, usually daily 6-MP and weekly methotrexate. This is effective in preventing relapse and improving survival in children.[121] Most adult maintenance therapies are based on pediatric studies, but the intensities vary. A combination of several antileukemic agents and 6-MP and methotrexate is generally used. The optimal drugs and dosage remain unknown.

Bone Marrow Transplantation

The role and timing of allogeneic (marrow harvested from a histocompatible donor) bone marrow transplantation (BMT) or peripheral blood stem cell (PBSC) transplantation in adult ALL is controversial. The survival benefit of BMT/PBSC transplantation needs to outweigh the greater expense and higher toxicities of treatment such as graft-versus-host disease. The graft-versus-leukemia effect is associated with a lower relapse rate, but the magnitude is unclear.[55] Patients with early pre–B-cell, CALLA-negative, Ph-positive ALL, chromosomal abnormalities [t(4;11), t(1;19)], or greater than 4 weeks to CR should undergo BMT/PBSC transplant.[55, 100] Patients with a high WBC count at diagnosis are also considered[114] (see Chapter 25). It is unclear whether BMT offers an advantage for ALL patients with a favorable prognosis. ALL patients with the Ph chromosome have had a 38% leukemia-free survival when they received BMT during first CR. Relapsed patients should also be considered for allogeneic BMT.

Autologous (marrow harvested from the patient) BMT or PBSC transplantation may be considered for patients too old for allogeneic BMT or without a matched donor. Results have been inferior to allogeneic BMT because of inability to effectively purge residual leukemic cells from the harvested bone marrow.[40, 114] A lack of graft-versus-leukemia effect may also play a part in lower long-term remission rates in autologous transplants.[55] In general, results are no better than for intensive chemotherapy alone. Clinical trials comparing allogeneic BMT (if a matched sibling is present), autologous BMT, and conventional maintenance therapy are underway that will answer crucial issues in management.[31] (See Chapter 25 for details on BMT.)

Therapy for Recurrent and Refractory Disease

Most ALL relapses occur within the first 2 years of remission.[97] As many as half of relapsed patients may achieve a second remission by repeating their original induction regimen; however, BMT is the only cure.[100] Patients who relapse after completing maintenance therapy have a better chance of attaining second remission than those patients who relapse while receiving therapy.[80, 100]

Patients with resistant disease who fail to achieve a first remission may respond to treatment with intermediate-dose to high-dose methotrexate and leukovorin rescue or with L-asparaginase.

Bone marrow transplantation may allow long-term survival for as many as 18% to 45% of those in second CR.[55] In pediatric and adult patients, it is common practice to offer allogeneic BMT for patients in second CR who have matched sibling donors.

Minimal Residual Disease

Methods of detecting minimal residual disease at levels below the sensitivity of morphologic evaluation are being used to determine the effects of antileukemia therapy. It may assist in identifying impending relapse of disease and allow for earlier treatment. Polymerase chain reaction (PCR) is the most sensitive method available and can assess for rearranged immunoglobulin heavy chain (IgH) and T-cell receptor (TCR) gene sequences. Monitoring for BCR-ABL fusion transcripts allow detection of the Ph chromosome. Results of this are used mostly in research settings in ALL therapy.[97]

Multidrug Resistance (MDR)

The MDR gene produces a glycoprotein p170 that functions as an efflux pump. This makes the ALL cell resis-

tant to chemotherapy drugs including vinca alkaloids, taxoids, anthracyclines, amsacrine, mitoxantrone, and epipodophylotoxins. This results in decreased chemotherapy levels in the malignant cells and affects the response rate. Glycoprotein p170 does not affect alkylating agents or antimetabolites. At diagnosis, 10% to 15% of patients express MDR and at relapse 15% to 60% do so. How to overcome MDR in ALL is not clear yet.[33, 149]

Acute Myeloid Leukemia

EPIDEMIOLOGY AND ETIOLOGY

Acute myeloid leukemia (AML) is also called acute nonlymphocytic leukemia and acute myelogeous leukemia. Specific risk factors have been identified in AML. People with certain genetic disorders, such as Down syndrome (trisomy 21), Bloom syndrome, Klinefelter's syndrome, and Fanconi's anemia, are at increased risk to develop AML.[130] Exposure to the hydrocarbon benzene also increases the risk of disease development. Benzene is an aromatic solvent and is present in unleaded gasoline, rubber cement, and cleaning solvents.[126] Farmers exposed to pesticides also have a higher rate of myeloid leukemias.[111, 140] Leukemia has been associated with exposure to ionizing radiation from nuclear reactions and from exposure to therapeutic and occupational radiation.[130] Because some RNA tumor viruses (retroviruses) cause myeloid leukemias in rodents, felines, and avians, a viral etiology of AML has been suspected in humans.[60] Cigarette smoking may be a risk factor for acute leukemia, with rates attributed to smoking as high as 7% to 14%[8] of leukemia cases in the United States.[16] Current smokers have the highest risk.[88, 129] Electromagnetic field (EMF) exposure has been implicated, but a review of all the literature to date reveals a doubtful link between EMF exposure and leukemia.[77] Others have called for more controlled studies.[3, 64]

Improvements in multimodality therapy over the past decade have resulted in increased survival and a potential cure for patients with a variety of cancers. Long-term survival now allows evaluation of late effects of cancer therapy. The incidence of secondary malignancies related to cytotoxic therapy and especially therapy-related acute myeloid leukemias (T-AMLs) has increased dramatically over the past decade. The median interval of occurrence of T-AML is 4 to 6 years after the original cancer treatment and is usually preceded by a preleukemic state detectable for 6 months.[39] Alkylating agents, especially prolonged use of melphalan in ovarian cancer,[48] multiple myeloma,[13] and breast cancer,[119] and nitrogen mustard for Hodgkin's disease,[116] are strongly implicated. The risk of leukemia rises with increasing doses of alkylating agents so that the rise is directly related to the total dose received. Chlorambucil, busulfan, and thiotepa are also associated with an increased risk of developing a later malignancy.

The pathophysiology of AML can be explained by genetic changes in bone marrow stem cells. Either a complete block or partial block in maturation occurs. The genetic changes in chromosomes lead to formation of growth-promoting oncogenes, inactivation of tumor suppressor genes, or changes in transcription factors. The natural history of AML arising de novo in young adults is believed to be a disease of committed stem cells, which is different from the same disease arising from a primitive stem cell typical of secondary AML.[76]

The incidence of AML is 3 cases per 100,000 population, with approximately 9700 new cases each year in the United States.[2] The median age at diagnosis is about 50 years.

CLINICAL FEATURES

As with ALL, AML symptoms are related to the rapidly expanding leukemic cell population. Symptoms of anemia are usually found in AML patients at presentation. A common finding is that of recurrent infections unresponsive to standard oral antibiotics. Reports of easy bruisability, epistaxis, or gingival bleeding reflect thrombocytopenia. Unlike ALL patients, virtually all AML patients are symptomatic at presentation.

Abnormal findings on physical examination are related to leukemic infiltration of an organ, granulocytopenia, or thrombocytopenia. A thorough and systematic physical examination confirms many of the patient's complaints and is an integral part of the diagnosis. Table 14–4 lists possible physical manifestations of both ALL and AML. Gingival infiltrates and skin nodules are frequently seen in acute myelomonocytic and monocytic leukemias and may precede other manifestations by 2 to 4 weeks.

DIAGNOSIS

A diagnosis of AML is highly suspect when the examination of peripheral blood smears shows an increased number of immature blast cells associated with anemia and thrombocytopenia. The presence of Auer rods suggests a diagnosis of AML before other diagnostic results are available. The total WBC count in AML may be normal, decreased, or increased. A small percentage of AML patients may present without peripheral blast cells. Platelet counts of less than 20,000/mm³ are common in AML. Abnormalities in one or more organ systems may result from leukemic cell infiltration or metabolic complications related to leukemia. Rarely a solid mass of leukemic cells will develop called a *granulocytic sarcoma or leukemic infiltrate.*

As with ALL, the marrow aspirate is used to obtain the differential count, and the biopsy is used to establish an assessment of cellularity and evaluate fibrosis. Myeloblasts comprise at least 30% of the nucleated cells in AML, and the marrow is hypercellular. A "packed" bone marrow with cellularity of 90% to 100% may be seen in AML patients.

A small sample of marrow aspirate is used for cytogenetics and immunophenotyping, which establishes the specific subclassification.

Table 14–1 compares physical findings and laboratory results of AML patients with those of ALL patients.

CLASSIFICATION

The degree of differentiation along different cell lines and the extent of cell maturation classify AML morphologically according to the FAB criteria.[61] Familiarity with this system is helpful for nurses caring for AML patients because it identifies the unique features of each subtype. Table 14–5 outlines the FAB classification for AML.[96]

PROGNOSIS

Oncology nurses should understand the factors affecting the prognosis of the patient with AML. In this disease, certain prognostic factors influence the rate of remission; other factors affect the duration of response. Patients over age 70 are less likely to survive the rigors of induction therapy, but those who do achieve remission generally survive as long as younger patients.

Age

In children, AML represents 20% of all cases of acute leukemia. Children younger than 1 year have a poor prognosis, probably related to their abnormal cytogenetics. Those aged 3 to 10 years have the best prognosis based on their favorable cytogenetics.[118] From 70% to 85% of patients achieve a CR, but more than half will relapse if treated only with chemotherapy.[121] In adults the frequency of AML increases with age, with up to a 10-fold increase compared with younger adults. The median age of AML patients is 60 years. In individuals older than 60 years, a combination of unfavorable cytogenetics, a higher incidence of previous myelodysplastic syndrome that has evolved into AML, and poor performance status of many elderly patients results in a poor prognosis.[53] Approximately 60% to 65% of adult AML patients achieve CR, with 20% maintaining a cure.[53]

Leukocyte Count

Of patients presenting with a WBC count greater than 100,000/mm³, significantly more die during the first week

TABLE 14-4
Clinical Features in Acute Leukemias

System/Region	Manifestation	Cause
Head/eyes/ears/nose/throat	Retinal capillary hemorrhage	Leukemic infiltration
	Fundic leukemic infiltration	Leukemic infiltration
	Papilledema	Leukemic infiltration
	Oropharyngeal infections	Secondary to immunocompromise
	Periodontal infections	Secondary to immunocompromise
	Gingival hypertrophy (AML)	Leukemic infiltration
	Dry mucous membranes	Overall systemic illness
	Dysphagia	Possible leukemic infiltration
	Cervical adenopathy	Leukemic infiltration
	Epistaxis	Thrombocytopenia
	Gingival bleeding	Thrombocytopenia
Cardiovascular/pulmonary	Possible tachycardia, tachypnea	Anemia or infection
	Conduction defects	Leukemic infiltration of bundle of His, valves, pericardium, or myocardium (rare)
	Murmurs	
	Pericarditis	
	Congestive heart failure	Fluid overload or underlying diagnosis
	Abnormal lung sounds	Possible bacterial pneumonia
Abdomen	Splenomegaly (ALL)	Leukemic infiltration
	Enlarged, tender kidneys (more common in pediatric ALL)	Leukemic infiltration
	Hepatomegaly	Leukemic infiltration
	Menorrhagia	Thrombocytopenia
Genitourinary	Renal failure or anuria	Uric acid nephropathy
Rectal	Perirectal abscesses	Decreased neutrophils
Extremities	Skin pallor	Anemia
	Ecchymosis, petechiae	Thrombocytopenia
	Leukemic skin infiltrates: small, raised, pinkish nodules	Leukemic infiltration
	Swollen joints or tenderness (most common in pediatric ALL)	Leukemic infiltration
Neurologic (CNS)	Headache, vomiting	Possible infiltration of CNS
	Visual disturbances	Possible CNS hemorrhage
	Cranial nerve VI, VII palsy	Infiltration of nerve sheath
Musculoskeletal	Bone or joint pain	Leukemic infiltration
	Swelling	Leukemic infiltration
	Osteolytic lesions	Leukemic infiltration
Other	Elevated temperature	Infection or tumor fever

of therapy, deaths from CNS hemorrhage are more common, overall remission is shorter, and fewer survive, compared with those presenting with lower WBC counts.[47] A very high WBC count can cause leukostatic lesion development in the microvasculature of the lungs or CNS. Leukostasis may lead to thromboembolic episodes and pulmonary or CNS bleeding. Presentation with an excessively high WBC count is a medical emergency, and the count must be reduced rapidly with hydroxyurea or leukapheresis or both.[112] Another poor prognostic factor in AML patients is prior treatment with chemotherapy or radiation therapy. This group includes patients with a treatment-related secondary leukemia and AML patients with recurring or resistant disease.

Immunophenotyping

The use of monoclonal antibodies to differentiate antigens aids in differentiating between AML and ALL. It is most useful in poorly differentiated AML and necessary to identify type M_0.[61] The different FAB classes are based on immunophenotyping and morphology.

Cytogenetics

As in ALL, the cytogenetic classification of AML is more indicative of prognosis than any other factors. As many as 60% to 90% of adults with AML have cytogenetic abnormalities. The cytogenetic breakpoints involved in balanced translocations form fusion proteins.

TABLE 14–5

French-American-British (FAB) Classification System of AMLs

FAB Type (% of Adult AMLs)	Bone Marrow Morphology	Clinical Features/Prognosis
M_0 (7%)	Myeloid lineage cannot be determined by conventional morphologic or cytochemical analysis; can be identified by immunophenotyping	Resistant to treatment. No distinctive cytogenetic pattern
M_1: myeloblastic (20%)	Without myeloid maturation, < 10% of cells are more mature than promyelocyte Auer rods present	M_1 and M_2 are most common adult AML diagnoses
M_2: myeloblastic (30%)	With maturation Blasts and promyelocytes > 50% of cells Auer bodies and/or granules t(8;21) in 20% of patients Promyelocytes, myelocytes and other mature myeloid elements	Most favorable prognosis High rate of cure (85–100%) with conventional chemotherapy, especially with t(8:21)

M_3: promyelocytic (APL) (10%)	Most cells abnormal promyelocytes
	Cells filled with large granules; may be microgranular
	Nucleus varies in size and shape
	Bundles of Auer bodies
	t(15;17)
		Median age 30–40 y; disseminated intravascular coagulation present in 80% of patients:
		    May occur after treatment initiation
		    Granules released as blasts die contain procoagulants and initiate coagulation cascade
		Good duration of remission
		WBC usually normal to low, < 3000/mm^3

M_3: variant (M_3V)	Granules detected only on electron microscopy (microgranular variant)	WBC high
M_4: myelomonocytic (15–20%)	> 20% of blasts must be monocytic Increased hyperleukocytosis Extramedullary leukemic involvement	Organomegaly Lymphadenopathy Gingival hyperplasias Soft tissue infiltration CNS leukemia Difficult to predict remission duration Median age higher
M_4E (5–10%)	Variable number of morphologically abnormal eosinophils present Inversion of chromosome 16	High rate of complete remission Median age 35–40 y
M_5: monocytic M_5a: *Subtype A*—poorly differentiated: all monoblasts (5%)	Monocytic cells exceed 80% Granulocytic component rarely exceeds 10% Abnormalities with chromosome 11	Organomegaly Lymphadenopathy Gingival hyperplasia
M_5b: *Subtype B*—differentiated: promonocyte predominant (5%)	Few cells may have Auer bodies	Soft tissue infiltration CNS leukemia Short remissions More common in older adults Higher blast count at diagnosis
M_6: erythroleukemia (Di Guglielmo syndrome [erythroleukemia]) (< 5%)	Erythropoietic component exceeds 50% of marrow cells Blasts have bizarre morphology Myeloblasts and promyelocytes > 30% of erythroid cells Complex karyotypes Loss of chromosome 5 and/or 7	Poor response to treatment Older adults Prolonged prodromal period May present with rheumatic disorder; 75% have positive Coombs' test; 30% have rheumatoid factor
M_7: megakaryocytic (< 5%)	Blasts resemble immature megakaryocytes or may be quite undifferentiated Increased marrow reticulin No consistent cyto abnormality	Marrow difficult to aspirate Increased lactate dehydrogenase Intense myelofibrosis Very poor prognosis

Other poor prognostic cytogenetic abnormalities: 5q-, -7, 7q-, and +8, 11q-. These patients have short durations of complete remission (median, 6 months). Interim prognosis: normal chrom, trisomy 8, abnormality of chrom 11, inv3.

These proteins result in disruption of transcription factors believed to be critical in myeloid differentiation. Some correspond to a specific FAB subtype: M_3 with t(15;17), M_2 with t(8;21), and M_4E_0 with inv(16), which are all favorable karyotypes; and M_6 and M_7 with complex karyotypes, which are unfavorable.[61] Monosomy 5 and 7 are frequently found in therapy related AML, which carries a poor prognosis. Plans for postremission therapy rely heavily on cytogenetic analysis at diagnosis.[40]

Other Risk Factors

A preexisting hematologic disorder, serious infection at diagnosis, CNS leukemia, organomegaly, and lymphadenopathy are clinical features indicative of poor prognosis.[60] Laboratory findings predictive of poor response include anemia, high peripheral blast count, thrombocytopenia, elevated blood urea nitrogen (BUN) and creatinine, increased LDH, or increased fibrinogen.[60] FAB M_5 carries a poor prognosis.

TREATMENT MODALITIES

The treatment goal of AML, as in ALL, is cure. Treatment is divided into two phases: induction and postremission therapy. Currently, maintenance therapy is not recommended in the treatment of AML. Postremission therapy options include the following:

1. Consolidation therapy with drug regimens almost as intensive as induction therapy. Consolidation is given over a period of months after the attainment of a complete remission.
2. Intensification with a dose-intensified schedule of drugs used during induction. The most frequently used agent is high-dose ARA-C (HIDAC) either alone or in combination with other antileukemic drugs. HIDAC is 2 to 3 g/m^2 for 8 to 12 doses and given for 2 to 3 cycles.[24, 148, 153]
3. Ablative therapy with allogeneic or autologous bone marrow or PBSC rescue.

A complete remission in AML is defined as less than 5% nucleated marrow blasts in a normocellular marrow. Peripheral blood counts must return to normal and preexisting adenopathy or organomegaly must be absent.

Induction Chemotherapy

Successful treatment of AML requires the control of bone marrow and systemic disease and specific treatment of CNS disease, if present. Cytarabine (ARA-C), 100 to 200 mg/m^2 continuous intravenous (IV) infusion for 7 days, plus daunorubicin, 45 to 60 mg/m^2 per day IV bolus for 3 days, is the standard treatment. This 3

+ 7 regimen results in a CR rate of 65% to 70%. Doxorubicin has been substituted but has more severe gastrointestinal toxicities.[40, 120]

Idarubicin has been substituted for daunorubicin, with reports of higher CR. Randomized trials have shown at least equal results with mitoxantrone and aclarubicin.[7, 73] Concerns have been raised that the doses of drugs were not biologically equivalent and therefore comparisons may not be accurate.[6, 148] HIDAC has been studied in various schedules, with no clear benefits over the 3 + 7 regimen.

The best anthracycline for younger patients appears to be idarubicin at 12 to 13 mg/m^2 for 3 days (daunomycin at 60–70 mg/m^2 may be equivalent). For older adults no regimen is superior.[4]

A bone marrow examination is repeated on days 10 to 14 from the first day of chemotherapy to assess for antileukemic response. A positive response is indicated by a hypocellular, aplastic marrow. Peripheral blood studies reflect marrow aplasia, with profound neutropenia and thrombocytopenia at the 14-day nadir. If the day 14 bone marrow shows persistent leukemia, a second induction is started despite severe pancytopenia. The marrow examination is repeated as the peripheral counts begin to recover. If evidence of leukemia persists 3 to 4 weeks after the start of induction and the marrow cellularity is recovered, the patient is reinduced with the same drugs and doses.

In previous studies, elderly patients were treated with reduced doses of chemotherapy. These trials showed a trend toward persistent leukemia with reduced doses. Further studies have supported the use of standard-dose chemotherapy for patients over age 60.[18]

Postremission Therapy

Median CR duration is 12 to 18 months with only 20% to 25% of complete responders remaining as long-term disease-free survivors. If further chemotherapy is not administered to the AML patient in remission, the survival time is much shorter and most patients will experience disease relapse within 6 to 8 months.[17, 25] The most effective postremission therapy and the program's optimal length are not known. Studies have shown no benefit from maintenance therapy over the shorter, more intense consolidation therapies.[120, 145] Other studies, however, found some benefit when comparing maintenance therapy with historical control studies.[28, 46] Because this conflicting information exists, patients should enter randomized clinical trials.

Consolidation is often cytarabine (ARA-C) 100 to 200 mg/m^2 per day continuous infusion times 5 days and 1 to 2 doses of an anthracyline times 2 to 4 courses.

Comparison between 100 mg, 400 mg, and 3 g (HIDAC) of ARA-C showed a higher 4-year disease-free survival rate in patients under age 60 compared with standard doses.[27, 107] HIDAC resulted in a significantly higher response in subgroups with favorable cytogenetics, that is, t(8;21). In intermediate-risk cytogenetics, HIDAC and ARA-C at 400 mg/m^2 were of equivalent benefit. Those with poor cytogenetics showed no difference between groups. Those older than 60 showed no benefit with higher doses plus they had an increased incidence of CNS neurotoxicity.[27, 127]

Bone Marrow Transplantation

Bone marrow transplantation may be the treatment of choice in certain AML patients in first remission. Autologous (auto) stem cell transplant allows higher doses of chemotherapy than intensification but lacks the graft-versus-leukemia effect of allogeneic (allo) stem cell transplant. It also has the potential complication of reinfusion of leukemic cells. Allotransplant has the graft-versus-leukemia effect but higher treatment-related mortality than the other two strategies.

Four recent studies have compared HIDAC, autotransplant, and allotransplant.[19, 27, 74, 156] The disease-free survival at 4 years was not significantly different among the three groups. Allotransplant had higher treatment-related mortality, whereas the other groups had higher rates of relapse. A substantial number of patients randomized to autotransplant in all the groups did not receive transplant and this has an effect on the interpretation. Certain subgroups definitely benefit from allotransplant, that is, those with prior myelodysplastic syndrome (MDS). Further identification of patients benefiting most still need to be identified. In addition, further decreases in treatment-related transplants may also favor allotransplant (see Chapter 25).

Recurrent Disease Therapy

Most patients who achieve CR later relapse with AML and die. Achieving remission after relapse is difficult, and patients who do achieve a second remission rarely survive more than a year. The likelihood of achieving a second CR depends on the length of the first CR. Those patients refractory to initial therapy or with a 6- to 12-month first remission achieves about 20% CR compared with 60% for those with a longer first CR. For patients eligible for allogeneic transplant, this is the first choice of treatment. Those not eligible for BMT should receive investigational treatment if the first CR is less than 1 year or should repeat the original induction if longer than 1 year.[61]

Hematopoietic Growth Factors (HGF)

The addition of granulocyte colony-stimulating factor (G-CSF) and granulocyte-macrophage CSF (GM-CSF)

has been studied in elderly patients in four large randomized studies. Myelosuppression was decreased in all four studies, but clinical benefits such as decreased infection rates were not always seen.[6] Benefits of HGF after induction are minimal.[106] It has greater value after consolidation, where a decrease in the duration of neutropenia is seen. GM-CSF has been approved for use during induction and consolidation therapy in elderly patients.

Multidrug Resistance

Multidrug resistance (MDR) to chemotherapy has been attributed to the MDR1 gene and its protein product, P-glycoprotein (P-gp). P-gp functions as a pump, transporting anthracyclines, *vinca* alkaloids, amsacrine, mitoxantrone, and etoposide in and out of malignant cells. This results in decreased chemotherapy levels in the malignant cells and affects response rate. P-gp does not affect alkylating agents or antimetabolites.[149]

A relationship between MDR1 expression and treatment outcome has been shown.[103] Newly diagnosed AML patients show expression of MDR-1 in 30% of patients less than 55 years and 70% in those older than 55 years.[98] Patients with a high level of P-gp have a poorer prognosis. Patients may also develop increased MDR-1 expression after treatment with chemotherapy. Many clinical trials require bone marrow aspirate specimens to determine MDR status.

Cyclosporin A (cyclosporine) has been shown to overcome MDR. List and coworkers[103] used cyclosporine in combination with ARA-C and daunorubicin in poor-risk AML patients and reported a complete response rate of 62%. Ongoing trials with cyclosporine and cyclosporine derivatives such as PSC 833 continue.

Therapy for Acute Promyelocytic Leukemia

Acute promyelocytic leukemia (APL), or FAB type M$_3$, is now treated differently than the other AMLs. Its unique t(15;17) forms a PML/RAR-fusion protein that blocks differentiation of hematopoietic precursor cells.[70] All-*trans*-retinoic acid (ATRA, tretinoin), when given, promotes cell differentiation.

Usually, APL presents with disseminated intravascular coagulation (DIC), which exacerbates with chemotherapy and has a mortality rate from hemorrhage ranging from 8% to 47%. Conventional chemotherapy produces CR in 60% to 80% of patients, with long-term survival of 35% to 45%.[150] Induction with ATRA at 45 mg/m^2 daily is given until no more APL blasts are seen in bone marrow smears, approximately 30 to 45 days.[38] Bone marrow aplasia is not necessary for normalization of counts. With the use of ATRA, CR rates greater than 90% and a quicker resolution of coagulopathy are seen. Induction mortality is decreased. A recent trial showed concurrent ATRA plus chemotherapy is superior to other methods and should be standard induction for all patients. An anthracycline and ATRA are generally sufficient.[54] Once CR is achieved, consolidation is mandatory for long-term cure. The best consolidation remains under investigation but must include anthracyclines, usually with ARA-C.

Complications of ATRA include retinoic acid syndrome (RAS) and hyperleukocytosis. RAS consists of fever and respiratory distress, weight gain, lower extremity edema, pleural or pericardial effusions, hypotension, and sometimes renal failure. Hyperleukocytosis can lead to pulmonary and CNS toxicity. Two different approaches are used to treat RAS. The addition of chemotherapy to patients with high WBC counts has decreased symptoms; leukapheresis may be used to control elevated counts. High-dose corticosteroids begun at the first sign of symptoms have alleviated symptoms. ATRA may be discontinued.[38]

For patients who relapse on ATRA, arsenic trioxide has proven to be effective and is in clinical trials.[138]

Future Trends

CD33 is an antigen expressed on most early myeloid cells and more than 90% of AML cells, but not on hematopoietic stem cells. Conjugates composed of anti-CD33 antibodies and the chemotherapy, calicheamicin, have shown promise in relapsed or refractory AML.[134]

In May 2000, American Home Products Corporation obtained FDA approval for the drug Mylotarg for the treatment of patients who are 60 years and older in first relapse with CD 33+ AML and not considered candidates for cytotoxic chemotherapy. The recommended dose is 9 mg/m^2 via a two-hour IV infusion once every 14 days for a total of two doses.

Chronic Leukemias

Chronic Myelogenous Leukemia

Chronic myelogenous leukemia (CML) is a myeloproliferative disorder characterized by proliferation of the granulocyte cell series. Chronic leukemias differ from acute leukemias in that the malignant WBCs appear mature and are well differentiated. A second unique difference is the progression of CML through three stages: chronic, accelerated, and blastic transformation, or blast crisis.

EPIDEMIOLOGY AND ETIOLOGY

The incidence of CML increases with exposure to high-dose ionizing radiation but is not clearly associated with any other factors.[105] CML occurs in less than 5% of pediatric leukemia cases. Two types of CML are seen in children. Juvenile CML occurs in children younger than 5 years and presents more like acute leukemia. It is not responsive to chemotherapy and should be treated with allogeneic BMT. If patients receive BMT, 30% to 50% become long-term disease-free survivors.[128] The adult form of CML is seen in the remainder of patients, with the same treatment options used.

The annual incidence of CML is 1 to 1.5/100,000 population; CML is less common than chronic lymphocytic leukemia (CLL) and is one fourth as common as acute leukemia. The incidence of CML increases with age: 4400 new cases are predicted for 2000.[68] The median age at presentation is 45 to 55 years.[69] Men have a rate 1.3 times higher than women.[51]

Significant advances have been made in understanding the biology of CML, and therapeutic improvements have increased the length of the chronic phase.

Philadelphia Chromosome

The hallmark of CML is the presence of a Philadelphia chromosome (Ph^1). Chromosome 22 is missing part of its long arm, which is translocated to the long arm of chromosome 9. A new hybrid BCR-ABL oncogene is formed. Most patients with CML express a 210-kd BCR-ABL protein. These BCR-ABL fusion proteins have increased protein tyrosine kinase activity compared to normal genes. This increased protein kinase activity is essential for the BCR-ABL protein to transform normal cells to CML.[109]

The CML progenitor cells undergo more divisions than their normal counterparts and continue to divide when normal cells stop. Therefore, there is a large increase in the number of granulocytes.[97]

The Ph chromosome is detected by cytogenetic analysis. Molecular analysis detects the BCR-ABL rearrangement and allows detection of minimal residual disease after therapy and can be used to detect early relapse.

In 5% to 10% of CML patients, the Ph chromosome is absent. These patients are generally older and have a shorter survival. Instead of blast transformation, an increased WBC, organomegaly, extramedullary infiltrates, and bone marrow failure without increased blasts is seen.[32]

CLINICAL FEATURES AND DIAGNOSIS

Chronic Phase

The presenting symptoms of *chronic phase* CML are related to expansion of the granulocytic mass. Symptoms may include fatigue, night sweats, pallor, dyspnea, anemia, anorexia, weight loss, and sternal tenderness. The most common finding at diagnosis is splenomegaly. The spleen may be only minimally enlarged or may be greatly enlarged, filling most of the abdomen. The splenomegaly is caused by infiltration of WBC and can cause left upper quadrant pain, early satiety, and abdominal fullness. Many patients may be diagnosed on routine blood work and are asymptomatic.

Most patients are diagnosed during the chronic phase, which has a median duration of 3 to 4 years. The chronic phase is the initial indolent form of CML. The presenting symptoms resolve as the patient responds to therapy. Patients usually feel well during this period.

A very high WBC count in CML generally does not lead to complications. An increase in WBC in chronic phase does not require emergency leukopheresis. If the patient presents in blast crisis, then leukostatic syndromes may occur as in AML. Rapid leukoreduction is not required. Rapid lowering can lead to tumor lysis syndrome. All patients should be placed on allopurinol until counts normalize.[97] Thrombocytosis is present in one third of patients, with platelet counts greater than 1 million/mm^3 in some patients. WBC and platelet counts may fluctuate in 30- to 60-day cycles without any therapy.[112]

Diagnosis of CML is established by hematologic evaluation. Table 14–6 describes blood and bone marrow findings. A bone marrow evaluation is required to assess cellularity, detect fibrosis, and obtain a specimen for cytogenetic analysis.

In addition to the presence of the Ph^1 chromosome in 95% of CML patients, the marrow is extremely hypercellular and may be devoid of fat. Myeloid elements are increased, and megakaryocytes may be excessive. Cytogenetic studies to detect the Ph^1 chromosome may be performed on peripheral blood if the WBC count is sufficiently elevated.[32, 97]

Accelerated Stage

The term *accelerated stage* is generally used to refer to patients who have been under treatment for some time and have shown a variety of signs of disease progression but who do not meet the criteria for blastic disease.[92] The cell generally acquires more chromosomal abnormalities and this leads to loss of differentiation with cells becoming more immature[97] (Table 14–6). Progression to the accelerated phase is characteristic of 75% to 80% of patients with CML. The time of progression to the accelerated phase is variable and greatly impacts length of survival. The leukocyte doubling time (LDT) shortens to 20 days or less during this stage. The first evidence of accelerated stage may be failure to respond to drugs effective during the chronic stage. Other evi-

TABLE 14–6
Chronic Myelogenous Leukemia

	Chronic	Accelerated	Blast
Peripheral blood	WBC often > 100,000→ Blasts < 5% Mature and immature granulocytes, segmented neutrophils predominate ↑ Basophils ↑ Eosinophils ↑ Megakaryocytes Mild anemia Normal or ↑ platelets	Basophils to > 20% Blasts > 15% Blast + promyelocytes > 30% Thrombocytopenia < 100,000 unrelated to toxicity Hgb < 7.0 WBC difficult to control after being stable	Blasts > 30% Plus all the same as accelerated phase
Bone marrow	Hypercellular Blasts < 5% ↑ Basophils ↑ Eosinophils ↑ Megakaryocytes in clusters	Blasts > 10% Basophils or eosinophils > 10% Cytogenetic—additional changes Fibrosis beginning	Blasts in clumps Blasts > 30% Fibrosis Leukemic infiltrates lymph nodes palpable
Fever	Resolves once WBC controlled	Symptoms recur after being previously controlled	Symptoms recur after being previously controlled
Night sweats	Resolves once WBC controlled	Symptoms recur after being previously controlled	Symptoms recur after being previously controlled
Weight loss	Resolves once WBC controlled	Symptoms recur after being previously controlled	Symptoms recur after being previously controlled
Splenomegaly	Resolves once WBC controlled	Symptoms recur after being previously controlled	Symptoms recur after being previously controlled
Bone pain	Resolves once WBC controlled	Symptoms recur after being previously controlled	Symptoms recur after being previously controlled
Survival	3–4 y	1 y	3–6 mo

dence shows peripheral blasts being 15% or more of cells, thrombocytopenia with a platelet count less than 100,000/mm³ unrelated to therapy, and cytogenetic clonal evolution.

Physical examination reveals increased fatigue, increasing anemia, recurrence of splenomegaly, and thrombocytopenia; occasionally, fever of unknown origin, lymphadenopathy, hepatomegaly, thrombocytosis, and basophilia are also noted. The patient may exhibit signs of hypermetabolism, including night sweats, decreased appetite, and weight loss. Periosteal infiltrates and lytic lesions may cause bony pain in addition to sternal pain.

Blood and bone marrow evaluation reveals increased promyelocytes and blasts. The onset of the accelerated phase is difficult to distinguish, and the diagnosis may be made retrospectively. Table 14–6 differentiates the clinical features in the chronic phase and the accelerated phase/blastic transformation.

Survival for patients in accelerated phase is difficult to describe because of disease heterogeneity but can be estimated at about a year.[135]

Blastic Phase

Patients with CML inevitably enter the *blastic stage,* an aggressive, rapidly terminal phase that is refractory to treatment (see Table 14–6).

Two thirds of patients have cells with predominantly myeloblastic characteristics; one third exhibit lymphoblastic features.[112] It is important to distinguish between myeloid or lymphoid transformation because patients with lymphoid disease respond better to treatment (with vincristine and prednisone) and live slightly longer. The blastic stage resembles a disease similar to AML or ALL.

Median survival after blastic transformation is usually less than 6 months.[139] At least 85% of patients die during the blast phase from complications such as bleeding, infections, and cerebral or pulmonary hemorrhages.[141]

TREATMENT MODALITIES

Treatment of CML is usually initiated when the diagnosis is established. At this stage, patients under age 55 should be considered for allogeneic BMT, the only curative treatment for this disease. For those without a donor, interferon therapy should be initiated.[90] Traditional therapies include busulfan and hydroxyurea.[90, 94]

Chemotherapy

Until 1980, busulfan (Myleran) and hydroxyurea (Hydrea) were the most effective agents in CML therapy. The usual busulfan dose is 0.1 mg/kg per day until the WBC count decreases by 50%, and then the dose is reduced by 50%. Therapy is stopped when the count is less than 20,000/mm³ and restarted when greater than 50,000/mm³. Busulfan therapy is associated with lung, marrow, and heart fibrosis and can cause Addison's disease.[34, 97]

Hydrea has a lower toxicity profile than busulfan but shorter control of WBC count and therefore needs more frequent follow-up. Starting doses of 40 mg/kg per day are adjusted based on the counts. Hydrea is the drug of choice to control WBC count before BMT. A randomized study between Hydrea and busulfan showed longer overall survival with Hydrea.[51]

Although treatment during the chronic phase with busulfan or hydroxyurea will improve marrow cellularity and decrease splenomegaly, it does not eliminate the Ph chromosome. It has a nonspecific manner to suppress hematopoiesis. Thus, even though these agents control the disease for an average of 3 years, all patients will progress to accelerated and blastic phases.

Intensive multidrug regimens are the treatments of choice for the blastic transformation phase of CML in patients who are not BMT candidates. These regimens include high doses of ARA-C (2 g/m²), possibly with anthracyclines. Overall response rates are low, ranging from 20% to 30%. Patients with lymphoid blast crisis, however, have a 60% response rate with ALL regimens based on vincristine and prednisone with remission duration of 9 to 12 months.[32, 51]

Interferon

Interferon (IFN) has been studied in the treatment of CML since 1981. It is the best nontransplant treatment currently proven to prolong survival. It has allowed for a complete hematologic response (CHR) in many patients and cytogenetic responses (suppression of the Ph¹-positive clone) in 10% to 15%. A randomized comparison between IFN alfa-2a (Roferon) and Hydrea showed that the overall survival of the IFN group was significantly better because of slowing of disease from chronic to accelerated or blastic phase.[81] A summary of ongoing trials shows median survival of 60 to 65 months, with 25% of patients being in durable cytogenetic remissions.[89]

Cytogenetic response is a prognostic factor for improved survival and is the target of many trials. Once cytogenetic response is obtained, IFN is continued for 2 to 3 years. The length of cytogenetic response is uncertain.[51] Combinations of IFN and daily low dose ARA-C show a complete hematologic response in most patients and a higher cytogenetic response than with IFN alone.[91] (See Chapter 24 for a complete discussion of IFN and its side effects.)

The target dose of IFN is 5 million IU/m² per day. These doses are often not achieved due to side effects. Decreasing the dosage also compromises the chance of a cytogenetic response.

Bone Marrow Transplantation

Bone marrow transplantation after high-dose chemotherapy and radiation therapy is the only potentially curative treatment for CML.[108] Best results occur when the transplant is performed early in the chronic phase. The 5-year survival for chronic phase patients is 60%, compared with 22% in the accelerated phase and 13% in the blast phase.[144]

The decision to treat young patients with an HLA-matched sibling clearly favors BMT. The decision to treat older patients with IFN versus BMT remains open to debate. BMT has the probability of cure but with high transplant-related mortality (TRM).[146] IFN prolongs chronic phase but without cure. Overall survival benefit for BMT versus IFN is significant for younger patients with a high-risk Sokol score. The choice for older, low-risk patients is not as clear due to TRM.[146] The graft-versus-leukemia effect with BMT is a significant factor in the efficacy of BMT. The use of minitransplants may lessen the risk for older adults in the future (see Chapter 25).

Autologous BMT has been tried either with purging the stem cells after collection or by giving intensive chemotherapy prior to collection of stem cells. Trials using various methods continue. Results remain inferior to allo-BMT.[51]

All patients younger than 55 years with an identical twin or with HLA-matched siblings should be considered for BMT early in the chronic phase. Many BMT centers now treat CML patients up to age 60.

Future Treatments

Homoharringtone (HHT) is a plant alkaloid derivative from the *Cephalotaxus fortuneii* tree. It has been used as low-dose continuous infusion, 2.5 mg/m² daily, in different regimens. Current studies combining HHT and IFN with or without low-dose ARA-C are underway. Early reports show a cytogenetic response in half the patients.[90]

A modified IFN attached to a polyethylene glycol (PEG-IFN) is being studied. PEG-IFN has a longer half-life and fewer side effects and should be in phase II trials soon.[90]

STI-571 is a tyrosine kinase inhibitor specific for cell lines that express BCR-ABL and cause CML. It is given once daily by oral administration. Phase I trials in patients refractory to IFN have shown normalization of blood counts with cytogenetic response in some pa-

tients.[45] Current phase II trials are ongoing with IFN refractory chronic phases patients and also with accelerated and blasts crisis patients.

Chronic Lymphocytic Leukemia

Chronic lymphocytic leukemia (CLL) is a malignant hematologic disorder characterized by proliferation and accumulation of relatively normal-appearing lymphocytes. The vast majority of cases (95%) are B-cell lymphoproliferative disorders with a single clone of B lymphocytes undergoing malignant transformation. The remaining 5% are T-cell lymphoproliferative disorders.[127] The following discussion focuses on B-cell CLL.

EPIDEMIOLOGY AND ETIOLOGY

The development of CLL is more a result of genetic predisposition than environmental influences. It is not associated with radiation or drug exposure. A familial tendency has been suggested but no pattern of inheritance has been reported. A strong correlation exists between CLL and autoimmune diseases such as autoimmune hemolytic anemia and immune thrombocytopenia purpura (ITP).[23] CLL has a variable clinical picture with many living a normal life span without treatment. Others will die of their disease within months to years of diagnosis.[157]

A defect in programmed cell death (PCD) or apoptosis rather than a change in cell cycle regulation causes CLL. Most cells are G_0 quiescent cells that gradually accumulate because they survive too long.[125] These cells are more resistant to the cytotoxic actions of anticancer therapies because of PCD defects and their G_0 stage of cell growth.[125]

Chronic lymphocytic leukemia is the most common leukemia in the United States, accounting for 25% of all newly diagnosed leukemias.[20] Estimated incidence for 2000 is 8100.[2] The median age of CLL patients is 60 years with one third less than age 60.[112] The disease affects twice as many men as women.[112]

CLINICAL FEATURES

Chronic lymphocytic leukemia is discovered on routine physical examination or routine laboratory work in the 25% of patients who are asymptomatic. Because CLL is a disease of immunoglobulin-secreting cells, recurrent skin and respiratory infections may be elicited from the patient history. Nearly 50% of the bone marrow is infiltrated before peripheral blood counts are compromised. Progressive accumulation of the abnormal lymphocytes into nodal structures and the advancing marrow involvement yield symptoms of malaise, anorexia, fatigue, and lymphadenopathy in the patient with advanced disease. Gastrointestinal and genitourinary complaints are related to enlarging abdominal lymph nodes. Splenomegaly may cause abdominal discomfort or early satiety.

Physical findings may be negative or positive only for splenomegaly in the patient with early stage disease. Advanced patients with anemia and thrombocytopenia display the typical findings of anemia and bruising or petechiae. Lymph node enlargement may be present on examination. Hepatomegaly may be seen in addition to splenomegaly if portal obstruction is related to abdominal adenopathy.

DIAGNOSIS

The NCI-sponsored working group (NCI-WG) has revised the guidelines for diagnosis of CLL[29]:

1. Peripheral blood lymphocytosis: an absolute lymphocyte count greater than 5000/mm³, with morphologically mature-appearing cells.
2. Immunophenotype of blood lymphocytes have B cells with CD19, CD20, CD23 positive in addition to CD5 positive, monoclonal expression of either kappa or gamma light chain, and low-density surface immunoglobulin secretion.
3. Bone marrow examination is not a requirement when the above are met but it is useful for prognostic information. Lymphoid cells must be more than 30% of cells.
4. The peripheral blood is sent for flow cytometry to assess the immunophenotype of the cells.

Lymph node biopsy if enlarged shows histology indistinguishable from that of well-differentiated lymphocytic lymphoma.[112]

CLASSIFICATION AND STAGING

There are several methods of classifying CLL and of distinguishing it from other lymphoid malignancies. The FAB group uses morphologic, cytochemical, and immunologic characteristics to separate chronic B- and T-cell leukemias from other disorders (i.e., lymphomas in leukemic phase).[10] The International Lymphoma Study Group proposed the Revised European-American Lymphoma (REAL) classification that has become widely accepted.[75]

The two most common staging systems are based on physical findings and lab abnormalities. They are the Rai (used in the United States) and the Binet (used in Europe) and are summarized in Table 14–7.[157] The Rai system has been modified because the original five stages segregated into the other risk groups. Both fail to identify subsets of early patients, that is, lymphocytosis alone in Binet stage A and splenomegaly alone in Rai O. They also do not identify subsets that will progress quickly.[85, 157]

PROGNOSIS

Clinical stage at time of diagnosis remains the strongest predictor of survival in patients with CLL. It must be remembered that CLL is a heterogeneous disease even for those with the same stage disease. Subsets of each stage may progress more quickly or have a more indolent course.[85, 157]

Age and Sex

Older age shows a poorer prognosis in CLL. When compared by stage, some of the differences may be attributed to comorbid conditions of the elderly. Women survive longer than men do.[157]

TABLE 14–7
The Rai and Binet Staging Systems

Staging System	Stage	Modified Three-Stage System	Clinical Features	Median Survival (y)
Rai	0	Low risk	Lymphocytes in blood and marrow only	>10
	I	Intermediate risk	Lymphocytosis + lymphadenopathy + splenomegaly ± hepatomegaly	7
	II			
	III	High risk	Lymphocytosis + anemia and/or thrombocytopenia	1.5
	IV			
Binet	A		<3 Node-bearing areas	>10
	B		≥3 Node-bearing areas	5
	C		Anemia and/or thrombocytopenia	2

From Zwiebel JA, Cheson BD: Chronic lymphocytic leukemia: staging and prognostic factors, Semin Oncol *25(1):43, 1998.*

Lymphocyte Doubling Time (LDT)

The rate at which the lymphocyte counts increases correlates with survival. Those with a LDT longer than 12 months have a better outcome.[122]

Bone Marrow Involvement

The bone marrow in CLL is generally diffusely infiltrated by mature-appearing lymphocytes. One third of patients exhibit a nondiffuse (nodular, interstitial, mixed) pattern of involvement and have a better prognosis.[29]

Immunophenotype

Because of the heterogeneity of CLL there is a difference in the frequency of expression of various resting and activation antigens. The distinctive characteristic is coexpression of CD5 with faint to virtually undetectable amounts of monoclonal surface immunoglobulins.[23]

β_2-Microglobulins (B2M)

Recent reports indicate that low or high serum B2M levels are associated with good and poor survival times, respectively, in the intermediate and high-risk groups.[93]

Cytogenetics

The most common alteration in B-cell CLL is deletions on chromosome 13 occurring in 65% to 75% of patients. The second most common is trisomy 12. Early studies show an association between prognosis and trisomy 12. Those with increased numbers of clonal abnormalities have shorter survival. No clinical impacts of chromosomal abnormalities have been identified.[87]

TREATMENT MODALITIES

Indications for Treatment

A significant percentage of B-cell patients have hypogammaglobulinemia leading to severe infectious complications. Cellular defects also lead to impaired immune responses to infections. Treatment requirements are often for complications (i.e., antibiotics, IV immunoglobulin) rather than the primary malignancy.[9]

One of the most difficult decisions in CLL is when to initiate treatment. At present, no cure exists for CLL. Treatment aims at alleviating symptoms. The absolute WBC count is not an indication for treatment. Patients with low-risk prognostic factors should not be treated. There is no survival advantage, and early treatment has had detrimental effects in some studies.

The NCI-WG recommends starting treatment when disease-related symptoms are present. These include B symptoms: weight loss greater than 10% in 6 months, profound fatigue, fever without infection, or night sweats, increase in anemia or thrombocytopenia, autoimmune anemia or thrombocytopenia, massively increased lymph nodes or spleen, repeated infections or rapid increase in WBC or high-risk Rai stage.[123]

Single-Agent Chemotherapy

Chlorambucil, an alkylating agent, is the earliest agent used in CLL patients. It is given orally in 6- to 14-mg doses every 2 to 4 weeks. The dose is reduced once the disease is controlled. Several months of treatment are required to obtain a complete response. Response rates range from 40% to 70%. Combinations with prednisone have given mixed results.[52]

Cyclophosphamide is as effective as chlorambucil, and its non–cross-resistance makes it useful in treating patients unresponsive to chlorambucil.[56]

Prednisone has been used to control leukocytosis and to treat immune-mediated hemolytic anemia and thrombocytopenia. Patients with extensive disease may be treated with steroids before initiating chemotherapy.[57] The use of steroids should be limited due to the increased risk of infection.

Combination Chemotherapy

Combination chemotherapy with cyclophosphamide, vincristine, and prednisone (CVP) has been used in patients with advanced CLL.[56] The addition of doxorubicin to this regimen (CHOP) resulted in a survival advantage.[58] No differences in survival were observed between patients randomized to CHOP or chlorambucil plus prednisone.[52] Currently there is little evidence of a role for maintenance chemotherapy in CLL once a response has been obtained. CVP has shown a response slightly better than chlorambucil and prednisone.[124]

Nucleoside Analogues

Fludarabine is the most studied nucleoside analogue. It has been proven to be effective after failure with alkylating agents. Clinical trials have shown fludarabine to be more effective in untreated patients than chlorambucil with 70% achieving either CR or partial response with fludarabine and 43% with chlorambucil.[123] Overall survival is the same although fludarabine has a prolonged remission with fewer infections. It is often used as front-line treatment, especially in younger patients. Cladribine (2-chlorodeoxyadenosine, 2-CdA) and pentostatin (Nipent) also have shown activity in CLL but there are fewer studies supporting their use. Their major toxicity is myelosuppression and patients must be monitored closely for infections. Current trials are investigating the use of fludarabine and alkylating agents as combination therapy.[123]

Splenectomy/Radiation Therapy

Splenectomy or radiation therapy has no influence on survival in CLL patients but may be beneficial in selected cases.[85, 123]

Bone Marrow Transplantation

Allogenic BMT has been increasingly tried as younger patients with high-risk disease are diagnosed. The chance for long-term survival is greater with allo (80%) than auto (48%) but treatment-related mortality is also higher (47% versus 12%). There appears to be evidence of a graft-versus-leukemia effect in CLL. The role of minitransplants is also being explored.[151] The final comparisons will depend on the outcome of randomized clinical trials, which have not been done thus far.

Future Therapies

Rituximab, a monoclonal antibody directed against CD20, is used in follicular lymphoma. It is in clinical trials in patients with CLL, but at much higher dose than used for lymphoma. Initial response rates are between 30% and 40%.[113]

Compath 1-H, a monoclonal antibody directed against CD52, has shown a remission response of 33% in CLL patients refractory to fludarabine. It is most effective on disease in the bone marrow and blood. Bulky lymphadenopathy does not respond well. Future studies will evaluate its use as postremission therapy to eliminate residual disease or as a method of purging bone marrow for possible autologous BMT.[93]

Bryostatin 1 is isolated from a marine bryozoan and in a phase II trial was able to cause CLL cells to differentiate into hairy cells in two of four patients. Further studies are now trying to differentiate CLL cells to hairy cells and then treat them with cladribine as described below.[147]

Hairy-Cell Leukemia

EPIDEMIOLOGY AND ETIOLOGY

Hairy-cell leukemia (HCL) is a rare chronic lymphoproliferative disorder of unknown etiology. There does not seem to be an association with ionizing radiation or other environmental factors. The disease is usually diagnosed in middle-aged patients and is quite rare,

representing less than 2% of adult leukemias, and approximately 500 to 600 new cases in the United States yearly.[82]

CLINICAL FEATURES

Clinical manifestations of HCL are related to excessive infiltration of the bone marrow or spleen or both with "hairy cells." This results in underproduction or excessive peripheral sequestration of circulating cells manifested as granulocytopenia, anemia, or thrombocytopenia.[15] The presenting complaints in more than half of patients are constitutional symptoms of weakness, lethargy, or fatigue. As many as one fourth of patients are diagnosed incidentally when a routine complete blood count reveals abnormalities. Physical findings are limited to splenomegaly, which is seen in as many as 90% of patients.[154] Patients are more susceptible to infections, usually gram-negative bacteria.[52]

DIAGNOSIS

The hallmark of HCL is the presence of the peculiar hairy cell in the blood, bone marrow, and reticuloendothelial organs. This cell is characterized morphologically by its hairlike projections. Cytochemical stains demonstrate the presence of tartrate-resistant acid phosphatase (TRAP). Patients are diagnosed based on the presence of cytopenias, hairy cells in the peripheral blood, splenomegaly, and bone marrow aspiration and biopsy. The bone marrow is frequently fibrotic and usually not aspirable. Splenomegaly is seen without peripheral lymphadenopathy.[85, 86]

CLASSIFICATION

Generally, no accepted staging system is useful for both prognosis and therapy. For the purpose of treatment decisions, it is best to consider this disease in two broad categories: untreated and progressive.

TREATMENT MODALITIES

Hairy-cell leukemia is a highly treatable and often a curable disease. Patients who are asymptomatic with acceptable blood counts can be observed until the disease progresses and requires treatment. Treatment is required when cytopenias become symptomatic, splenomegaly increases, or infectious complications exist.

The standard therapy for HCL was originally splenectomy. This procedure normalizes the peripheral blood in most patients, but virtually no change occurs in the bone marrow, and all patients have progressive disease in 12 to 18 months.[132] Splenectomy is now rarely required in HCL except in splenic rupture.

Interferon-alfa in low, well-tolerated doses is effective in HCL.[63, 101, 132, 133] IFN is administered subcutaneously three times a week for 1 year and yields a 10% CR rate and an 80% overall response rate.[63] This treatment is not curative, however, and retreatment is necessary in most patients whose therapy is stopped.[137] Reinitiating of IFN therapy can induce second responses in at least some patients. Treatment-related side effects occur as with all IFN therapy.

Deoxycoformycin (dCF), also called pentostatin, is a purine analogue first reported to have activity in HCL in 1984. This drug is given as a short infusion every other week for 3 to 6 months and produces a 57% complete response rate and an overall 83% response rate. CRs are of substantial duration, and some patients appear to be cured by this agent.[26, 63]

Cladribine (2-CdA), another purine analogue, has similar activity to dCF. The drug is given intravenously daily for 1 week and produces a total response rate of 97%, with 85% CR and 12% partial remission. Both previously treated and newly diagnosed patients have had the same results. Fever is common. Recovery of blood counts has ranged from 11 to 268 days.[49, 117] Initial therapy with dCF or 2-CdA has now become standard therapy.[85]

Long-term follow-up of 165 patients receiving either dCF or cladribine showed 5-year survival for all patients to be 97% with low treatment-related toxicity. Those who relapsed achieved a durable second remission with either dCF or cladribine.[37]

Myelodysplastic Syndromes

EPIDEMIOLOGY AND ETIOLOGY

The myelodysplastic syndromes (MDSs) are a heterogeneous group of disorders previously referred to as "oligoblastic leukemia," "smoldering acute leukemia," or "preleukemia."[30] *Myelodysplasia* is a disease of elderly persons. More than 80% of persons with MDS are older than 60 years of age. In persons greater than age 70, the incidence is three times that of AML.[8] The incidence of MDS may be increasing, especially secondary or treatment-related MDS. Men are affected more frequently than women.

Although the etiology of MDS is unclear, it is a common clonal (due to a cytogenetic abnormality) stem cell disorder with a much higher incidence than AML.[11] Myelodysplasia is noted for chromosomal deletions, whereas AML generally has balanced chromosomal translocations. The initial abnormality occurs at the level of the multipotent (pluripotent) stem cell and accounts for the dysplastic changes seen in all three cell lines.[83] Some studies have implicated exposure to ben-

zene, radiation, chemotherapy, and alkylating agents in particular as initiating factors in the development of myelodysplasia.[102]

CLINICAL FEATURES

Presenting symptoms depend on the subtype of MDS. Those with early disease will have minimal symptoms, whereas those with advanced subtypes can have symptoms indistinguishable from AML. Severe pancytopenia and all of its related problems can be present.[36] Infections, particularly respiratory or gram-negative septicemias, are frequently the presenting symptom. Bleeding may be present as a result of either thrombocytopenia or poorly functioning circulating platelets.[22] Splenomegaly is present in 10%, especially in chronic myelomonocytic leukemia (CMML).[115]

DIAGNOSIS

Bone marrow aspiration and biopsy establish the diagnosis of MDS. Particular morphologic changes can be seen in both the marrow and the peripheral blood as described below. Chromosomal studies are also performed because approximately 70% to 80% of all patients with MDS display chromosomal abnormalities.[143] Vitamin B_{12} and folate levels should be evaluated in the elderly to rule out the cause of anemia.[115]

CLASSIFICATION

The FAB classification system developed in 1982 is used to classify MDS into five subgroups. It is based on the percentage of blasts and ring sideroblasts (immature red cells with iron granules arranged in a ring around the nucleus) in the bone marrow and the presence or absence of a raised peripheral blood monocyte count. Patients may pass through several stages as the disease progresses. The distinct pathologic entities are: (1) refractory anemia (RA), (2) refractory anemia with ringed sideroblasts (RARS), (3) chronic myelomonocytic leukemia (CMML), (4) refractory anemia with excess blasts (RAEB), and (5) refractory anemia with excess blasts in transition (RAEB-t). These disorders vary from relatively indolent hematologic disorders to conditions indistinguishable from acute leukemia. Table 14–8 lists their percentages.

Because prognosis was difficult to predict based on the FAB classification alone, the International Prognostic Scoring System (IPPS) was developed. It includes bone marrow blast percentage, chromosomal abnormalities, and the number and severity of peripheral cytopenias. Based on the score, a rating of high-intensity, intermediate-intensity, or low-intensity is reached. Decisions regarding treatment can be made using the score.

TABLE 14-8
Myelodysplastic Syndrome Subtypes

	Peripheral Blood Blasts	Bone Marrow Blasts	Survival Months
RA	<1%	<5%	18–64
RARS	<1%	<5%	14–76+
		>15% ring sideroblasts	
RAEB	<5%	5–20%	7–16
RAEB+	≥5%		
	+Auer rods	21–30%	2.5–11
CMML	<5%		
	Monocytes > 1000/mm³	≤20%	9–60+

Adapted from Third MIC Cooperative Group Study: Morphologic, immunologic and cytogenetic working classification of the primary myelodysplastic syndromes and therapy-related myelodysplasia and leukemias, Cancer Genet Cytogenet 32:1, 1988; and List AF, Doll DC: The myelodysplastic syndromes. In Lee GR and others, editors: Wintrobe's clinical hematology, Philadelphia, Williams & Wilkins, 1999:2320.

PROGNOSIS

Because of the heterogeneity of MDS, prognosis varies widely. Both FAB and IPPS are used to assess risk. Approximate survival times are listed in Table 14–8.

Patients older than 60 years have poorer outcomes in the low-intensity and intermediate-intensity groups. Patients older than 70 years have an even worse survival than those between 60 and 70 years. Coexisting diseases in the elderly contribute to their poorer survival. There is no difference in the high-intensity groups in terms of survival.[65]

TREATMENT MODALITIES

Because of the elderly age of MDS patients, various treatment approaches have been used, including no therapy, pyridoxine, androgens, and steroids. These options are rarely effective.[50] Patients with only RA may have an indolent disease course and can be supported by transfusion therapy for many years. Iron chelation therapy should be considered in these patients.

Supportive care is the standard treatment for many of the elderly population. Transfusions of PRBCs and platelets, along with antibiotic treatment for infections are indicated.[115]

Hematopoietic growth factors work in selected patients but often are not as effective in advanced subtypes. It can decrease PRBC transfusion requirements and may stimulate WBC production. HGFs in various combinations are undergoing clinical trials. Therapy with GM-CSF plus low-dose ARA-C was evaluated, with equal thirds of patients improving, remaining stable, or declining.[66] Another multicenter phase III study randomized RAEB/RAEB-t patients to observation versus long-term G-CSF therapy. Improved neutrophil counts were observed in most G-CSF patients without side effects. No difference in the incidence of or time of progression to AML was noted. The incidence of infections is being evaluated.[67, 104]

Erythropoietin (EPO) alone has shown limited effect. However, in combination with G-CSF, 40% to 45% of patients had decreased transfusion requirements and increased hemoglobin levels. Most had neutrophil responses.[66]

Amifostine (Ethyol) potentiates the growth of multipotent (pluripotent) progenitors and erythroid cells in vitro. It is thought to act on the myelodysplastic clone. Phase I/II trials have shown improvements in all three cell lines. Phase II multicenter trials are underway, some evaluating the interaction with chemotherapy and growth factors.[102]

Differentiating agents can transform nonfunctional immature blasts and promyeloblasts into functional mature granulocytes.[22] Various agents have been studied, including retinoic acids, low-dose cytarabine, tretinoin, interferon-alfa, and hexamethylmelamine bisacetamide. Thus far, none of these agents has achieved a measure of success substantial enough to consider these differentiating agents to be standard therapy for MDS. A pyrimidine analog, 5-azacytidine (5-Aza), is a new pharmacologic differentiating agent. Phase II studies showed hematologic improvement in 40% of MDS patients.[110, 136]

Because of the older age of patients, low-dose treatments have been investigated. Low-dose cytarabine yielded responses in approximately 15% to 25%.[110] Topotecan (1.25 mg/m² daily) and cytarabine (1 g/m² per day times 5 days) showed response in 63% of patients.[12]

Patients less than 60 years with a matched donor are referred for allogeneic BMT, as in AML. Allogeneic BMT studies have shown disease-free survival rates of 41% and 55%, with a median patient age of 30 years.[50] Autologous BMT is a treatment option for younger patients in CR after intensive chemotherapy. One fourth of patients were in remission for more than 3 years in one trial.[41] Again, most patients are over age 60 and will not be eligible for these therapies.

Future clinical trials will continue to build on the results of current studies of MDS therapy.

CONCLUSION

Great progress has been made in the knowledge of the biologic nature and treatment of leukemia during the past decade. Advances in supportive care of the immunosuppressed patient have dramatically improved survival in leukemia patients. Much research is still required to define more effective therapies to increase disease-free survival and decrease relapse rates.

The challenges and opportunities for nurses are numerous in the field of leukemia. The acuity level of patient care for those with leukemia depends on the disease variables and practice setting. Hospital-based nurses provide care for the leukemic patient who is acutely ill. The intensity and complexity of the nursing care required for many of these patients rival those of intensive care units. Other patients with leukemia, such as those in chronic phase CML, early CLL, AML, or ALL in remission or those receiving milder continuation therapy, are seen in the clinic or outpatient setting.

Another practice setting is the BMT unit, where intensive acute care and ambulatory care are required. Historically, most leukemia patients were transferred to major metropolitan centers for treatment. In recent years, however, with improved mechanisms to transfer medical technology into the community, more patients are cared for locally. The NCI's Cooperative Group Outreach Program (CGOP) and, since 1983, the Community Clinical Oncology Program (CCOP) provide the opportunity to enroll leukemia patients in cooperative group clinical trials. The number of institutions performing BMT has also increased dramatically and will continue to increase over the next decades as BMT becomes a promising treatment option for many types of cancer.

The nurse in clinical practice may easily feel overwhelmed by the complexity and intensity of both learning about the disease of leukemia and providing care to the patient with leukemia. A useful strategy for learning this information and integrating it into one's nursing practice is to focus on one type of leukemia at a time. The nurse should select a patient newly diagnosed with leukemia and review the individual patient's presenting symptoms, results of the diagnostic evaluation, prognostic indicators, and treatment plan. The nurse should monitor this treatment plan, the selected drug regimen, blood counts, marrow results, and the potential side effects experienced by the patient as a result of the disease or treatment. These concepts should be incorporated into an individualized nursing plan of care. Depending on the practice setting, the nurse may want to collaborate with another inpatient or outpatient nursing colleague to follow the patient's progress. After completing this exercise a few times, the nurse will gain confidence in the knowledge of the leukemias and their treatment and thereby improve clinical practice expertise in caring for patients with leukemia.

The intensity and complexity of caring for leukemic patients are both rewarding and frustrating. Providing direct care to an acutely ill patient in a life-threatening situation fosters very close relationships with both the patient and the members of his or her support system. These relationships can be intensely rewarding. At the same time the intensity of care can lead to frustration and exhaustion when the patient does not respond to therapy or dies. Sudden and unexpected medical crisis and death do occur in this population of patients. Nurses caring for patients with leukemia must be cognizant of their own feelings and needs. The most valuable support system oncology nurses have is the support and understanding of their peers. These are the people who experience the same joys, fears, pain, and frustration of caring for the acutely ill patient. The most important self-care aspect of the nurse caring for the patient with leukemia is recognizing the level of investment and acknowledging the emotional peaks and valleys that accompany this investment.

Nursing Management

The medical and nursing management of lymphocytic and myeloid leukemia patients is similar and is detailed here. The intensity of therapy and resultant side effects will differ for acute versus chronic leukemias. Supportive care of the leukemic patient is a major contributor to increased survival and improved quality of life. The talents and resources of all members of the interdisciplinary team are required to support the patient and family through all phases of this disease process. The nurse, relying on a strong knowledge of the disease and the potential complications, uses systematic assessments to monitor physiologic homeostasis. For the person with leukemia, medical and nursing support is required in three areas: (1) to prevent or correct expected side effects of the disease and treatment, (2) to anticipate and treat unexpected or potential complications, and (3) to facilitate psychosocial adaptation of the patient and family.[1, 84]

Nursing Diagnosis

- *Knowledge deficit related to new leukemia diagnosis, disease process, treatment plan, side effects*

Outcome Goal

Patient and family will be able to:

- Verbalize and demonstrate understanding of disease treatment and goals.

Interventions

- Review disease process, treatment regimen, management and prevention of complications, and goals of treatment.[21]
- Assess patient's preferred style of learning; identify any existing barriers to learning, including language and cultural beliefs; teach in short sessions; involve family members and significant others in teaching sessions; question patient to evaluate understanding of new information; and continue to reinforce information.
- Participate in informed consent process if patient is eligible for a clinical trial (see Chapter 26).
- Assess and discuss patient's desired level of information; explain common terminology.
- Orient patient and family to hospital unit and services (e.g., parking, accommodations, and meals).
- Explain role of multidisciplinary team members and how to access their services.
- Provide information about insertion of venous access devices, and promote self-care of line after insertion.
- Provide information regarding available community resources and link where possible.
- Assist patient in developing system of treatment management through use of calendars, schedules, etc.
- In fertile patients, discuss issues of fertility (sperm banking, egg retrieval).
- Discuss issues of sexuality.
- Explain purpose of baseline testing.
- Provide a calendar of planned treatments and tests.

Nursing Diagnosis

- *Anxiety related to new diagnosis, uncertain outcome of potentially fatal disease, loss of control in hospital environment, alteration in body image, alteration in interpersonal relationships*

Outcome Goal

Patient and family will be able to:

- Verbalize and/or demonstrate manageable anxiety throughout course of illness and seek out appropriate resources.

Interventions

- Perform psychosocial assessment of patient/family;

identify strengths, weaknesses, coping skills, and cultural preferences.
- Recognize increased anxiety levels that may occur while awaiting an official diagnosis, before painful or frightening procedures, before major treatments, on learning of relapse, and on anniversary dates.[99]
- Administer/offer antianxiety medications as ordered; assess effectiveness.
- Use therapeutic and healing touch.
- Use guided imagery, relaxation training, and cognitive distraction to alleviate anxiety before painful or stressful procedures.
- Assist patient/family to set realistic goals concerning level of activity, work schedule, and self-care activities.
- Encourage patient/family to verbalize questions, fears, and concerns.
- Involve chaplaincy services, social workers, psychologists, psychiatry, and support volunteers as needed.
- Inform patient/family of available community resources (e.g., Leukemia Society of America, American Cancer Society).

PRETREATMENT PHASE

The nurse caring for the patient with leukemia must have a thorough knowledge of the medical management of treatment-related toxicities and potential disease complications to provide effective nursing care.

The following assessments and medical interventions are performed before initiating antileukemia therapy. The nurse must incorporate the rationale for these studies into the patient teaching plan to help orient the patient and family to the plan of care.

- Assessment of serum chemistries:
  Renal function: elevated creatinine may limit use of aminoglycoside antibiotics.
  Hepatic function: doses of anthracyclines or vincristine may require reduction for elevated liver enzymes.
  Electrolytes: normal electrolytes may minimize risk of certain drug side effects.
- Blood typing should be performed to ensure the availability of RBC and platelet transfusions.
- HLA typing should be performed on admission for patients who are possible bone marrow transplantation (BMT) candidates.
- Baseline coagulation profile should be performed on patients with acute promyelocytic leukemia. These patients have an increased incidence of disseminated intravascular coagulation (DIC) (see Chapter 20). Patients with DIC may require heparinization or fresh-frozen plasma and platelet sup-

port before treatment initiation although with the use of ATRA, DIC is less of a problem.

- Baseline chest x-ray film eliminates later confusion and assesses presence of possible pulmonary complications before treatment.
- Radionucleotide ventriculogram ensuring an adequate left ventricular ejection fraction before treatment requiring anthracyclines is important in patients with a questionable cardiac history or before enrollment in clinical trials.
- It is important to establish central venous access, preferably with a multilumen catheter, before treatment. If patient is thrombocytopenic at diagnosis, platelet transfusion may be required before invasive procedure to reduce risk of bleeding. Catheter site must be monitored closely for postoperative bleeding.
- Decision to delay chemotherapy initiation to resolve an infection is determined by status of leukemia, severity of infection, and number of circulating granulocytes.
- Acute tumor lysis syndrome occurs more often in high WBC greater than 100,000 (less of a problem in CML). Patients at risk should receive high doses of allopurinol before treatment and urinary alkalization, with sodium bicarbonate added to IV solutions.
- Although uncommon, uric acid deposits in the urinary tract may occur in patients with very high WBC counts. Again, allopurinol, 300 mg orally daily, should be instituted before starting treatment.

By monitoring the results of these studies, the nurse can assess potential patient complications. For example, an abnormal coagulation profile in a patient with acute promyelocytic (M_3) leukemia should signal the nurse to incorporate bleeding precautions and assessment for shocklike symptoms into the patient care and teaching plan.

CHEMOTHERAPY SIDE EFFECTS

Regardless of the chemotherapy regimen chosen, infection and bleeding are the most common side effects of acute leukemia therapy. Induction chemotherapy not only kills the malignant clone of leukemia cells in the marrow, but also suppresses the production of normal hematologic elements. Thus, as the platelets, WBCs, and to a lesser extent RBCs in the peripheral blood die, there are no new cells to replace them. The patient is severely immunocompromised until the normal marrow components begin to regenerate. Chemotherapy for CML and CLL with Hydrea will usually decrease WBCs without a significant effect on

RBCs and platelets. Once more intensive chemotherapy is used, then more intense side effects will occur. For care of patients receiving monoclonal antibodies, see Chapter 24.

One of the most important considerations in the care of the leukopenic patient is the lack of the normal host responses to infection (see Chapter 31 for care of the immunosuppressed patient).

In patients who receive high-dose ARA-C (HIDAC) or regimens aimed at overcoming multidrug resistance, the period of myelosuppression may last 3 to 4 weeks. Infection risk increases when the *absolute neutrophil count* (ANC) falls below 500 cells/mm^3 and exceeds 1 week. The ANC is calculated by multiplying the percentage of segmented and bands neutrophils by the total WBCs.

Therapy with HIDAC increases the risk for ocular problems and neurotoxicity. Corneal damage, burning, photophobia, decreased acuity, and conjunctivitis are reported. Corticosteroid eye drops are thought to help prevent these side effects.[149]

Increased neurotoxicity is seen in elderly patients receiving HIDAC, especially cerebellar toxicities, and is not recommended in patients over age 60. Doses are often decreased to 1.5 to 2.0 g/m.² Nursing interventions include a pretreatment assessment of the patient's neurologic status, gait, speech, eye movements, and ability to perform alternating movements rapidly. These assessments should be repeated prior to each dose of HIDAC.[149]

Neurotoxicity can occur with several chemotherapies used in the treatment of leukemia. Methotrexate given intrathecally can cause both acute and delayed reactions. Acutely, meningeal irritation can occur. Myelopathy or encephalopathy can occur within days to a week after therapy and is thought to be related to increased CSF levels. Leukoencephalopathy is a delayed reaction that can occur years later and is seen mostly in children. Use of concurrent cranial irradiation increases the risk.[59]

Vincristine produces peripheral sensorimotor neuropathies. Numbness and tingling in the hands and feet are early signs. With further doses the patient can develop motor weakness, gait changes and inability to write or hold objects. Constipation is common, related to autonomic neuropathy. Toxicity depends on dosage and frequency. Giving further medication when toxicities have not resolved increases the risk for further problems that may be irreversible.

Corticosteroids are used in the treatment of ALL and sometimes CLL with prednisone being the most commonly used. Common side effects include depression, mania, difficulty sleeping, mood swings, and increased appetite with possible delirium in rare instances. Increased appetite and weight gain can be disturbing to a patient's self image. Myopathy, especially of the lower extremities, can make stair climbing and even walking difficult. Steroids also act on the immune system as a suppressant and can increase the risk of infection. At the same time, it will mask an increase in body temperature.

Asparaginase, used in ALL, often produces hypersensitivity reactions. It may occur with the first injection but generally occurs after repeated exposure. The patient must be observed for signs of an allergic reaction for one hour after injection. Anaphylaxis may occur, and appropriate medications should be available. Cerebellar dysfunction can also occur with asparaginase. Hepatotoxicity resulting from asparaginase may contribute to CNS findings.[59]

An increased temperature may be the only indication of an infectious process. Other indications may include chills, cough, burning and frequency on urination, diarrhea, or a sore that will not heal. It is important to note that corticosteroid therapy may suppress the febrile response. Also, with few WBCs, pus will not always be present in infected wounds. Astute nursing assessment is required to monitor potential sites of infection and provide appropriate interventions. The nurse, caring for the leukemic patient on a daily basis, is also in the best position to detect subtle changes that may be the earliest indicators of impending septic shock. Patients are often at home with neutropenia after chemotherapy and along with family members needed to be taught the importance of monitoring their temperatures.

Mucositis secondary to chemotherapy is most often seen with cytarabine, doxorubicin, bleomycin, etoposide, 5-fluorouracil, mercaptopurine, and methotrexate. Ulcers can be minimal or involve the entire oral and gastrointestinal mucosa. Effects generally occur within a few days after starting chemotherapy. Secondary effects are oral infections, pain and decreased oral intake.[44]

A randomized study comparing chlorhexidine versus plain water shows water to be just as effective.[43] Another showed sodium bicarbonate-normal saline gargling to be more effective against mucositis than chlorhexidine.[95]

With the availability of platelet transfusion support, hemorrhage is less of a problem than in past years. Prophylactic transfusions are usually administered in asymptomatic patients when the platelet count is below 10,000 to 20,000/mm^3. Platelet counts should be checked 15 minutes to 1 hour after transfusion to assess the increment of platelet increase. This also enables evaluation of possible alloimmunization and the need for a different platelet product. Alloimmunization occurs because the antigens on the trans-

fused platelets react with the patient's antibodies, and the platelets are destroyed. Using platelets that have been leukoreduced and/or irradiated can decrease the risk. If a poor response still occurs, single-donor or HLA-matched platelets may be used. When patients develop fever, chills, or hives during transfusions, they may be premedicated with diphenhydramine and hydrocortisone and/or acetaminophen.

Transfusion of packed RBCs may be required to control anemia. Patients are usually transfused when their hemoglobin concentration falls between 7 to 8 g/dL. Elderly patients may require transfusions sooner to preserve cardiopulmonary function. An average 70-kg adult should increase 1 g/dL (hematocrit 2–3%) with each unit of packed RBC.[152] Nursing assessment includes monitoring for paleness, dyspnea, dizziness, headache, and irritability. Tachycardia and tachypnea indicate cardiac hypoxia.

Nursing Diagnosis

- *Risk for infection related to alteration in immune function secondary to leukemia and immunosuppressive chemotherapy*

Outcome Goals

Patient will be able to:

- Demonstrate an understanding of the precautions to take to avoid infections and the signs and symptoms of possible infection.
- Seek appropriate treatment when demonstrating signs and symptoms of infection.

Interventions

- Teach patient/family the purpose and importance of neutropenic precautions.
- If appropriate, encourage patient to keep a chart of daily blood counts.
- Monitor temperature and vital signs every 4 hours when patient is neutropenic. Assess for changes in blood pressure, urine output, and mental status that may be early signs of septic shock. Patients at home should monitor their temperature while awake every 4 hours. Intravenous antibiotics should be initiated for temperature greater than 101 or with shaking chills.
- Have patient avoid fresh fruits and vegetables and pepper.
- Do not allow fresh flowers in patient's room.
- Avoid rectal manipulation.
- Ensure consistent handwashing by all people entering patient's room.
- Ensure consistent handwashing by patient before eating and after toileting.

- Limit number of visitors to two at a time; no visitors with colds, influenza, herpes, or recent vaccinations.
- Avoid trauma to skin and mucous membranes.
- Do not administer intramuscular injections.

Nursing Diagnosis

- Risk for injury associated with bleeding related to alteration in clotting factors, thrombocytopenia secondary to leukemia and/or treatment

Outcome Goals

Patient will be able to:

- Verbalize/demonstrate an understanding of the precautions to prevent bleeding so that risks of bleeding will be minimized.
- Seek appropriate treatment when demonstrating signs and symptoms of occult bleeding.

Interventions

- Teach patient/family the significance of platelet function and bleeding precautions.
- Check platelet counts at least every other day during immunosuppressive leukemia therapies.
- Monitor results of coagulation studies; assess for signs and symptoms of DIC.
- Assess for petechiae, bruising, epistaxis, hematuria, hematochezia, and oral, rectal, or vaginal bleeding.
- Monitor platelet transfusions.
- Apply pressure on bone marrow or venipuncture sites for 3 to 5 minutes.
- Do not administer intramuscular injections.
- Avoid rectal manipulation.
- Use only electric razors.
- Do not administer aspirin-containing medications.
- Ensure safe environment: no sharp objects, bed rails up, ambulate with assistance.
- Prevent trauma to skin and mucous membranes.
- Use soft toothbrush.

Nursing Diagnosis

- Altered nutrition less than body requirements, related to treatment-induced nausea, vomiting, stomatitis, anorexia

Outcome Goals

Patient will be able to:

- Maintain adequate body weight and muscle mass throughout treatment.

- Verbalize/demonstrate an understanding of measures to prevent treatment-induced side effects.

Interventions

- Monitor patient's weight.
- Refer to nutritionist if ongoing pattern of weight loss or history of eating disorder, obesity, or diabetes.
- Record intake and output every shift.
- Record calorie counts.
- Administer antiemetics for nausea, and assess effectiveness.
- Assess for diarrhea and constipation, and medicate as needed.
- Constipation is very common with vincristine.
- Perform daily assessment of lips and oral mucosa for mucositis.
- Teach patient the purpose of oral care protocol and evaluate technique.
- Evaluate and document compliance to oral care protocol.
- Use topical analgesics in mouth and on lips if open ulcers are present.
- Encourage small, frequent meals with high-calorie, high-protein foods.
- Encourage intake of culturally preferred foods from home if unable to obtain at hospital.

DISEASE-RELATED COMPLICATIONS

Leukostasis

Patients with exceptionally high circulating blast counts are at risk to develop leukostasis. Leukemic blasts aggregating and invading capillary walls, causing rupture and bleeding causes this syndrome. This occurs most often in the brain because of its vascularity and limited space. Intrapulmonary bleeding can also result from this "sludging syndrome." These complications are associated with significant morbidity and mortality, and this medical emergency necessitates immediate reduction of the circulating leukocytes. High doses of hydroxyurea or high-dose chemotherapy may be instituted, or leukapheresis with a filtered, continuous-flow cell separator may help reduce the cell burden. Once the danger of leukostasis is eliminated, definitive antileukemia therapy is initiated.

Interventions

- Monitor for changes in level of consciousness; perform neurologic examinations as ordered.
- Monitor respiratory status.

- Administer high-dose chemotherapy as ordered.
- Monitor leukapheresis process.
- Monitor absolute blast counts.

$$\text{absolute blast count} = \frac{\text{total WBC count} \times \text{blasts}}{100}$$

Disseminated Intravascular Coagulation

Diffuse or disseminated intravascular coagulation (DIC) is a complex syndrome characterized by the activation of coagulation and formation of fibrin within the general circulation (see Chapter 20). Patients with acute promyelocytic leukemia (APL, FAB type M_3) are at high risk of developing DIC after the initiation of chemotherapy as the granules from the promyelocytes are released and initiate the coagulation cascade. The use of ATRA decreases the incidence of DIC.

Interventions

- Ensure systematic assessment for occult, overt, or sudden massive bleeding.
- Begin therapy with ATRA according to protocol for M_3 (APL).
- Initiate antileukemia therapy to correct the underlying disease pathology.
- Administer antibiotics for sepsis.
- Administer blood products (platelets, fresh-frozen plasma) as ordered.
- Apply pressure to venipuncture sites.
- Administer heparin if ordered.

Treatment for DIC must focus on eliminating the underlying cause and instituting supportive therapy with the appropriate blood products.

Typhlitis

Typhlitis, or inflammation of the cecum, is thought to be related to *Clostridia* sepsis or other bacteria, including *Pseudomonas, Escherichia coli,* or *Klebsiella.* This diagnosis should be considered in the neutropenic patient who develops severe abdominal pain. Bloody diarrhea, absence of bowel sounds, rebound tenderness, and fever may accompany the pain. An abdominal x-ray film may reveal a right lower quadrant soft tissue mass, dilated colon, or pericecal edema. The pathologic diagnosis is established by stool culture, and the identified pathogen is treated with appropriate antibiotics.

Interventions

- Put patient on bedrest.
- Maintain IV fluids.

- Assess fluid and electrolyte balance.
- Ensure patient has no oral intake.
- Administer and evaluate analgesics.

Renal Failure

Renal failure in leukemia patients may result from urate nephropathy, aminoglycoside toxicity, sepsis, or leukemic infiltration of the kidneys.

Interventions

- Hydration and urine alkalinization are used with certain regimens (e.g., high-dose methotrexate) or with a high WBC count during induction therapy.
- Monitor BUN and creatinine values.
- Record accurate intake and output.
- Monitor vital signs and mental status.
- Assess for signs of alteration in tissue perfusion.

PATIENT AND FAMILY TEACHING

As with other types of cancer care, the teaching of leukemic patients should begin at the time of diagnosis and continue throughout the disease course. In acute leukemia, teaching is required in both the inpatient setting during the induction phase and intensive supportive care period and in the outpatient setting during continuation therapy and long-term follow-up.

A leukemia diagnosis may be a shock to patients experiencing few if any symptoms at the time of diagnosis. Some patients, experiencing an acute illness or a lengthy period of medical evaluation before the discovery of the diagnosis, may feel a sense of relief to know finally a definitive diagnosis. Certainly the diagnosis of any potentially fatal disease is a time of crisis for the entire family. The boxes list geriatric considerations and patient teaching priorities.

GERIATRIC CONSIDERATIONS

Leukemia

Perform cardiovascular evaluation, including radionucleotide ventriculogram to assess left ventricular ejection fraction.
Monitor for signs and symptoms of fluid overload.
Maintain a safe environment: bed rails, call light within reach, assistance with ambulating.
Assess potential barriers to learning: decreased visual acuity, poor hearing, decreased concentration.
Assess previous bowel routines.
Assess over-the-counter drug use.
Assess visual and auditory status before treatment.
Drugs causing neurotoxicities, i.e., vincristine, ARA-C, need to have dose adjustments

---

PATIENT TEACHING PRIORITIES

Leukemia

Normal hematopoiesis, purpose of red blood cells, white blood cells, and platelets

Pathophysiology of leukemia

Goals of planned treatment

Treatment schedule and method of administration

Expected side effects and related interventions

Plan for symptom management

Neutropenia and bleeding precautions

Plan for patient/family participation in treatment and shared decision-making

Explanation of any procedures, i.e., bone marrow biopsy, catheter insertion[1]

Exploration of patient coping methods and assistance as needed

---

To provide effective care, the nurse must always be sensitive to the patient's feelings of isolation and loss of control. The patient may display the need to regain control, especially during lengthy hospitalizations. Addressing this need for control early in the hospitalization is important. Control issues can be divided into three areas as follows:

Patient Controlled	*No Control*	*Nurse Controlled*
Antibiotic skin care regimen	Disease process	Scheduled medications
Time to bathe	Administration of blood products	Vital signs
Time for dressing change	X-ray films	Mealtimes
Oral care	Laboratory work	Weights
Dietary choices		
Analgesia		
Visiting times		

The main point to remember is that many aspects of nursing care can be flexible and items such as when the patient will bathe can be negotiated.

Chapter Questions

1. The specific leukemia that has a defect in programmed cell death allowing an accumulation of cells is:
   a. AML
   b. ALL
   c. CML
   d. CLL

2. The French-American-British (FAB) classification system is based on the following criteria:
   a. Cytogenetic abnormalities, immunophenotypic features
   b. Cytogenetic abnormalities, cellularity ratio
   c. Cellular morphology, cytogenetic abnormalities
   d. Cellular morphology, immunophenotypic features

3. Important prognostic factors in ALL remission duration include:
   a. Cytogenetic abnormalities, time to achieve remission, age, WBC count after treatment
   b. Cytogenetic abnormalities, time to disease relapse, age, initial WBC count
   c. Cytogenetic abnormalities, time to achieve remission, age, initial WBC count
   d. Cytogenetic abnormalities, time to disease relapse, age, WBC count after treatment

4. The usual treatment modality progressions for ALL include:
   a. Induction, postremission, CNS treatment, BMT, recurrent/refractory disease
   b. Induction, CNS treatment, postremission, BMT, recurrent/refractory disease
   c. Induction, BMT, CNS treatment, postremission, recurrent/refractory disease
   d. Induction, BMT, CNS treatment, recurrent/refractory disease, postremission

5. The most frequently used drug for dose intensification in treatment of AML is:
   a. High-dose ARA-C (cytarabine)
   b. High-dose Cytoxan (cylophosphamide)
   c. High-dose doxorubicin (Adriamycin)
   d. High-dose idarubicin (Idamycin)

6. A complete remission in AML is defined as:
   a. Less than 1% nucleated marrow blasts in a normocellular marrow
   b. Less than 10% nucleated marrow blasts in a normocellular marrow
   c. Less than 5% nucleated marrow blasts in a normocellular marrow
   d. Less than 15% nucleated marrow blasts in a normocellular marrow

7. All-*trans*-retinoic acid (ATRA) used in treatment of APL promotes:
   a. Cell differentiation
   b. Cell destruction
   c. Cell cycling
   d. Cell coagulation

8. Treatment modalities used in *curative* treatment of CML include:

a. Chemotherapy, biotherapy, autologous bone marrow transplantation

b. Chemotherapy, biotherapy, allogeneic bone marrow transplantation

c. Chemotherapy (high-dose), autologous bone marrow transplantation, biotherapy

d. Chemotherapy (high-dose), radiation therapy, allogeneic bone marrow transplantation

9. All the following are true regarding chronic lymphocytic leukemia (CLL) *except:*

a. Are usually diagnosed via routine physical exams and/or laboratory tests

b. FAB classification is used for disease staging

c. Approximately 95% of CLL are B-cell lymphoproliferative disorders

d. CLL accounts for 25% of all newly diagnosed leukemia cases in the United States

10. All of the following are true regarding myelodysplastic syndrome *except:*

a. MDS is a heterogeneous group of disorders

b. MDS is more common in young adults

c. MDS etiology is unclear, note for chromosomal abnormalities

d. Various treatment approaches are used

BIBLIOGRAPHY

1. Alcoser PW, Burchett S: Bone marrow transplantation: Immune system suppression and reconstitution, *AJN* 99(6):26, 1999.

2. American Cancer Society: *Cancer facts and figures—2000,* Atlanta, The Society, 2000.

3. Angelillo IF: Residential exposure to electromagnetic fields and childhood leukemia: a metaanalysis, *Bull World Health Organ* 77:906, 1999.

4. Appelbaum FR, Gilliland DG, Tallman MS: The biology and treatment of acute myeloid leukemia. *Hematology 1998,* p. 15.

5. Appelbaum FR: Progress in adult acute lymphoblastic leukemia, *WJM* 164(2):180, 1996.

6. Applebaum FR, Downing J, William C: The biology and therapy of AML, *Hematology 1995,* p. 22.

7. Arleen A and others: Randomized multi-center trial of cytosine arabinoside with mitoxantrone or daunorubicin in previously untreated adult patients with acute nonlymphocytic leukemia, *Leukemia* 4:177, 1990.

8. Aul C, Gattermann N, Schneider W: Age-related incidence and other epidemiological aspects of myelodysplastic syndromes, *Br J Hematol* 82:358, 1992.

9. Bartik MM, Welker D, Kay NE: Impairments in immune cell function in B cell chronic lymphocytic leukemia, *Semin Oncol* 25:27, 1998.

10. Bennett JM and others: Proposals for the classification of chronic (mature) B and T lymphoid leukemias, *J Clin Pathol* 42:567, 1989.

11. Bennett JM and others: Proposals for the classification of the myelodysplastic syndromes, *Br J Haematol* 51:189, 1982.

12. Beran M and others: Results of combination chemotherapy with topotecan and high-dose cytosine arabinoside (ara-C) in previously untreated patients with high-risk myelodysplastic syndrome (MDS) and chronic myelomonocytic leukemia (CMML), *Blood* 90(suppl 1):583a, 1997 (abstr).

13. Bergsagel DE, Bailey MB, Langley GR: The chemotherapy of plasma-cell myeloma and the incidence of acute leukemia, *N Engl J Med* 301:743, 1979.

14. Bondurant MC, Koury MJ: Origin and development of blood cells. In Lee GR, Foerster J, Lukens J, and others, editors: *Wintrobe's clinical hematology,* Philadelphia, Williams & Wilkins, 1999:2342.

15. Bouroncle BA: Leukemic reticuloendotheliosis, *Blood* 53:412, 1979.

16. Brownson RC, Novotny TE, Perry MC: Cigarette smoking and adult leukemia: a metaanalysis, *Arch Intern Med* 153:469, 1993.

17. Buchner T and others: Intensified induction and consolidation with or without maintenance chemotherapy for AML: two multicenter studies of the German AML Cooperative Group, *J Clin Oncol* 3:1583, 1985.

18. Buchner T: Management of acute myeloid leukemia in the elderly, *Cancer Control,* March/April 1995.

19. Burnett A and others: Randomized comparison of addition of autologous bone-marrow transplantation to intensive chemotherapy for acute myeloid leukaemia in first remission: Results of MRC AML10 trial, *Lancet* 351:700, 1998.

20. Byrd JC, Flinn IW, Graver MR: Introduction: chronic lymphocytic leukemia, *Semin Oncol* 25:4, 1998.

21. Caguioa PB, Tansan S, McCaffrey RP: Chronic lymphocytic leukemia, *Am J Med Sci* 308:196, 1994.

22. Cain J and others: Myelodysplastic syndromes: a review for nurses, *Oncol Nurs Forum* 18:113, 1991.

23. Caligans-Cappio F: New insights into the biology of B-chronic lymphocyte leukemia. In: *Hematology 1999,* p. 249.

24. Cassileth P and others: Comparison of autologous bone marrow transplantation (AutoBMT) with high-dose cytarabine (HiDAC) in adult acute myeloid leukemia (AML) in first remission (CR1): an ECOG Intergroup study, *Proc Am Soc Clin Oncol* 16:89a, 1997 (abstr).

25. Cassileth PA and others: Maintenance chemotherapy protocols remission duration in adult acute nonlymphocytic leukemia, *J Clin Oncol* 6:583, 1988.

26. Cassileth PA and others: Pentostatin induces durable remissions in HCL, *J Clin Oncol* 9:243, 1991.

27. Cassileth PA and others: Varying intensities of postremission therapy in acute myeloid leukemia, *Blood* 79:1924, 1992.

28. Champlain R and others: Postremission chemotherapy for adults with acute myelogenous leukemia: improved survival with high-dose cytarabine and daunorubicin consolidation treatment, *J Clin Oncol* 8:1199, 1990.

29. Cheson BD and others: National Cancer Institute-sponsored working group guidelines for chronic lymphocytic leukemia: revised guidelines for diagnosis and treatment. *Blood* 87:4990, 1996.

30. Cheson BD: The myelodysplastic syndromes: current approaches to therapy, *Ann Intern Med* 112:932, 1990.

31. Copelan EA, McGuire EA: The biology and treatment of acute lymphoblastic leukemia in adults, *Blood* 85:1151, 1995.

32. Cortes JE, Kantarjian H: Acute lymphocytic leukemia. In Pazdur R, editor: *Medical oncology: a comprehensive review,* ed 2, New York, Huntington, 1996.

33. Cortes JE, Kantarjian HM: Acute lymphoblastic leukemia. A comprehensive review with emphasis on biology and therapy, *Cancer* 76:2393, 1995.

34. Cortes JE, Talpaz M, Kantarjian H: Chronic myelogenous leukemia: a review, *Am J Med* 100:555, 1996.

35. Cortes JE, Talpaz M, Kantarjian H: Chronic myelogenous leukemia. In Pazdur R, editor: *Medical oncology: a comprehensive review,* ed 2, New York, Huntington, 1996.

36. Dang CV: Myelodysplastic syndrome, *JAMA* 267:2077, 1992.

37. Deardon CE and others: Long-term follow-up of patients with hairy cell leukaemia after treatment with pentostatin or cladribine, *Br J Haematol* 106:515, 1999.

38. Degos L and others: All-*trans*-retinoic acid as a differentiating agent in the treatment of acute promyelocytic leukemia, *Blood* 85:2643, 1995.

39. DeGramont A and others: Preleukemic changes in cases of non-lymphocytic leukemia secondary to cytotoxic therapy: analysis of 105 cases, *Cancer* 58:630, 1986.

40. Devine SM, Larson RA: Acute leukemia in adults: recent developments in diagnosis and treatment, *CA Cancer J Clin* 44:326, 1994.

41. De Witte, T, Van Biezen A, Hermans J, et al: Autologous bone marrow transplantation for patients with myelodysplastic syndrome (MDS) or acute myeloid leukemia following MDS, *Blood* 90:3853, 1997.

42. DiJulio J: Hematopoiesis: an overview, *Oncol Nurs Forum* 18(suppl):3, 1991.

43. Dodd MJ, Larson PJ, Dibble SL et al: Randomized clinical trail of chlorhexidine versus placebo for prevention of oral mucositis in patients receiving chemotherapy, *Oncol Nurs Forum* 23:921, 1996.

44. Dreizen S: Descriptions and incidence of oral complications, *HCI Monogr* 9:11, 1990.

45. Drucker B: Status of BCR-ABL tyrosine kinase inhibitors in CML, *Hematology 1999,* p. 169.

46. Dutcher JP and others: Intensive maintenance therapy improves survival in adult nonlymphocytic leukemia: an eight-year follow-up, *Leukemia* 2:413, 1988.

47. Dutcher JP, Schiffer CA, Wiernik PH: Hyperleukocytosis in adult nonlymphocytic leukemia: impact on remission rate, duration, and survival, *J Clin Oncol* 5:1364, 1987.

48. Einhorn N: Acute leukemia after chemotherapy (Melphalan), *Cancer* 41:444, 1978.

49. Estey EH and others: Treatment of hairy cell leukemia with 2-chlorodeoxyadenosine (2-CdA), *Blood* 79:882, 1992.

50. Estey EH: Treatment of acute myelogenous leukemia and myelodysplastic leukemia and myelodysplastic syndromes, *Semin Hematol* 32:132, 1995.

51. Faderl S and others: Chronic myelogenous leukemia: biology and therapy, *Ann Intern Med* 131:207, 1999.

52. Fayad L, O'Brien S: Chronic lymphocytic leukemia and associated disorders. In Pazdur R, editor: *Medical oncology: a comprehensive review,* ed 2, New York, Huntington, 1996.

53. Feldman EJ: Acute meylogenous leukemia in the older patient, *Semin Oncol* 22(supp 1):21, 1995.

54. Fenaux P and others: ATRA followed by chemotherapy (CT) vs ATRA plus CT and the role of maintenance therapy in newly diagnosed acute promyelocytic leukemia (APL): first interim results of APL93 trial, *Blood* 90:122a, 1997 (abstr).

55. Finiewicz KJ, Larson RA: Dose-intensive therapy for adult acute lymphoblastic leukemia, *Semin Oncol* 26:6, 1999.

56. Foon KA, Gale RP: Biology of chronic lymphocytic leukemia, *Semin Hematol* 24:209, 1987.

57. Foon KA, Gale RP: Staging and therapy of chronic lymphocytic leukemia *Semin Hematol* 24:264, 1987.

58. French Cooperative Group on Chronic Lymphocytic Leukemia: Effectiveness of "CHOP" regimen in advanced untreated chronic lymphocytic leukemia, *Lancet* 1:1346, 1986.

59. Furlong TG: Neurologic complications of immunosuppressive cancer therapy, *Oncol Nurs Forum* 20:1337, 1993.

60. Gale RP, Foon KA: Acute myelogenous leukemia. In Gale RP, editor: *Acute leukemia,* Boston, Blackwell, 1986.

61. Ghaddar HM, Estey EH: Acute myelogenous leukemia. In Pazdur R, editor: *Medical oncology: a comprehensive review,* ed 2, New York, Huntington, 1996.

62. Giona F and others: Adult acute lymphoblastic leukemia: description and analysis of long-term survivors, a retrospective study, *Haematologica* 74:475, 1989.

63. Golomb HM, Ellis E: Treatment options for hairy cell leukemia, *Semin Oncol* 18(suppl 7), 1991.

64. Green LM and others: Childhood leukemia and personal monitoring of residential exposures to electric and magnetic fields in Ontario, Canada, *Cancer Causes Control* 10:233, 1999.

65. Greenberg P and others: International scoring system for evaluating prognosis in myelodysplastic syndromes. *Blood* 89:2079, 1997.

66. Greenberg P and others: Myelodysplastic syndromes and myeloproliferative disorders: clinical, therapeutic and molecular advances. In: *Hematology 1995,* p. 18.

67. Greenberg P and others: Phase III randomized multicenter trial of G-CSF vs. observation for MDS, *Blood* 82(suppl 1):196a, 1993.

68. Greenlee RT and others: Cancer statistics 2000, *CA Cancer J Clin* 50:7, 2000.

69. Griffin JD: Management of chronic myelogenous leukemia, *Semin Hematol* 23(suppl):20, 1986.

70. Grignani F and others: Acute promyelocytic leukemia: from genetics to treatment, *Blood* 83:10, 1994.

71. Gulati GL, Ashton JK, Hyun BH: Structure and function of the bone marrow and hematopoiesis, *Hematol Oncol Clin North Am* 2:495, 1988.

72. Gunz FW: Leukemia in the past. In Gunz FW, editor: *Leukemia,* Orlando, FL, Grune & Stratton, 1983.

73. Hansen OP and others: Aclarubicin plus cytosine arabinoside versus daunorubicin plus cytosine arabinoside in previously untreated patients with acute myeloid leukemia: a Danish National Phase III trial, *Leukemia* 5:510, 1991.

74. Harousseau J-L and others: Comparison of autologous bone marrow transplantation and intensive chemotherapy as postremission therapy in adult acute myeloid leukemia, *Blood* 90:2978, 1997.

75. Harris NL and others: A revised European-American classification of lymphoid neoplasms: a proposal from the International Lymphomas Study Group [per comments], *Blood* 84:1361, 1994.

76. Head DR: Revised classification of acute myeloid leukemia, *Leukemia* 10:1826, 1996.

77. Heath CW: Electromagnetic field exposure and cancer: a review of epidemiologic evidence, *CA Cancer J Clin* 46:29, 1996.

78. Hernandez JA, Land KJ, McKenna RW: Leukemias, myeloma, and other lymphoreticular neoplasms, *Cancer Suppl* 75:381, 1995.

79. Hoelzer DF: Therapy of the newly diagnosed adult with acute lymphoblastic leukemia, *Hematol Oncol Clin North Am* 7:139, 1993.

80. Hoezler D, Gale RP: Acute lymphoblastic leukemia in adults: recent progress, future directions, *Semin Hematol* 24(1):27, 1987.

81. Italian Cooperative Study Group on Chronic Myeloid Leukemia: Interferon alpha-2a as compared with conventional chemotherapy for the treatment of chronic myeloid leukemia, *N Engl J Med* 330:820, 1994.

82. Jaiyesimi IA, Kantarjian HM, Estey EH: Advances in therapy for hairy cell leukemia, *Cancer* 72:5, 1993.

83. Janssen JWG and others: Clonal analysis of myelodysplastic syndromes: evidence of multipotent syndromes: Evidence of multipotent stem cell origin, *Blood* 73:248, 1989.

84. Johnson BL: Leukemias. In Groenwald SL, editor: *Cancer nursing: practice and principles,* Boston, Jones & Bartlett, 1987.

85. Johnston JB: Chronic lymphocytic leukemia. In Lee GR and others, editors: *Wintrobe's clinical hematology,* Philadelphia, Williams & Wilkins, 1999:2405.

86. Johnston JB: Hairy cell leukemia. In Lee GR and others, editors: *Wintrobe's clinical hematology,* Philadelphia, Williams & Wilkins, 1999:2428.

87. Juliasson G, Merup M: Cytogenetics in chronic lymphocytic leukemia, *Semin Oncol* 25:19, 1998.

88. Kane EV, Roman E, Cartwright RE, et al: Tobacco and the risk of acute leukemia in adults, *Br J Cancer* 81:1228, 1999.

89. Kantarjian HM and others: CML: a concise update, *Blood* 82:691, 1993.

90. Kantarjian HM and others: Treatment of Philadelphia chromosome-positive early chronic phase chronic myelogenous leukemia with daily doses of interferon alpha and low-dose cytarabine, *J Clin Oncol* 17:284, 1999.

91. Kantarjian HM, Talpaz M: Interferon alpha plus low-dose cytarabine and other promising treatment modalities for chronic myelogenous leukemia, *Hematology* 1999, p. 152.

92. Kantarjian HM: Adult acute lymphocytic leukemia: critical review of current knowledge, *Am J Med* 97:176, 1994.

93. Keating M and others: Multicenter study of Campath 1-H in patients with chronic lymphocytic leukemia (B-CLL) refractory to fludarabine. *Proceedings of the 4th Congress of the European Hematology Association,* June 9-12, 1999, Barcelona, Spain.

94. Keating MJ and others: The serum $\beta 2M$ level is more powerful than stage in predicting response and survival in CLL, *Blood* 86(suppl 1):606a, 1995.

95. Kim YH, Choi JS: Prevention of chemotherapy induced oral mucositis in patients with acute leukemia by the two oral care protocols: the comparison of sodium bicarbonate-normal saline gargling and chlorhexidine gargling, *Oncol Nurs Forum 98 Congress* 101, 1998.

96. Kinney MC, Lukens JN: Classification and differentiation of the acute leukemias. In Lee GR and others, editors: *Wintrobe's clinical hematology,* Philadelphia, Williams & Wilkins, 1999:2209.

97. Laport GF, Larson RA: Treatment of adult lymphoblastic leukemia, *Semin Oncol* 24:70, 1997.

98. Leith CP and others: Acute myeloid leukemia in the elderly: assessment of multidrug resistance (MDR1) and cytogenetics distinguishes biologic subgroups with remarkably distinct responses to standard chemotherapy. A Southwest Oncology Group study, *Blood* 89:3323, 1997.

99. Levenson JA, Lesko LM: Psychiatric aspects of adult leukemia, *Semin Oncol Nurs* 6:76, 1990.

100. Levit L, Lin R: Biology and treatment of adult acute lymphoblastic leukemia, *West J Med* 164:143, 1996.

101. Lill MC, Golde DW: Treatment of hairy cell leukemia, *Blood Rev* 4:238, 1990.

102. List AF and others: Stimulation of hematopoiesis by amifostine in patients with myelodysplastic syndrome, *Blood* 90:3364, 1997.

103. List AF and others: Phase I/II trial of cyclosporin as a chemotherapy-resistance modifier in acute leukemia, *J Clin Oncol* 11:1652, 1993.

104. List AF and others: The myelodysplastic syndromes: biology and implications for management, *J Clin Oncol* 8:1424, 1990.

105. Lord BI, Hendry JH: Radiation toxicology: bone marrow and leukaemia. In Hendry JJ, Lord BI, editors: *Radiation toxicology. Bone marrow & leukaemia,* London, Taylor & Francis, 1995:1.

106. Lowenberg B and others: Use of recombinant GM-CSF during and after remission induction chemotherapy in patients aged 61 years and older with acute myeloid leukemia: final report of AML-11, a phase III randomized study of the Leukemia Cooperative Group of European Organisation for the Research and Treatment of Cancer and the Dutch Belgian Hemato-Oncology Cooperative Group, *Blood* 90:2952, 1997.

107. Mayer RJ and others: Intensive postremission chemotherapy in adults with acute myelogenous leukemia, *N Engl J Med* 331:896, 1994.

108. McGlave P and others: Therapy of chronic myelogenous leukemia with allogeneic bone marrow transplantation, *J Clin Oncol* 5:1033, 1987.

109. Melo JV: Insights into the molecular patho-physiology of chronic myeloid leukemia: targets for therapeutic strategies? *Hematology 1999,* p. 143.

110. Miller KB and others: The evaluation of low-dose cytarabine in the treatment of myelodysplastic syndromes: a phase III intergroup study, *Ann Hematol* 65:162, 1992.

111. Mills PK: Correlation analysis of pesticide use data and cancer incidence rates in California counties, *Arch Environ Health* 53:410, 1998.

112. Mitus AJ, Rosenthal DS: The adult leukemias. In Murphy GP, Lawrence W Jr, Lenhard RE Jr, editors: *American Cancer Society textbook of clinical oncology,* ed 2, Atlanta, American Cancer Society, 1995.

113. O'Brien S and others: Phase I/II study of Rituxan in chronic lymphocytic leukemia, *Blood* 92:105a (abstract 431), 1998.

114. Ong ST, Larson RA: Current management of acute lymphoblastic leukemia in adults, *Oncology* 9:433, 1995.

115. Oscier DG: The ABC of clinical haematology. The myelodysplastic syndromes. *BMJ* 314:883, 1997.

116. Papa G and others: Acute leukemia in patients treated for Hodgkin's disease, *Br J Haematol* 309:1079, 1984.

117. Piro LD, Douglas JE, Saven A: The Scripps Clinic experience with 2-chlorodeoxyadenosine in the treatment of hairy cell leukemia, *Leuk Lymphoma* 13(suppl 1):121, 1994.

118. Poplack DG and others: Leukemias and lymphomas of childhood. In Devita VT Jr, Hellman S, Rosenberg SA, editors: *Cancer principles and practice,* ed 4, Philadelphia, Lippincott, 1993.

119. Portugal MA and others: Acute leukemia as a complication of advanced breast cancer, *Cancer Treat Rep* 63:177, 1979.

120. Preisler H and others: Comparison of three remission induction regimens and two postinduction strategies for the treatment of acute nonlymphocytic leukemia: a Cancer and Leukemia Group B study, *Blood* 69:1441, 1987.

121. Pui C: Childhood leukemias, *N Engl J Med* 332:1618, 1995.

122. Rai KR, Kipps TJ, Barlogie B: Chronic lymphocytic leukemia and myeloma: update on the biology and management. *Hematology 1996,* p. 62.

123. Rai KR and others: Chronic lymphocytic leukemia. *Hematology 1998,* p. 313.

124. Raphael B and others: Comparison of chlorambucil and prednisone versus cyclophosphamide, vincristine, and prednisone as initial treatment for chronic lymphocytic leukemia: long-term follow-up of an Eastern Cooperative Oncology Group randomized trial, *J Clin Oncol* 9:770, 1991.

125. Reed JC: Molecular biology chronic lymphocytic leukemia, *Semin Oncol* 25:11, 1998.

126. Rinsky RA and others: Benzene and leukemia, *N Engl J Med* 316:1044, 1987.

127. Rozman C, Montserrat E: Chronic lymphocytic leukemia, *N Engl J Med* 333:1052, 1995.

128. Sanders JE: Bone marrow transplantation for pediatric leukemia, *Pediatr Annu* 20:671, 1991.

129. Sandler DP and others: Cigarette smoking and risk of acute leukemia: associations with morphology and cytogenetic abnormalities in bone marrow, *J Natl Cancer Inst* 85:1994, 1993.

130. Sandler DP, Ross JA: Epidemiology of acute leukemia in children and adults. *Semin Oncol* 24:3, 1997.

131. Saven A, Piro L: Newer purine analogues for the treatment of hairy cell leukemia, *N Engl J Med* 330:691, 1994.

132. Saven A, Piro LD: Treatment of hairy cell leukemia, *Blood* 79:1111, 1992.

133. Schiffer CA: Interferon studies in the treatment of patients with leukemia, *Semin Oncol* 18(suppl 7):1, 1991.

134. Sievers EL and others: Selection ablation of acute myeloid leukemia using an anti-CD33 calicheamicin immunoconjugate, *Blood* 90:504a, 1997.

135. Silver RT: Chronic myeloid leukemia: a perspective of the clinical and biologic issues of the chronic phase, *Hematol Oncol Clin North Am* 4:319, 1990.

136. Silverman LR and others: Effects of treatment with 5-azacytidine on the in vivo and in vitro hematopoiesis in patients with myelodysplastic syndromes, *Leukemia* 7(suppl 1):21, 1993.

137. Smith JW and others: Prolonged continuous treatment of hairy cell leukemia patients with recombinant interferon-alpha 2a, *Blood* 78:1664, 1991.

138. Soignet SL and others: Complete remission after treatment of acute promyelocytic leukemia with arsenic trioxide, *N Engl J Med* 339:1341, 1998.

139. Sokal JE and others: Staging and prognosis in chronic myelogenous leukemia, *Semin Hematol* 25(1):49, 1988.

140. Sperati A and others: Mortality among male licensed pesticide users and their wives, *Am J Med* 36:142, 1999.

141. Talpaz M and others: Therapy of chronic myelogenous leukemia: chemotherapy and interferons, *Semin Hematol* 25:62, 1988.

142. Thandla S, Aplan PD: Molecular biology of acute lymphocytic leukemia, *Semin Oncol* 24:45, 1997.

143. Third MIC Cooperative Group Study: Morphologic, immunologic and cytogenetic working classification of the primary myelodysplastic syndromes and therapy-related myelodysplasia and leukemias, *Cancer Genet Cytogenet* 32:1, 1988.

144. Thomas ED: Marrow transplantation for chronic myelogenous leukemia. In Gale RP, Champlin R, editors: *Bone marrow transplantation: current controversies,* San Diego, Academic, 1988.

145. Toronto Leukemia Study Group: Survival in acute myeloblastic leukemia is not prolonged by remission maintenance or early reinduction chemotherapy, *Leuk Res* 12:195, 1988.

146. Tura S: α-Interferon versus allogeneic stem cell transplantation in early chronic phase chronic myelogenous leukemia: strategies by age and risk group, *Hematology 1999,* p. 156.

147. Varterasian ML and others: Phase II trial of Bryostatin 1 in patients with relapsed low-grade non-Hodgkins

lymphoma and chronic lymphocytic leukemia, *Clin Cancer Res* 6:825, 2000.

148. Vogler WR and others: A phase III trial comparing idarubicin and daunorubicine in combinations with cytarabine in acute myelogenous leukemia. A Southeastern Cancer Group Study, *J Clin Oncol* 10:1103, 1992.

149. Waldman AR: High-dose post remission therapy. In Wujcik D, editor: *Nursing care issues in adult acute leukemia,* New York, Huntington, 1995.

150. Warrell RP and others: Acute promyelocytic leukemia, *N Engl J Med* 329:177, 1993.

151. Waselenko JK, Flynn JM, Byrd JC: Stem cell transplantation in chronic lymphocytic leukemia: the time for designing randomized studies has arrived, *Semin Oncol* 26:48, 1999.

152. Webb IJ, Anderson KC: Transfusion support in acute leukemias, *Semin Oncol* 24:141, 1997.

153. Weick JK and others: A randomized investigation of high-dose versus standard-dose cytosine arabinoside with daunorubicin in patients with previously untreated acute myeloid leukemia: a Southwest Oncology Group study, *Blood* 88:2841, 1996.

154. Westbrook CA, Golomb HM: Hairy cell leukemia, *Curr Concepts Oncol,* Winter, 1984.

155. Whitlock JA, Gaynon PS: Acute lymphocytic leukemia. In Lee GR and others, editors: *Wintrobe's clinical hematology,* Philadelphia, Williams & Wilkins, 1999:2241.

156. Zittoun RA and others: Autologous or allogeneic bone marrow transplantation compared intensive chemotherapy in acute myeloid leukemia, *N Engl J Med* 332:217, 1995.

157. Zwiebel JA, Cheson BO: Chronic lymphocytic leukemia: staging and prognostic factors, *Semin Oncol* 25:42, 1998.

15 CHAPTER

Lung Cancers

Shirley E. Otto

Lung cancer is the leading cancer-related death for both men (32%) and women (25%), surpassing breast, prostate, and colon cancer combined for the year 2000 in the United States. Despite all the changes in diagnostics and treatment modalities, lung cancer remains the number one cancer disease treatment problem. Recently lung cancer achieved the status of being dubbed "the invisible cancer" because of the lack of attention and research funding it receives relative to these other diseases. At the third annual Lung Cancer Awareness Day, a speaker stated "the number of people living at risk for lung cancer is in the *tens of millions,* yet there are NO famous spokesperson, no races for a cure, and no movies of the week about people living with lung cancer." A longtime established perception from the public regarding lung cancer is "smokers have brought the cancer on themselves and are therefore less deserving of compassion." Recent data regarding lung cancer found that approximately 50% of the newly diagnosed patients are former *smokers, those who were able to kick the habit and who may not have smoked for many years.*[34, 92, 96, 108]

Although lung cancer mortality continues to rise among American men, the incidence of lung cancer among men has leveled off or slightly declined for the first time. A *downturn* in the incidence of lung cancer in men began in the late 1980s; between 1990 and 1996, incidence rates decreased significantly—2.6% per year, and for the year 2000 the same trend continues. Despite research and public education efforts, however, lung cancer incidence and mortality continue to rise among American women, an increase of more than 400% during the last 30 years. Incidence rates among women are stabilizing and have begun to decline among women aged 40 to 59. The dismal statistics and poor survival outcomes for lung cancer are related to the fact that the majority of all new cancer cases are at an advanced stage at the time of diagnosis. Clinical trials using multimodality therapies or new agents are attempting to reverse this trend. In the meantime, smoking prevention and cessation remains the key to reducing lung cancer deaths.[34, 92, 96, 108]

EPIDEMIOLOGY

An estimated 164,100 new cases of lung cancer are projected and 156,900 deaths are expected to occur in the United States in 2000. More men than women develop lung cancer, but the gap is narrowing. New reported data from 1994 to 1996 predict the birth to death probability of developing invasive lung cancer for men: birth to 39 years, 1 in 2592; 40–59 years, 1 in 78; 60–79 years, 1 in 16; and risk over the life span birth to death 1 in 12; for women: birth to 39 years, 1 in 2894; 40–59 years, 1 in 106; 60–79 years, 1 in 25; and risk over the life span birth to death 1 in 18.[34, 96, 108]

ETIOLOGY AND RISK FACTORS

Smoking

Death from lung cancer was relatively rare until the twentieth century. In 1912, Adler found only 374 cases of lung cancer described in world literature and questioned the value of writing about such an insignificant problem. Little did he expect the abrupt increase in deaths related to lung cancer beginning around 1935 (4300 deaths) and continuing until now (156,900 deaths estimated in 2000). The increased incidence in men in the 1930s and in women in the 1960s followed the pattern of increased acceptance of smoking behavior, first in men and then in women. A prospective study by Hammond in 1954 first demonstrated the relationship between smoking and the risk of developing lung cancer. Tobacco use (smoking active and passive) accounts for 90% of all the lung cancer diagnoses. Observers note that lung cancer mortality rates in people who have smoked two packs a day for 10 years (20 pack-years) are 15 to 25 times higher than in nonsmokers. The latency period between initiation of smoking and the development of lung cancer is about 15 to 20 years. The World Health

Organization (WHO) estimates that *10 million* people will die annually from *diseases linked to smoking by 2020,* compared to *4 million in 2000.*[18, 24, 34, 90]

Air Pollution

Air pollutants have been incriminated in the etiology of lung cancer (e.g., sulfur dioxide). Nevertheless, although high rates of lung cancer occur in major cities such as Los Angeles and New York where high levels of air pollution are a problem, no definite correlation to lung cancer incidence has been proved.

Race and Socioeconomics

Among African American men of all ages in the United States, incidence of lung cancer has decreased since 1980 and this may be associated with a corresponding drop in mortality rates. Smoking prevalence among African Americans is also on the decline (from 41% in the mid-1970s to 34% in the late 1980s to 26.5% in 1992). Based on the decreasing number of new lung cancer diagnoses and the decreasing number of lung cancer deaths in men, there continues to be a decreasing trend for smoking in African American men similar to that of 1992. Nevertheless, cancer mortality is higher among nonwhites than whites and may be related to the increased smoking and use of nonfilter cigarettes by African Americans. Socioeconomic factors (e.g., workplace conditions, poor nutrition) might contribute to this difference, but this is only speculation. Unconfirmed studies suggest, however, that there is an increased risk of squamous cell and small-cell lung cancers in men with diets low in vitamin A.[24, 34, 70, 104, 106]

Geography

Geographic clustering of lung cancer among men has been noted along the Gulf of Mexico and the southeastern Atlantic coast. Whether this is related to industrial asbestos exposure from industries such as shipbuilding is not known. Mortality rates are lowest in farming areas and lower in rural versus urban counties.

Industry

Industrial exposure to the following agents is believed to place persons at greater risk of lung cancer: mustard gas, radon, asbestos, radioisotopes, polycyclic aromatic hydrocarbons (present in crude petroleum, coal, tars, combustion products of most organic materials), nickel, chromium, haloethers, iron ore, inorganic arsenic, wood dust, and isopropyl oil. Certain occupational groups at

---

BOX 15-1

Occupational Groups at Risk for Lung Cancer

Asbestos workers
Atomic energy workers
Automobile maintenance
Chemical workers
Chloromethyl ethyl workers
Copper smelter workers
Foundry workers
Gas workers
Glass, pottery, linoleum workers
Insecticide workers
Insulation workers
Metal material workers
Nickel workers
Petroleum workers
Radon exposure
Shipyard workers
Spray painters
Steel workers
Uranium miners

Data from references 24, 29, 38, 42, 45, 47, 50, 66, 88.

---

risk because of potential exposure to the above agents have been identified (Box 15–1).[18, 24, 29, 34, 38, 45, 47]

Family and Health History

The risk of lung cancer is increased in persons with a prior history of lung disease or a family history of lung cancer. Recent research supports the theory that lung cancer risk is an inherited trait. A specific gene that predisposes to early age onset of lung cancer may account for as many as 47% of cases by age 60. In a recent analysis of 337 lung cancer families, a mendelian codominant inheritance that predisposed those exposed to smoking to the development of lung cancer was the best explanation of the data. If this genetic predisposition proves true, it could mean that lung cancers occur uniquely among gene carriers and would help explain why all smokers do not develop lung cancer. This would have a major impact on approaches to lung cancer prevention, screening, and early detection.[24, 29, 47, 55, 66, 93]

PREVENTION, SCREENING, AND DETECTION

Primary Prevention

Smoking. Of the 552,200 estimated cancer deaths in 2000, about 156,900 (28.5% of all cancer deaths) were caused by lung cancer. The majority (at least 85%) of lung cancer deaths are smoking related and thus preventable. As many as one third of heavy smokers (25 cigarettes or more a day) who are 35 years old will experience premature death from a smoking-related disease. WHO declared May 31, 2000 as the World No Tobacco Day, in an effort to educate people about smoking issues and to take a stand regarding smoke-free air. In 1990, the U.S. government designated all federal buildings become smoke free, all airline flights within the United States 2 hours or less in duration were designated smoke-free flights, and in June 2000, all flights within the United States and international flights entering the United States were designated smoke-free flights.[34, 42, 92]

Primary lung cancer prevention focuses on decreasing the number of new smokers and helping present smokers to quit. It may involve decreasing the hazards of smoking through use of low-tar and filtered cigarettes for those who continue to smoke. The risk of developing and dying from lung cancer correlates directly with the number of cigarettes smoked, and lung cancer incidence can be reduced by as much as 20% by use of low-tar and filter cigarettes, assuming no increase in number of cigarettes smoked.[94]

Studies show that the spouse of a smoker can be at increased risk of developing lung cancer, because the National Research Council reports that as many as 8000 people die annually from passive cigarette smoke. Sidestream smoke contains as many, if not more, carcinogens than inhaled smoke. Many worksites where extensive smoking occurs (e.g., bars and restaurants) may also place people at risk. In a population-based case-control study of cancer risk secondary to passive smoking, the only individuals found to be at increased risk (twice the risk of an unexposed nonsmoker) were those exposed during childhood or adolescence to the secondary smoke of more than one smoker in the home.[18, 21]

Although smokers are encouraged to stop smoking, a smoker's risk of developing lung cancer may never equal that of one who has never smoked, perhaps because of the prolonged lag time in the development of lung cancer. One study found no benefit from smoking cessation at 10 years; others found lung cancer risk dropping to 5.9 times by 10 years. Smokers who quit for at least 15 years may still have twice the risk of developing lung cancer as those who never smoked. It may take 20 years before the risks are similar.[34]

Smoking Cessation and Public Education. The overall prevalence of smoking among high school seniors has decreased from 27% when programs were instituted in the 1970s but has now leveled off at about 20% of students. By age 18, 75% of smokers have tried their first cigarette and 50% are regular smokers. The trend toward recruitment of smokers in adolescence, especially among teenage girls, needs to be broken. Programs found most successful in preventing initiation of smoking among youth are school based, using peer leaders and role-playing. Because more than half of female smokers begin smoking before age 13, prevention efforts must be aimed at the junior high age group or younger.

Among adults, many avenues are available to encourage smoking cessation, but 95% of smokers who quit do not seek outside help, preferring methods that can be done on their own. Factors that distinguish those smokers who quit from those who do not include a strong motivation to quit, use of behavioral techniques, and good social support to quit. Physician advice, even if minimal, fosters quitting, particularly when the patient is experiencing increased symptoms or a new smoking-related illness, such as emphysema.[71, 72]

Radon. Identification of risk groups helps to establish safety guidelines. Much media coverage has been given to the risk of lung cancer resulting from exposure to radon or asbestos. Radon has been implicated as a significant cause of lung cancer. However, even in uranium miners with high cumulative radon exposure, most lung cancers can be attributed to synergism between radon and cigarette smoking. Extrapolating risks from high-level, industrial radon exposure (uranium mining) to low-level, nonindustrial exposure (home, worksite) is met with conflicting opinions. A recent review of published studies found inconsistencies in results and methodology, leaving the correlation between residential radon exposure and lung cancer weak at best. There is some agreement, however, that most lung cancers attributed to indoor radon probably occur among smokers; only about 2000 of the 13,000 estimated annual lung cancer deaths attributed to nonindustrial radon exposure occur in nonsmokers.[24, 47, 88]

Asbestos. Before the establishment of the 1971 Occupational Safety and Health Administration (OSHA) asbestos exposure guidelines, studies done on workers in the asbestos industry (e.g., automobile maintenance, insulation, shipyard work) showed clearly that lung cancer was vastly increased if workers also smoked. Numerous studies have shown a strong synergism between smoking and asbestos exposure in the development of lung cancer. Asbestos workers who did not smoke had a risk of lung cancer about five times that of nonsmokers who worked in other industries. This compared with a 10 times greater risk for smokers not working in the asbestos industry and an 87 times greater risk for asbestos workers who were smokers. Again, extrapolating the risk from industrial to low-level asbestos exposure (school, worksite) is controversial. It appears that the risk of lung cancer related to exposure to the levels of asbestos left intact in public buildings is very small. If primary prevention priorities are based on the numbers of persons expected to die of lung cancer caused by environmental exposure, efforts should focus on elimination of passive smoking, which results in about 6000 lung cancer deaths per year in Americans, rather than on reducing low-level radon, which is associated with the deaths of about 2000 nonsmokers per year, or low-level asbestos exposure, which causes far fewer deaths.[24, 29, 38, 45, 47]

Secondary Prevention

Secondary prevention is aimed at early diagnosis of lung cancer in populations at high risk. Populations considered at high risk generally include persons older than 45 years who have smoked heavily, that is, one or more packs per day. Patients who claim to be nonsmokers need to be queried as to past smoking history.[34]

The National Cancer Institute (NCI) sponsored three large randomized, controlled trials beginning in the early 1970s to examine the benefit of radiologic examinations and sputum cytology as lung cancer screening tools in asymptomatic, high-risk individuals. None of the studies has shown a difference in the lung cancer mortality rates among screened versus control groups. It is possible that patients who undergo regular screening eventually die of their lung cancer at the same rate as others, having only been diagnosed earlier in the natural history of their disease (lead-time bias). The NCI began a large-scale study in late 1992 at 15 U.S. centers and will continue over 16 years to assess the value of screening in reducing mortality in prostate, lung, and colorectal cancers. There will be 37,000 men in both the screened and the control groups. It is hoped this study at last will answer the important questions about lung cancer screening. The Patient Teaching Priorities box lists prevention and early detection teaching priorities.[24, 29, 47, 94]

In persons with symptoms, a history of lung disease, a family history of lung cancer, or a heavy smoking history, chest x-ray films and sputum cytology are the primary tools used to screen for lung cancer. Monoclonal antibodies may prove to be a valuable tool in the detection of early lung cancer by sputum cytology. Early findings showed that cells in sputum specimens that stained positive with antilung cancer antibodies were 91% predictive of the development of lung cancer within 2 years. Carcinoembryonic antigen (CEA), elevated in only 50% of lung cancer patients, may be useful in postoperative follow-up, but it is not useful in lung cancer screening or for prognostic purposes.[24, 29, 47, 94]

Chemoprevention Strategies

A number of biochemical markers that reflect the highly proliferative state of bronchial premalignancy and non–small-cell lung cancer (NSCLC) cells are being tested as biomarkers of lung cancer risk and of response to chemoprevention intervention. This includes epidermal

---

PATIENT TEACHING PRIORITIES

Lung Cancer: Prevention and Early Detection

1. Avoid use of tobacco.

Risks increase according to number of cigarettes/day, number of years smoking, and tar and nicotine content of cigarettes. Secondary smoke increases the risk of lung cancer in nonsmokers, especially children and adolescents. Parental smoking habits influence children. Pipe, cigar smoking, or smokeless tobacco is not an acceptable alternative. Smoking cessation clinics and programs and medications are available to help those who desire to quit. Women, youth, blacks, and uneducated persons should be the focus of smoking cessation efforts.

2. Know environmental carcinogens that increase risk.

High-risk occupations have been identified that expose persons to high levels of carcinogens. Certain toxic substances increase risk. The synergistic effects of environmental carcinogens (especially radon or asbestos) and cigarette smoking increase risk.

3. Personal and family history are important risk factors.

Lung cancer risk may be inherited and is greater in those with a history of lung disease. Lung cancer is difficult to detect early, and symptoms do not appear until disease is advanced. Best advice is to *quit smoking now.* There are currently no effective screening methods for detecting cancer early enough to improve cure rates, even in high-risk populations.

Data from references 21, 24, 29, 36, 38, 45, 47, 50, 66, 71, 72, 88, 90, 104.

---

growth factor receptor (EGFR), proliferating cell nuclear antigen (PCNA), and Ki-67. EGFR to date has shown the most activity regarding cell proliferation and a reversal of bronchial neoplasia with decreased EGFR levels. PCNA activity suggests that increased levels may correlate with a shortened survival. The most recent data available show that in 1991, approximately 30% of adult men and 19% women were estimated to be former smokers, representing a 77% change since 1965. This translates into approximately 44 million adult former smokers nationwide, of whom 15 million are aged 45 to 64 years, and 11 million now older than 65 years. This group of people (former smokers) will be the target population for the lung cancer chemoprevention trials. Some of these trials will explore the use of retinoids (vitamins A and E), p53 gene mutations, and growth factors on the human bronchial epithelial cells.[36, 55, 106, 108]

CLASSIFICATION

The WHO has identified numerous categories of lung tumors or lesions, but the overwhelming majority (90%) consists of one of five types: (1) small-cell anaplastic carcinoma, (2) squamous cell carcinoma, (3) adenocarcinoma, (4) large-cell anaplastic carcinoma, and (5) mixed cell types. The clinical signs and symptoms at presentation often suggest the histology of a lung cancer; adequate tissue for cytologic or pathologic examination is essential for diagnosis. This section describes some of the clinical and histologic features of the five main types of lung cancer. It is now believed that all lung cancers arise out of a common stem cell gone awry.[24, 29, 47, 108]

Small-Cell Lung Cancer

Small-cell anaplastic carcinoma behaves biologically and clinically so differently from all other cell types that the latter are referred to as non–small-cell lung cancers (NSCLCs). Although usually metastatic at the time of diagnosis (more than two thirds of the time) because of its large growth fraction and aggressive nature, small-cell lung cancer (SCLC) is the most sensitive of all lung cancers to both single-agent and combination chemotherapy and radiation therapy. It is thought to arise from the basal cell lining of the bronchial mucosa called a *Kulchitsky-type cell.* Because it most often arises in the central part of the chest, postobstructive pneumonia and atelectasis often occur (Fig. 15–1). Frequent sites of distant metastasis are the brain, liver, and bone marrow. SCLC has sometimes been referred to as *oat cell carci-* noma or lymphocyte tumor because of its small round spindle shape microscopic resemblance to oats. SCLC accounts for about 20% to 25% of all lung cancers.[24, 47]

Paraneoplastic syndromes in SCLC patients include Eaton-Lambert syndrome (proximal muscle weakness), syndrome of inappropriate antidiuretic hormone (SIADH, from ectopic arginine vasopressin [AVP]), and Cushing's syndrome (from ectopic adrenocorticotropic hormone [ACTH]). Although the incidence of ectopic ACTH production and Cushing's syndrome in association with SCLC may be low (4.5% in one series), its appearance has been associated with a poor response to chemotherapy, a shortened survival time, and an increase in therapy-related complications. Other hormones produced by SCLCs include calcitonin and gastrin-releasing peptide (GRP), or bombesin. That SCLC cells contain neurosecretory granules and are capable of hormone production was once thought to result from neural crest embryologic origin. The term *dispersed neuroendocrine cells* is now used to describe the variety of cells (carcinoid, some large-cell, and small-cell undifferentiated carcinomas) that share similar morphologic and immunohistochemical features and are capable of peptide hormone production.[24, 27, 47, 66]

Non–Small-Cell Lung Cancer

Squamous cell carcinoma may be described as well, moderately, or poorly differentiated. These cells differentiate toward stratified columnar (squamous) epithelium lining the airway and have receptors for epidermal growth factor, which stimulates the growth of epidermal tissues and is perhaps critical to malignant cell growth. This carcinoma may not be visualized easily on chest x-ray films because it tends to arise in the central (medial) portion of the lung. This may delay diagnosis (Fig. 15–2). Squamous cell is the most likely lung cancer to present as a *Pancoast's tumor,* which is high in the lung apex with extension to the chest wall, causing a classic shoulder pain that radiates down the ulnar nerve distribution (Fig. 15–3). It is often associated with sudden onset of hypercalcemia resulting from the production of a parathyroid hormone-like substance and is not associated with the presence of bone metastases.[24, 29, 66, 94]

Adenocarcinoma is increasing in frequency, perhaps as a result of the increasing incidence of women with lung cancer. This type is often recognized microscopically by its glandular appearance and mucin production and includes acinar, papillary, solid, and bronchioalveolar types. Along with large-cell carcinoma, adenocarcinoma is easily seen on chest x-ray films because it usually arises in radiographically visualized, peripheral lung tissue (Fig. 15–4). Because of adenocarcinoma's highly metastatic nature, patients may present with or develop brain, liver, adrenal, or bone metastasis. Para-

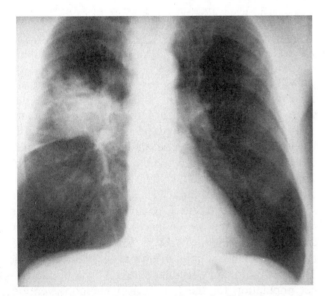

FIGURE 15–1 Patient with small-cell lung cancer in which large tumor mass is centrally located and adjacent pleura is thickened. There is fluid in fissure and possible postobstructive signs of atelectasis. (Courtesy Dr. Norman Martin, Diagnostic Radiology, University of Kansas Medical Center.)

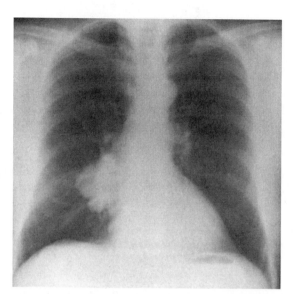

FIGURE 15-2 Patient with squamous cell carcinoma that developed centrally (right middle lobe) with left hilar prominence showing regional lymph node spread. (Courtesy Dr. Norman Martin, Diagnostic Radiology, University of Kansas Medical Center.)

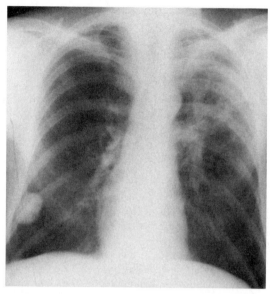

FIGURE 15-4 Adenocarcinomas can present as clearly defined peripheral lesions. Patient with right lower lobe lesion. (Courtesy Dr. Norman Martin, Diagnostic Radiology, University of Kansas Medical Center.)

neoplastic syndromes frequently associated with adenocarcinomas are hypercoagulability syndromes (marantic endocarditis, disseminated intravascular coagulation [DIC], migratory thrombophlebitis), and clubbing of the fingers with hypertrophic pulmonary osteoarthropathy.[24, 29, 68]

Large-cell anaplastic carcinoma is so named because it appears microscopically as large cells lacking any dis-

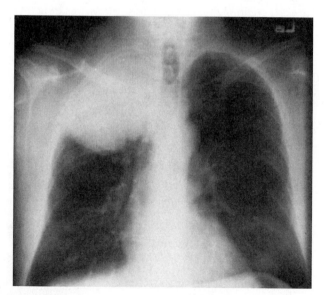

FIGURE 15-3 Classic Pancoast tumor in patient with squamous cell carcinoma of lung. Large right upper apex mass with nearly complete right first rib bony destruction and right supraclavicular fullness. (Courtesy Dr. Norman Martin, Diagnostic Radiology, University of Kansas Medical Center.)

tinguishing features. Clinical signs and symptoms are similar to those seen in adenocarcinoma, such as pain from pleural or chest wall invasion and lung abscesses, but this lesion is less likely to spread beyond the chest cavity.

Mixed cell types is the last major lung cancer category. The theory that all lung cancers have the same stem cell origin helps explain the existence of mixed cell tumors. In a review of 100 lung cancer cases, 45% showed two different major histologic cell types. Multiple cell lines are seen in 10% to 20% of specimens. In a given patient, any combination of cell types is possible within a single lesion or specimen, although the predominant cell type in different metastatic lesions may vary. Of all the combined categories (squamous cell, adenocarcinoma, large cell, and mixed cell), NSCLC accounts for about 75% to 80% of all lung cancer.[24, 29]

BIOLOGY OF LUNG CANCER AND CLINICAL SIGNIFICANCE

Multiple genetic lesions and events may be necessary in the development of lung cancer. Chromosomal mutations or deletions that appear to play a role in malignant transformation and growth involve both the activation of "up-regulating" genes (*proto-oncogenes*) and the inactivation or deletion of "down-regulating," suppressor genes (*antioncogenes*). Recent research demonstrates a deletion in the 3p chromosome region of 100% of SCLCs and up to 74% of NSCLCs. This chromosome region has become the focus of intense research to determine the exact gene and its function. Whether the deletion

COMPLICATIONS

Lung Cancer: Disease Related

Direct Spread or Metastases

Bone marrow involvement (pancytopenia)
Bone metastasis (pain, pathologic fractures)
Brain metastasis
Spinal cord compression (paralysis)
Superior vena cava syndrome (respiratory distress)
Pleural effusion
Pericardial effusion (tamponade, dysrhythmias)
Endobronchial lesion (cough, hemoptysis)
Postobstructive atelectasis and/or pneumonia
Liver metastasis
Regional spread

Indirect Effects or Paraneoplastic Syndromes

Syndrome of inappropriate antidiuretic hormone
    (SIADH) (small cell) and hyponatremia
Hypercalcemia (squamous cell)
Cushing's syndrome and ectopic adrencorticotropic hor-
    mone (ACTH)
Anorexia, taste changes, weight loss, cachexia
Degenerative neuropathies
Fever of unknown origin (multiple cultures and
    work-ups)
Disseminated intravascular coagulopathies (bleeding,
    deep vein thromboses)
Clubbing and hypertrophic osteoarthropathy
Anemia
Granulocytosis, thrombocytosis

Data from references 24, 25, 29, 36, 47, 66.

mass, and hilar and mediastinal changes suggestive of regional lymphadenopathy or pleural effusions; all of these suggest possible malignancy.

3. Computed tomography (CT) scans are used for detection of nodes less than 1 cm in diameter, local invasion of the primary tumor to the chest wall, bony structure, and pleura. Spiral CT scanning shows that a different imaging picture of the lung tissue is being used in some instances.

4. Magnetic resonance imaging (MRI) is used to investigate changes in the bone marrow of the verte-

CLINICAL FEATURES

Lung Cancer

Most Common Symptoms at Presentation

Change in cough (most have chronic smoker's cough)
Chest pain
Recurrent bronchitis or pneumonia unresponsive to an-
    tibiotics
Dyspnea or wheezing
Stridor
Hemoptysis
Weight loss
Fatigue
Dysphagia

Symptoms of Regional Tumor Spread

Superior vena cava syndrome (SVCS)
Hoarseness from recurrent laryngeal nerve paralysis
Phrenic nerve paralysis with elevated hemidiaphragm
    and dyspnea
Horner's syndrome (unilateral ptosis, miosis, loss of fa-
    cial sweat)
Pancoast's syndrome (shoulder pain radiating down
    arm along ulnar nerve distribution)
Tracheal or esophageal obstruction
Pericardial effusion and tamponade
Pleural effusion
Hypoxia and dyspnea related to lymphangitic spread

Evidence of Metastatic Disease or Paraneoplastic Syndrome

Bone pain related to bone involvement
Headaches, mental status changes, or other neurologic
    findings resulting from brain metastasis or SIADH
    with hyponatremia
Abdominal pain, elevated liver function tests, enlarged
    liver, gastrointestinal disturbances (anorexia, cache-
    xia), jaundice, hepatomegaly related to liver
    involvement
Pancytopenia secondary to bone marrow involvement
Weight loss
Other paraneoplastic syndromes

Data from references 24, 29, 36, 47, 64, 66.

is the same in both SCLC and NSCLC is not known. Other chromosomal deletions common in lung cancer are in the regions of 11p, 17p (p53 gene), and the retinoblastoma (Rb) gene. The p53 gene is frequently mutated or inactivated in all types of lung cancer. Reincorporating some of these genes in malignant cell cultures has halted cell growth, suggesting these genes control or down-regulate cellular growth[24, 29, 47, 66] (see Complications box).

DIAGNOSIS

When a patient is suspected of having lung cancer based on clinical features, a definitive histologic or cytologic diagnosis is essential, as an estimate of the stage of the disease to determine the desired treatment(s) approach.[24, 29, 47, 68]

1. History and physical examination (see Clinical Features box)
2. Chest x-ray films (anteroposterior and lateral), which may reveal peripheral nodules, a definitive

bra suggestive of carcinoma as well as spinal cord invasion.

5. Complete blood count (CBC) with differential and platelet count, as well as blood chemistries

6. Histologic diagnosis, which may be as simple as collecting early morning sputum 3 days in a row (diagnostic 80% of the time), is most valuable in squamous cell carcinoma. However, *bronchoscopy* is frequently used today because it expedites diagnosis, provides a better specimen for histologic evaluation, and aids in staging. Efforts to obtain adequate tissue for diagnosis become increasingly more invasive and can involve the following:

- Fiberoptic bronchoscopy with biopsy or bronchial brushings or washings for cytology (90% efficient)
- Percutaneous transthoracic needle aspiration or biopsy under fluoroscopy or CT guidance for peripheral lung lesions
- Biopsy of supraclavicular or scalene lymph nodes
- Mediastinoscopy (or mediastinotomy, if left upper chest lesions) to biopsy nodes or tissues, which aids in staging
- Biopsy of accessible metastatic sites (e.g., bone)
- Thoracentesis for cytology or pleural biopsy
- Thoracotomy as a last resort

STAGING

Once the diagnosis of lung cancer has been made, and before the definitive treatment is considered, a clinical extent of the disease process is required. Obtaining a tissue diagnosis usually includes using various staging procedures. The histology (SCLC versus NSCLC) will then determine how to proceed with staging. Histology and stage of disease help dictate prognosis and treatment options. When discussing treatment options with the patient, prognosis is an important consideration because risks and toxicities associated with the treatment must be balanced against potential survival benefits. Prognostic factors in lung cancer are discussed later in this chapter.[24, 29, 47]

In general, a CT scan or MRI of the chest down through the adrenal glands obtained earlier for SCLC or NSCLC is evaluated. Some argue that further staging in asymptomatic patients is unwarranted because it rarely reveals metastatic disease. The incidence of "silent" metastases in asymptomatic patients who appear to be clinically stage I or II disease is low; the incidence of metastases to the brain is 2.7%; to bone, 3.4%; and to the liver, 9.3%. Others note that 50% of patients with NSCLC have metastatic disease, and because of inadequate staging, as many as one fourth of patients

who undergo so-called curative therapy will eventually die as a result of metastatic disease. In many cases, nonresectability will still be demonstrated by the time these studies are done. If patients with NSCLC have evidence of bone pain, weight loss, or abnormal liver function or calcium levels, further work-up might require the following[24, 29, 47]:

Bone scan
CT scan of the abdomen or liver
CT scan or MRI study of the head
Liver or bone marrow biopsy (or both)
Plain films of bone
Pulmonary function studies
Vascular studies

One of the greatest current controversies in the treatment of NSCLC is the resectability of stage IIIA disease (based on mediastinal lymph node involvement) with curative intent. Therefore preoperative staging of these patients has become more critical. CT scans and MRI are often inadequate in diagnosing chest wall and mediastinal involvement, essential determinants of resectability and likelihood of cure. Although CT or MRI scans guide decisions regarding the necessity of invasive procedures and which procedure to perform, mediastinoscopy, mediastinotomy, and thoracotomy frequently are required after the scans (at least in the study setting) to document involvement histologically.[24, 29, 47]

If the cancer is deemed resectable, pulmonary function and blood gas studies are required to determine if the patient is able to undergo pneumonectomy or pulmonary resection.

Because two thirds of SCLC patients have metastatic disease, initial staging routinely includes the following:

Bone scan
CT scan of the abdomen
Bone marrow biopsy
CT or MRI study of the head
With or without liver biopsy
Pulmonary function studies
Vascular studies

The American Joint Committee on Cancer (AJCC) tumor, node, metastasis (TNM) cancer staging system has been useful in prognosis and planning treatment for NSCLC. The TNM system classifies cancers according to the following staging designations (Table 15–1):

Primary Tumor (T)*

TX   Primary tumor cannot be assessed or tumor proved by the presence of malignant cells in sputum or bronchial washings but not visualized by imaging or bronchoscopy

---

*From Beahrs OH and others, editors: *Manual for staging of cancer,* ed 5, Philadelphia, Lippincott-Raven, 1997.

TABLE 15–1

Stage Grouping for Lung Cancers

Stage	Tumor	Node	Metastasis
Occult carcinoma	TX	N0	M0
0	Tis	N0	M0
I	T1	N0	M0
	T2	N0	M0
II	T1	N1	M0
	T2	N1	M0
IIIA	T1	N2	M0
	T2	N2	M0
	T3	N0, N1, N2	M0
IIIB	Any T	N3	M0
	T4	Any N	M0
IV	Any T	Any N	M1

From Beahrs OH and others, editors: Manual for staging of cancer, ed 5, Philadelphia, Lippincott-Raven, 1997.

T0   No evidence of primary tumor

Tis   Carcinoma in situ

T1   Tumor 3 cm or less in greatest dimension, surrounded by lung or visceral pleura, without bronchoscopic evidence of invasion more proximal than the lobar bronchus (i.e., not in the main bronchus)

T2   Tumor with any of the following features of size or extent:
- More than 3 cm in greatest dimension
- Involvement of main bronchus 2 cm or more distal to the carina
- Invasion of the visceral pleura
- Associated with atelectasis or obstructive pneumonitis that extends to the hilar region but does not involve the entire lung

T3   Tumor of any size that directly invades any of the following: chest wall (including superior sulcus tumors), diaphragm, mediastinal pleura, parietal pericardium; or tumor in the main bronchus less than 2 cm distal to the carina; or associated atelectasis or obstructive pneumonitis of the entire lung

T4   Tumor of any size that invades any of the following: mediastinum, heart, great vessels, trachea, esophagus, vertebral body, carina; or tumor with a malignant pleural effusion

Regional Lymph Nodes (N)

NX   Regional lymph nodes cannot be assessed

N0   No regional lymph node metastasis

N1   Metastasis in ipsilateral peribronchial and/or ipsilateral hilar lymph node(s), including direct extension

N2   Metastasis in ipsilateral mediastinal and/or subcarinal lymph node(s)

N3   Metastasis in contralateral mediastinal, contralateral hilar, ipsilateral or contralateral scalene, or supraclavicular lymph node(s)

Distant Metastasis (M)

MX   Presence of distant metastasis cannot be assessed

M0   No distant metastasis

M1   Distant metastasis

For the most part, the TNM system is not useful in SCLC. TNM takes on clinical significance only when surgery for stage I SCLC is a consideration. The Veterans Administration Lung Cancer Study Group's two-stage system is typically used for SCLC because it correlates with prognosis. Controversy exists regarding what constitutes limited versus extensive disease.

Limited—Disease is restricted to one hemithorax with regional lymph node metastases, including hilar, ipsilateral, and contralateral mediastinal and/or supraclavicular nodes, and including ipsilateral pleural effusion regardless of cytology.

Extensive—Disease is beyond the above definition and may involve metastasis to liver, bone, bone marrow, brain, adrenals, and lymph nodes.

Other authors maintain that limited disease is that which is confined to one hemithorax and can be encompassed in a single radiation port. They therefore continue to assign pleural effusions to the extensive stage category because of the large volume of tissue requiring radiation to treat the pleural surface. Because pleural effusions are a poor prognostic factor, variations in staging SCLC can make comparisons of treatment response rates and survival data by stage confusing and possibly misleading.[2, 69]

METASTASIS

Metastasis to any site, as a consequence of lung cancer, can seriously interfere with the patient's ability to accomplish simple activities of daily living. Depending on where the metastatic lesion is located, clinical manifestations can lead to critical oncologic emergencies. Cancers of the lung find many distant sanctuaries, including bone marrow, pericardium and heart, kidney, and adrenal gland. The most common sites of metastasis of lung cancer are to the other lung and pleura, brain, bone, liver, and lymph nodes. Because of its relevance to staging of NSCLC, only intrathoracic spread is addressed here. Other sites of metastasis are discussed later in conjunction with their treatment.[24, 29, 47]

Intrathoracic Spread

Various methods are used to assess lymph node involvement. In patients with SCLC, if there is a definite diagnosis, further invasive procedures to determine lymph node involvement is usually not done. Work-up will continue to ascertain brain, bone, and liver metastasis. Even in limited disease, local thoracic extension may account for chest pain, wheeze, hemoptysis, dysphagia, and hoarseness. If a pleural effusion or an abnormal lactate dehydrogenase (LDH) level is present, long-term survival is not likely. The usual consensus is that a primary NSCLC tumor is incurable if nodes (high paratracheal, subcarinal, or contralateral) are replaced with tumor. When evaluating NSCLC for mediastinal involvement, some literature notes that on CT scan (1) nodes less than 1 cm are considered normal; (2) nodes from 1 to 1.5 cm in diameter are considered suspicious; and (3) nodes greater than 1.5 cm in diameter are considered abnormal. Nodes considered normal may harbor disease, and nodes considered abnormal may just be reactive to pneumonia or other disease.

Controversy surrounds what constitutes a "normal" node. Study results disagree on the accuracy of CT or MRI staging. Of patients with a negative CT scan, 10% to 20% will prove to have positive mediastinal lymph nodes at the time of thoracotomy, whereas 30% of those with enlarged nodes on CT will be negative on biopsy. Mountain[69] recommends mediastinoscopy or mediastinotomy (or both) for patients who might otherwise be denied curative resection based on the radiologist's interpretation. Based on examination of the mediastinum by mediastinoscopy, Mountain[69] cites the following criteria for incurable and unresectable NSCLC: (1) tumor involvement of "contralateral paratracheal lymph nodes or ipsilateral paratracheal lymph nodes in the upper half of the intrathoracic trachea," (2) direct invasion of the trachea, and (3) evidence of gross perinodal disease. If surgery is to be performed for NSCLC, Feld and others recommend extensive nodal dissection for accurate postoperative staging. Obvious clinical contralateral lymph node involvement is associated with a much poorer 5-year survival than when only microscopic nodal involvement is discovered.[24, 29, 47, 69, 93]

TREATMENT MODALITIES

Non–Small-Cell Lung Cancer

Surgery. Surgery is the treatment of choice for stages I and II NSCLC, representing 25% of all lung cancers, and the primary hope for cure. Some selected stage IIIA patients may benefit from surgical resection in terms of improved survival. Stage IIIB patients are not surgical candidates. Pneumonectomy for stage II and some stage I patients may be required unless precluded by preexisting cardiopulmonary disease. During the past two decades, lung-conserving operations including sleeve-lobotomy, segmentectomy, wedge resection, and sleeve-pneumonectomy have been used as resections of choice in selected patients with lung cancer.[29] Some surgeons advocate wedge or segmental resection for small, peripheral lung lesions; others find the incidence of local recurrence too high with this limited procedure when a more aggressive approach could be curative. At the very least, lobectomy with regional lymph node dissection is most optimal for early stage disease whenever possible. Criteria for nonresectability include T4, N3, and M1 lesions (stages IIIB and IV); the presence of small-cell histology; or inability of the patient to tolerate the procedure clinically. A "complete" resection should mean (1) the surgeon is certain the procedure removed all known disease, (2) the proximal margins of the resected specimen are microscopically free of tumor, (3) the most distant lymph nodes within each lymphatic drainage area are microscopically free of tumor, and (4) the resected lymph node capsules are intact.[24, 29, 93]

Patients with squamous cell cancer have the best survival rates, perhaps because of earlier diagnosis and because the disease exhibits less of a tendency to metastasize and has a slower growth rate. More than 70% of patients relapse after "curative" surgery because of distant metastases rather than local lesions (<25%). This argues for improved methods of early detection and good systemic adjuvant therapy. Five-year survival after curative therapy is excellent for stage I patients (60–80%) but drops dramatically to 28% for the best stage IIIA patients. Thus the potential benefit of surgery must be weighed against the risks of operative morbidity and mortality. The incidence of lung resection complications increases with age (over 70 years). However, age alone is not a contraindication to surgery because age may not reflect other important risk factors, such as coexisting diseases, low forced expiratory volume, weight loss, disease stage, and extent of resection. Surgical resection for palliation of NSCLC metastases can help maintain a decent quality of life in patients with rapidly progressing or recurrent spinal cord compression or solitary brain metastasis[24, 47] (see Complications box). Table 15–2 lists the estimated survival rates following complete surgical resection.

Laser Therapy. Patients with lung cancer may experience distressful symptoms or complications from endobronchial lesions, including postobstructive atelectasis and pneumonia, hemoptysis, irritating and uncontrolled cough, and hypoxemia and self-care deficit. If the endobronchial lesions involve the trachea or mainstem bronchi, laser therapy may be successfully used with palliative intent. The laser is less effective in treating

COMPLICATIONS

Lung Cancer: Surgical Treatment

Airway obstruction, dyspnea, hypoxemia, respiratory
failure
Anesthesia side effects (nausea and vomiting)
Bleeding (hypotension, cardiogenic shock)
Cardiac dysrhythmias, congestive heart failure, fluid
overload
Fever, sepsis (empyema, fistula formation)
Pneumonia
Pneumothorax
Pulmonary embolus
Wound dehiscence
Prolonged hospitalization
Death

Data from references 24, 25, 29, 46, 47, 48, 53, 57.

obstructions of smaller airways. Treatment may be repeated and can be done entirely on an outpatient basis. The procedure has been associated with a 75% success rate in advanced lung cancer. Effectiveness of the procedure is independent of other modes of therapy, patient's age, or performance status. Patients whose airway is obstructed by an exophytic lesion of squamous cell origin may derive the greatest benefit.[24, 29, 47] (See Chapter 21 for more information regarding varied surgical procedures for diagnosis, staging, and treatment.)

TABLE 15–2
Estimated Survival Following Complete Surgical Resection

Stage	Grouping	Estimated 5-Year Survival Following Complete Surgical Resection
0	TisN0M0	100%
IA	T1N0M0	75%
IB	T2N0M0	55%
IIA	T1N1M0	50%
IIB	T2N1M0	40%
	T3N0M0	
IIIA	T1-3N2M0	15%
	T3N1M0	35%
IIIB	T1-3N3M0	5-10%
	T4 Any NM0	5-10%
IV	Any t, Any N, M1 (Solitary M1)	5-10%

Reprinted with permission from Feld R and others: Lung. In Abeloff MD and others, editors: Clinical oncology, ed 2, New York, Churchill Livingstone, 1999:1411.

Radiation Therapy. Optimal doses of external beam radiation for NSCLC are now believed to be about 60 Gy. Best tumor control occurs with five fractions (treatments) per week over 6 to 7 weeks without interruption (no midtherapy "rests" as in treatment known as a "split course"). Hyperfractionation schedules (more than one treatment per day) are currently under study, and preliminary findings suggest these achieve better responses than standard schedules. A hyperfractionated dose-response relationship to survival appears to plateau at 69.9 Gy. Because doses in this range can be delivered by standard radiation with comparable survival, studies are now comparing hyperfractionated with standard schedules to answer the question of superior method. However, tumors of greater than 6 cm are not effectively destroyed by external beam therapy, whereas tumor size less than 3 cm is associated with a favorable prognosis.[10, 24, 27, 29, 37, 47]

Brachytherapy. High-dose rate (HDR) endobronchial brachytherapy (EBBT) to quickly alleviate airway obstruction or hemorrhage followed by definitive surgery or external beam radiation therapy with or without induction or concurrent chemotherapy is becoming one of the important modalities in managing patients with NSCLC. Additionally, HDR is used often in combination with laser therapy to treat recurrent and obstructing lung lesions. This technology allows for careful placement of catheters close to the tumor. Then, using computerized remote control, HDR iridium (^{192}Ir) is introduced into the catheter. Within a few minutes, while caregivers are safe from exposure, a very high dose of radiation (5–10 Gy/session) can be delivered to select tissue without injury to adjacent healthy tissue, which is especially critical at this anatomic site. Sessions may be repeated every 1 to 2 weeks for a cumulative dose in the range of 20 to 43.6 Gy. Symptoms (cough, hemoptysis, and dyspnea) can be relieved 30% to 80% of the time with minimal risk in properly selected patients.[10, 24, 27, 29, 37, 47]

Brachytherapy, based on the known dose-response relationship to tumor control, is being used to treat local disease recurrence that relapses within 15 months, in approximately 60% of patients who receive standard radiation therapy to the primary chest tumor. It is also indicated for the patient who cannot undergo resection because of the tumor's location, medical contraindications, or refusal of surgery. In the two previous clinical cases, patients with otherwise resectable NSCLC could be offered radiation therapy with curative intent; 5-year survival rates may be as high as 25%. In some cases, brachytherapy radiation implants with iodine 125 are used to sterilize tumors 7 to 8 cm in size by delivering doses of 160 to 250 Gy to the tumor without significant damage to surrounding tissue. These treatments require hospitalization while the radioactive implants are in place.[24, 29, 47]

For inoperable, locally advanced NSCLC in patients with poor prognosis, radiation alone is usually reserved for palliation of symptoms such as painful bone metastases, superior vena cava syndrome (SVCS), or those previously mentioned. Symptoms are relieved in 24% to 100% of these patients. Some studies have shown comparable symptom relief with lower than standard radiation doses at considerably less cost and inconvenience for these terminally ill patients.

The use of definitive radiotherapy at an unresectable early stage (stages I–IIIA) remains controversial. Some recognize improved median or 5-year survival in the clinical setting. The median survival in stage IIIA or IIIB NSCLC treated with radiation alone is less than 1 year. Results of trials comparing chemotherapy plus radiation with radiation alone in unresected, locally advanced NSCLC have been contradictory. One author notes a modest survival benefit if the chemotherapy regimen is cisplatin based and no difference in survival if it is not. The combined research groups, the Radiation Therapy Oncology Group (RTOG), the Eastern Cooperative Oncology Group (ECOG), and the Southwest Oncology Group (SWOG), are implementing a randomized comparative trial to determine the role of surgery compared to chemotherapy and radiotherapy for NSCLC patients with marginally resected tumors. All patients will receive combination chemotherapy (cisplatin 50 mg/m^2 on days 1, 8, 29, 36 and etoposide 50 mg/m^2 on days 1–5 and 29–33) concurrent with radiation therapy (45 Gy at 1.8 Gy/fraction, 5 days per week for 5 weeks). Half the patients will proceed to surgical exploration after an interval of 2 to 4 weeks, and half the patients continue without interruption with combination chemotherapy (cisplatin 50 mg/m^2 on days 1, 8, 29, 36 and etoposide 50 mg/m^2 on days 1–5 and 29–33) and radiation therapy (total 61.0 Gy in 33 fractions). Outcomes are inconclusive at this time.[10, 77, 83, 91]

Chemotherapy. As many as 75% to 80% of all lung cancers are NSCLC; of these, 70% of patients will present with regional or advanced disease. Even in the best of cases involving surgical resection (stage I), about 20% to 40% of patients will have relapse. Relapse occurs in 70% of patients with more advanced disease. Thus the majority of lung cancer patients have frank or occult metastatic NSCLC and could benefit from effective systemic therapy. Response rates with single agents have been notoriously low (9–27%). The most active single agents in NSCLC include mitomycin C, vindesine, vinblastine, etoposide, ifosfamide, cisplatin, carboplatin, cyclophosphamide, vincristine, doxorubicin, bleomycin, vinorelbine (Navelbine), and paclitaxel. Among newer single agents showing promise are epirubicin, docetaxel,

irinotecan, and gemcitabine (Gemzar). Docetaxel has shown significant activity in advanced NSCLC, producing response in both untreated patients and those previously treated with a platinum-based regimen. Navelbine, in controlled randomized studies, has produced an increase in survival; therefore in newly diagnosed stage IV NSCLC, this should be considered as a first-line therapy option* (Tables 15–3, 15–4, and 15–5).

Most clinical researchers concur that phase II and phase III randomized trials patient response rates vary accordingly: (1) With few exceptions, response rates rarely exceed 40% (usually ranging from 20% to 30%); (2) complete responses are almost never observed and, for almost all patients, chemotherapy is only palliative; (3) combinations containing cisplatin usually produce the best responses; (4) the overall impact of combination chemotherapy regimens on improved survival is modest (for all NSCLC patients, the median length of survival remains at 8–12 months, and the majority of patients rarely survive longer than 1 year); and (5) most combination chemotherapy regimens are associated with moderate toxicity (including alopecia and nausea and vomiting) and frequent hospital admissions for administration of chemotherapy or the evaluation of chemotherapy-induced side effects.[†]

Performance status has become a major factor in deciding who should undergo chemotherapy. Patients are pathologically staged before therapy if mediastinal nodes are greater than 1 cm on CT. An SWOG study (9019), closed December 1995, assessed the role and necessity of surgery in select stage IIIA and IIIB patients when concurrent preoperative chemotherapy and radiation therapy are compared with chemotherapy and radiation alone. Outside a protocol setting, some will recommend chemotherapy to patients with NSCLC only if the patient (1) is informed of the limitations of therapy, (2) is clearly incurable by surgery or radiation, (3) has no significant symptoms that radiation could palliate, (4) has a good performance status, and (5) has measurable disease to assess any response so that treatment can be continued appropriately.[‡]

Quality of life studies are added to most lung cancer clinical research trials. For many patients weighing the benefits versus the risks of clinical trials is an essential component. Each patient/family needs to consider what are the potential outcomes for pursuing the clinical trial as well as what is important to them regarding quality of life issues.

Combination Chemotherapy and Radiation Therapy. For inoperable, locally advanced NSCLC, cisplatin-

---

* References 10, 24, 28, 29, 32, 35, 47, 54, 83.

† References 10, 24, 28, 29, 32, 35, 47, 54, 83.

‡ References 10, 24, 28, 29, 32, 35, 47, 54, 83.

TABLE 15-3

Chemotherapy Regimens in Non–Small-Cell Lung Cancer

Drug Regimen	Dose	Schedule
ICE		
Ifosfamide (+Mesna)	4 g/m² IV day 1	Every 4 wk
Cisplatin	250 mg/m² IV days 1–3	Every 4 wk
Etoposide (VP-16)	100 mg/m² IV days 1–4	Every 4 wk
or		
Ifosfamide (+Mesna)	1500 mg/m² IV days 1–3	Every 4 wk
Carboplatin	300 mg/m² IV day 1	Every 4 wk
Etoposide (VP-16)	60–100 mg/m² IV days 1–3	Every 4 wk
MIP		
Mitomycin-C	6 mg/m² IVP day 1	Every 3–4 wk
Ifosfamide (+Mesna)	4 g/m² IV day 1	Every 3–4 wk
Cisplatin	100 mg/m² IV day 2	Every 3–4 wk
or		
Mitomycin C	6 mg/m² IVP day 1	Every 4 wk
Ifosfamide (+Mesna)	3 g/m² IV day 1	Every 4 wk
Cisplatin	50 mg/m² IV day 1	Every 4 wk
TAXOL		
	200–250 mg/m² IV over 24 h day 1	Every 3 wk
TAXOL-CISPLATIN		
Taxol	135–170 mg/m² IV over 6 h day 1 followed by	Every 3 wk
Cisplatin	75 mg/m² IV day 1	Every 3 wk

IV, intravenous; IVP, IV push.

Data from references 9, 24, 28, 29, 33, 35.

based regimens in combination with radiotherapy may improve median but not long-term survival. Postoperative cisplatin-based regimens plus radiotherapy in incompletely resected or fully resected stage II and IIIA patients are associated with improved median survival and a decrease in distant relapses (except for brain) but have not reduced mortality rates. Because of an apparent synergism when cisplatin is combined with radiation, studies continue to investigate this combination to achieve improved cure rates.

The best inroads seem to be occurring in the treatment of stage IIIA NSCLC with preoperative adjuvant (also known as *protoadjuvant* or *neoadjuvant*) chemo-

TABLE 15-4

Single-Agent Chemotherapy Drugs for Non–Small-Cell Lung Cancer

Paclitaxel	175–250 mg/m² (via 24-h infusion)
Docetaxel	75–100 mg/m²
Vinorelbine	30 mg/m²
Gemcitabine	1000–1250 mg/m²
Irinotecan	100 mg/m²

ALL the above drugs are used in combination for phase I and II clinical trials.

Data from references 9, 24, 28, 29, 32, 86, 87, 99.

therapy with or without radiation therapy. Although results are difficult to compare because of inconsistencies in staging (lack of pretreatment pathologic staging) and absence of multi-institutional trials, preliminary findings indicate a prolonged survival for patients receiving adjuvant therapy. Preoperative chemotherapy alone or in combination with radiotherapy is apparently rendering some patients pathologic complete remissions (CRs) at thoracotomy (9–11% in one series). Three-year survival rates ranged from 26% to 45%. Although findings provide hope, preoperative chemotherapy in stage IIIA NSCLC is still investigational and is appropriate only in a clinical trial setting. Patients should be informed of this option. If recent and upcoming trials demonstrate a survival advantage to preoperative chemotherapy and radiotherapy, those most likely to benefit are the 20% of patients having a normal CT but who are found to have positive mediastinal nodes after biopsy.[24, 29]

Future Concerns. New, more effective chemotherapy agents and combinations are needed, especially if they are associated with a low toxicity profile. Randomized phase III trials should be carried out only in clearly defined patient groups (e.g., pathologic staging and performance status). Immunohistochemical analysis may

TABLE 15-5

Common Chemotherapy Regimens in Advanced Non–Small-Cell Lung Cancer

Drug Regimen	Dose	Schedule
CAP		
Cyclophosphamide	500 mg/m^2 IV day 1	Every 3–4 wk
Doxorubicin	50 mg/m^2 IV day 1	Every 3–4 wk
Cisplatin	50 mg/m^2 IV day 1	Every 3–4 wk
CE		
Caboplatin	100 mg/m^2 IV day 1	Every 3–4 wk
Etoposide	3 mg/m^2 IV days 1–3	Every 3–4 wk
	300–375 mg/m^2 IV day 1	
	100–120 mg/m^2 IV days 1–3	
BEP		
Bleomycin	25 mg/m^2 IV days 1–3	Every 4 wk
Etoposide	100 mg/m^2 IV days 1–3	Every 4 wk
Cisplatin	25 mg/m^2 IV days 1–3	Every 4 wk
EP		
Etoposide (VP-16)	80–120 mg/m^2 IV days 1–3	Every 3–4 wk
Cisplatin	80–120 mg/m^2 IV day 2	Every 3–4 wk
MVbP		
Mitomycin C	10 mg/m^2 IV day 1	Every 6–12 wk
Vinblastine	6 mg/m^2 IV day 1	Every 2–3 wk
Cisplatin	40–100 mg/m^2 IV day 1	Every 3–6 wk
VbP		
Vinblastine	6 mg/m^2 IV days 1 and 2	Every 3 wk
Cisplatin	120 mg/m^2 IV day 1	Every 3 wk
VdP		
Vindesine	3 mg/m^2 IV every week for 5 weeks	Every other week
Cisplatin	120 mg/m^2 IV days 1 and 29	Every 6 wk

IV, intravenous.

Data from references 24 and 29.

help to identify that subgroup of NSCLCs with neuroendocrine features that may benefit from adjuvant chemotherapy. Examination of chromosomes for K-*ras* mutations may also delineate patients with adenocarcinoma of the lung who may benefit from more aggressive treatment or else should not be subjected to treatment because of the aggressive nature of their disease and guaranteed short survival. Biotherapy research includes phase I studies with use of growth factors and monoclonal antibodies and their impact on lung cancer disease and treatment. Outcomes are yet undetermined for the impact of this modality.[67, 78, 84, 105]

Small-Cell Lung Cancer

Surgery. In the 1960s and 1970s most surgical attempts to treat SCLC (stages I and II) met with dismal results, with less than 1% surviving at 5 years. The Veterans Administration and Armed Forces Cooperative Group found an amazing 36% 5-year survival among SCLC patients who had an unknown diagnosis and a single pulmonary lesion preoperatively. However, less than 5% of SCLC patients are diagnosed in the early stages of disease when it is resectable, and the chest is still the most common site of relapse. Adjuvant chemotherapy after surgical resection for stage I disease results in about a 45% 5-year survival rate.[12, 24, 47]

Current recommended treatment of SCLC presenting as a single pulmonary nodule is surgery followed by adjuvant chemotherapy with or without radiation to the chest. Prophylactic cranial irradiation may be considered, but studies have not proved any survival benefit. The Lung Cancer Study Group (LCSG) and ECOG completed a prospective randomized study to examine the benefit of surgery in patients with stages I to IIIA SCLC. Patients were randomized to receive either preoperative chemotherapy plus surgery and radiotherapy or chemotherapy and radiotherapy alone. Preliminary results show no survival benefit with surgery. Unless randomized trials can demonstrate an advantage to chemotherapy plus surgery in early stage disease, the exact role of surgery will remain unclear. However, there appears to be a small group of SCLC patients (<1%) with true stage I disease who may be cured by surgery with or without chemotherapy.[24, 47]

Radiation Therapy. In limited-disease (LD) SCLC, trials combining chest radiation and chemotherapy have now shown improved long-term survival rates (26–56% at 2 years; 7–20% at 4 years) and a decrease in local recurrences. Concurrent radiotherapy with chemotherapy or alternating chemotherapy with radiotherapy seems to produce the best results. It is too early to know whether long-term survival will translate to cures. Before etoposide-cisplatin (EP) regimens, organ toxicities from combined-modality approaches were too severe (e.g., congestive heart failure, dyspnea) and without survival benefit. Toxicities noted with EP plus radiation were myelosuppression, esophagitis, and some reports of pulmonary toxicity (possibly from the radiation port size), but none was life-threatening. Use of CT guidance in radiation treatment planning, individually designed blocks, and a shrinking field help protect surrounding healthy lung, esophagus, and spinal cord tissues from unwanted radiation.[24, 37, 47, 49]

With the combined-modality approach, the most common site of failure is the chest in about 30% of LD SCLCs. When chemotherapy is given alone in LD SCLC, however, the incidence of local chest relapse is 80%. Some note that the intensity of the first chemotherapy dose may predict survival. Current trials are examining the role of dose intensity and timing of modalities in preventing local recurrences and in improving long-term survival. Research in this area has increased because of the availability of hematopoietic growth factors and peripheral blood stem cell (PBSC) support. In extensive SCLC, there is no advantage to combining radiation therapy with chemotherapy. The main role for radiation therapy in these patients is palliation of symptoms.[15, 20, 24, 35, 47, 102]

The brain is a frequent site of metastasis, and the effect of most systemic chemotherapy on the central nervous system (CNS) is extremely limited. Whole-brain irradiation (WBI) is often necessary. If brain metastasis has occurred, 40 Gy is needed to prevent relapse. Unlike treatment in NSCLC, *prophylactic cranial irradiation* (PCI) has often been done to prevent CNS failure. PCI can reduce the incidence of CNS relapse from 25% to 6% and has generally been reserved for patients achieving a CR to chemotherapy. PCI may be used during systemic therapy in a clinical trial involving a potential cure. However, authors are questioning the value of PCI because of the high incidence and severity of CNS toxicities. Late toxicities from PCI in long-term survivors are only now being realized and may be underreported in some studies because of only incidental and retrospective reporting. Among the 7% of patients surviving beyond 5 years in one retrospective review, 22% were found to have developed probable CNS toxicity that surfaced 2 to 5 years after combination chemotherapy and radiotherapy. Patients had neurologic complaints, abnormal neurologic findings, and abnormal CT scans. In some patients, progressive clinical deterioration from neurologic deficits required life-style changes or extended care. Because of late toxicities, PCI is usually limited to no more than 30 Gy and is not given concurrently with chemotherapy to avoid synergistic injury to brain tissue. Many still reserve PCI until treatment of the primary tumor is completed.[12, 20, 28, 37, 49]

Radiation to other common sites of metastasis (e.g., liver, spine) will not prevent tumor spreading to those sites. Prompt therapy (chemotherapy or radiation) for known meningeal carcinomatosis and spinal metastases is useful and necessary, but no preventive therapy exists for these complications. Patients with extensive disease (ED) who present with SVCS should be spared radiation because they usually will respond adequately to chemotherapy.[24, 47]

Chemotherapy. Before chemotherapy, half of SCLC patients with LD died within 12 to 14 weeks, and half of those with ED died within 6 weeks without treatment. Combination chemotherapy became the cornerstone of treatment in the 1980s for SCLC patients, with overall responses of up to 90% and CRs of 40% to 50%. Long-term survival depends on achieving a CR, usually within the first months of treatment.[24, 47]

Since the mid-1970s, many single agents have shown response rates from 15% to 50%. These include cyclophosphamide, ifosfamide, doxorubicin, epirubicin, etoposide, teniposide, cisplatin, carboplatin, vincristine, methotrexate, and the nitrosureas. Etoposide appears to produce a very dose-dependent and schedule-dependent response. There are improved response rates in SCLC when etoposide is given in multiple daily intravenous (IV) doses (for 3–5 days) rather than as a single bolus. A study has demonstrated excellent response rates and minimal toxicities (primarily mild myelosuppression) when etoposide is given as a daily oral dose (50 mg/m^2) for 5 to 21 consecutive days every 4 weeks. Carboplatin, with a 60% response rate in untreated patients, has shown to be highly active as a single agent as well as in combination regimens. Paclitaxel, topotecan, and irinotecan (the topoisomerase I inhibitors), gemcitabine, topotecan and oral preparations of etoposide and platinum have shown some promise and warrant further investigation. Combination chemotherapy appears to be improving survival statistics in SCLC patients (Tables 15–6 and 15–7).[24, 47, 49]

TABLE 15-6
Common Chemotherapy Regimens in Small-Cell Lung Cancer

Drug Regimen	Dose	Schedule
CAV		
Cyclophosphamide	750–1500 mg/m² IV day 1	Every 3 wk
Doxorubicin	40–50 mg/m² IV day 1	Every 3 wk
Vincristine	2 mg IV day 1	Every 3 wk
CAE		
Cyclophosphamide	1000 mg/m² IV day 1	Every 3 wk
Doxorubicin	45 mg/m² IV day 1	Every 3 wk
Etoposide	50 mg/m² IV days 1–5	Every 3 wk
CEV		
Cyclophosphamide	1000 mg/m² IV day 1	Every 3 wk
Etoposide (VP-16)	50 mg/m² IV day 1	Every 3 wk
Etoposide	100 mg/m² PO days 2–5	Every 3 wk
Vincristine	2 mg IV day 1	Every 3 wk
CAVE		
Cyclophosphamide	1000 mg/m² IV day 1	Every 3 wk
Doxorubicin	50 mg/m² IV day 1	Every 3 wk
Etoposide (VP-16)	60 mg/m² IV days 1–5	Every 3 wk
Vincristine	1 mg/m² IV days 1 and 8	Every 3 wk
CMCcV		
Cyclophosphamide	700 mg/m² IV day 1	Every 4 wk
Lomustine	70 mg/m² PO day 1 HS	Every 4 wk
Vincristine	1.3 mg/m² IV days 1, 8, 15, 22 first cycle, then day 1 only in subsequent cycles	Every 4 wk
Methotrexate	20 mg/m² PO days 18 and 21	Every 4 wk
EP		
Etoposide	100 mg/m² IV days 1–3	Every 3 wk
Cisplatin	25 mg/m² IV day 1–3	Every 3 wk

CAV and EP Cycle of CAV as above alternating every 3 wk with cycle of EP as above

IV, Intravenous; PO, oral; HS, at bedtime.
Data from references 12, 19, 20, 24, 47, 49, 62, 80, 102, 103.

TABLE 15-7
New Chemotherapy Drugs Used in Small-Cell Lung Cancer

Ifosfamide	1–2 g/m² IV 30 min infusion daily for 5 days
Oral etoposide	Dose is two times the IV dose rounded to nearest 50 mg
Oral platinum	JM216 (bisacetato-amine-dichloro-cyclohexylamine-platinum) 120 mg/m² for 5 days
Paclitaxel	250 mg/m² IV infusion over 24 h
Topotecan	1.5 mg/m² IV 30 minute infusion daily for 5 days

Data from references 13, 26, 49, 52, 75, 83.

Etoposide plus cisplatin (EP) has proved superior to cytoxan, doxorubicin (Adriamycin), and vincristine (CAV) regimens for both LD and ED in regard to responses, survival, and reduced toxicities. Large cooperative group and single institution studies found improved median survival (18–19 months) in LD patients receiving regimens containing VP-16 plus cisplatin with or without radiation therapy to the primary tumor. Current practice is to give intense chemotherapy of short duration (fewer than six cycles) with active agents. Restaging should include bronchoscopy and all initial staging studies to determine response. No study has shown a survival benefit for prolonged (1–2 years) maintenance chemotherapy in patients achieving a CR with induction therapy. In LD patients, late dose intensification after a CR was achieved during induction therapy proved a superior treatment to maintenance therapy. The only current maintenance studies are those evaluating the role of biologic response modifiers.[24, 47, 49, 91]

Overall, 80% to 90% of SCLCs will respond to chemotherapy. Of patients who respond to chemotherapy, 50% will begin to relapse within 10 to 12 months. From 30% to 64% of SCLCs that relapse after an initial response will subsequently respond to either the same or another type (second-line) of chemotherapy. About 20% to 25% of ED patients will achieve a CR with combination chemotherapy, usually without radiation therapy. Trials using combination chemotherapy regimens have reported survival rates of 23% at 1 year and 4% at 2 years in ED SCLC. Perhaps 1% of ED patients survive beyond 5 years and may be cured, although relapse is possible beyond 5 years. Current clinical trials using combinations of new and active agents are underway to try to improve long-term survival and reduce toxicity. One SWOG study (9216) compares CODE (cisplatin, vincristine, doxorubicin, and etoposide) plus thoracic radiation therapy versus alternating CAV and VP-16 in extensive-stage SCLC. Another study (LUN-11) investigates the use of paclitaxel/carboplatin with extended oral VP-16 in limited-stage or extensive-stage SCLC. Efforts to overcome drug resistance by use of alternating non–cross-resistant regimens or high-dose regimens with or without autologous bone marrow transplant in ED have not generally improved disease-free survival, although initial CRs are impressive. Aggressive chemotherapy is currently not warranted outside a protocol setting for these SCLC patients with poor prognosis. Most patients, however, can achieve some quality time by means of standard chemotherapy regimens, with mild toxicities before eventual death as a result of their disease.[12, 20, 26, 37, 49]

Delayed Effects of Treatment. Only now are there sufficient numbers of SCLC survivors to appreciate the late effects of treatment. The late toxicity of PCI with or without chemotherapy depends on total dose of radiation, port size, and concurrent therapies. Findings include cerebral atrophy, dementia, confusion, and personality changes. Efforts to decrease these effects are already in place, and research is focused on whether late toxicity from PCI is worth any survival benefit. Secondary leukemias (e.g., acute myelogenous leukemia) can occur, presumably resulting from chemotherapy. This problem may be resolved by avoiding maintenance regimens and alkylating agents. Patients cured of SCLC who continue to smoke tobacco have a greater risk of developing a second primary lesion than of experiencing a relapse from SCLC. These people need to be so advised and encouraged to stop smoking.[24, 47]

Future Concerns. Controversial issues that need to be addressed focus on the best schedule and dose of etoposide and the role of radiation therapy in the long-term survival of patients with LD SCLC. Whether chemotherapy dose intensification will lead to improved long-term survival and whether the survival benefit of PCI is worth the toxicities remain to be seen. Insights gained through genetic engineering and the discovery of genetic variations unique to SCLC (i.e., *myc*-oncogene amplification and gene deletions in chromosome 3p) may lead to improved early detection or treatment by genetic manipulation. Two trials (SWOG no. 8991 and an Intergroup study with ECOG) are currently being analyzed related to survival data with variant versus classic SCLC subtypes to assess the prognostic significance of these histologies. Use of granulocyte-macrophage colony-stimulating factor (GM-CSF) or granulocyte CSF (G-CSF) to prevent the frequent dose-limiting side effect of neutropenic sepsis with chemotherapy is being tested in clinical trials. Preliminary results of a SWOG study (8812) in LD SCLC suggest that patients who were randomized to the combined chemotherapy-radiotherapy plus GM-CSF group had more severe toxicity (e.g., infection, thrombocytopenia) than those who did not receive GM-CSF.[11–13, 20, 26, 37, 54, 75]

TREATMENT OF METASTASIS

Patients with lung cancer frequently develop varied metastatic disease processes. Some of the most common sites include brain, bone, liver, pleural effusions, or cardiac complications via cardiac tamponade. Each of these metastatic disease sites with their clinical features and diagnostic and treatment interventions are discussed below.

Brain Metastasis

Distant metastasis rather than local chest recurrence is the most common reason for disease treatment failure after curative surgery for NSCLC, and the predominant site of metastasis is the brain. Lung cancer accounts for the majority of all primary cancers (lung, 64%; breast, 14%; unknown primary, 8%; melanoma, 4%; colorectal, 3%; other, 7%) that metastasize to the brain. Therefore, even the most vague CNS symptoms suggest the need for follow-up with CT, MRI, or arteriography. Lumbar puncture (LP) should be avoided if cerebral metastasis is suspected. Studies using CT scan data indicate that metastases of the brain are multiple in slightly more than 50% of the cases (Fig. 15–5). Increased intracranial pressure (ICP) and cerebrospinal fluid (CSF) obstruction cause generalized symptoms such as change in level of consciousness (LOC), papillary changes and papilledema, headache and seizures, vomiting, and change in vital signs (wide pulse pressure, increased blood pressure, bradycardia, irregular pulse). Local compression or destruction of tissue from edema or encroachment

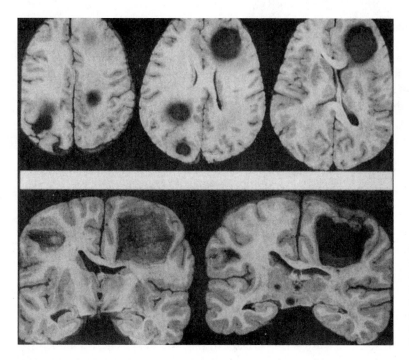

FIGURE 15–5 Brain metastases. *Top,* Gross specimens show metastatic deposits of an undifferentiated large cell lung carcinoma. The metastases form essentially necrotic masses with peripheral enhancement and peritumoral edema. *Bottom,* Occasionally, extensive necrosis transforms metastases into cysts lined by only a thin rim of viable tumor.

of the mass can cause a multitude of problems depending on location. *Aphasia* (inability to express or understand verbal symbols), *agnosia* (inability to recognize objects), and *apraxia* (inability to execute purposeful movements) result from pressure on the right parietal lobe. A tumor in the left parietal lobe can cause difficulty with the simplest of tasks, such as reading or adding up the grocery bill. Other subtle mental changes, such as recent memory loss, can occur if the limbic system is involved.[24, 40, 47, 59, 79]

Treatment should be palliative to correct the patient's neurologic deficits, which, in turn, enhances quality of life. Almost all patients with brain metastases should be started on corticosteroid therapy at the time of diagnosis. Usual starting dosage is 4 mg four times daily given either orally or intravenously, with the clinical effects noticeable within 6 to 24 hours after the first dose, and reaching maximum effect in 3 to 7 days. Corticosteroid therapy is followed by radiation therapy. WBI therapy increases the median survival to 3 to 6 months. Currently typical radiation treatment schedules consist of short courses (7–15 days) of WBI (150–400 cGy/d) with total doses in the range of 3000 to 5000 cGy. Surgical therapy is usually not an option for most patients with brain metastases because of the presence of multiple lesions or extensive systemic cancer. In some patients with limited metastatic disease sites combination surgical treatment followed by postoperative radiotherapy may be more effective than radiation therapy alone.[24, 40, 47, 79]

Coping with brain and neurologic complications poses a dilemma for both the patient and family. The goal of treatment is to control the neurologic deficits and promote an optimal life-style. The nurse can facilitate better communication to and with the patient and family using the following inventions for patients with alterations in thought processes*:

- Introduce self and face the patient while speaking.
- Inform patient of date, day, and time on awakening and as needed.
- Keep verbal communication simple and direct without shouting or being condescending.
- Remember that the patient is thinking in slow motion, therefore:
    Speak slowly because it takes patient a long time to process what is being said and how to respond.
    Use short, simple sentences.
    Present only one idea at a time.
    Ask affirmative questions rather than negative ones. "Do you want a drink?" is better than "Don't you want a drink?"
    Do not ask questions that require patient to make a choice, e.g., "Do you want to stay up awhile or would you like to go back to bed?"
- Encourage the use of appropriate greetings and social exchanges.
- Do not tease or encourage patient to respond inappropriately.
- Encourage gestures and talking with hands whenever possible. Ask the patient to describe or show you

---

* References 2, 3, 7, 17, 36, 39, 94, 95, 98.

what he means; frequently this will enable the patient to say the word itself.

- Be prepared for bizarre, inaccurate use of language and swearing. Such responses are very common with the brain-injured patient. Accept this without amusement or anger. Help the patient by providing the correct word without emotion.
- Decrease noise level and refrain from talking to other people over the patient.
- Keep the patient's bed rails up, and avoid restraints unless necessary for patient safety.
- Supervise activities to allow as much autonomy as possible.
- Provide simple, step-by-step instructions for tasks.
- Provide positive reinforcement for accomplished tasks (e.g., bathing, self-care, eating).
- Minimize energies used in clothing changes by selecting simplistic style and comfort wear.
- Provide for rest and naps; reduce mental activity late in the day.
- Observe the patient on a scheduled frequency.
- Include family/caregiver in teaching and management of patient; refer to community resources or social services as needed.

Bone Metastasis

Bone metastasis contributes significant morbidity for most patients with cancer. Lung, liver, and bone are the most common sites for metastases for all the cancer diseases. Characteristically, pain that becomes progressively worse over weeks or months is frequently associated with bone metastasis in the patient with lung cancer. This complication, though not life-threatening, can be disabling if pathologic fractures occur or extradural spinal disease results in spinal cord compression. Bone provides structural support and a site for the hematopoiesis; therefore, it acts as a reservoir to maintain homeostasis of calcium, magnesium, phosphorus, and sodium. When the cancer cells migrate (metastasize) from the anatomic cancer disease site (lung) to other tissues (bone), an imbalance of homeostasis occurs. The cancer cells now in the bone cause an alteration in the osteoblastic activity (bone reconstruction) and osteoclastic activity (bone destruction). This alteration results in clinical complications for the patient.[6, 14, 24, 47]

The disruption of the osteoblastic and osteoclastic activity results in an imbalance of calcium and phosphorus levels (e.g., elevated alkaline phosphatase and serum calcium [hypercalcemia]), and urinary markers are positive for bone resorption. As the bone destruction process increases, further alterations in serum electrolytes occur, and the patient develops multiple clinical symptoms of increased pain, thirst, polyuria, anorexia, fatigue, changes in mental status (confused, irritable), dehydration, and constipation. Diagnostic tests usually ordered to diagnose, monitor, and evaluate treatment responses include bone scans, x-rays, CT scans, MRI, serum calcium levels, alkaline phosphatase levels, and complete blood count[6, 14, 57] (see Chapter 20).

Skeletal metastasis usually occurs in the vertebra (70%), pelvis (41%), femur (25%), and skull (14%). The appearance on x-ray film can vary greatly. Osteolytic lesions have ragged margins, can infiltrate an entire bone, and are more vulnerable to pathologic fractures than osteoblastic lesions. Osteoblastic lesions are sclerotic metastatic foci characterized by increased radiographic density (Fig. 15–6). Occasionally, both sclerotic and lytic patterns emerge. Patients with widespread bony metastasis, compared with a single bony lesion, usually have decreased survival time.

Management for this complication is directed toward patient comfort and prevention of additional complications such as sensory and motor dysfunction. Multiple medications (analgesics, nonsteroidal anti-inflammatory drugs [NSAIDs]), bisphosphonates, and chemotherapy are used for pain management and hypercalcemia, and to improve mobility and bone structure status. Additionally, radiation therapy and surgical intervention are used to promote comfort and increase ambulation and mobility. Orthopedic management can be attempted to

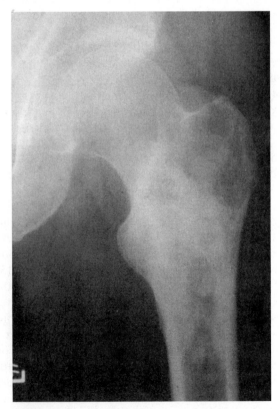

FIGURE 15-6 Osteoblastic metastatic lesion to hip from adenocarcinoma of lung.

promote spinal stabilization and prevent cord compression. Prophylactic fixation of metastatic lesions in the long bones with rods (Enders) or implants (Zickel, Moore, bipolar, total hip) can prevent pathologic fractures and ensure ambulation or upper extremity control (Figs. 15–6 and 15–7). Combination chemotherapy may also help alleviate or modify this painful process. Although most lung cancer patients will not experience prolonged survival, control of painful bony metastasis remains essential.[14, 24, 40, 46, 65, 94]

Liver Metastasis

Liver metastasis occurs in approximately 15% of the patients with lung cancer and for this patient population the added diagnosis of liver metastasis is a poor prognostic sign. Patients with solitary metastatic sites generally survive longer than those with widespread liver metastasis. Diagnostic methods, such as CT scans with angiography (noncontrast, contrast, delayed, imaging), MRI, positron emission tomography, and intraoperative ultrasonography, and biochemical laboratory tests, such as alkaline phosphatase, gamma-glutamyl transpeptidase (GGTP), serum aspartate aminotransferase (AST, SGOT), lactate dehydrogenase (LDH), and prothrombin time, have led to increased sensitivity and specificity in the diagnosis of liver metastases. Innovative surgical treatments (hepatic resection, micrometastasectomies); chemotherapy (systemic and regional), chemoembolization (local entrapment of a drug in the embolization agent), cryosurgery (destruction of tissues using a freezing probe), and radiation therapy (whole-liver external beam) have improved the overall response rates for multiple patients with liver metastases.[24, 29, 47]

Because many patients with lung cancer have moderate to advanced disease at the time of diagnosis, and a limited prolonged survival outcome, the added burden of liver metastasis further compromises their status. Many of the diagnostic and treatment interventions have potential risks or complications. Based on the patient's lung cancer stage, overall health wellness (presence of weight loss, cachexia), and other lung cancer metastatic disease processes, the diagnostic and treatment interventions may be limited to palliative care. Pain management, ascites management, dietary interventions, and hygiene with prudent skin care to minimize skin breakdown are the usual nursing interventions at this disease stage.[57, 95, 98, 107]

Cardiac Metastasis

Malignant involvement of the cardiac muscle produces pericardial effusion; if enough fluid accumulates in the pericardium to obstruct blood flow to the ventricle, cardiac tamponade will result. The symptoms induced by pericardial effusion often mimic the cancer's overall systemic effects and include dyspnea and cyanosis, orthopnea, venous distention, leg edema, and cardiac enlargement. Additional symptoms may include hiccups, coughing, and weak or absent apical pulse. Cardiac tamponade may develop slowly or quickly, and the onset of severe symptoms depends on how rapidly the fluid accumulates. Medical management generally consists of pericardiocentesis (cardiac window procedure performed using local anesthesia), systemic chemotherapy, or intrapericardial administration of various other agents. Palliative care interventions such as these can improve the quality of the patient's remaining life. If the patient's mean life expectancy is 9 to 13 months, varied other treatment modalities could be pursued[24, 25, 47, 98] (see Chapter 20).

PLEURAL EFFUSIONS AND CHEST TUBES

The pleural cavity consists of the space between the parietal pleura and the visceral pleura. The *parietal pleura* lines the chest, and the *visceral pleura* covers the lung. The two pleura, lubricated by a thin layer of fluid, glide over each other during inspiration and expiration. A vacuum is created by the fluid and causes the surfaces to adhere to each other. In the normal lung, no true

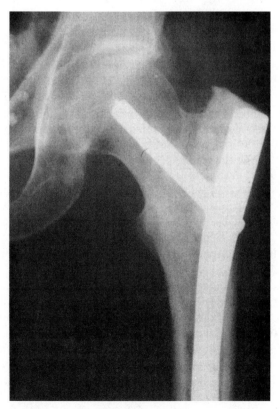

FIGURE 15–7 Example of a prophylactic Zickel hip nailing from metastatic adenocarcinoma of lung.

space exists between the two pleura, and if one develops, it alters respiratory function and the lungs can no longer expand properly. A pleural effusion has thus been created.[24, 47, 61]

Approximately half the patients with breast or lung cancer will develop pleural effusion sometime during the course of their illness. As a result pleural fluid can accumulate and obstruct lymphatic drainage and increase capillary permeability. Lung expansion is impaired with poor gas exchange, and respiratory embarrassment is the outcome. Other consequences include atelectasis and recurrent infections. Pleural effusions are classified as symptomatic (mild, moderate, severe) or secondary to a responsive or nonresponsive malignancy; the presence of pleural effusion translates to a prognosis of survival of less than 6 months.[24, 47, 61]

Various methods of treatment for pleural effusion are available, including repeated thoracentesis, intrapleural instillation of chemotherapy, intracavitary radioactive colloids, and pleurectomy. Due to the limited life expectancy for patients with lung cancer, treatment should be implemented promptly. Thoracentesis can provide immediate relief of symptoms but fluid reaccumulation is common. Pleural sclerosis after draining of the fluid is the most commonly used form of treatment to achieve long-term control.[24, 56, 61, 101]

The patient with pleural effusion who is to be sclerosed has a chest tube, and providing care to patients with chest tubes in place is cause for concern. The nurse should provide scheduled, skilled, ongoing assessments, interventions, and evaluations of the patient with a chest tube for the duration of the chest tube placement and for a period of time following removal of the chest tube. When a chest tube is inserted, placement depends on whether it is to drain air only, such as pneumothorax (second or third intercostal space), or fluid, such as an effusion (fourth or sixth intercostal space). Because air rises, tube placement will be higher for a pneumothorax.[22, 23, 31, 56, 60]

Once the chest tube has been inserted and sutured in place, it is connected to underwater-seal drainage (e.g., Pleur-Evac; Fig. 15–8). The principle is to keep the chest tube under sterile fluid (usually water) to prevent air from going back up the tube into the pleural cavity. If a pleural effusion is present, suction will remove the fluid from the pleural space. However, as the lung contracts during expiration, it is important to prevent air and the effusion fluid from returning to the chest cavity. This process is minimized because the chest tube tip is under water.[22, 23, 31, 60]

When a commercial drainage system such as the Pleur-Evac is used, three separate chambers (formerly bottles) are usually visible. The first compartment collects the fluid from the chest, the second is the water-seal chamber, and the third is the suction control chamber. It maintains proper suction and limits the negative pres-

sure applied to the pleura. This is usually set at 20 cm H_2O, negative pressure for adults. If turning up the suction regulator increases the flow rate, more vigorous bubbling will occur in the suction control chamber, and air or fluid will be pulled more quickly from the chest. Because the water level is set at 20 cm H_2O, however, no increase will occur in the negative pressure applied to the pleural cavity.[22, 23, 31, 60]

Specific factors must be assessed and monitored after the chest tube system is in place. If the patient has a pleural effusion rather than a pneumothorax, bubbling in the water-seal chamber could indicate a leak in the system. The nurse should clamp the drainage tube near the patient with a padded hemostat, and if the bubbling stops, there is probably a leak at the insertion site or inside the pleural cavity. If the bubbling does not stop when the tube is clamped, a leak is present in the system itself; the most likely place is the link between the chest tube and the drainage system. This chest tube area must always be secured with adhesive tape to reduce the risk of air leakage. Great *caution* must be exercised when using clamps on a chest tube. If air or fluid can no longer come out of the pleural space but is still entering the space through the lung, a tension pneumothorax can ensue. This situation is serious because, with increased tension in the pleural space, the mediastinum is shifted to the opposite side and blood return to the heart is dangerously impaired. If no blood is available for cardiac output, the blood pressure is unobtainable and the patient will be in respiratory distress.*

It is *rarely necessary* to clamp a chest tube. Even if the chest tube becomes disconnected from the system, it is easier to reconnect the tubing rather than to clamp the tubing. In certain instances, the clamp may be forgotten and tension pneumothorax may result. Patients can be easily transported for diagnostic tests, assisted to the bathroom, or ambulated with no problem as long as the underwater seal is kept intact.[22, 23, 31, 60]

Stripping and milking the chest tube can also be dangerous because suction is created, affecting the pleural space. This procedure may be done ONLY if a blood clot or other material obstructs the tube. Pressure as "high" as 350 cm H_2O has been recorded with stripping. Milking the chest tube is a more gentle form of stripping; both forms use manual compression between the chest tube and drainage system. To prevent obstruction, the nurse must ensure that there is adequate gravity drainage from the patient to the unit. Any dependent loop of tubing or tubing located on the bed can create back-pressure or a flow resistance in the tubing. Unless fluid is within the drainage tube, raising the system above the chest causes no problem. Even if drained fluid were within the tubing, the only harm would be fluid returning

---

* References 22, 23, 31, 47, 48, 52, 57, 60, 61, 94.

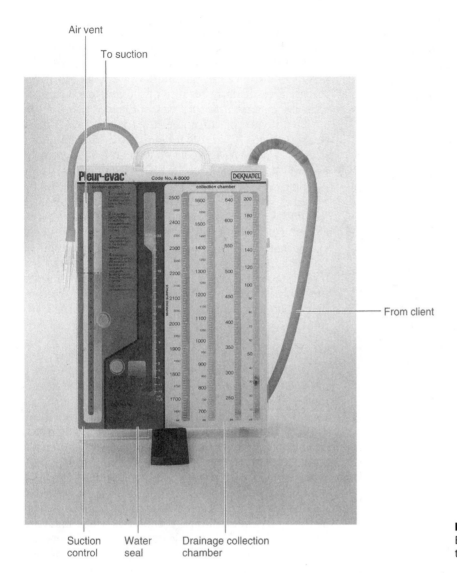

Air vent

To suction

From client

Suction control

Water seal

Drainage collection chamber

FIGURE 15 – 8 Example of Pleur-Evac drainage system. (Courtesy of DeKnatel, Inc.)

to the pleural space. This may not be pleasant, but it is not an emergency. Other minor problems can develop, but usually these are not life-threatening.[22, 23, 31, 60]

Because malignant pleural effusion carries a poor prognosis in lung cancer (two thirds of patients will die within 3 months), the primary management goal is to control symptoms. As previously stated, an agent such as the antibiotic doxycycline can be used to sclerose the patient's lung with relatively good results. Although more expensive, some physicians prefer to use bleomycin as a sclerosing agent because little or no pain is associated with its instillation. More important than any antineoplastic activity is the sclerosis of the pleura that the agent produces to prevent fluid reaccumulation.[24, 47, 61]

Instilling doxycycline or talc through a thoracostomy tube accomplishes sclerosing. Closed-tube thoracostomy attached to water-seal drainage with gentle suction (usually 20 cm H_2O) should be in place 24 to 48 hours before pleural sclerosing to promote chest drainage.

Sclerosis is usually done when the total chest tube output for 24 hours is less than 100 mL. Patients are usually premedicated with an analgesic (morphine), antipyretic (Tylenol), and antihistamine (Benedryl) to minimize the pain and hypersensitivity reactions. Lidocaine (150 mg) can be added to the doxycycline medium, and the solution is instilled through the chest tube to sclerose the pleura. The chest tube is then clamped for 2 hours, and the patient is turned side to side, back to abdomen, and in Trendelenburg and reverse Trendelenburg positions every 15 minutes to ensure equal distribution of the sclerosing agent. The tube is then unclamped, left to drain for 12 to 24 hours, and removed if chest tube drainage is minimal. Sclerosing can be repeated again in 24 hours, if necessary.[8, 24, 47, 61]

ELDERLY PATIENTS WITH LUNG CANCER

The incidence and risk of developing cancer increase with age because of several related factors, including accumulation of, or repeated contact with carcinogens, decreased immunologic resistance, hormonal imbalance, and age-related cell alterations that influence susceptibility to cancer. Lung cancer, in particular, may be ignored because the vague symptoms can be linked with the aging process, such as fatigue, decreased appetite, nonspecific aches and pains, and even a cough.

Treatment modalities associated with lung cancer can be devastating to older persons, especially if they are already debilitated. Chemotherapy not only suppresses the bone marrow, but also causes severe compromise to the patient's nutritional status (Box 15–2). Many clinicians automatically reduce chemotherapy doses based on a patient's age. Others examine factors such

as the physiologic rather than the chronological age and the likelihood of cure when making decisions about doses. Intensity of chemotherapy correlated with the quality of life in elderly patients have become a focus for research, particularly because of the shortened survival time associated with a lung cancer diagnosis. In a retrospective review of chemotherapy for SCLC in elderly patients (age 70 or older), intensive chemotherapy (CAV regimen) was associated with more severe toxicities and deaths compared with less intensive therapy (single agent, radiation alone). However, those who received more intense treatment survived about 5 months longer. The authors concluded that the small survival advantage did not justify the severe toxicities of intense chemotherapy. Many elderly people have compromised cardiovascular, hepatic, neurologic, renal and respiratory systems that result in a diminished homeostasis in the body. Alterations in drug metabolism, excretion, fluid/electrolyte balance, and sensory and motor functions are critical issues to address in the disease and treatment process.[76, 83, 89, 102]

Radiation therapy is notorious for causing increased fatigue, which further compromises the energy levels in patients who have other chronic diseases. One important related consequence of lung cancer in elderly persons is decreased physical and psychological comfort. Attitudes held by professional caregivers regarding pain management (elderly patients do not have as much pain, automatically assumes patient has a compromised respiratory and sensory status) potentially may cause them to withhold dosing amounts or delay dosing schedule of routine analgesic and sedative medications. All patient medication interventions need to be individualized based on the patient's disease status, age, weight, current and previous medication usage, reported patient pain level, anxiety level, and alterations in sleep.[53, 65]

Often the elderly population is compromised in financial, social, physical, and family resources. Psychosocially they may desire to participate in self-care but the family member/caregiver has a compromised health status and is not able to perform the required patient care activities. Many of these issues encompass all patients with cancer; however, the concern with patients with lung cancer is their usually limited survival time after diagnosis. For elderly patients, adjustments to change often come with greater difficulty and the adjustment to lung cancer and its treatments must be made rapidly. Consequently, the nurse must be alerted to these particular problems to provide timely interventions for these patients' rapidly increasing nursing care needs[95, 98] (see Chapters 28 and 30).

REHABILITATION

Activity Maintenance

Limited information is available on long-term survival of patients with lung cancer. Those who survive and

---

BOX 15–2

Impact of Cancer, Cancer Treatment, and Aging on Nutrition

Cancer and Cancer Treatment

Tumor/host competition
Increased requirements
Malabsorption/obstruction
Taste alteration (dysgeusia)
Anorexia
Nausea/vomiting
Mucositis/esophagitis
Depression/fatigue
Early satiety
Fluid and electrolyte imbalance

Aging

Impaired ability to plan/prepare meals
Psychologic/social/sensorimotor factors
Impaired taste
Decreased salivation
Slowing of digestive process
Mastication difficulties
Altered hormonal secretions
Other chronic illnesses (arthritis, diabetes, hypertension)

Increased Risk of

Weight loss
Malnutrition
Cachexia
Muscle wasting
Impaired wound healing
Susceptibility to infection
Depression, anxiety
Treatment-related complications (immunosuppression, radiation esophagitis and pneumonitits)
Poor prognosis

Data from references 24, 47, 64, 86, 94.

complete their course of treatment may experience problems with radiation pneumonitis and pulmonary fibrosis, second malignancies, and neurologic complications (e.g., memory loss, confusion, ataxia, vision loss, and dysphagia) from PCI. It is important to encourage patients and family members with supportive counseling, but the nurse must also offer some concrete suggestions for maintaining activities of daily living in the face of an altered life-style[2, 3, 36, 94] (Box 15–3).

Pulmonary Program. Patients with pulmonary fibrosis may experience exacerbation of dyspnea that is usually frightening for both the patient and the family. Anticipated assessments and prompt interventions should be taught to the family member/caregiver that will diminish the physical sensations, to reduce their fear and anxiety regarding the event. Family members or significant others must be aware of what to expect and what to do if breathing difficulties ensue. Most people become agitated, diaphoretic, and pale, and gasp for breath. They may speak with short, staccato words and have a frozen appearance with large, staring eyes. Patients must be educated in strategies for managing dyspnea (Box 15–4).

BOX 15–3

Modifications of Activities of Daily Living for Patient/Family Experiencing Lung Cancer

Do not treat patient as an invalid just because her activity tolerance has decreased.

Encourage the spouse/children to include patient in family decision-making.

Help patient establish a new daily routine with realistic goals:

- Patient can assist with small tasks (e.g., fold clothes, assist children with homework, pay bills if mentally alert).
- Patient should try to accomplish one major task every day, every other day, or every week.

Encourage patient to have some small activity to anticipate (e.g., visit from a friend, ride in the car, attending church, eat out at a restaurant, call a friend long distance, participate in a support group [patient can help others as well as herself], enjoy nature).

If larger-scale activities are possible, encourage them but caution patient to use moderation (e.g., take a trip to visit out-of-town family or friends), participate in a hobby or activity she has always wanted to do.

Data from references 36, 39, 63, 97.

BOX 15–4

Strategies for Managing Dyspnea

Breathing

Teach new breathing pattern:
  Take slow, deep breaths.
  Use diaphragm.
  Exhale through pursed lips.
  Exhale longer than inhale.

Positioning

Have patient assume comfortable position:
  Sit on bedside, fold arms over pillow on bedside table.
  Sit on chair, feet wide apart, elbows resting on knees.
  Lean on wall, feet apart, shoulders relaxed and bent forward.
  Elevate head of bed.

Emotional Support

Do not leave patient in distress alone:
  Observe patient frequently.
  Place frequent phone call to patient on home care.
  Teach coaching and support to family or caregiver.

Relaxation

Remember that relaxation conserves oxygen:
  Place hands on patient's shoulders and press downward.
  Dangle arms and rotate shoulders.

Planned Activity

Have patient conserve energy and get adequate rest:
  Assess normal life-style and activities of daily living.
  Plan chores around rest period.
  Establish support for household activities and recreation.

Oxygen Therapy

Provide oxygen supply and implement safety precautions.
Provide instructions regarding smoking, storage, heat, and use of equipment.

Pharmacologic Agents

Some agents relieve dyspnea, especially in patients who are terminally ill: sedatives, narcotics, steroids, scopolamine.

From Haylock P: *Semin Oncol Nurs,* 3:293, 1987; and Haylock P: Cancer metastasis: an update, *Semin Oncol Nurs* 14(3):172, 1998.

A grading scale for dyspnea may be helpful for the patient to describe the severity of current symptoms. If instructed to grade the dyspnea on a scale from 0 to 10, with 0 being no difficulty and 10 being unable to breathe, patients can more accurately relate the problem. Critical nursing assessment and identification of specific management techniques can prevent a crisis.[5, 36, 57, 94]

Exercise and Relaxation Techniques. Most patients who have been successfully treated for lung cancer or are presently undergoing treatment realize intellectually that they must begin exercising gradually, but many do not comply. Exercise is a positive reinforcement for patients in that it helps them feel well and increases their activity tolerance, but the nurse must caution the patient against too much exercise and activity too soon. An assessment should be made of anticipated activities and activity tolerance. The patient's overall state of health will dictate level of functioning and ability to maintain an exercise program. Relaxation techniques and guided imagery also are helpful during stressful treatment regimens and the anxiety-producing posttreatment period. Multiple self-help audiotapes, compact disk, and videotapes for meditation, relaxation, guided imagery are available at the local library, bookstores, and discount stores. The effective management of short-term and long-term side effects from lung cancer treatment is essential for patient rehabilitation. Overcoming as many treatment barriers as possible will motivate the patient and family toward achieving increased and sustained psychological and physical independence.[94, 97]

HOME HEALTH AND HOSPICE

Most patients with lung cancer will experience progressive disease with increasing symptoms and consequently increased dependency on others for self-care needs. Inherent in such a downhill trajectory is the need for frequent interventions or hospitalizations. Patients who are frequent emergency department visitors or who have frequent readmissions to the hospital due to exacerbations of chronic illnesses are often patients who could or should have received home health care at an earlier time. Elderly patients are more at risk for hospitalization and recurrent hospitalizations and home health care does reduce the number of hospital readmissions. The early discharge process limits the time during hospitalization for health professionals to instruct the patient in the self-care practices necessary to enhance their recovery in the home[39, 43, 44, 63] (see Chapter 29).

Nurses caring for lung cancer patients in the home setting today may be involved in their actual therapy through chemotherapy administration and management of side effects. The nurse's knowledge base must include use of present technology (e.g., management of various central venous catheters, patient-controlled analgesia [PCA] pumps, epidural catheters, oxygen and suction equipment). Nursing expertise to assist patients in understanding chronic pain management (e.g., use of scheduled versus PRN opioids, oral dosing in preference

to use of pumps when appropriate, prophylactic bowel regimens to prevent constipation) may obviate trips to the emergency department or hospitalizations. The patient and family may need assistance to understand the important role of low-dose morphine (2.5–5 mg every 4 hours) because it acts centrally in the brain to relieve severe dyspnea and "air hunger" associated with end-stage respiratory compromise. Compassionate nursing can assist families to know what to expect and how to deal with these events, particularly when death may be that event. Death from fatal hemoptysis, although sometimes feared, is rare; only 3.3% of patients in one large series died of exsanguination from tumor eroding through a major pulmonary vessel. Historically, 60% of lung cancer patients die from the tumor causing airway obstruction, postobstructive pneumonia, and sepsis. Caring and knowledgeable home health and hospice nurses can do much to reduce the suffering and anxiety associated with lung cancer.[36, 43, 44, 63, 94, 97]

PROGNOSIS

Prognostic Factors

Three factors play a major role in the prognosis of lung cancer: extent of disease, cell type, and patient's performance status. The survival rate for patients with localized disease is 37%; however, survival at 5 years is 13% for all patients regardless of stage at diagnosis. This represents a slight improvement in overall survival since the early 1970s. Prognosis is best for patients with well-differentiated squamous cell lung cancer, and those with SCLC have the poorest survival rate. Performance status is critical in determining the patient's treatment regimen and therefore the prognosis. Patients who are ambulatory tolerate treatment better than those who are not fully ambulatory but are out of bed 50% of the time. Prognosis continues to decline as the patient becomes more debilitated. Age, gender, weight loss, and immune status also affect the patient's response to treatment. Physiologic rather than chronological age is the important assessment factor when making treatment decisions, and age may influence treatment options and prognosis in elderly patients, as discussed earlier.[16, 17]

Adenocarcinoma is more predominant in women with lung cancer, whereas squamous cell cancer is more prevalent in men. Overall, women with lung cancer survive longer than their male counterparts in the United States.[44] In addition to the previous prognostic factors, weight loss of greater than 10 lb in 6 months is not a favorable sign. Patients with an intact immune system, as evidenced by a normal reaction to an immunologic challenge, will respond better. Patients with SCLC have an immune deficit that may contribute to the rapid growth of this cancer. Because any lung cancer patient will be exposed to multimodality treatment, it is important to be able to predict tolerance to such intense therapy.

Correlation with Histologic Cell Type and Stage

Non–Small-Cell Lung Cancer. The AJCC classification system and new international staging system are used to determine the best therapy modalities for NSCLC. Successful treatment with surgery or radiation therapy is possible in most patients with stage I disease; however, only 25% to 30% of patients present with stage I or II NSCLC. Adjuvant chemotherapy is currently being investigated for use in patients with early stage disease. For patients who present with widespread advanced disease, the administration of new combinations of chemotherapy has shown only a slight survival benefit.

Even with new treatment combinations, benefits and cure rates are modest. Five-year survival rates after resection for early stage NSCLC are reasonably good and have continued to improve as the result of stricter patient selection and progressive nursing support. These patients with later stage disease (stage IIIa) have a better prognosis if mediastinal lymph nodes are not involved.

Patients with squamous cell cancer survive longer than those with adenocarcinoma and large-cell undifferentiated carcinoma. Also, patients with stage I squamous cell cancer do significantly better than those with stage II or III tumors.

Depending on the TNM status and cell type of stage IIIA patients, survival ranges from 18% to 40%. The outlook for stage IIIB and IV patients remains bleak, but therapeutic strategies, including biologic response modifiers and monoclonal antibodies, are continually being pursued. More successful treatments for NSCLC are being discovered, although slowly.

Small-Cell Lung Cancer. Given the great biologic and clinical difference from other lung cancer types, SCLC is also staged differently. Patients with limited-stage disease who are treated with combination chemotherapy experience a 12- to 16-month median survival time and a 15% to 35% 2-year disease-free survival rate. Recent combined radiation-chemotherapy approaches show 24% to 54% survival at 2 years in LD. Unfortunately, patients with SCLC may still relapse 5 years after treatment. Without treatment, SCLC results in death in about 3 months. The best approach for long-term survival in limited-stage SCLC appears to be combination chemotherapy and radiation therapy to the chest. Researchers advocate alternating chemotherapy treatment cycles to prevent resistance to the drugs. However, clinical trials have failed to demonstrate improved survival by this technique, perhaps because of the inability to define truly non–cross-resistant regimens.[50]

In stages I and II LD, patients without mediastinal node involvement who underwent surgical resection and received combination chemotherapy after surgery had a 5-year survival rate of 35%. These patients represent less than 5% of SCLC patients. For patients with stage III disease, preoperative chemotherapy followed by surgery was attempted without dramatic results. Many randomized prospective studies have incorporated all the treatment modalities both alone and in combination. Although investigations continue to search for the best combination, preliminary data suggest benefit from combined therapy in limited SCLC if full doses of chemotherapy and radiation therapy are given.

The majority of patients (70%) with SCLC have ED, and the outlook for their survival is dismal. From 7% to 20% of these patients will be alive 2 years after diagnosis. Radiation plays a major role in local control and in symptom management to limit or modify cranial and bone metastasis and SVCS. Many patients with ED respond to therapy involving a combination of drugs and achieve notable palliation.

In a review of SWOG trials, one versus multiple metastatic sites was a predictor of survival. For patients with a single site, median survival was 12 months versus only 7 months for those with multiple metastatic sites. Other factors predictive of survival are a normal LDH and absence of a pleural effusion.

Patients with ED who experience a CR will usually survive beyond the median time frame. Although initial responses can be dramatic for both limited and extensive SCLC, long-term survival is worse than that seen with NSCLC. SCLC overall survival rate at 2 years is less than 10%. More knowledge about this disease and new agents or treatment combinations are needed to obtain better outcomes.

CONCLUSION

Lung cancer remains the most common cause of cancer death for both women (25%) and men (32%). Significant numbers of these patients have metastatic disease at the time of diagnosis; therefore, the overall 5-year survival rate is approximately 12%. Tobacco use remains the key factor in reducing lung cancer disease and death. Because of the many complications (e.g., brain, bone, liver, and pleural effusions), elderly population related issues, and physical/psychosocial needs, nursing care for all patients with lung cancer can be very challenging. Compassionate and knowledgeable nursing care is of great importance to the patient with lung cancer and the family.

Nursing Management

Nursing diagnoses related to lung cancer listed below are followed by nursing interventions for various treatments and rehabilitation.

Nursing Diagnoses: *Primary*

- *Knowledge deficit related to prevention of lung cancer* (see Patient Teaching Priorities box for suggested educational guidelines)
- *Breathing pattern, ineffective, related to loss of adequate ventilation (actual or potential)*
- *Gas exchange, impaired, related to decreased passage of gases between alveoli of lungs and vascular system (actual or potential)*
- *Knowledge deficit related to a new medical condition, new treatments, surgical procedures (preoperative and postoperative), medications*
- *Nutrition, altered: less than body requirements, related to anorexia*
- *Pain related to liver and/or bone metastasis (actual or potential)*
- *Thought processes, altered, related to brain metastasis (actual or potential)*
- *Fatigue related to treatment and treatment sequelae*

Nursing Diagnoses: *Secondary*

- *Anxiety related to dyspnea*
- *Powerlessness related to hospitalization and feelings of lack of control*
- *Noncompliance (potential) related to negative side effects of prescribed treatments*
- *Grieving, dysfunctional, related to loss of function of body system*
- *Body image disturbance related to loss of body functions*
- *Sexual dysfunction related to change of body part, physiologic limitations*
- *Coping, ineffective individual, related to rapidly progressive disease process*
- *Coping, ineffective family: compromised, related to rapidly progressive disease process*

Outcome Goals: *Surgery*

Patient will be able to:

- State which surgical diagnostic and operative procedures will be done (e.g., mediastinoscopy, lobectomy) and why.
- Communicate surgical discomfort and request adequate medication for relief.
- Understand the different modalities for medication administration (e.g., IV, epidural).
- Consume appropriate foods and liquids to maintain nutritional status.
- Relate importance of pulmonary hygiene and comply with necessary maintenance (cough and deep breathe [C&DB], exercise).
- Understand importance of smoking cessation before surgery and attempt to quit.
- Understand that mechanical ventilation and chest tubes may be necessary and why.
- Express concerns related to body image, life-style changes, and sexuality issues.

SURGERY

Surgical nursing care begins during the diagnostic period for those patients requiring *mediastinoscopy* (small suprasternal incision) or *mediastinotomy* (small parasternal incision that allows direct visualization of lymph nodes or through which left mediastinal lymph nodes or even a primary lung tumor may be biopsied) for tissue diagnosis or staging purposes. Monitoring blood pressure, pulse, and respirations and observing dressings for indication of internal or external bleeding are necessary in the immediate postoperative period. Fever can indicate mediastinitis; crepitus can indicate air leakage into subcutaneous tissues; and the development of dyspnea, cyanosis, or decreased breath sounds can be signs of pneumothorax. Postoperative local pain requires analgesics (see Complications box).

In patients who undergo thoracotomy for wedge resection, lobectomy, or pneumonectomy, nursing care is more complex. Standard nursing concerns with these patients are the same as for other cancer surgeries (e.g., adequate nutritional state, coping mechanisms, risk of postoperative emboli)[57, 58, 100] (see Chapter 21).

Malnutrition, hypoalbuminemia, smoking history, and chronic obstructive pulmonary disease (COPD) place patients with lung cancer at higher risk of postoperative complications such as pneumonia, fistula formation, and respiratory or congestive heart failure. Preoperative or postoperative total parenteral nutrition (TPN) may be necessary to improve nutritional status and promote recovery from thoracotomy. If surgery is delayed, smokers should be advised to stop smoking at least a few weeks before surgery. Although preoperative pulmonary function studies should predict patients' ability to undergo surgery, they need to know before thoracotomy that they may be placed on a ventilator and will have one or more chest tubes after the procedure.[4, 57, 58, 61, 68, 93, 100]

The most common postoperative complication is *cardiac dysrhythmia.* Often asymptomatic, it is responsive to appropriate drugs. The nature of drainage from chest tubes placed after partial pulmonary resection can reveal bleeding complications or development of empyema. In patients who become agitated, confused, and then dyspneic and hypoxic, serious alterations in ventilation and respiration are likely, and monitoring vital signs, breath sounds, and blood gases is important. Diligent aspiration of the tracheobronchial tree with frequent deep breathing and coughing can prevent mechanical obstruction and pneumonia resulting from the accumulation of secretions. However, deep suctioning that could cause trauma to the suture line must be avoided.[4, 29, 57, 94, 100]

The need for good pulmonary toilet cannot be overemphasized. Patients may experience much fear and discomfort associated with chest tubes or a ventilator, for which medication may be required. Good pain management, a major nursing concern after thoracotomy, can enhance mobility, coughing, and deep breathing. An epidural catheter to control pain may be placed during surgery; this enables the patient to recover more comfortably. Some patients may need narcotic analgesics for several months after the procedure to ease persistent pain. For prolonged postoperative pain, nerve blocks or other interventions should be considered. Depending on the amount of healthy lung tissue remaining after surgery, most patients will not experience severe respiratory compromise affecting life-style activities. See Patient Teaching Priorities box.[4, 29, 57, 61, 74, 100]

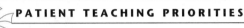

PATIENT TEACHING PRIORITIES

Surgery for Lung Cancer

Preoperative

Have patient relate knowledge of reason for surgery preoperatively.

Describe the type of procedure to be done (e.g., wedge resection, lobectomy, pneumonectomy).

Discuss need for optimal ventilation (stop smoking, cough, take deep breaths immediately after surgery).

Explain need for leg and arm exercises. Shoulder on affected side will be very sore and must be moved to prevent frozen shoulder.

Discuss different methods of pain relief (IM, IV, epidural) with patient. Encourage patient to ask for medication when needed. This promotes coughing and deep breathing.

Explain postoperative routine and that patient will most likely have a chest tube in place.

Postoperative

Reinforce need for early ambulation despite chest tube and also need to cough and deep breathe.

Reinforce all postoperative routines previously taught.

Review surgical results with patient and ensure proper follow-up.

Explore with patient the implications of altered body image:

Changes in life-style

Verbalization of fear of rejection and reaction of others

Changes in relationships

Problems with sexuality

Data from references 48, 57, 64, 93, 100, 107.

RADIATION THERAPY

Outcome Goals

Patient will be able to:

- State which acute, site-specific side effects will occur after chest or brain radiation therapy (e.g., possible nausea/vomiting, radiation pneumonitis, fatigue, skin reaction, myelosuppression, difficulty swallowing, headache, hair loss) and how to treat them.[30, 41]
- State which long-term side effects may occur after radiation therapy (e.g., pulmonary fibrosis, sexuality concerns, and radiation recall with chemotherapy, memory loss, confusion, and weakness).
- Consume appropriate foods and liquids to maintain nutritional status.
- State procedure for radiation therapy treatment (e.g., simulation, blocks, and treatment time).
- Communicate discomfort with swallowing and request adequate medication for relief.

Radiation to the Chest

Side effects experienced during or after radiation therapy will vary depending on (1) the organ systems or normal tissue within the radiation port (field), (2) the amount and duration of radiation, and (3) the type of concurrent or recent chemotherapy. When radiation is given to the primary tumor in the chest, portions of normal lung tissue, heart, skin, and contents of the mediastinum (major vessels, trachea, esophagus) may also receive radiation, although the dose will be much lower. By noting the tattoos or marks delineating the radiation port on the patient's chest, the nurse can make some predictions about the effects of radiation on normal tissues. Although efforts are made to block vital organs, some side effects are unavoidable. Nursing interventions focus on avoidance, relief, or management of side effects (see Patient Teaching Priorities box).[41, 48, 53, 74, 94]

Skin alterations related to radiation are much less severe than in the past. Equipment has been improved so it can deliver the radiation beneath the surface of the skin and more directly to the desired depth and location. Nursing assessment of skin integrity, the patient's complaints, and knowledge of anticipated side effects form the basis of interventions. Skin damage may be only mild erythema or can progress to dry and then moist desquamation. If moist desquamation occurs, radiation treatments will likely be interrupted. Therefore teaching should highlight preventive care: avoid constrictive clothing over irradiated areas; avoid tape, perfume, deodorants, iodine, talcum, or other irritating substances on irradiated skin; wear soft cotton clothing over skin; and avoid heat, cold, or sunlight on these areas. The skin should be kept dry and open to the air when possible. For tender or dry skin, use

---

PATIENT TEACHING PRIORITIES

Radiation Therapy for Lung Cancer

General Side Effects of Radiation Therapy

Explain measures to limit, as necessary, patient's activities during treatment to conserve energy.

Discuss measures to maintain adequate nutritional intake.

Explain measures to control radiodermatitis if necessary.

Describe rationale and measures to take following a decrease in hematopoietic function.

Discuss reasons for and measures to deal with sexuality concerns.

Site-Specific Side Effects

Describe signs and symptoms of pneumonitis, esophagitis, and cough.

Discuss measures to maintain adequate oxygenation.

Instruct patient to drink 2 to 3 liters of fluid a day, unless contraindicated.

Administer antiemetics for nausea/vomiting.

Caution patient to avoid tobacco and alcohol.

Note availability of patient information booklets.

Emotional Support

Educate patient/family regarding radiation therapy procedures to decrease anxiety.

Explain that side effects may last for 2 to 4 weeks after treatment completion.

Ensure understanding of anxiety or grief process because of illness and reassure patient that this is normal response.

Data from references 41, 48, 53, 57, 64, 86.

---

water-based ointments (e.g., A&D Ointment, hydrous lanolin) rather than oil-based creams or ointments, which may contain heavy metals. Vigorous scrubbing or rubbing is to be avoided, but use of gentle soaps (e.g., Aveeno, Dove) is usually allowed. If moist desquamation occurs, the area may be cleansed with quarter-strength hydrogen peroxide and normal saline, rinsed gently with saline and patted dry. Areas of skin breakdown should be monitored for infection. Moisture vapor-permeable dressings (Op-site, Tegaderm) may offer protection to these areas. Most patients have skin reactions by their last week of therapy. Administration of certain chemotherapeutic drugs (e.g., dactinomycin, doxorubicin) during therapy or close to the initiation of radiation therapy can lead to radiation recall, and erythema or skin breakdown may occur.[41, 48, 53, 64, 74, 94]

Sore throat resulting from esophagitis can develop by the third week of radiation therapy. If the pain is severe, food and fluid intake may be decreased because of difficulty swallowing. Patients should be advised that, if this occurs, they should contact the nurse or physician. A nasogastric feeding tube or a percutaneous endoscopic gastrostomy (PEG) may be placed to assist the patient with nutrition intake. Not only can nutrition be impaired, but esophagitis may also become a source for infection. If signs of candidiasis (white, adherent plaques) are present in the oral cavity, an antifungal agent should be prescribed (Mycelex troches, nystatin, ketoconazole). A soft, bland diet (noncitrus) and nutritional supplements (e.g., Ensure, Instant Breakfast) can be beneficial. If weight loss resulting from esophagitis occurs, the patient should be weighed daily and evaluated for dehydration. A mixture of diphenhydramine elixir, viscous lidocaine, and Mylanta or Amphojel (depending on the consistency of the patient's stools) in a 1:1:1 ratio can be administered as a swish-and-swallow remedy when esophagitis is painful (5 mL before meals and as needed). Systemic analgesics may be required.[53, 64, 94]

Nutritional status can be further compromised by *anorexia*, which occurs in most patients by the fourth week of treatment. Anorectic patients should be encouraged to eat small amounts frequently. The book *Eating Hints* by the NCI may aid patients and their families in discovering types of food more tolerable to these patients. The addition of small amounts of powdered milk to appropriate foods will also increase protein intake. Good nutrition is essential to repair and heal normal tissues during radiation therapy.[64, 85, 86, 107]

Fatigue is a major problem in more than 90% of patients by the third week of treatment. Patients should be so warned and guided into planning any activities with scheduled rest periods. Symptoms may persist for months after completion of radiation therapy.

If more than 25% of active bone marrow is in the radiation port, *myelosuppression* may occur. Complete blood counts should be done weekly during therapy. Neutropenia and thrombocytopenia precede a drop in hemoglobin. Packed red blood cells may be transfused if the hemoglobin drops below 10 g because effective radiation treatment depends on an adequate oxygen supply to the tumor. If the white blood cell count drops below 3000/mm³ or the platelets drop below 40,000/mm³, radiation therapy may be temporarily discontinued.[24, 30, 41, 81, 82]

Radiation pneumonitis occurs infrequently but is dose limiting if it develops during radiation treatments. Because it is dose dependent, it can occur 3 to 24 weeks after therapy. In acute radiation pneumonitis, a hacking cough or mild chest pain might be the first symptom. Signs and symptoms also include dyspnea and hypoxia, fever, and night sweats; evidence of interstitial or alveolar infiltrates is seen on chest x-ray films; and the sputum is negative for pathogens. The severity of symptoms correlates with the dose and lung volume irradiated. In severe cases, pneumonitis may be associated with hemoptysis, fever, chills, or abscess and may even result in death. Usually, doses of 45 Gy or less will not lead to severe toxicity, and pneumonitis will resolve, often within 3 to 4 weeks. Patients may require temporary hospitalization for administration of oxygen, steroids, antibiotics, sedatives, and cough suppressants. Cultures are obtained to rule out infection, but antibiotics may be given empirically. Steroids are the cornerstones of therapy for radiation pneumonitis. At the start of therapy, patients should be given at least 60 mg prednisone per day. Tapering is carried out very gradually, and the patient must be monitored for any recurrence of symptoms.[5, 24, 41, 53]

Coping strategies for *dyspnea* are often self-taught but may include position changes, moving slowly, and planning in advance for activities. If pneumonitis leads to subsequent scarring and tissue changes (pulmonary fibrosis), chest auscultation will reveal muffled and diminished vesicular sounds, rhonchi, and wheezes from air flow across narrowed airways. Late fibrotic changes resemble severe COPD and can lead to anxiety and fear with dyspnea.[41, 65]

Cardiac toxicities, although minimal today because of blocking techniques, can include pericarditis, the classic symptom for which is chest pain, or a pericardial effusion and tamponade, which involve increased central venous pressure, evidenced by jugular venous distention followed by tachycardia, dyspnea, and cough (see Chapter 20). Cardiac toxicities usually depend on delivery of at least 40 Gy to the heart.[24, 41, 94]

Radiation to the Brain

Radiation to the brain can lead to hair loss, but the severity of hair loss is usually dose dependent. At doses of 15 to 30 Gy, the degree of hair loss is variable. At a dose of 50 Gy or more, permanent loss is likely. Because PCI in SCLC is usually no more than 30 Gy, hair will begin to regrow about 3 to 4 weeks after the completion of radiation therapy. However, hair loss after PCI will be temporarily complete, including the eyebrows.[24, 41, 53] (See Chapter 31 for resources and ways to deal with hair loss.)

During brain irradiation, patients receive dexamethasone to reduce the resultant edema of brain tissue. However, symptoms of neurologic impairment related to edema should be monitored and may include irritability, confusion, restlessness, headaches, memory loss, a change in personality or mental status, nausea, unequal or decreased pupil reactivity to light, elevated blood pressure, sensory or motor changes, or a drop in pulse rate. Cerebral edema can lead to obstruction of the eustachian tube with resultant local ear pain or infection.[24, 41, 53, 94]

Late effects of WBI in long-term survivors may be even more severe when it is given concurrently with chemotherapy. Findings reflecting neurologic injury can include memory loss, problems in judgment, parkinsonian symptoms, weakness, confusion, depression, dizziness, organic brain syndrome, abnormal gait, ataxia, intention tremors, inability to concentrate, and cerebral atrophy. Symptoms have become so severe that one patient had to quit work and another was placed in an extended care facility. Any sequelae such as these should be documented, and the physician should be notified for possible CT or MRI evaluation. Any such changes could also herald a CNS relapse.[24, 25, 41, 46, 53, 57] The Complications box lists potential radiation treatment-related complications of lung cancer.

Radiation Implant

Implants may be used to treat large and otherwise inaccessible tumor masses in the lung. Nursing care of these patients follows guidelines discussed in the Complications box (Lung Cancer: Surgical Treatment). Patient teaching related to radiation therapy should include the information given in the Complications box (Radiation Treatment).

Combined Radiation and Chemotherapy

Normal radiation therapy toxicities on organ systems are increased to varying degrees by concomitant or consecutive (within weeks of) administration of cer-

Radiation Treatment for Lung Cancer*

Irradiation to Chest

Skin erythema to wet desquamation

Esophagitis, dysphagia, strictures, weight loss

Acute pneumonitis or pulmonary fibrosis (dyspnea, hypoxemia, chronic or temporary oxygen and steroid dependency)

Pericarditis, dysrhythmias, pericardial effusion, congestive heart failure

Myelosuppression (sepsis, bleeding, fatigue)

Fatigue

Irradiation to Brain

Early and usually temporary effects: hair loss, skin erythema, and nausea

Signs of cerebral edema that need immediate attention during radiation: irritability, confusion, restlessness, headaches, nausea, changes in personality, sensory or motor changes

Late and permanent effects: memory loss, problems in judgment, parkinsonian symptoms, weakness, confusion, depression, dizziness, organic brain syndrome, abnormal gait, intention tremor, inability to concentrate, loss of self-care or work capability, cerebral atrophy[30, 48, 53, 57]

* Concurrent chemotherapy and radiation can augment all these effects.

Data from references 24, 41, 48, 53, 57, 64, 86.

Chemotherapy Drugs with Related Organ Toxicity

Bleomycin: *lung, *skin, mucosa

Carboplatin: kidney, bone marrow

Cisplatin: kidney, bone marrow, neurologic, hearing loss

Docetaxel: bone marrow, *lung, neurologic

Doxorubicin: *lung, *heart, *skin, mucosa, esophagus

Etoposide (VP-16): bone marrow, *heart, neurologic

5-Fluorouracil: lung, heart, skin, mucosa

Gemcitabine: bone marrow, *lung, liver and renal compromise

Hydroxyurea: lung, skin, mucosa, esophagus

Ifosfamide: kidney, neurologic

Irinotecan: bone marrow, *lung

Methotrexate: bone marrow, *lung, kidney, skin, mucosa

Mitomycin C: lung, heart, kidney

Paclitaxel: bone marrow, *lung, neurologic

Procarbazine: gastrointestinal tract

Topotecan: bone marrow, *lung, neurologic

Vinblastine: neurologic

Vincristine: lung, neurologic

Vinorelbine: neurologic, kidney

* Drugs/organ systems with potential for increased toxicity if chemotherapy given in combination with radiation.

Data from references 5, 9, 19, 76.

---

tain chemotherapy drugs. The severity of the toxicity depends on the drug and its dose, the radiation dose, and the timing of each in relation to the other. Damage to the target organ may be short term, permanent and life changing, or fatal. Because radiation therapy ports for lung cancer patients can involve the heart, lungs, brain, and other contents of the mediastinum, the potential severity of any synergistic drug-radiation toxicity is great. Specifically, esophagitis can lead to a stricture, CNS damage can include leukoencephalopathy or necrosis, or fatal interstitial fibrosis of large lulng volumes can occur. Nursing knowledge of chemotherapy agents can help predict toxicities resulting from their concomitant administration during radiation therapy. Combination chemotherapy regimens involving any of the drugs listed in the accompanying box may enhance and broaden the spectrum of usual organ system toxicities. Neither intrathecal therapy nor systemic chemotherapy with these agents should be given during radiation therapy to the associated target organ unless part of a specific protocol or investigational study, in which the rationale for combined radiation and chemotherapy is clearly stated and the patient understands the risks before therapy is begun.*

CHEMOTHERAPY

Patients with lung cancer, especially small-cell carcinoma, may receive several chemotherapy drugs having multiple potential toxicities and, in some cases, synergistic toxicities because two or more treatment modalities are being used sequentially or simultaneously (see Complications: Chemotherapy box). These toxicities include myelosuppression, nausea and vomiting, renal damage, cardiac insult, pneumonitis/ fibrosis, hemorrhagic cystitis, neurotoxicities, stomatitis, extravasation, and phlebitis.[76]

---

* References 5, 30, 41, 49, 54, 53, 76, 83.

Nursing assessment and management of these toxicities can help to greatly improve the patient's quality of life and are discussed in depth in Chapter 23.

COMPLICATIONS

Chemotherapy for Lung Cancer

Myelosuppression (sepsis, bleeding, weakness, fatigue)
Nephrotoxicity (compromised renal function, magnesium wasting)
Hemorrhagic cystitis
Neurotoxicity
  Peripheral neuropathies (paresthesias, jaw pain, sensory loss, motor weakness, constipation or ileus, tinnitus, permanent hearing loss)
  CNS toxicity (confusion, hallucinations, somnolence, coma)
Cardiac (myopathy, dysrhythmia, congestive heart failure, myocardial infarction)
Pneumonitis or pulmonary fibrosis
Nausea and vomiting (dehydration, weight loss)
Taste changes (anorexia, weight loss)
Mucositis (pain, difficulty swallowing, weight loss, diarrhea)
Anaphylaxis (death) or hypotension
Alopecia
Tissue damage and pain if vesicant extravasation
Syndrome of inappropriate secretion of antidiuretic hormone (SIADH) and hyponatremia

Data from references 5, 25, 46, 76.

Tables 15–4 and 15–5 list some of the newer or investigational regimens used in small-cell and non–small-cell lung cancer. Some of these have been associated with significant toxicity. Tables 15–6 and 15–7 list doses and schedules of common chemotherapeutic regimens. These tables are not intended to be a comprehensive summary of all available regimens, but merely a sample of current therapies.

See the Patient Teaching Priorities box.

Outcome Goals: Chemotherapy

Patient will be able to:

- Verbalize importance of monitoring bleeding, infection, and fatigue when myelosuppressed and reporting to physician.
- Monitor intake and output.
- Monitor and report side effects (e.g., peripheral neuropathies, sensorimotor weakness, constipa-tion, confusion, uncontrolled dry cough, mucositis).
- Understand and comply with prevention and intervention of side effects.
- Communicate concerns related to body image, alopecia, and sexuality.
- Describe and use appropriate stress reduction techniques (e.g., relaxation therapy, guided imagery).

PATIENT TEACHING PRIORITIES

Chemotherapy

Chemotherapeutic Agents

Review patient knowledge of chemotherapy and explain the therapeutic effects.
Provide patient/family with written information regarding all chemotherapeutic agents used.
Explain immediate and late (7–14 days) side effects of specific drug regimen.
Describe potential treatment schedule with usual drug administration routes

General Side Effects

Provide information for patient/family on self-management of stomatitis, nausea/vomiting, diarrhea and constipation, alopecia, myelosuppression, fatigue, and sexuality concerns.
Discuss which side effects must be reported to the physician/nurse immediately.

Specific Side Effects

Discuss specific side effects with patient/family according to prescribed drug regimen.
Explain which side effects are reversible.
Explain which medications/foods are to be avoided, if any.
Review how patient makes contact with appropriate health care team member should side effects occur that cannot be managed at home.
Review community resources available to patient.

Emotional Support

Encourage patient/family to verbalize needs and questions concerning chemotherapy and its side effects.
Encourage patient to maintain activities and relationships to promote self-worth.
Encourage patient to verbalize feelings, frustrations, anger, and thoughts regarding changed life-style.
Teach patient/family problem-solving techniques.
Discuss methods of handling and addressing stress and coping with family/friends.

Data from references 5 and 76.

Chapter Questions

1. In 2000, approximately how many Americans were diagnosed with lung cancer?
   a. 300,000
   b. 200,000
   c. 175,000
   d. 157,000

2. Prognostic factors most often associated with survival outcome for patients with lung cancer include:
   a. Extensive versus limited disease, weight loss, performance status, histology cell type
   b. Extensive versus limited disease, tumor marker, performance status, and histology cell type
   c. Extensive versus limited disease, weight loss, treatment regimens, histology cell type
   d. Extensive versus limited disease, tumor marker, treatment regimens, and histology cell type

3. Current single chemotherapy agents showing promise in the treatment of NSCLC are:
   a. Docetaxel, paclitaxel, gemcitabine, doxorubicin, and vinorelbine
   b. Docetaxel, paclitaxel, 5-fluorouracil, irinotecan, and vinorelbine
   c. Docetaxel, paclitaxel, gemcitabine, irinotecan, and vinorelbine
   d. Docetaxel, paclitaxel, gemcitabine, methotrexate, and vinblastine

4. Approximately 80% of all new lung cancer cases are NSCLC. What percent of this patient population has regional to advanced disease at time of diagnosis?
   a. 80%
   b. 70%
   c. 50%
   d. 35%

5. Patient teaching priorities for prevention and detection of lung cancer include:
   a. Avoid tobacco use, know environmental carcinogens that increase risk, and personal and family history
   b. Limit tobacco use, know environmental carcinogens that increase risk, and personal and family history
   c. Limit tobacco use, know work-related carcinogens that increase risk, and personal and family history
   d. Avoid tobacco use, know work-related carcinogens that increase risk, and personal and family history

6. Common diagnostic methods used in a lung cancer diagnostic work-up include:
   a. Bone, CT, and brain scans; bronchoscope; 3 sputum cytology specimens
   b. Bone, CT, and liver scans; bronchoscope; 3 sputum cytology specimens
   c. Bone, CT, and brain scans; bronchoscope; laboratory studies
   d. Bone, CT, and liver scans; bronchoscope; laboratory studies

7. The most common anatomic site for lung cancer metastasis is:
   a. Bone
   b. Brain
   c. Heart
   d. Liver

8. Bone metastasis related to lung cancer is most often treated with:
   a. Analgesia, biphosphates, radiation therapy, and surgery
   b. Analgesia, biotherapy, chemotherapy, and radiation therapy
   c. Analgesia, biphosphates, biotherapy, and radiation therapy
   d. Analgesia, biphosphates, hormonal therapy and radiation therapy

9. Pleural effusion management usually involves chest tube insertion with connection to underwater-seal drainage system. Which of the following is applicable to prudent care of the chest tube?
   a. All tubing connections should be tightly secured, taped, and clamps placed nearby.
   b. Clamps are always used on the chest tube when transporting and/or assisting with patient ambulation.
   c. Unless fluid is within the tube, raising the drainage system above the chest causes no problem.
   d. Stripping and milking the chest tube have minimal patient complications

10. Rehabilitation modifications that can facilitate quality of life for patients with lung cancer include:
    a. Cardiac program, activity maintenance, and exercise/relaxation techniques
    b. Cardiac program, activity maintenance, complementary/alternative therapies
    c. Pulmonary program, activity maintenance, complementary/alternative therapies
    d. Pulmonary program, activity maintenance, and exercise/relaxation techniques

11. Nursing interventions for patients with lung cancer surgery are essential to prevent the most common postoperative complication of:
    a. Pneumonia
    b. Cardiac dysrhythmia

c. Congestive heart failure

d. Fistula formation

12. Education regarding the side effects related to radiation therapy should include the following:

    a. Skin reactions are usually severe and take months to heal.

    b. Radiation pneumonitits occurs and requires frequent hospitalization.

    c. Fatigue rarely occurs, and the patient is encouraged to do as much as possible each day.

    d. Pain related to esophagitis can interfere with swallowing food and fluids.

BIBLIOGRAPHY

1. Beahrs OH and others, editors: *Manual for staging of cancer,* ed 5, Philadelphia, Lippincott-Raven, 1997.

2. Bernhard J, Ganz P: Psychosocial issues in lung cancer patients. Part I, *Chest* 90:216, 1991.

3. Bernhard J, Ganz P: Psychosocial issues in lung cancer patients. Part II, *Chest* 90:480, 1991.

4. Brenner ZR: Preventing postoperative complications: what's old, what's new, what's tried and true, *Nursing* 29(10):39, 1999.

5. Camp-Sorrell D: Surviving the cancer, surviving the treatment: acute cardiac and pulmonary toxicity, *Oncol Nurs Forum* 26:983, 1999.

6. Camp-Sorrell D, Hawkins R: Clinical decisions for assessing and managing bone metastasis, *Oncology, 2000,* East Hanover, NJ, Novartis.

7. Cella D: Measuring quality of life in palliative care, *Semin Oncol* 22(2, suppl 13):73, 1995.

8. Chamberlein MC, Korman KP: Carcinoma meningitis secondary to non-small-cell lung cancer: combined modality therapy, *Arch Neurol* 55:506, 1998.

9. Choy H, Akerley W, Devore R: Paclitaxel, carboplatin and radiation therapy for non–small-cell lung cancer, *Oncology Huntingt* 12(1 suppl 2):80, 1998.

10. Choy H and others: Multi-institutional phase II trial of paclitaxel, carboplatin, and concurrent radiation therapy for locally advanced non–small-cell lung cancer, *J Clin Oncol* 16:3316, 1998.

11. Chouaid C and others: Routine use of granulocyte colony-stimulating factor is not cost-effective and does not increase comfort in the treatment of small-cell lung cancer: an analysis using a Markov model, *J Clin Oncol* 16:2700, 1998.

12. Chute JP and others: Twenty years of phase III trials for patients with extensive-stage small-cell lung cancer: perceptible progress, *J Clin Oncol* 17:1794, 1999.

13. Clark PI: Current role of oral etoposide in the management of small cell lung cancer, *Drugs* 58(suppl 3):17, 1999.

14. Coleman RE, Rubens RD: Bone metastasis. In Abeloff MD and others, editors: *Clinical oncology,* ed 2, New York, Churchill Livingstone, 1999.

15. Cotton V and others: Small-cell lung cancer: patients included in clinical trials are not representative of the patient population as a whole, *Ann Oncol* 10:809, 1999.

16. Dahlin CM: Care and compassion in conveying bad news, *Clin J Oncol Nurs* 3:73, 1999.

17. Damaron BI: Nurse-physician-patient communication: the vital triangle. Fairfield, CT, Medical Education Resources, Inc., Wyeth Genetics Institute, Logical Communications, 2000.

18. Damber L, Larsson S: Combined effects of mining and smoking in the causation of lung carcinoma, *Acta Radiol Oncol* 21:305, 1982.

19. DeVita VT Jr: Principles of cancer management: chemotherapy. In DeVita VT Jr, Hellman S, and Rosenberg SA, editors: *Cancer principles and practice of oncology,* ed 5, Philadelphia, Lippincott-Raven, 1997.

20. Elias A and others: Dose-intensive therapy for limited-stage small cell lung cancer: long-term outcome, *J Clin Oncol* 17:1175, 1999.

21. Eriksen M, Lemaistre C, Newell GR: Health hazards of passive smoking, *Annu Rev Public Health* 9:47, 1988.

22. Erickson R: Mastering the in's and out's of chest drainage. Part 1, *Nursing 89,* 19:36, 1989.

23. Erickson R: Mastering the in's and out's of chest drainage. Part 2, *Nursing 89,* 19:46, 1989.

24. Feld R and others: Lung. In Abeloff MD and others, editors: *Clinical oncology,* ed 2, New York, Churchill Livingstone, 1999.

25. Finley JP: Metabolic emergencies. In Itano JK, Taoka KN, editors. *Core curriculum for oncology nursing,* ed 3, Philadelphia, Saunders, 1998.

26. Fokkema E and others: Phase II study of oral platinum drug JM216 as first-line treatment in patients with small-cell lung cancer, *J Clin Oncol* 17:3822, 1999.

27. Friedberg JS: Clinical presentation of stage IIIA (N2) non–small cell lung: role of multimodality therapy, *Chest* 116(6 suppl):497S, 1999.

28. Gandara DR and others: Activity of docetaxel in platinum-treated non–small-cell lung cancer: results of a phase II multicenter trial, *J Clin Oncol* 18:131, 2000.

29. Ginsberg RJ, Vokes EE, Raben A: Non–small cell lung cancer. In DeVita VT Jr., Hellman S, Rosenberg SA, editors: *Cancer principles and practice of oncology,* ed 5, Philadelphia, Lippincott-Raven, 1997.

30. Gordon GS, Vokes EE: Chemoradiation for locally advanced unresectable, NSCLC. New standard of care, emerging strategies, *Oncology Huntingt* 13:1075, 1999.

31. Gordon PA, Noron JM, Merrell R: Refining chest tube management: analysis of the state of practice, *Dimen Crit Care Nurs* 14:6, 1995.

32. Gralla R and others: Single-agent therapy and in combination with cisplatin, *Ann Oncol* 10(suppl 5):S41, 1999.

33. Greco FA, Hainsworth JD: Paclitaxel-based therapy in non-small-cell lung cancer: improved third generation chemotherapy, *Ann Oncol* 10(suppl 5):S63, 1999.

34. Greenlee RT and others: Cancer Statistics 2000, *CA Cancer J Clin* 50:7, 2000.

35. Grunberg SM: Cyclophosphamide and etoposide for non-small cell and small cell lung cancer, *Drugs* 58(suppl 3):11, 1999.

36. Haas BK: Focus on health promotion: self-efficacy in oncology nursing research and practice, *Oncol Nurs Forum* 27:89, 2000.

37. Halme M and others: Tumor response and radiation-induced lung injury in patients with recurrent small cell lung cancer treated with radiotherapy and concomitant interferon-alpha, *Lung Cancer* 23:39, 1999.

38. Hammond E, Selikoff I, Seidman H: Asbestos exposure, cigarette smoking and death rates, *Ann NY Acad Sci* 330:473, 1979.

39. Harris KA: The informational needs of patients with cancer and their families, *Cancer Pract* 6(1):39, 1998.

40. Haylock PJ: Cancer metastasis: an update, *Semin Oncol Nurs* 14(3):172, 1998.

41. Hellman S: Principles of cancer management: radiation therapy. In DeVita VT Jr, Hellman S, Rosenberg SA, editors: *Cancer principles and practice of oncology,* ed 5, Philadelphia, Lippincott-Raven, 1997.

42. Henschke CI and others: Early lung action project: overall design and findings and from baseline screening, *Lancet* 354:99, 1999.

43. Highfield MEF: Providing spiritual care to patients with cancer, *Clin J Oncol Nurs* 4:115, 2000.

44. Hospice and Palliative Nurses Association: *Hospice and palliative nursing practice review,* ed 3, Arlington, VA, Kendal/Hunt Publishing Co. The Society, 1999.

45. Hughes J, Weill H: Asbestos exposure—quantitative assessment of risk, *Am Rev Respir Dis* 133:5, 1986.

46. Hunter JC: Structural emergencies. In Itano JK, Taoka KN, editors: *Core curriculum for oncology nursing,* ed 3, Philadelphia, Saunders, 1998.

47. Ihde DC, Glatstein E, Pass HI: Small cell lung cancer. In DeVita VT Jr, Hellman S, Rosenberg SA, editors: *Cancer principles and practice of oncology,* ed 5, Philadelphia, Lippincott-Raven, 1997.

48. Ingle RJ: Lung cancers. In Groenwald SL and others, editors: *Cancer nursing: principles and practice,* ed 4, Boston, Jones & Bartlett, 1997.

49. Johnson DH: Management of small cell lung cancer: current state of the art, *Chest* 116(6 suppl):525S, 1999.

50. Kirschling RJ and others: Paclitaxel and G-CSF in previously untreated patients with extensive stage small-cell-lung cancer: a phase II study of the North Central Cancer Treatment Group, *Am J Clin Oncol* 22:517, 1999.

51. Kirton CA: Assessing breath sounds, *Nursing* 25:50, 1995.

52. Knopp JM: Lung cancer. In Dow KH and others, editors: *Nursing care in radiation oncology,* ed 2, Philadelphia, Saunders, 1999.

53. Komaki R, Cox JD: Combinations of radiation therapy and chemotherapy for NSCLC. In Roth JA, Cox JD, Hong WK, editors: *Lung cancer,* Malden, MA, Blackwell Science, 1998.

54. Komaki R: Combined chemotherapy and radiation therapy in surgically unresectable regionally advanced non-small-cell lung cancer. *Semin Radiat Oncol* 6(2):86, 1996.

55. Khuri FR: Chemoprevention of cancer. *Highlights in Oncology Practice* 16(4):100, 1999.

56. Lazzara D: Why is the Heimlich chest device making a comeback? *Nursing* 26(12):50, 1996.

57. Lind J: Nursing care of the client with lung cancer. In Itano JK, Taoka KN, editors: *Core curriculum for oncology nursing,* ed 3, Philadelphia, Saunders, 1998.

58. LoCicero J: Role of thoroscopy in the diagnosis and treatment of lung cancer. In Roth JA, Cox JD, Hong WK: *Lung cancer,* Malden, MA, Blackwell Science, 1998.

59. Looney M: Death, dying, and grief in the face of cancer. In Burke CC, editor: *Psychosocial dimensions of oncology nursing care,* Pittsburgh, Oncology Nursing Press, 1998.

60. Macey RA, Landstrom LL: Replacing a chest-tube drainage-collection device, *AJN* 93(3):95, 1993.

61. Maghfoor I, Doll DC, Yarbro J: Effusions. In Abeloff MD and others, editors: *Clinical oncology,* ed 2, New York, Churchill Livingstone, 1999.

62. Masutani M and others: Dose-intensive weekly alternating chemotherapy for patients with small cell lung cancer: randomized trial, can it improve survival of patients with good prognostic factors? *Oncol Rep* 7:305, 2000.

63. Mayer D: Cancer patient empowerment, *Oncol Nurs Updates* 6(4):1, 1999.

64. Miller SE: Stomatitits and esophagitis. In Yasko JM, editor: *Nursing management of symptoms associated with chemotherapy,* Bala Cynwyd, PA, Pharmacia & Upjohn, Meniscus Health Care Communications, 1998.

65. Miaskowski C, Lee RK: Pain, fatigue, and sleep disturbances in oncology patients receiving radiation therapy for bone metastasis: a pilot study. *J Pain Symptom Manage* 17(5):320, 1999.

66. Minna JD and others: Molecular biology of lung cancer. In DeVita VT Jr, Hellman S, Rosenberg SA, editors: *Cancer principles and practice of oncology,* ed 5, Philadelphia, Lippincott-Raven, 1997.

67. Moran TA, Viele CS: *Liposomal technologies,* Mountain View, CA, Medical Education Resources, Alza Pharmaceuticals, 2000.

68. Morice RC: Preoperative evaluation of the patient with lung cancer. In Roth JA, Cox JD, Hong WK, editors: *Lung cancer,* Malden, MA, Blackwell Science, 1998.

69. Mountain CF, Libshitz HI, Hermes KE: *Lung cancer, a handbook for staging, image, and lymph node classification,* Houston, TX, Charles P. Young Company, 1999.

70. National Cancer Institute: *Cancer statistics review: 1973–87,* NIH Publication No. 90-2789, Bethesda, MD, US Department of Health and Human Services, 1990.

71. National Cancer Institute: *School programs to prevent smoking: the National Cancer Institute guide to strategies that succeed,* NIH Publication No. 90-5000, Bethesda, MD, US Department of Health and Human Services, 1994.

72. National Cancer Institute: *Self-guided strategies for smoking cessation: a program planner's guide,* NIH Publication No. 91-3104, Bethesda, MD, US Department of Health and Human Services, 1994.

73. North American Nursing Diagnosis Association: *Nursing diagnosis: definitions and classification,* Philadelphia, The Association, 1999.

74. Olson K, Tkachuk L, Hanson J: Preventing pressure sores in oncology patients, *Clin Nurs Res* 7:207, 1998.

75. Ormrod D, Spencer CM: Topotecan: a review of its efficacy in small cell lung cancer, *Drugs* 58:533, 1999.

76. Oncology Nursing Society: *Cancer chemotherapy guidelines and recommendations for practice,* Pittsburgh, Oncology Nursing Press, 1999.

77. Orton CG and others: Study of lung density corrections in a clinical trial (RTOG 88-08). Radiation Therapy Oncology Group. *Int J Radiat Oncol Biol Phys* 41:787, 1998.

78. Pass HL: Photodynamic therapy and thoracic malignancies. In Roth JA, Cox JD, Hong WK, editors: *Lung cancer,* Malden, MA, Blackwell Science, 1998.

79. Patchell RA: Brain metastasis and carcinomatous meningitis. In Abeloff MD and others, editors: *Clinical oncology,* ed 2, New York, Churchill Livingstone, 1999.

80. Postmus PE, Smit EF: Small-cell lung cancer: is there a standard therapy? *Oncology Huntingt* 12(1 suppl 2):25, 1998.

81. Rieger PT: *Clinical handbook of biotherapy,* Boston, Jones & Bartlett, 1999.

82. Rieger PT: Management of cancer in the next millennium: DNA holds the key, *Highlights Oncol Pract* 16(4):110, 1999.

83. Roberts JR: Trimodality therapy for non-small-cell lung cancer, *Oncology Huntingt* 13(100 suppl 6):101, 1999.

84. Ross DJ, Mohsenifar Z, Koerner SK: Survival characteristics after neodymium: YAG laser photoresection in advanced stage lung cancer, *Chest* 98:581, 1990.

85. Ruckdeschel JC: Future directions in non-small-cell lung cancer: a continuing perspective, *Oncology Huntingt* 12(1 suppl 2):90, 1998.

86. Sandler A, Ettinger DS: Gemcitabine: single-agent and combination therapy in non-small-cell lung cancer, *Oncologist* 4(3):241, 1999.

87. Sandler A, van-Oosterom AT: Irinotecan in cancers of the lung and cervix, *Anticancer Drugs* 10(suppl 1):S13, 1999.

88. Samet J, Nero A: Indoor radon and lung cancer, *N Engl J Med* 320:591, 1989.

89. Satoh H and others: Management of small lung cancer in elderly, *Anticancer Res* 19(5C):4507, 1999.

90. Satoh H and others: Smoking and smoking-related lung cancer in female patients, *Anticancer Res* 19(6C):5627, 1999.

91. Sause W and others: Final results of phase III trial in regionally advanced unresectable non-small-cell lung cancer: Radiation Therapy Oncology. Eastern Cooperative Group. Southwest Oncology Group, *Chest* 117(2):358, 2000.

92. Seffrin JR: An endgame for cancer, *CA Cancer J Clin* 50:7, 2000.

93. Shields TW, Karrer K: Surgery for small-cell lung cancer. In Roth JA, Cox JD, Hong WK, editors: *Lung cancer,* Malden, MA, Blackwell Science, 1998.

94. Shell J, Bulson KR, Vanderlugt LF: Lung cancers. In Otto SE, editor: *Oncology nursing,* ed 3, St. Louis, Mosby, 1997.

95. Sivesind DM, Rohaly-Davis JA: Coping with cancer: patient issues. In Burke CC, editor: *Psychosocial dimensions of oncology nursing care,* Pittsburgh, Oncology Nursing Press, 1998.

96. Smith RA and others: American Cancer Society Guidelines for early detection of cancer, *CA Cancer J Clin* 50:7, 2000.

97. Snyder M, Chlan L: Music therapy. *Annu Rev Nurs Res* 17:23, 1999.

98. Socci M: Palliative nursing in advanced cancer care, *Nurs Intervent Oncol* 12:19, 2000.

99. Steagall A: *New advances in the treatment of advanced non-small lung cancer.* Bala Cynwyd, PA, New Horizons in Solid Tumor Chemotherapy, Meniscus Educational Institute, 2000.

100. Szopa TJ: Nursing implications of surgical treatment. In Itano JK, Taoka KN, editors: *Core curriculum for oncology nursing,* ed 3, Philadelphia, Saunders, 1998.

101. Taubert J, Wright S: Malignant pleural effusion: nursing interventions using an indwelling pleural catheter with intermittent drainage, *Nurs Intervent Oncol* 12:8, 2000.

102. Teng M, Choy H, Ettinger D: Combined chemotherapy for limited-stage small-cell lung cancer, *Oncology Huntingt* 13(10 suppl 5):107, 1999.

103. Urban T and others: Standard combination versus alternating chemotherapy in small cell lung cancer: a randomized clinical trial including 394 patients. *Lung Cancer* 25(2):105, 1999.

104. US Environmental Protection Agency: *A citizen's guide to radon: what it is and what to do about it,* OPA-86-004, Washington, DC, USDHHS Office of Air and Radiation, 1986.

105. Viele CS, Iwamoto RR: *The clinical application of cytoprotectants,* Mountain View, CA, Medical Education Resources, Alza Pharmaceuticals, 2000.

106. Virtamo J: Vitamins and lung cancer, *Proc Nutr Soc* 50:329, 1999.

107. Wickham R: *Surviving the cancer experience: managing nausea and vomiting,* Pittsburgh, Oncology Education Services, Glaxo Wellcome, 2000.

108. Woolam GL: Cancer statistics: a benchmark for the new century, *CA Cancer J Clin* 50:7, 2000.

Malignant Lymphoma

Betty Thomas Daniel

Malignant lymphoma is a diverse group of neoplasms that originate in the lymphatic system. Included in this system are organs and tissues such as the thymus, lymph nodes, spleen, bone marrow, blood, and lymph. Lymph is derived from interstitial fluid and flows through lymphatic vessels so that it is eventually returned to the circulatory system by way of the thoracic duct. Along its course, lymph is filtered of particulate through lymph nodes, which are small, encapsulated organs located along the lymphatic vessels (Fig. 16–1). Lymph nodes have a very specific architecture (Fig. 16–2) that allows for areas of lymphocyte maturation and differentiation. Lymphocytes are the predominant cell present in lymph nodes and are the cellular element involved in malignant lymphoma.

Lymphocytes originate in the bone marrow and, through the process of maturation and differentiation, develop into several different types of mature lymphocytes (Fig. 16–3). At any stage of this maturation and differentiation, the normal cell may transform into a malignant cell, giving rise to a malignancy that is specific to the stage in which the cell became transformed.

Based on the characteristics of the malignant lymphocytes, malignant lymphomas are divided into two major subgroups: Hodgkin's disease and non-Hodgkin's lymphoma. This chapter discusses the incidence, etiology, classifications, clinical manifestations, diagnosis, and treatment of Hodgkin's disease and non-Hodgkin's lymphoma and also provides guidelines for care of patients with malignant lymphoma.

Hodgkin's Disease

HISTORICAL BACKGROUND

In 1832 Thomas Hodgkin described a progressively fatal disease characterized by enormous lymph node swellings that he believed to be one disease.[26] Characteristic cells involved in this disease were identified microscopically by Sternberg and Reed in 1898 and 1902, respectively.[4] The identification of these cells, now known as *Reed-Sternberg cells,* allowed for the initial classification of Hodgkin's disease. Reed-Sternberg cells are characterized as binucleated or multinucleated in a background of inflammatory cells. It is unusual as a malignancy in that the tumor cells are in the minority, and the normal inflammatory cells predominate.[31] In the past two decades advances in histology and immunohistology have revealed that the Reed-Sternberg cell is of B-cell lineage, and that Hodgkin's disease is not a single disease, but instead two separate diseases.[27] The classic Hodgkin's disease, which accounts for about 95% of cases, includes the subsets of nodular sclerosis, mixed cellularity, lymphocyte rich, and lymphocyte depletion. The other disease entity is the rare nodular lymphocyte predominance Hodgkin's disease.[11, 27]

The potential curability of Hodgkin's disease was first recognized in 1920, when patients with localized tumors treated with radiation were shown to have 10% survival.[13] By the 1960s about one third of the patients were being cured with radiation. In 1970, the National Cancer Institute (NCI) reported that patients with advanced Hodgkin's disease could attain complete remission and long-term survival using a combination chemotherapy of nitrogen mustard, Oncovin (vincristine), procarbazine, and prednisone, known as MOPP.[13] These advances resulted in a standard approach to the diagnosis and treatment of Hodgkin's disease. Since the mid-1970s, development and research efforts have focused on more accurate ways of staging, initial therapies for various stages, treatment of resistant and relapsed disease, and the long-term effects of treatment regimens.

EPIDEMIOLOGY AND ETIOLOGY

In the United States in 2000, the estimated number of new cases of Hodgkin's disease was 7400, with an estimated 1400 deaths.[8] This represents an incidence of less than 1% of all cancers. However, Hodgkin's disease

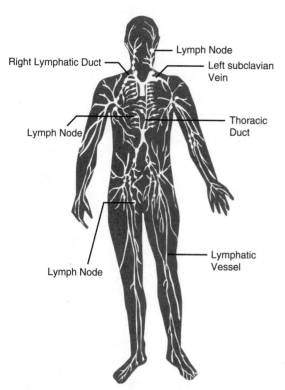

FIGURE 16 – 1 The lymphatic system. (From Sompayrac L: *How the immune system works,* Malden, MA, Blackwell Science, 1999.)

is the most common cancer of young adults. Median age of diagnosis is 26 to 31 years; however, a bimodal pattern of incidence has been seen in the United States. One peak is seen between 20 and 29 years, then there is a gradual decline between 40 and 59 years, followed by another peak after 60 years. It has now been determined that the second peak is more the result of misclassification. The most recent data from the NCI indicate many of these cases are aggressive non-Hodgkin's lymphoma. Hodgkin's disease is also slightly more common in men, who may have a poorer prognosis. About 90% of all cases in the United States occur in whites.[19]

The cause of Hodgkin's disease remains elusive. No strong evidence for specific etiologic factors exists. However, clinical manifestations and epidemiologic studies have suggested a viral etiology or disturbance of the immune system. The infectious agent most frequently implicated is the *Epstein-Barr virus* (EBV). Epidemiologic studies of clusters of Hodgkin's disease cases suggest the possibility that the disease occurs as a rare consequence of EBV infection. However, no conclusive evidence for a relationship between EBV and Hodgkin's disease exists.[4, 20]

Genetic and occupational predispositions for Hodgkin's disease may also exist. Epidemiologic studies have identified an increased risk of disease among siblings of persons with Hodgkin's disease, following tonsillectomy

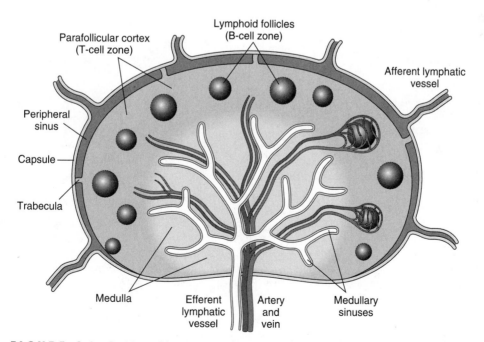

FIGURE 16 – 2 Normal lymph node architecture. Schematic diagram of a lymph node illustrates the blood and lymphatic supply and the distribution of B- and C-cell zones. (From Cotran RS, Kumar V, Collins T: *Robbins pathologic basis of disease,* ed 6, Philadelphia, Saunders, 1999.)

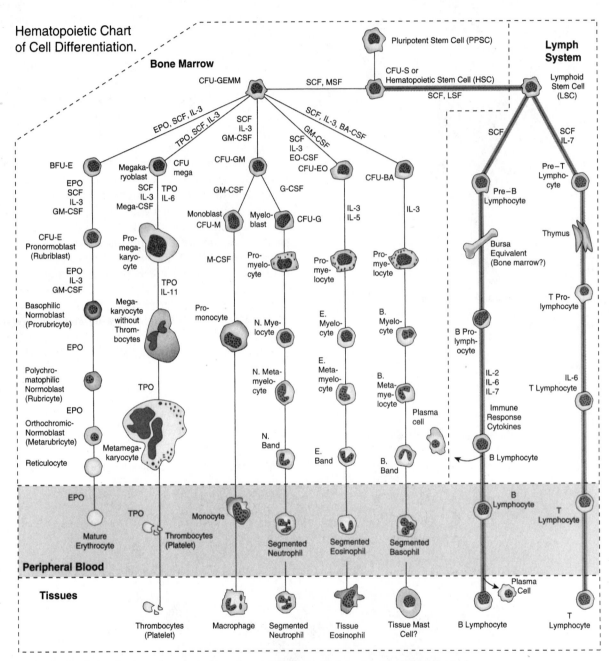

FIGURE 16-3 Lymphopoiesis. Hematopoietic chart with lymphopoiesis highlighted. (From Stevens ML: *Fundamentals of clinical hematology*, Philadelphia, Saunders, 1997.)

and appendectomy, a linkage with certain HLA antigens, and among persons in the occupation of woodworking. Evidence to support these ideas is inconclusive.[4]

PREVENTION, SCREENING, AND DETECTION

Prevention of Hodgkin's disease is not applicable because there are no identified preventable risks. Early detection is important but may be hampered by the vagueness of the common symptoms. Patients should be encouraged to seek medical attention for persistent common signs and symptoms.

CLASSIFICATION

In 1995, the World Health Organization (WHO) convened a group of leading pathologists and hematopathologists, with a clinical advisory committee of hematologists and oncologists to develop a new classification of hematologic malignancies. In November 1997, this group accepted the "Revised European-American Classification of Lymphoid Neoplasms" (REAL). The *WHO Classification of Neoplastic Diseases of the Hematopoietic and Lymphoid Tissues* (Table 16–1) identifies two types of Hodgkin's disease with four subtypes based primarily on the microscopic features of the involved tissues.[10] Table 16–2 summarizes characteristics of the different histopathologic classifications of Hodgkin's disease.

CLINICAL FEATURES

The most common signs and symptoms of Hodgkin's disease are lymphadenopathy, fever, night sweats, weight loss, pruritus, and alcohol-induced pain.[19] Generally lymph nodes are present above the diaphragm, and only later is there generalized lymphatic and extranodal disease. Mediastinal nodes may become enlarged to greater than 10 cm, and the patients may complain of dry cough or shortness of breath, especially when lying down, and substernal pain.[5, 19] Unexplained fever of greater than 38°C during the past month, drenching and recurrent night sweats, and unexplained weight loss greater than 10% in less than 6 months usually signify advanced disease. Other presenting signs include generalized pruritus and pain in the enlarged nodes after the ingestion of alcohol. Neither pruritus nor alcohol-induced pain has known prognostic significance[19, 31] (see Clinical Features box).

Other rare occurrences are superior vena cava syndrome (SVCS), upper extremity thrombosis, phrenic nerve or laryngeal nerve entrapment, ureteral obstruction, lymphedema, venous thrombosis of the lower extremities, and splenomegaly. Almost all these signs and

TABLE 16–1

Proposed WHO Classification of Lymphoid Neoplasms*

B-CELL NEOPLASMS

Precursor B-Cell Neoplasm
- Precursor B-lymphoblastic leukaemia/lymphoma (precursor B-cell acute lymphoblastic leukaemia)

Mature (Peripheral) B-Cell Neoplasms†
- B-cell chronic lymphocytic leukaemia/small lymphocytic lymphoma
- B-cell prolymphocytic leukaemia
- Lymphoplasmacytic lymphoma
- Splenic marginal zone B-cell lymphoma (+/− villous lymphocytes)
- Hairy cell leukaemia
- Plasma cell myeloma/plasmacytoma
- Extranodal marginal zone B-cell lymphoma of MALT type
- Nodal marginal zone B-cell lymphoma (+/− monocytoid B cells)
- Follicular lymphoma
- Mantle cell lymphoma
- Diffuse large B-cell lymphoma
    Mediastinal large B-cell lymphoma
    Primary effusion lymphoma
- Burkitt lymphoma/Burkitt cell leukaemia

T AND NK-CELL NEOPLASMS

Precursor T-Cell Neoplasm
- Precursor T-lymphoblastic lymphoma/leukaemia (precursor T-cell acute lymphoblastic leukaemia)

Mature (Peripheral) T-Cell Neoplasms†
- T-cell prolymphocytic leukaemia
- T-cell granular lymphocytic leukaemia
- Aggressive NK-cell leukaemia
- Adult T-cell lymphoma/leukaemia (HTLV1+)
- Extranodal NK/T-cell lymphoma, nasal type
- Enteropathy-type T-cell lymphoma
- Hepatosplenic $\gamma\delta$ T-cell lymphoma
- Subcutaneous panniculitis-like T-cell lymphoma
- Mycosis fungoides/Sezary syndrome
- Anaplastic large cell lymphoma, T/null cell, primary cutaneous type
- Peripheral T-cell lymphoma, not otherwise characterized
- Angioimmunoblastic T-cell lymphoma
- Anaplastic large cell lymphoma, T/null cell, primary systemic type

HODGKIN'S LYMPHOMA (HODGKIN'S DISEASE)
- Nodular lymphocyte predominance Hodgkin's lymphoma
- Classical Hodgkin's lymphoma
    Nodular sclerosis Hodgkin's lymphoma (Grades 1 and 2)
    Lymphocyte-rich classical Hodgkin's lymphoma
    Mixed cellularity Hodgkin's lymphoma
    Lymphocyte depletion Hodgkin's lymphoma

* *Only major categories are included.*

† *B- and T/NK-cell neoplasms are grouped according to major clinical presentations (predominantly disseminated/leukaemic, primary extranodal, predominantly nodal).*

From Harris NL and others: The World Health Organization classification of neoplastic diseases of the haematopoietic and lymphoid tissues: report of the Clinical Advisory Committee meeting, Airlie House, VA, November 1997, Histopathology 36(1):69, 2000.

CLINICAL FEATURES

Hodgkin's Disease and Non-Hodgkin's Lymphoma

Hodgkin's Disease	Non-Hodgkin's Lymphoma
Painless lymphadenopathy	Generalized painless lymphadenopathy
Fever	Vague abdominal discomfort
Night sweats	Back pain
Weight loss	Gastrointestinal complaints
Pruritus	
Alcohol-induced pain	

---

symptoms can be attributed to enlarged nodes or lymph tissue compressing other structures. These signs and symptoms are more commonly seen in non-Hodgkin's lymphomas.[19]

DIAGNOSIS AND STAGING

When a patient presents with clinical manifestations suggestive of Hodgkin's disease, a thorough history and physical examination must be performed. Diagnosis is confirmed with a biopsy and histopathology of the enlarged node.[19] However, if there is evidence of a recent infectious process, a lymph node biopsy may be delayed a short period to observe the clinical course. When feasible, the most accessible and most abnormal node should be biopsied. The entire node should be removed to ensure adequate histologic examination. Needle aspiration is not adequate for diagnosis because the architecture of the lymph node is important for diagnosis and histologic subclassification.[31]

After a tissue diagnosis of Hodgkin's disease has been established, the extent of disease involvement must be determined. This process of staging is critical for selection of the proper strategy. The *Cotswold Staging Classification for Hodgkin's Disease,* a modification of the traditional Ann Arbor Staging system, is found in Table 16–3. To stage the extent of the disease accurately, it is recommended that the following procedures be initiated as soon as possible after a definitive diagnosis of Hodgkin's disease[4, 5, 31]

1. Detailed history and physical examination with emphasis on history of fever, night sweats, weight loss (B symptoms), and pruritus and assessment of lymph node regions, inspection of Waldeyer's ring, palpation of liver and spleen, and evaluation cardiac and pulmonary status
2. Laboratory work-up, including complete blood count (CBC), differential, platelet count, erythro-

cyte sedimentation rate (ESR), liver and renal function tests, and serum uric acid
3. Radiology work-up, including a chest x-ray (posteroanterior and lateral with measurement of mass/thoracic ratio); computed tomography (CT) scans of the chest, abdomen, and pelvis (magnetic resonance imaging [MRI] is not considered as useful as CT); bipedal lymphangiogram (if presents with inguinal or iliac Hodgkin's disease)
4. Bilateral bone marrow biopsy and aspirate
5. Skeletal survey if bone tenderness is noted on history and physical examination
6. A gallium scan is useful in determining extent of mediastinal or chest disease
7. Percutaneous needle biopsy of any suspicious extranodal lesions (e.g., hepatic, bone, pulmonary, or cutaneous)
8. Staging laparotomy only if identification of abdominal disease will significantly affect treatment decisions. Laparotomy includes splenectomy; biopsy of celiac, splenic, hilar, porta hepatic, para-aortic and iliac nodes; wedge or needle (or both) biopsy of liver; and open iliac crest bone marrow biopsy if not done previously.

The laboratory studies performed as a part of the staging work-up are not indicative of Hodgkin's disease. They provide baseline blood values, indications for further studies, and prognostic indicators. CBCs and routine chemistry evaluations are generally within normal limits. The exceptions to this are leukocytosis, a mild thrombocytosis, and anemia.[19] An elevated alkaline phosphatase may also indicate bone involvement that would require further evaluation with a bone scan. A significantly elevated lactate dehydrogenase (LDH) is considered an indication of bulky disease and carries a poor prognosis.[19, 31] An elevated ESR is considered to be a prognostic indicator because it is associated with advanced disease and B symptoms. It may also be used to monitor disease after treatment.[5]

During and after treatment, many of the same staging procedures are repeated to document response to treatment and then to document complete remission. When recurrence is suspected, the diagnostic and staging process is repeated. It is important to document disease recurrence by node biopsy and to determine the site and extent of recurrence. All these factors are as important for effective treatment of recurrence as they are for the management of new diagnoses.

METASTASIS

Hodgkin's disease spreads contiguously from one lymph node chain to another. Strong evidence indicates that Hodgkin's disease begins in one lymph node, then

TABLE 16-2
Summary of Characteristics of Classifications of Hodgkin's Disease

NODULAR LYMPHOCYTE PREDOMINANCE HODGKIN'S DISEASE (NLPHD)

1. Atypical cells are CD45$^+$ and express B-cell associated antigens (CD19, CD20, CD22, and CD79a), but lack the Hodgkin's disease antigens CD15 and CD30
2. They do not have the bcl-2 rearrangement common to NHL
3. Accounts for 5–6% of cases of HD
4. Male:female ratio 3:1 or greater
5. Median age is mid-30s but seen in both children and the elderly
6. 75% patients stage I or II at time of diagnosis
7. 90% patients have 10-y survival
8. Higher risk of developing NHL than other types of HD
9. Cause of death is often NHL or other cancers, not HD

CLASSIC HODGKIN'S DISEASE

1. Presence of classic Reed-Sternberg cells in a background of either nodular sclerosis, mixed cellularity, or lymphocyte depletion
2. Cells are CD15$^+$ and CD30$^+$; B cell antigens usually negative

NODULAR SCLEROSIS HODGKIN'S DISEASE (NSHD)

1. Partially nodular pattern with fibrous bands separating nodule; diffuse area are common, and necrosis present
2. Characteristic cell is lacunar-type Reed-Sternberg, which may be abundant
3. Diagnostic Reed-Sternberg cells present, but rare
4. Subdivided into grade 1 and grade 2 based on the number and atypia of Reed-Sternberg cells (grade 2 similar to lymphocyte-depleted variant; associated with worse prognosis than grade 1; increased rate of relapse shorter survival and worse response to initial therapy)
5. 60–80% of cases of HD
6. Most common in adolescents and young adults; but can occur at any age
7. Incidence equal in males and females
8. Mediastinum and other supradiaphragmatic sites are common

MIXED-CELLULARITY HODGKIN'S DISEASE (MCHD)

1. Infiltrate usually diffuse or at most vaguely nodular, without sclerosis
2. Diagnostic Reed-Sternberg cells present in background of inflammatory cells (lymphocytes, eosinophils, plasma cells, and histiocytes)
3. 15–30% cases of HD
4. Seen at any age; lacks early peak of NSHD
5. Mediastinal involvement less common than NSHD; abdominal and splenic involvement more common
6. Characterized by B symptoms (weight loss, fever, night sweats)
7. Most present with stage III or IV disease

LYMPHOCYTE-RICH CLASSIC HODGKIN'S DISEASE (LRCHD)

1. Classic Reed-Sternberg cells in an background of predominantly lymphocytes
2. Confused at times with LPHD which does not have the classic Reed-Sternberg cells
3. CD15$^+$ and CD30$^+$ antigens
4. Clinical features and survival pattern same as MCHD

LYMPHOCYTE-DEPLETION HODGKIN'S DISEASE (LDHD)

1. Infiltrate is diffuse and often appears hypocellular, with diffuse fibrosis and necrosis
2. Large numbers of Reed-Sternberg cells, and few inflammatory cells
3. Least common variant of HD (approximately 5% of HD)
4. Most common type associated with AIDS
5. More common in elderly
6. Widespread disease at time of diagnosis with abdominal lymphadenopathy, liver involvement, and bone metastasis

Data from DeVita VT, Mauch PM, Harris NL: Hodgkin's disease. In DeVita VT, Hellman S, Rosenberg SA, editors: Cancer: principles and practice of oncology, *ed 5, Philadelphia, Lippincott-Raven, 1997.*

TABLE 16-3
The Cotswolds Staging Classification

Stage I   Involvement of a single lymph node region or lymphoid structure (e.g., spleen, thymus, Waldeyer's ring).

Stage II   Involvement of two or more lymph node regions on the same side of the diaphragm (the mediastinum is a single site, hilar lymph nodes are lateralized). The number of anatomical sites should be indicated by a suffix (e.g., II).

Stage III Involvement of lymph node regions or structures on both sides of the diaphragm.
　　　　　 III_1 With or without splenic hilar, coeliac, or portal nodes
　　　　　 III_2 With para-aortic, iliac, mesenteric nodes.

Stages IV Involvement of extranodal site(s) beyond that designated "E"
　　　　　 A   No symptoms
　　　　　 B   Fever, drenching sweats, weight loss
　　　　　 X   Bulky disease:
　　　　　　　 >1/3 widening of mediastinum
　　　　　　　 >10 cm maximum dimension of nodal mass
　　　　　 E   Involvement of a single extranodal site, contiguous or proximal to known nodal site
　　　　　 CS Clinical stage
　　　　　 PS Pathological stage

From Canellos GP: Hodgkin's disease. In Freireich EJ, Kantarjian HM, editors: Medical management of hematological malignant diseases. New York, Marcel Dekker, 1998.

spreads to adjacent nodes, until eventually the malignant cells invade the blood vessels and spread to other organs. Involvement of retroperitoneal nodes, lungs, liver, spleen, and bone marrow usually occurs after Hodgkin's disease is generalized. Mesenteric lymph nodes and any organ can be involved in advanced cases.[4]

TREATMENT MODALITIES

As a result of the advances in precise staging, knowledge of prognostic factors, the development of supervoltage radiation therapy, and effective combination chemotherapy, survival rates for Hodgkin's disease have improved greatly. All patients of all stages should be treated aggressively with a curative intent. The goal of treatment is to achieve the highest overall cure rate with minimal side effects to ensure quality of life and survival of patients cured of their disease.[2, 19, 31, 32]

Early Stage Disease

Stage I/II A or B (with or without symptoms) is defined as early stage Hodgkin's disease. However, there is con-

TABLE 16-4
Prognostic Factors in Localized Hodgkin's Disease (EORTC* Criteria)

Very Favorable (6% of patients)
Clinical stage IA, female, < 40 years of age, ESR < 50 mm, lymphocyte predominant or nodular sclerosis; mediastinal/thoracic ratio < 0.35.

Favorable (45% of patients)
CS I/II A/B; 1–3 sites; mediastinal/thoracic ratio < 0.35; < 50 years of age; stage A/ESR < 50 or stage B/ESR < 30 mm/h.

Unfavorable (45% of patients)
Age > 50; or A/ESR ≥ 50 or B/ESR ≥ 30; or CS II ≥ 4 sites or mediastinal/thoracic ratio ≥ 0.35.

* European Organization for Research and Treatment of Cancer.

From Canellos GP: Hodgkin's disease. In Freireich EJ, Kantarjian HM, editors: Medical management of hematological malignant diseases. New York, Marcel Dekker, 1998.

siderable variation diseasedisvariation in the presentation of early stage Hodgkin's. Therefore, proper staging, prognostic indicators, and knowledge of the toxicities of the treatment regimens are important factors required in the selection of the most appropriate therapy.[2, 4, 19, 31] The European Organization for Research and Treatment of Cancer have grouped negative prognostic factors into very favorable, favorable, and unfavorable criteria (Table 16–4) for use in early stage Hodgkin's disease.[2] Negative prognostic factors include male gender, systemic symptoms and elevated ESR, bulky disease (usually >10 cm), mixed cellularity histology, four or more nodal sites above the diaphragm, and age greater than 50 years. Toxicities associated with treatment of Hodgkin's disease are listed in Table 16–5.

TABLE 16-5
Treatment-Related Complications in Hodgkin's Lymphoma Survivors

Pneumonitis	Melanoma
Pericarditis	Sarcoma
Pericardial fibrosis	Sterility
Pulmonary fibrosis	Hypothyroidism
Cardiomyopathy	Myelodysplasia
Atherosclerotic heart disease	Acute nonlymphocytic leukemia
Peripheral neuropathy	
Breast cancer	Acute myelogenous leukemia
Lung cancer	
Thyroid cancer	Non-Hodgkin's lymphoma
Stomach cancer	

Data from references 4, 27, and 31.

There are generally three treatment options for early stage Hodgkin's disease: radiation therapy, chemotherapy, or combined chemotherapy and radiation therapy. Figure 16–4 illustrates standard fields for radiation used to treat Hodgkin's disease. Table 16–6 lists chemotherapy regimens. The choice of regimen depends on the clinical circumstances regarding toxicities to avoid. The most common protocol used today is the ABVD because of the demonstrated efficacy and lower toxicity to bone marrow and germ cells.[2, 4, 19, 31] Patients meeting the very favorable criteria or with documented minimal stage IIA disease following laparotomy are offered mantle radiation. Patients with pathologic stage I/II A or B disease should received mantle and para-aortic radiation therapy. Patients who have not had a laparotomy would receive subtotal lymphoid irradiation with a splenic field. Combined modality therapy is recommended for patients with favorable criteria without a laparotomy and required for those presenting with unfavorable criteria. Chemotherapy alone is given to pa-

TABLE 16–6
Selected Chemotherapy Regimens in the Treatment of Hodgkin's Lymphoma

MOPP	Mechlorethamine
	Vincristine
	Procarbazine
	Prednisone
ABVD	Cytarabine
	Bleomycin
	Vinblastine
	Dacarbazine
MOPP Alternating with ABVD	
Ch1VPP	Chlorambucil
	Vinblastine
	Procarbazine
	Prednisone
MVPP	Mechlorethamine
	Vinblastine
	Procarbazine
	Prednisone
CABS	CCNU
	Doxorubicin
	Bleomycin
	Streptozotocin
Stanford V	Doxorubicin
	Vinblastine
	Mechlorethamine
	Vincristine
	Bleomycin
	Etoposide
	Prednisone

Data from references 24, 26, and 31.

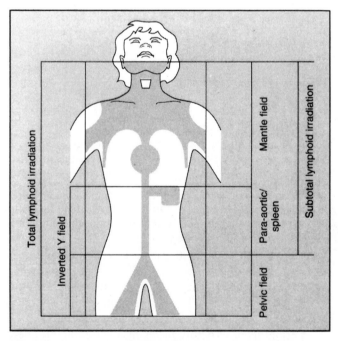

FIGURE 16–4 Standard radiation fields for Hodgkin's disease. *Mantle field,* From mandible to diaphragm; lungs, heart, spinal cord, and humeral heads are shielded. *Inverted Y field,* From diaphragm to ischial tuberosities, including the spleen if not removed; spinal cord, kidneys, bladder, rectum, and gonads are shielded. *Subtotal lymphoid irradiation,* Involves mantle zone and uppermost inverted Y zone (*para-aortic/spleen zone*); does not include the pelvic, inguinal, or femoral nodes. *Total lymphoid irradiation,* Mantle zone and complete inverted-Y zone. (From Portlock CS, Yahalom J: Hodgkin's disease. In Goldman L, Bennett JD, editors: *Cecil textbook of medicine,* ed 21, Philadelphia, Saunders, 2000.)

tients with unfavorable features, but who do not have bulky disease (>10 cm).[2, 31, 32]

Advanced Disease

Advanced Hodgkin's disease is considered to be stage III and IV. Current therapy for this group of patients remains chemotherapy alone using any of the regimens listed in Table 16–6. The treatment of choice is considered to be ABVD or ABVD alternating with MOPP.[2, 19, 31] Controversy remains regarding the value of radiation therapy for advanced disease. Consolidation with radiation therapy following chemotherapy has not demonstrated any survival advantage. For patients presenting with a bulky mediastinal mass, a combined modality therapy using radiation may be beneficial.[2]

Relapsed or Recurrent Disease

After initial therapy, 40% to 50% of patients with stage III/IV disease and 20% to 30% with stage I/II disease will have residual or recurrent disease.[2] The optimal treatment regimen for these patients continues to be controversial. Patients who relapse after radiation alone are generally treated with standard chemotherapy with excellent complete remission rates and 50% to 80% long-term survival rates.[31] For patients relapsing after chemotherapy, several treatment approaches have been used, with varying degrees of success.

When relapse occurs after chemotherapy, the length of disease-free survival is important in planning further treatment. Patients experiencing relapse after long disease-free survival have a 70% to 90% complete response rate to standard chemotherapy regimens.[31] Those who relapse less than 12 months after initial therapy are less likely to achieve a complete remission using standard dose chemotherapy.[31] This group should be offered high-dose chemotherapy with or without radiation therapy followed by autologous bone marrow or stem cell support.[4, 19, 31] Complete response rates reported range from 50% to 80%.[31] Conditioning regimens vary, however, BEAM (BCNU, etoposide, Ara-C, and melphalan) and CBV (cyclophosphamide, BCNU, and etopside) are commonly used.[2] Allogeneic transplantation has not shown any advantage to autologous and has had a poorer outcome in many studies.[2, 31] (See Chapter 25 for further information.)

When autologous stem cell transplant is not possible, patients should be offered clinical trials using new drug or biologic therapies.[4] Clinical trials in progress include studies using radiolabeled immunoglobulin therapy. Antiferritine antibody labeled with either yttrium-90 or iodine-131 was used with a 30% complete response rate and a 60% overall response rate. Other trials include work with antibodies to CD25 and CD30 to generate anti-idiotypic antibodies to serve as vaccines and the use of monoclonal antibodies to CD25 and CD30. These are all exciting possibilities for use in recurrent/refractory Hodgkin's disease.[4] Table 16–7 lists protocols that have been effective as salvage treatment for Hodgkin's disease.

PROGNOSIS

Hodgkin's disease is considered to be very a curable cancer. For patients with stage I/II A disease treated with radiation therapy alone, the 20-year survival rate is 70% to 80%, and the overall survival rate after salvage therapy for those with relapse is 80% to 95%.[4] Even those with stage III/IV advanced disease are able to achieve remission after chemotherapy with a complete remission rate of 89% with ABVD. Patients with relapsed or resistance disease have a less favorable prognosis. Stage I/II disease with relapse has a 57% to 62% disease-free survival rate at 10 years. Relapses after chemotherapy with remissions less than 12 months are projected to have less than 17% survival at 20 years.[4]

TABLE 16–7
Salvage Chemotherapy Regimens for Hodgkin's Lymphoma

CAV	CCNU
	Melphalan
	Etoposide
ABDIC	Doxorubicin
	Bleomycin
	Dacarbazine
	CCNU
	Prednisone
MINE	Mitoguazone
	Ifosfamide
	Vinorelbine
	Etoposide
EVA	Etoposide
	Vinblastine
	Doxorubicin
MIME	Mitoguazone
	Ifosfamide
	Methotrexate
	Etoposide
EPOCH	Etoposide
	Vincristine
	Doxorubicin
	Cyclophosphamide
	Prednisone

Data from references 2, 4, and 27.

Even after surviving Hodgkin's disease, patients face possible complications from their treatment, which can occur years after diagnosis and treatment. The major long-term complications of Hodgkin's disease and its treatment are second malignancies and gonadal dysfunction.[4] Sterility occurs in almost 80% of men and is often a permanent side effect of chemotherapy, especially the MOPP regimen. Radiation scatter from pelvic radiation can also significantly affect testicular function. Patients should be made aware of these possible effects before treatment. The testicles should be shielded during pelvic radiation.[31] Sperm banking may be offered, but many men with Hodgkin's disease have impaired spermatogenesis before receiving any treatment. Therefore, use of sperm banking is limited. Infertility in women is less common and is usually seen in older patients. In women, reproductive dysfunction after radiation or chemotherapy is usually related to primary ovarian failure. Women older than 25 years and those who are treated with chemotherapy and pelvic radiation have the highest incidence of premature ovarian failure (80–100%).[31] These possible effects should be discussed with patients, and when feasible, the ovaries should be shielded during pelvic radiation. (See Chapter 33 for further information.)

COMPLICATIONS

Non-Hodgkin's Lymphoma

Disease Related

Superior vena cava syndrome
Central nervous system involvement
Spinal cord involvement

Treatment Related

Radiation therapy
Pulmonary fibrosis
Pericardial fibrosis
Hypothyroidism
Secondary malignancies
Infertility
Sterility
Chemotherapy
Myelodysplasia
Acute leukemia
Infertility
Cardiac dysfunction

The most common second malignancies are acute myeloid leukemia, non-Hodgkin's lymphoma, thyroid cancer, breast cancer, and lung cancer. Acute myeloid leukemia is the most common second malignancy and generally occurs anytime within the first decade after treatment. The treatment regimen most often implicated as the risk factor for developing secondary acute myeloid leukemia is combined modality therapy.[19] The incidence of non-Hodgkin's lymphoma as a secondary malignancy is slightly less than that of acute myeloid leukemia and usually is not observed until 15 years after treatment.[31] The risk of thyroid cancer after irradiation is 16 times that of the general population. Children have an even greater risk than adults (67 times the risk).[5] Breast cancer usually occurs about 15 years after irradiation and is significantly more common in young girls and women who received mantle radiation. Lung cancer is more common in patients who smoke and the risk is about four times that of the normal population. It is thought that radiation potentiates the cellular changes already initiated by smoking.[5] Other less common sites of solid tumors include the stomach, soft tissue, bones, and skin.

Non-Hodgkin's Lymphoma

EPIDEMIOLOGY AND ETIOLOGY

As a group of neoplasms, non-Hodgkin's lymphoma (NHL) is morphologically and clinically different from Hodgkin's disease. After the Reed-Sternberg cell was identified as the characteristic cell of Hodgkin's disease, all other lymphomas were classified as non-Hodgkin's. Basically, NHL became a term to identify diseases with similarities to Hodgkin's but without the characteristic Reed-Sternberg cell.

In 2000 there were an estimated 54,900 new cases of NHL and 26,100 deaths attributed to NHL.[8] NHL represents the sixth most common cause of cancer deaths in the United States.[24] The incidence over the past 15 years has increased 50%, partly due to an increase in lymphomas related to human immunodeficiency virus (HIV) and an unexplained increase in older adults.[9, 24] Men are at slightly higher risk than women. It is more common in adults than children; however, there is a steady increase from childhood through 80 years of age. The average age at diagnosis is 45 to 55 years.[9, 24] Due to the number of years of life lost to this disease, it is ranked fourth in economic impact among cancers.[23]

Although the etiology of NHL remains unknown, a variety of factors have been associated with increased risk (Table 16–8). These include a number of immunodeficiency conditions, autoimmune disorders, infectious diseases, and environmental factors. Immunodeficiency conditions can be divided into congenital and acquired disorders. These disorders have in common defects in immunoregulation, particularly in cell-mediated immunity, resulting in decreased cytokine production, and uncontrolled B-cell proliferation, often associated with EBV genome.[9] Lymphomas that develop under these conditions are usually highly aggressive B-cell NHL that are widely disseminated.[23] Ataxia telangiectasia (AT) is an autosomal recessive disorder associated with chronic EBV infections. Patients with AT have an increased risk of developing NHL, Hodgkin's disease, gastric carcinomas, and dysgerminomas.[9, 23] Approximately 10% of children with AT develop NHL.[23] Wiskott-Aldrich syndrome (WAS) is an X-linked recessive disorder that involves a progressive decline in cell-mediated immunity. NHL occurs in approximately 15% of these children, with the primary site in the central nervous system (CNS) in one third of the cases.[9, 23] Other congenital immune disorders include severe combined immune deficiency (SCID), common variable immunodeficiency (CVID), IgA deficiency, IgM deficiency, hyper-IgM syndrome, and X-linked hypogammaglobulinemia. All of these disorders are associated with a high incidence of NHL. There is also an increased incidence of NHL that occurs in patients receiving long-term immunosuppression (e.g., organ transplant recipients), and in patients with rheumatoid arthritis or celiac disease.[7, 29]

Infectious agents may also be etiologic factors by virtue of contributing to the chronic stimulation of the immune system. *Helicobacter pylori, Borrelia burgdorferi,* hepatitis C virus, EBV, human T-cell leukemia virus type 1 (HTLV-1), and human herpes virus 8 (HHV-8)

TABLE 16-8
Risk Factors Associated with Non-Hodgkin's Lymphoma

IMMUNODEFICIENCY DISORDERS

Acquired
Immunosuppression post-transplantation
Acquired immunodeficiency syndrome

Congenital
Ataxia-telangiectasia
Wiscott-Aldrich syndrome
Severe combined immunodeficiency
Common variable immunodeficiency
IgA and IgM deficiency
Hyper IgM syndrome
X-linked hypogammaglobulinemia
X-linked lymphoproliferative disorder

AUTOIMMUNE DISORDERS

Hashimoto's thyroiditis
Sjogren's syndrome
Rheumatoid arthritis
Systemic lupus erythematosus

INFECTIOUS AGENTS

Epstein-Barr virus (EBV)
Human T-cell leukemia virus type I (HTLV-I)
Human herpes virus-8 (HHV-8)
Helicobacter pylori
Hepatitis C virus

ENVIRONMENTAL FACTORS

Diphenylhydantoin (dilantin)
Phenoxyherbicides
Organophosphates
Benzene
Styrene
1-3 Butadiene
Trichloroethylene
Perchloroethylene
Creosote
Lead arsenate
Formaldehyde
Paint thinner
Hair dyes

OTHERS

Immunosuppressive therapy
Chemotherapy
Radiation therapy
Castleman's Disease

Data from references 7, 9, 23, and 29.

have been linked to NHL. *H. pylori* infection of the stomach leads to chronic inflammation and is associated with the development of mucosa-associated lymphoid tissue (MALT lymphomas).[7, 9, 22, 23, 29] *B. burgdorfferi,* Lyme disease, is associated with some forms of skin lymphoma.[29] EBV is associated with many different forms of NHL as well as Hodgkin's disease.[7, 9] HTLV-1 is implicated in the etiology of adult T-cell lymphoma/leukemias.[7, 22, 23, 29] HHV-8 was identified as a new herpes virus through the use of polymerase chain reaction-based technique studying Kaposi sarcoma tissue. This virus was found to be present in a number of patients with acquired immunodeficiency syndrome (AIDS) presenting with lymphomas located in body cavities (pleural, pericardial, and peritoneal). Today HHV-8 is a recognized risk factor for body cavity-based lymphomas in patients with HIV infection and in multicentric Castleman's disease.[9, 14, 16] Hepatitis C has also been implicated with increased risk of NHL.[9, 29]

Exposure to some chemicals and physical agents has also been associated with an increased incidence of NHL. Phenytoin (Dilantin) has been associated with both pseudolymphoma and malignant lymphoma.[9] Other drugs implicated by some epidemiologic studies include aspirin, antibiotics, steroid, digitalis, estrogen, and tranquilizers.[9] Occupations that place people at higher risk include agriculture, forestry, fishing, construction, and leather workers. The chemicals implicated in these jobs include chlorophenols and phenoxyacetic acids.[9] Other controversial factors include hair dyes, ultraviolet light, and nutritional factors. Nutritional factors have also been investigated and results are conflicting. Milk, butter, liver, meat, coffee, and cola have been implicated.[9, 29] NHL has occurred as a secondary malignancy after chemotherapy and radiation therapy for Hodgkin's disease.[23, 29]

PREVENTION, SCREENING, AND DETECTION

Prevention of NHL is not applicable because there are no identified preventable risks. Early detection is important but may be hampered by the vagueness of the common symptoms. Patients should be encouraged to seek medical attention for persistent common signs and symptoms.

CLASSIFICATION

This is a group of diseases with diverse histologies. Over the years, it was noted that the histology of the tumor has a significant influence on treatment and prognosis of the disease; however, controversy over the classification system has continued. In the 1956, Rappaport introduced a classification system based on growth pattern, cell type, and degree of differentiation. This system was widely accepted and used throughout the United States.[9, 12, 21, 23] The competing systems at that time were the Kiel system, widely used in Europe, and the Lukes and Collins system.[9, 12, 21, 23] In 1982, a group of hematopathologists and oncologists who specialized in lymphomas published a modification of the three classifications known as the *Working Formulation for Clinical*

Usage.[9, 21, 23] The Working Formulation divided the lymphomas into histologic grades based on the aggressiveness of the cell type and the observed growth pattern. The histologic grades—low, intermediate, and high—generally correspond with the expected clinical course. Problems developed with the Working Formulation in terms of omitted disease entities and exceptions to the prognostic categories.[9, 12] In 1994, the *Revised European-American Lymphoma Classification* (REAL) was published by the International Lymphoma Study Group. It attempted to overcome some of the deficiencies of earlier systems and incorporate the increased knowledge in the areas of morphology, immunophenotype, genetic features, and clinical features of lymphomas.[12] Unfortunately, it was met with opposition because it was not considered usable outside of major medical centers. This led to the newest system, the *WHO Classification of Neoplastic Diseases of the Hematopoietic and Lymphoid Tissues,* proposed by 10 committees of pathologists, as well as a Clinical Advisory Committee of international hematologists and oncologists in 1997 (see Table 16–1).[10] This group agreed to adopt the REAL classification as the classification of lymphoid neoplasms. The REAL classification system recognizes three major categories of lymphoid malignancies: B-cell lymphomas, T/natural killer (NK)-cell lymphomas, and Hodgkin's disease.[23] The B-cell and T-cell lymphomas can be grouped according to their natural (untreated) history for clinical purposes: indolent, aggressive, and highly aggressive (Table 16–9).[23, 29]

TABLE 16–9
Clinical Classification of Non-Hodgkin's B-Cell Lymphomas

INDOLENT B-CELL LYMPHOMAS
Lymphoplasmacytic lymphoma
Splenic marginal zone lymphoma
B-cell small lymphocytic lymphoma
Extranodal marginal zone B-cell (MALT) lymphoma
Nodal marginal zone B-cell lymphoma
Follicle center lymphoma (follicular lymphoma)
Mantle cell lymphoma

AGGRESSIVE B-CELL LYMPHOMAS
Diffuse large B-cell lymphoma
Primary mediastinal (thymic) large B-cell lymphoma
Anaplastic large B-cell lymphoma

VERY AGGRESSIVE B-CELL LYMPHOMAS
Burkitt's lymphoma
Precursor B-cell lymphoblastic leukemia/lymphoma

Data from Shipp MA, Mauch PM, Harris NL: Non-Hodgkin's lymphoma. In DeVita VT, Hellman S, Rosenberg SA, editors: Cancer: principles and practice of oncology, ed 5, Philadelphia, Lippincott-Raven, 1997.

CLINICAL FEATURES

The most common symptom of NHL unrelated to AIDS is painless lymphadenopathy, often in the cervical chain or supraclavicular region.[9] However, the various subgroups of lymphoma are associated with specific signs and symptoms.[29] *Nodal indolent lymphomas* are typically seen in middle-aged or older adults, who complain of painless lymphadenopathy, but are otherwise healthy.[17, 29] They often report a long history of waxing and waning of adenopathy. B symptoms are uncommon in indolent lymphomas.[29] Most patients present with bone marrow involvement *Extranodal indolent lymphomas* are found in the stomach, parotid gland, thyroid, or lung. They are usually localized stage I or II disease. Patients may complain of abdominal discomfort relating to splenomegaly and may have neutropenia or thrombocytopenia.[29]

Aggressive lymphomas are more often symptomatic at presentation. Patients present with pain, obstructive symptoms such as swelling in legs or SVCS, or B symptoms. T-cell lymphomas present more frequently with extranodal involvement and severe B symptoms. Extensive retroperitoneal adenopathy is more common than peripheral adenopathy. The site of disease is often indicative of the histology. For example nasopharyngeal lymphoma is usually an EBV-associated T-cell or NK-cell lymphoma. Patients present with varying stages of disease; however, the more extensive disease is associated with a worse prognosis.[29] *Very aggressive lymphomas* are more commonly found in younger adults and children, and occasionally in older adults. Bone marrow and peripheral blood involvement is common. CNS involvement is not uncommon. Very high LDH levels are common; however, this is not true of other lymphomas.[29]

DIAGNOSIS AND STAGING

A biopsy of an abnormal lymph node or mass is necessary to diagnose NHL. After a diagnosis of NHL, the clinical stage of the disease must be determined. After diagnosis is made through excisional or incisional biopsy, it is important to stage the disease and identify the presence of prognostic factors to make a decision regarding treatment strategies. Table 16–10 describes the typical staging work-up. The staging begins with a complete history and physical. The history focuses on the presence of B symptoms and duration and rate of lymph node enlargement. The physical examination includes assessment of lymph node chains including measurement of enlarged nodes.[16, 23, 24, 29] Subsequent diagnostic studies are indicated by the specific disease entity or presentation of the disease. Like Hodgkin's disease, no specific laboratory studies are indicative of NHL;

T A B L E 1 6 – 1 0
Staging Work-up for Non-Hodgkin's Lymphoma

1. Excisional biopsy of lymph node reviewed by hematopathologist
2. History and physical (include B-symptoms, autoimmune disorders, congenital/acquired immune disorders, infections, chemical or environmental exposures, assessment of nodal areas and common extrandoal sites, splenomegaly and hepatomegaly)
3. Blood work
   a. Complete blood count, differential, and platelet count
   b. LDH
   c. Alkaline phosphate
   d. Uric acid
   e. BUN/Creatinine
   f. Calcium
   g. Albumin
   h. β-2 microglobulin
   i. Cytokines (IL-2 receptor, tumor necrosis factor)
4. CT chest (if abnormal chest x-ray), CT abdomen, pelvis, and neck
5. MRI (patients with neurological/CNS symptoms)
6. Bone marrow aspiration and biopsy
7. Lumbar puncture with cytology (patients with risk of CNS involvement or neurological symptoms)
8. GI endoscopy
9. Cytology of pleural effusion or ascites
10. Immunophenotype of pathological specimens
11. Gallium scan
12. MRI
13. Bone scan
14. PET scan

Data from references 4, 6, 7, 9, and 24.

---

however, they do provide additional prognostic and site-specific information.[23] In addition to routine blood tests, it is important to obtain serum LDH and β_2-microglobulin levels. These are important indicators of prognosis and indirect indicators of tumor burden.[6, 24] Other blood tests should include hepatitis B and C titers, and HIV, HTVL-1, and EBV serology, because these have important implications for treatment.[16, 29] Cytogenetic and molecular analyses of bone marrow and peripheral blood are also obtained. With the advent of polymerase chain reaction technology it is possible to identify specific immunoglobulin gene rearrangements or chromosomal translocations with high specificity and to evaluate the significance of minimal residual disease in a variety of subtypes of lymphomas. Although it is early to base treatment recommendation on the molecular analysis, in the future these techniques will likely affect treatment strategies.[6, 22, 24]

Imaging studies should include routine chest x-ray and CT of the abdomen and pelvis. Chest x-ray may reveal hilar or mediastinal adenopathy, pleural effusion,

or parenchymal involvement.[6, 24] If there is an abnormality on the chest x-ray, a CT of the chest is indicated. CT of the abdomen and pelvis is necessary to evaluate mesenteric and retroperitoneal involvement.[16, 23, 29] Patients with indolent lymphomas should have a lymphangiogram because this procedure is more sensitive in assessing lower abdominal and pelvic adenopathy, which is important in considering treatment options.[29] Gallium scans are positive in nearly all aggressive and highly aggressive lymphomas and approximately 50% of indolent lymphomas. They are used to identify initial sites of disease, monitor response to treatment, and detect early recurrence.[16, 24]

Bone marrow biopsy should be routine for staging NHL. Many institutions routinely do bilateral biopsies because these have about 15% higher yield than unilateral.[16, 29] For patients with highly aggressive lymphomas, mantle cell lymphoma, HIV-related lymphoma, primary CNS lymphoma, and large-cell lymphoma with bone marrow involvement, a lumbar puncture is recommended. If liver involvement is suspected, a liver biopsy may be indicated.[29] For patients with head and neck involvement and those with a gastrointestinal (GI) primary, an upper GI series with small bowel follow-through and endoscopy are indicated. Staging laparotomies and splenectomies are no longer routinely performed in patients with NHLs.

Although originally designed for staging of Hodgkin's disease, the Cotswold modification of the Ann Arbor staging system has been routinely applied to NHL (see Table 16–3). The staging system is based on the number of sites of involvement, the presence of disease above or below the diaphragm, evidence of systemic symptoms, and extranodal disease.[9, 24] However, due to the differences in the patterns of disease spread in Hodgkin's disease and NHL it has been necessary to identify additional prognostic clinical factors to more accurately reflect NHL.[6, 29] Clinical prognostic factors enable the clinician to choose the optimal treatment strategy and accurately predict outcomes.[29] Table 16–11 shows two systems currently used to predict the prognosis of patients prior to initiating therapy: the International Prognostic Index (IPI) and the M. D. Anderson Tumor Score System. The IPI is based on five parameters: age, performance status, serum LDH, involvement of more than one extranodal site, and stage of disease. A point is assigned to each factor, then points summed for a total score according to risk.[9, 15, 16, 24, 29] The M. D. Anderson Tumor Score System is also based on five parameters and a score is given for presence or absence of the parameters. A score greater than 3 identifies the patient as a poor risk/prognosis and would be treated on investigational protocols. Those with a score of less than 3 have an 80% disease-free survival rate when treated with conventional regimens.[15, 16, 29]

TABLE 16-11
International Index and Tumor Score System

A. INTERNATIONAL INDEX

Parameter	Criteria	Score
Age	< 60 y	0
	> 60 y	1
Ann Arbor Stage	I–II	0
	III–IV	1
Serum LDH	Normal	0
	> normal	1
Performance status	0–1	0
	> 1	1
Extranodal sites	0–1	0
	> 1	1

Total Score	Risk
0, 1	Low
2	Low intermediate
3	High intermediate
4, 5	High risk

B. TUMOR SCORE SYSTEM

Parameter	Adverse Feature
Ann Arbor stage	III–IV
Symptoms	Presence of B symptoms
Tumor bulk	Mass > 7 cm or CXR detectable mediastinal mass
β-2M	≥3.0
LDH	≥685

Each adverse feature scores one point. Totals of 3 or greater define poor-risk patients.

From Marlton P, Cabanillas F: Therapy of aggressive lymphoma. In Freireich EJ, Kantarjian HM, editors: Medical management of hematologic malignant diseases. *New York, Marcel Dekker, 1998.*

METASTASIS

The metastatic process varies with the type of lymphoma: *follicular* has bone marrow involvement and *diffuse* disseminates rapidly and involves areas such as the CNS, bone, and GI tract.

TREATMENT MODALITIES AND PROGNOSIS

Treatment approaches to NHLs are based on the specific histology of the neoplasm, stage of disease, and the prognosis and physiologic status of the patient. Many institutions will use either the IPI or the M. D. Anderson Tumor Score System, which use these parameters to aid in the planning of treatment.

Indolent Non-Hodgkin's Lymphoma

Controversy surrounds whether treatment of indolent or low-grade NHL can induce long-term disease-free survival and actually alter the disease's natural history.

Because the natural history of indolent lymphomas is such that they grow very slowly and rarely invade normal structures, the controversy is understandable. They are very responsive to a variety of treatments; however, multiple relapses are the rule. Patients generally have a long survival after diagnosis, but indolent NHLs are unlikely to be cured with current therapies.[9, 17, 23] Indolent NHL are unique in that they are known to transform into more aggressive forms, and they may undergo spontaneous regression.[9] After undergoing transformation, indolent NHLs have a reported survival of less than a year.[9, 17]

Early stage indolent NHL generally refers to Ann Arbor stages I and II. They are generally uncommon.[9] Radiation therapy to the involved field or total nodal radiation produces up 85% disease-free survival with follow-up over 10 years.[9] Although these numbers may suggest that some limited number of patients may be curable, the survival curves do not reflect relapses after 10 years.[9, 17] Most relapses occur outside of the radiation field. The role of chemotherapy in the treatment of early stage indolent lymphoma has not been greatly explored. Small studies report fewer relapses by combining radiation and chemotherapy; however, no improved survival has been shown.[9, 23]

The majority of patients with indolent NHL have advanced (stage III or IV) disease at diagnosis. The optimal treatment regimen for these patients is controversial and ranges from watchful waiting to intensive chemotherapy and autologous bone marrow transplantation.[9, 16, 23, 29] Unfortunately, no treatment option has been shown to improve survival. Treatment options tend to be determined by the patient and physician preference or by investigational protocols.[29] Treatment may be deferred until symptoms become bothersome or the disease has transformed into a more aggressive type of lymphoma.[17, 23] Patients may be offered conventional chemotherapy, such as CVP or CHOP, but there is no convincing survival benefit shown for this group.[9, 29] Interferon has been effective in producing remissions, especially in patients with follicular lymphoma. It has

been used mainly with combination chemotherapy, either in the induction phase or as maintenance therapy.

Nucleoside analogs such as fludarabine and cladribine (2-CDA) have been active in treating indolent lymphomas.[9, 29] They are associated with profound immunosuppression and treatment may be complicated by opportunistic infections such as *Pneumocystis carini* pneumonia, herpes infections, and fungal pneumonias.[29] Topoisomerase I inhibitors, topotecan, irinotean (CPT-11), and campotothecin have shown some effectiveness in heavily treated patients, and may have synergy with topoisomerase II inhibitors such as etoposide.[9] These are in early phase of study and the optimal placement of these newer agents is uncertain. Monoclonal antibodies have also been used in the treatment of NHL. Idec-C2B8 (Rituximab) is a chimeric anti-CD20 antibody. The CD20 antigen is expressed in 95% of B-cell lymphomas. This antibody has minimal toxicity and a short treatment schedule that make it very tolerable for patients.[29] High-dose chemotherapy and autologous or al-

T A B L E   1 6 – 1 2

Selected Chemotherapeutic Regimens to Treat Non-Hodgkin's Lymphoma

CAP-BOP	Cyclophosphamide Doxorubicin Procarbazine Bleomycin Vincristine Prednisone	MACOP-B	Methotrexate Leucovorin Doxorubicin Cyclophosphamide Vincristine Prednisone Bleomycin
CHOP	Cyclophosphamide Doxorubicin Vincristine Prednisone	m-BACOD	Methotrexate Leucovorin Bleomycin Doxorubicin Cyclophosphamide Vincristine Dexamethasone
CHOP-Bleo	Cyclophosphamide Doxorubicin Vincristine Prednisone Bleomycin	ProMACE-CytaBOM	Cyclophosphamide Etoposide Doxorubicin Cytosine Arabinoside Bleomycin Vincristine Methotrexate Leucovorin Prednisone
CMED	Cyclophosphamide Etoposide Decadron Methotrexate Leucovorin		
COPP	Cyclophosphamide Vincristine Procarbazine Prednisone		
CVP	Cyclophosphamide Vincristine Prednisone		

Data from references 4, 9, 16, and 18.

logeneic bone marrow transplantation have been used as clinical trials with encouraging results.[17, 29]

Aggressive Non-Hodgkin's Lymphoma

The most common aggressive lymphoma type is diffuse large B-cell lymphoma. More is known and more treatments have been tried for this group of lymphomas. Once the diagnosis and stage of disease is determined then a decision is made whether the disease is curable with the CHOP regimen. The IPI or M. D. Anderson Tumor Score is used to determine this. If the chance of cure with CHOP is greater than 75%, then it should be used if at all possible. It is well tolerated, simple to administer, and has a disease-free survival rate at 10 years of 82% in stage I patients and 64% in stage II patients.[9, 15, 29] If the patient has poor cardiac function, then a regimen without anthracycline should be used.[29] The value of radiation therapy is uncertain. In some centers it is used as consolidation for bulky disease in early and advanced stages.[9]

Patients with a tumor score of greater than 2 or an IPI of greater than 3 are considered to have an unfavorable prognosis and would not benefit from the CHOP regimen. The cure rate with CHOP is less than 30%. However, the best treatment for this group of patients is still undetermined. Varying combinations of chemotherapy have been studied (Table 16–12). The novel approach to treating high-risk patients consists of alternating triple therapy with ASHAP (doxorubicin, methyprednisolone, cytarabine, and cisplatin), M-BACOS, and MINE. The results show a superior benefit to the CHOP regimens. This group of patients may also be offered high-dose chemotherapy followed by autologous bone marrow transplant. One study showed a 59% 5-year disease free-survival following transplant.[29]

Forty percent of the patients with aggressive NHL will not respond to conventional induction therapy, and approximately 50% of those who respond will relapse.[29] This makes salvage regimens critically important. Most regimens are based on non–cross-resistant agents, or at least different agents than those used initially.[9, 15, 29] Table 16–13 lists selected salvage regimens. With the approval of Idec-C2B8 (Rituximab) by the Food and Drug Administration for refractory or relapsed B-cell NHL, most of the protocols now give this monoclonal antibody on day 1 of each cycle of chemotherapy. High-dose chemotherapy with growth factor support is among the new regimens. Patients who respond to the salvage chemotherapy regimens are often offered autologous bone marrow transplantation.

Highly Aggressive Non-Hodgkin's Lymphoma

Highly aggressive lymphomas are almost always either T-cell lymphoblastic or B-cell (Burkitt) lymphomas.[29]

TABLE 16–13
Salvage Chemotherapy Regimens for Non-Hodgkin's Lymphoma

ESHAP	Etoposide Methylprednisolone Cytarabine Cisplatin
EPOCH	Etoposide Vincristine Doxorubicin Cyclophosphamide Prednisone
DHAP	Cisplatin Cytarabine Dexamethasone
CEPP	Cyclophosphamide Etoposide Procarbazine Prednisone
IMVP-16	Ifosfamide Methotrexate Etoposide
MIME	Methyl-gag Ifosfamide Methotrexate Etoposide
MINE	Mesna Ifosfamide Mitoxantrone Etoposide

Data from references 9, 16, and 18.

The lymphoblasitc lymphomas are histologically and cytologically the same as the lymphoblasts of acute lymphoblastic leukemia.[16] Therefore treatment of highly aggressive lymphomas requires an intense chemotherapy regimen similar to those used to treat acute leukemia.[29] The treatment regimen should provide prophylactic treatment to the CNS (methotrexate or cytarabine intrathecally) because lymphoblastic lymphoma is associated with high risk of CNS involvement. An effective treatment regimen commonly used is Hyper-CVAD alternating with methotrexate-Ara-C. Courses are alternated every 3 weeks for 8 cycles.[29] Maintenance therapy consists of 6-mercaptopurine, methotrexate, vincristine, and prednisone. If complete remission is not achieved with initial therapy, the chance of any significant disease-free survival is dismal. After aggressive treatment, more than 90% of patients with good prognostic features can experience a 5-year relapse-free survival.[23] Because of the increased risk of relapse in this patient population, clinical trials are now investigating the use of high-dose chemotherapy with or without total body irradiation

TABLE 16–14
Summary of Hodgkin's Disease and Non-Hodgkin's Lymphoma

	Hodgkin's Disease	Non-Hodgkin's Lymphoma
Epidemiology/etiology	Bimodal incidence pattern, predominantly males, under 40 y Higher risk associated with Epstein-Barr virus, (EBV), woodworking; familial association, linked to certain HLA antigens	Predominantly female, increased incidence in whites; median age at diagnosis, 55 y Etiology unknown; association with viral infection, ionizing radiation, immunosuppression, other environmental factors
Clinical features	Cervical, supraclavicular, and mediastinal lymphadenopathy B symptoms in 40% of patients: fever, night sweats, weight loss Occasionally pruritus and alcohol-induced pain	Superficial lymphadenopathy, usually cervical and/or mediastinal involvement B symptoms less common than in Hodgkin's disease (most patients are asymptomatic)
Diagnosis/staging	Lymph node biopsy Staging laparotomy if considering radiation therapy Histology: Reed-Sternberg cells WHO Classification Cotswold modified Ann Arbor Staging System	Biopsy of involved lymph node Biopsy of extrandoal lymph nodes if no lymphadenopathy WHO classification (REAL) Cotswold modified AnnArbor Staging System,
Treatment*	Stages I and IIa (no mediastinal mass): radiation therapy Stages I and IIA (large mediastinal mass), stages I and IIB (no mediastinal mass), and stages IIIa with upper abdominal disease: radiation therapy and ABVD or MOPP Stages IIIA with lower abdominal disease, stage IIIB, and stage IV:MOPP/ABV, or MOPP/ABVD hybrid, and MOPP/ABV hybrid	Indolent lymphomas: "watch and wait" for older adults with good risks, radiation therapy for early stage, aggressive combination chemotherapy for advanced stages Aggressive and highly aggressive lymphomas: aggressive combination chemotherapy (CHOP [C, cyclophosphamide; H, doxorubicin HCl; O, Oncovin vincristine; P, prednisone] standard)
Salvage treatment	Failed radiation therapy: standard chemotherapy Failed complete remission (CR) within months after standard chemotherapy: high-dose chemotherapy with autologous bone marrow transplant (BMT) or peripheral blood stem cell (PBSC) transfusion Fail CR more than 1 year: re-treatment with same standard chemotherapy	High-dose chemotherapy with autologous or allogeneic BMT or PBSC transfusion Investigational combination chemotherapy

* See Tables 16–6 and 6–12 for chemotherapy regimens.

Data from DeVita VT Jr, Hellman S, Rosenberg SA: Cancer: principles and practices of oncology, ed 5, Philadelphia, Lippincott-Raven, 1997; and from Hoffman R and others: Hematology: basic principles and practice, ed 3, New York, Churchill Livingstone, 2000.

with autologous or allogeneic bone marrow support for poor prognosis patients.[23]

Table 16–14 summarizes and compares Hodgkin's disease and NHL.

CONCLUSION

To provide the best patient care, nurses must be knowledgeable about the disease process and the principles of chemotherapy and radiation therapy. Nurses need to be able to provide patients and families with information regarding the disease process, treatment options, possible side effects of treatment, and consequences of treatment. This information is necessary for patients and families to make informed choices and to monitor signs and symptoms on a routine basis. Providing consistent repetition of information can help patients and families understand the abstract concepts of the disease and treatment regimen.

Psychosocial issues, such as coping, sexuality, and survivorship, also must be addressed. Malignant lymphomas, particularly Hodgkin's disease, have peak incidences in young to middle adulthood, affecting most patients at a very productive, goal-oriented time of life. Caring for lymphoma patients offers the nurse varied and exciting challenges.

Nursing Management

Patients with malignant lymphoma can experience a broad range of physical conditions, from being mildly symptomatic to acutely ill. Patients with localized or indolent disease may be relatively asymptomatic from the disease and treatment. The majority of these patients are treated as outpatients, and the side effects from their treatments are generally not severe. Patients with extensive or aggressive disease are more often acutely ill and at risk for potentially severe side effects of therapy.

Several potential complications are specific to patients with malignant lymphoma. Nurses should monitor these so nursing care can be planned appropriately and nursing interventions can be implemented promptly. These potential complications are lymphadenopathy, myelosuppression, and CNS involvement.

Lymphadenopathy is the primary symptom of malignant lymphoma. The enlarged nodes usually are nontender. However, they can cause pain or dysfunction by compressing neighboring tissues or organs. Lymphadenopathy can also cause a decrease in lymph and venous return to the heart. The flow of lymph through the affected lymph nodes is blocked because the disease process has destroyed the architecture of the nodes. Because the lymphatic system is close to the venous system, enlarged nodes may mechanically obstruct venous blood flow. The blockage of lymph and venous flow creates lymphedema in the tissues distal to the affected node region. When assessing a patient with lymphadenopathy, it is important to note the function of the surrounding tissues and organs and the presence of lymphedema. A plan must be implemented that provides for optimal mobility and drainage of the affected limb.

Myelosuppression is a common complication of cancer treatment. Patients experiencing myelosuppression are at increased risk for infection, bleeding, and anemia. As in the leukemias, myelosuppression in lymphoma can be caused by the disease as well as by the treatment regimens. This is significant in this population because patients may experience marked and prolonged myelosuppression that results in increased morbidity. Patients who have compromised bone marrow function before treatment will experience a more rapid and generally prolonged myelosuppressive period. Patients who are myelosuppressed must be monitored closely for signs and symptoms of infection, bleeding, and anemia. Thorough assessment and prompt treatment are essential to decreasing the morbidity and mortality of the myelosuppressed patient.

The degree and length of myelosuppression may also affect the treatment plan. Treatment may be delayed until bone marrow function recovers, and future chemotherapy doses may be decreased to prevent severe myelosuppression. In both instances, optimal treatment is being compromised and may affect disease response. In addition to protecting patients from infection, bleeding, and anemia, nurses must assist patients in coping with possible changes in their treatment plans.

Lymphomatous involvement of the CNS is another potential complication of malignant lymphoma. It is more common in the aggressive and highly aggressive types of NHL. The involvement can occur as a space-occupying lesion in the brain or spinal cord or as an infiltration of the cerebrospinal fluid that causes irritation to the meninges. Cord compression, seizures, altered mental status, or cranial nerve palsies can occur as a result. Nurses therefore must be alert to subtle changes in patients' neurologic functioning. Nursing care must include assessment of mobility, sensory deficits or enhancements, cognitive abilities, and self-care abilities. Interventions must be appropriate to the patient's level of functioning. The ultimate goal is to assist the patient to achieve optimal functioning.

More than 50% of patients diagnosed with malignant lymphoma today will be alive in 5 years. However, complications can occur years after diagnosis and successful treatment and can have a significant impact on psychosocial functioning. Patients generally have an increased sense of vulnerability, fear of recurrence, and distress over changes in physical condition. Patients may have no apparent body changes secondary to disease and treatment but may feel less adequate, physically damaged, and less in control.

Patients and families all bring their history, experiences, and preconceived ideas into new situations. For teaching to be effective, these factors need to be identified and incorporated into the teaching plan. Because the malignant lymphomas are such a diverse group of diseases, they are often confusing. This is also a stressful time for patients and families, and it can be difficult for them to understand the abstract concepts of the disease and treatment. Consistent repetition and varying ways of providing information generally increase the ability to understand new concepts. Community resources often provide educational, emotional, or financial support and assistance. An assessment of patients' support systems, resources, and ability to communicate needs and feelings is important for nurses to be able to assist patients in maintaining or reestablishing roles and identities in school, work, and interpersonal relationships. The patient teaching priorities and geriatric considerations are listed in the boxes.

Examples of nursing care plans for malignant lymphoma follow.

Nursing Diagnosis

- *Ineffective individual coping, related to new diagnosis, potential life-style changes*

Outcome Goals

Patient will be able to:

- Demonstrate evidence of adjustment to psycho-emotional stressors related to new diagnosis and life-style changes.
- Demonstrate positive problem-solving behaviors.

Interventions

- Assess patient's level of distress and anxiety related to:
    Uncertainty of future
    Bothersome symptoms
    Changes in self-concept
    Effect of past experiences
- Assess for signs of maladaptive or risky behaviors that interfere with responsible health practices:
    Missed appointments
    Failure to attend to symptoms
    Chronic attention to symptoms
    Loss of future orientation

PATIENT TEACHING PRIORITIES

Hodgkin's Disease and Non-Hodgkin's Lymphoma

Signs and symptoms of disease: fever, night sweats, weight loss, painless lymphadenopathy, generalized vague gastrointestinal discomfort, back pain

Signs and symptoms of infection: fever, chills, cough, erythema, malaise

Sexual dysfunction: infertility, sterility; discuss options for contraception and ovary and sperm banking

Discuss treatment options: chemotherapy, radiation therapy, surgery, bone marrow transplant (BMT); purpose, schedule, simulation plan for radiation therapy; monitoring weekly blood counts; chemotherapy drug side effects and schedule; BMT types (allogeneic/autologous); before, during, and after transplant care components

---

GERIATRIC CONSIDERATIONS

Hodgkin's Disease and Non-Hodgkin's Lymphoma

Chemotherapy dose and schedule may be altered related to compromised cardiac, hepatic, renal, respiratory, and/or neuromuscular function.

Radiation therapy side effects: excessively dry skin, early skin reactions; increased fatigue; medication dose adjustment to minimize side effects; consider facilitation with transportation.

Financial considerations: fixed income—consider consultation with social services regarding housing, Meals on Wheels, medication prescriptions, and self-care needs.

- Identify patient's support system, resources, and communication patterns.
- Assess patient's problem-solving capabilities.
- Assess patient's level of knowledge regarding recurrence, development of secondary malignancy, and long-term effects of treatment.
- Listen attentively and provide support.
- Encourage verbalization of fears and concerns.
- Assist patient to recognize stressors, and assist with problem-solving.
- Provide reassurance that anxiety or distress about health are common feelings among cancer survivors.
- Initiate referrals to social work, psychology, or community resources, as appropriate.

Nursing Diagnosis

- *Ineffective family coping: compromised, related to new diagnosis*

Outcome Goals

Family will be able to:

- Identify stressors.
- Demonstrate effective use of coping strategies.
- Verbalize adjustments necessary in activities and roles.

Interventions

- Assess past family relationships and coping patterns.
- Provide opportunities for expression of feelings.
- Include family/significant other in teaching sessions.
- Assist family/significant other in meeting adaptations and changes in activities and roles, as needed.

- Initiate referrals to social work, psychology, or community resources, as appropriate.

Nursing Diagnosis

- *Risk for infection, related to myelosuppression*

Outcome Goals

Patient will be able to:

- Verbalize knowledge of high risk for infection.
- Demonstrate appropriate measures to minimize risk for infection.

Interventions

- Assess for presence of risk factors:
    Bone marrow involvement
    Decreased white blood cell count
- Assess for signs and symptoms of infection:
    Fever
    Cough
    Erythema
- Institute measures to prevent exposure to potential sources of infection:
    Meticulous handwashing
    Meticulous hygiene
    Avoidance of people with colds, flu
    Good oral hygiene after meals
- Monitor laboratory values:
    Blood counts
    Electrolytes
    Liver enzymes
- Minimize invasive procedures.
- Reassure patient and family that increased susceptibility to infections is temporary.

Nursing Diagnosis

- *Knowledge deficit related to disease process, treatment, and complications*

Outcome Goals

Patient will be able to:

- State diagnosis and explain disease process.
- State rationale for treatment and identify treatment protocol.
- Identify potential treatment complications.

Interventions

- Evaluate patient and family readiness to learn.
- Identify barriers to learning, such as language, physical deficiencies, psychological deficiencies, and intellectual development.

- Determine patient and family level of knowledge of:
    Function of lymph system
    Signs and symptoms of lymphoma
    Chemotherapy and radiation therapy
    Side effects of treatment
- Review information patient and family have already been given. Reinforce and clarify misconceptions.
- Explain basic anatomy and physiology of lymphatic system and of specific body systems affected by location of disease.
- Review and reinforce information regarding recurrence, secondary malignancy, and long-term effects of treatment.
- Individualize information for subtype of lymphoma and extent of disease.
- Explain symptoms of potential complications.
- Explain radiation therapy fields and possible side effects (see Chapter 22).
- Explain principles of chemotherapy, names of specific agents, and possible side effects (see Chapter 23).
- Provide written materials to reinforce teaching.
- Encourage verbalization of questions, fears, and concerns.
- Listen attentively and provide support.
- Initiate referrals to other health care professionals and community resources as needed.

Nursing Diagnosis

- *Impaired physical mobility, related to CNS involvement, lymphadenopathy*

Outcome Goals

Patient will be able to:

- State rationale for potential mobility problems.
- List signs and symptoms of impaired physical mobility.
- Verbalize/demonstrate measures to prevent/minimize mobility problems.

Interventions

- Assess range of motion and strength of hands, arms, and legs.
- Assess mobility for ambulation and for self-care activities.
- Take steps to reduce environmental hazards.
- Encourage patient to perform active range of motion, perform moderate exercise, and receive adequate rest.
- Assist patient with ambulation as needed.

Nursing Diagnosis

- *Feeding self-care deficit; bathing/hygiene self-care deficit; dressing/grooming self-care deficit, related to CNS involvement, disease progression*

Outcome Goals

Patient will be able to:

- Verbalize rationale for potential self-care deficit.
- Verbalize/demonstrate measures to prevent/minimize deficits.
- Perform activities of daily living within limits of functional capacity.

Interventions

- Assess patient's abilities for:
  Self-feeding
  Self-bathing and self-grooming
  Self-dressing
- Assess patient's motivation and endurance for self-care.
- Promote patient's maximum involvement in self-care activities.
- Provide assistance with self-care activities as appropriate to patient's level of functioning.

Nursing Diagnosis

- *Sensory/perceptual alterations (specify) related to CNS involvement*

Outcome Goals

Patient will be able to:

- Verbalize rationale for potential sensory alterations.
- Identify signs and symptoms related to sensory changes.

Interventions

- Assess patient for level of orientation and level of activity.
- Orient patient to all three spheres as needed.
- Provide meaningful sensory input (e.g., clock, calendar, familiar objects).
- Explain all activities and request patient's perception of situation.
- If patient becomes confused, direct back to reality.

Nursing Diagnosis

- *Altered sexuality patterns, related to disease process, treatment*

Outcome Goals

Patient will be able to:

- Verbalize impact of disease and treatment on sexuality.
- Maintain satisfying sexual role.

Interventions

- Assess for physical symptoms that may affect libido:
  Fatigue
  Nausea and vomiting
  Anorexia
  Pain
- Assess for fear, anxiety, depression, and diminished self-concept.
- Promote open communication about sexual issues by bringing up the subject.
- Discuss possible effects of disease and treatment regimen on libido and sexual functioning (see Chapter 33).

Nursing Diagnosis

- *Altered tissue perfusion, related to lymphadenopathy*

Outcome Goals

Patient will be able to:

- Verbalize rationale for potential lymphedema.
- State signs and symptoms of lymphedema.
- Maintain usual functional status.

Interventions

- Assess for signs and symptoms of lymphedema:
  Redness
  Warmth
  Swelling
- Assess function of surrounding tissues and organs.
- Encourage mobility of affected limb.
- Elevate affected limb.
- Assess for infection secondary to lymphedema.

Chapter Questions

1. Which is the *true* statement regarding incidence of Hodgkin's disease?
   a. Incidence peaks in the 20s and 30s.
   b. Incidence peaks in the 60s and 70s.
   c. Incidence gradually increases after age 20, then decreases after age 50.
   d. Incidence has two peaks, between ages 20 and 29 and again after age 60.

2. According to the WHO classification system, Hodgkin's disease is divided into which two major groups:
   a. Nodular lymphocyte predominance Hodgkin's disease and classical Hodgkin's disease
   b. Mixed cellularity Hodgkin's disease and nodular sclerosis Hodgkin's disease
   c. Lymphocyte depletion Hodgkin's disease and nodular lymphocyte predominance Hodgkin's disease
   d. Nodular sclerosis Hodgkin's disease and classical Hodgkin's disease

3. Which of the following types of Hodgkin's disease has the best prognosis?
   a. Lymphocyte predominance Hodgkin's disease
   b. Mixed cellularity Hodgkin's disease
   c. Lymphocyte depletion Hodgkin's disease
   d. Nodular sclerosis Hodgkin's disease

4. What are B symptoms?
   a. Lymphadenopathy, weight loss, fever
   b. Pruritus, weight loss, fever
   c. Weight loss, fever, night sweats
   d. Lymphadenopathy, fever, night sweats

5. Which of the following is a *true* statement regarding treatment for a patient with Hodgkin's disease relapsing after a long disease-free survival?
   a. Treatment of choice is radiation and combination chemotherapy.
   b. Treatment of choice is standard combination chemotherapy.
   c. Treatment of choice is radiation and ABMT.
   d. Treatment of choice is chemotherapy and ABMT.

6. Which is the most frequently used classification system for non-Hodgkin's lymphoma?
   a. Rappaport system
   b. NCI clinical schema
   c. Ann Arbor system
   d. WHO Classification of Neoplastic Diseases of the Hematopoietic and Lymphoid Tissues

7. The most common presenting symptom of NHL is:
   a. Mediastinal lymphadenopathy
   b. Painless generalized lymphadenopathy
   c. Painful lymph nodes
   d. Retroperitoneal lymphadenopathy

8. Treatment plan for stage I and II indolent NHL would include:
   a. Radiation therapy
   b. Single-agent chemotherapy
   c. Combination chemotherapy
   d. Radiation therapy and chemotherapy

9. Your patient was admitted last night with pain and swelling of the right leg and groin. The night nurse reports that the patient's diagnosis is lymphoblastic lymphoma. To what might you attribute the painfully swollen leg?
   a. Deep vein thrombosis
   b. Infection
   c. Lymphedema
   d. Radiation therapy

10. Your friend's mother has been diagnosed with indolent lymphoma. She is very distressed and asks if her mother will die soon. What is the prognosis for this disease?
    a. Prognosis is grim; patients may live only weeks untreated.
    b. Prognosis is fair; patients may live several months untreated.
    c. Prognosis is fair; patients may live many months untreated.
    d. Prognosis is good; patients may live years untreated.

BIBLIOGRAPHY

1. Bilodeau BA, Fessele KL: Non-Hodgkin's lymphoma, *Semin Oncol Nurs* 14:273, 1998.
2. Canellos GP: Hodgkin's disease. In Freireich EJ, Kantarjian HM, editors: *Medical management of hematological malignant diseases,* New York, Marcel Dekker, 1999.
3. Cotran RS, Kumar V, Collins T: *Robbins pathologic basis of disease,* ed 6, Philadelphia, Saunders, 1999.
4. DeVita VT, Mauch PM, Harris NL: Hodgkin's disease. In DeVita VT, Hellman S, Rosenberg SA, editors: *Cancer: principles and practice of oncology,* ed 5, Philadelphia, Lippincott-Raven, 1997.
5. Fine NMH, Scallion LE: Hodgkin's disease. In Miaskowski C, Bushsel P, editors: *Oncology nursing: assessment and clinical care,* St. Louis, Mosby, 1999.
6. Freedman AS, Nadler LM: Malignancies of lymphoid cells. In Fauci AS and others, editors: *Harrison's principles of internal medicine,* ed 14, New York, McGraw-Hill, 1998.
7. Gil-Delgado MA, Khayat D, Johnson SAN: Lymphomas. In Pollock RE, editor: *Manual of clinical oncology,* ed 7, New York, Wiley-Liss, 1999.
8. Greenlee RT and others: Cancer statistics, 2000, *CA Cancer J Clin* 50:7, 2000.
9. Greer JP, Macon WR, McCurley TL: Non-Hodgkin's lymphoma. In Lee GR and others, editors: *Wintrobe's*

Clinical hematology, ed 10, Baltimore, Williams & Wilkins, 1999.

10. Harris NL and others: The World Health Organization classification of neoplastic diseases of haematopoietic and lymphoid tissues: report of the Clinical Advisory Committee meeting, Airlie House, VA, November 1997, *Histopathology* 36:69, 2000.

11. Jox A and others: Hodgkin's disease—new treatment strategies toward the cure of patients. *Cancer Treat Rev* 25:269, 1999.

12. Koeppen H, Vardiman JW: New entities, issues and controversies in the classification of malignant lymphoma, *Semin Oncol* 25:421, 1998.

13. Lister A: The management of Hodgkin's disease, *Cancer genesis of lymphomas, Curr Opin Oncol* 11:351, 1999.

14. Lyons SF, Leibowitz DN: The roles of human viruses in the pathogenesis of lymphoma, *Semin Oncol* 25:461, 1998.

15. Marlton P, Cabanillas F: Therapy of aggressive lymphoma. In Freireich EJ, Kantarjian HM, editors: *Medical management of hematological malignant diseases,* New York, Marcel Dekker, 1999.

16. Molina A, Pezner RD: Non-Hodgkin's lymphoma. In Pazdur R and others, editors: *Cancer management: a multidisciplinary approach,* ed 3, Melville, NY, PRR, Inc., 1998.

17. Morgan DS, Horning SJ: The indolent lymphomas. In Freireich EJ, Kantarjian HM, editors: *Medical management of hematological malignant diseases,* New York, Marcel Dekker, 1999.

18. Moskowitz CH, Portlock CS: Non-Hodgkin's lymphoma. In Kirkwood JM, Lotze MT, Yasko JM, editors: *Current cancer therapeutics,* ed 3, Philadelphia, Churchill Livingstone, 1998.

19. Portlock CS, Glick J: Hodgkin's disease: clinical manifestation, staging, and treatment. In Hoffman R and others, editors: *Hematology: basic principles and practice,* ed 3, New York, Churchill Livingstone, 2000.

20. Portlock CS, Hahalom J: Hodgkin's disease. In Goldman L, Bennett JC, editors: *Cecil textbook of medicine,* ed 21, Philadelphia, Saunders, 2000.

21. Pugh WC, McBride JA: The pathologic basis for the classification of non-Hodgkin's lymphoma. In Hoffman R and others, editors: *Hematology: basic principles and practice,* ed 3, New York, Churchill Livingstone, 2000.

22. Sarris A, Ford R: Recent advances in the molecular pathoeditors: *Wintrobe's clinical hematology,* ed 10, Baltimore, Williams & Wilkins, 1999.

23. Shipp MA, Mauch PM, Harris NL: Non-Hodgkin's lymphoma. In DeVita VT, Hellman S, Rosenberg SA, editors: *Cancer: principles and practice of oncology,* ed 5, Philadelphia, Lippincott-Raven, 1997.

24. Shipp MA, Harris NL: Non-Hodgkin's lymphomas. In Goldman L, Bennett JC, editors: *Cecil textbook of medicine,* ed 21, Philadelphia, Saunders, 2000.

25. Sompayrac L: *How the Immune system works,* Malden, MA, Blackwell Science, 1999.

26. Stein H: Hodgkin's disease: biology and origin of Hodgkin and Reed-Sternberg cells, *Cancer Treat Rev* 25:161, 1999.

27. Stein RS: Hodgkin disease. In Lee GR and others, editors: *Wintrobe's clinical hematology,* ed 10, Baltimore, Williams & Wilkins, 1999.

28. Stevens ML: *Fundamentals of clinical hematology,* Philadelphia, Saunders, 1997.

29. Van Besien K, Cabanillas F: Clinical manifestations, staging, and treatment of non-Hodgkin's lymphoma. In Hoffman R and others, editors: *Hematology: basic principles and practice,* ed 3, New York, Churchill Livingstone, 2000.

30. Vose JM: Current approaches to the management of non-Hodgkin's lymphoma, *Semin Oncol* 25:483, 1998.

31. Yahalom J, Straus D: Hodgkin's disease. In Pazdur R and others, editors: *Cancer management: a multidisciplinary approach,* ed 3, Melville, NY, PRR, Inc., 1998.

32. Yuen AR, Horning SJ: Hodgkin's disease. In Kirkwood JM, Lotze MT, Yasko JM, editors: *Current cancer therapeutics,* ed 3, Philadelphia, Churchill Livingstone, 1998.

Multiple Myeloma

Shirley E. Otto

CHAPTER 17

EPIDEMIOLOGY

Multiple myeloma is a rare malignancy of plasma cells that accounts for only 1.1% of all hematologic malignancies diagnosed in the United States. The disease accounted for an estimated 13,600 new cases and 11,200 deaths in the year 2000. An increase in the incidence rate over the past decades is partially attributable to an improvement in diagnostic techniques.[16]

Multiple myeloma is diagnosed in an equal number of men and women and occurs 14 times more frequently in African Americans than in whites. However, the death rate among African Americans is approximately twice that of whites. Multiple myeloma is diagnosed primarily in individuals over 40 years of age, with a peak incidence at about 70 years of age.[36]

ETIOLOGY AND RISK FACTORS

The etiology of multiple myeloma is not understood. Basic research in animal models has identified cellular factors such as chromosomal abnormalities, host-genetic factors, chronic antigenic stimulation, viruses, and growth factors as possible contributors to the development of plasma cell dyscrasias. Other host factors, such as increasing age, race, and occupational exposure to petroleum products, rubber, farming-related chemicals, asbestos, and radiation, may contribute to increasing risk for the disease.[3, 6, 36]

PREVENTION, SCREENING, AND DETECTION

No recommendations exist for the prevention or screening of asymptomatic individuals for multiple myeloma. Detection of multiple myeloma in symptomatic individuals is based on a thorough history, physical examination, laboratory findings, and radiographic studies.

CLINICAL FEATURES

Although some individuals may be asymptomatic, most patients present to the clinician with a history of weakness, anorexia, weight loss, and fatigue. Symptoms of more advanced disease include bone pain, particularly in the back, and anemia. Depending on the sites of involvement, additional symptoms may include recurrent infection, changes in urinary patterns, and cognitive, sensory, or motor changes. Findings on physical examination are related to the sites of involvement. Fever, redness, swelling, tenderness, and pus formation associated with bacterial infections may be present. Peripheral neuropathies may be noted. The skin may be pale, and petechiae or ecchymoses may be present. See the Clinical Features and Complications boxes.[6, 9, 21, 36]

DIAGNOSIS AND STAGING

The diagnosis of multiple myeloma is based on findings obtained from laboratory and radiographic studies. Serum and urine electrophoretic and immunologic studies reveal elevations in IgG, IgA, and light-chain levels. Additional laboratory studies may demonstrate anemia, thrombocytopenia, and leukopenia in the presence of bone marrow involvement, hypercalcemia in the presence of lytic bone lesions, and proteinuria, hyperuricemia, azotemia, and elevated blood urea nitrogen (BUN), creatinine, and Bence-Jones urine protein levels with renal involvement. Radiographic studies typically include skeletal x-ray films, bone surveys, and magnetic resonance imaging (MRI) to detect the presence of osteoporosis, osteolytic lesions, or pathologic fractures. For a diagnosis of multiple myeloma to be made, one or more of the following criteria must be met: (1) plasma cell infiltration of the bone marrow of at least 10%, (2) a monoclonal spike on serum or urine electrophoresis, (3) radiographic confirmation of osteoporosis and osteolytic lesions, and (4) soft-tissue plasma cell tumors (Figs. 17–1 and 17–2).[6, 9, 12, 21, 29, 36]

No universal staging system for multiple myeloma currently exists. Box 17–1 outlines one example of a frequently used staging system based on tumor burden.

> ### CLINICAL FEATURES
> #### Multiple Myeloma
>
> Anorexia, fatigue, weight loss
> Back and bone pain
> Recurrent infections
> Changes in cognitive, sensory, and motor function and urinary pattern

TREATMENT MODALITIES

Treatment of multiple myeloma in the early stages of the disease consists of observation if patients are asymptomatic. Patients are monitored with interval clinical examinations and laboratory and radiographic studies for signs of progressive disease such as severe anemia, thrombocytopenia and leukopenia, bone pain, osteolysis, or renal failure. Once progression of disease is documented, active treatment with antineoplastic agents or radiation therapy is initiated.

Chemotherapy

Chemotherapy usually consists of intermittent melphalan and prednisone and results in a 70% response rate. Responses are generally short-term, and some patients experience progression of the disease with drug resistance. Clinicians have used combinations of prednisone, high-dose melphalan, vincristine, carmustine (BCNU), cyclophosphamide, and doxorubicin. Examples of combination chemotherapy regimens include: VMCP—vincristine, melphalan, carmustine, prednisone; VBAP—vincristine, carmustine, doxorubicin, and prednisone; and VCAP—vincristine, chyclosphosphamide, doxorubicin, and prednisone. Systemic combination chemotherapy has demonstrated a survival ranging from 18 months to 36 months, with an over median survival of 24 months. The use of biologic therapy with interferon-alfa and interleukin-2 has shown advantages when used in combination with antineoplastic agents.[6, 12, 18, 36]

Radiation Therapy

Radiation therapy may be used to treat patients with chemotherapy-resistant disease, to relieve bone pain, and to treat spinal cord compression. It has been estimated that 70% of all patients eventually require and potentially benefit from radiation therapy as a palliative agent. Although radiation therapy can greatly improve the quality of life for patients with multiple myeloma, the length of survival is not enhanced.[36]

Peripheral Blood Stem Cell Transplantation

Recently, the role of autologous peripheral blood stem cell transplantation (PBSCT) in the treatment of patients with multiple myeloma is being used for selected patients—age less than 65, stage of disease, and having a favorable response to initial chemotherapy. Success has been limited by the inability to eradicate the malignant plasma cell clone. However, researchers continue to evaluate the effectiveness of high-dose antineoplastic therapy followed by autogolous PBSCT with marrow that has been purged with an antibody specific for plasma cells. In addition, researchers are exploring the application of autologous PBSCT earlier in the course of the disease.[1, 32, 36, 38] (see Chapter 25).

The use of allogeneic PBSCT in the treatment of multiple myeloma is limited by age (<55 years) and the lack of an appropriate marrow donor. Only a small number of patients are eligible for allogeneic PBSCT. As associated high mortality rate occurs, with more than half the patients dying in the first year after transplants due to disease- and treatment-related complications. Approximately 44% of patients achieve a complete remission with autologous and allogeneic PBSCT.[36, 38]

Biologic Response Modifiers

Recently, interferon-alfa has been used alone and in combination with conventional chemotherapy to treat patients with multiple myeloma. Response rates among patients previously untreated and among patients who were refractory to conventional therapy make interferon-alfa a promising second-line treatment. Given the results of recent studies on the effect of

> ### COMPLICATIONS
> #### Multiple Myeloma
>
> **Disease Related**
>
> Thrombocytopenia
> Severe anemia
> Leukopenia and renal failure
> Spinal cord compression
> Hypercalcemia
> Dehydration
> Lytic bone lesions
> Pathologic fractures
> Repeated infections
>
> **Treatment Related**
>
> Myelosuppression
> Renal insufficiency
> Mental status changes
> Neuropathy
> Cardiopulmonary toxicities

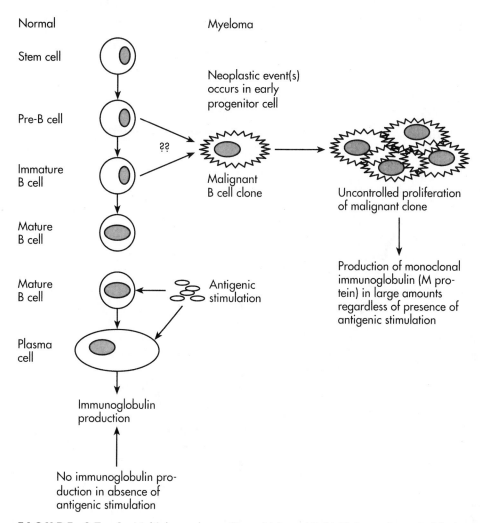

FIGURE 17-1 Multiple myeloma. (From Malamed S: Multiple myeloma. In Miaskowski C, Buchsel P, editors: *Oncology nursing assessment and clinical care,* St. Louis, Mosby, 1999.)

interleukin-2 and interleukin-6 on disease progression, the role of biologic therapy in the treatment of patients with multiple myeloma is only beginning to be explored.[36]

Colony-stimulating factors such as Epogen for anemia; Neupogen for granulocyte recovery; sargramostin for granulocyte, eosinophil, and monocyte recovery; and oprelvekin prevent thrombocytopenia following combination chemotherapy, high-dose chemotherapy, and allogeneic and autologous marrow transplantations. These drugs have lessened the myelosuppressive effects related to the associated therapies and have improved the overall survival outcomes.[4, 8, 10, 26, 27, 31, 35]

PROGNOSIS

Multiple myeloma is an incurable disease. The course of disease progression for patients is determined by the severity of organ involvement at the time of diagnosis and response to active treatment. Asymptomatic patients may live with the disease for months to years without active treatment. For symptomatic patients requiring treatment, a pattern of response has been described. During the initial 2 to 3 years of treatment, patients respond well to antineoplastic therapy. A plateau phase follows when the disease remains stable but does not respond as well as in the initial phase. During the third phase the disease becomes resistant to the antineoplastic therapy and progresses at a rapid rate. Survival can range from a few months to more than 10 years, with a median survival of 2.5 to 3 years. A statistically significant improvement in the relative 5-year survival rate, from 12% to 28%, occurred from the 1960s to 1990s. For the year 2000 survival rates include 32% at 4 years, 28% at 7 years, and for stage I disease 52% at 4 years

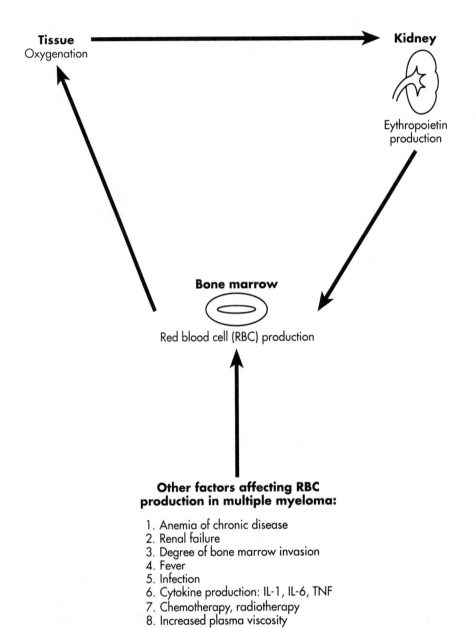

**Other factors affecting RBC
production in multiple myeloma:**

1. Anemia of chronic disease
2. Renal failure
3. Degree of bone marrow invasion
4. Fever
5. Infection
6. Cytokine production: IL-1, IL-6, TNF
7. Chemotherapy, radiotherapy
8. Increased plasma viscosity

FIGURE 17 – 2 Development of normal and myeloma B cells. (From Malamed S: Multiple myeloma. In Miaskowski C, Buchsel P, editors: *Oncology nursing assessment and clinical care,* St. Louis, Mosby, 1999.)

BOX 17-1

Myeloma Staging System

I. Multiple myeloma
  Major criteria
  A. Plasmacytoma on tissue biopsy
  B. Bone marrow plasmacytosis with >30% plasma cells
  C. Monoclonal globulin spike on serum electrophoresis exceeding 3.5 g/dL for G peaks or 2.0 g/dL for A peaks, ≥ 1.0 g/24 hours of κ- or λ-light-chain excretion on urine electrophoresis in presence of amyloidosis
  Minor criteria
  1. Bone marrow plasmacytosis 10–30% plasma cells
  2. Monoclonal globulin spike present, but less than the level defined above
  3. Lytic bone lesions
  4. Residual normal IgM < 50 mg/dL, IgA < 100 mg/dL, IgG < 600 mg/dL. Diagnosis confirmed when any of following features are documented in symptomatic patients with clearly progressive disease. Diagnosis of myeloma requires a minimum of one major + one minor criterion or three minor criteria that must include A + B, that is,
    a. A + 2, A + 3, A + 4 (A + 1 not sufficient)
    b. B + 2, B + 3, B + 4
    c. C + 1, C + 3, C + 4
    d. 1 + 2 + 3, 1 + 2 + 4

II. Indolent myeloma
  Same as myeloma except:
  A. No bone lesions or only limited bone lesions (≤3 lytic lesions); no compression fractures
  B. M-component levels: (1) IgG < 7 g/dL; (2) IgA < 5/dL
  C. No symptoms or associated disease features, that is,
    1. Performance status > 70%
    2. Hemoglobin > 10 g/dL
    3. Serum calcium normal
    4. Serum creatinine < 2.0 mg/dL
    5. No infections
III. Smoldering myeloma
  Same as indolent myeloma except:
  A. No bone lesions
  B. Bone marrow plasma cells ≥ 30%
IV. Monoclonal gammopathy of undetermined significance (MGUS)
  A. Monoclonal gammopathy
  B. M-component level
    1. IgG ≤ 3.5 g/dL
    2. IgA ≤ 2.0 g/dL
    3. BJ protein ≤ 1.0 g/24 hours
  C. Bone marrow plasma cells < 10%
  D. No bone lesions
  E. No symptoms

IgA, Immunoglobulin A; *IgG,* immunoglobulin G; *IgM,* immunoglobulin M; *BJ,* Bence-Jones light chain.
Modified from Salmon SE, Cassady JR: Plasma cell neoplasms. In DeVita VT Jr, Hellman S, Rosenberg SA, editors, *Cancer: principles and practice of oncology,* ed 5, Philadelphia, Lippincott-Raven, 1997.

---

for patients receiving autologous or allogeneic (or both) stem cell transplantation.[6, 9, 17, 22, 36]

CONCLUSION

The patient with multiple myeloma presents many challenges to the health care team during the course of the disease. Because no cure for the disease is available and its course is protracted over several years for most patients, the team's focus is to plan with the patient and significant others care that will maintain independence in activities of daily living, provide a safe living and treatment environment, and preserve an acceptable level of patient comfort. The care demands cooperation and support from significant others and members of the health care team in acute care, community, and home settings.

Nursing Management

Nursing care for the patient with multiple myeloma centers on educating the patient and significant others about the disease and treatment, teaching self-care skills to minimize threats to quality of life, monitoring for signs and symptoms of complications of the disease and treatment, and coordinating implementation of an interdisciplinary plan of care that addresses complications of the disease and treatment. The teaching plan for patients with multiple myeloma and their significant others includes information about the chronic nature of the disease, rationale for observation in patients without symptoms, and health-enhancing strategies such as maintaining an adequate fluid intake of 3000 mL each day, maintaining mobility to decrease the risk of bone destruction from inactivity, and instituting safety precautions to minimize the risk of injury from thrombocytopenia, anemia, and leukopenia. Specific nursing interventions to address common nursing diagnoses among patients with multiple myeloma are presented in other chapters in this text (see Chapters 30 and 31).

Because bony destruction is a common effect of multiple myeloma and pathologic fractures can alter the quality of life significantly, safety precautions are

Nursing Assessments for Complications of Multiple Myeloma

Complication	Nursing Assessments
Renal insufficiency	Monitor BUN, creatinine, uric acid, calcium, potassium, glucose, and phosphorus levels as ordered by the physician.
	Assess for changes in the character of the urine: volume, color, and odor.
Hyperviscosity syndrome	Monitor for intermittent claudication and changes in the skin color of the extremities.
	Assess for neurologic changes, such as headache or visual disturbances.
	Monitor for changes in mental status, such as irritability, drowsiness, confusion, or coma.
	Assess for signs and symptoms of congestive heart failure.
Dehydration	Monitor intake and output every 8 hours. Assess skin turgor each day. Evaluate subjective symptoms by patient, such as thirst and dry skin.

Data from references 2, 5, 7, 14, 23, 27, 33, and 34.

PATIENT TEACHING PRIORITIES

Multiple Myeloma

In teaching the patient with multiple myeloma, the nurse must consider critical aspects of the disease and treatment that potentially affect the quality of life for the patient. Teaching must be reinforced verbally, with written materials that are culturally sensitive, and with appropriate audiovisual resources.

Self-Care Activities

Create a safe environment: remove throw rugs, install safety equipment in bathrooms, keep frequently used articles within reach, and remove articles from frequently traveled paths.
Maintain range of motion, muscle strength, and endurance within limitations of bony involvement.
Monitor dietary calcium intake.
Monitor oral intake and urine output.

Symptoms to Report to Health Care Team

Signs of infection: fever, chills, pain, erythema, swelling, pus formation
Signs of dehydration: thirst, lethargy, decreased skin turgor, decreased urine output, increased urine concentration
Increased lethargy, mental confusion, apathy

Demands of Treatment

Routine appointments for treatment and follow-up at regular intervals
Estimate of direct costs (e.g., drugs, supplies) and indirect costs of therapy (e.g., transportation, time away from work).

stressed in developing a long-term plan of care.[9, 20, 28, 33, 34, 35, 37]

Nursing Diagnosis

- *Injury, risk for, related to bony destruction by plasma cell tumors*

Outcome Goal

Patient will be able to:

- Participate in strategies to decrease risks of pathologic fractures.

Assessment

- Identify personal risk factors for injury: extent and sites of bony involvement, muscle strength of extremities, changes in sensation, difficulty in ambulating, type of shoes worn when ambulating, knowledge of proper body mechanics, mental status.

- Identify environmental risk factors for injury: crowded rooms, throw rugs, proximity of needed articles, or bathroom.
- Assess perceived threats to safety from patient's perspective.

Interventions

- Consult physical therapy for instruction in proper body mechanics, transfer techniques, positioning, and use of assistive devices for development of an exercise program to maintain muscle strength and range of motion without jeopardizing risk of pathologic fractures.
- Arrange hospital room environment to decrease the risks to safety: telephone, call light, and personal articles within easy reach and clear pathway to the bathroom.
- Refer to home health agency to evaluate home environment for safety risk factors and recommended modifications before discharge.
- Encourage patient to ask for assistance from health care team or significant others, as needed, with ambulation or activities of daily living.
- The nurse also assumes responsibility for monitoring the patient with multiple myeloma for signs and symptoms of complications of the disease and treatment, such as hypercalcemia, pain, spinal cord compression, renal insufficiency, hyperviscosity

---

GERIATRIC CONSIDERATIONS

Multiple Myeloma

Peak incidence of disease: 70 years of age

Issues regarding occupation and potential for early retirement

Social and recreational activities may need adjustment to conserve energy and minimize injury risks

Potential for mental status changes

Consider environmental safety factors and abilities to meet self-care needs for hygiene, nutrition, elimination, and comfort

Data from references 17, 20, 21, 24, 33, and 35.

---

syndrome, and dehydration. Often, early recognition and treatment of these complications will result in improvement in the patient's ability to tolerate treatment and in quality of life. Specific nursing assessments and interventions for patients at risk for or experiencing hypercalcemia, spinal cord compression, and pain are detailed in Chapters 20 and 30. Nursing assessments to monitor for renal insufficiency, dehydration, and hyperviscosity syndrome are presented in detail in the table on page 444. Presence of any of the signs and symptoms should be reported to the physician.

- See also Patient Teaching Priorities and Geriatric Considerations boxes.

Chapter Questions

1. Multiple myeloma occurs in approximately __% of the U.S. population.
   a. 1%
   b. 5%
   c. 10%
   d. 15%

2. Multiple myeloma is diagnosed primarily in individuals ages __ with a peak incidence __ years.
   a. Over 30 years of age, peak incidence about 60 years
   b. Over 50 years of age, peak incidence about 65 years
   c. Over 60 years of age, peak incidence about 75 years
   d. Over 40 years of age, peak incidence about 70 years

3. Clinical features associated with multiple myeloma include:

   a. Anorexia, nausea, headaches, cardiac and hepatic function, and urinary pattern
   b. Anorexia, nausea, leg pain, respiratory and endocrine function, and urinary pattern
   c. Anorexia, fatigue, bone pain, sensory and motor function, and urinary pattern
   d. Anorexia, fatigue, leg pain, cardiac and hepatic function and urinary pattern

4. Chemotherapy drugs commonly used in combination treatment for multiple myeloma include:
   a. Melphalan, prednisone, vinblastine, danorubicin, cyclophosphamide, and BCNU
   b. Melphalan, prednisone, vincristine, doxorubicin, cyclophosphamide, and BCNU
   c. Melphalan, prednisone, vinblastine, doxorubicin, ifosfamide, and BCNU
   d. Melphalan, prednisone, vincristine, daunorubicin, ifosfamide, and BCNU

5. Which of the following symptoms is the most important for the patient with multiple myeloma to report to the nurse and/or physician?
   a. Increase in the severity of pain with movement

b. Presence of edema in the lower extremities

c. Increase in the level of fatigue with activity

d. Loss of sensation to pain in the lower extremities

BIBLIOGRAPHY

1. Alcoser PW, Burchett S: Bone marrow transplantation: immune system suppression and reconstitution, *AJN* 99:26, 1999.

2. Alexander J: Nursing care of the client with lymphoma and multiple myeloma. In Itano JK, Taoka KN, editors: *Core curriculum for oncology nursing,* ed 3, Philadelphia, Saunders, 1998.

3. Berger A, Portenoy R, Weissman D: *Principles and practices of supportive oncology,* Philadelphia, Lippincott-Raven, 1998.

4. Boyle DA and others: Quality improvement initiatives in bone marrow transplant nursing, *Innovations in Breast Cancer* 3:57, 1998.

5. Brophy L: Immunology. In Itano JK, Taoka KN, editors: *Core curriculum for oncology nursing,* ed 3, Philadelphia, Saunders, 1998.

6. Bubley GJ, Schnipper LE: Multiple myeloma. In Holleb AI, Fink DJ, Murphy GP, editors: *American Cancer Society textbook of clinical oncology,* Atlanta, American Cancer Society, 1995.

7. Camp-Sorrell D: Myelosuppression. In Itano JK, Taoka KN, editors: *Core curriculum for oncology nursing,* ed 3, Philadelphia, Saunders, 1998.

8. Cella D, Bron D: The effect of epoetin alfa on quality of life in anemic cancer patients, *Cancer Practice* 7:177, 1999.

9. Clark JC: Multiple myeloma. In Otto SE, editor: *Oncology nursing,* ed 3, St. Louis, Mosby, 1997.

10. Comley AL and others: Effect of subcutaneous granulocyte colony-stimulating factor injectate volume on drug efficacy, site complications, and client comfort, *Oncol Nurs Forum* 26:87, 1999.

12. DeVita VT Jr: Principles of cancer management: chemotherapy. In DeVita VT Jr, Hellman S, Roseman SA, editors: *Cancer: principles and practice of oncology,* ed 5, Philadelphia, Lippincott-Raven, 1997.

13. Ehrenberger H, Murray PJ: Issues in the communications technologies in nursing research. *Oncol Nurs Forum* 25:4, 1999.

14. Ferrell BR, editor: Pain management. *Quality of Life: A Nursing Challenge* 4(4):85, 1997.

15. Gahart BL, Nazareno AR: *Intravenous medications,* ed 16, St. Louis, Mosby, 2000.

16. Greenlee RT and others: Cancer statistics 2000, *CA Cancer J Clin* 50:7, 2000.

17. Harris KA: The informational needs of patients with cancer and their families, *Cancer Practice* 6:39, 1998.

18. Haylock PJ: Cancer metastasis: an update, *Semin Oncol Nursing* 14:172, 1998.

19. Johnson BL, Gross J: *Handbook of oncology nursing,* ed 3, Boston, Jones and Bartlett, 1998.

20. Levitt SH: Managing pain in elderly patients, *JAMA* 281:605, 1999.

21. Malamed S: Multiple myeloma. In Miaskowski C, Buchsel P, editors: *Oncology nursing assessment and clinical care,* St. Louis, Mosby, 1999.

22. Mayer D: Cancer patient empowerment, *Oncology Nursing Updates* 6:1, 1999.

23. McCaffery M, Pasero C: *Pain clinical manual,* St. Louis, Mosby, 1999.

24. Miaskowski C, Lee KA: Pain, fatigue, and sleep disturbances in oncology outpatients receiving radiation therapy for bone metastasis: a pilot study, *J Pain Symptom Manage* 17:320, 1999.

25. McCorkle R and others: *Cancer nursing: a comprehensive textbook,* ed 2, Philadelphia, Saunders, 1997.

26. Moldawer N, Carr E: The promise of recombinant interleukin-2, *AJN* 100:35, 2000.

27. Myers JS: Supportive care in preventing and reducing cancer therapy-induced toxicities, *New Therapies Symposia Highlights* 10, Bala Cynwyd, PA, Meniscus, 1999.

28. Oncology Nursing Society: *Cancer chemotherapy guidelines and recommendations for practice,* Pittsburgh, Oncology Nursing Press, 1999.

29. Pagana KD, Pagana TJ: *Mosby's diagnostic & laboratory test reference,* St. Louis, Mosby, 1998.

30. Phipps WJ, Sands JK, Marek JF: *Medical-surgical nursing: concepts and clinical practice,* ed 6, St. Louis, Mosby, 1999.

31. Rieger PT: *Clinical handbook of biotherapy,* Boston, Jones and Bartlett, 1999.

32. Rieger PT: Management of cancer in the next millennium: DNA holds the key, *Highlights in Oncology Practice* 16:110, 1999.

33. Pearce JD: Alterations in moblility, skin integrity, and neurologic status. In Itano JK, Taoka KN, editors: *Core curriculum for oncology nursing,* ed 3, Philadelphia, Saunders, 1998.

34. Peterson PG: Sepsis and septic shock. In Chernecky C, Berger B, editors: *Advanced and critical care oncology nursing,* Philadelphia, Saunders, 1998.

35. Petursson CT: Bleeding due to thrombocytopenia. In Yasko JM: *Nursing management of symptoms associated with chemotherapy,* Bala Cynwyd, PA, Pharmacia & Upjohn, Meniscus Health Care Communications, 1998.

36. Salmon SE, Cassady JR: Plasma cell neoplasms. In DeVita VT Jr, Hellman S, Rosenberg SA, editors: *Cancer: principles and practice of oncology,* ed 5, Philadelphia, Lippincott-Raven, 1997.

37. Van Gulick AJ: Anemia. In Yasko JM: *Nursing management of symptoms associated with chemotherapy,* Bala Cynwyd, PA, Pharmacia & Upjohn, Meniscus Health Care Communications, 1998.

38. Wagner ND, Quiones VW: Allogeneic peripheral blood stem cell transplantation: clinical overview and nursing implications, *Oncol Nurs Forum,* 25:1049, 1998.

Skin Cancers

Martha Langhorne

Skin cancer is the most common cancer in the United States and accounts for more than one third of all malignancies.[21] Cancer is diagnosed in the skin more often than anywhere else in the body, and half the population will probably develop at least one skin cancer by the time they reach age 65.[2] During the last two to three decades, the incidence of skin cancer has increased alarmingly. This increase parallels the changing lifestyles of most Americans, which permits increased, mostly recreational, exposure to the harmful effects of sunlight.[26] Table 18–1 lists the major risks for skin cancers.

Arguably, there are reports that look favorably on sun exposure. These sources proclaim that the sun is instrumental in deterring or containing other serious life-threatening illnesses. Some studies report on the seasonal patterns of an increase in cardiovascular mortality and cardiovascular risk factors partly explained by reduced exposure to the sun during the winter months. Very subjectively, a heightened sense of "well being" for those suffering with mental illness or depression is often said to be derived from lying or sitting in the sun. It is known that sun exposure increases vitamin D production, reduces the risk of rickets in childhood, and is used to treat some forms of psoriasis. It has been suggested, based on the ecologic association with latitude, that exposure to sunlight reduces the incidence of multiple sclerosis.[29] This information, and in light of the fact that we are in a "self-care/holistic/herbal remedies" era of treating ourselves, may make the message of sun avoidance a hard one to accept.

Skin cancer is classified into two basic groups: nonmelanoma and malignant melanoma. Both nonmelanoma and melanoma skin cancers increase exponentially with age.[8] Nonmelanoma skin cancer is the term used to describe basal cell carcinoma (BCC) and squamous cell carcinoma (SCC).[14] These two cancers accounted for the approximately 1.3 million new cases of skin cancers in the United States in the year 2000. These cancers are highly curable and are more common among individuals with lightly pigmented skin.[1] A diagnosis of BCC or SCC does not, and should not, raise the kind of alarm signals associated with melanoma. Make no mistake, however, if left untreated SCC and BCC can result in serious morbidity and death.[14] It is estimated that the nonmelanoma skin cancers will account for nearly 30% of the 9600 deaths attributable to skin cancers in the year 2000.[1]

Malignant melanoma is the least common and most deadly of these three types of skin cancers.[7] It is estimated that 47,700 new cases of melanoma will occur in the United States and 7700 people will die from the disease in the year 2000. For the past 30 years the incidence rate of melanoma has risen at a rate of 4% per year. The incidence rate is 10 times higher in whites than in African Americans, and malignant melanoma is one of the most common cancers in young adults.[1, 8]

Nonmelanoma Skin Cancers

Basal Cell Carcinoma

EPIDEMIOLOGY

Basal cell carcinoma (BCC) is the most common cutaneous tumor, with more than a half-million cases diagnosed in the United States annually.[11] Comprising 60% of the primary skin cancers, BCC is characterized by a slow-growing lesion that invades local tissue.[41] Metastases are occasionally associated with cutaneous SCC, but only rarely with BCC.[46] Those metastases that do occur usually do so to local nodes.[37] BCC can be found on any area of the body, including those not exposed to the sun. It is most commonly found on the face, head, and neck but may be missed if situated behind the ear.[15, 48] Because it is primarily caused by sun exposure, it is unusual for BCC to be seen on the dorsal surface of the hand.[15] Table 18–2 lists the common sites of nonmelanoma skin cancers.

TABLE 18-1
Major Risk Factors for Skin Cancers

Risk Factor	Skin Cancer Risk
Personal factors	Excessive exposure to sunlight Easily burned Increasing age Premalignant states
Life-style	Outdoor work Outdoor recreational activities Chronic exposure to chemical agents
Drugs	Treatment for psoriasis (psoralen ultraviolet A [PUVA])
Immunologic factor	Organ transplant recipients

From Itano JK, Taoka KN, editors: Core curriculum for oncology nursing, ed 3, Philadelphia, Saunders, 1998:557.

The BCCs can grow in size and result in significant cosmetic and functional morbidity.[11] Although they can be any size, lesions typically range between 3 and 15 mm in diameter at initial presentation. A large BCC can become very destructive. Larger lesions are more likely to erode into muscle, cartilage, or bone.[14] This morbidity has profound socioeconomic consequences, such as increased hospitalizations and time missed from work.[15]

This form of skin cancer is named such because these cancer cells resemble the round cells found in the lower part or base of the epidermis.[3] Other names for this form of cancer include basal cell epithelioma, Jacob's ulcer, and rodent carcinoma.[15, 48] BCC derives from the same cell line as SCC, the keratinocytes. These basal cells/keratinocytes are situated at the lowest layer of the epidermis, just above the basement membrane that attaches the epidermis to the dermis. When one basal cell divides, one daughter cell advances slowly upward through the epidermis as a squamous cell, while the other remains along the basal layer to reproduce again.

This tumor is most commonly found in whites and rarely occurs in dark-skinned persons.[31] Unlike whites, African Americans who do get skin cancer are more likely to have SCC than BCC. When BCC occurs in African Americans, it is usually found on the face, head, or neck, and the lesions are clinically similar to those found in whites, although they are more likely to be of the pigmented type.[15]

CAUSAL FACTORS

The primary cause of skin cancer is the sun. Sun exposure causes skin cancer through the effects of ultraviolet (UV) radiation, which penetrates into the dermis and damages DNA. UV radiation is divided into three different wavelengths: UVA, UVB, and UVC.[18, 31] UVA radiation causes changes in blood vessels, contributes to aging, and is linked to carcinogenesis. UVA radiation waves are longer than UVB waves and are thought to be more damaging. Approximately 1000 times more UVA waves reach the earth's surface than UVB waves. UVB waves are shorter and cause redness to the skin, some DNA damage, and aging. Exposure to UVB radiation is associated with the development of malignant melanoma. UVC waves are the shortest and rarely reach the earth's surface because of the blocking effect of the ozone layer and offer little threat.[18, 31]

Exposure to solar radiation is increasing worldwide because the protective ozone layer is thinning.[18] Clear evidence indicates that ozone depletion is occurring over Antarctica, presumably as a result of the use of chlorofluorocarbons in the populated regions of the world.[5] Discussions of and opinions regarding changes in the ozone layer and the relationship of that phenomenon to skin cancer are both complicated and numerous.[31] Obviously, any factor that increases the overall amount of UVB radiation will lead to an increase in skin cancer.[5]

The bulk of the ozone lies within the stratosphere, the atmospheric level about 10 to 50 km (6–30 miles) above sea level. The ozone layer effectively blocks all UVC radiation and most UVB radiation, but UVA radiation will pass through unaffected.[5] Although it has been shown that UVB radiation is related to both melanoma and nonmelanoma skin cancers, it has not definitely been shown that stratospheric ozone depletion is translating into increasing penetrating UV radiation. Further studies are needed to determine the varying effects that ozone layer depletion may have on skin cancer development and trends.[31]

TABLE 18-2
Common Sites of Nonmelanoma Skin Cancers

Type of Skin Cancer	Common Sites
Nodular basal cell carcinoma	Face, head, neck
Superficial basal cell carcinoma	Trunk, extremities
Pigmented basal cell carcinoma	Face, head, neck
Morpheaform basal cell carcinoma	Head, neck
Squamous cell carcinoma	Head, nose, border of lips, hands

From Itano JK, Taoka KN, editors: Core curriculum for oncology nursing, ed 3, Philadelphia, Saunders, 1998:553.

ETIOLOGY AND RISK FACTORS

The risk of BCC increases with age; this type of skin cancer is relatively uncommon (although it is becoming more common) in persons younger than age 40. The higher incidence of BCC in older persons is most likely related to cumulative exposure to carcinogens, decreased capacity for DNA repair, and reduced density of melanocytes.[15] Individuals who freckle easily or have fair skin, red or blond hair, and blue or green eyes are at greatest risk for the development of BCC at a younger age. Several inherited syndromes make early onset of BCC more likely; these include albinism, xeroderma pigmentosum, or albinism and nevoid BCC syndrome. Other risk factors include a family history of BCC and being a farmer, sailor, or other worker who spends more than 3 hours a day outdoors, even in winter.[15]

Most tanning booths emit UVA radiation. Indoor tanning with UVA radiation is frequently promoted as providing protection against UVB sunburns. The deeper penetration of UVA waves into the dermis causes melanin production; however, the melanosomes are not transferred to the superficial layer of the skin, the epidermis. Persons with a UVA tan who are exposed to UVB radiation receive skin damage in the form of sunburns. The erythema associated with the sunburn is not visible because of the masking effect of the UVA suntan. Exposure to UV radiation from tanning beds should be avoided. Up to 23% of the light from tanning devices is in the UVB range, but even with pure UVA DNA damage, cancer, vascular damage, and melanocyte stimulation can occur.

Because BCC can be found on areas of the body not exposed to sun, factors other than sun exposure may play a part in its development. These include genetic determinants and exposure to chemical cocarcinogens, arsenic, or excessive amounts of ionizing radiation. Scars, burns, and chronic venous stasis ulcers may also create a predisposition to the development of BCC.[15]

There is conflicting information being examined regarding those who have basal cell skin cancer being at an increased risk for other cancers, primarily non-Hodgkin's lymphoma and salivary gland and lip cancer, although breast, larynx, leukemia, kidney, and testis are mentioned in some studies. These findings are limited because studies to date do not account for patterns of life-style, occupational exposure to carcinogens, family history of cancer, or comorbidities, particularly those associated with immunosuppression. Chronic sun exposure is felt to decrease the ability of DNA to repair itself and therefore increases the likelihood of immunosuppression, which could be linked to the reported rise in non-Hodgkin's lymphoma in those with BCC.[10, 29]

In the future we may see the development of a BCC skin cancer test. Currently, in the genetic revolution taking place, scientists working with frog embryos have identified the gene pathway for development of BCC. A particular gene, named Sonic Hedgehog by researchers, activates other genes in the development of BCC.[17] Also, within the Sonic Hedgehog pathway a protein called Gli1 is expressed. Scientists believe that Gli1 is present in 98% of BCCs and adjacent tissue areas. Gli1 could become an important marker and diagnostic tool. A simple chemical test to detect Gli1 in skin cancer could eliminate the need for painful biopsies.[17] Scientists are now trying to develop a new breed of mice whose skin is more similar to humans that would be genetically programmed to develop BCC in adulthood. Further understanding as to how this protein expresses itself could lead to new treatments and eventually a cure. The task would then be to develop topical agents, which could be applied to the skin to inhibit the function of the pathway.[17]

PREVENTION, SCREENING, AND DETECTION

Primary Prevention

Skin cancer may be the ideal cancer for prevention because risk factors for its development are well known, most notably UV radiation; thus, there are many opportunities for primary prevention. Sun exposure is the only risk factor that can be modified and has therefore been the target of most primary prevention programs. No clinical trials to date have evaluated whether or not limiting exposure to solar radiation is effective in reducing the risk of malignant melanoma and nonmelanoma skin cancer. This strategy would appear to be beneficial because multiple studies have linked sun exposure to both malignant melanoma and nonmelanoma skin cancer.[21] The primary prevention message for health care providers and the public is to stay away from the sun. This is primarily done through sun avoidance and the use of sunscreens.

Sun Avoidance. Skin cancers are unique in that UV exposure and susceptibility cause 90% of these malignancies. Therefore, methods that protect against this exposure should help in reducing the incidence of skin cancer.[38] The most effective way to prevent BCC is to protect skin from the sun.[15] Sun avoidance is felt to be far superior to sun protection. However, a certain amount of sun exposure is unavoidable.[11] Avoidance of long or excessive exposure through shelter or protective clothing has long been the mainstay of skin cancer protection.[12] Preventive measures to reduce sun exposure include sun avoidance, particularly between the hours of 10 AM and 3 PM, physical barriers such as hats and summer clothing, and sunscreens that offer a sun protective factor (SPF) of up to 30.[31]

Histologic changes from sun damage precede obvious clinical changes by at least a decade, and there is a 10- to 20-year latency period between UV exposure and clinical appearance of a tumor. Therefore, sun protection early in life is essential. Most exposure to the sun occurs during childhood. Children receive three times the annual sun exposure of adults.[18] It is estimated that 80% of a person's lifetime exposure to the sun occurs before age 18.[2, 40] Minimizing sun exposure for children is recommended.[40]

For residents of the southern areas of the country or high altitudes, the damaging effects of the sun's rays are especially strong.[45] The incidence of BCCs in the United States is highest in geographic areas where solar radiation is strongest, especially the Southeast coast, Florida, Texas, and Southern California.[32] Reflection of sunlight by water, sand, concrete, or snow intensifies the rate at which skin will burn. Skin is vulnerable even on a cloudy day; up to 80% of the sun's radiation still penetrates through the clouds.[45]

Outdoor activities, such as walking, gardening, and other hobbies, should be planned for the early morning or late afternoon. Prolonged sunbathing or outdoor activities for any longer than *2½ hours per day* puts an individual at risk for skin cancer.[31] There is also a misconception that a tan, obtained naturally or with the use of self-tanning products, will protect the skin from the harmful effects of the sun. However, a suntan does not provide enough protection against UV radiation, and a sunscreen should be used at all times.

Sunscreens. The use of sunscreens and sun protection in the middle and later years will prevent further photo damage; however, health care providers, patients, and the public alike must understand that there is no such thing as a "healthy tan." *Tanning indicates that excessive sun exposure has occurred.*[11]

The literature reflects varying opinions as to the benefit of sunscreen products. Sunscreens are important, but not a substitute for the avoidance measures.[22] Because evidence indicates that repeated short-term exposures to sun have a cumulative effect, patients should be advised to apply sunscreen to chronically sun-exposed areas of the face and forearms any day they will be leaving the house.

Due to the long lag time between the UV exposure and the development of cancer, the efficacy of sunscreen use is difficult to determine in humans.[21] Although recommended, it has been determined that sunscreens do block sunburn, but there is no definite proof that sunscreen actually prevents skin cancer. Studies often cited to support the view that sunscreen might not be of benefit were conducted prior to the 1980s, when the high-SPF 15+ became available. Most did not control for skin phenotype. Because fair-skinned persons are

more likely to use sunscreens, and more likely to get skin cancers, the cross-correlation of all these factors confounds these conclusions.[39]

To further complicate the issue, some sources feel the availability of high-SPF sunscreens can lead to increased time spent in the sun.[13] Therefore, patients using these sunscreens may prolong their exposure and actually increase their risk of developing skin cancer.[21] In one long-term Australian study results showed that there was no harmful effect of daily use of sunscreen and SCC rather than BCC was amenable to prevention through sunscreen use.[12] Patients should be advised to avoid sunbathing. Those who insist on sunbathing should be advised to avoid midday sun and to apply a high-SPF sunscreen.

There are two types of sunscreen agents, chemical and physical. *Chemical sunscreens* work by absorbing UV rays and should be applied at least 30 minutes before sun exposure. *Physical sunscreen* forms a protective coating that reflect or scatter UV rays away from the skin. These physical, "chemical-free" sunscreens can be used by those with very sensitive skin.[43]

Sunscreen classifications are based on an index of protection against skin erythema called "sun protective factor" or SPF, which quantifies protection against UVB.[18] The term SPF is a measure of protection against sunburn, which allows for rating the effectiveness of a product. Higher SPF values indicate that the product offers more protection against sunburning. SPF describes protection against UVB radiation only.[43] UVA radiation has not been quantified.

There are now broad-spectrum sunscreens that absorb UVA and UVB. The purchase of a broad-spectrum sunscreen, which protects against both UVA and UVB radiation, is important.[43] Sunscreens may also be classified as either water-resistant or waterproof. Water-resistant sunscreens retain sun protection for at least 40 minutes in the water. Waterproof sunscreens retain sun protection for at least 80 minutes in the water. Therefore, even waterproof sunscreens must be reapplied frequently to maintain labeled SPF value.[43]

Nonmelanoma skin cancers are associated with cumulative sun exposure. Persons with fair skin are at higher risk of adverse effects from UV radiation.[18] Sunscreens with a SPF of 30 or more are preferred over those with lower ratings (<15).[18, 31] A person with very sun-sensitive skin may need a sunscreen product of 35 or more.[45]

Children above the age of 6 months can benefit from the use of sunscreen.[45] It has been shown that the regular use of an SPF 15 sunscreen during the first 18 years of life could reduce the lifetime incidence of skin cancer by 78%.[43] Sunscreens should be applied 15 to 30 minutes before exposure and at least every 2 to 3 hours during exposure, depending on the product. The 30 minutes prior to exposure allows the sunscreen to bind to the skin.[45] Sunscreens may need to be applied more often because of heat, humidity, and perspiration combine to decrease their effectiveness.[31] Sunscreens should be worn year round.[45] When applying sunscreens use liberally to sun-exposed areas of the body, particularly the head and neck region (*frequent sites of BCC*) plus the rims of the ears, cheeks, forehead, bald spots, under the tip of the nose, behind the knees, and inside the arches.[31, 45] Lips should be covered with a lip balm containing sunscreen.[45]

The nose is the site of approximately 25% of all BCCs. Photo protection here is critical. It is important to protect the nose from as many harmful UV rays as possible. This is only possible with the use of a sun block. Only physical sun blocks, such as a nose guard, which attaches to sunglasses, or zinc oxide or talc, block all solar rays.[21, 22]

Raising Awareness. The public health message becomes a simple one of suggesting an overall reduction in exposure to sunlight, initially concentrating on telling people how to reduce the risk of sunburn when outdoors.[25] Numerous national groups and community organizations have created intensive public education efforts to promote skin cancer prevention. Most suggest a stepped approach to reduce unprotected sun exposure: (1) limit exposure to the sun during the midday hours, (2) if out in the sun, cover exposed area with clothing (long-sleeved shirts) and hats, and (3) for areas of the skin not adequately covered, use a waterproof, broad-spectrum sunscreen with an SPF of at least 15.

Minimized sun exposure for children is recommended. It is important to educate children, parents, and teachers about the importance of sun protection, for example, taking advantage of shade provided by trees, canopies, and umbrellas. Some school districts ban the use of hats by children, feeling the practice lends to gang identification; however, this would be another protective measure against the UV rays of the sun.[22, 40]

Public education messages for primary prevention of skin cancer can be carried out in a number of ways, including the use of the media, informational pamphlets, lectures, videotapes, and discussions between patients and health care providers during regular office visits.[21] Several such programs exist. One is, *"Slip! Slop! and Slap!"* with Sid the Seagull demonstrating Slip! on a shirt, Slop! on some sunscreen, and Slap! on a hat. "Sun Smart" is a teaching resource to be used with primary school children. Counseling of patients, especially those at highest risk, to use the triad of behaviors will make "WAR" on their skin cancer risk:

*W*ear protective clothing
*A*void the midday sun
*R*egular use of sun screen[38]

In four Texas cities, a unique program called the "Under Cover Skin Cancer Prevention Project" was initiated. This program was designed to change knowledge and attitudes about UV radiation while promoting risk reduction strategies. Media partners in each city announced daily UV readings four times each day along with educational and behavior change messages, which resulted in a change in behavior in these four locations.[21]

Secondary Prevention

Prevention methods for nonmelanoma skin cancers and malignant melanoma are similar.[31] Skin cancer screening is a major modality used for their prevention. The American Cancer Society recommends screening for skin cancer every 3 years for persons 20 to 40 years old and annually after the age of 40. Such screening is defined as any process of examining the skin for early detection of malignancy.[21]

Three criteria must be met for cancer screening to be effective. *First,* and perhaps most importantly, the early detection resulting from a screening intervention should positively affect outcomes. This measure is easily met because the influence of early treatment on survival is probably more evident with skin cancer than with any other tumor. *Secondly,* the screening process needs to be straightforward. Because skin cancer is on the body surface, no invasive tools are required, and the process is rapid and simple.[39] These exams can be incorporated into an office visit in which the health care provider is examining the person for another illness, or a planned and scheduled examination purposely for the examination of the skin.[21] *Thirdly,* the marginal cost of screening compared to the cost treating an advanced melanoma seems to be economically well worth the investment of a screening program.[39] Office settings and clinics can offer patients and families patient information guides as to "How to Examine Your Skin," to improve compliance and increase awareness regarding the importance of self-examination of the skin.

Barriers to Screening

Although the value of skin cancer screening seems evident, in the United States and Australia, two countries with the highest levels of skin cancer, primary care physicians do not routinely examine the skin for skin cancer. Barriers are numerous and include lack of diagnostic skills effective in recognizing early skin cancer, lack of time, lack of positive feedback, distraction by other health issues, failure to remember recommendations, patient embarrassment from undressing, or inadequate physician reimbursement.[21, 39]

With the obvious endpoint of screening being reduced mortality and the optimal follow-up time 5 to 10 years later, it is extremely difficult to determine whether or not a skin cancer screening has produced a successful outcome.[21] High-risk individuals should be screened periodically, either individually or through mass screening. Risk factors include family history, fair skin, multiple nevi, and a history of other skin cancers. Physicians and health care providers conducting total cutaneous exams should receive adequate training to ensure high-quality examinations, with high sensitivity and specificity. Further research efforts, especially prospective studies, are needed to define the role of screening in variable risk populations to define better optimal periodicity for screening.[18]

CLASSIFICATION AND CLINICAL FEATURES

The clinical presentation of BCC is discussed in five categories. Among these five categories, plus recurrence, some are easily recognized and others are less obvious. BCC may start as a translucent growth that has pink and white tones, a shiny border, giving it a "pearly" appearance, and a tendency to crust.[2, 14] This "pearl-like lesion" can have an overlying telangiectasis.[14]

About two thirds of BCCs occur on the face; the remainder usually involve the scalp, neck, or trunk.[14] Often these nodules tend to become quite friable and may develop a hemorrhagic ulceration. If left untreated, they can severely damage underlying tissue and the skin.[2] The most common types listed are *nodular,* most often appearing on the face, particularly the cheeks, forehead, eyelids, and nasolabial folds, followed by superficial, morpheaform, and pigmented.[14, 31] Of these three latter types of BCC, *superficial,* usually appears as a scaling erythematous plaque; *morpheaform* often has clinical elements of a typical or superficial BCC combined with a scarlike appearance and a indistinct margin; and *pigmented* can be confused with melanoma.[14]

DIAGNOSIS

A complete skin examination is the key diagnostic component. Once suspected clinically, BCC must always be definitely diagnosed by histology.[32] If the physical examination is normal, no additional evaluation is generally necessary. Evaluate any suspicious cutaneous lesions or lymph adenopathy with biopsy to rule out metastases or new primary lesions.[14]

Typical techniques used to perform the biopsy include a small punch biopsy or shave biopsy.[14] A *shave biopsy* (top lesion into depth of middermis) is performed using local anesthesia. *Punch* biopsy (sharp, small circular "punch" similar to a cookie cutter approach) is used if the tumor is suspected to be in the deeper layers of

CLINICAL FEATURES

Basal Cell Carcinoma (BCC)

Nodular BCC

Bulky, nodular growth caused by lack of keratinization
Characteristics include a thinning epidermis, producing a shiny pink, translucent, pearly hue over the lesion
Early stages resemble a smooth pimple that fails to heal
As the tumor enlarges, the border edge raises and the center becomes necrotic
Lesion bleeds easily from mild injury and doubles in size every 6 to 12 months at the rate of 5 mm per year

Superficial BCC

Tends to develop in multiple sites, growing peripherally across the skin surface, becoming as large as 10 to 15 cm
Appears most frequently on the trunk as a well-demarcated, erythematous, scaly patch with discreet nodules
Often confused with psoriasis

Pigmented BCC

Contains melanin in the epidermis, dermis, and within the tumor itself
Often mistaken clinically as melanoma
Colors include blue, black, or brown appearance with a raised pearly border
Found in dark-complexioned persons such as Latin Americans or Japanese (not African Americans)

Morpheaform or Sclerotic BCC

More aggressive lesion that appears as a flat, depressed scarlike plaque, pale yellow or white in color
Margins indistinct with nodules, ulcerations, or bleeding occurring within the plaque
Often undetected or misdiagnosed with a lower cure rate than nodular BCC

Keratonic BCC

Appears clinically similar to nodular ulcerative form
Located in the preauricular and postauricular sulcus
Aggressive in its growth
Often recurs locally
Type most likely to metastasize

Data from references 10, 18, 28, 46.

the skin. The tissue sample is examined to determine the clinical diagnosis and identifying features of the various classifications. On determination of the clinical diagnosis, classification, and histopathologic grading, specific treatment modalities are recommended.

The American Joint Committee on Cancer (AJCC) recommends the following stage grouping:

Primary Tumor (T)

TX	Primary tumor cannot be assessed
T0	No evidence of primary tumor
Tis	Carcinoma *in situ*
T1	Tumor 2 cm or less in greatest dimension
T2	Tumor more than 2 cm but not more than 5 cm in greatest dimension
T3	Tumor more than 5 cm in greatest dimension
T4	Tumor invades deep extradermal structures (i.e., cartilage, skeletal muscle, or bone)

Note: In the case of multiple simultaneous tumors, the tumor with the highest T category will be classified and the number of separate tumors will be indicated in parentheses, e.g., T2 (5).

Regional Lymph Nodes (N)

NX	Regional lymph nodes cannot be assessed
N0	No regional lymph node metastasis
N1	Regional lymph node metastasis

Distant Metastasis (M)

MX	Distant metastasis cannot be assessed
M0	No distant metastasis
M1	Distant metastasis

STAGE GROUPING

Stage 0	Tis	N0	M0
Stage I	T1	N0	M0
Stage II	T2	N0	M0
	T3	N0	M0
Stage III	T4	N0	M0
	Any T	N1	M0
Stage IV	Any T	Any N	M1

Used with the permission of the American Joint Committee on Cancer (AJCC®), Chicago, Illinois. The original source for this material is the AJCC® Cancer Staging Handbook, 5th edition (1998) published by Lippincott-Raven Publishers, Philadelphia, Pennsylvania.

Clinical staging is based on the physical examination and palpation of lymph nodes. Pathologic staging requires resection of the entire site and confirmation of any lymph node involvement. Underlying bony structures should be imaged, especially if these lesions occur on the scalp. Complete excision of the site and microscopic verification are necessary to determine histologic type.[31] It is important to avoid very thin shave biopsies that do not penetrate through the full thickness of the epidermis; such incomplete specimens will not enable the pathologist to differentiate in situ tumors from invasive ones.[14, 32]

Histologic grading for BCCs and SCCs is similar to the grading system for other cancers. G1 signifies well-differentiated tumor cells, G2 refers to moderately well-differentiated cells, G3 signifies poorly differentiated cells, and G4 signifies undifferentiated cells. Confirmation of the extent of disease by biopsy of the suspected cutaneous or subcutaneous spread is imperative.[31]

METASTASES AND RECURRENCE

Metastatic BCC is extremely rare. However, when this occurs it is usually via hematologic or lymphatic spread. The malignant character of the tumor depends on the destructive growth of the primary tumor rather than on metastasis.[4]

In a literature review regarding metastatic BCC, men experience metastases more frequently than women. The most common sites for primary tumors were on the head and neck, whereas the most common sites of metastasis, in decreasing order of frequency, were regional lymph nodes, lung, bone, skin, liver, and pleura. The average time elapsed between diagnosis of the primary tumor and the appearance of metastasis was 9 years. Median age at the first sign of metastasis was 59 years, and median survival time after initial diagnosis of metastasis was 8 months.[15]

A patient who develops one BCC has nearly a 35% to 50% chance of developing a second BCC lesion within the next 3.5 to 5 years, in addition to other skin cancers. Therefore, close observation of the patient for recurrence is recommended.[15, 22, 24, 32] In one study tumor location was found to be of prognostic significance: primary lesions on the head or neck were more likely to recur than those on the trunk or extremities, particularly those located around the ear.[4, 15] In addition, being older than 60, being male, having severe acitinic skin damage, and having sun exposure all increased the risk of recurrence.[15]

TREATMENT MODALITIES

Treatment for both BCC and SCC depends on many factors: the size and location of the lesion, histologic type of cancer, extension into nearby structures, presence of metastases, previous treatment, anticipated cosmetic results, and the patient's age and condition. Multiple modalities exist for the treatment of BCC: surgery, for example, surgical excision, cryosurgery, Mohs' surgery, laser; electrodesiccation and curettage; radiation therapy; chemotherapy; and biotherapy.[15, 31] No single treatment is ideal for all lesions. The goal of therapy is permanent cure with the best cosmetic results.[15] Substantial disfigurement can occur if the BCC is located on the face.[4]

Surgery

Surgical intervention is used to treat about 90% of BCCs. The goal is the complete removal of the tumor. Most of the procedures require local anesthesia and minimal equipment and can be performed in an ambulatory setting.[31]

Excisional Surgery. Surgical excision is an effective form of therapy for BCC, particularly for large lesions or those with poorly defined margins in high-risk sites such as the cheeks, forehead, trunk, and legs.[15, 31] Often a simple ellipse with suturing is feasible; however, in more difficult anatomic locations, the use of skin flaps and grafts may be necessary. In 95% of cases, for tumors smaller than 2 cm, the minimal margin necessary to eradicate the entire cancer is 4 mm.[15] Surgical excision may also be indicated when metastasis is present.[31]

Cryosurgery. Cryosurgery involves tissue destruction by freezing. Liquid nitrogen is administered by a spray or the use of cryoprobes. Rapid freezing results in intracellular and extracellular ice crystallization. Cell destruction is potentiated by a rapid freeze and slow thaw cycle. This method is useful in small to large nodular and superficial BCCs but is *not* indicated for deeply invasive tumors or BCCs of the scalp. Cryosurgery is recommended for BCCs of the eyelid because the procedure preserves normal tissue and obviates the need for reconstructive surgery.[31] The advantages of cryosurgery are that it is cost effective, fast, and easy and does not cause blood loss or require anesthesia. Disadvantages include patient discomfort with therapy, delayed healing time, and occasionally hypopigmentation. Cryosurgery should not be used for patients who have recurrent BCC or a history of cryoglobulinemia, cold agglutinin syndrome, or Raynaud's phenomenon.[15]

Electrodesiccation and Curettage. This is a more efficient and more cost-effective method of treating BCC than surgical excision, Mohs' surgery, or radiation therapy. However, the success of the procedure depends on the skill of the health care provider performing it. Considerable experience is necessary to acquire proper technique and learn how to identify the lesions for which the treatment is appropriate.[15]

This surgical method uses heat to destroy tissue. After the tumor is marked and anesthetized, a debulking process is used to scrape abnormal tissue within 1 to 2 mm. The base of tumor is then electrodesiccated. Curettage of the base is performed using both a large and tiny curette to track any extension of the tumor. The procedure is repeated as necessary until a normal plane of tissue is reached.[31] This form of tumor debulking should not involve tissue below the dermis.[15] These interventions are useful with small (<2 cm) to medium nodular and superficial BCCs with well-defined margins.

BCCs larger than 2 cm in diameter, those located in zones at high risk for recurrence, and all high-risk SCCs are best treated by other methods.[31]

Electrodesiccation and curettage is not a satisfactory procedure for lesions adjacent to the lips, nasal orifices, or eyelids, because the healing process results in significant retraction of the surrounding tissues. It also has a lower cure rate than excision and, consequently, is less appropriate for removal of those tumors with higher risk for metastasis or deep invasion because of their location.[14]

Mohs' Micrographic Surgery. Mohs' micrographic surgery involves surgical removal of the tumor layer by layer until all margins are free of the tumor on microscopic examination. Mohs' microsurgery permits the best histologic verification of complete removal and allows for maximum conservation of tissue. This is the treatment of choice for invasive SCCs and primary BCCs that are larger than 2 cm in diameter, have indistinct clinical margins, are located on zones of the face with a known high recurrence rate, occur in a cosmetic or functional area, such as the nose or eyelid, or are aggressive, such as morpheaform BCC.[31] This surgery should also be considered for immunosuppressed patients, in whom BCC may be more likely to metastasize.[15]

Present day Mohs' surgery uses fresh frozen tissue instead of tissue fixed with zinc chloride paste.[15] A unique feature is that specimens are sectioned and color coded in a manner that permits microscopic examination of the entire surgical margin simultaneously.[14] This allows for repeated sectioning and microscopic examination until all the cancer is removed; immediate repair can then be performed. Using Mohs' surgery, a tumor can be completely excised in 1 day without removing more than 1 to 2 mm of normal skin. The overall cure rate with this technique is 99% for primary BCC and 96% for recurrent lesions.[15] Regardless of the surgical treatment used, the cure rate for BCC after surgical intervention is nearly 95%.[31]

Lasers. The carbon dioxide laser has advantages over conventional surgery by sealing small blood vessels and nerves. It provides a relatively bloodless surgical field and reduced postoperative pain.[31]

Postsurgical Care. The appropriate follow-up interval depends on the details of the individual case. Patients with a superficial BCC and little other evidence of sun exposure may only need to be seen once a year, whereas those with a high-risk SCC might need to be initially seen every 1 to 2 months. Follow-up care focuses on identifying recurrent and new primary tumors. A complete skin examination should be done and regional lymph nodes checked for evidence of possible metastasis, particularly if the patient was treated for SCC.[14]

Radiation Therapy

The indications for ionizing radiation therapy for nonmelanoma skin cancer are continually being modified, as alternative treatments become more accessible. Radiation therapy may be used when surgery is not feasible or surgical destruction is not desirable.[15] Radiation therapy is a viable and effective alternative when surgical interventions are contraindicated and in elderly or debilitated persons who are unable to tolerate a surgical procedure. Tissue conservation is a benefit of radiation therapy, especially when dealing with lesions on the nose, eyelids, or lips. Cosmetic results are good with this type of treatment because surgical scars and skin grafting are eliminated.[31] A combined approach of preoperative and postoperative radiation and surgery may be indicated for extensive tumors.

Radiation is fractionated over multiple treatment sessions (usually 450 Gy/3 weeks in 300 cGy daily fractions) to reduce radiation-induced side effects. Disadvantages of this treatment method are related to the administration schedule because it may pose problems for patients and their families who must travel a distance to reach the treatment center.[31]

Radiation therapy should not be used for the following:

- Lesions in areas such as the inner canthus, where recurrences might be catastrophic
- Lesions in patients younger than 50, who would be subject to long-term sequelae such as carcinogenesis and chronic radiation dermatitis
- Lesions in previously radiated areas
- Morpheaform BCC[15]
- Tumors located on the trunk, extremities, and dorsum of the hands or scalp
- Those tumors arising in sweat and sebaceous glands
- Morpheaform basal cell tumors or verrucous squamous cell tumors
- For tumors larger than 8 cm
- For tumors located on the upper lip growing into the nostril[31]

Chemotherapy and Biotherapy

Topical chemotherapy, usually using topical 5-fluorouracil (5-FU; Efudex, Fluroplex), is an effective modality for superficial multicentric BCCs but is ineffective for other histologic types. 5-FU destroys the surface tumor without affecting deeper cells, thus allowing invasion to continue at the base of the tumor.[31] Treatment must continue for 6 weeks. Patient compliance is sometimes problematic because of the severe degree of inflammation that usually accompanies treatment.[15] Other agents such as cisplatin, bleomycin, cyclophosphamide, 5-FU, and vinblastine have been studied; cisplatin has been the most effective and is associated with the longest remission.[31]

The lack of an established systemic therapy for recurrent or advanced local, regional, or metastatic disease has led to the use of *biologic response modifiers* (BRMs), especially interferon-alfa. Systemic interferon-alfa has produced a 50% objective response rate in clinical testing. A study of 172 patients receiving intralesional injections of interferon alfa-2b reported an 81% cure rate after a follow-up period of 1 year. Other agents, specifically retinoids, have also shown some activity against BCC. Topical retinoid therapy and systemic retinoid therapy have both produced objective response rates greater than 50% in both BCCs and SCCs.[31]

PROGNOSIS

Metastatic disease is rarely seen with BCC, even though it tends to be a locally aggressive tumor. If left untreated, the tumor will locally invade vital structures such as blood vessels, lymph nodes, nerve sheaths, cartilage, bone, lungs, and the dura mater.[31] BCC is highly curable with early detection and treatment. Cure rates are close to 100% in persons with lesions less than 1 cm. When surgical intervention is used, the overall 5-year survival rate is approximately 99% for primary lesions and 96% with recurrent lesions.[31] It is imperative that persons with BCC continue defined scheduled follow-up examinations by a physician. Follow-up examinations should be performed at 6-month intervals during the first 2 years and then yearly for 5 years to detect the recurrence of previously treated or new primary BCCs while they are small enough to remove without significant cosmetic loss.[31]

Squamous Cell Carcinoma

EPIDEMIOLOGY

Squamous cell cancer (SCC) is less common than BCC but its rate of increase is higher. SCC accounts for 20% of all nonmelanoma skin cancers and has a mortality rate of 1% to 2%. The actual morbidity and mortality rates of SCC equal those of melanoma.[16, 23, 31] SCC occurs more frequently in persons with light complexions. Persons at greatest risk sunburn easily, tan poorly, and have red or blonde hair and blue eyes.[16] SCC is also more common in men, and the incidence increases with advancing age. The average age of onset for SCC is approximately 60 years.[31] Unlike BCC, this tumor frequently occurs on the hands and forearms as well as on the head and neck region, especially the ears, lower lip, scalp, and upper face.[31]

Although skin cancer is relatively uncommon in African American patients, SCC is found 20% more often in this population than is BCC. Nonsun-exposed sites, often a preexisting scar, leg wound, or old burn area, are affected most often in African American patients. Most common on the face and lower extremities, these tumors are very aggressive and the mortality rate is about 18.4%[16] (see Table 18–2).

ETIOLOGY AND RISK FACTORS

Squamous cell carcinoma is most often found in sun-damaged skin previously affected by actinic keratoses. All the predisposing risk factors mentioned in regard to BCC have also been associated with the development of SCC.[31] The correlation between the incidence of SCC of the skin and exposure to UV light is well established.[16] Sun exposure and the use of chewing tobacco increase the risk of SCC of the lips and mucous membranes. The male/female ratio of patients with SCC of the lip is 12:1. The lower lip is affected far more often than is the upper lip. Lesions occurring in these locations are very aggressive and carry higher rates of metastasis, morbidity, and mortality than do lesions in other sites (the only exceptions being the penis, scrotum, and anus). Preexisting scars, ulcers, sinus tracts, and some chronic dermatoses also give rise to this disease. When SCC develops in nonhealing ulcers, persistent sinus tracts, or old scars, it is more aggressive than usual and carries higher metastasis and mortality rates.[16]

Additional factors that increase the risk of a new SCC within 5 years of an original diagnosis of SCC include male sex, age greater than 60, three or more prior skin cancers, a history of severe actinic keratoses, and being a former or current smoker.[16] Among causal factors are ionizing radiation, arsenic, or industrial chemicals; oncogenic viral infection; immunosuppression, and particular genodermatoses.

Ionizing Radiation

Radiation is used for the treatment of many diseases, including those of the skin (e.g., acne, dermatitis, hemangiomas, skin cancer) as well as those caused by occupational exposure. The most important risk factor for radiation-induced SCC is the total accumulated dose. The latency period for presentation of disease ranges from 7 weeks to 60 years.[16]

Arsenic

The association between exposure to arsenic and the development of cancer was recorded as early as 1820.

Patients may be exposed to arsenic through smelting of ore, certain insecticides, cattle and sheep dips, certain medicaments, and drinking water from contaminated wells. Exposure occurs through ingestion or inhalation and may manifest as *hyperkeratotic papules,* also known as arsenic keratoses, on the palms and soles. The likelihood of transformation to skin cancer correlates directly with the amount of exposure.[16]

Viral Infection

Human papillomavirus (HPV) infection has been implicated in the development of cutaneous SCC, most commonly HPV types 16 and 18.[16]

Industrial Chemicals

Coal tar, pitch, paraffin oil, lubricating oils, creosote, soot, and fuel oils have been implicated in the development of SCC. Cancer of the scrotum is particularly common in men who work with pitch or cutting oils.[16]

Immunosuppression

Organ transplant recipients have an increased incidence of SCC. It is more common than BCC in these patients. Tumors usually occur on sun-exposed skin areas and the risk of metastasis is high. The average latency period is 1 to 7 years after transplantation, depending on the type and duration of immunosuppression. Earlier onset, lower incidence, and lower rate of metastasis are noted with use of cyclosporine (Sandimmune) alone versus treatment with the conventional immunosuppressive regimen of azathioprine (Imuran), cyclosphosphamide (Cytoxan, Neosar), and prednisone.[16] According to one theory, immunosuppressive therapy potentiates the carcinogenic effects of UV radiation. In addition, an impaired immune surveillance system may be incapable of destroying potentially malignant mutant cells.[16]

Genodermatoses

Patients with xeroderma pigmentosum or albinism, particularly oculocutaneous albinism, are at increased risk for SCC. In xeroderma pigmentosum, patients lack the enzyme needed to repair DNA after UV exposure; in albinism, patients lack the pigment (melanin) that protects against radiation.[16] Patients presenting with SCC are also at risk of cancer of the respiratory organs, lip, buccal cavity, and pharynx, small intestine (in men), non-Hodgkin's lymphoma, and leukemia.[10]

PREVENTION, SCREENING AND DETECTION

Prevention and detection methods are similar for both SCC and BCC. The avoidance of UV light and the use of sunscreens and protective clothing are important.[31] Regular use of sunscreen with an SPF of 15 or greater throughout childhood and adolescence significantly reduces the lifetime risk of nonmelanoma skin cancer.[16] In addition to the head and neck area, sunscreens should also be liberally applied to the hands and forearms.[31]

Actinic Keratoses

Actinic (solar) keratoses are the most common precancerous lesion of the skin. Actinic keratoses usually develop in fair-skinned persons, sometimes in those in their twenties to mid-thirties but more often among the middle aged or elderly, who have had excessive exposure to the sun with little or no protection by a sunscreen.[16] Lesions are usually found on sun-exposed areas of the body, such as the face, ears, and dorsa of the hands and forearms. Typically, they are small lesions, 3 mm to 1 cm; however, larger lesions may be found. They appear as discrete, red or flesh-colored papules, often covered by a white, gray, or yellow adherent lamellar scale. The scale periodically falls off but re-forms. It is painful to remove the scale prematurely.[16, 37] The clinical course of actinic keratoses is varied: lesions may disappear spontaneously, remain stable, or progress to SCC. In about 25% of the these cases lesions resolve spontaneously within 1 year, especially in persons who reduce their exposure to the sun.[16, 37]

The exact relationship between actinic keratoses and SCC is unknown. Estimates of malignant transformation vary from 1% to 20%; more recently, less than 1 patient of 1000 per year with actinic keratoses is said to transform to SCC.[16, 37]

Some authorities note that to treat all lesions to prevent the morbidity and mortality could result in SCC is unjustifiable based on cost-benefit analysis. Opinions vary and the issue at present is not completely settled. Some physicians advocate only close observation of the lesions, whereas others treat actinic keratoses early to avoid any potential risk of malignant transformation. Most, however, consider actinic keratosis a precancerous lesion.[16]

CLASSIFICATION AND CLINICAL FEATURES

Squamous cell carcinoma has a more indiscriminate method of classification. Because of the varying general characteristics and the source of tissue presentation, it is classified by presenting symptoms, tissue source, and histologic difference. SCC should be suspected whenever clinical features are noted. Presentations vary. Lesions may be superficial, discrete, and hard, and have

an indurated, rounded base. They may be dull red and contain telangiectasias, or they may be dome-shaped nodules with ulcerations and crusting.[16] If SCC is suspected, special attention should be paid to the regional

---

CLINICAL FEATURES

Squamous Cell Carcinoma (SCC)

General Characteristics

Occurs anywhere on sun-damaged skin and on mucous membrane with squamous epithelium

Appears as a round to irregular shape, with a plaque-like or nodular character covered by a warty scale, indistinct margins, and firm erythematous dome-shaped nodule with corelike center that ulcerates

Dull red in color

Grows by expansion and infiltration as well as by tracking along various tissue planes

Invades below the level of the sweat gland and has a higher degree of malignant potential

Overall invasiveness and depth of neoplasm are significant when determining risk of recurrence

Ischemic Ulceration

Occurs in varicose ulcers, chronic ulcers, and poorly healed fistulas/tracks with old scars

Accompanied by increased drainage, pain, and bleeding

Bowen's Disease

Associated with arsenic ingestion

Occurs on sun-exposed and nonsun-exposed areas of the skin, including mucous membrane of vulva, vagina, nose, and conjunctiva

Nodular reddish brown plaque with areas of scales and crusts

Actinic Cheilitis

Rapidly growing progressive invasive lesion that occurs on the lip, often a result of smoking

Lower lip is primary site in 95% of patients

Early appearance is local thickening, progressing to a firm nodular lesion with destructive ulceration

Diagnosis is frequently missed (2 years after onset) and lesion is usually 1 to 2 cm in diameter at initial biopsy

Reported risk of metastasis from SCC of lip has ranged from 5% to 37%

Verrucous

Well-differentiated lesion frequently seen on glans penis, vulva, scrotum, sole, back, or buttock and appears as a slowly growing, warty lesion

Surgical excision is treatment of choice

Data from references 14, 26, 33, 37.

lymph node chains, particularly if the lesion is located on the hands, ear, or lip.[14]

DIAGNOSIS AND STAGING

Diagnosis and staging for SCC are the same as for BCC described earlier in this chapter.[31]

METASTASIS

The frequency of metastasis of SCC of the skin is higher than that seen in the less aggressive BCC and ranges from 0.3% to 3.7%, with death resulting in 75% of these patients.[16, 31] The occurrence and degree vary according to morphologic characteristics and size and depth of penetration of the tumor.[31] Metastasis occurs late via the lymphatics (within 2 years) after the tumor has invaded the subcutaneous lymph nodes and the lymphatics of the deeper structure.[31]

TREATMENT MODALITIES

Squamous cell carcinoma can be treated by procedures similar to those used with BCC with some exceptions. For example, a slightly larger excisional margin should be performed surgically, and it is important to examine the regional lymph nodes for the presence of tumor.[31] The therapeutic approach will depend on the size and location of the carcinoma, the extent of local involvement, and potential for metastasis. Primary tumors respond best to treatment; recurrent tumors have a 25% to 45% chance of metastasis, depending on their location.[16] The occurrence and degree of metastasis vary according to morphologic characteristics, size, and depth of penetration of the tumor.[31]

Treatments can be divided into those providing *local, regional,* and *distant* control of spread.[16] For example, the treatment of high-risk SCC with no palpable lymph nodes may involve one of the following: local control alone, regional control with prophylactic lymph node dissection, radiation to draining nodes, or combined therapy. Metastatic SCC lymph nodes are treated surgically, with adjuvant radiation therapy given preoperatively or postoperatively.[31]

Local Control

Local control is used for low-risk tumors, which have a high cure rate, are small, and usually occur in actinically damaged skin.[16]

Cryotherapy. Cryotherapy for SCC is useful in selected patients. Lesions with a diameter of 0.5 to 2.0 cm and well-defined borders are amenable to this modality. This technique boasts exceptional cosmetic results and has achieved 5-year cure rates as high as 96%.[31]

Chemotherapy. Topical 5-FU is recommended for treatment of premalignant actinic keratoses. (See BCC section on chemotherapy.) Sunscreen should be used during therapy to minimize photosensitization and after therapy to prevent further sun damage.[16] An alternative to topical 5-FU is topical masoprocol (Actinex), which was effective in treating actinic keratoses on the head and neck.[16] In advanced SCC, systemic retinoids have produced response rates greater than 70%.[31]

Radiation Therapy. Radiation therapy is recommended for treatment of primary SCC using a variety of fractionation regimens, ranging from 22 Gy in a single fraction to 70 Gy in multiple fractions.[31]

Regional Control

The presence of palpable lymph nodes necessitates regional control consisting of radiation therapy and lymph node dissection.[16]

Chemotherapy. Chemotherapy regimens in preliminary clinical trials have demonstrated some efficacy.[16] Although future clinical trials are needed to better define cure rates, high-risk lesions may be treated with surgery, adjuvant radiotherapy to the primary site, and nodal drainage.

Distant Control

The decision to treat a lesion as a *low-risk tumor* is based on knowledge of the characteristics of *high-risk tumors.* The metastatic potential depends on anatomic site, size, histologic features, and etiology of the tumor, host immunosuppression, and prior treatment.[16] In general, lesions greater than 2 cm in diameter have double the local recurrence rate (15.2% versus 7.4%) and triple the metastatic rate (30.3% versus 9.1%) compared with lesions less than 2 cm in diameter.[16] Therefore, poorly differentiated and large SCCs carry an increased frequency of metastasis and a poor prognosis.[16]

Mohs' Surgery. The treatment of choice for high-risk tumors is Mohs' surgery (see BCC under surgical intervention). This technique is particularly useful for lesions greater than 2 cm in diameter, those with poor histologic differentiation, and those located on the ear, lip, and penis.[16]

PROGNOSIS

For the first 5 years after diagnosis and treatment of SCC, patients should have frequent follow-up examinations to ensure early detection of recurrences and metastasis. More than 75% of local recurrences are noted within 2 years after surgery, and 80% of metastases occur within 2 years after diagnosis. In addition, 95% of all local recurrences and metastases take place within 5 years after treatment.[16] Of the two nonmelanoma skin cancers, metastasis is seen more often in SCC. Ordinarily, primary SCC localized to the skin has an incidence of metastasis of approximately 3%. Primary lesions of the lip metastasize more frequently, at a rate greater than 10%.[31]

Squamous cell carcinoma also has high cure rates (75–80%) when either surgery or radiation is used. Because this lesion has the ability to metastasize as well as recur, it is generally considered a higher-risk skin cancer. Most deaths resulting from nonmelanoma skin cancer can be attributed to SCC.[31]

Malignant Melanoma

EPIDEMIOLOGY

Malignant melanoma is estimated to affect 47,700 people in the United States in 2000 and cause 7700 deaths.[1, 8] Malignant melanoma is the least common of the three types, but it is the most deadly form of skin cancer. Melanoma accounts for 3% of all cancer in the United States each year. Its incidence ranks sixth among men and seventh among women.[7] The incidence of melanoma is rising at a rate of 4% per year, exceeding the rate of any other tumor.[1, 2, 6, 7] In 1935, only 1 in 1500 Americans developed melanoma. It is estimated that by the year 2000, 1 in 75 Americans will develop melanoma during his or her lifetime.[7, 35, 36, 38, 40]

Melanoma is unique among serious malignancies in that it is visible, can be readily detected, and, in its early stages, can be cured.[42] Trouble begins in melanocytes when an undefined collaboration between aberrant genes and environmental factors spurs the growth of cancerous cells. Because most of the pigment-producing cells are lodged in the basal layer of the epidermis, telltale signs generally appear on the skin. However, melanocytes are scattered at other sites as well. This accounts for the fewer than 10% of melanomas that occur in more obscure locations, such as the eyes, the oral and anogenital mucosa, the esophagus, and the meninges.[6]

Similar to the nonmelanoma skin cancers, malignant melanoma most frequently affects whites. Most African Americans, because of their dark skin, are far less likely to develop melanoma than whites.[2] When dark-skinned persons and Asians do get melanoma, it tends to occur at sites not exposed to the sun, such as palms, soles, nailbeds, fingers, toes, and mucous membranes.[8, 31]

TABLE 18–3
Common Sites of Malignant Melanoma

Type of Melanoma	Common Sites
Lentigo maligna melanoma	Face, neck, trunk, dorsum of hands
Superficial spreading melanoma	Backs of men; legs of women
Nodular melanoma	Trunk, head, neck
Acral-lentiginous melanoma	Palms of hands, soles of feet, nailbeds, mucous membranes

From Itano JK, Taoka KN, editors: Core curriculum for oncology nursing, *ed 3, Philadelphia, Saunders, 1998:554.*

Unlike BCC and SCC, melanoma may occur in persons in their teens and early twenties or thirties.[31] It has become one of the most common cancers in young adults and is most likely to appear between the ages of 30 and 60, the highest incidence rates occurring in persons over 60.[2, 8] Although the risk of melanoma does increase with age, about 50% of patients with malignant melanoma are under age 55.[31, 40] In men, the upper back and trunk are the most common sites of occurrence; the back and lower extremities are the most common sites in women.[31] Table 18–3 lists the common sites of malignant melanoma.

ETIOLOGY AND RISK FACTORS

Two important environmental factors are sun exposure and geographic latitude.[31] The incidence of melanoma among whites is inversely related to latitude of residence and latitude gradient.[11] The closer one lives to the equator, the higher the risk for developing melanoma.[31] The risk of developing melanoma is highest in countries with a high ambient solar radiation.[21] For every 1000 feet above sea level, there is a compounded 4% increase in UV radiation exposure.[31] In addition, the risk for developing melanoma in those countries tends to be greater with native-born people than with immigrants to that country. The risk decreases with increasing age of immigration to the host country for both melanoma and nonmelanoma skin cancers.[21]

The world's highest incidence is in Australia, a subtropical country with a largely Celtic population.[8] In the United States, the occurrence of melanoma is greatest in the "Sun Belt" states, such as California, Arizona, and Texas.[7] A single blistering sunburn before the age of 20 increases the risk of melanoma later in life.[40, 42] The greatest risk is associated with a history of multiple blistering sunburns in childhood.[7, 42] Unlike the more common skin cancers, which are associated with total cumulative exposure to UV radiation, melanomas are associated with intense intermittent exposure, although the disease also develops in people who have had regular, cumulative exposure.[2, 7, 8] A person's ability to tan seems to be a factor. Persons who burn easily and are poor tanners have an increased risk.[31, 42] Persons who are fair skinned are at higher risk although malignant melanoma can occur in persons of any skin type.[7, 31, 40] Other risk factors, such as blond or red hair color, are risk factors for the development of both nonmelanoma skin cancers and melanoma.[7, 8, 31, 42]

Melanoma is at least five times more likely to occur in someone who has already had melanoma.[40] Additional risk factors include: persons with 20 or more moles,[7] a familial history of melanoma, a personal or familial history of *clinically atypical moles* (CAMs; formerly known as dysplastic nevi), congenital nevi, immunodeficiency due to Hodgkin's lymphoma, organ transplantation, and possibly human immunodeficiency virus infection.[6, 31, 42] First-degree relatives of patients with melanoma are about two to eight times more likely than the general public to be diagnosed with melanoma[31] (see Chapter 2).

Just one abnormal mole—such as a large, flat spot with varying color, asymmetric shape, and indistinct borders—doubles a person's chance of getting melanoma. The increase was 12-fold in people with 10 or more atypical moles; those who also had considerable freckling from exposure to sunlight had a 20-fold risk.[2]

PREVENTION, SCREENING, AND DETECTION

Prevention methods for nonmelanoma skin cancers and malignant melanoma are similar. The avoidance of intense sun exposure and the use of protective clothing and sunscreens are important. Children should also be protected from sunburns because an increased risk for melanoma exists in persons who have experienced traumatic sunburns as children.[31]

Early detection and prompt treatment are essential. Warning signs of melanoma are any unusual skin condition: scaliness, oozing, or bleeding of a mole or other pigmented growth; a change in color or size of a mole or any other pigmented growth or spot; a spread of the pigment beyond the normal border; a change in sensation, itchiness, tenderness, or pain; and the development of a new lesion or nodule.[31] The early warning signs of malignant melanoma can be easily remembered by thinking of the acronym ABCD: *asymmetry, border, color,* and *diameter.* Malignant melanomas are usually asymmetric (i.e., one half of the mole does not match the other half). Early malignant melanomas tend to have irregular borders. The edges become ragged, notched, or blurred, unlike smooth margins. Pigmentation in malignant melanomas is not uniform. Colors may range from various hues of tan and brown to black, with red and white intermingled. Malignant melanomas are

often greater than 5 to 6 mm when first identified. A sudden or continued increase in the size of a mole should be reported.[2, 31, 35, 38, 40, 42]

A complete skin examination by primary care providers would almost certainly result in earlier diagnosis of many melanomas. Such screening may also detect persons who are at increased risk for melanoma.[42] The best outcomes depend on the provider's ability to identify hazardous lesions, and get rid of them, before they have a chance to flourish. Patients who have had one melanoma are at increased risk of a second primary lesion and should remain under surveillance for the rest of their lives.[6]

However, inducing people to visit a health professional for skin examination requires one to rely on the ability of the professional to be able to recognize abnormalities and to know the correct procedure to deal with them. An imperative of any public health program or screening clinic that relies on professional services to provide diagnosis and management of abnormalities detected by the public, therefore, is to train professionals first, prior to the public education or screening program.[25] Examination of the skin once a month by inspecting all skin surfaces for any of the above changes is imperative for those persons at risk of developing malignant melanoma. Persons previously diagnosed with malignant melanoma should also perform skin self-examination once a month because of the increased likelihood for recurrence.[31, 42]

Any patient who has had melanoma needs to be seen regularly for a skin check and physical examination. Appointments should be scheduled every 3 months in the first year after an occurrence and every 6 months thereafter. Patients who have had very thin melanomas can probably be examined on a yearly basis after several uneventful years. Again, the objective is to make sure there are no signs of metastasis and no new tumors. Lymph nodes, liver, and spleen should be palpated.[6]

The educated patient or family member is often the first person to detect changes in skin conditions. In one study, 53% of 216 incident cases of melanoma in Massachusetts were self-discovered, whereas the remaining cases were detected by medical providers (26%), family members (17%), and others (3%). Compared with men, women were more likely to discover their own lesions and those of their spouses.[31]

CLASSIFICATION AND CLINICAL FEATURES

Malignant melanomas may arise from three types of moles, or nevi: CANs, *the common acquired nevus;* CAMs, *clinically atypical moles* (formerly dysplastic nevi); or *congenital melanocytic nevus.*[6, 31] The number and types of moles on a person's body are strong predictors of melanoma susceptibility.[2] The most frequently encountered benign pigmented lesion is the *CAN, commonly acquired nevus,* better known as the "normal mole." CANs are absent at birth. Nevus production begins in childhood with increased development during puberty. Production begins to taper off at about 35 to 40 years of age. Most adults have about 20 to 40 nevi on their bodies. CAN are usually small (< 5 mm), exhibiting uniformity in color, surface, symmetry, and regularity of borders. The risk that any one CAN will develop into a malignant lesion is small.

CAMs are *clinically atypical moles.* CAMs are acquired pigmented lesions, considered to be precursors of melanoma as well as the markers of persons at risk for melanoma.[31] CAMs possess one or more of the physical traits of melanoma. A CAM can be both asymmetric and bigger than a CAN, approximately 5 mm or more, with ragged, ill-defined borders, an uneven surface, or variegated coloring. If the CAM is indeed a melanoma the abnormalities it displays are usually more striking. For example, sometimes melanomas undergo partial spontaneous regression, so those portions of a lesion appear to have been bleached.[6]

Though not malignant, CAMs are a significant harbinger. People who have CAMs are at an increased risk of developing melanoma, particularly if they have a large number of them (>50). This was formerly called *dysplastic nevus syndrome* (*DNS*). In some people CAMs can develop on the body throughout the life span. CAMs may run in families or be sporadic. Although the CAM itself is usually benign, a person who has a large number of CAMs (>50) and a familial or personal history of melanoma is at increased risk for developing melanoma. In addition, if the person has CAMs and two first-degree relatives with melanoma, the lifetime risk for developing melanoma will rise to 50% to 100%.[6, 31] CAMs can appear anywhere on the body but are typically found on the trunk, back, breasts, buttocks, genitals, and scalp.[31]

Congenital melanocytic nevi appear as raised, dark-brown to black, oval or round macules that may contain coarse hairs. These congenital nevi are present at birth and are classified by size in diameter as small (<1.5 cm), medium (1.5–19.9 cm), and large (>19.9 cm). Most congenital nevi are small or medium. The risk of developing malignant melanoma from congenital nevi is controversial, with estimates as high as 22 times. Persons with congenital nevi larger than 3 to 5 cm are thought to be at even greater risk of developing malignant melanoma.[31]

TYPES OF MELANOMA

Early primary melanoma, characterized by a radical growth phase that is confined to the epidermis or to the superficial dermis (or both), can evolve into advanced melanoma that has a vertical growth phase with competence for invasion of the deep dermis and development of metastasis. Early stage melanoma is curable, but the prognosis for individuals with metastatic disease is dismal, with a 5-year survival rate of only 12%.[36] It metastasizes to remote sites early, and its metastases are characteristically unresponsive to treatment.[41]

There are four types of malignant melanoma: *superficial spreading, nodular, lentigo maligna, and acral lentiginous.*

Superficial spreading malignant melanoma is the most common form and has the best chance of being cured.[2] About 70% of all cutaneous melanomas are of this type, which occurs more often in women than in men, usually seen between the ages of 40 and 50.[2, 31] These lesions

---

CLINICAL FEATURES

Common Benign Pigmented Lesions

Simple Lentigo

Small, 1 to 5 mm, macular, pigmented lesion
Precursor to common mole
Sharply defined, round
Smooth or jagged edges that may appear on the surface of skin
More concentrated on sun-exposed areas

Junctional Nevus

Small, less than 6 mm, well-circumscribed, pigmented lesion with smooth surface
Relatively uniform pigmentation that ranges from dark brown to black

Compound Nevus

Well-circumscribed, less than 6 mm, raised papule
Uniform in pigmentation
Skin colored tan to various shades of brown

Solar Lentigo

Small to somewhat larger macule known as a "liver spot"
Found on sun-exposed people with significant sun damage: face, chest, back, dorsa of hands
Uniform tan to brown

Seborrheic Keratosis

Sharply demarcated purple that ranges in diameter
Few millimeters to several centimeters
Verrucous, round, ovid, variably raised
Surface "dull" or "warty"
Common on face, neck, trunk
Variably raised
Light brown to dark brown

Data from references 7, 14, 21, 28, 32, 41, 48.

CLINICAL FEATURES

*Malignant Melanoma
Pigmented Lesions*

Superficial Spreading Melanoma

Variegated in color with areas appearing blue, black,
  gray, white, or pink

Irregular pigmented plaque with areas of regression
  and notched borders; horizontal or radial extension

May appear scaly and crusty and itch

Increasingly more common among young adults

Nodular Melanoma

Often resembles a ''blood blister''

Appears as a symmetric, raised, dome-shaped lesion;
  vertical growth patterns

Blue-black in color

Can be amelanotic

Lentigo Malignant Melanoma

Appears as a large, flat, irregular lesion resembling a
  stain

Variegated in color, ranging from tan to black with
  areas of regression

Located on face and neck of elderly, severely sun-
  tanned whites

Acral Lentiginous Melanoma

Usually flat, irregular, with an average diameter of
  3 cm

Blue or black discoloration or a tan and brown stain

Occurs on palms and soles or under nailbeds

Data from references 2, 3, 6, 7, 8, 33, 38.

usually occur on the back in men and on the lower legs
in women.[31, 42]

Nodular malignant melanoma is the next most frequently occurring melanoma.[31] These represent 10% to
20% of melanomas occurring in whites and manifests
vertical growth early in their inception.[42] Nodular melanomas may occur anywhere on the body; however, common sites of occurrence are the head, neck, and trunk
regions.[31] Most nodular melanomas appear as a blue
or black nodule although 5% have no pigmentation.
Containing the ''hallmark characteristics of melanoma,''
lack of marked asymmetry, border irregularity, and
color variegation, nodular melanomas are usually detected late, after extensive invasion has occurred.[42]

Lentigo maligna melanoma is a rare form of melanoma accounting for 5% to 12% of melanomas.[31, 42]
These lesions occur after age 60, primarily on the sun-
exposed areas of the body, most often the head and
neck. There is a prolonged growth phase for this slow-
growing melanoma during which time the lesion is called
lentigo maligna. The term ''lentigo maligna melanoma''
is reserved for invasive lesions.[42]

Acral lentiginous melanoma is the least common, accounting for less than 10% of all melanomas.[31] This type
of melanomas is the most common in African Americans, Hispanics, and Orientals. It is frequently found on
the palms, soles, and periungual and subungual surfaces.
It frequently has a short radical growth phase, resulting
in late detection and a poor prognosis.[42]

DIAGNOSIS AND STAGING

Melanoma has two subsequent growth phases: radical
and vertical. During the radical growth phase, the tumor
spreads laterally along the skin surface. During the vertical growth phase the melanoma extends downward
through the layers of the epidermis and dermis and
into the subcutaneous tissue. As it continues to grow
downward, it invades the lymphatic and vascular systems. This results in local and regional disease, as well
as spread to distant lymph nodes and visceral organs.[7]

When a lesion is suspected to be melanoma, a biopsy
should be performed. The technique of choice is a total
excisional biopsy with narrow margins.[31] Overall prognosis and treatment are based on the stage of disease
using the AJCC's staging classification.

Primary Tumor (pT)

pTX	Primary tumor cannot be assessed
pT0	No evidence of primary tumor
pTis	Melanoma *in situ* (atypical melanocytic hyperplasia, severe melanocytic dysplasia), not an invasive malignant lesion (Clark's Level I)
pT1	Tumor 0.75 mm or less in thickness and invades the papillary dermis (Clark's Level II)
pT2	Tumor more than 0.75 mm but not more than 1.5 mm in thickness and/or invades to papillary-reticular dermal interface (Clark's Level III)
pT3	Tumor more than 1.5 mm but not more than 4 mm in thickness and/or invades the reticular dermis (Clark's Level IV)
pT3a	Tumor more than 1.5 mm but not more than 3 mm in thickness
pT3b	Tumor more than 3 mm but not more than 4 mm in thickness
pT4	Tumor more than 4 mm in thickness and/or invades the subcutaneous tissue (Clark's Level V) and/or satellite(s) within 2 cm of the primary tumor
pT4a	Tumor more than 4 mm in thickness and/or invades the subcutaneous tissue
pT4b	Satellite(s) within 2 cm of the primary tumor

Regional Lymph Nodes (N)

NX	Regional lymph nodes cannot be assessed
N0	No regional lymph node metastasis
N1	Metastasis 3 cm or less in greatest dimension in any regional lymph node(s)

N2   Metastasis more than 3 cm in greatest dimension in any regional lymph node(s) and/or in-transit metastasis

      N2a   Metastasis more than 3 cm in greatest dimension in any regional lymph node(s)

      N2b   In-transit metastasis

      N2c   Both (N2a and N2b)

Note: In-transit metastasis involves skin or subcutaneous tissue more than 2 cm from the primary tumor but not beyond the regional lymph nodes.

Distant Metastasis (M)

MX   Distant metastasis cannot be assesesd

M0   No distant metastasis

M1   Distant metastasis

      M1a   Metastasis in skin or subcutaneous tissue or lymph node(s) beyond the regional lymph nodes

      M1b   Visceral metastasis

STAGE GROUPING			
Stage 0	pTis	N0	M0
Stage I	pT1	N0	M0
	pT2	N0	M0
Stage II	pT3	N0	M0
Stage III	pT4	N0	M0
	Any pT	N1	M0
	Any pT	N2	M0
Stage IV	Any pT	Any N	M1

Used with the permission of the American Joint Committee on Cancer (AJCC®), Chicago, Illinois. The original source for this material is the AJCC® Cancer Staging Handbook, 5th edition (1998) published by Lippincott-Raven Publishers, Philadelphia, Pennsylvania.

Pathologic staging of the primary melanoma is based on a microscopic assessment of thickness and level of invasion (Clark's levels I–V). Therefore, evaluation of the entire tumor is advised rather than a wedge or a punch biopsy. Regional nodes should be evaluated by a physical examination. Histopathologic grading for melanoma is identical to the grading system used for BCC and SCC.

Diagnostic work-up should include a complete physical, with a full skin check to rule out a second primary. Special note should be made of symptoms suggestive of metastatic disease such as abdominal pain, bone pain, weight loss, double vision, headaches, malaise, seizures. A chest film should be ordered to exclude the possibility of a silent lung metastasis. The liver, spleen, and regional lymph nodes should be palpated for lymphadenopathy.[6]

Further diagnostic testing includes routine laboratory tests—complete blood count, lactate dehydrogenase, blood urea nitrogen, partial thromboplastin time, liver enzyme studies, urinalysis, serum creatinine, and blood chemistries. Other essential studies, for example, computed tomography (CT) scan or magnetic resonance imaging (MRI) are guided by the symptomatology reported by the patient and outcome of the above tests.[31]

Lesion thickness largely dictates how exhaustive the search for signs of metastatic disease will be.[6] Clark's level and Breslow's depth are two methods to predict prognosis of melanoma, which is related to the depth of invasion of the primary tumor.[7]

Clark's Level and Breslow's Thickness

In 1989, Clark and colleagues in the Pigmented Lesion Study Group (PLSG) published results of a prospective study of a large cohort with long term follow-up in an effort to identify criteria predictive of prognosis for a given patient with stage 1 primary invasive malignant melanoma. An analysis of 6 of 23 attributes studied were shown to have the greatest independent predictive strength: (1) *tumor cell mitotic rate per mm²*, (2) *presence of tumor infiltrating lymphocyte*, (3) *tumor thickness*, (4) *anatomic location of the primary lesion*, (5) *sex of the patient, and* (6) *histologic regression.* Results of this seminal work were expanded and further validated these predictive attributes.[36] This investigative research led to the use of Clark's level and Breslow's depth as prognostic indicators of primary malignant melanoma.

Clark's level is a qualitative description of the increasing levels of penetration through the dermis to the subcutaneous fat, whereas Breslow's depth is a direct measurement of the primary tumor depth or thickness.[7, 35] A reading of *Clark's level* is comprised of four histopathologic attributes identified as being predictive of clinical outcome: tumor thickness, mitotic rate, histologic regression, and presence of tumor infiltrating lymphocytes[36] (Fig. 18–1).

Breslow's thickness is the crucial parameter of vertical tumor thickness, from the top of the granular layer to the base of the tumor. The *Breslow thickness* reflects the observation that prognosis worsens with increasing ranges of tumor thickness. To date, *the single attribute best predictive of clinical outcome for a given patient is the depth of tumor invasion, the Breslow level, or Breslow thickness,* considered the gold standard for stratifying patients according to risk of metastatic disease.[36] Although the Breslow gauge is currently the most trustworthy tool available, it is not foolproof.[6] Many individuals with deeply invasive tumors cured by simple excision and some individuals with superficially invasive lesions die from metastasis.[36]

ADDITIONAL PROGNOSTIC FACTORS

An assortment of other prognostic elements are often considered: women seem to have a better survival rate than men, probably due to hormonal factors[20, 35]; patients with melanoma of the head, neck, or trunk tend to fare worse than those with a tumor on the extremities;

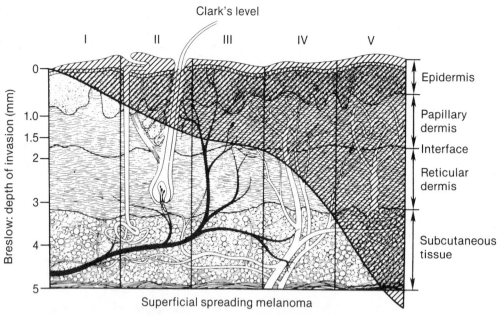

FIGURE 18 – 1 Anatomic landmarks and Clark's level of invasion. (From DiSaia PJ, Creasman WT: *Clinical gynecologic oncology*, ed 5, St. Louis, Mosby, 1997.)

and a lesion on the hands or feet carries a worse prognosis than one on the arms or legs.[6, 36]

Lymph Node Involvement

A part of the surgical treatment of melanoma is actually an extension of the diagnostic process of staging the patient's disease. Historically, staging was first done through elective lymph node dissection (ELND).[34] Regional lymph nodes are a common site for the first appearance of metastatic tumor.[7, 35, 47] Therefore, the presence or absence of node involvement is a second powerful predictor of outcome.[7]

The ELND procedure is the complete dissection of the lymphatic basin draining the site of the primary melanoma in patients with clinically negative nodes.[47] The rationale for this procedure was based on the following hypothesis:

1. That most metastases in melanoma progress through the lymph nodes and then on to distant sites
2. That some patients with clinically negative nodes will have occult micrometastases to regional nodes
3. That these regional metastases will result in distant metastases if not treated
4. That treatment of patients with regional micrometastases will result in improved survival rates as compared with survival rates of patients with clinically positive nodal disease[47]

Patients with regional lymph node involvement at the time of diagnosis or with recurrent disease in the re-

gional lymph node basin have high relapse rates of 50% to 90%.[7]

One of the ongoing controversies regarding melanoma care has been the management of lymph nodes that are normal on physical examination.[35] Three decades ago prophylactic lymph node dissection was warranted in everyone. At that time however, the thin melanomas that so characterize the disease in North America today was unheard of. The vast majority of patients with melanoma had thick, nodular, recurrent cancers with nodal metastasis.[35] It was and is essential to examine the risk/reward ratio of lymph node dissection, controlling for the risk of complications such as chronic lymphedema and the occasional mortality. ELND therefore, remains controversial.[7]

Retrospective analyses of clinical data have shown there is no survival advantage for ELND when patients have tumors less than 1 mm in thickness because the cure rate from local excision alone is very high. On the opposite end of the spectrum, patients with tumors greater than 4 mm in thickness have a very high incidence of distant as well as local and regional metastasis. Therefore, this group also would not benefit from ELND. It was in the intermediate thickness group (1–4 mm) that ELND was felt to be useful because the incidence of regional metastasis was significantly greater than the incidence of distant metastasis.[47]

In the Melanoma Intergroup Trial, the group of patients younger than 60 years with tumors 1 to 2 mm in thickness did achieve a significantly improved survival after ELND compared with observed patients. End results showed the prognosis for patients with regional lymph node metastasis is proportional to the number of nodes involved. Survival for patients undergoing resection of lymph nodes containing clinically occult melanoma is significantly longer than patients who undergo resection of palpably enlarged nodes.[7, 47]

Sentinel Lymph Node Techniques

The concept of sentinel lymph node (SLN) biopsy was introduced when work with lymphoscintigraphy demonstrated that lymph node basins draining from a specific site could be defined by injection of a radionuclide. Animal and then human studies demonstrated that there are well-defined pathways from each cutaneous site to a specific regional lymph nodes or node.[47] *This rationale assumes that for every site, the lymphatic drainage is not only to a specific basin, but first to a specific node within that basin and then to other nodes sequentially. Thus, if the sentinel (first) node is negative, the remaining distal nodes will be negative also.* Complete node dissection then would not be indicated.[34]

The ability to identify preoperatively the regional nodal basins at greatest risk and the first or SLNs within those basins would provide maximum benefit to those patients at greatest risk for metastases, while sparing other patients the morbidity and cost of complete node dissections. In addition, following SLN dissection, side effects are few and patients can use their arm immediately.[30] This is the rationale for lymphatic mapping and SLN biopsy (see Chapter 21).

Preoperative Lymphoscintigraphy. Preoperative lymphoscintigraphy, SLN biopsy, and intraoperative radiolymphatic mapping have greatly improved our ability to accurately assess the status of the regional lymph nodes and decrease the morbidity of ELND.[7] Introduced in 1992 by Morton and colleagues, *"sentinel lymph node technology"* is a common concept today.[34, 35, 47] Lymph nodes draining from a specific site can be defined by injection of a radionuclide (sulfur colloid or technetium-labeled human serum albumin) into the skin at the primary site before a wide local excision is performed.[7, 47] As the radionucleotide is absorbed by the lymphatics, radiographic images are taken. These identify the lymph node basin that drains the primary lesion.[7] This is a definite advantage because these results were not always consistent with the classic anatomic drawings of lymphatic pathways, particularly those for truncal, head, and neck tumors. Initially, this technique was used as a guide for ELND.[34]

Sentinel Lymph Node Mapping and Biopsy. First used by Morton and coworkers in 1992,[34, 47] in addition to preoperative lymphoscintigraphy, a vital blue dye is injected intradermally around the primary site. This allows for intraoperative visualization of the lymphatics and

the SLN.[34] The SLN receives drainage directly from the primary tumor site.[19] The first lymph node, the SLN, is surgically removed and wide excision is performed. Both specimens are sent for thorough histologic examination. The SNL has been found to reflect the histologic status of the whole basin. If the SNL is negative for metastatic disease the remainder of the nodes are usually negative and lymph node dissection is not indicated.[7] This technique does require a large flap incision over the nodal basin and meticulous dissection to identify all of the blue-stained lymphatic channels.[34]

Intraoperative Lymphoscintigraphy. In this staging procedure, after injection of the radiocolloid, a hand held gamma-detecting probe is used intraoperatively to identify nodes containing the radiocolloid. Often favored, it requires less dissection and can often be done under local anesthesia. Gershenwald and coworkers found that combining techniques significantly improved SLN localization from 87% using dye only to 99% using dye and radioactive colloid together.[34] SLN mapping is a rational alternative to routine ELND. It provides accurate staging data of the nodes and is a relatively low morbidity technique that identifies patients most likely to benefit from lymph node dissection. Mapping also identifies patients at risk for recurrence who may have potential benefit from some adjuvant therapies.[30]

Strong evidence indicates the SLN accurately reflects the pathology of the regional node basin. The National Cancer Institute is currently conducting the Multicenter Selective Lymphadenectomy Trial. This ongoing prospective study, which randomly allocates patients to either wide local excision (WLE) or WLE and SLN biopsy, will give the first indication of the degree to which sentinel lymphadenectomy affects survival rates. Results of this study are expected in the year 2001.[34]

Sentinel node mapping should not be used when palpable nodes are present or when wide excision or skin graft closure of the primary tumor is done. The latter procedure alters the lymphatic drainage pattern. Mapping is also not done if the primary melanoma is not still intact.[30]

Immunohistochemical and Polymerase Assays. The advent of immunohistochemical markers of cell proliferation profoundly influenced tumor pathology.[44] Currently there are studies underway using melanoma-specific immunohistochemical and polymerase chain reaction (PCR) assays to detect occult melanoma micrometastasis in lymph node tissue that has been removed by biopsy. One such assay is reverse transcriptase (RT)-PCR, which detects the presence of tyrosinase messenger RNA. Tyrosinase, which is involved in the production of melanin, is expressed almost exclusively by melanocytes and melanoma cells. Its presence in an SLN found to be histologically negative for melanoma might point to patients who have a more guarded prognosis and may be candidates for more complete lymph node dissection or adjuvant therapy or both. Currently several RT-PCR assays are being studied to detect circulating melanoma cells in the blood. If proven to be specific for melanoma and not normally detected in those without melanoma, these assays may be used to improve staging and management of malignant melanoma.[7, 34, 44]

Vaccine Therapy. Early vaccine studies in some animal models showed a protective benefit using bacillus Calmette-Guerin (BCG) and levamisole. There was evidence of spontaneous regression of melanomas, which suggested the vaccine's ability to launch a natural immunity to the tumor. Today, current vaccine therapy for melanoma is progressing in conjunction with the advances in biotechnology. Some specific melanoma antigens have been identified, which induce specific cell line antibody and T-cell responses (e.g., vaccina or detox). Newer vaccines including genetically engineered and peptide models are in the preliminary stages of investigation. Although research reports anticipate great progress in melanoma using vaccine therapy, these advances are being closely monitored in clinical trial settings.[7, 34]

METASTASES

Malignant melanoma may spread to any organ or remote viscera. Common sites for disseminated disease are the skin (intracutaneous or subcutaneous metastasis), bone, brain, lung, and liver.[31] Malignant melanoma may grow radially or vertically. All melanomas except the nodular type have an initial radical growth phase, which may last more than a decade. During this phase the melanoma cells remain confined to the epidermis. The lesion expands horizontally with only a slight increase in the tumor's depth.

Dermal penetration and invasion of the dermis and subcutaneous tissue by the melanoma cells characterize the vertical phase. The lesions may then metastasize by way of the vascular or lymphatic channels. The melanoma cells then spread rapidly to other parts of the body. Nodular malignant melanoma has no radical growth phase. These lesions are usually convex and are palpable because of growth elevation above the level of the normal skin.[31]

TREATMENT MODALITIES

Surgery

Surgical resection remains the mainstay of melanoma treatment for stage I and II disease. Historically, and up until the 1970s, most melanoma patients were treated with local excisions using a 3- to 5-cm margin. Often

surgeons used smaller margins though to avoid resection of major anatomic structures and improve cosmesis; in some situations the location of the tumor might make it impossible to adhere to recommended perimeters.[6, 47] It was later determined that patients with smaller margins experienced recurrence rates equal to those patients with larger margins. Retrospectively, it was determined that the incidence of local recurrence was related to tumor thickness and similar factors related to survival.[47]

The Melanoma Trial of the World Health Organization also demonstrated that tumors less than 1 mm in thickness could be excised with a 1-cm margin, after which no recurrences were seen. Although patients with tumors greater than 4 mm in thickness have a relatively high risk of local recurrence, little evidence supports extending the width of local excision beyond 2 cm. Wider excisions may reduce the incidence of recurrence but are unlikely to have a survival benefit when the risk of preexisting systemic metastasis is so high.[47] Wide local excision is defined as a dissection extending down through the subcutaneous tissues to, but not including, the fascia.

Excisional biopsy with a 3- to 5-mm margin is appropriate for in situ melanoma.[47] Patients with stage III disease include those with primary lesions more than 4 mm in depth and those with disease contained in, but not confined to, the regional lymph nodes. For patients with known disease in the regional lymph node basin, a lymph node dissection is indicated. Even after surgical resection, these patients face a high rate of recurrence. In stage IV disease the melanoma has spread beyond the regional lymph nodes and into other tissues and organs. Surgical resection for the most part is not indicated, with the possible exception of a single metastatic lesion or to palliate painful lesions[7, 34, 47] (see Chapter 21).

Elective Regional Node Dissection (ERLAND)

Issues concerning and parameters for elective lymph node dissection were discussed previously. Cutaneous melanoma primarily spreads to four main lymph node basins: intraparotid, cervical, axillary, and ilioguinal. If metastatic disease first appears in intraparotid nodes, superficial parotidectomy in conjunction with nodal dissection is usually performed. If cervical nodes are extensively affected, a radical neck dissection is the procedure of choice. Axillary node dissection with an en bloc of pectoralis minor muscle is the standard procedure.[31]

Elective lymph node dissection for patients with stage I disease has been a hotly debated topic. The argument whether regional dissection improves prognosis in patients who have tumors of "intermediate thickness" (1.5–4.0 mm) remains undecided. Those in favor suggest that removal of lymph nodes that feel normal captures microscopic disease. Opponents say that removing the lymph nodes only alters the time disease will manifest itself.[6]

The dilemma becomes more complicated if the lesion has access to more than one lymph node basin. For instance, a lesion on the lower leg would most often metastasize to inguinal lymph nodes on the same side. However, if the tumor were in the middle of the back, which nodes would be considered for dissection? For these reasons and others, SLN identification may reduce the percentage of patients who must endure nodal dissection only to find the nodes are negative.[6]

Radiation Therapy

Historically, melanoma was felt to be radioresistant.[7, 31] Primary melanoma is seldom treated with radiotherapy with the exception of lentigo maligna. Two methods of radiation therapy are used for lentigo maligna. The first is fractionated radiation therapy, and the second, the Meischer technique, primarily used in Europe, uses a contact machine that delivers large doses of radiation that penetrate superficially.[34] Adjuvant radiation therapy to the nodal basins of high-risk tumors may prolong survival or reduce subsequent metastasis. Radiation has been used to treat nodal basins where surgery has shown multiple positive nodes, extracapsular tumor, or a single node fully replaced by tumor. Radiation therapy has decreased regional recurrence but has not improved long-term survival rates.[34]

While total brain radiation therapy has increased survival time, particularly when combined with surgical resection. Radiation is also beneficial for patients who are in pain due to bone metastasis, but full regression of the tumor is rare.[7]

Chemotherapy

DTIC. On the whole, chemotherapy has not been that useful in the treatment of disseminated malignant melanoma, and in some sources has been used as a palliative approach.[6] Primarily used in stage IV with metastatic disease, DTIC is the most readily recognized Food and Drug Administration approved agent for that purpose. Several other chemotherapy agents have been studied (vincristine, vinblastine, cisplatin, carboplatin, BCNU, and CCNU) and none have consistently shown better response rates than DTIC.[7, 34] The most common dosage schedule has been 250 mg/m^2 daily for 5 days every 4 weeks.[31] Used singly, the response rate with DTIC is between 10% and 20%, with a median duration of 3 to 6 months. Response is better for metastasis to soft-tissue areas—lymph node, skin, and lung generally fare better than bone, brain, or liver.

The well-known adverse side effects of DTIC, myleosuppression and gastrointestinal distress, are somewhat lessened with the 5-HT$_3$ antiemetics. These products provide for a higher single dose, which could be repeated every 3 weeks.[9, 34] Ongoing clinical trials at both the Cancer Community Oncology Program (CCOP) study comparing DTIC alone with cisplatin/ vinblastine/DTIC and the Memorial Sloan Kettering Cancer Center study comparing DTIC alone against BCNU/DTIC/tamoxifen (called chemohormonal therapy) will reveal whether overall response rate and survival is improved with DTIC in combination with a particular agent.[34]

Two new agents currently under investigation may also improve response rates. The first, *temozolomide,* is an analogue of DTIC, which has the ability to cross the blood–brain barrier, which will be efficacious in those patients who develop brain metastasis or those who have central nervous system involvement. Currently under phase II clinical trials, one advantage is that the drug is administered orally and secondly, temozolomide is not dependent on metabolic activation in the liver. Response rates thus far are comparable to DTIC.[34] *Fotemustine,* a nitrosourea that has been studied in France and not yet available in the United States, also has the benefit of crossing the blood–brain barrier. A multicenter phase II study of 153 patients reported an overall response rate of 24% and a response rate of approximately 20% in persons with brain metastases.[34] High-dose chemotherapy followed by autologous bone marrow transplantation is another option for patients being explored in clinical studies. These regimens require intensive hospitalization and are associated with significant morbidity.[31]

Hyperthermic Regional Perfusion

This technique, also called *isolated limb perfusion* (ILP), was developed in the 1950s to treat various cancers, but is most effective in treating melanoma of the limbs.[34] It is the perfusion of chemotherapeutic agents directly into an extremity. This technique is most often used with melphalen or cisplatin, although nitrogen mustard, and DTIC have also been used.[31, 34] This procedure is most often used for *in transit metastasis,* which involves skin or subcutaneous tissue more than 2 cm from the primary tumor but not beyond the regional lymph nodes.[7]

The limb is usually perfused for 1 hour with a high concentration of drug at 39° to 41°C (102.2°–105.8°F) with a perfusion pump and extracorporeal circulator. The hyperthermia enhances the cytotoxic effect so that the total dose of drug may be reduced. This modality delivers a high concentration of drug to areas of locoregional recurrences in an extremity and produces minimal side effects.[31] This procedure must be performed in a specialized setting.

Although this technique eliminates most adverse systemic effects associated with chemotherapy, some systemic toxicity from perfusate leakage has been reported. Regional toxicity is more common and varies from blistering erythema and limb edema, to myopathy and peripheral neuropathy that can be long term in 5% to 8% of the patients. Vascular events, including arterial and venous thrombosis, and tissue necrosis have been reported with melphalan.[34] Other complications include nerve and muscle damage and rarely, the loss of the extremity.[31] Objective data regarding the benefits of ILP are still limited. The majority of studies conducted to date have been retrospective, comparing a variety of histologic findings, staging systems, dosages, and temperature elevations. Prospective studies to date are limited by small number of participants. The best supported indication for ILP is as therapeutic treatment for unresectable disease, primarily stage III disease, in transit metastasis. In recent years, complete remission rates for therapeutic ILP are over 50%. Although recurrences after ILP have remained high (40%), the possibility of salvaging a limb makes the use of ILP a significant alternative.[34]

Over time modifications of the traditional technique have led to improvements for therapeutic limb perfusion. Multiple schedules and combinations have been attempted. One of the most promising has been the synergistic combination of melphalan with cytokine tumor necrosis factor-α (TNF-α) and interferon-gamma (IFN-μ). Results in the literature show that complete remission rates for this triple regimen are significantly better than for ILP using melphalan alone.[34] Larger prospective studies are needed to delineate the appropriate applications and benefits of limb perfusion. Based on current information, those patients with aggressive nonresectable primary or recurrent disease are those most likely to benefit from ILP and should be strongly considered for this treatment.[34]

Biotherapy

Interferon-alfa-2b. For patients with known disease in the regional lymph node basin, a lymph node dissection is indicated. Even after surgical resection, these patients face a high risk of recurrence. Because adjuvant chemotherapy has not proved beneficial in improving disease free survival or life expectancy, much of the research has focused on biotherapy.[7] Biotherapy uses agents normally produced in the body in small amounts to stimulate the immune system's normal ability to recognize and fight cancer.[7] These agents are also referred to as *biologic response modifiers or BMRs.*

Recombinant interferon alfa-2b, a BRM, was the first approved as adjuvant therapy to surgery for patients with malignant melanoma. At its inception it was indicated in adults 18 years and older who were free of disease postoperatively but likely to experience a recurrence. Although survival differences were not monumental, they were significant enough to prove that interferon alfa-2b could influence the course of disease.[6] Through recombinant DNA technology, these agents can be produced in large quantities, making them available for clinical use.[7]

The treatment of melanoma was significantly changed in January 1996, when Kirkwood and coworkers from the Eastern Cooperative Oncology Group (ECOG) reported that high doses of interferon alfa-2b significantly prolonged both relapse-free and overall survival following surgical resection of high-risk primary melanoma (AJCC stage II-B) or regional lymph node metastasis (AJCC stage III). This important study was the first randomized, controlled trial to show a significant benefit of adjuvant therapy in prolonging relapse-free and overall survival of high-risk melanoma patients.[27]

Recombinant interferon alfa-2b has recently been approved for use in persons who are at risk for recurrence, in whom improved survival rates have been demonstrated. Such patients include those with melanoma thickness that exceeds 4 mm or who have primary or recurrent nodal involvement.[42] After early reports of longer remissions with interferon-α (IFN-α) alone, *biochemotherapeutic* regimens were studied with hope of achieving further increases in efficacy. Initial investigations, involving DTIC plus IFN-α, did not show consistently improved response or survival rates. Numerous other combinations were tested, such as IFN with DTIC, bleomycin, cisplatin and tamoxifen (DBCT), which increased toxicities without improving efficacy.[34]

At least one phase II study of IFN plus the four-drug regimen of DTIC/vincristine/bleomycin/lomustine, however, shows a substantially higher response rate of 62%. Further studies need to confirm this finding. The majority of the data suggest that adding IFN-α alone does not provide benefit over chemotherapy alone.[34]

Interleukin-2 (IL-2). Recombinant IL-2 is a cytokine that stimulates the immune system to produce T cells, lymphokine-activated killer cells, and natural killer (NK) cells that may target and kill cancer cells. Recombinant IL-2 also promotes the creation and release of other cytokines and activates B cells to produce immunoglobulins.[9] Positive results have more consistently been reported with the use of IL-2 in biochemotherapeutic regimens.[34] Although responses of 13% to 33% have been reported with the IL-2/DTIC, these rates do not vary significantly from results with DTIC alone. However, when both IL-2 and interferon alfa-2 were combined with cisplatin/vinblastine/DTIC (CVD) in the study by Legha and colleagues at the M. D. Anderson

Cancer Center, the response rates were as high as 60% with 21% of patients having a complete response.[34] These therapeutic benefits were not obtained without distress, however. Severe toxicities occurred with early BRMs and still do today.[34]

Each combination of BRM and chemotherapy brings its own set of drug interactions.[9] Melanoma patients who receive concurrent biochemotherapy must be in relatively good health, have a performance status of 0, 1, or 2 on the ECOG scale, normal white blood cell and platelet counts, normal serum creatinine and serum bilirubin levels, and be free of all other serious diseases other than cancer.[9] All patients are hospitalized because of the toxic side effects that most patients encounter with concurrent biochemotherapy. The major side effects for these patients can be grouped into the following categories: hematologic, cardiovascular, renal, hepatic, gastrointestinal, pulmonary, neurologic, integumentary, and general flulike symptoms[9] (see Chapter 24).

Hormonal Therapy

Estrogen and progesterone receptors found on melanoma cells signify a relationship between hormones and malignant melanoma. Some sources report women "do better" with malignant melanoma and attribute that advantage to hormonal factors.[6, 20] Hormonal therapy for malignant melanoma is under investigation. Tamoxifen and diethylstibesterol are being explored.[31]

Long-Term Follow-up

A patient who has had melanoma must be seen for regular skin checks and physical exams. These should take place every 3 months for the first year and every 6 months thereafter. Melanoma is not considered to be cured after 5 years without recurrence. It is quite common for patients to develop evidence of metastasis 5 to 10 years after the primary lesion was removed and sometimes more than a decade or two later. The objective is to make sure there are no signs of metastasis and no new tumors.[6]

In addition to complete blood count, blood chemistries and an annual chest film should be obtained. Regular liver function studies should be ordered; alkaline phosphatase and alanine aminotransferase are recommended for patients who had thicker melanomas. If these are elevated, a CT of the liver should be ordered. One study of 145 patients who had recurrences after surgical resection of an intermediate or high-risk melanoma indicated that patient history or physical examination identified 94% of new episodes. The remaining 6% were discovered by chest film.[6] Patients may also present with an unknown primary tumor. That is, a metastasis is revealed in the brain or the lung with now prior evidence of the source. It is felt that the initial tumor regressed. Lifelong vigilance is essential.[6]

PROGNOSIS

The single attribute best predictive of clinical outcome for a given patient is depth of tumor invasion, the Breslow level, considered the gold standard for stratifying patients according to risk of metastatic disease.[6] The overall 5-year survival rate for persons with melanoma is 88%.[1] Surgery is curative in more than 90% of instances when the melanoma is thin (< 1 mm) and has not spread beyond the initial area of growth. Cure with surgery is 70% to 80% when a melanoma lesion is greater than 1 mm but less than 3 mm thick. Lesions more than 4 mm in depth are considered deep melanomas, and about 42% will recur after surgical resection.[7] The presence or absence of lymph node involvement is a second powerful predictor of outcome. Patients with regional lymph node involvement at time of diagnosis or with recurrent disease in the regional lymph node basin have relapse rates of 50% to 90%.[7]

CONCLUSION

Skin cancers are the most common forms of cancer and no individual escapes the risk of developing one of these three diseases. Although BCCs and SCCs are readily preventable, treatable, and to some extent curable, we still have an uphill battle convincing the public and fellow health care providers of the efficacy of sun avoidance, sun protection, screening, and detection. Malignant melanoma is a devastating disease. Although recognizing that the genetic revolution has offered several new possibilities for treatment and improved survival outcomes, we still have to develop measures of identifying those at increased risk, teach avoidance and protective measures, develop protocols to combat treatment toxicities and side effects, and emphasize long-term follow-up. "Skin cancer writes its message on the skin with its own ink and is there for all of us to see. Unfortunately, some see but do not comprehend," according to Dr. Neville Davis of Australia.[39]

Nursing Management

Nursing diagnoses, assessments, and interventions are similar for both nonmelanoma and malignant melanoma. Some variations may be necessary depending on type and location of skin cancer and method of treatment. A complete nursing history includes information regarding risk factors, previous treatment, and a thorough skin examination focusing on all moles for any suspicious changes. Nursing management of side effects of treatment methods are discussed in detail in Chapters 21 to 24. Skin grafting is common after surgical treatment of melanoma.[4, 8, 9, 21]

Postsurgical interventions include instructing patients and families on the management of a surgical wound. Keeping the area clean and dry and observing for signs and symptoms of infection are imperative. If skin grafting is required, patients and their families should be instructed to keep the graft immobile to prevent stress on the edges of the wound. Limbs should be elevated to minimize edema. Mineral oil or lanolin may be used to remove superficial crusts, moisten the site of the skin graft, and stimulate circulation.

The results of treatment of both nonmelanoma and malignant melanoma may lead to rehabilitation problems. Disfigurement may occur as a result of surgical interventions. Nonmelanoma skin cancers tend to occur in sun-exposed areas of the body, especially the head and neck regions. Surgical interventions to this area of the body may affect a person's body image and self-esteem. Assisting patients to cope with alterations in body image is a prime responsibility of the nurse.*

Immobility may also occur as a result of surgical interventions. The wider margins necessary in malignant melanoma coupled with skin grafting may lead to problems of immobility. Assisting patients to maintain their level of functioning is also an important responsibility of the nurse.

Patient/family teaching for malignant melanoma is similar to the teaching for nonmelanoma skin cancers. The importance of early detection should be emphasized to both patients and family members. Patients and family members should be instructed on the importance of monthly, systematic skin self-examination. Individuals should be instructed to check the entire skin surface, paying special attention to all moles for suspicious changes. Family members can be taught to assist patients by checking the scalp and back region. Patients diagnosed with melanoma

and those at risk of developing melanoma should be encouraged to keep regularly scheduled appointments with their physician.

Methods of prevention, primarily the importance of avoiding intense sunlight and the use of protective clothing and sunscreens, should also be taught. Parents should be instructed on the above-mentioned prevention measures for their children. Both patient and family members should be instructed about the ABCD rules for remembering the warning signs of melanoma.

Nursing diagnoses for basal cell carcinoma (BCC) and squamous cell carcinoma (SCC) are similar. Some variations may be necessary depending on type and location of skin cancer and method of treatment.

*Nursing Diagnoses**

- *Knowledge deficit related to prevention and early detection of skin cancer, disease process, treatment (surgery, radiation therapy, chemotherapy, biotherapy), home care management of surgical wound*
- *Skin integrity, impaired, related to skin cancer and surgical treatment*
- *Infection, risk for, related to surgical wound*
- *Mobility, impaired physical, related to surgical treatment and possible skin graft*
- *Body image disturbance related to location and surgical treatment for skin cancer*
- *Social interaction, impaired, related to location and surgical treatment of skin cancer*
- *Anxiety related to diagnosis of cancer, fear of recurrence, death, pain, disfigurement, changes in lifestyle*

Assessment and Intervention

- Nursing assessment and intervention should focus on prevention, detection, and treatment methods.
- The nursing history should include a thorough skin assessment, which consists of information regarding patient risk factors, and a complete skin examination.
- Patient teaching priorities should include the prevention and detection methods discussed in this chapter (see Patient Teaching Priorities).
- See Geriatric Considerations box.
- Postsurgical interventions include instructing patients and families on the management of a surgical wound.

---

* References 21, 24, 25, 29, 31, 35, 36, 44.

* Data from references 1–3, 5, 10, 13, 18, 25, 28, 29, 33, 38.

PATIENT TEACHING PRIORITIES

Skin Cancers

Risk Factors for Development of Malignant Melanoma

Family history of malignant melanoma
Presence of blond or red hair
Presence of marked freckling on upper back
History of three or more blistering sunburns before age 20
History of 3 or more years of an outdoor summer job as a teenager
Presence of actinic keratosis

Prevention of Skin Cancer Measures

Avoid excessive sun exposure, particularly the hours between 10 AM and 3 PM.
Wear sunscreens and lip balm with a sun protection factor of 30 or greater.
Use available shade.
Wear protective clothing.
Refrain from using manufactured tanning devices.

Skin Cancer Screening and Detection

Perform monthly self-examination of skin or with other person.
With good lighting, use two mirrors to visualize the abdomen, perineal area, and back.
Use blow hair dryer and mirror to visualize scalp.
Observe each body part carefully, especially hidden areas such as between toes and folds of skin.
Use of body chart facilitates documentation of changes and suspected lesions to report.
Persons with two or more family members with a history of malignant melanoma should be examined by a dermatologist every 6 months.
Recognize and report symptoms or changes in skin characteristics promptly to physician, such as:
  A, Asymmetry of shape
  B, Border irregularity
  C, Color variegation (black, brown, white, blue, red)
  D, Diameter larger than 5 mm

Data from references 2, 3, 6, 11, 13, 18, 22, 25, 28, 33, and 40.

- Keeping the area clean and dry and observing for signs and symptoms of infection are imperative.
- If skin grafting is required, patients and their families should be instructed to keep the graft immobile to prevent stress on the edges of the wound. Limbs should be elevated to minimize edema.
- Mineral oil or lanolin may be used to remove superficial crusts, moisten the site of the skin graft, and stimulate circulation. See Complications box.

GERIATRIC CONSIDERATIONS

Skin Cancers

Geriatric population has greatest incidence of precancerous and cancerous skin lesions.
Average age of onset for squamous cell, lentigo malignant melanoma, and acral lentiginous melanoma is 60 years.
Age-related sensory and muscle deficits require assistance of other person for monthly skin self-examination.
Age-related changes in skin characteristics include fair skin and easily bruised superficial tissue.
Limited access to health care system and limited health care resources may inhibit preventive health care.
Senior citizen centers should be targeted to reach those who participate in organized activities

Data from references 11, 13, 18, 33, 39, 43, 45, and 48.

COMPLICATIONS

Skin Cancers

Surgery and Radiation Therapy

Scarring of affected tissue
Skin discoloration
Alterations in cosmetic appearance
Chronic skin ulcerations
Limited use of limb if extensive treatment

Chemotherapy and Biotherapy

Nausea and vomiting
Flulike syndrome
Myelosuppression
Paresthesia
Necrotic tissue as result of drug extravasation
Pulmonary fibrosis
Renal damage
Hot flashes
Hypersensitivity
Ototoxicity
Alopecia
Allergic reaction

General

Alteration in cosmetic appearance and body image
Loss of functional use of extremity
Scarring and skin discoloration
Metastatic disease process resulting in invasive treatment and potential ultimate death

Data from references 5, 9, 15, 19, 23, 34, 35, 47, and 49.

- Nursing management of complications of other treatment methods, such as radiation therapy, chemotherapy, and biotherapy, are discussed in detail in Chapters 22, 23, and 24, respectively.*
- The importance of early detection should be stressed with both patients and families. BCC is almost always curable. Recurrent lesions or new lesions can be successfully treated when detected early for BCC and SCC.
- Patients and family members should be instructed on the procedure and the importance of periodic skin self-examination. Patients should be encouraged to keep appointments for regular follow-up examinations with their physician. Methods of prevention should also be taught, primarily the importance of avoiding intense sunlight and using protective sunscreens and clothing.

Outcome Goals

Patient/family will be able to:

- Define basal cell, squamous cell, and melanoma skin cancer.
- Describe risk factors: skin color, hair color, exposure to UV radiation, and chemical carcinogens.
- Recognize signs and symptoms of disease: sore that does not heal; persistent lump or swelling; bleeding from mole; freckle, birthmark, or other preexisting lesions; changes in moles or birthmarks—size, shape, outline, elevation, surface, sensation, surrounding skin changes, and color.
- State prevention measures: avoid prolonged exposure to sunlight; minimize sun burning and sun tanning; and use sunscreens appropriately.

Interventions

- Define and describe risk factors: fair complexion, sunburn easily, red or blond hair, reside in geographic region that receives high levels of UV radiation, and history of nonmelanoma/melanoma skin cancer.
- Describe and discuss methods to minimize sun exposure: wear lip balm/sunscreen with SPF of 15 or higher, avoid exposure to sun between hours of 10 AM and 3 PM; wear protective clothing, maximize use of available shade, keep infants and children out of the sun, and teach and practice sun protection measures early in children's growth and developmental process.

- Discuss importance of and procedure for routine skin self-examination: cover entire skin in a methodic fashion; use good lighting, mirrors, hair dryer, and another person to examine difficult-to-see areas (scalp, perineum, back); and document and report promptly any changes and/or new conditions.

Nursing Diagnosis

- *Knowledge deficit related to disease process*

Outcome Goals

Patient/family will be able to:

- Verbalize signs and symptoms to report to physician/nurse.
- Verbalize signs and symptoms of altered skin integrity.

Interventions

- Discuss clinical features related to expectations for basal cell, squamous cell, and malignant melanoma (see Clinical Features boxes).
- Discuss potential procedures to be used in diagnosis and treatment of the specific skin cancer.
- Discuss symptoms to report to physician regarding disease process and/or a change in recovery, such as pain, fever, redness, swelling, and drainage at the biopsy/treatment site.

Nursing Diagnosis

- *Knowledge deficit related to method of treating disease (surgery, radiation therapy, chemical therapy, chemotherapy, biotherapy, isolated limb perfusion)*

Outcome Goals

Patient/family will be able to:

- Verbalize selected treatment and specific side effects.
- Identify signs and symptoms to report to physician and nurse (e.g., nausea and vomiting, pain, fever, pruritus, rash, swelling, lymph node tenderness).

Interventions

- Discuss schedule of specific therapy.
- Discuss treatment-related side effects.
- Discuss signs and symptoms related to complications from the various therapies.
- Discuss resources/alternative plans to facilitate compliance in the treatment of the disease (travel

---

* References 4, 9, 19, 27, 30, 35, 38, 47.

to/from physician/radiation therapy, dressings, supplies, home care assistance).
- Provide written materials explaining disease and treatment of disease.

Nursing Diagnosis

- *Knowledge deficit regarding home care management of surgical wound*

Outcome Goals

Patient/family will be able to:

- Perform necessary dressing procedure.
- Demonstrate proper knowledge of medication administration.
- Identify potential complications (e.g., fever, chills, erythema, increased wound drainage).
- Demonstrate proper body mechanics for mobility purposes.

Interventions

- Demonstrate dressing change with return demonstration of procedure.
- Have patient/family state place for purchase of supplies, resource to contact for assistance and to report symptoms, and signs and symptoms that may indicate infection.
- Ensure patient/family know procedure and can demonstrate proper body mechanics for mobility purposes, understand limitations and restrictions for elevation of extremity, and practice general hygiene.

Nursing Diagnosis

- *Skin integrity, impaired, related to skin cancer and surgical treatment*

Outcome Goals

Patient/family will be able to:

- Verbalize/demonstrate appropriate hygiene measures.
- Maintain adequate food and fluid intake.
- Maintain normal body weight.
- Maintain normal level of activity.
- Identify protection measures to avoid sources of infection.

Interventions

- Discuss/demonstrate hygiene (wash affected area with tepid water, pat dry); avoid pressure and irritating clothing.

- Discuss nutrition and hydration needs.
- Explain need to avoid exposure to infection.

Nursing Diagnosis

- *Infection, risk for, related to skin cancer and surgical treatment*

Outcome Goals

- Patient remains infection free, as evidenced by:
    Temperature within normal limits
    Laboratory values within normal limits
    Absence of inflammation, tenderness, or purulent drainage
    Maintenance of skin integrity

Interventions

- Discuss signs and symptoms of infection: pain, redness, swelling, drainage, and fever of 38°C (100.4°F); patient/family identifies when, where, and to whom to report information regarding infection risk.
- Provide prescribed therapies (antibiotics, analgesics, dressings).
- Implement measures to protect skin and affected area from trauma and bleeding.

Nursing Diagnosis

- *Mobility, impaired physical, related to surgical treatment and possible skin graft*

Outcome Goals

Patient will be able to:

- Demonstrate measures to prevent skin breakdown.
- Maintain optimal mobility sufficient to manage activities of daily living and independent transfers.
- Demonstrate measures to promote adequate circulation to tissues.

Interventions

- Discuss/teach proper body mechanics when transferring to/from bed/chair/commode and when walking.
- Discuss/demonstrate restrictions and limitations for affected extremity.
- Discuss/demonstrate rationale for body position changes if immobilized in bed.
- Discuss/demonstrate body mechanics for daily hygiene, and state any restrictions on shower/tub bath.

Nursing Diagnosis

- *Body image disturbance related to location and surgical treatment for skin cancer*

Outcome Goals

Patient/family will be able to:

- Identify/use appropriate community resources.
- Communicate feelings about changes in body image.
- Participate in care and ongoing decision making.

Interventions

- Encourage patient to share feelings with physician/nurse/family regarding changes in body image.
- Arrange and/or consult with professional/lay resources (cancer survivor) if requested by patient/family.
- Provide materials and pictorial images regarding invasive procedures and reconstruction process.
- Discuss/arrange cosmetic resources to enhance positive feelings about body image changes.

Nursing Diagnosis

- *Social interaction, impaired, related to location and surgical treatment of skin cancer*

Outcome Goals

Patient/family will be able to:

- Identify/use appropriate community resources.
- Participate in decision-making.
- Verbalize/demonstrate necessary life-style adaptations.

Interventions

- Discuss/plan selected activities patient can pursue (e.g., music, movies, reading, hobbies, crafts).
- Discuss/plan with family/significant other/home care agency resources to utilize in the community (e.g., Meals on Wheels, social contacts appropriate to age and developmental needs).
- Discuss/arrange for rehabilitation resources (e.g., physical therapy, occupational therapy).

Nursing Diagnosis

- *Anxiety related to diagnosis of cancer, fear of recurrence, death, pain, disfigurement, changes in lifestyle*

Outcome Goals

Patient will be able to:

- Discuss feelings and concerns with family members/health care team.
- Identify positive coping strategies.
- Identify specific concerns related to disease and treatment.

Interventions

- Discuss feelings and concerns related to these topics and ask what these experiences mean to patient.
- Identify patient's previous/present coping strategies when encountering difficult situations.
- Identify specific concerns and fears patient may be experiencing.
- Encourage patient to share feelings with family/friends/health care team.
- Demonstrate/encourage patient to use relaxation/distraction/meditation exercises to aid in other coping strategies.

Chapter Questions

1. Currently under study at Memorial Sloan Kettering is a combination chemotherapy-hormonal therapy protocol consisting of:
   a. BCNU/DTIC/tamoxifen
   b. DTIC/diethylstibesterol/BCNU
   c. Etoposide/DTIC/thiotepa
   d. Doxorubicin/semustine/megace
2. The difficulty of measuring decreased mortality as an outcome of skin cancer screening programs is primarily due to:
   a. fact of optimal follow-up time being 5 to 10 years later
   b. Cost of program set up and follow through
   c. Decreased access
   d. Failure of participants to do monthly skin self-examinations
3. Basal cell carcinoma (BCC) types include:
   a. Nodular, superficial, pigmented, keratonic, and verrucous
   b. Nodular, superficial, pigmented, morpheaform, and keratonic
   c. Composed nevus, seborrheic keratosis, nodular, pigmented, and actinic chelitis
   d. Morpheaform, keratonic, superficial, junctional nevi, and simple lentigo
4. Additional names for basal cell carcinoma are:
   a. Acitinic keratoses
   b. CAM or clinically atypical mole

c. Pickling skin

d. Jacob's ulcer or rodent carcinoma

5. Which of the following are true for SCC metastatic disease?

a. 6–10% of patients develop metastatic disease, occurrence and degree vary according to size and depth of invasion, and metastasis occurs early via the lymphatics

b. 10–12% of patients develop metastatic disease, occurrence and degree vary according to depth of invasion, metastasis occurs early via hematologic spread

c. 2–4% of patients develop metastatic disease, occurrence and degree vary according to the depth of invasion, metastasis occurs late via the hematologic spread

d. 0.3–4% of patients develop metastatic disease, occurrence and degree vary according to morphologic characteristics, and size and depth of the tumor. These metastases occur late via the lymphatics.

6. Ultraviolet (UV) radiation is divided into three stages: UVA, UVB, and UVC. Which of the following is true regarding the risk of developing skin cancer from UVA, UVB, and UVC?

a. UVB radiation produces the most damage to skin.

b. UVB waves are longer and penetrate into the epidermis more than UVA waves.

c. UVC waves are the longest and cause the most severe sunburn

d. UVA waves are shorter and do not penetrate the dermis.

7. Skin cancer prevention measures include:

a. Avoid all sunlight, use sunscreens with a higher than 15 SPF, wear comfortable attire, perform weekly skin self-exams

b. Avoid afternoon sunlight, use sunscreens with a higher than 30 SPF, wear comfortable attire, perform monthly skin self-exams

c. Avoid intense sunlight, use sunscreens with a higher than 30 SPF, wear protective attire, perform monthly skin self-exams

d. Avoid intense sunlight, use sunscreens with a higher than 10 SPF, wear cool attire, perform weekly skin self-exams

8. The most important prognostic factors in melanoma include:

a. Clark's level and regional lymph node involvement

b. Breslow's level or Breslow's thickness and presence of node involvement

c. Location of primary lesion, and depth of lesion

d. Melanoma type, diagnostic evaluation, and treatment modality

9. ELND, *elective lymph node dissection,* is a useful technique for tumors of the following thickness:

a. < 0.5 mm

b. 0.5–1.0 mm

c. 1.0–4.0 mm

d. > 4.0 mm

10. The incidence and mortality figures for malignant melanoma in the year 2000 are estimated at:

a. Incidence 45,000, mortality 10,000

b. Incidence 46,500, mortality 8,000

c. Incidence 47,700, mortality 7,700

d. Incidence 50,000, mortality 7,500

BIBLIOGRAPHY

1. American Cancer Society: *Cancer facts and figures, 2000.* Atlanta, The Society, 2000.

2. Anonymous: Melanoma: vigilance saves lives, *Harvard Health Lett* 2:6, 1997.

3. Anonymous: *What you need to know about skin cancer.* US National Institutes of Health. National Cancer Institute, United States Department of Health & Human Services Publications. Public Health Service #NIH95-1564:1-13, 1995.

4. Apgar B: A comparison of treatments for basal cell carcinoma, *Am Fam Physician* 61:1460, 2000.

5. Browder J, Beers B: Photoaging cosmetic effects of sun damage, *Postgrad Med* 93:74, 1993.

6. Edwards L and others: Melanoma a strategy for detection and treatment, *Patient Care* 30:126, 1996.

7. Gale D, Richards J: An overview of malignant melanoma, *Dev Supportive Care* (*Meniscus*) 2:113, 1999.

8. Gilchrist B and others: Mechanisms of disease: the pathogenesis of melanoma induced by ultraviolet radiation, *N Engl J Med* 340:1341, 1999.

9. Gilmore M: Nursing management of patients receiving concurrent biochemotherapy for melanoma, *Nurs Intervent Oncol, M.D. Anderson Case Reports & Review* 9:3, 1997.

10. Goldberg L: Basal cell carcinoma as predictor for other cancers (commentary), *Lancet* 349:664, 1997.

11. Gordon M, Hecker M: Care of the skin at midlife: diagnosis of pigmented lesions, *Geriatrics* 52:56, 1997.

12. Green A and others: Daily sun screen and beta-carotene supplementation in prevention of basal-cell and squamous-cell carcinomas of the skin: a randomized controlled trial, *Lancet* 354(9180):723, 1999.

13. Green A and others: Can sun screens reduce skin cancer? *AJN* 99:14, 1999.

14. Gross E: Non-melanoma skin cancer: clues to early detection, keys to effective treatment, *Consultant* 39:829, 1999.

15. Hacker S, Browder J, Ramos-Caro F: Basal cell carcinoma: choosing the best method of treatment for a particular lesion, *Postgrad Med* 93:101, 1993.

16. Hacker S, Flowers F: Squamous cell carcinoma of the skin—will heightened awareness of risk factors slow its increase? *Postgrad Med* 93:115, 1993.

17. Henderson C: Scientists closer to developing BCC skin cancer test, *Cancer Weekly Plus,* November 3, 1997:24.

18. Hill L, Ferrini R: Skin cancer prevention and screening: summary of American College of Preventive Medicine's practice policy statements, *CA Cancer J Clin* 48:232, 1998.

19. Jansen L and others: Sentinel node biopsy for melanoma in the head and neck region, *Head Neck* 22:27, 2000.

20. Kemeny M, Stewart A: Superior survival of young women with melanoma, *Am J Surg* 177:176, 1999.

21. Kirsner R, Federman D: The rationale for skin cancer screening and prevention, *Am J Managed Care* 4:1279, 1998.

22. Koch S, Miller S: Basal cell carcinoma in a teenage boy, *Clin Pediatr* 36:113, 1997.

23. Kraus D, Carew J, Harrison L: Regional lymph node metastasis from cutaneous squamous cell carcinoma, *Arch Otolaryngol Head Neck Surg* 124:582, 1998.

24. Levi F and others: What is the risk of a second invasive cancer following basal cell carcinoma? *Arch Dermatol* 135:1531, 1999.

25. Marks R: Prevention and control of melanoma: the public health approach, *CA Cancer J Clin* 46:199, 1996.

26. McDonald C: American Cancer Society perspective on the American College of Preventative Medicine's policy statements on skin cancer prevention and screening, *CA Cancer J Clin* 48:229, 1998.

27. Morton D, Barth A: Vaccine therapy for malignant melanoma, *CA Cancer J Clin* 46:225, 1996.

28. Naik N, Brodell R, Fatteh S: When to suspect superficial basal cell carcinoma, *Postgrad Med* 104:157, 1998.

29. Ness A and others: Are we really dying for a tan? *BMJ* 319(7202):114, 1999.

30. Oncology Nursing Society: Sentinel lymph node biopsy: current status, *1999 Annual Congress-Symposia Highlights,* P 1-2, 1999.

31. Otto S: Skin cancers. In Otto S, editor: *Oncology nursing,* ed 3, St. Louis, Mosby, 1997.

32. Pariser D, Phillips P: Basal cell carcinoma: when to treat it yourself, and when to refer, *Geriatrics* 49:39, 1994.

33. Patient Information from Your Doctor: How to examine your skin, *Patient Care* 30:116, 2000.

34. Pitts J, Maloney M: Therapeutic advances in melanoma, *Dermatol Clin* 18:157, 2000.

35. Polk H: Surgical progress and understanding in the treatment of the melanoma epidemic, *Am J Surg* 178:443, 1999.

36. Reed J, Albino A: Update of diagnostic and prognostic markers in cutaneous malignant melanoma, *Dermatol Clin* 17:631, 1999.

37. Reeves J, Maibach H: Basal cell carcinoma and squamous cell carcinoma. In Reeves JRT, Mailbach HI, editors, *Clinical dermatology illustrated: a regional approach,* ed 3, Philadelphia, Davis, 1998.

38. Rigel D: Malignant melanoma: perspectives on incidence and its effect on awareness, diagnosis and treatment, *CA Cancer J Clin* 46:195, 1996.

39. Rigel D: Is the ounce of screening and prevention for skin cancer worth the pound of cure? *CA Cancer J Clin* 48:236, 1998.

40. Robins P: Malignant melanoma: guidelines for prevention and early detection, *Consultant* 36:2027,1996.

41. Rose L: Recognizing neoplastic skin lesions: a photo guide, *Am Fam Physician* 58:873, 1998.

42. Roth M, Grant-Kels J: Pigmented skin lesions: how to distinguish the benign from malignant melanoma, *Consultant* 36:1516, 1996.

43. Shah R: Sun screens and sun protection: what you should know, *Dev Supportive Cancer Care* 2:141, 1999.

44. Shea C, Prieto V: Recent developments in the pathology of melanocytic neoplasia, *Dermatol Clin* 17:615, 1999.

45. Smoots E: Tips on saving your skin from the sun, *Consultant* 36:1527, 1996.

46. Tavin E, Persky M, Jacobs J: Metastatic basal cell carcinoma of the head and neck, *Laryngoscope* 105(part 1): 814, 1995.

47. Urist M: Surgical management of primary cutaneous melanoma, *CA Cancer J Clin.* 46:217, 1996.

48. Walling A: Basal cell carcinoma, *Am Fam Physician* 59:1042, 1999.

49. White W, Loggie B: Sentinel lymphadenectomy in the management of primary cutaneous malignant melanoma, an update, *Dermatol Clin* 17:645,1999.

Pediatric Cancers

Shirley E. Otto

Great strides have been made in the treatment of children with cancer, resulting in vastly improved survival and reduced mortality. As survival rates have improved during the past decades, the significance of delayed effects of treatment has become apparent. An estimated 12,400 children will be diagnosed with cancer in the year 2000, and despite advances in treatment, 2300 children will die of cancer. Ongoing research encompasses multiple topics: cancer etiology studies, early detection and screening programs, multiresearch group cancer treatment trials, and long-term quality of life issues.[43, 56, 125] This chapter provides a basic overview of the most common childhood cancers.

Leukemia

Leukemia is the most common malignancy in children, representing 33% of all childhood cancers under age 15 years and 25% under the age of 20 years. The majority of leukemias in children are *lymphoblastic* (75.5%), with myeloid leukemias accounting for 15% to 40% and the largest group of these being the acute myeloid leukemias (11.4%). The cause of leukemia remains unknown and is most likely a result of a combination of factors. Possible causative agents under investigation include viruses, radiation, chemical and drug exposures, chromosomal aberrations, electromagnetic fields, and familial predisposition.[45, 56, 82, 120, 130, 131]

Acute Lymphoblastic Leukemia

The incidence of acute lymphoblastic leukemia (ALL) is 40/1 million white children and 20/1 million African American children in the United States annually, with 2600 cases diagnosed for the year 2000. There is a male predominance of 3 : 1 over females and a peak incidence at 4 years of age. Five-year relative survival has dramatically improved from 4% in the early 1960s to nearly 80% for the year 2000. This dramatic difference is related to the availability of newer and more effective chemotherapy treatments for children with cancer.[11, 56, 66, 88]

CLASSIFICATION

Based on the French-American-British (FAB) classification system, 80% of childhood cases of ALL are L1 type, 17% L2, and 3% L3.[4] Of the immunophenotypes, 57% of childhood ALL are early pre-B cell, 25% pre-B cell, 1% transitional pre-B cell, 2% B cell, and 15% T cell.[88] (See Chapter 14 for a further discussion of the FAB subtypes and immunophenotypes.)

CLINICAL PRESENTATION

Clinical manifestations depend on the degree to which the bone marrow has been compromised as well as the location and the extent of extramedullary infiltration. Common presenting signs and symptoms are fever, pain, bleeding, petechiae, purpura, fatigue, pallor, recurrent infection, and lymphadenopathy. These symptoms may have been present for days or weeks or, rarely, months before diagnosis. These nonspecific symptoms must be distinguished from many nonmalignant conditions and other malignant diseases that involve the bone marrow.[88]

PROGNOSIS

Multiple factors have been used to predict outcome in children with ALL and are now also used to direct treatment. Only age (younger than 1 year or older than 15 years) and hyperleukocytosis have consistently been associated with a poor outcome. In general, the more mature the cell of origin, the less favorable is the prognosis, with early pre-B cell having the best prognosis and mature B cell the poorest. Early pre–B-cell leukemia is more likely to have initial features predictive of a good outcome. With improvements in treatment, the prognostic distinctions among immunophenotypes decrease or disappear.[40, 135]

The presence of the common ALL antigen (CALLA) is associated with a positive outcome, and 75% to 80% of B-cell ALL patients are CALLA positive. Hyperdiploidy is also associated with a good prognosis. Some chromosomal aberrations are associated with a poor outcome, such as Philadelphia-positive cells, t8;14, t1;19, and 14;11.[45, 82]

TREATMENT MODALITIES

All protocols now include some form of four phases of therapy: induction for remission, a phase of intensification/consolidation, treatment directed toward the central nervous system (CNS), and continuation therapy. Over the past decade the use of intensive induction therapy has greatly improved survival in children with ALL, resulting in a remission rate of 97% to 98% in children with ALL. It has been recognized that some form of intensification is necessary in the prevention of bone marrow relapse, even for those considered low risk.[80]

The need for CNS treatment was recognized in the 1960s. The use of radiation and intrathecal methotrexate is associated with adverse effects. It is now common practice to omit radiation for those at low risk for CNS disease but to provide CNS treatment through the use of intrathecal methotrexate or triple intrathecal therapy (cytarabine, hydrocortisone, and methotrexate). Radiation is reserved for those with CNS disease or at high risk for a CNS relapse (high white blood cell count [WBC], T-cell ALL with high WBC, and Philadelphia-positive ALL). Under investigation is the benefit for use of a second induction/intensification phase before the continuation or maintenance phase for some subgroups of patients. The length of treatment has not been established but in general continues for 2.5 to 3 years after diagnosis.*

Most relapses occur either during treatment or within 2 years after completion of therapy. Treatment of recurrent leukemia remains under investigation. Although achievement of a second remission is possible in more than 90% of patients, long-term survival remains a challenge for those patients with a bone marrow relapse. For those with an isolated CNS or testicular relapse, 50% are long-term survivors with a second course of therapy. Many investigators now recommend the use of allogeneic bone marrow transplantation (BMT) for those that have a bone marrow relapse on or shortly after the completion of therapy. BMT with conventional and alternative donor sources continues to show promise. The apparent success using related, partially matched and unrelated, matched donors has provided options to an increasing number of children.[78, 88, 91, 135, 153]

Late Effects

A major delayed effect of therapy has been the development of second malignancies. One estimate is that 2.5% of patients will develop a second cancer 15 years after diagnosis. Brain tumors were the most common second malignancy occurring in those who received cranial radiation, followed by a second leukemia associated with the use of epipodophyllotoxins and lymphomas. Declines in intelligence quotient (IQ) and cognitive dysfunctions, decreased reading and mathematic levels, and memory deficits have been noted. These problems are thought to be related to the use of methotrexate and radiation for CNS prophylaxis and treatment (Table 19-1).*

Acute Myelogenous Leukemia

Acute myelogenous leukemia (AML) is less common in children than in adults, representing 15% to 25% of leukemias in children. Approximately 400 new cases are diagnosed annually in the United States. AML is more common in whites and boys, with a slight peak incidence in adolescence and in those younger than 2 years of age.

ETIOLOGY

The cause of leukemia in children remains unclear, but those with certain genetic disorders such as Down syndrome are at higher risk for the development of AML. A statistically significant risk was found for children who had a parent exposed to pesticides and petroleum products and those with mothers who used marijuana while pregnant. Other contributing risk factors include exposure to ionizing radiation and drugs such as benzene, alkylating agents, nitrosureas, and epipodophyllotoxins.[52, 82, 130, 131, 135, 151]

CLASSIFICATION

Several subtypes of AML become important when determining treatment and prognosis. The subtypes according to the FAB classification system are M1, myeloblastic undifferentiated; M2, myeloblastic differentiated; M3, promyelocytic; M4, myelomonocytic; M5, monoblastic; M6, erythroblastic; and M7, megakaryoblastic[52] (see Chapter 14).

* References 12, 15, 40, 50, 88, 91, 135, 153.

* References 41, 43, 61, 66, 88, 115, 125.

TABLE 19–1
Organ-Specific Late Effects of Cancer Therapy and Screening Methodology

Organ	Therapy	Screening Test
Musculoskeletal	Radiotherapy (RT)	Physical exam, scoliosis exam (annually if growing) x-ray prn
Breast	Mediastinal RT	Breast exam, mammography beginning age 25–30
CNS	Cranial RT	Neurocognitive testing (baseline, q 3–5 y prn) MRI baseline
Neuroendocrine	Hypothalamic-pituitary RT	Growth curve every year. Bone age (age 9) GH stimulation test, TSH, free T_4, T_3 (baseline 3–5 y prn) LH, FSH, test/est, prolactin (baseline, prn) 8 AM cortisol baseline
Cardiac	Anthracyclines Mediastinal/t-spine RT	ECHO/ECG (baseline for all; q 3–5 y after anthracycline) Holter q 5 y prn (high-dose anthracycline) Stress test/dobutamine stress. Echo prn (after RT)
Pulmonary	RT Bleomycin, CCNU/BCNU	PFT baseline, q 3–5 y prn
Ovary	Alkylating agents RT	Menstrual history annually LH, FSH, estradiol baseline (age > 12) and prn
Testes	Alkylating agents RT	LH, FSH, testos baseline (age > 12) and prn Sperm analysis
Renal	Cisplatin (carboplatin) Ifosfamide	Creatinine, Mg q 1–2 y Creatine clearance baseline and q 3–5 y prn Urinalysis (RT, ifosfamide) Ifosfamide: serum phosphate, urine glucose, protein
Bladder	Cyclophosphamide Ifosfamide, RT	Urinalysis annually for heme
Thyroid	RT to neck, mediastinum	TSH, Free T_4, T_3 q y × 10 Scans (U/S) prn
Liver	6-MP, MTX, Act-d, RT	Liver function tests q 1–3 y
GI	Intestinal RT	Stool guiac every year, colonoscopy (ACS)

RT, radiation therapy; MTX, methotrexate; Mg, magnesium; prn, whenever necessary; MRI, magnetic resonance imaging; GH, growth hormone; TSH, thyroid-stimulating hormone; LH, luteinizing hormone; FSH, follicle-stimulating hormone; test/est, testosterone/estrogen; ECHO/ECG, echocardiography/electrocardiography; PFT, pulmonary function tests; T_4, thyroxine; T_3, triiodothyronine; 6-MP, 6-mercaptopurine; U/S, ultrasound; ACS, American Cancer Society.
Reprinted with permission from Schwartz CL: Long-term survivors of childhood cancer: the late effects of therapy, Oncologist 4:45, 1999.

CLINICAL PRESENTATION

As in ALL, the primary presenting symptoms with AML is a result of bone marrow disease: pallor, anemia, fever, infection, headache, tinnitus, petechiae, and bruising or bleeding. The presenting signs and symptoms usually reflect diminished production of red blood cells, granulocytes, and platelets, leading to the anemia, infection, and bleeding. In addition, children with AML may have symptoms of organ involvement. Splenomegaly and hepatomegaly are present in 50%, lymphadenopathy in 25%, and CNS disease in 5% to 15% of children at diagnosis. Approximately 2% of patients with CNS symptoms report additional complaints of nausea, vomiting, photophobia and papilledema.[22, 52]

PROGNOSTIC FACTORS

Prognostic indicators have been extensively studied in ALL but have not been as clear-cut as in AML. Only WBC and the FAB subtype M5 have consistently been identified with a poor prognosis. Young age (<2 years) has also been associated with a poor prognosis, but whether this is related to age or the most common subtypes in infants (M5, M4) is not known.[51, 135]

TREATMENT MODALITIES

Induction protocols vary, but remission rates are 75% to 85%, and those who do not achieve remission die of infection, bleeding, leukostasis, or resistant disease. CNS prophylaxis is often included in treatment regimens to prevent CNS relapse and consists of intrathecal cytosine arabinoside (cytarabine). Consolidation or continuation therapy is far from standardized. Some centers recommend BMT, either allogeneic or autologous, in the first remission, whereas others wait for a relapse to occur. Studies are ongoing regarding the efficacy of intensive chemotherapy versus BMT. Current 5-year survival rates from AML range from 25% to 40% for all treatment regimens.[11, 52, 78, 80]

Chronic Myelogenous Leukemia

Chronic myelogenous leukemia (CML) is an uncommon disease in children, representing 1% to 5% of all childhood leukemias. The two forms of CML are the *adult type,* which is usually seen in older children and adolescents but seldom seen in children younger than 6 months, and the *juvenile form,* which is almost always seen in infants younger than 24 months. The cause of CML is unknown, as is the case with other childhood leukemias.[4]

ADULT CHRONIC MYELOGENOUS LEUKEMIA

Adult CML is usually associated with the presence of the Philadelphia chromosome, which is directly attributed to the disease process. Three phases of adult CML have been identified: chronic, accelerated, and blast. The chronic phase is an indolent phase lasting from 3 to 4 years. Most children are diagnosed in this phase either through an abnormal complete blood count (CBC) during a routine physical examination or through the development of symptoms. Common symptoms include fever, pallor, weight loss, and bone pain. Patients often have splenomegaly or hepatomegaly or both, which can be mild or severe, and an elevated WBC, eosinophilia, and basophilia. Treatment with oral hydroxyurea or busulfan provides adequate control in the chronic phase but does not reduce the number of cells containing the Philadelphia chromosome.[4, 52]

Eventually the chronic phase leads to the accelerated phase, with an increasing WBC and redevelopment of the presenting symptoms. Patients usually progress rapidly to the blast phase, with symptoms of bone marrow disease resembling ALL. This phase is very resistant to therapy. Multiagent regimens are used in an attempt to obtain a second chronic phase.[4]

JUVENILE CHRONIC MYELOGENOUS LEUKEMIA

Juvenile CML is very rare and presents as well as follows a more acute course. The median survival is less than 10 months with or without treatment. Presenting symptoms include bleeding, malaise, lymphadenopathy, and fever. A small number of patients have pulmonary symptoms caused by leukemic infiltrates. Abdominal distention and pain result from a rapidly enlarging spleen. Many patients have skin manifestations similar to an eczematous rash and caused by cutaneous infiltrates.[4]

TREATMENT MODALITIES

No real cure exists for either type of CML, and the only possible curative therapy is BMT. With the adult form the ideal time to transplant is in the chronic phase. The juvenile form is very resistive to treatment, but intensive multiagent regimens have been used to obtain short remissions, during which BMT is then performed.

Brain Tumors

Brain tumors are the most common solid tumor of childhood and are second in frequency only to leukemia. These tumors account for about 20% of all childhood malignancies under age 15. The highest incidence rates occur among infants and children through age 7. Approximately 2400 new cases will be diagnosed for the year 2000 in the United States. More than half of all CNS cancers in children and adolescents are astrocytomas.[20, 56]

CLASSIFICATION

No uniform classification system exists for brain tumors because there is no uniform grading system. The histologic types differ from those in adults. The majority of tumors in children older than 1 year are infratentorial (60%), in contrast to adults, who have primarily supratentorial tumors. Supratentorial tumors predominate in those younger than 1 year and begin to increase in the adolescent years.[20]

HISTOLOGY

Approximately 50% of brain tumors in children are *astrocytomas,* with 11% high grade, 13% cerebellar astrocytomas, and 23% cerebral astrocytomas. Of the remaining tumors in children, 25% are medulloblastomas, 10% brain stem gliomas, 9% ependymomas, and 9% other subtypes.[20]

ETIOLOGY

The cause of brain tumors in children is unknown. Both hereditary and environmental factors have been implicated. Prior radiotherapy is a known cause of brain tumors. Parental occupation in the chemical or aircraft industry and organic compounds such as nitrosamines and nitrosureas has also been suspected as a risk factor. Fifteen percent of those with neurofibromatosis develop brain tumors, and in patients with acquired immunodeficiency syndrome (AIDS) the Epstein-Barr virus (EBV) may initiate an aggressive form of non-Hodgkin's lymphoma of the brain.[20, 25, 59, 83]

CLINICAL PRESENTATION

The presenting symptoms of a child with a brain tumor depend on the site and size. These signs and symptoms can range from nonspecific to characteristically localizing. The presenting symptoms are often related to increased intracranial pressure (ICP) and are often worse in the morning, improving as the child is upright with improved cephalic venous return. In one series, 86% of children with brain tumors had signs of increased ICP. The child may complain of a headache, which can be diffuse, frontal, or occipital. Vomiting can be projectile or nonprojectile in nature. Lethargy, irritability, and behavior changes often occur. In school-age children academic performance and personality changes may be observed. An increased head circumference may be noted in the infant, possibly with separation of the sutures. Papilledema is often found, and the child may also experience diplopia and strabismus.

Symptoms often provide clues to the tumor's location. These symptoms include ataxia, gait disturbances, seizures, focal motor or sensory abnormalities, decreased visual acuity, nystagmus, and strabismus. Growth retardation, diabetes insipidus, delayed puberty, hormonal deficits, and visual disturbances may result if the hypothalamic-pituitary axis is involved.[20, 30, 101]

DIAGNOSTIC EVALUATION

The diagnostic evaluation of a child with a suspected brain tumor begins with a thorough physical and neurologic examination. Magnetic resonance imaging (MRI) or computed tomography (CT) scan with and without contrast is the major radiologic examination. A lumbar puncture and gadolinium-enhanced MRI are necessary for detection of dissemination of tumor into the cerebrospinal fluid (CSF).[20, 102, 104]

TREATMENT MODALITIES

The management of children with brain tumors involves the use of surgery, chemotherapy, and radiation. The goal of surgery is to decrease the tumor burden, thereby decreasing symptoms, and to obtain tissue for histologic evaluation. The exception is with diffuse gliomas of the brain stem, in which case MRI is usually diagnostic. In general, the better the resection, the better is the prognosis. Advances in neurosurgery have increased the cure rate, decreased perioperative complications, and decreased the postsurgical deficits. Stereotactic needle biopsies of deep-seated tumors allow diagnosis in delicate regions.[58, 32, 93, 94]

The use of radiation has long been the major approach to management of brain tumors in children and is usually initiated as soon as the diagnosis is confirmed and the surgical wound is healed. Total doses as low as 2000 to 3000 cGy or as much as 7000 cGy are given, depending on the tumor's pathology and location and the child's age. The use of hyperfractionated radiation has allowed the delivery of higher doses without increasing the adverse effects. Radiosensitizers have been used to increase cellular radiosensitivity, thereby increasing tumor cell kill and minimize host side effects. Multiple agents are under investigation for their appropriate clinical efficacy. The use of radiation in young children often requires sedation to obtain complete immobility, along with casts or molds individually designed for positioning. Radiation is not without risks, and it is now standard procedure to defer radiation by the use of postoperative chemotherapy in those younger than 2 or 3 years.[20, 81, 93, 94, 101, 125] (See Table 19–1 and Chapter 22.)

Chemotherapy has proved to be a valuable addition to radiation and surgery in the management of brain tumors, increasing median survival. Chemotherapy protocols that include nitrosureas, alkylating agents, and vinca alkaloids vary according to the drugs used, route, schedule, and dosing regimens. The use of chemotherapy before radiation is becoming increasingly common as a method to evaluate tumor response separate from the response caused by the effects of radiation. The use of autologous BMT or peripheral blood stem cell (PBSC) rescue is currently under investigation as a method to intensify therapy with high-grade or recurrent tumors.[20, 58, 81, 90, 101]

PROGNOSIS

Prognostic signs include the amount of resection, child's age, and tumor's grade. Survival depends on tumor histology, tumor cell ploidy (a diploid DNA content is associated with a poor prognosis), amount of surgical resection, age, neurologic and physical status, and presence or absence of dissemination. The 5-year survival rate for all children with brain tumors ranges from 10% to 70%.[90, 93, 129, 143]

LATE EFFECTS

Problems with decreased cognitive function, and in some cases mental retardation, are seen after the diagnosis and successful treatment of brain tumors in children. Young age at diagnosis is an important risk factor for long-term sequelae. Possibly 68% of children younger than 6 years treated for brain tumors may experience intellectual deterioration. The effects of cranial radiation have long been recognized as a risk, especially in the young child. Children with infratentorial tumors are at higher risk for long-term adverse effects than those with supratentorial tumors. Endocrine deficiencies, including growth problems and hypothyroidism, are typically seen. Finally, children treated for brain tumors are at risk for the development of secondary brain neoplasms, most often from radiation.*

Lymphoma

Lymphomas represent the third most common cancer in children and, along with other reticuloendothelial neoplasms, account for more than 10% of cases among children under age 15 and more than 15% of cases under age 20. These malignancies of the lymphatic system have long been thought to have an infectious etiology. The main integrating factors in these diseases include infection with EBV, genetic predisposition, and exposure to toxins.[56]

Hodgkin's Disease

Hodgkin's disease in children is now considered similar to that in adults regarding biology, etiology, natural history, and response to treatment. (See Chapter 16 for a complete discussion of Hodgkin's disease, because this section refers only to those aspects pertinent to the disease in children.)

EPIDEMIOLOGY

Hodgkin's disease accounts for just slightly more childhood cases (approximately 1860 in the year 2000) than does non-Hodgkin's lymphoma (NHL). Incidence rates of Hodgkin's increase throughout childhood but over all total cases have declined slightly between 1975 and 1995. Over this same period, the 5-year survival rate for Hodgkin's disease has risen to 91%. It is rarely seen in those younger than 5 years, with two peaks in incidence, ages 15 to 40 years and after age 50 years. Hodgkin's disease has a higher incidence in males until the adolescent years, when a slight female predominance occurs.[56, 69]

Of the four subtypes of Hodgkin's disease, 77% of those occurring in adolescents and 45% of those in children younger than 10 years are the nodular sclerosing subtype. The lymphocytic depletion subtype is rare under the age of 10 years, but the lymphocytic predominant subtype occurs more often in this age group than in adults. Thirty-two percent of children younger than 10 years are diagnosed with the mixed cellularity subtype.[69]

CLINICAL PRESENTATION

The diagnosis of lymphoma in a child is difficult because of the common finding of enlarged lymph nodes in chil-

dren, which are most often a benign reactive process. Ninety percent of children with Hodgkin's disease present with an unusual lump, which varies in size and may have been present for weeks or months. Nonspecific systemic symptoms may include fatigue, anorexia, and slight weight loss. Unexplained fever with temperatures above 38.0°C orally and weight loss of more than 10% within the previous 6 months with drenching night sweats are of prognostic significance.[22, 69]

Lymph nodes involved with Hodgkin's disease are usually not tender, are firm and rubbery, and are fixed or minimally movable. Location can also be a clue to malignancy in that enlarged nodes in the upper half of the neck (anterior and posterior chains or submandibular region) are often associated with upper respiratory infections in children. These nodes should be biopsied if the enlargement has not resolved within 3 to 6 weeks. The nodes of the lower cervical and supraclavicular chains are more often involved with Hodgkin's disease and should be biopsied without delay. In one review, 48% of nodes biopsied from the supraclavicular and lower neck regions were involved with Hodgkin's disease. From 20% to 30% of children present with the classic B symptoms of weight loss, fevers, and night sweats. Almost 60% of children have mediastinal involvement[22, 69] (see Chapter 16).

DIAGNOSTIC EVALUATION

An extensive diagnostic evaluation is necessary for staging, which plays an important role in determining treatment. (See Chapter 5 for a discussion of diagnosis and staging, which is approached the same in children as in adults.) Alkaline phosphatase is a nonspecific indicator of disease activity but is less useful in children because of normal elevated levels from bone growth, but if elevated, a bone scan is done to detect bone disease. Serum copper levels may be elevated because of normal hormonal activity in children and is not related to the malignancy. Splenectomies are controversial in children, but it is now generally believed that they are necessary when radiation is used alone. When chemotherapy is used, however, either alone or in combination with radiation, splenectomies are not necessary and clinical staging is sufficient. The most effective timing of radiotherapy and chemotherapy is not yet established.[69, 102, 104].

TREATMENT MODALITIES

Treatment for children is similar to that for adults. Radiation doses may be reduced in young children to decrease the negative effects on bone and soft tissue growth. The traditional MOPP (mechlorethamine, vincristine, procarbazine, prednisone) is used, along with other regimens that have been developed. The use of

---

* References 47, 58, 61, 66, 110, 115, 125.

MOPP alternating with ABVD (Adriamycin [doxorubicin], bleomycin, vinblastine, dacarbazine) is still being evaluated in clinical research trials. Various chemotherapeutic regimens are being investigated for resistant or relapsed disease, including autologous BMT. Chemotherapy is considered the primary treatment for patients with advanced-stage disease. Most clinicians agree that radiotherapy is a useful supplement for patients who present with bulky disease.[11, 32, 69, 70, 123]

Late Effects

Patients with Hodgkin's disease are at risk for multiple complications related to chemotherapy and radiation to the chest, including cardiac, pulmonary, and gonadal dysfunctions and abnormalities in development of bone and soft tissue in the radiation field. The development of second malignancies is similar to that in other children who have received radiation and chemotherapy, especially with alkylating agents. A relationship between splenectomy and the development of leukemia has also been reported[9, 16, 34, 61, 125, 144] (see Table 19-1).

PROGNOSIS

Young age is clearly a positive prognostic sign, as is early diagnosis. Both those younger than 10 years and those 11 to 16 years old, regardless of stage, have a projected survival of 74%, versus 34% in those age 17 years or older. From 1975 to 1995 the 5-year survival rate for Hodgkin's disease has risen to 91% overall. Most relapses in patients with Hodgkin's disease occur within the first 3 years. Patients with limited-stage disease who have a relapse after radiotherapy have a good long-term survival rate ranging from 50% to 80% after retreatment with chemotherapy regimens used for advanced stage disease.[16, 17, 56, 69]

Non-Hodgkin's Lymphoma

Sixty percent of all lymphomas are of the non-Hodgkin's type and represent 10% of all childhood malignancies. Non-Hodgkin's lymphoma (NHL) in children is often widespread at diagnosis.

EPIDEMIOLOGY

Non-Hodgkin's lymphoma has a peak incidence in the 7- to 11-year-old age group, a low incidence in adolescence, and a male predominance. Viruses, genetic factors, and radiation have been implicated as causative factors in several studies, along with an increased risk in those with primary immunodeficiency syndromes, immunosuppression, connective tissue diseases, and anticonvulsant therapy. NHL has been increasing as a secondary malignancy after multimodal therapy.[56, 72, 120, 126, 151]

HISTOLOGY

This lymphoma can be divided into three groups: lymphoblastic, small noncleaved cell (Burkitt's or non-Burkitt's), and large-cell lymphomas. Lymphoblastic lymphomas are usually T cell in origin. Small noncleaved cell and large-cell lymphomas are usually of B-cell origin. Various chromosomal abnormalities have been associated with NHL.[126]

CLINICAL PRESENTATION AND STAGING

The child with NHL often has an acute onset of symptoms and rapid progression. Lymphoblastic lymphomas typically arise in the anterior superior mediastinum, and 75% of these children have a mediastinal mass at diagnosis. They often present with symptoms of dysphagia, dyspnea, wheezing, or stridor. Additional symptoms may include pain, swelling of the neck, face, and upper extremities from superior vena cava obstruction. Other sites of involvement may include the skin, tonsils, lymph nodes, bone, bone marrow, CNS, and testes. Eighty percent of nonlymphoblastic lymphomas originate in the abdomen, often presenting as an acute abdomen.[22, 126, 151]

Many different staging systems exist, and all are based on the extent of disease: localized disease, extensive thoracic or intra-abdominal disease, widespread disease without bone marrow involvement, and disease with bone marrow involvement. Controversy exists regarding whether lymphoma with bone marrow involvement is a true lymphoma or is actually a leukemia, but regardless of the classification, it is an aggressive disease requiring aggressive treatment[87, 126] (see Chapter 16).

DIAGNOSTIC EVALUATION

The diagnostic and staging evaluation is based on tissue samples from any bulky disease, bone marrow aspirates and biopsies to evaluate bone marrow involvement, and CSF to detect CNS involvement. Appropriate radiographic studies, including CT and gallium scans, angiograms, and ultrasound should be done to evaluate the extent of bulky disease, and laboratory studies should include EBV titers.[102, 104, 126]

TREATMENT MODALITIES AND PROGNOSIS

All children receive chemotherapy, with the exact combination and therapy duration depending on the type and extent of disease. Those with extensive disease, especially the Burkitt's and lymphoblastic types, are at high risk for tumor lysis syndrome (see Chapter 20). The overall survival rate for patients with localized disease is almost 90%, with a 60% to 70% rate for those with advanced disease. Efforts are being made to tailor the chemotherapy to maximize dose intensity and minimize organ toxicities. When it occurs, relapse is usually early in treatment, although relapse toward the end or after the completion of therapy is also possible. The most common sites of relapse are the primary site, bone marrow, and CNS. Those who relapse or have resistant disease have a very poor survival rate, and autologous or allogeneic BMT is often pursued.[8, 11, 19, 61, 126]

Wilms' Tumor (Nephroblastoma)

Wilms' tumor, an embryonic neoplasm, is the most common renal tumor of childhood and the fifth most common childhood cancer, representing 6% of all childhood cancers. Wilms' tumor predominantly occurs in the first 5 years of life, with incidence rates slightly higher among girls, and for African Americans compared with whites. Approximately 400 new cases are diagnosed each year at a median age of 2 to 3 years.[54, 56]

ETIOLOGY

Most cases are sporadic, but a small number are familial and are inherited in an autosomal dominant manner. An association exists between Wilms' tumor and deletion or inactivation of the short arm of chromosome 11, band 13. Children with Wilms' tumor may have associated congenital anomalies, including aniridia (congenital absence of iris), hemihypertrophy, cryptorchidism, hypospadias, and Beckwith-Wiedemann syndrome. The possible role of parental environment exposures in the etiology of Wilms' tumor is unknown.[18, 26, 71, 134]

CLINICAL PRESENTATION

Typically an otherwise healthy-appearing child has an asymptomatic abdominal mass, often noted by the parent or primary health care professional on a routine examination. Other presenting symptoms include hematuria, dysuria, hypertension, abdominal pain, fever, anemia, and malaise. Wilms' tumor is usually a nontender, firm, flank mass that is confined to one side. The lungs are the primary sites of distant metastasis and recurrent disease, with 25% of patients showing metastasis at diagnosis. Other sites of metastasis include the collateral kidney, liver, bones, or brain. Lymphatic spread to regional nodes is associated with advanced disease.[54, 112]

DIAGNOSTIC EVALUATION

Initially a flat plate of the abdomen will identify the primary mass, followed by an ultrasound, which can identify the site of origin. The other kidney is also examined to rule out bilateral involvement and detect extension into renal veins and the inferior vena cava. An abdominal CT scan or MRI has become the imaging modality of choice for evaluating the extent of disease before surgery. Identification of biologic and genetic characteristics as risk factors for the specific tumor facilitates the process for a template treatment approach. Chest CT scan and chest x-ray films are done preoperatively to detect pulmonary metastasis.[18, 54, 57, 112]

A bone marrow aspirate, biopsy, and skeletal survey should be done if bone metastasis is suspected. Laboratory tests should include a serum and 24-hour urine creatinine clearance. Control of hypertension is important preoperatively, and although it resolves in most children after surgery, some may require long-term antihypertensive therapy. Definitive diagnosis is made at surgery, usually involving removal of the involved kidney. In bilateral disease the most involved kidney is removed and the other resected as much as possible.[54, 55, 57, 134]

STAGING AND PROGNOSIS

Wilms' tumor is generally staged according to the classification system identified by the National Wilms' Tumor Study Group (Box 19–1). Staging is based on surgical findings, pathology, and the presence or absence of distant metastasis. Wilms' tumor is further stratified by histologic type, designated favorable or unfavorable. Treatment and prognosis are based on stage and histologic type. Most patients with Wilms' tumor have favorable histology and survive after nephrectomy and chemotherapy, but 10% have a poor prognostic variables, including unfavorable (anaplastic) histology, chromosomal loss and diploidy.[49, 54, 57, 134]

The overall 5-year survival rate for patients with Wilms' tumor at all stages and with any histology type is approximately 92%. Those with favorable histology (renal embryoma without anaplasia) and without metastatic disease currently have a 90% rate of long-term survival. Those with an unfavorable histology (anaplastic, clear cell sarcoma) or those with metastatic disease have an 80% chance of long-term survival. The exception is those with rhabdoid tumors, who have a poor prognosis and a greater than 80% mortality. Twenty-five percent of those with stage IV disease and favorable histology have recurrence of their disease, and 50% of those with unfavorable histology and stage II or IV disease experience a relapse.[23, 55, 57, 106, 127]

TREATMENT MODALITIES

Through the cooperative work of the Children's Cancer Group and the Pediatric Oncology Group in the

---

BOX 19 – 1

Staging of Wilms' Tumor

Stage I Tumor limited to kidney and completely removed

Surface of renal capsule intact

No rupture before or during removal

No apparent residual tumor beyond margins

Stage II Tumor extends beyond kidney but completely removed

Regional extension of tumor (i.e., penetration of renal capsule)

Vessels outside kidney infiltrated or contain tumor thrombus

Tumor may have been biopsied, or there has been spillage of tumor confined to flank

No residual tumor apparent at or beyond the margins of excision

Stage III Residual nonhematogenous tumor confined to abdomen

Occurrence of any of the following:

Lymph nodes found to be involved in hilus, periaortic chains, or beyond

Diffuse peritoneal contamination by tumor (e.g., spillage of tumor beyond flank before or during surgery or tumor growth that has penetrated through peritoneal surface)

Implants on peritoneal surface

Tumor extends beyond surgical margins grossly or microscopically

Tumor not completely resectable because of local infiltration into vital structures

Stage IV Hematogenous metastases (e.g., lung, liver, bone, brain)

Stage V Bilateral renal tumors; attempt to stage both sides separately according to disease extent before biopsy

---

National Wilms' Study Group trials, advances have been made regarding treatment intensity and duration. Four national Wilms' tumor trials have been completed, and a fifth study is currently accepting patients for treatment.[83] Treatment involves chemotherapy alone with or without radiation, depending on the stage and histologic type. Autologous stem cell transplantation is considered for consolidation therapy of high-risk relapsed patients who have achieved complete remission. Recurrent disease is treated with an aggressive, multimodal approach, and many patients are cured,

especially those who have an isolated pulmonary relapse.*

Late Effects

Follow-up for late effects include (1) surveillance of function of the remaining kidney, scoliosis and soft-tissue growth problems related to radiation, and thyroid abnormalities after lung irradiation and (2) monitoring for second malignancies, usually in the radiation field.[17, 57, 125, 128]

Neuroblastoma

Neuroblastoma originates from neural crest tissue anywhere along the craniospinal axis and is one of the small, round, blue cell tumors of childhood. Neural crest tissue is the precursor for the adrenal medulla and sympathetic nervous system, and the tumor can present wherever nervous tissue is found. It is the most common malignant tumor in infancy and second only to brain tumors as the most frequent solid tumor in the first decade of life.[20]

EPIDEMIOLOGY

Neuroblastoma accounts for 14% of all cancers in children younger than 5 years of age. In contrast with CNS malignancies, survival is highest among infants and declines with increasing age. The annual incidence is 8.0/1 million white children and 8.7/1 million African American children in the United States, with approximately 550 cases diagnosed annually. Neuroblastoma is embryonic tumors with bizarre behavior that can regress, mature, or rapidly progress; therefore, the exact incidence remains unknown. More than 50% of patients are diagnosed before 2 years of age and more than 80% before age 5 years. Most patients have advanced disease at diagnosis. There is a slightly higher frequency in boys.[20, 24, 45, 56, 57]

ETIOLOGY

The etiology of neuroblastoma remains unknown. Although most cases are probably sporadic, some evidence indicates that neuroblastoma may have an autosomal dominant pattern of inheritance. However, the risk for development of neuroblastoma in siblings or offspring is less than 6%.[57, 100]

GENETICS

Several genetic abnormalities have been found associated with neuroblastoma and have prognostic implica-

---

* References 29, 31, 44, 55, 57, 83, 106, 116, 119, 122, 128, 146.

tions. The *N-myc* oncogene is an amplified gene present in human neuroblastomas. The higher the number of *N-myc* copies present, the poorer is the prognosis. A deletion or rearrangement on the short arm of chromosome 1 has been described, and some evidence suggests that this is associated with a very poor prognosis. Neuroblastoma is associated with loss of heterozygosity on chromosome 1p36 and occasionally deletions on 14q and 17q. DNA content has also been analyzed, with diploid neuroblastoma carrying a poorer prognosis then aneuploid.[20, 45, 57]

CLINICAL PRESENTATION

Because neuroblastoma can arise from any site along the sympathetic nervous system chain, the locations of primary tumors at the time of diagnosis are varied and change with age. The presenting clinical symptoms depend on the location of the tumor and the stage of the disease. Neuroblastomas most often arise in the retroperitoneum (65%) and present as hard, nontender abdominal masses. Other common sites include the mediastinum (15%), pelvis (5%), and neck (< 5%). Paraspinal tumors tend to grow through the intervertebral foramina, and patients often have paralysis. Those with cervical or high thoracic ganglia involvement may have Horner's syndrome. Metastatic extension of neuroblastoma occurs in two patterns: lymphatic and hematogenous.[20] Approximately two thirds of these tumors have metastasis at diagnosis, most often to the cortical bone, bone marrow, lymph nodes, liver, or subcutaneous tissue. Sphenoid bone or orbital soft tissue involvement results in the distinctive ecchymotic orbital proptosis or "raccoon eyes." Characteristic of neuroblastoma in neonates is hepatic and skin metastasis.[20, 57, 100]

DIAGNOSTIC EVALUATION

Serum ferritin and neuron-specific enolase are useful for prognostic purposes, with elevations indicating a poorer prognosis. More than 90% of children with neuroblastoma have elevated urine catecholamines (vanillylmandelic acid [VMA] or homovanillic acid [HVA] or both). Positive uptake by meta-iodo-benzyl-guanidine (MIGB) also help confirm the diagnosis of neuroblastoma.[100] The primary tumor should be evaluated with a CT scan or MRI, with MRI especially useful for intraspinal extension. Bilateral bone marrow aspirates and biopsies, bone and MIBG scans with radiographic films of abnormal sites, and a CT scan or MRI of the head and orbits, chest, abdomen, and pelvis are necessary to detect and evaluate metastatic disease.[20, 100]

STAGING AND PROGNOSIS

Currently, four staging systems are in use, one by each of the major cooperative groups (Pediatric Oncology Group [POG], Childrens Cancer Group [CCG], and one used by St. Jude's Children's Research Hospital [SJCRH]). The fourth was proposed by a group of international experts to standardize staging and direct treatment (Box 19–2).

Age and stage at diagnosis are important prognostic factors, with young age (<1 year) and low stage (I, II, or IVS) associated with a favorable prognosis. A number of biologic features of neuroblastoma are associated with a poor prognosis: amplified *N-myc* copies, chromosomal ploidy, elevated serum ferritin (>150 ng/mL) and neuron-specific enolase (1000 ng/mL), and a low urine VMA/HVA ratio. Those with poorly differentiated tumors have a poor prognosis, and those with the more highly differentiated tumors have a better prognosis.[57, 100]

BOX 19–2

International Neuroblastoma Staging System

Stage I	Localized tumor with complete gross resection, with or without microscopic disease
	Representative ipsilateral and contralateral lymph nodes microscopically negative
Stage IIA	Unilateral localized tumor with incomplete gross resection
	Representative ipsilateral and contralateral lymph nodes microscopically negative
Stage IIB	Unilateral localized tumor with or without complete gross resection
	Positive ipsilateral regional lymph nodes and enlarged contralateral lymph nodes negative microscopically
Stage III	Tumor crossing midline with or without regional lymph node involvement
	or
	Unilateral tumor with contralateral regional lymph node involvement
	or
	Midline tumor with bilateral regional lymph node involvement
Stage IV	Dissemination of tumor to distant lymph nodes, bone, bone marrow, liver, and/or other organs (except as defined for stage IVS)
Stage IVS	Localized primary tumor (as defined in stages I, IIA, and IIB), with dissemination limited to liver, skin, and/or bone marrow
	Younger than 1 year of age

TREATMENT MODALITIES AND SURVIVAL

Survival for patients with stage I disease is approaching 100%. For this group and others with localized disease (stage II), surgery may be the only treatment required. Stage IVS occurs almost exclusively in those younger than 1 year. Treatment varies: no surgery, awaiting spontaneous regression; surgery alone; and low-dose chemotherapy. Neuroblastoma is one of the few tumors that may demonstrate spontaneous regression. The survival rate among these treatment groups is not statistically significant and ranges from 70% to 80%. For patients with stage III disease, survival has improved dramatically to 60% to 72% with the use of intensive therapy, including radiation, surgery, and chemotherapy. The survival for stage IV patients has not improved significantly in the past 20 years and remains at 11% to 17%. New approaches, including autologous and allogeneic BMT, are under investigation. Survival is affected by age and stage of disease at time of diagnosis. Overall survival for all the stages combined has improved to 64%.[57, 100, 106, 122]

BOX 19-3

Clinical Group Staging System for Rhabdomyosarcoma

Group I Localized disease, completely resected
  A: Confined to site of origin
  B: Infiltration beyond site of origin

Group II Total gross resection with evidence of regional spread
  A: Gross resection with microscopic disease
  B: No microscopic disease, regional disease with involved nodes
  C: Regional disease with involved nodes, gross resection with microscopic disease

Group III A: Localized or locally extensive tumor, gross residual after biopsy only
  B: Localized or locally extensive tumor, gross residual after major resection

Group IV Distant metastasis at diagnosis

Rhabdomyosarcoma

Rhabdomyosarcoma is the third most common extracranial solid tumor in childhood. It is the most common soft-tissue sarcoma in children and accounts for 5% to 8% of all childhood malignancies.[27, 139]

EPIDEMIOLOGY

The annual incidence of rhabdomyosarcoma in the United States in children 15 years of age or younger is between 4 and 7 cases per million children, with approximately 250 new cases diagnosed each year.[56, 139] Almost two thirds of cases are diagnosed in children aged 6 years or younger, with a smaller incidence peak in early to middle adolescence. There is a male predominance, with a male/female ratio of 1.4:1. Although most cases of rhabdomyosarcoma are sporadic, it has been associated with neurofibromatosis and with familial cancer syndromes. Rhabdomyosarcoma is included in the family cancer syndrome known as *Li-Fraumeni syndrome,* which has been associated with mutations in the p53 gene. Mothers of children with rhabdomyosarcoma have an increased risk of developing breast cancer, and an increased incidence of adrenocortical cancer and brain tumors has been reported in first-degree relatives.[7, 14, 27, 56, 73, 139]

HISTOLOGY

Rhabdomyosarcomas are highly malignant tumors that originate from mesenchymal cells, the precursors to stri-

ated skeletal muscle cells, and are included in the category of small, round, blue cell tumors of childhood. No uniform histologic classification system exists, but efforts are underway to evaluate data from the Intergroup Rhabdomyosarcoma Studies (IRS) to establish a common histologic and clinical staging criteria for classification. For the purposes of determining treatment strategies, the IRS classifies rhabdomyosarcoma as favorable histology (mixed, undifferentiated, embryonal, botryoid, other) or unfavorable histology (alveolar). Box 19–3 summarizes the clinical grouping system. Development and testing of a new, nonsurgical-based staging system are being done with IRS-IV.[73, 139]

CLINICAL PRESENTATION

The most common presenting symptom is the presence of a mass, usually found by the patient or parent, but symptoms vary according to the site of origin and the presence of metastasis. The most common site of occurrence is the head and neck (38%), followed by the genitourinary tract (21%), extremity (18%), trunk (7%), and retroperitoneum (7%). Rhabdomyosarcoma most often metastasizes to the lungs (40–50%), bone marrow (20–30%), bone (10%), and depending on the site of the primary tumor lymph node (20%), brain, spinal cord, and heart.[14, 139]

DIAGNOSTIC EVALUATION

The diagnostic evaluation is also determined by the site and includes radiologic imaging of the primary tumor through plain films and a CT scan or MRI. Bone scans and skeletal surveys are useful for detection of metastatic disease, followed by a CT scan or MRI of any identified areas of concern. Ultrasounds are used for tumors such as abdominal masses. A bone marrow aspirate and biopsy should be done to rule out bone marrow metastasis. A biopsy is necessary to confirm the diagnosis.[7, 104, 139]

TREATMENT MODALITIES AND PROGNOSIS

Rhabdomyosarcoma is both a local and systemic disease, with most patients having metastasis at diagnosis; thus treatment must be aimed at local control and eradication of metastasis. Treatment is based on the site of origin and extent of disease but often includes surgery, chemotherapy, and radiation.[2, 139] Surgical removal of the tumor is indicated when it will not compromise function and may reduce the amount of radiation necessary for local control. It is not indicated when there is extensive disease, because it does not improve the outcome, probably because of micrometastasis. If only partial surgical removal is possible, the initial approach should be biopsy alone.[57, 14, 139, 143, 152]

Various drugs have been used in the treatment of rhabdomyosarcoma in multiple combinations, with more intensive therapy and additional drugs for patients with more extensive disease or unfavorable histology. The treatment duration depends on the extent of disease and the primary site. Radiation is used to eradicate residual cells at the primary site or to reduce bulk disease. New methods of delivery are being used, such as brachytherapy to decrease the long-term cosmetic effects of radiation, especially to the head and neck.[139]

Patients with distant metastatic disease and those with resistant or recurrent disease remain a challenge, with few significant improvements in treatment in recent years. Currently, overall survival is 60% to 70%, but of those with metastatic disease, only 20% to 25% are curable even with the most aggressive therapy. New, more intensive therapeutic regimens are being investigated, including the use of growth factors and BMT.[122, 137, 139]

Bone Tumors

Malignant bone tumors represent 5% of all malignancies in children and 10% of all malignancies in adolescence. Peak incidence is at age 15, a trend that coincides with adolescent growth spurts. *Osteosarcoma (osteogenic sarcoma)* is the most common bone malignancy in childhood, accounting for 56% of bone tumors. *Ewing's sarcoma represents* 34% of these tumors, and the remaining 20% are of a variety of malignancies.[56]

Osteogenic Sarcoma

Incidence rates are similar in boys and girls until after age 13, when disease in boys becomes more common. Osteosarcoma incidence is slightly higher in African Americans than whites, but Ewing's sarcoma is almost 6 times more common in whites than African Americans. Only half the bone tumors in children are malignant; of these osteosarcoma is the most common, accounting for 34% of all primary sarcomas of bone and approximately 56% of malignant bone tumors in the first two decades of life.[56, 86]

ETIOLOGY

The etiology of osteosarcoma is unclear. A relationship appears to exist between the growth spurt of adolescence and the development of osteosarcoma. It has also been reported that those who develop osteosarcoma are taller than their peers. There is an increased risk for the development of osteosarcoma in children with the hereditary form of retinoblastoma and for those treated with radiation, especially in doses greater than 6000 cGy. Almost all cases of osteogenic sarcoma in those over age 40 years are associated with Paget's disease, a precursor to osteosarcoma. Trauma was thought at one time to be associated with the development of osteosarcoma, but the occurrence of an injury brings the person to medical attention and the lesion is found coincidentally. Other reported causes contributing to the development of osteosarcoma include viruses and exposure to alkylating agents.[83, 86]

CLINICAL PRESENTATION

In order of frequency, the most common sites of occurrence are femur, tibia, humerus, fibula, scapula, ileum, radius, mandible, and clavicle. Pain in the affected site is the most frequent presenting complaint. The pain can be severe, may have been present for a short time or for months, and increases with activity, often resulting in a limp. Other symptoms may include tenderness, swelling, erythema, or limited range of motion. Metastasis is present in 15% to 20% of patients at diagnosis, with 90% occurring in the lungs. Other possible sites of metastasis include bone, kidney, and brain.[22, 83, 86] Table 19–2 lists common clinical presentations.

HISTOLOGY

Osteosarcoma is a malignant sarcoma of bone that originates from osteon. The histology subtype is important. No uniformly accepted classification system exists, but the categories used most often are conventional (osteo-

TABLE 19–2
Four Clinical Presentations of Neoplasms

1. *Pain*
   Character
   Length of time present
   Relief and how obtained
   Inflammatory signs
      Pain is proportional to inflammatory response
         Severe pain: Abscess or infection
         Modest pain: Active neoplastic process
         No pain: Quiescent process
   Neurologic symptoms and signs
      Reactive zone involves nerve sheath
      Sharp pain
      Paresthesia
2. *Soft-tissue mass*
   Duration present
   Rate of growth
      Measure and record size
   Changes in consistency
      Mass or swelling
      Firm or soft
   Mobility
      Fixed or free
3. *Incidental radiologic findings*
   Prior symptoms
   Why radiologic obtained
4. *Pathologic fracture*
   Prior symptoms and signs
   Mechanism of fracture
   Characteristic of fracture

Reprinted with permission from Letson GD, Greenfield GB, Heinrich SD: Evaluation of the child with a bone or soft-tissue neoplasm, Orthop Clin North Am 27(3):432, 1996.

blastic, chondroblastic, fibroblastic), telangiectatic, parosteal and periosteal, multifocal, and miscellaneous. The conventional subtype is that seen most often in adolescents and children.[8, 22, 83, 86]

DIAGNOSTIC EVALUATION

Although a biopsy is required to confirm the diagnosis of osteosarcoma, all imaging studies should be completed before biopsy. Plain radiographic films are usually the first indication of the presence of a tumor. MRI and CT scans of the primary lesion provide information regarding extent of disease and the presence of "skip" lesions. The MRI diagnostic findings are enhanced when using dynamic contrast-enhanced imaging with the MRI studies.[8] The initial evaluation should include a bone scan to determine extent of disease and areas of metastasis. A chest x-ray film and chest CT scan are also necessary to rule out lung metastasis. These radiographic examinations are also helpful in measuring response to treatment, progression of disease, or the development of metastatic disease.[1, 8, 10, 36, 83, 86, 100]

TREATMENT MODALITIES

Surgery

Treatment of osteosarcoma incorporates both surgery and chemotherapy. Advances in radiographic imaging, the use of preoperative chemotherapy to reduce the size of the primary lesion, and improvements in surgical techniques have revolutionized the treatment of osteosarcoma. The extent of surgery depends on the location and degree of tumor involvement, with amputation no longer necessary for all patients. Limb salvage is possible only if a clear margin of 6 to 7 cm can be maintained and if the extremity will be functional postoperatively. Limb salvage procedures are not used when a pathologic fracture exists or when there is skeletal immaturity. Boxes 19–4 and 19–5 review common terms and techniques used in limb salvage surgery. Regardless of the procedure used, both physical rehabilitation and psychological rehabilitation are necessary.[83, 86, 100]

Chemotherapy

Surgery only provides local control of the tumor. Eighty percent of those treated with surgery alone will develop and die of metastatic disease. Prior clinical trials have documented the efficacy of a variety of drugs in various combinations. With the use of adjuvant chemotherapy and the improvement in surgical technique, survival rates are now 65%. Intra-arterial infusions directly to the tumors, thus avoiding systemic effects of the drugs, are now possible. For the majority of patients, neoadjuvant chemotherapy should be initiated as soon as possible after the biopsy and staging studies and should be

---

BOX 19–4

Terminology for Limb Salvage Surgery

Allograft—graft from another individual (usually a cadaver)
Autologous graft—graft taken from patient
Vascularized graft—graft implanted with vessels supplying it intact, usually from fibula or iliac crest
Arthroplasty—surgical formation or reformation of a joint
Arthrodesis—surgical fusion of a joint
Endoprosthesis—artificial replacement of a joint or bone by a metallic implant (chrome, steel, titanium)

Modified from Hockenberry MJ, Lane B: Limb salvage procedures in children with osteosarcoma, *Cancer Nurs* 11:2, 1988. Updated from Link MP, Eilber F: Osteosarcoma. In Pizzo PA, Poplack DG, editors: *Principles and practice of pediatric oncology*, ed 3, Philadelphia, Lippincott-Raven, 1997.

BOX 19–5

Limb Salvage Techniques

Distal Femur

Autologous arthrodesis (with tibia or femur intermedullary rod graft)

Segmental prosthesis to restore skeletal continuity

Prosthetic knee replacement for lesions involving diaphysis

Tibial rotation plasty

Proximal Femur

Endoprosthesis—long-stem Moore prosthesis with acrylic cement

Total joint prosthesis—hip replacement or arthroplasty

Proximal Tibia

Resection arthrodesis

Proximal Humerus

Tikhoff-Linberg procedure

Total shoulder replacement

Endoprosthesis

Proximal humerus allograft

Modified from Hockenberry MJ, Lane B: Limb salvage procedures in children with osteosarcoma, *Cancer Nurs* 11:2, 1988.

---

continued approximately 9 to 12 weeks prior to definitive surgery of the primary tumor.[100] Preoperative chemotherapy provides not only reduction in tumor sizes before resection, but also evaluation of tumor response, allowing for changes in therapy if efficacy is unsatisfactory. Osteosarcoma is highly radioresistant, and radiotherapy is reserved primarily for reduction before surgery or for palliation for those with unresponsive disease.[33, 83, 86, 100]

Late Effects

In addition to long-term follow-up to detect adverse effects resulting from chemotherapy, osteogenic sarcoma patients need ongoing evaluation regarding limb or prosthesis function. In general, osteosarcoma patients have less risk of second malignancies than those with other childhood tumors.[83, 86, 100]

PROGNOSIS

Tumors localized to the axial skeleton (e.g., trunk and pelvis) and the presence of symptoms for more then 6 months are considered poor prognostic signs. In general, the more distal the lesion, the better is the prognosis, which corresponds to the likelihood of complete surgical resection. The most important prognostic factor is the extent of disease at diagnosis, and metastasis is a poor sign. Other relevant factors include age (younger than 10 years, worse; older than 20 years, better), tumor size (< 15 cm, negative factor), gender (female more favorable), elevated alkaline phosphatase and lactate dehydrogenase (LDH) levels (both poor prognostic signs), and histology, with telangiectatic associated with the poorest outcome. Despite promising new approaches, patients with axial skeleton primaries continue to fare poorly because local control cannot be achieved in the most cases. The outcome for patients with metastatic disease remains unsatisfactory.[83, 86, 100]

Ewing's Sarcoma

Ewing's sarcoma is second only to osteosarcoma as the most common malignant bone tumor in children and adolescence, representing 1% of all childhood cancers. The differential diagnosis includes all the common solid tumors of childhood when they present in their primitive or undifferentiated form. These small, round, blue cell tumors of childhood include small-cell osteosarcomas, rhabdomyosarcomas, neuroblastomas, lymphomas, and primitive neuroectodermal tumors. The extraosseous origin of some Ewing's sarcoma is consistent with current evidence that suggests the cell of origin of most tumors is neural and not mesenchymal as previously believed.[3, 10, 36, 68]

EPIDEMIOLOGY

Ewing's sarcoma occurs in 2 or 3/1 million white children, with a low incidence in African American children. There is a slight male predominance, with girls having a slightly better prognosis. Sixty-five percent of patients are diagnosed in the second decade of life, and the disease is rarely seen before age 5 years or after age 30. As in osteosarcoma, there is a slightly increased incidence in taller adolescents, with the typical patient 15 years old, tall, white, and male.[68, 72]

CLINICAL PRESENTATION

The most common symptom is pain with or without swelling at the primary site. Two thirds of patients have a palpable mass, and one fifth have fever and leukocytosis, leading to a misdiagnosis of osteomyelitis. Presenting symptoms are also related to site of occurrence. The duration of symptoms can be days, months, or even years as in those with pelvic tumors. Systemic symptoms of weight loss, fatigue, and fever are present in only one third of patients and are most often associated with metastatic disease. The most common sites of occurrence are the pelvis, tibia, fibula, and femur, but Ewing's can occur in any bone[8, 10, 22, 68, 83] (see Table 19–2).

DIAGNOSTIC EVALUATION

The most important step in the diagnosis of Ewing's sarcoma is the biopsy, securing adequate tissue for evaluation. The diagnostic work-up includes plain films of the primary lesion, and MRI or CT scan of the primary tumor site allows for detection of extent of soft tissue involvement. A chest x-ray film and CT scan are necessary to rule out metastatic lesions. To detect distant metastasis, a bone scan is usually included in the initial work-up. Bilateral bone marrow aspirate is used to detect bone marrow involvement.[8, 10, 22, 36]

STAGING AND PROGNOSIS

No widely accepted staging system exists for Ewing's sarcoma. The tumors are often characterized by site of presentation, size, and the presence or absence of metastasis. Twenty-five percent of patients have metastasis at diagnosis, most often to the lung, bone, and bone marrow. The most important prognostic indicator is extent of disease and metastasis. Large tumor size and volume are also associated with a poor prognosis. Most primary lesions in unfavorable sites tend to be large. An elevated LDH level is a poor sign and correlates to the extent of disease. Tumors of the proximal extremities, pelvis, and axial skeleton carry the poorest prognosis. Histologic response to therapy is also a prognostic indicator, with less than 10% viable tumor at the time of surgery a positive sign.[68, 83]

TREATMENT MODALITIES

Marked progress has occurred in the treatment of Ewing's sarcoma since the late 1960s, resulting in a 2-year disease-free survival rate of 70% for those with localized tumors. Ewing's sarcoma has been described as a systemic disease that initially presents as a local problem, making it necessary to use not only local control with radiation and surgery, but also systemic treatment with chemotherapy. Large doses of radiation are necessary, with 5000 to 6000 cGy to the whole bone and a 1000 cGy boost to the primary lesion, which can be associated with functional impairment of the extremity. Portal radiation is being investigated to spare limb function further. Surgery is usually done if the bone is resectable and expendable or for children in whom radiation will cause unacceptable morbidity.[1, 3, 68, 89, 92, 124]

The Intergroup Ewing's Sarcoma Study (IESS) protocols have documented the efficacy of a variety of drugs in varying combinations and doses. Chemotherapy often is given, followed by radiation and resection of the primary lesion, and then further chemotherapy. For those with localized disease treated in this way, the 2-year survival rate is 60% to 70%.[33, 68]

Historically the survival for those considered high risk has been 20%. Under examination is a more intensive therapy using autologous BMT in the treatment regimen, with a projected disease-free survival at 2 years of 80%. Those with metastasis and recurrence still have a bleak prognosis, and late relapse continues to be a problem.

Long-term surveillance includes issues similar to those associated with osteogenic sarcoma. In addition, radiation-induced malignancies constitute a risk, especially for those who have received multiagent therapy.[33, 68, 122]

SURVIVORSHIP

As we enter this new millennium, we are encountering higher numbers of survivors from the disease of cancer. For the year 2000, approximately 1 in every 900 individuals will be a survivor of childhood cancer and predictions for the year 2010 state 1 in every 250 young adults will be long-term survivors.[17, 47] Multiple issues concern these survivors that include long-term or delayed effects from multiagent chemotherapy and radiation therapy. The most commonly reported long-term effects of cancer and the associated treatments are second malignancies; cardiac, gastrointestinal, hepatic, neurocognitive, and renal dysfunction; pulmonary disease; and psychological consequences. Additional concerns include the ability to have healthy children and complications that may occur during pregnancy or childbirth.

To address the above concerns an important multi-institutional study is being coordinated by the University of Minnesota, the Childhood Cancer Survivor Study (CCSS), known by participants as the Long-Term Follow-up Study. The current registration has 13,650 registered people from 25 different institutions in the United States and Canada. Issues that will be explored include mortality, secondary malignancies, long-term cardiopulmonary toxicity, reproductive endocrinology, cancer genetics, health-related behaviors, and patterns of childhood survivorship.[47]

Childhood survivors of cancer need to pursue an ongoing life-style that encompasses an annual health evaluation that includes screening for specific risk factors for each person (see Table 19–1).[115, 125] Additional life-style behaviors include abstinence from tobacco, limited exposure to alcohol, sun protection, reduced fat intake, and maximal intake of fruits and vegetables. Surveillance techniques for early detection of some cancers (testicular and breast self-examination, mammography, examination of stools for blood with evaluation of rectum and colon) should be performed on a scheduled frequency. Health care providers have a responsibility to keep abreast of the changes regarding childhood cancer survivorship to provide ongoing, competent, optimal care.[47, 113, 115, 125]

CONCLUSION

Nurses have a major role in caring for the child and family with cancer. Multimodality diagnostics and therapies may be used, which creates a substantial need for education and psychosocial support. Many of these patients are treated in multiple settings, so it is imperative that ongoing communication exits between all the health care staff in these various settings. Great strides have been made in the past decade with imaging techniques; laboratory diagnostics; combination chemotherapy regimens; radiation therapy; peripheral blood stem cell, cord blood, and bone marrow transplantations; and innovative surgical interventions. Significant advances have been made with some diseases, such as leukemia, Hodgkin's disease, and Wilms' tumor, whereas others have been more disappointing. Continued research and commitment to providing conscientious care for the child with cancer and the families are essential to their quality of life.

Nursing Management

Nursing Diagnoses

- *Coping, ineffective individual, related to situational crisis, ineffective coping methods, inadequate support systems*
- *Anxiety related to unmet informational needs about health condition and treatment*
- *Self-esteem disturbance related to life-threatening, acute or chronic illness*

Outcome Goals

The patient/family will be able to:

- Ask for assistance.
- Participate in decision-making with regard to health care, activities of daily living, and family interaction.
- Identify, cultivate, and use available resources.
- Openly communicate feelings related to disease, treatment, and prognosis.[133, 140, 150]
- Identify alternative resources when present coping strategies do not provide support.

Interventions

- Recognize individual needs and developmental level of child:
    Infant: dependent on parents' presence and support
    Toddler: separation from parent is major issue; fear of bodily injury and pain; loss of control related to loss of routine, physical restriction, and dependency; benefits from play therapy
    Preschooler: parents' presence of primary importance; fear of mutilation related to surgery or injections; hospital viewed as punishment or rejection, treatment as punishment or hostile; benefits from play therapy

    School-age child: concerned with lack of body control and mastery; anxiety handled through knowledge
    Adolescent: focus on peers and separation from them/family; hospital/treatment a threat to independence; anxiety handled through knowledge and participating in decision-making
- Determine patient/family learning needs and knowledge levels pertaining to specific disease process, treatment modalities, and diagnostic testing.*
- Assess patient's/family's views and beliefs about cancer.
- Observe patient's/family's coping mechanisms.
- Assess cultural background and belief systems.
- Assess readiness of patient/family to learn.

 PATIENT TEACHING PRIORITIES

Pediatric Cancers

Assess patient/family learning needs for:
    Specific disease process (e.g., leukemia, lymphoma, Wilms' tumor, osteosarcoma)
    Specific diagnostic testing (e.g., arteriography, bone marrow biopsy, MRI)
    Specific treatment modalities (e.g., chemotherapy, radiation therapy, surgery)
Assess and monitor developmental and psychosocial responses to cancer.
Initiate referrals to multidisciplinary health care team: physical therapist, dietitian, social services, occupational therapist, rehabilitation services, and school system.

---

*References 12, 63, 65, 77, 79, 97, 105, 110, 111, 140, 149.

- Determine what patient/family believe is important to know.
- Provide and discuss information related to specific type of cancer, diagnostic testing, and treatment.
- Educate the family about emotional reactions to cancer and possible developmental regression.
- Initiate referrals to other health team members: child life therapy, physical therapy, dietitian, and social services.

- Promote normalcy through attending in-hospital classroom, maintaining schoolwork, and providing opportunities for play and recreation.
- Foster maintenance of peer relationships and reentry into the community through school reentry intervention and continued contact while hospitalized or at home.
- The Patient Teaching Priorities box lists priorities for the pediatric patient with cancer and the family.

Chapter Questions

1. Four common clinical presentations for pediatric musculoskeletal cancers include:
   a. Pain, pathologic fracture, incidental radiograph findings, mass in abdomen
   b. Pain, pathologic fracture, MRI, soft-tissue mass
   c. Pain, pathologic fracture, MRI, mass in abdomen
   d. Pain, pathologic fracture, incidental radiograph findings, soft-tissue mass
2. The most common cancer in children is:
   a. Brain tumors
   b. Bone tumors
   c. Hodgkin's disease
   d. Leukemia
3. Late effects of radiation therapy include all the following *except*:
   a. Taste alterations
   b. Learning and development problems
   c. Potential secondary malignancy
   d. Thyroid abnormalities
4. The following disease included in the family cancer syndrome associated with mutations in the p53 gene is:
   a. Burkitt's lymphoma
   b. Brain tumors
   c. Osteosarcoma
   d. Rhabdomyosarcoma
5. The most common *solid tumor* in children is:
   a. Brain tumor
   b. Neuroblastoma
   c. Rhabdomyosarcoma
   d. Wilms' tumor
6. All the following are classified as small, round, blue cell tumors of childhood *except*:
   a. Ewing's sarcoma
   b. Neuroblastoma
   c. Rhabdomyosarcoma
   d. Wilms' tumor
7. Which of the following diseases most often clinically presents with a mediastinal mass at time of diagnosis?
   a. Brain tumors
   b. Lymphoblastic lymphoma
   c. Osteogenic sarcoma
   d. Rhabdomyosarcoma
8. CNS prophylaxis is necessary for which of the following diseases?
   a. Acute lymphoblastic leukemia
   b. Ewing's sarcoma
   c. Lymphoma
   d. Neuroblastoma
9. Chemotherapy drugs most often associated with organ-specific (ovary, testes) toxicity are:
   a. Antitumor antibiotics
   b. Alkylating agents
   c. Antimetabolites
   d. Nitrosureas
10. Presenting symptoms of child with a brain tumor often include clinical features relating to the tumor's:
   a. Site, blood supply, intracranial pressure
   b. Site, blood supply, extracranial pressure
   c. Site, size, intracranial pressure
   d. Site, size, extracranial pressure

BIBLIOGRAPHY

1. Abudu A and others: Tumor volume as a predictor of necrosis, after chemotherapy in Ewing's sarcoma, *J Bone Joint Surg Br* 81:317, 1999.
2. Abramson DH and others: Implant brachtherapy: a novel treatment for recurrent orbital rhabdomyosarcoma, *J AAPOS* 1:154, 1997.
3. Aherns S and others: Evaluation of prognostic factors in a tumor volume-adapted treatment strategy for localized Ewing sarcoma of bone: the CESS 86 experience. Cooperative Ewing Sarcoma Study, *Med Pediatr Oncol* 32: 186, 1999.
4. Altman AJ: Chronic leukemias of childhood. In Pizzo PA, Poplack DG, editors: *Principles and practice of pediatric oncology,* ed 3, Philadelphia, Lippincott-Raven, 1997.
5. American Association of Blood Banks: *Technical manual,* ed 13, Bethesda, MD, 1999.
6. American Association of Blood Banks: *Standards for blood banks and transfusion services,* ed 18, Sections

J8.1000, J8.3000, J6000-J8000, Bethesda, MD, The Association, 1998.

7. Anderson J and others: Genes, chromosomes, and rhabdomyosarcoma, *Genes Chromosomes Cancer* 26:275, 1999.

8. Andrassy RJ, Hays RJ: General principles of surgery. In Pizzo PA, Poplack DG, editors: *Principles and practice of pediatric oncology,* ed 3, Philadelphia, Lippincott-Raven, 1997.

9. Atahan IL and others: Thyroid dysfunction in children receiving neck irradiation for Hodgkin's disease, *Radiat Med* 16:359, 1998.

10. Bacci G and others: Delayed diagnosis and tumor stage in Ewing's sarcoma, *Oncol Rep* 6:465, 1999.

11. Balis FM, Holcenberg JS, Poplack DG: General principles of chemotherapy. In Pizzo PA, Poplack DG, editors: *Principles and practice of pediatric oncology,* ed 3, Philadelphia, Lippincott-Raven, 1997.

12. Ball J, Bindler R: *Pediatric nursing: caring for children,* ed 2, Stamford, CT, 1999.

13. Bean CA and others: High-tech homecare infusion therapies, *Crit Care Nurs Clin North Am* 10:287, 1998.

14. Beech TR and others: What comprises appropriate therapy for children/adolescents with rhabdomyosarcoma arising in the abdominal wall? A report from the Intergroup Rhabdomyosarcoma Study Group, *J Pediatric Surg* 34:668, 1999.

15. Belasco JB and others: Hypofractionated moderate dose radiation, intrathecal chemotherapy, and repetitive reinduction/consolidation systemic therapy for central nervous system relapse of acute lymphoblastic leukemia in children, *Med Pediatr Oncol* 34:125, 2000.

16. Bhatia S, Meadows AT, Robinson LL: Second chances after pediatric Hodgkin's disease, *J Clin Oncol* 16:2570, 1998.

17. Blatt J: Pregnancy outcome in long-term survivors of childhood cancer, *Med Pediatr Oncol* 33:29, 1999.

18. Bove KE: Wilms' tumor and related abnormalities in the fetus and newborn, *Semin Perinatol* 23:310, 1999.

19. Boyle DA and others: Quality improvement initiatives in bone marrow transplant nursing, *Innovations in Breast Cancer Care,* 3:57, 1998.

20. Brodeur GM, Castleberry RP: Neuroblastoma. In Pizzo PA, Poplack DG, editors: *Principles and practice of pediatric oncology,* ed 3, Philadelphia, Lippincott-Raven, 1997.

21. Burkett S: The child with cancer. In Ashwill JW, Droske SC, editors: *Nursing care of children principles and practice,* Philadelphia, Saunders, 1999.

22. Cabral DA, Tucker LB: Malignancies in children who initially present with rheumatic complaints, *J Pediatr* 134:53, 1999.

23. Capra ML and others: Wilms' tumor: a 25-year review of the role of preoperative chemotherapy, *J Pediatr Surg* 34:579, 1999.

24. Christensen J, Akcasu N: the role of the pediatric nurse practitioner in the comprehensive management of pediatric oncology patients, in the outpatient setting, *J Pediatr Oncol* 16:58, 1999.

25. Collins VP: Glioma, *Cancer Survivor* 32:37, 1998.

26. Coppes MJ, Egeler RM: Genetics of Wilms' tumor, *Semin Urol Oncol* 17:2, 1999.

27. Dagher R, Helman L: Rhabdomyosarcoma: an overview, *Oncologist* 4:34, 1999.

28. Davies and others: Multiple roles for the Wilms' tumor suppressor, WT1, *Cancer Res* 59(suppl 7):1747s, 1999.

29. Davies-Johns T, Chidel M, Macklis RM: The role of radiation therapy in the management of Wilms' tumor, *Semin Urol Oncol* 17:46, 1999.

30. Debinski W and others: Receptor for interleukin 13 is abundantly and specifically over-expressed in-patients with glioblastoma multiforme, *Int J Oncol* 15:481, 1999.

31. Desai D, Nicholls G, Duffy PG: Bench surgery with auto-transplantation for bilateral synchronous Wilms' tumor: a report of three cases, *J Pediatr Surg* 34:632, 1999.

32. DeVita VT Jr, Hellman S, Rosenberg SA, editors: *Cancer principles and practice of oncology,* ed 5, Philadelphia, Lippincott-Raven, 1997.

33. Diaz MA, Vicent MG, Madero L: High-dose busulfan/melphalan as conditioning for autologous PBPC transplantation in pediatric patients with solid tumors, *Bone Marrow Transplant* 24:1157, 1999.

34. Dolgin MJ and others: Quality of life in adult survivors, of childhood cancers, *Social Work in Health Care* 28:31, 1999.

35. Dugger B: Intravenous nursing competency: why is it important? *INS* 20(6):287, 1997.

36. Durbin M and others: Ewing's sarcoma masquerading as osteomyelitis, *Clin Orthop* 357:176, 1998.

37. El-Khasdrawy AM, Hoffer FA, Reddick WE: Ewing's sarcoma recurrence Vs radiation necrosis in dynamic contrast-enhanced MR imaging: a case report, *Pediatr Radiol* 29:272, 1999.

38. Fanos V, Cataldi T: Antibacterial-induced nephrotoxicity in the newborn, *Drug Safety* 20:245, 1999.

39. Fann BD: Fluid and electrolyte balance in the pediatric patient, *INS* 21:153, 1998.

40. Finiewicz KJ, Larson RA: Dose-intensive therapy for adult acute lymphoblastic leukemia, *Semin Oncol* 26:6, 1999.

41. Fletcher JC, Dorn LD, Waldron P: Ethical considerations in pediatric oncology. In Pizzo PA, Poplack DG, editors: *Principles and practice of pediatric oncology,* ed 3, Philadelphia, Lippincott-Raven, 1997.

42. Forchielli ML, Paolucci G, Lo CW: Total parenteral nutrition and home parenteral: an effective combination to sustain malnourished children with cancer, *Nutr Rev* 57:15, 1999.

43. Foley F: Children, teens, and cancer; going forward, slipping back, *Cancer Practice* 7:4, 1999.

44. Fortney JT and others: Anesthesia for pediatric external beam radiation therapy, *Int J Radiat Oncol Biol Phys* 44:587, 1999.

45. Fraser MC, Calzone KA, Goldstein AM: Familial cancers: evolving challenges for nursing practice, *Oncol Nurs Updates* 4:1, 1997.

46. Frey AM: When a child needs peripheral IV therapy, *Nursing* 28:18, 1998.

47. Friedman DL: The childhood cancer survivor study: an important research initiative for childhood cancer survivors, *J Pediatr Oncol Nurs* 16:172, 1999.

48. Fruhwald MC and others: High expression of somatostatin receptor subtype 2 (sst2) in medulloblastoma, *Pediatr Res* 45(5 Pt 1):697, 1999.

49. Gidding CE and others: Vincristine pharmacokinetics after repetitive dosing in children, *Cancer Chemother Pharmacol* 44:203, 1999.

50. Giona F and others: Management of advanced acute lymphoblastic leukemia in children and adults: results of the ALL R-87 protocol. AIEOP and GIMEMA Cooperative Group, *Leuk Lymphoma* 32:89, 1998.

51. Goddard AG and others: Growth hormone deficiency following radiotherapy for orbital and parameningeal sarcomas, *Pediatr Hematol Oncol* 16:23, 1999.

52. Golab TR, Weinstein HJ, Grier HE: Acute myelogenous leukemia. In Pizzo PA, Poplack DG, editors: *Principles and practice of pediatric oncology,* ed 3, Philadelphia, Lippincott-Raven, 1997.

53. Gorski LA, editor: *Best practices in home infusion therapy,* Frederick, MD, Aspen, 1999.

54. Green DM and others: Wilms' tumor. In Pizzo PA, Poplack DG, editors: *Principles and practice of pediatric oncology,* ed 3, Philadelphia, Lippincott-Raven, 1997.

55. Green DM and others: Effect of duration of treatment on treatment outcome and cost of treatment for Wilms' tumor: a report from the National Wilms' Tumor Study Group, *J Clin Oncol* 16:3744, 1998.

56. Greenlee RT and others: Cancer statistics 2000, *CA Cancer J Clin* 50:7, 2000.

57. Grosfeld JL: Risk-based management: current concepts of treating malignant solid tumors of childhood, *J Am Coll Surg* 189:407, 1999.

58. Grovas AC and others: Regimen-related toxicity of myeloablative chemotherapy with BCNU, thiotepa, and etoposide followed by autologous stem cell rescue for children with newly diagnosed glioblastoma multiforme: report from the Children's Cancer Group, *Med Pediatr Oncol* 33:83, 1999.

59. Hardell L, Nasman A, Pahlson A, Hallquist A, and Hansson-Mild K: Use of cellular telephones and the risk for brain tumors: a case-control study, *Int J Oncol* 15:113, 1999.

60. Harmening DM: *Modern blood banking and transfusion practices,* ed 4, Philadelphia, Davis, 1999.

61. Harpham W: Long-term survivorship. In Berger A, Portenoy RK, Weissman DE, editors: *Principles and practice of supportive oncology,* Philadelphia, Lippincott-Raven, 1998.

62. Harris JL, Maguire D: Developing a protocol to prevent and treat pediatric central venous catheter occlusions, *INS* 22:194, 1999.

63. Harris KA: The informational needs of patients with cancer and their families, *Cancer Pract* 6:39, 1998.

64. Harvey J and others: Providing quality care in childhood cancer survivorship: learning from the past, looking to the future, *J Pediatr Oncol Nurs* 16:117, 1999.

65. Hazinski MF: *Manual of pediatric critical care,* St. Louis, Mosby, 1999.

66. Hobbie WL: Survivorship in the 21st century: "cure is not enough," *J Pediatr Oncol Nurs* 16:115, 1999.

67. Hockenberry-Eaton M, Kline NE: Nursing support of the child with cancer. In Pizzo PA, Poplack DG, editors: *Principles and practice of pediatric oncology,* ed 3, Philadelphia, Lippincott-Raven, 1997.

68. Horowitz ME and others: Ewing's sarcomas family of tumors: Ewing's sarcoma of bone and soft tissue and the peripheral primitive neuroectodermal tumors. In Pizzo PA, Poplack DG, editors: *Principles and practice of pediatric oncology,* ed 3, Philadelphia, Lippincott-Raven, 1997.

69. Hudson MM, Donaldson SS: Hodgkin's disease, *Pediatr Clin North Am* 44:891, 1997.

70. Hudson MM and others: Increased mortality after successful treatment for Hodgkin's disease, *J Clin Oncol* 16:3592, 1998.

71. Huff V: Wilms' tumor genetics, *Am J Med Genet* 79:260, 1998.

72. Hum L, Krieger N, Finklestein MM: The relationship between parental occupation and bone cancer risk in offspring, *Int J Epidemiol* 27:766, 1998.

73. Humphrey G and others: Expression of CD44 by rhabdomyosarcoma: a new prognostic marker? *Br J Cancer* 80:918, 1999.

74. Intravenous Nurses Society: Peripherally inserted central catheters, *INS* 20:172, 1997.

75. Intravenous Nurses Society: The registered nurses' role in vascular access device selection, *INS* 20:71, 1997.

76. Intravenous Nurses Society: Revised Intravenous Nursing Standards of practice, *INS* 21(1 Suppl), 1998.

77. Jacob E: Making the transition from hospital to home, caring for the newly diagnosed child with cancer, *Home Care Provider* 4:67, 1999.

78. Kline NE: Investigational cancer treatment for children, *J Pediatr Oncol Nurs* 16:1, 1999.

79. Kozachik SL, Given BA, Given CW: Cancer patients at home: activating nurses to assist patients and to involve families in care at home, *Oncol Nurs Updates* 6:1, 1999.

80. Kubota M and others: Second malignancy following treatment of acute lymphoblastic leukemia in children, *Int J Hematol* 67:397, 1998.

81. Lassen U and others: Treatment of newly diagnosed glioblastoma multiforme with carmustine, cisplatin and etoposide followed by radiotherapy. A phase II study, *J Neurooncol* 43:161, 1999.

82. Lea DH, Jenkins J: Cancer genetics for nurses: part I. The genetics basis for cancer, *Oncol Nurs Updates* 4:1, 1997.

83. Letson GD, Greenfeld GB, Heinrich SD: Evaluation of the child with a bone or soft-tissue neoplasm: *Orthop Clin North Am* 27:525, 1996.

84. Levien MG, Bringelsen KA: Postoperative chemotherapy in the National Wilms' Tumor Studies, *Semin Urol Oncol* 17:40, 1999.

85. Linet MS and others: Residential exposure to magnetic fields and acute lymphoblastic leukemia in children, *N Engl J Med* 337:1, 1997.

86. Link MP, Eilber F: Osteosarcoma. In Pizzo PA, Poplack DG, editors: *Principles and practice of pediatric oncology,* ed 3, Philadelphia, Lippincott-Raven, 1997.

87. Magrath IT: the treatment of pediatric lymphomas: paradigms to plagiarize? *Ann Oncol* 8(suppl 1): 7, 1997.

88. Margolin JF, Poplack DG: Acute lymphoblastic leukemia. In Pizzo PA, Poplack DG, editors: *Principles and practice of pediatric oncology,* ed 3, Philadelphia, Lippincott-Raven, 1997.

89. Marina NM and others: Chemotherapy dose-intensification for pediatric patients with Ewing's family of tumors and desmoplastic small round-cell tumors: a feasibility study at St. Jude Children's Research Hospital, *J Clin Oncol* 17:180, 1999.

90. Matthay KK and others: Treatment of high-risk neuroblastoma with intensive chemotherapy, radiotherapy, autologous bone marrow transplantation, and 13-cis-retinoic acid. Children's Cancer Group, *N Engl J Med* 341:1165, 1999.

91. Melnick SJ: Acute lymphoblastic leukemia, *Clin Lab Med* 19:169, 1999.

92. Merchant TE and others: Effect of low-dose radiation therapy when combined with surgical resection for Ewing's sarcoma, *Med Pediatr Oncol* 33:65, 1999.

93. Merchant TE and others: High-grade pediatric spinal cord tumors, *Pediatr Neurosurg* 30:1, 1999.

94. Mittelman A and others: Phase II clinical trial of didemnin B in patients with recurrent or refractory anaplastic astrocytoma or glioblastoma multiforme, *Invest New Drugs* 17:179, 1999.

95. Moore K: Out-of-pocket expenditures of outpatients receiving chemotherapy, *Oncol Nurs Forum* 25:1615, 1998.

96. Murray JS: The lived experience of childhood cancer: one sibling's experience, *Issues in Comprehensive Pediatric Nursing* 21:217, 1998.

97. Murray JS: Siblings of children with cancer: a review of the literature, *J Pediatr Oncol Nurs* 16:25, 1999.

98. Oeffinger KC and others: Programs for adult survivors of childhood cancer, *J Clin Oncol* 16:2864, 1998.

99. Oncology Nursing Society: *Cancer chemotherapy guidelines and recommendations for practice,* Pittsburgh, Oncology Nursing Press, 1999.

100. O'Reilly R and others: NCCN pediatric osteoscarcoma practice guidelines, *Oncology* 10:1799, 1996.

101. Osmak M, Vrhovec I, Skrk J: Cisplatin resistant glioblastoma cells may have increased concentration of urokinase plasminogen activator and plasminogen acitvator inhibitor type I, *J Neurooncol* 42: 95, 1999.

102. Pagana KD, Pagana TJ: *Mosby's diagnostic & laboratory test reference,* St. Louis, Mosby, 1998.

103. Palumbo JS, Zwerdling T: Soft tissue sarcomas of infancy, *Semin Perinatol* 23: 299, 1999.

104. Parker BR: Imaging studies in the diagnosis of pediatric malignancies. In Pizzo PA, Poplack DG, editors: *Principles and practice of pediatric oncology,* ed 3, Philadelphia, Lippincott-Raven, 1997.

105. Peacock A, Bechtel GA, Lillis PP: Case management of the pediatric oncology patient, *J Case Manage* 5:46, 1999.

106. Perentesis J and others: Autologous stem cell transplantation for high-risk pediatric solid tumors, *Bone Marrow Transplant* 24:609, 1999.

107. Perry AG and Potter PA: *Clinical nursing skills & techniques,* ed 4, St. Louis, Mosby, 1998.

108. Pession A and others: Phase I study of high-dose thiotepa with busulfan, etoposide, and autologous stem cell support in children with disseminated solid tumors, *Med Pediatr Oncol* 33:450, 1999.

109. Phipps WJ, Sands JK, Marek JF: *Medical-Surgical nursing: concepts and clinical practice,* ed 6, St. Louis, Mosby, 1999.

110. Pillitteri A: Nursing care of the child with cancer. In Pillitteri A: *Maternal and child health nursing,* ed 3, Philadelphia, Lippincott-Raven, 1999.

111. Pillitteri A: *Child health nursing: care of the child and family:* Philadelphia, Lippincott-Raven, 1999.

112. Pye S: Diagnosis and referral of Wilms' tumor, *Nurse Pract* 24:121, 1999.

113. Pyke-Grimm KA and others: Preferences for participation in treatment decision making and information needs of parents of children with cancer: a pilot study, *J Pediatr Oncol Nurs* 16:13, 1999.

114. Raney RB and others: Late complications of therapy in 213 children with localized, nonorbital soft-tissue sarcoma of the head and neck: a descriptive report from the Intergroup Rhabdomyosarcoma Studies (IRS) II and III. IRS Group of the Children's Cancer Group and the Pediatric Oncology Group, *Med Pediatr Oncol* 33:362, 1999.

115. Richardson RC, Nelson MB, Meeske K: Young survivors of childhood cancer: attending to emerging medical psychosocial needs, *J Pediatr Oncol Nurs* 16:136, 1999.

116. Ritchey ML: The role of preoperative chemotherapy for Wilms' tumor: the NWTSG perspective. National Wilms' Tumor Study Group, *Semin Urol Oncol* 17:21, 1999.

117. Rodriguez RP: Amputation surgery and prostheses, *Orthop Clin North Am* 27:525, 1996.

118. Rogers JS, Soud TE: *Manual of pediatric emergency nursing,* St. Louis, Mosby, 1998.

119. Ross JH, Kay R: Surgical considerations for patients with Wilms' tumor, *Semin Urol Oncol* 17:33, 1999.

120. Ross JA and others: Seasonal variations in the diagnosis of childhood cancer in the United States, *Br J Cancer* 81:549, 1999.

121. Sallee D and others: Primary pediatric cardiac tumors: a 17 year experience, *Cardiol Young* 9:155, 1999.

122. Saunders JE: Bone marrow transplantation in pediatric oncology. In Pizzo PA, Poplack DG, editors: *Principles and practice of pediatric oncology,* ed 3, Philadelphia, Lippincott-Raven, 1997.

123. Schellong G: Pediatric Hodgkin's disease: treatment in the late 1990's, *Ann Oncol* 9(suppl 5): S115, 1998.

124. Schindler OS and other: Use of extendible total femoral replacements in children with malignant bone tumors, *Clin Orthop* 357:157, 1998.

125. Schwartz CL: Long-term survivors of childhood cancer: the late effects of therapy, *Oncologist* 4:45, 1999.

126. Shad A, Magrath IT: Malignant non-Hodgkin's lymphoma in children. In Pizzo PA, Poplack DG, editors: *Principles and practice of pediatric oncology,* ed 3, Philadelphia, Lippincott-Raven, 1997.

127. Shamberger RC: Pediatric renal tumors, *Semin Surg Oncol* 16:105, 1999.

128. Shamberger RC and others: Surgery-related factors and local recurrence of Wilms' tumor in National Wilms Tumor Study 4. *Ann Surg* 229:292, 1999.

129. Shankar SM and others: Pharmacokinetics of single daily dose gentamicin in children with cancer, *J Pediatr Hematol Oncol* 21:284, 1999.

130. Smith M: Considerations on a possible viral etiology for B-precursor acute lymphoblastic leukemia of childhood, *J Immunother* 20:89, 1997.

131. Smith MA and others: Evidence that childhood acute lymphoblastic leukemia is associated with an infectious agent linked to hygiene conditions, *Cancer Causes Control* 9:285, 1998.

132. Springfeld D: Autograft reconstruction, *Orthop Clin North Am* 27:483, 1996.

133. Terzo H: The effects of childhood cancer on siblings, *Pediatr Nurs* 25:309, 1999.

134. Tomlinson GS, Cole CH, Smith NM: Bilateral Wilms' tumor: a clinicopathologic review, *Pathology* 31:12, 1999.

135. Van-den-Berg H and others: Favorable outcome after 1-year treatment of childhood T-cell acute lymphoblastic leukemia, *Med Pediatr Oncol* 30:46, 1998.

136. Vlasek R, Sim FH: Ewing's sarcoma, *Orthop Clin North Am* 27:591, 1996.

137. Walterhouse DO and others: High-dose chemotherapy followed by peripheral blood stem cell rescue for metastatic rhabdomyosarcoma: the experience at Chicago Children's Memorial Hospital, *Med Pediatr Oncol* 32:88, 1999.

138. Ward WG, Yang RS, Eckardt JJ: Endoprosthetic bone reconstruction following malignant tumor resection in skeletally immature patients, *Orthop Clin North Am* 27:493, 1996.

139. Wexler LH, Helman LJ: Rhabdomyosarcomas and the undifferentiated sarcomas. In Pizzo PA, Poplack DG, editors: *Principles and practice of pediatric oncology,* ed 3, Philadelphia, Lippincott-Raven, 1997.

140. Whaley LF, Wong DL: *Nursing care of infants and children,* ed 6, St. Louis, Mosby, 1999.

141. Wheeler C, Frey AM: Intravenous therapy in children. In Terry J and others, editors: *Intravenous therapy: clinical principles and practice,* Philadelphia, Saunders, 1995.

142. Wiener ES, Albanese CT: Venous access in pediatric patients, *INS* 21(5S):S122, 1998.

143. Whitlock JA, Holcenberg JS: Phase I study topotecan administered as a 21 day continuous infusion in children with recurrent solid tumors: a report from the Children's Cancer Group. *Clin Cancer Res* 5:3956, 1999.

144. Wolden SL and others: Second cancers following pediatric Hodgkin's disease, *J Clin Oncol* 16:536, 1998.

145. Wolf RE, Enneking WF: The staging and surgery of musculoskeletal neoplasms, *Orthop Clin North Am* 27:473, 1996.

146. Woo MH and others: Pharmacokinetics of paclitaxel in anephric patient, *Cancer Chemother Pharmacol* 43:92, 1999.

147. Wood D: A comparative study of two securement techniques for short peripheral intravenous catheters, *INS* 20:280, 1997.

148. Wong DL and others: *Whaley and Wong's nursing care of infants and children,* ed 6, wwwmosby.com Merlin/peds__wong__ncic: The child with cancer, St. Louis, Mosby, 1999.

149. Wong DL, Perry SE: *Maternal child nursing,* St. Louis, Mosby, 1998.

150. Woodgate RL: Conceptual understanding of resilience in the adolescent with cancer: part I, *J Pediatr Oncol Nurs* 16(1):35, 1999.

151. Workman ML: The lymphoid system and its role in maintaining immunocompetence, *Semin Oncol Nurs* 14:248, 1998.

152. Young RF: The role of the gamma knife in the treatment of malignant primary and metastatic tumors, *CA Cancer J Clin* 48:177, 1998.

153. Yule SM and others: Cyclosphamide and ifosfamide metabolites in the cerebrospinal fluid of children, *Clin Cancer Res* 3:1985, 1997.

Oncologic Complications

Jamie S. Myers

Oncologic complications occur frequently in patients with cancer and may be a direct result of the disease. In these cases, presentation of the oncologic complications may be what precipitates the work-up and diagnosis of the malignancy. However, they are more frequently an indication of progressive or advancing disease. Oncologic complications also occur as a result of treatment for cancer. Acute, life-threatening oncologic complications are often referred to as oncologic emergencies.

Oncologic emergencies may be categorized in different ways. Woodard and Hogan[159] group them as follows: neurologic, cardiopulmonary, metabolic, hematologic, infectious, gastrointestinal, genitourinary, and infusion-related. They define *oncologic emergencies* as "clinical situations in which the condition is secondary to a malignancy or its treatment, and when there are potentially immediate catastrophic consequences in the absence of successful intervention" (Table 20–1).

The Oncology Nursing Society (ONS) *Core Curriculum for Oncology Nursing* (3rd edition, 1998) divides oncologic emergencies into two main categories: metabolic and structural. This chapter will be organized according to the ONS categories, with the addition of hypersensitivity (anaphylaxis) and tumor lysis syndrome (Table 20–2).

Management of an oncologic complication depends on many important factors related to the patient and the underlying disease (Box 20–1). These factors must be given thorough consideration before the initiation of treatment.

Once the oncologic complication is analyzed, decisions about the aggressiveness of treatment can be made. Aggressive treatment may be appropriate when the potential exists for a cure or prolonged survival. However, in advanced disease palliative treatment may be given to reduce symptoms and restore functional status. Finally, withholding treatment and providing supportive care may be the most appropriate decision in the presence of disseminated metastatic disease.[52, 95] Quality of life should always be the driving force in any decision regard-

ing care of the patient with cancer. The overall goal is to prevent, reverse, or minimize life-threatening oncologic complications through prophylactic measures, early detection, and effective management.

Use of critical care interventions for patients with cancer has increased for a variety of reasons: new hope for cure or long-term remission, increased ability to treat certain complications, and consumer demands. Due to the urgent nature of oncologic complications, prevention, early recognition, adequate decision-making, and prompt treatment are of paramount importance when delivering care to patients with cancer. Nurses are in a key role to accurately assess patients who are at high risk for complications.

Assessment is essential because a change in the patient's condition may be subtle or dramatic. Two key concepts when caring for people with cancer are (1) the identification of patients at risk for developing an oncologic complication and (2) the involvement of the family and significant others. The patient and family require considerable education and support. The time limitations for patient and family education present a great challenge. Explanations of tests and procedures and the rationale for changes in patient care or setting must be kept simple. Treatment options and goals of therapy must be explained and discussed. This is especially important when the realistic outcome is palliation. Nurses with demonstrated expertise in oncology are a vital component in the care of the patient with an oncologic emergency.

Structural Oncologic Complication

Cardiac Tamponade

DEFINITION

Neoplastic cardiac tamponade is the compression of the cardiac muscle by pathologic fluid accumulation under

TABLE 20-1
Categories of Oncologic Emergencies

NEUROLOGIC
Spinal cord compression
Intracranial malignancy
Seizures

CARDIOPULMONARY
Superior vena cava syndrome
Cardiac tamponade
Massive hemoptysis
Airway obstruction
Large pleural effusion

METABOLIC
Hypercalcemia
Tumor lysis syndrome
Hyponatremia
Hypoglycemia
Adrenal failure

HEMATOLOGIC
Thrombocytopenia
Thrombosis
Increased viscosity syndromes

INFECTIOUS
Neutropenic sepsis
Vascular access device-related sepsis

GASTROINTESTINAL
Obstruction
Hemorrhage

GENITOURINARY
Obstruction
Hemorrhage

INFUSION-RELATED
Allergic-reactions
Extravasation

Data from Woodard WL III, Hogan DK: Oncologic emergencies: implications for nurses, J Intravenous Nursing 19(5):257, 1996.

pressure within the pericardial sac. Fluid accumulates because of pericardial constriction by a tumor or postirradiation pericarditis.[13, 65, 94, 99, 134] Compression of the myocardium interferes with dilation of the heart chambers, which prevents adequate cardiac filling during diastole. This in turn reduces blood flow to the ventricles and reduces stroke volume, which results in decreased cardiac output. Other pressures are then affected, including an elevated central venous pressure (CVP) and a lowered left atrial pressure (Fig. 20–1). Two compensatory mechanisms, initiated by adrenergic stimulation, attempt to counteract these pressures to increase cardiac output and maintain peripheral perfusion.[39] An increase in heart rate (tachycardia) helps maintain cardiac output at low stroke volumes and increases systolic emptying. Peripheral vasoconstriction maintains arterial pressure

and venous return. If cardiac output is not increased by compensatory mechanisms, this can cause circulatory collapse, which is fatal if untreated.[10, 52]

ETIOLOGY AND RISK FACTORS

A variety of nonmalignant or malignant conditions may be responsible for the development of cardiac tamponade. Nonmalignant causes include[49, 101, 128]:

Cardiovascular causes: heart surgery, chest trauma, aneurysm, rupture of the great vessel, cardiac procedures (angiography, insertion or removal of pacer wires), insertion of central venous catheter
Infectious pericarditis; bacterial, fungal, viral, or tubercular infections
Connective tissue disorders: systemic lupus erythematosus (SLE), scleroderma, rheumatoid disease
Myxedema
Uremia
Pharmacologic therapy: anthracyclines (doxorubicin, daunomycin, and others), anticoagulants (heparin, sodium warfarin), hydralazine (Apresoline), procainamide (Procaine SR, Pronestyl)

Malignant causes include the following[49, 72, 78, 99, 111]:

Neoplastic pericarditis with effusion: primary tumors of the pericardium (mesotheliomas, sarcomas, malignant teratomas), metastatic tumors of the pericardium (lung cancer, breast tumors, leukemias, lymphomas, melanomas, and sarcomas)
Neoplastic constrictive pericarditis (metastatic tumor infiltration)

TABLE 20-2
ONS Core Curriculum
Oncologic Emergency Categories

STRUCTURAL
Cardiac tamponade
Increased intracranial pressure
Spinal cord compression
Superior vena cava syndrome

METABOLIC
Disseminated intravascular coagulation
Hypercalcemia
Hypersensitivity reaction (anaphylaxis)
Malignant pleural effusion
Sepsis
Syndrome of inappropriate antidiuretic hormone
Tumor lysis syndrome

Data from Finley JP: Metabolic emergencies. In Itano JK, Taoka KN, editors: Oncology Nursing Society core curriculum for oncology nursing, ed 3, Philadelphia, Saunders, 1998:315; and Hardy J: Clinical management. Corticosteroids in palliative care, Eur J Palliative Care 5:46, 1998.

Radiation pericarditis (exposure of the heart to 400 Gy or more)[99]

Pericardial effusion with tamponade is a life-threatening problem whether the cause is malignant or nonmalignant. Cancer and open-heart surgery are the leading causes of cardiac tamponade. Malignant pericardial tamponade occurs in approximately 5% to 15% of patients with a neoplasm that involves the heart.[78] The high estimates of this complication are based on compilations of autopsy data regarding cardiac (including pericardial) metastasis, which range from 0.1% to 21%.[72] The majority of these patients are asymptomatic, with only 20% to 30% showing clinical evidence of cardiac disease before death.[94]

Most cases of neoplastic cardiac tamponade represent metastatic invasion of the pericardium. Pericardial metastasis is unusual without documentation of other metastases. Only rarely is the cause primary disease of the myocardium (mesothelioma, angiosarcoma, fibrosarcoma, and malignant teratoma).[71, 78] Any cancer has the potential for metastatic spread to the pericardium via direct tumor extension, lymphatic invasion, or hematogenous dissemination. Patients with pericardial effusions are at risk for tamponade. Pericardial effusions caused by metastatic disease are present in 5% to 50% of patients with cancer.[111] However, cancers at greatest risk for the development of neoplastic cardiac tamponade include breast cancer, lung cancer, lymphoma, and leukemia, which account for 80% of this complication.[13, 65, 105, 106] Other malignant causes are melanoma, gastrointestinal (GI) cancers, and sarcomas.[49, 108] Approximately 5% of patients who receive radiation therapy to the mediastinum (400 Gy or more) develop acute pericarditis with or without pericardial effusion during treatment or chronic constrictive pericarditis up to 20 years after treatment. More than 90% of the cases occur in the first year after radiation treatment.[99, 109]

PATHOPHYSIOLOGY

The heart and a portion of the great vessels are encased in a thin, tough, double-layered fibrous sac called the *pericardium,* which contains little elastic tissue. The inner layer, or sheath, is known as the *visceral pericardium.* It is a delicate serous membrane that lines the interior of the fibrous sac and is continuous with the surface of the heart.[94, 99] The outer layer of the pericardium is called the *parietal pericardium.* This sheath is fibrous and provides strength and protection. The left sternal portion is in direct contact with the chest wall. Between the two layers of the pericardium is a cavity that contains 10 to 20 mL of a clear serous lubricating fluid, originating from the lymphatic channels surrounding the heart, and serves to cushion the myocardium.[94, 99]

The pathophysiology of pericardial tamponade is a progressive accumulation of fluid in the pericardial sac (Fig. 20–2), which leads to compression of the heart, hampering dilation of its chambers and thus limiting diastolic atrial filling; intrapericardial pressure rises, and bilateral ventricular stroke volume decreases. Initially the sac will stretch to accommodate increases in fluid, and compensatory mechanisms—an increased heart rate (tachycardia) and increased peripheral vascular tone (peripheral vasoconstriction)—maintain adequate cardiac output. However, as these temporary adaptive responses begin to fail, a vicious cycle of increased fluid with decreased atrial pressure, decreased cardiac output, and decreased venous return will progress to circulatory collapse and, if untreated, to shock, cardiac arrest, and death.

B O X   2 0 - 1

Management Factors in the Evaluation and Treatment of an Oncologic Emergency

Symptoms and Signs

Are the symptoms and signs caused by the tumor or by complications of treatment?

How quickly are the symptoms of the oncologic emergency progressing?

Natural History of the Primary Tumor

Is there a previous diagnosis of malignancy?

What is the disease-free interval between the diagnosis of the primary tumor and the onset of the emergency?

Has the emergency developed in the setting of terminal disease?

Efficacy of Available Treatment

No prior therapy versus extensive pretreatment

Should treatment be directed at the underlying malignancy and/or the urgent complication?

Will the patient's general medical condition influence the ability to administer effective treatment?

Treatment and Goals

Potential for cure

Is prompt palliation required to prevent further debilitation?

What is the risk versus benefit ratio of treatment?

Should treatment be withheld if the patient is terminal with minimal chance of response to available antitumor therapies?

From Glover D, Glick JH: Oncologic emergencies. In Holleb AI, Fink DJ, Murphy GP, editors: *American Cancer Society textbook of clinical oncology,* ed 2, Atlanta, American Cancer Society, 1995. Reprinted with permission of the American Cancer Society, Inc.

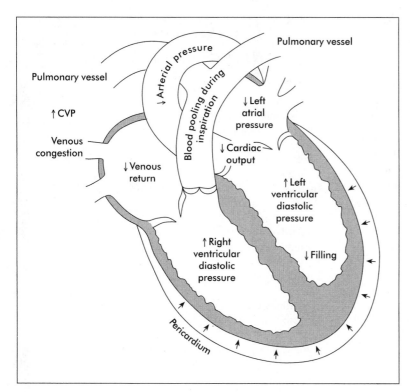

FIGURE 20-1 Cardiovascular effects of increased intrapleural pressure. Intraventricular diastolic pressure rises as a result of higher intrapericardial pressure. This prevents adequate filling of the ventricle, causing venous congestion, decreased cardiac output, lowered left atrial pressure, and elevated central venous pressure (*CVP*). ↑, Increased; ↓, decreased. (From Dietz KA, Flaherty AM: Oncologic emergencies. In Groenwald SL and others, editors: *Cancer nursing: principles and practice,* ed 2, Boston, Jones & Bartlett, 1990. Reprinted with permission.)

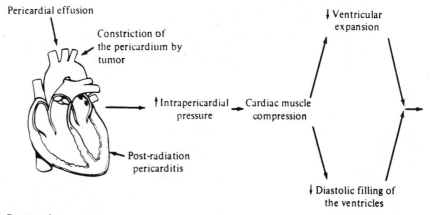

FIGURE 20-2 Development of neoplastic pericardial tamponade. (From Yasko JM, Schafer SL: Neoplastic pericardial tamponade. In Yasko JM, editor: *Guidelines for cancer care: symptom management,* Reston, VA, Reston, © 1983. Reprinted with permission of Prentice-Hall, Inc., Upper Saddle River, NJ.)

The severity of cardiac tamponade depends on the amount of fluid in the pericardium, the rate of accumulation, and the degree of pericardial and organic compromise. Usually there will be no change in cardiac activity with the addition of 50 mL or less of fluid in the pericardial space. Gradual fluid accumulation permits the pericardium to stretch and accommodate. As much as 2 liters or more can accumulate without producing signs of cardiac compromise.* However, 100 to 200 mL fluid may cause severe cardiac impairment if the accumulation occurs rapidly.[71, 134, 72, 78, 94] Whether gradual or acute, the fluid accumulation that leads to cardiac tamponade in the presence of malignant disease is the result of one of the following mechanisms[65, 111]:

- Direct tumor (primary or metastatic) extension and blockage of the lymphatic drainage
- Malignant lymphatic engorgement and impairment of drainage
- Tumor (primary or metastatic) implantation in or around the pericardium with inflammation and fluid production
- Radiation-induced pericarditis of the pericardium with fluid accumulation

Retrograde lymphatic dissemination is thought to be the main pathway of pericardial metastasis, creating fluid seepage through the visceral pericardium and into the pericardial space.[72] Neoplastic cardiac tamponade related to malignant pericardial effusion, whether resulting from a constricting tumor, lymphatic dissemination, or postirradiation pericarditis, is a medical emergency and must be recognized and treated promptly.

CLINICAL FEATURES

Patients with neoplastic cardiac tamponade manifest a wide variety of non-specific clinical signs and symptoms. These are directly related to the amount and rapidity of onset of fluid accumulation and the resultant disruption of normal hemodynamics.[72, 105] Small or slowly developing effusions may be asymptomatic. As fluid increases, the most common symptoms are dyspnea, tachycardia, retrosternal chest pain (usually relieved by sitting up and leaning forward) and a nonproductive cough.[49, 72, 105, 108] Other symptoms can include fatigue, weakness, dizziness, palpitations, and orthopnea.[72, 105] Tamponade due to radiation pericarditis may also exhibit fever and pleuritic chest pain.[49] The progression of pericardial effusion to cardiac tamponade can be categorized into three stages (Table 20-3).

Other classic signs of cardiac tamponade are pulsus paradoxus and jugular venous distention from increased

---

*References 52, 65, 71, 78, 91, 94, 101, 134, 140.

CLINICAL FEATURES

Neoplastic Cardiac Tamponade

Clinical Signs[13, 140]

Tachycardia
Low systolic blood pressure
Tachypnea with normal breath sounds
Vasoconstriction
Thready, diminished pulse pressure or pulsus paradoxus
Increased central venous pressure (CVP)
Arterial hypotension
Cardiomegaly
Precordial dullness to percussion
Distant weak heart sounds
Pericardial friction rub
Engorged neck veins
Ascites
Hepatomegaly
Hepatojugular reflux
Peripheral edema
Cool, clammy extremities or peripheral cyanosis
Oliguria secondary to decreased renal perfusion
Apprehension, anxiety
Clouded sensorium or impaired consciousness

Symptoms

Dyspnea or shortness of breath
Retrosternal chest pain
Diaphoresis
Anxiety
Cough
Hoarseness, hiccups
Nausea, vomiting
Abdominal pain

---

venous pressure (see Diagnosis section).[49] Beck's triad has also been considered a hallmark of cardiac tamponade.[78] These three signs include an elevated CVP, distant or muffled heart sounds (due to the encasement of the heart by fluid), and arterial hypotension. The point of maximal impulse may shift laterally from the fifth intercostal space due to cardiac enlargement.[134] As with the other symptoms described above, no one cardinal sign is consistently present and a sufficient clinical indicator to diagnose cardiac tamponade.

DIAGNOSIS

Identification of neoplastic cardiac tamponade depends greatly on a clinical diagnosis based on a detailed history and thorough physical examination. The presence or absence of any of the signs and symptoms depends on the stage of cardiac tamponade. A current or past history of cancer and cancer treatments should be noted.

TABLE 20-3
Stages of a Progressive Pericardial Effusion

Stage I		Stage II		Stage III	
Clinical Findings	Pathophysiologic Correlates	Clinical Findings	Pathophysiologic Correlates	Clinical Findings	Pathophysiologic Correlates
SUBJECTIVE					
Asymptomatic	Hemodynamic compensatory mechanisms effective	Dyspnea, shortness of breath with exertion, fatigued, lightheaded	Decreased cardiac output and arterial blood pressure	Dyspnea, short of breath at rest, orthopnea	Decreased cardiac output
		Fullness, heaviness felt in chest	Compression of heart	Cough, hoarseness, dysphagia	Impingement of effusion on bronchi, esophagus, and laryngeal nerves
		Abdominal discomfort	Increased right ventricular pressure causes venous stasis in liver and splanchnic veins	Retrosternal chest pain	Compression of heart
				Anxiety, apprehension	Progressive hypoxia
OBJECTIVE					
Mild tachycardia (100 beats/ min)	Maintaining cardiac output	Tachycardia (> 100 beats/min)	Maintaining cardiac output	Tachycardia (> 100 beats/min)	Decreased cardiac output
		Occasional pulsus paradoxus	Inspiratory fall in arterial systolic pressure	Pulsus paradoxus	Inspiratory fall in arterial systolic pressure
		Mild peripheral edema and abdominal distension	Venous/visceral congestion	Jugular venous distension, ascites	Venous congestion
				Hypotension	Decreased systolic pressure and increased diastolic pressure
				Impaired consciousness	Progressive hypoxia
				Pale, cyanotic appearance	Peripheral vasoconstriction
				Muffled heart sounds, friction rub	Distension of pericardial cavity

Data from Mangan CM: Malignant pericardial effusions: pathophysiology and clinical correlates. Oncol Nurs Forum, *19(8):1217, 1992.*

For a patient with no known history of cancer, other possible diagnoses must be ruled out, such as right ventricular heart failure, hydropericardium, rapid blood volume expansion, congestive heart failure (CHF), and pulmonary edema. Patients with cancer may also be at risk for cancer-related or treatment-related processes, such as radiation fibrosis, heart muscle metastases, coronary artery occlusion, or drug-induced CHF.

Two clinical findings that are classic features of cardiac tamponade are pulsus paradoxus and hepatojugular reflux. Testing for these two manifestations can be performed at the bedside.

Pulsus paradoxus (Fig. 20–3) is an abnormal finding of a weaker pulse during inspiration, resulting from a greater than normal (10 mm Hg) decrease in systolic blood pressure during the inspiratory phase of normal respiration. Cardiac tamponade constricts the myocardium, and during inspiration the diaphragm exerts additional pressure on the pericardial sac. The left ventricle receives less blood, and stroke volume is decreased,

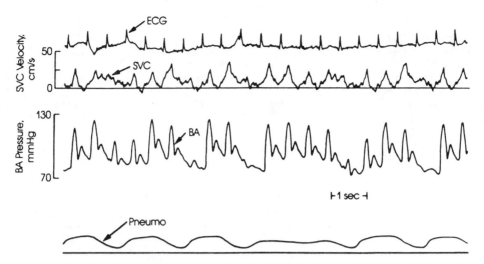

FIGURE 20-3 Simultaneous recording of electrocardiogram (*ECG*), blood flow velocity in the superior vena cava (*SVC*), brachial arterial (*BA*) pressure, and the pneumogram (*Pneumo*) in a patient with cardiac compression and paradoxic pulse (pulsus paradoxus). A downward deflection of the pneumogram denotes inspiration, when SVC blood velocity rises and arterial pressure falls (paradoxic pulse). Arterial pressure is maintained during prolonged expiratory pause. (From Braunwald E: Pericardial disease. In Braunwald E and others, editors: *Harrison's principles of internal medicine,* ed 11, New York, McGraw-Hill, 1987. Reproduced with permission of the McGraw-Hill Companies.)

which is seen as a decrease in systolic blood pressure during inspiration. The arterial pulse may also be absent during inspiration.[71, 91, 101]

Pulsus paradoxus can be determined in one of two ways (see Fig. 20-3). Patients with an indwelling arterial catheter can have their blood pressure monitored during inspiration. Patients without invasive equipment can have their blood pressure evaluated by routine sphygmomanometry. A blood pressure cuff is placed around the arm and inflated to greater than 20 mm Hg above systolic pressure. The cuff is deflated slowly until the first systolic sound (Korotkoff sound) is auscultated, and the reading is noted. This occurs during expiration, and the sounds disappear during inspiration. The cuff is further deflated until sounds can be heard throughout the respiratory cycle (expiration and inspiration). This reading is also noted. The difference in mm Hg between the two readings is the value of the paradox. If the difference is more than 10 mm Hg between the two readings, pulsus paradoxus is present.[91]

Inaccurate results may occur when assessing for pulsus paradoxus. Mechanical ventilation can artificially mimic paradoxic pulse. If hypotension is present, pulsus paradoxus may not be found by auscultation. In this situation the inspiratory decline in blood pressure can be noted by close examination of the carotid or femoral pulse. Pulsus paradoxus may disappear during extreme tamponade, when the systolic pressure may decrease below 50 mm Hg. Finally, other conditions may be manifested with pulsus paradoxus. These include obesity, severe obstructive respiratory disease, acute cor pulmo-

nale, right ventricular infarction, and hypovolemic shock.[91, 71]

Hepatojugular reflex is an elevation in jugular venous pressure by 1 cm or more. Testing for this abnormal condition is accomplished by placing the patient in the supine position with the head of the bed elevated to a level where jugular venous pulsations are visible. Pressure is then exerted continuously over the right upper quadrant of the abdomen for 30 to 60 seconds, and jugular pressure is observed. An increase in the pressure represents a positive reflex arising from venous congestion associated with a prolonged elevation of the CVP.[91]

Tests ordered by the physician will include a chest x-ray film, electrocardiogram (ECG), and an echocardiogram. A routine chest x-ray film is not a specific diagnostic tool, because it cannot differentiate among possible causes of an enlarged heart shadow. Fluid accumulation of 100 mL will not change the cardiac silhouette on a film, but this amount of fluid can produce tamponade if onset is rapid. More than 250 mL fluid within the pericardial sac will enlarge the cardiac silhouette. A "water bottle heart" is seen on the x-ray film as a result of the disappearance of the normal contours between the great vessels and the cardiac chambers.[47, 72, 91, 94, 108] More than half the patients with cardiac tamponade have cardiac enlargement, mediastinal widening, or hilar adenopathy.[94] Lung fields on chest x-ray films are usually normal because pulmonary bed capacity has not been impaired.

The ECG provides a limited amount of useful information. Elevated ST segments, nonspecific T-wave changes, decreased QRS voltage, and sinus tachycardia may be seen.[91, 101] *Electrical alternans,* which is the alternation of amplitude and direction of the P wave and QRS complexes on every other beat, is the most specific although infrequent abnormality in patients with neoplastic cardiac tamponade. This heart block, appearing at every other beat, is thought to result from variations in cardiac position at the time of electrical depolarization. In rare cases, atrial fibrillation has been present.[47, 134]

Two-dimensional echocardiography is the most specific and sensitive technique for establishing the presence of pericardial effusion.[65, 111] This noninvasive, reliable test should be done whenever possible if cardiac tamponade is suspected. The presence, location, and approximate quantity of fluid can be determined by the cardiac ultrasound. Normal findings on the echocardiogram show the posterior left ventricular wall in contact with the posterior pericardium and pleura and the anterior right ventricular wall in close approximation to the chest wall.[10, 22] In tamponade, echo-free spaces that separate the moving walls from the immobile pericardium indicate the presence of fluid.[47] The spaces appear first posteriorly and then anteriorly. The absence of pericardial fluid usually rules out cardiac tamponade. Findings consistent with tamponade include swinging of the heart, right atrial compression, right ventricular collapse with inspiration, and left ventricular diastolic compression.[128] Although an echocardiogram cannot determine the cause of the pericardial fluid, it is extremely helpful in the evaluation of an effusion, as well as in site selection for pericardiocentesis.

Recent advances in echocardiography have added new dimensions to diagnostic testing, including transesophageal echo (TEE), stress echo, and intra-arterial echo. TEE has been used in critically ill patients as a diagnostic tool in hypotensive crisis. Pericardial tamponade has been correctly diagnosed in these patients. The esophagus is the closest structure to the heart. Positioning the TEE scope with its transducer in that location permits high-resolution images of the cardiac structure. The TEE scope is a modification of the endoscope, and its tip can be moved antegrade, retrograde, and laterally to obtain tomographic views of cardiac structures using a biplane or omniplane transducer. This procedure can be done at the bedside, in the operating room, or as an outpatient procedure.[12, 76]

Other testing that may be performed during a diagnostic work-up for neoplastic cardiac tamponade includes cardiac catheterization, various types of scanning, and laboratory blood work. Catheterization of the heart can confirm a diagnosis of tamponade and determine the size and exact location of the pericardial fluid. In the presence of tamponade, intracardiac pressure is increased, and diastolic pressures are abnormal but almost equal in all chambers of the heart (10–25 mm Hg), as measured during catheterization.

Recent improvements in technology have assisted in the diagnosis of cardiac tamponade. Computed tomography (CT) and magnetic resonance imaging (MRI) have been useful in the assessment of a thickened pericardium and the diagnosis of constrictive pericarditis with effusion versus radiation fibrosis. The CT scan of the chest can be used to visualize and confirm lesions that are difficult to detect.[94] These specific differential diagnoses are crucial because treatment differs in each situation.

Laboratory blood tests ordered during the diagnostic work-up for neoplastic cardiac tamponade may include hematocrit, potassium (K^+), calcium (Ca^{++}), and arterial blood gases (ABGs). These tests are not conclusive for cardiac tamponade, but they can support a differential diagnosis. Pericardial fluid sent for cytologic examination has been diagnostic in about 80% of patients, but there are a significant percentage of false-negative reports. Certain malignancies make cytologic diagnosis more difficult. Late effusive constructive pericarditis in lymphoma patients treated with radiation and mantle radiation-related effusion in Hodgkin's disease may present with negative cytologic evaluations.[111]

Testing for neoplastic cardiac tamponade varies greatly in scope and depth, as determined by the patient's clinical appearance, including tolerance for various procedures. Time is of the essence. Clinically evident neoplastic effusions are usually large enough to be evaluated by echocardiography.[139]

TREATMENT MODALITIES

Neoplastic cardiac tamponade is a life-threatening situation that requires immediate medical intervention as soon as the diagnosis is confirmed. The immediate goal of treatment is the removal of pericardial fluid to relieve impending circulatory collapse. After symptomatic relief of tamponade, the longer-range goal is management of the underlying disease and prevention of reaccumulation.

Pharmacologic Therapy

Mild neoplastic cardiac tamponade may be treated with drug therapy using corticosteroids and diuretics. Supportive measures during cardiac tamponade are aimed at maintaining blood pressure and cardiac functioning.[71] Common prescriptions include prednisone (40–60 mg/d) with furosemide (Lasix: 40 mg/d) or Aldactazide (spironolactone and hydrochlorothiazide, 25–200 mg/d). Radiation pericarditis is often effectively treated with high-dose steroids or nonsteroidal anti-inflammatory drugs (NSAIDs). However, when these drugs are discontinued, the pericarditis often recurs. If an effusion recurs or tamponade becomes acute, more aggressive treatment is indicated.[58] Infusions of blood products and intravenous (IV) fluids will expand volume and increase ventricular filling pressures. Vasoactive drugs (e.g., nitroprusside, isoproterenol, dopamine) may be useful.[128] Isoproterenol can increase heart rate and contractility, and low-dose dopamine may improve contractility. However, α-adrenergic medications will likely increase afterload and adversely affect cardiac output. The use of diuretics at this point will decrease volume and further impair ventricular filling.[71]

Fluid Removal

Immediate withdrawal of fluid from the pericardium is done for both therapeutic and diagnostic reasons. Indications include a slow leak, diagnostic confirmation, rapid relief of acute tamponade, or symptomatic relief when deterioration of the patient's condition is evidenced by cyanosis, dyspnea, changes in mental status, or shock.[71] Another indicator for an aggressive approach to relieve tamponade is the "rule of 20," or a decrease in pulse pressure of more than 20 mm Hg, pulsus paradoxus greater than 20 mm Hg, and CVP greater than 20 cm water before intervention. Temporary measures such as administration of volume expanders, vasoactive drugs, and oxygen therapy are often continued prior to and during surgical intervention.

Pericardiocentesis is a percutaneous needle pericardiotomy with aspiration. It is considered an emergency treatment option for cardiac tamponade. It is ideally performed with guidance by cardiac catheterization or two-dimensional echocardiogram. Unguided approaches should only be done in extreme emergency situations.[78]

The technique most often used for pericardiocentesis is the introduction of a large-bore needle into the pericardial space through a small stab incision by a subxiphoid approach. The needle is angled toward the left shoulder. The safety of this procedure depends on attention to the underlying disease and the amount and exact location of the fluid present. An echocardiogram done before pericardiocentesis can be of great assistance in site selection. There is less risk with larger volumes of fluid accumulation because of the increased distance between the pericardium and the surface of the heart. To reduce the risks associated with pericardiocentesis, the procedure is performed with continuous monitoring of CVP and ECG using the V lead directly attached to the metal hub, or shaft, of the needle.[128]

The complications rate of pericardiocentesis range from 10% to -25% and include puncture of the right atrium or ventricle, laceration of the coronary artery, accidental introduction of air into the chambers of the

heart, dysrhythmias, vasovagal reaction with bradycardia, and infection.[94] Although the subxiphoid approach avoids the pleural space, pneumothorax or other injury to the lungs can occur.[47] Throughout the procedure, equipment must be available for emergency surgery and cardiopulmonary resuscitation.

Successful penetration of the pericardial sac during pericardiocentesis is often confirmed by a palpable "pop." This is accompanied by an increase in the QRS-complex voltage on the ECG, resulting when the pericardium is touched. If there is an acute elevation of the ST and PR segments, premature atrial contractions (PACs), or premature ventricular contractions (PVCs), there has been contact between the needle and the myocardium, and the needle should be withdrawn. After confirmation of needle location, fluid is aspirated slowly over 10 to 30 minutes. Although there is dramatic improvement in the patient with the removal of 25 to 50 mL fluid, as much of the fluid as possible should be removed.[10]

Pericardial effusion fluid can be classified as a transudate (low-protein fluid leaked from blood vessels due to non-malignant mechanical factors such as cirrhosis) or an exudate (protein-rich fluid leaked from blood vessels with increased permeability). Malignant effusions are typically exudates from the irritation of serous membrane caused by sloughed cancer cells or tumor implants.[94] Fluid return from the pericardium is normally clear and straw colored. In the presence of a malignancy, it is often bloody. This fluid should be immediately tested for hematocrit and fibrinogen to distinguish between a bloody effusion and penetration of the heart. Bloody effusions have lower levels of hematocrit and fibrinogen than circulating blood.

Although malignant effusions are usually serosanguineous, clear fluid does not rule out a neoplastic disease. Fluid studies include specific gravity, protein, cell count, stains, cultures, and cytologic analysis. Cytologic examination of pericardial fluid is essential to assist with diagnosis. With metastatic cancer the cytologic identification is 80% to 90% accurate, with essentially no false-positive results.[111] The results with lymphomas, sarcomas, and primary mesotheliomas of the pericardium are much less sensitive. Although a positive cytology may define the histopathology of the neoplastic disease, it may not identify the primary site.

Pericardiocentesis is usually effective in relieving signs and symptoms of neoplastic cardiac tamponade, but fluid generally reaccumulates in 24 to 48 hours. In some instances the elevated venous pressure associated with cardiac tamponade may remain despite pericardiocentesis. This situation may result from superior vena cava syndrome (SVCS), CHF, or effusive-constrictive pericardial disease caused by radiation therapy (400 Gy or more), tuberculosis, or extensive malignancy. This condition can be confirmed by measuring simultaneous pressures in the pericardial sac and the right atrium. Therefore, further local or systemic therapy is required after any pericardiocentesis. The choice of treatment depends on the etiology and extent of the underlying disease and the patient's overall condition.

Multiple taps and placement of an indwelling catheter have been helpful in controlling fluid accumulation; however, these measures are temporary. Long-term catheter placement is contraindicated because of the high risk of infection. A short-term indwelling pericardial catheter with multiple holes for drainage can be easily inserted with an introducer over a flexible guidewire. Once it is in place, a stopcock is placed at the distal end of the catheter. The catheter is drained each shift and may be irrigated daily with a small volume (5–10 mL) of saline or heparinized saline (100 U/mL). Irrigation may be useful if the tamponade is caused by a coagulopathy. In the presence of neoplastic fluid it is probably not necessary because fibrinogen levels of the fluid are low. Complications may include catheter infection, catheter blockage, dysrhythmias, and infective pericarditis.[134]

Percutaneous balloon pericardiotomy is done following the pericardiocentesis. A guide wire is inserted in to the pericardium. A balloon catheter is then placed, and the balloon inflated to create a window through which fluid may drain more freely into the pleural space. Adhesions may form between the parietal and visceral pericardium. This prevents reaccumulation of fluid.[13, 78, 94]

Subxiphoid pericardiotomy (pericardial window) is performed under local or general anesthesia. A small segment of the pericardium is resected and fluid withdrawn.[13]

Surgical pericardiectomy involves a thoracotomy or median sternotomy under general anesthesia. A large portion of the pericardium is resected, thus allowing continued drainage into the pleural space. This aggressive measure is reserved for patients for whom a significant long-term survival is anticipated.[13, 71, 111] It provides excellent visualization of the pericardium. The pathology can be observed and biopsied. Large rectangular pieces of the pericardium are removed from both the left and right sides. The phrenic nerves define the boundaries of the procedure and remain intact. For several days a chest tube is left in each side to assist with drainage.

Total pericardiectomy is the treatment of choice for patients with radiation-induced effusive-constrictive pericardial disease, or fibrosis, and also for those with pericardial mesothelioma. It is usually contraindicated in patients with extensive metastatic disease.

Surgical procedures are usually effective in controlling pericardial effusions by allowing the pericardial fluid to drain into the pleural cavity, which provides greater surface area for reabsorption. Pericardial effusions and tamponade rarely recur after these surgical procedures. However, in some instances the windows have closed. Several potential complications are associated with these procedures, including the usual risks associated with general anesthesia and the possibility of dysrhythmias, bleeding, infection, and hemothorax. Pulmonary edema can occur with postoperative diuresis in patients who were heavily hydrated before surgery. Figure 20–4 illustrates pericardiectomy through the median sternotomy approach.

Sclerotherapy may be done for patients with recurrent or persistent pericardial effusion. A short-term catheter is left in place following one of the procedures outlined above. The catheter may be left in place to facilitate continued short-term drainage until drainage has slowed enough to allow the successful instillation of a sclerosing agent. Instillation of such agents irritates the pericardial sac, causing the two linings to adhere to one another and obliterate the pericardial space where fluid accumulates.[134] Complications may include localized pain, fever, premature ventricular contractions, atrial arrhythmias, pericarditis, and myelosuppression.[134] Sclerosing is considered successful when there is no drainage for a 24-hour period.

Agents may include bleomycin, tetracycline, doxorubicin, 5-fluorouracil (5-FU), methotrexate, nitrogen mustard, radioactive phosphorus, talc, and thiotepa radioactive gold or phosphorus, quinacrine, thiotepa, doxycycline, cisplatin, and minocycline.[13, 49, 94, 111, 134]

Radiation Therapy

Radiation therapy may be the treatment of choice for neoplastic cardiac tamponade of gradual onset caused by a radiosensitive tumor of the lung or breast or a hematopoietic malignancy. Generally, external beam radiation therapy (200–400 Gy) is delivered to a port that includes the heart and pericardial structures and the lower mediastinum. Careful assessment of any previous radiation therapy is important to establish tissue tolerance. Cardiac tolerance is 350 to 400 Gy, beyond which a complication of pericarditis may develop.[101] External beam radiotherapy is most often used, but internal radiation therapy has been done using radioactive phosphorus, yttrium, or gold instilled into the pericardial space.[163]

Chemotherapy

Systemic chemotherapy may be given to responsive tumors such as lymphoma, breast cancer, or small (oat) cell carcinoma of the lung. This may be the initial treatment of a pericardial effusion when it is slow and the patient is asymptomatic. However, in acute neoplastic

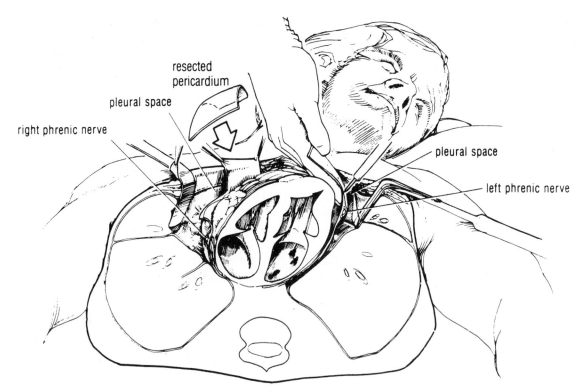

FIGURE 20–4 Pericardiectomy through a median sternotomy approach. (From Miller SE, Campbell DB: Malignant pericardial effusions. In Polomano RC, Miller SE, editors: *Understanding and managing oncologic emergencies,* Monograph, Columbus, OH, Adria Laboratories, 1987.)

cardiac tamponade, systemic chemotherapy is done when the patient is clinically stable after pericardiocentesis.

PROGNOSIS

Survival of the patient with neoplastic cardiac tamponade depends on the cause of the primary malignancy, the stage of cancer at the time of intervention, tumor responsiveness to radiation therapy or chemotherapy, hemodynamic significance of the tamponade, effectiveness of therapy, and general medical condition of the patient. The mortality rate for cardiac tamponade has been reported to be 25%. However, this rate increases to 65% if the tamponade goes unrecognized.[99] Although the overall prognosis of the patient may be poor, the spectacular response that is usually seen with the removal of pericardial fluid warrants aggressive action.

Nursing management of the patient with cardiac tamponade is outlined in the accompanying box.

Nursing Management

CARDIAC TAMPONADE

Nursing interventions for the patient with neoplastic cardiac tamponade are multifaceted and highly variable, depending on the acuteness of the patient's condition. Onset of tamponade may be impending and insidious or rapid and life-threatening. Knowledge of the patient's current and past history, coupled with astute physical assessment skills, is necessary.

Patients may be on a medical oncology unit or in the critical care area. Close monitoring of vital signs is of paramount importance. Nursing care is directed at maintaining optimal cardiopulmonary function and preventing circulatory collapse through immediate identifications and treatment of neoplastic cardiac tamponade.

Nursing Diagnoses

- *Decreased cardiac output, related to diastolic filling of the ventricles from compression of the heart*
- *Altered tissue perfusion, peripheral, related to decreased cardiac output*

Outcome Goal

Patient will be able to:

- Maintain optimal cardiac output, as evidenced by relief of chest pain, vital signs within patient's normal limits, cardiac rhythm without dysrhythmias, central venous pressure (CVP) and pulmonary capillary wedge pressure (PCWP) within patient's normal limits, adequate intake and output, and laboratory values and diagnostic tests approaching normal levels.

Interventions

- Assess hemodynamic and cardiovascular status:
  Monitor blood pressure, pulse, CVP, and cardiac output.
  Observe for increased jugular venous pressure.
  Observe cardiac rhythm continuously (note abnormalities associated with cardiac tamponade: ST segment elevation, T-wave inversion, and electrical alterations).
  Monitor heart sounds.
  Assess extremities for color, temperature, and pulses.
- Assess respiratory status:
  Observe breathing patterns (note abnormalities associated with cardiac tamponade: pulsus paradoxus, respiratory alkalosis, Kussmaul's sign, and hypoxemia).
  Auscultate lungs for breath sounds.
- Observe skin temperature, color, and turgor.
- Monitor intake and output.
- Assess neurologic status:
  Determine orientation to person and place.
  Assess responses to verbal and tactile stimuli.
  Report any changes in level of consciousness.
- Monitor laboratory values and test results:
  Electrolytes, with attention to Ca^{++} and K^+ because of the risk of cardiac dysrhythmias
  ECG for changes
  Echocardiogram
  Chest x-ray film
- Reposition patient to enhance circulation. This must be done slowly to allow compensation for decreased cardiac output.
- Perform measures to reduce the workload of the heart:
  Assist with all activities.
  Schedule rest periods.
  Use comfort measures (analgesics, repositioning, relaxation techniques, antianxiety medications).

- Administer vasoactive drugs as ordered.
- Be prepared for cardiac arrest and emergency resuscitation.

Nursing Diagnosis

- *Impaired gas exchange, related to decreased circulation and pulmonary congestion*

Outcome Goal

Patient will be able to:

- Achieve/maintain adequate pulmonary function, as evidenced by vital signs within patient's normal limits, breath sounds and respiratory stable/improved, and activity tolerance within patient's normal limits.

Interventions

- Monitor respiratory status:
  Observe for signs and symptoms of respiratory difficulty (dyspnea, tachypnea, Kussmaul's sign, shortness of breath, air hunger).
  Auscultate chest for breath sounds.
  Monitor laboratory values (arterial blood gases, electrolytes, chest x-ray film).
- Assist with breathing and pulmonary toilet:
  Position for comfort and enhanced chest expansion
  Deep breathing and coughing every 2 hours
  Frequent mouth care
  Suctioning if needed
- Administer oxygen therapy and mechanical ventilation as prescribed.

Nursing Diagnosis

- *Risk for injury, related to invasive procedures/surgery*

Outcome Goal

Patient will be able to:

- Experience minimal side effects related to invasive procedure, as evidenced by adequate skin integrity, absence of or minimal bleeding, adequate respiratory function, and absence of infection.

Interventions

- Assess patient for complications: bleeding, infection, atelectasis, pneumothorax, and pleural effusion.
- Obtain vital signs every 15 minutes for the first hour after procedure/surgery and continue frequently as indicated.

- Monitor respiratory status closely:
  Observe respirations for rate, rhythm, and depth. Note any difficulties.
  Auscultate chest for breath sounds and expansion.
- Observe monitoring equipment frequently for changes.

- Assess all catheters for patency and drainage, and observe site for signs of infection.
- Assess patient with care but encourage as much independence as possible.

Data from references 65, 68, 71, 78, 99, 101, and 134.

Increased Intracranial Pressure

DEFINITION

Increased intracranial pressure (IICP) is also referred to as intracranial hypertension.[4] IICP results when the volume of any of the three components within the skull and meninges is increased. These components include the brain, cerebrospinal fluid (CSF), and cerebral blood volume.[14] IICP, if not successfully treated, can lead to brain herniation and death.

ETIOLOGY AND RISK FACTORS

The most common oncologic etiology for IICP is brain metastases. Twenty to 40% of cancer patients develop brain metastases.[136] Metastatic brain tumors are four to five times more common than primary lesions.[14] Lung and breast cancers are the solid tumors that most frequently metastasize to the brain in adults.[136] Colon, breast, and renal cell carcinomas often spread to the brain as single lesions. Lung cancer and melanoma often produce multiple intracranial metastases.[136] The most common site for brain metastases is the cortico-medullary junction, probably due to the amount of blood flow.[108] Brain tumors cause IICP by obstruction of CSF or cerebral blood flow, increasing the volume of brain tissue and edema.[14]

Other causes of IICP that may occur in oncology patients are hematomas, hemorrhage, cerebral irritation, or infection with exudate. Patients with thrombocytopenia or platelet dysfunction are at risk for cerebral bleeding. Patients receiving radiation therapy to the brain may experience cerebral irritation. Patients with lymphoma, leukemia, central nervous system (CNS) tumors, or an Ommaya reservoir are at some risk for CNS infection. Syndrome of inappropriate diuretic hormone (SIADH) and CNS infections can cause cellular or cytotoxic edema resulting in IICP. Patients with head and neck cancer may experience IICP from compression of the internal jugular veins. Patients with severe hyponatremia from SIADH may develop IICP from increased intracellular fluid in brain cells due to increased extracellular hypoosmolality.[74]

PATHOPHYSIOLOGY

The skull and meninges form a rigid covering that contains the brain tissue (80%), blood (10%), and CSF (10%). Normal intracranial pressure (ICP) is 4 to 15 mm Hg or 80 to 10 cm of water. Brain metastases cause vasogenic cerebral edema by disrupting the blood–brain barrier. This allows fluid and protein to leak out of the capillaries into the extracellular space primarily in the white matter of the brain.[4]

The Monro-Kellie hypothesis states that the cranial contents are maintained in a dynamic equilibrium. An increase in the volume of any one component must cause a decrease in volume of the other two.[4, 14] This volume decrease is called *compensation*. Compensatory mechanisms include movement of the CSF from around the brain tissue to the spinal cord, decreased CSF production by the choroid plexus, increased CSF absorption by arachnoid villi, or shunting of venous blood to other sites.[14] The compensatory mechanisms will eventually be depleted and very small increases in the volume of the cranial contents will cause significant IICP. Autoregulation is the ability to maintain a constant rate of cerebral blood flow regardless of variations in systemic arterial pressure and venous drainage.[4, 14] This occurs through constriction or dilation of cerebral blood vessels. Autoregulation failure occurs with the exhaustion of the compensatory mechanisms, as well as severe hypotension or hypertension. Slight increases in systemic blood pressure will then cause IICP. Diminished cerebral blood flow leads to tissue hypoxia and reduced removal of carbon dioxide and lactic acid. Build-up of these metabolic by-products causes vasodilation leading to edema and exacerbating the IICP.[14]

Because cerebral veins have no valve, anything that restricts cerebral venous outflow can cause an increased cerebral volume. Actions that increase intrathoracic or intra-abdominal pressures can restrict outflow. Such actions include the Vasalva maneuver, bending over, coughing, sneezing, extreme neck flexion or extension, hip flexion, lying on the abdomen, and positive end-expiratory pressure (PEEP) treatments.[14]

When compensatory mechanisms and autoregulation fail, IICP can displace brain tissue from one cranial compartment to another. This herniation moves brain tissue from the area of high pressure to an area of lower pressure, compressing other neural tissue, blood vessels, CSF pathways, and increasing edema. Depending on the location and severity of the herniation, the patient can suffer loss of consciousness, and respiratory and cardiac arrest.[14]

CLINICAL FEATURES

General symptoms for IICP include headache, nausea, vomiting, change in level of consciousness, impaired cognitive function, changes in personality, hemiparesis, language difficulty, dysphagia, ataxia, and seizures.[14, 108] Seizures are common with metastases from melanoma due to their hemorrhagic nature.[14] They are the presenting symptom in 15% to 20% of patients, probably because melanoma is the systemic cancer with the highest incidence of intracranial metastases.[23] Headaches are commonly most severe on waking. This may be due to carbon dioxide retention during sleep that causes cerebral vessel dilatation and enhances cerebral edema.[108] Visual findings of IICP include blurring, changes in pupil size and light accommodation, visual field deficits, and papilledema (a late sign).[14] Advanced IICP can cause hemiparesis, hemiplegia, decreased reflexes, and decorticate and decerebrate posturing.[14] Cushing's triad, another late sign of IICP, is a combination of hypertension, bradycardia, and irregular or slow respirations.[14] Posturing and Cushing's triad are generally associated with the terminal phase of herniation.[14]

DIAGNOSIS

Patients with cancer who develop neurologic changes should be evaluated immediately for brain metastases.[23] Both CT scanning with contrast and gadolinium contrast-enhanced MRI are used to evaluate brain metastases.[136] MRI has been found to be the most sensitive tool and is the preferred diagnostic method.[14] Lumbar puncture should be avoided with IICP due to the risk of exacerbation and herniation.[106]

TREATMENT MODALITIES

Rapid reduction of cerebral edema and decompression of the ICP is the immediate treatment goal.

Pharmacologic Management

Corticosteroids can rapidly decrease peritumoral edema. Improvement in symptoms may be seen within 24 hours. Steroids are continued for at least 3 to 7 days until definitive treatment can be initiated and effective or as long as needed to manage the symptoms of IICP.[116, 136] Patients at risk for herniation are started on high doses, such as 100 mg dexamethasone IV. Maintenance doses may be as high as 30 mg four times a day.[23] Corticosteroids are thought to decrease capillary permeability and promote extracellular fluid resorption.[23]

Osmotic diuretics (such as mannitol) may also be needed to decrease cerebral edema by increasing plasma osmolarity and drawing extracellular fluid back into the plasma where it can be excreted by the kidneys.[4] A typical starting dose of mannitol is 1 mg/kg IV followed by 0.25 to 0.50 g/kg every 4 to 6 hours. *Loop diuretics* (such as furosemide) are used to decrease CSF production and enhance the excretion of sodium and water from the brain. Side effects of diuretics may include arrhythmias, and fluid and electrolyte imbalances. Diuretics may be combined with fluid restrictions.[18] Electrolytes and hemodynamics must be closely monitored.

Anticonvulsants (such as phenytoin, carbamazepine, phenobarbital, and valproic acid) are given to manage seizures when appropriate.[23]

Surgery

Emergent surgical intervention is needed for the patient with life-threatening IICP. When IICP is due to cerebral edema obstructing the flow of CSF, insertion of a ventriculoperitoneal shunt or temporary ventriculostomy can provide immediate drainage of CSF and relief of IICP while interventions are initiated to treat the underlying cause of the edema.[4, 14] Partial or complete resection of tumor is necessary for rapidly enlarging brain lesions. This is most quickly accomplished by a craniotomy. Remaining tumor can then be treated with radiation therapy or chemotherapy depending on the histology and tumor responsiveness. Resection provides the benefit of tissue diagnosis in addition to reducing tumor volume. Risks of surgery include post-operative edema, further neurologic deficit, bleeding, and infection.[14]

Radiation and Chemotherapy

Radiation and chemotherapy are primarily used to treat brain metastases and primary tumors that can cause IICP. They are most effective for tumor histologies that are sensitive to radiation and chemotherapy (lymphoma, small-cell lung carcinoma [SCLC], choriocarcinoma).[136] Acute symptoms of IICP must be addressed immediately with medications to decrease edema and surgical intervention. Once the acute symptoms are controlled, radiation or chemotherapy can be used to address the underlying cause of IICP (see Chapter 6).

PROGNOSIS

Prognosis for the patient with IICP initially depends on the severity and rapidity of the symptoms as well as the early recognition and prompt initiation of appropriate treatment. Ultimate survival depends on the type and stage of cancer and response to overall treatment of the underlying disease. Patients with untreated brain metastases survive an average of 1 month.[108]

Nursing management of the patient with IICP is outlined in the accompanying box.

Nursing Management

INCREASED INTRACRANIAL PRESSURE[61]

As with most oncologic emergencies, the prompt recognition of the signs of increasing intracranial pressure (IICP) is critical to initiating the appropriate interventions before the damage is irreparable.

Nursing Diagnoses

- Altered tissue perfusion, cerebral related to increased ICP from tumor expansion, edema, obstruction of CSF flow, or bleeding.
- Altered thought processes related to neurologic changes secondary to IICP

Outcome Goals

Patient will be able to:

- Exhibit stable neurologic and vital signs within 24 hours of diagnosis.
- Maintain normal fluid and electrolyte balance.

Interventions

- Assess baseline neurologic status and reassess every 1 hour and as needed.
- Position patient with head of bed elevated 30 to 45 degrees and prevent extreme neck flexion, extension, or rotation.
- Assess airway and maintain patency.
- Monitor intake and output.
- Monitor serum electrolytes, osmolality and creatinine.
- Administer steroids, osmotic agents, and diuretics as prescribed.
- Avoid, if possible, activities that aggravate IICP, such as endotracheal suctioning.

- Monitor temperature and maintain afebrile state with antipyretics as needed.
- Provide as calm and quiet an environment as possible.
- Prepare patient/family for procedures or surgical intervention.
- Provide patient/family with education about radiation or chemotherapy as needed.
- Be prepared to transfer patient to ICU if necessary for mechanical respiration and hemodynamic monitoring.

Nursing Diagnosis

- Risk for injury secondary to altered mental status and/or seizure activity

Outcome Goal

Patient will be able to:

- Remain free from injury secondary to confusion or seizure activity.

Interventions

- Monitor for mental status changes and seizure activity.
- Administer steroids and anticonvulsants as prescribed.
- Monitor blood levels of anticonvulsants.
- Frequently reorient patient to time and place.
- Encourage family members to remain at bedside if patient is confused.
- Pad side rails and remove any hard items that could injure patient in the event of tonic/clonic manifestations.
- Assess respiratory status and maintain patent airway.

Spinal Cord Compression

DEFINITION

A neoplasm in the epidural space can encroach on the spinal cord or cauda equina and result in spinal cord compression (SCC).[82] SCC is a medical emergency requiring early detection and prompt treatment. Although it is rarely fatal, it can result in permanent neurologic deficits such as paralysis and loss of bowel and bladder control.

ETIOLOGY AND RISK FACTORS

Spinal cord compression is the second most common neurologic complication of cancer following brain metastases.[24, 50] It occurs in 5% to 10% of patients with cancer.[14, 50, 77, 108] Primary tumors of the spinal cord account for a very small percentage of SCC. Metastatic disease is the most common cause. Patients with cancer that metastasizes to the bone and those with existing bony disease are at the greatest risk for SCC. Lung, breast, and prostate cancers are associated with about 50% to 60% of SCC cases.[14, 24, 50, 106, 136] Other cancers commonly associated with SCC include multiple myeloma, lymphoma, melanoma, renal cancer, and sarcoma.[28, 77, 106, 108, 136]

PATHOPHYSIOLOGY

The adult human vertebral column, or backbone, is a versatile arrangement of 33 vertebrae joined in series and supported by ligaments. The 33 vertebrae include 7 cervical, 12 thoracic, 5 lumbar, 5 sacral, and 5 coccygeal. The sacral and coccygeal vertebrae are fused into the sacrum and coccyx, respectively.[14] The vertebrae support the body by strength and rigidity while also providing flexibility and mobility. In addition, the column surrounds and protects the spinal cord, which is enlarged in the cervical and lumbar areas. The cord itself is covered by three protective meninges (also called leptomeninges) or membranes[14] (Figs. 20–5 and 20–6).

These *meninges* originate as coverings for the brain and extend downward over the spinal cord. The outermost membrane is the *dura mater* (hard mother), which is made up of dense fibrous connective tissue. The space between the walls of the vertebral column and the outer surface of the dura mater is referred to as the *epidural,* or *extradural, space.* Within that space can be found blood vessels and connective and adipose tissue. No lymph nodes are located within this space. The *subdural space* follows next, between the inner surface of the dura mater and the underlying arachnoid membrane. Below the arachnoid membrane is the *subarachnoid space.* It lies between the arachnoid membrane and the

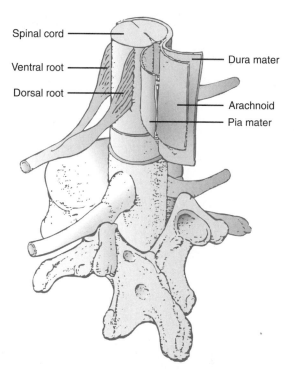

FIGURE 20–5 The spinal meninges. (From Hickey JV: *The clinical practice of neurological and neurosurgical nursing,* ed 3, Philadelphia, Lippincott, 1992.)

innermost membrane, the *pia mater* ("gentle mother"), which is closely attached to the spinal cord. The subarachnoid space contains liquid referred to as spinal fluid. However, it is more accurately called *cerebrospinal fluid* (CSF), because the subarachnoid space begins in the brain and follows down the cord.[39]

Metastatic disease to the vertebrae typically occurs in the anterior extradural space and causes SCC from compression to the cord as opposed to tissue invasion.[14, 136] Tumor involvement of the spinal cord may be classified according to the cell of origin (primary spinal cord tumors versus metastatic disease) and the site of anatomic presentation related to the spinal dura (Table 20–4).[90] Primary tumors arising in the spinal cord are intramedullary and directly invade and destroy the cord.[14] Primary tumors of the meninges or nerve roots are extramedullary. Most oncologic SCC is caused by metastatic disease. Twenty-five percent spreads to the extradural space and can displace the spinal cord, irritate spinal nerve roots, or obstruct the flow of CSF[14]; 75% causes vertebral destruction and collapse that forces bony fragments into the extradural space[50] (Fig. 20–7).

The epidural space may be invaded by tumor in a variety of ways. Hematogenous spread of malignant cells, through Batson's parapsinal venous plexus, to the vertebral body is the most frequent route.[50] It is estimated to lead to 85% of oncologic SCC.[82] Tumor growth from the marrow invades the bone matrix and destroys

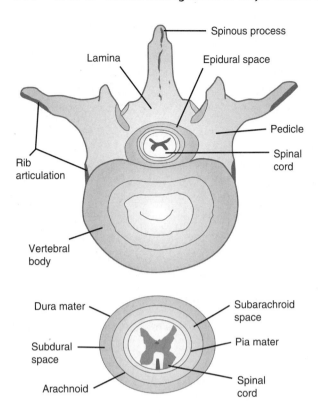

FIGURE 20–6 Cross section of vertebra and spinal cord.

the vertebral body. Vertebral body destruction allows tumor to directly invade the extradural space and compress the cord. Vertebral body destruction may also allow vertebral body collapse, forcing bony fragments into the extradural space and mechanically compressing the cord. Paraspinal tumors grow through the intervertebral foramen to cause cord compression.[50] Non-

T A B L E   2 0 – 4
Anatomic Presentation of Spinal Cord Tumors

EXTRADURAL	INTRADURAL
Metastatic solid tumors (breast, lung, prostate)	*Extramedullary*
	Schwannoma
Sarcoma	Meningioma
Lymphoma	*Intramedullary*
Myeloma	Ependymoma
Chordoma	Astrocytoma
	Oligodendroglioma
	Hemangioblastoma
	Mixed glioma

Modified from Belford K: Central nervous system cancers. In Groenwald SL, Frogge MH, Goodman M, Yarbro CH, editors: Cancer nursing: principles and practice, ed 4, Boston, Jones & Bartlett, 1997:980; and data from Maher De Leon ME, Schnell S, Rozental JM: Tumors of the spine and spinal cord. Semin Oncol Nurs 14:43, 1998.

Hodgkin's lymphomas cause SCC in this way in about 10% of cases.[24]

Ascending and descending nerve fiber tracts are located in the white matter of the spinal cord (outer portion). Damage to ascending tracts causes pain or sensory deficits or both. Descending tract damage causes motor deficits, bowel and bladder dysfunction, and impaired sexual function.[130] Neurologic deficits are caused by three different processes:

- Direct compression of the spinal cord or cauda equina by the tumor itself
- Interruption of the vascular supply to neural structure by the tumor
- Compression caused by vertebral collapse resulting from a pathologic fracture or dislocation. The bone may extrude onto the cord and produce pressure that compresses the nerve roots.

The severity of the compression can increase in the presence of edema from obstruction of the venous plexus, which supplies the spinal cord.

CLINICAL FEATURES

The clinical presentation of SCC is similar in all patients, regardless of the origin of the tumor. Symptomatology is directly related to the location of the compression.

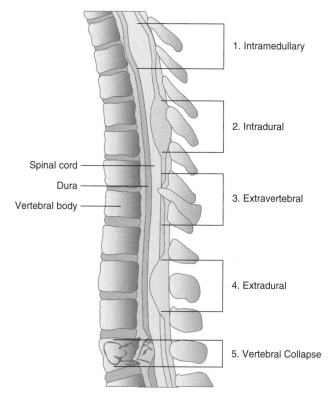

1. Intramedullary

2. Intradural

Spinal cord

Dura

Vertebral body

3. Extravertebral

4. Extradural

5. Vertebral Collapse

FIGURE 20 – 7 Malignant invasion of the spinal cord.

CLINICAL FEATURES

Spinal Cord Compression

Clinical Signs[28, 50]

Muscle weakness (unsteadiness, footdrop, paralysis)

Sensory impairment (paralysis, loss of bowel and bladder control, paraplegia)

Symptoms

Pain

Tingling and/or numbness in extremities

Diminished pain and temperature sensation

Sexual dysfunction

The distribution of spinal metastases with SCC correlates with the number of vertebrae and size of the epidural space in each segment, with 10% in the cervical area, 70% in the thoracic, and 20% in the lumbosacral.[37, 66, 106, 108, 158]

The cardinal signs and associated symptoms of SCC are well documented and usually follow an established pattern of appearance, which includes pain, motor weakness, sensory loss, and finally autonomic dysfunction (see Clinical Features box).

Back pain is the presenting complaint in 97% of patients.* It is related to SCC and may occur weeks or months before neurologic deficits occur. However, fast-growing tumors can rapidly progress to irreversible paraplegia in a matter of hours to days after neurologic deficit appears.[24] The pain is either localized or radicular. Localized pain, along the spinal axis, is classically the initial symptom and results from stretching of the periosteum of the afflicted bone, vertebral collapse, invasion of spinal tracts, tension on spinal nerve roots, or tumor attachment to the proximal dura.[130, 136] Pain that is radicular in nature is caused by nerve root compression from a pathologic fracture and compression of the verte-

brae. The distribution of radicular pain depends on the level of spinal involvement. It may move along the dermatomal distribution and is aggravated by movement such as coughing, sneezing, straining as with the Valsalva maneuver, or straight leg raising.[106, 136] Thoracic radicular pain, which is most common, radiates in a band around the chest or abdomen.[130]

The pain associated with SCC is usually intense, persistent, and progressive, although thoracic compression is often felt as a constriction.[152, 158] Any pain of SCC may be accompanied by vertebral tenderness on percussion at or near the level of compression. It is often unilateral when the compression is in the cervical or lumbosacral area and usually bilateral in the thoracic region. The pain is usually worse at night because the spine lengthens when recumbent and the abdominal contents place pressure against the spine and cord.[77] A key to early detection is a detailed assessment for any changes in pain. Patients may have been suffering with pain from bony metastasis for a time. With the onset of SCC, the pain often changes its location and intensity.

Weakness is only a presenting complaint in 2% of cases. However, 75% to 86% of patients have subtle evidence of motor defect on initial clinical examination.[77] Initially, motor symptoms are asymptomatic. The time frame for motor weakness to develop following the onset of is variable, from hours to days, weeks, or months.[52, 158] The location of weakness is usually restricted to the lower extremities but may vary based on the location of the tumor.[77] Common patient complaints include stiffness and heaviness of the affected extremity. It may manifest itself as an unsteady gait or ataxia with a favoring or dragging of the affected extremity or extremities. Patients experience difficulty walking or climbing stairs.[106] Symptoms often associated with

*References 37, 39, 40, 56, 66, 77, 106

weakness include hyperreflexia, spasticity, and a positive Babinski sign.[14]

Sensory loss usually follows motor weakness but precedes actual motor loss. These sensory losses progress in the same pattern as motor symptoms. Symptoms of sensory loss include numbness, tingling, paresthesia, and feelings of coldness in the affected area. Loss of sensation to light touch first, then loss of pain, followed by loss of thermal sensation, occur in 80% of patients. Concurrent loss of proprioception, deep pressure, vibratory sense, and position sense indicates a severe compression. After the release of SCC, neurologic functions return in the reverse order of how the dysfunctions appeared. If the motor weakness and sensory loss progress rapidly to motor loss, the prognosis is poor.

Autonomic dysfunction appears if the compression progresses. Urinary disturbances include hesitancy and retention, followed by overflow and incontinence. Early changes may be as subtle as an increased post-voiding residual volume. Lack of urge to defecate and inability to bear down are initial bowel disturbances, which may lead to constipation, obstipation, and finally incontinence. Loss of sphincter control is a later sign and is associated with a poorer prognosis. Sexual dysfunction may be manifested as impotence.[77, 118, 158]

DIAGNOSIS

When SCC is suspected in any patient, a diagnosis should be confirmed immediately because of the potential for rapid progression and possible permanent neurologic dysfunction. A good history and physical examination should be accompanied by thorough neurologic testing. Physical findings include percussion tenderness at the level of compression. If radicular pain is present, it will increase with spinal movement on straight leg raises. Motor and sensory involvement is manifested by hyperactive reflexes, positive Babinski signs, variable spastic weakness, and bilateral sensory loss below the level of the compression. Absence of sweating below the level of involvement may be noted. Bowel and bladder dysfunction may also be detected. Corresponding subjective data should be elicited because differences could be significant.

Testing for a patient with suspected SCC begins with plain x-ray films. Plain films are positive in 85% of patients with SCC.[52, 118, 108, 130, 136] Radiographic findings reveal osteolytic lesions with loss of a pedicle, vertebral body destruction, or collapse of vertebral body. Intervertebral disks are not affected by neoplastic disease because they have an insufficient blood supply. A problem with plain x-ray films is that if the tumor grows paraspinal, with invasion of the epidural space through the foramina, the bone film may be normal. This is common with lung tumors and lymphoma. Another concern is that a tumor can be present for 6 months without x-ray changes. A bone scan is often more sensitive and may be positive 6 months before plain films.[130] Osteoblastic lesions show new bone formation that may extend into the epidural space.[158]

The diagnostic method of choice to evaluate SCC is the MRI scan.[90] It can identify compression, soft-tissue lesions, cord lesions, as well as bone destruction. MRI also distinguishes between extradural, intradural, and extramedullary lesions.[82] The major benefits of MRI are as follows:

- It is sensitive to neurologic tissue.
- It is noninvasive.
- It is helpful in patients with severe contrast allergies.
- It images the entire spine, providing various views.
- It is helpful in patients with brain metastasis.
- It may show multiple epidural deposits of tumor that may not be obvious on initial myelogram.
- It avoids the risk of neurologic deterioration after lumbar puncture.
- New open MRI machines have provided an option for people with claustrophobia and those who are too large to fit into a closed machine.

The disadvantages of MRI are:

- The need for the patient to lie still in one position, which may be difficult for someone with central back pain.
- Claustrophobia has been a common problem.

Myelography is reserved for cases where MRI does not explain neurologic deficits. Myelography is an invasive examination. It requires a needle puncture to withdraw CSF and instill contrast media into the subarachnoid space. Two lumbar punctures may be needed to visualize upper and lower margins of the block. CSF sampling can be done to rule out meningeal carcinomatosis or when unable to do MRI due to lack of access, severe scoliosis, presence of hardware such as a pacemaker, or the patient's inability to tolerate lying in one position for the procedure.[24, 82, 136] CSF protein elevations greater than 100 mg/mL have been noted in most patients with SCC. Glucose is normal, cell count is unremarkable, and cytology is usually negative. A 16% to 24% risk of neurologic deterioration has been reported if the lumbar puncture is done below the tumor site.[108] There is risk of neurologic deterioration with a complete subarachnoid block.[37, 50] Other risks include infection and bleeding.

Computed tomography may identify early destructive lesions not seen on plain films, differentiate tumor from osteoporosis, and define paraspinal tumors that may extend epidurally.[158] CT is superior to MRI in evaluation of vertebral stability and bone destruction prior to a surgical intervention.[50]

TREATMENT MODALITIES

The choice of treatment for patients with SCC depends on the primary tumor, the rapidity of onset of the compression, and the level, severity, and duration of the blockage. The most frequent treatment modalities for SCC are steroids, radiation therapy, and surgery. The goals of therapy are to preserve or restore neurologic function, maintain spinal stability, control tumor growth, and relieve pain.[136] Symptom relief from metastatic disease facilitates the improvement of quality of life.

Steroids

The use of corticosteroids is indicated for cord and nerve root compression; however, there is controversy over the appropriate dose and schedule.[24, 28, 50, 58, 63] Rapidly progressive symptoms are typically treated with high-dose steroids, such as dexamethasone, 100 mg IV bolus. This is followed by 16 to 24 mg orally four times a day until definitive treatment is begun and symptoms resolve.[106] Steroid administration is frequently begun prior to the completion of the diagnostic work-up to rapidly decrease pain and swelling. A slower progression of symptoms may be managed with an initial IV bolus of 10 mg, followed by 4 mg orally every 6 hours. Most patients will receive pain relief within a few hours. Doses are carefully tapered by reducing the dose by one third every 3 to 4 days after treatment is initiated.[24] Patients are closely observed for neurologic deficits during the taper so that higher doses may be resumed if needed. Too rapid of withdrawal can precipitate symptoms of acute adrenal insufficiency.[14] Patients are also observed for the short-term side effects and toxicities associated with steroid use, such as fluid retention, blood glucose alterations, and mood alterations.[14] Patients who require long-term steroids for symptom control are at risk for GI bleeding, opportunistic infections, and osteoporosis.[14]

Radiation Therapy

Radiation is the treatment of choice for SCC in most cases and is typically started within 24 hours of diagnosis.[136] Radiation portals are planned to extend two vertebral bodies above and below the site of cord compression. Adjacent sites of bony disease and paravertebral masses are also included in the treatment field.[50] Standard doses range from 200 to 300 cGy/fraction to a total dose of 3000 to 4000 cGy over 2 to 4 weeks. Controversy exists over the benefits of using higher treatment fractions for the first 3 days of therapy. Smaller fractions may be used for patients with the best long-term prognosis to decrease damage to the spinal cord.[24] Radiation therapy has been shown to reduce pain, compression, and tumor size in 70% to 80% of patients.[24, 50, 136] It improves motor function and reverses paralysis in 11% to 16% of cases and can prevent local recurrence.[50]

Long-term effects to the spinal cord may include myelopathy. This may occur anywhere from 3 to 28 months after radiation therapy. Symptoms range from reversible paresthesias to complete functional loss below the radiation field.[14]

Surgery

Surgery has been replaced by radiation therapy in all but the following[14]:

- Spinal instability or bony collapse into spinal canal
- Rapid neurologic deterioration
- The cause for SCC is questionable, or there is no known primary malignancy.
- Prior maximum-tolerance radiation at the site of compression precludes further irradiation.
- Neurologic deterioration occurs during radiation therapy.
- Radioresistant tumor

Surgical stabilization of the spinal column requires intact bone above and below the site of compression.[14] Most tumors present in the vertebral body and invade the epidural space anteriorly. A posterior decompression laminectomy relieves compression of the spinal cord by removing the spinous processes and the lamina one level above and below the compression. It allows relaxation of the cord, but cannot remove tumor that is anterior to the cord. Posterior laminectomy may cause spinal instability and is reserved for posterior tumors.[50]

Anterior decompression with spinal stabilization is performed for tumors in the vertebral body that produce anterior compression. It is now the surgical procedure of choice. Anterior decompression allows total removal of the involved vertebral body. A thoracotomy or retroperitoneal approach is used. The vertebral body is replaced with methylmethacrylate and supplemented with metal prostheses that are attached to the adjacent vertebrae.[50]

Surgical interventions for SCC are not appropriate for multiple levels of disease, complete paralysis, or patients who are poor risks for anesthesia.[50]

Chemotherapy

Chemotherapy has a role as adjuvant therapy in the treatment of SCC. In most instances, it is combined with radiation therapy to treat SCC resulting from lymphoma.[39, 118] Chemotherapy may be given concomitantly or after radiation therapy as systemic treatment for the primary underlying malignancy. Chemosensitive tumors include lymphoma, myeloma, breast, prostate, and germ cell tumors.[50]

Prevention

Recent research has demonstrated a role for certain biphosphonates, particularly pamidronate, in decreasing the skeletal complications of bony metastases. Patients with advanced multiple myeloma treated monthly with infusions of 90 mg pamidronate exhibited a decreased incidence in bone pain, pathologic fractures requiring surgery and radiation therapy, and cord compression.[15] Use of pamidronate is expanding to patients with other cancers that spread to the bone, such as breast and prostate cancers.

PROGNOSIS

The degree of neurologic dysfunction at the time of diagnosis is the greatest predictor of outcome. Eighty percent of patients with little or no ambulatory dysfunc-tion will remain ambulatory. Twenty to 60% of patients with partial paralysis will regain function.[50] Ten to 16% of patients with paraplegia improve.[108] Patients with favorable histology (lymphoma, myeloma, breast, prostate, seminoma, SCLC) and those with a slower progression of symptoms have a better chance of functional improvement with treatment.[39, 50] Prompt recognition and treatment cannot be over stressed for patients with SCC. Patient/family education is also vital to facilitate the early report of the signs and symptoms associated with SCC. Paraplegia and incontinence are preventable when treatment is begun in time.[50]

Nursing management of the patient with SCC is outlined in the accompanying box.

Nursing Management

SPINAL CORD COMPRESSION

Spinal cord compression (SCC) is a true oncologic emergency requiring immediate attention. The primary aspect of nursing care is early detection because response to therapy is directly related to the patient's functional status at diagnosis. An in-depth history and data collection are essential in those patients who are at risk for SCC. Nursing assessment should focus on pain, motor and sensory status, and bowel and bladder functions. The nursing care of these patients is extremely variable, depending on the presence and severity of the compression and the medical treatment. Very subtle changes in patient status are significant and should be reported.

Nursing Diagnosis

- *Impaired physical mobility, related to spinal cord compression*

Outcome Goals

Patient will be able to:

- Demonstrate measures to maintain optimal mobility and prevent complications.
- Identify factors that influence maintenance or disruption in mobility.
- Cooperate with necessary treatments and procedures.
- Demonstrate necessary life-style changes.
- Demonstrate safety measures.
- Achieve/maintain optimal mobility consistent with disease process.

Interventions

- Assess patient's level of function/mobility:
  Check for the presence of sensory loss and paresthesia by noting sensation and deep tendon reflexes in extremities.
  Monitor serum calcium level for potential increase from immobility.
  Determine motor weakness and dysfunction by checking gait, range of motion (ROM), and coordination.
  Determine bowel, bladder, and sexual function.
- Check for evidence of venous thrombosis from immobilization:
  Determine the presence of redness, swelling, warmth, positive Homans' sign (pain on dorsiflexion), and venous streaking and erythema.
  Use antiembolic stockings as ordered.
  Measure calves each day and note any edema.
- Implement pain management program as indicated.
- Establish activity regimen according to patient's physical status and physician order:
  Institute passive ROM exercises as ordered.
  Assist patients with transfer and ambulation as needed.
  Provide back brace for patients with unstable spines as ordered.
  Move bedridden patients with extreme care and maintain proper body alignment. Use lift sheets and assistive devices (e.g., trapeze, Hoyer lift). Support joints. Turn patient by log-rolling method.
- Obtain consultations with physical and occupational therapy for evaluation and assistance.

- Implement safety measures as appropriate:
    Place all articles within patient's reach.
    Keep bed rails up and pad them if necessary.
    Assist patient with all movements or encourage use of assistive devices.
- Encourage and assist patient to perform self-care when possible.
- Discuss and teach the use of assistive and supportive devices.
- Arrange consultation or referral to rehabilitative services as needed.

Nursing Diagnosis

- *Ineffective breathing pattern, related to the level of compression and/or immobility*

Outcome Goal

Patient will be able to:

- Demonstrate absence of complications of impaired mobility, as evidenced by respiratory status and vital signs within normal limits and skin integrity intact.

Interventions

- Assess respiratory status:
    Observe breathing for distress (respiratory rate, rhythm, amplitude).
    Auscultate lungs for breath sounds every shift.
    Obtain arterial blood gases (ABGs) as ordered.
- Encourage and assist patient with pulmonary hygiene every 2 hours:
    Reposition every 2 hours.
    Facilitate deep breathing and coughing.
- Consult with physician regarding need for more aggressive pulmonary measures (incentive spirometry, ultrasonic nebulizer, chest physical therapy).
- Provide mechanical respiratory support, if necessary.

Nursing Diagnosis

- *Risk for impaired skin integrity, related to immobility*

Outcome Goals

Patient will be able to:

- Maintain good skin integrity and optimal level of physical activity.
- Identify/demonstrate measures to promote skin integrity.
- Verbalize/demonstrate appropriate hygiene measures.

- Identify signs and symptoms to report to the health care team.
- Verbalize/demonstrate adequate nutritional and fluid intake.
- Verbalize/demonstrate position change and transfer techniques.

Interventions

- Assess skin integrity, with special attention to areas over bony prominences; note any redness, discoloration, swelling, or breakdown.
- Culture any suspicious drainage.
- Institute skin care protocol specific to assessment.
- Modify bed surface with approved pressure-reducing mattress.
- Change patient's position every 2 hours and massage pressure areas.

Nursing Diagnosis

- *Constipation related to decreased activity or immobility*

Outcome Goals

Patient will be able to:

- Demonstrate measures to promote adequate bowel elimination.
- Verbalize/demonstrate adequate nutritional and fluid intake.
- Use prophylactic stool softeners as indicated.
- Follow schedule for defecation.
- Demonstrate knowledge of bowel training program techniques.
- Show absence of fecal impaction.

Interventions

- Obtain history of bowel elimination, including laxative use and other aids for elimination.
- Assess abdomen each day (observe for distention, auscultate for bowel sounds, perform rectal examination for impaction).
- Monitor bowel movements (frequency, amount, odor, consistency).
- Encourage fluids as appropriate.
- Increase bulk and fiber in diet as indicated.
- Administer stool softeners, laxatives, bulk products, and lubricants as ordered.
- Initiate bowel training program as necessary, and encourage compliance.

Nursing Diagnosis

- *Altered urinary elimination, related to neurogenic bladder, loss of voluntary control of micturition*

Outcome Goals

Patient will be able to:

- Maintain adequate urinary control and elimination.
- Express desire to void.
- Follow pattern of fluid intake and voiding.
- Void before activities that are prolonged.
- Check bladder for distention when appropriate.
- Use appropriate measures to initiate voiding when necessary.
- Maintain socially acceptable bladder-emptying program.
- Verbalize signs and symptoms of bladder distention.
- Identify signs and symptoms to report to the health care team.

Interventions

- Obtain history of bladder elimination patterns.
- Assess abdomen (observe for distention, percuss area above symphysis pubis).
- Monitor urine output (frequency, amount, odor, color).
- Check for residual after each voiding as ordered.
- Monitor laboratory values (urinalysis, serum BUN, creatinine).
- Assess for signs and symptoms of a urinary tract infection (elevated temperature, changes in odor or color of urine, frequency and dysuria, complaints of burning and/or urgency).
- Culture urine as ordered.
- Observe for presence of hyperreflexia (reaction that occurs with blocks at the sixth thoracic vertebra or above in which there is increased production of norepinephrine in an attempt to cause evacuation of the bowel or bladder). Signs and symptoms include increased blood pressure, pounding headache, vasodilation, flushing, increased temperature, profuse sweating, chest pain, bradycardia, nausea.
- Obtain order for indwelling urinary catheter if repeated catheterization is necessary to relieve distention or continued urinary residual teach appropriate patients self-catheterization procedure.
- Initiate bladder training program as necessary and encourage compliance.

Nursing Diagnosis

- *Sexual dysfunction related to disease process and treatment*

Outcome Goals

Patient will be able to:

- Demonstrate knowledge related to alteration in sexuality.
- Identify alterations in sexual function.
- Identify factors that influence sexual identity.
- Identify/demonstrate behaviors and measures to promote acceptance of self as sexual being.

Interventions

- Examine own attitudes, knowledge, and skills in the area of sexuality, sexual function, and sexual counseling.
- Provide a therapeutic environment that demonstrates acceptance of sexual behavior and allows patient to feel comfortable to discuss sexual concerns.
- Elicit a sexual history as appropriate.
- Be respectful of social, cultural, and religious factors that may influence patient's perceptions of sexuality, sexual function, and sexual identity, and ensure confidentiality.
- Use the Plissit model to develop relevant nursing interventions. Use levels with which you feel comfortable:

    P, Permission: convey permission to have (or not have) sexual thoughts, concerns, feelings (assure patient that concerns regarding sexual function after cancer diagnosis are legitimate).

    LI, Limited information: provide limited information relative to patient's problem while acknowledging that other individuals experience similar concerns (e.g., many individuals have concerns about type of birth control recommended while receiving chemotherapy).

    SS, Specific suggestions: offer specific suggestions relevant to patient's problems (e.g., use of pillows and coital positions that minimize or allay threat of pathologic fractures).

    IT, Intensive therapy: refer to appropriate resource for longer-term therapy or rehabilitation (e.g., sex therapist for continued erectile dysfunction, surgeon for reconstructive surgery).

- Discuss the potential impact of disease and treatment on sexuality and sexual function.
- Identify available resources, and make referrals as appropriate.

Nursing Diagnoses

- *Body image disturbance related to physical dysfunction, disease process, immobility*
- *Altered role performance related to physical dysfunction, disease, mobility*

Outcome Goals

Patient will be able to:

- Demonstrate successful positive coping and adaptation.

- Recognize when current coping mechanisms are not working.
- Ask for assistance.
- Initiate and perform self-care tasks.
- Identify, cultivate, and use available resources.

Interventions

- Assess patient's past and present coping abilities through interview, observation of physical and verbal participation in self-care, and discussion.
- Promote and observe interaction with family, friends, and staff.

- Encourage verbalization of feelings and concerns.
- Assist and support the establishment of goals and adaptive coping mechanisms.
- Make referrals as appropriate for counseling and rehabilitative services.

Nursing care of a patient with SCC is complex and challenging, reflecting the extreme variability among patients. Situations exist along a continuum from early detection and alarm through emergency and rehabilitation. The role of the oncology nurse in coordinating care is crucial.

Data from references 24, 28, 82, 90, and 99.

Superior Vena Cava Syndrome

DEFINITION

The superior vena cava is a major venous vessel that returns blood to the right atrium of the heart from the head, upper thorax, and upper extremities. Obstruction of the venous flow through this vessel results in impaired venous drainage, with engorgement of the vessels from the head and upper body torso. As the venous pressure rises in the superior vena cava, blood is shunted to collateral venous pathways to facilitate return to the right atrium. The result is a characteristic constellation of physical findings known as superior vena cava syndrome (SVCS).[39, 72, 87]

ETIOLOGY AND RISK FACTORS

The causes ascribed to SVCS have changed over the years as information has increased regarding the cancer process. William Hunter first described SVCS in 1757 in a patient with a syphilitic aneurysm.[57, 65] Over the years, benign conditions such as aortic aneurysms, thyroid goiter, tuberculous mediastinitis, and infectious diseases were most frequently considered to be the cause of SVCS.[134] Today, only 3% of the cases of SVCS have a benign cause (Table 20–5). Cancer is responsible for more than 97% of all cases.[65, 134] Any tumor, primary

or metastatic, can block the blood flow of the superior vena cava (SVC). Three fourths of all malignant cases of SVCS are caused by bronchogenic cancer, particularly SCLC. Squamous cell cancer of the lung is the second most common lung histology to cause SVCS.[72] Lung cancers occurring on the right side are four times more likely to be associated with SVCS due to the proximity to the SVC.[57] Lymphomas account for approximately 15% to 20% of SVCS cases.[65] This includes both Hodgkin's disease and non-Hodgkin's lymphoma (usually involving right-sided perihilar adenopathy).[57] Other mediastinal presentations of malignancies associated with SVCS have been Kaposi's sarcoma, thymoma, and germ cell tumors.[72] Breast cancer is the most common metastatic disease to cause SVCS.[72] Other metastatic diseases causing SVCS include esophageal, colon, and testicular cancers.[92] Fibrous mesothelioma has also been associated with SVCS.[57] SVCS may be the presenting symptomatology in patients with lung cancer.[57]

Innovations in therapeutic interventions for cancer have added two new causes. Venous thrombosis related to indwelling central venous catheters has been observed in patients with SVCS. Several authorities ascribe this to be the most common nonmalignant cause of SVC obstruction.[39, 52] Radiation-induced fibrosis can result in the narrowing of the SVC and produce the same clinical picture. SVCS occurs in approximately 3% to 4% of patients with cancer.[57] Most patients with SVCS are in the fourth to seventh decades of life. The ratio of men to women is approximately 3:1.[57] However, as lung cancer incidence and death rates change, especially among women, so will the incidence and age and gender distribution of SVCS.

PATHOPHYSIOLOGY

The SVC is a thin-walled, low-pressure vessel about 7 cm in length (Fig. 20–8). It extends from the junction of the right and left innominate veins to the right atrium. Location in the thorax is to the right of the arteries of

TABLE 20–5
Nonmalignant Causes of SVCS

Aortic aneurysm
Infectious agents
Substernal thyroid
Central venous catheters

Data from Miaskowski C: Oncologic emergencies. In Miaskowski CM, Buchsel P, editors: Oncology nursing assessment and clinical care, St. Louis, Mosby, 1999:221.

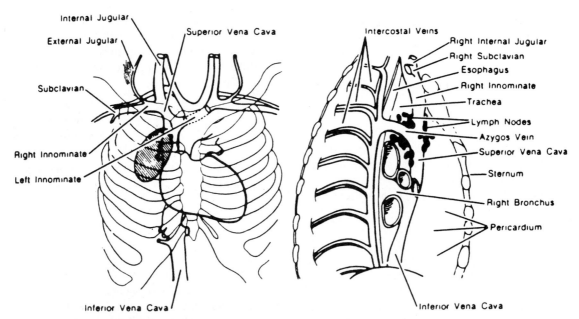

FIGURE 20–8 Schematic representation of the thorax, frontal and lateral views. Shaded areas indicate typical site of obstruction. (From Lockich J, Goodman R: Superior vena cava syndrome, *JAMA* 231:58, 1975. Copyrighted 1975, American Medical Association.)

the trachea and right mainstem bronchus and posterior to the sternum. The thorax is a rigid anatomic compartment with little ability for expansion. In its space within the thorax/mediastinum, the SVC is extremely vulnerable to displacement and compression because it has a thin wall, and low venous pressure, and is surrounded by the rigid structures of the sternum, trachea, vertebrae, lymph nodes, aorta, pulmonary artery, and right bronchus.[57, 67] Therefore obstruction of the SVC can be a consequence of three physiologic events[65, 99, 101]:

1. External compression by an extrinsic mass, solid tumor, or enlarged lymph node
2. Intravascular obstruction by tumor or thrombosis
3. Intraluminal reaction to tumor invasion or inflammation

Impedance of venous flow through the SVC and subsequent development of SVCS depends on several factors: the degree and location of the blockage, growth rate of the tumor, patency of the azygos vein, and proliferation of collateral circulation. The azygos vein (see Fig. 20–8) plays a pivotal role in the flow of blood through the SVC, entering it just above the pericardial reflection and making it a major tributary. The azygos vein system is the most important alternative pathway for collateral circulation. Other collateral systems include the internal mammary, lateral thoracic, paraspinous, and esophageal venous networks.[160]

Impairment of the venous circulation through the SVC reduces blood flow to the right atrium, which results in venous hypertension with venous stasis and a decrease in cardiac output. If untreated, the syndrome progresses from vascular congestion to thrombosis, cerebral edema, pulmonary complications, and death (in weeks to months).[57] Death may occur from brain stem herniation or tracheal obstruction.[134]

CLINICAL FEATURES

The clinical picture seen in SVCS is directly related to obstruction of venous drainage in the upper body (see Fig. 20–8). Compression of intrathoracic structures, vascular congestion, and venous hypertension present distinguishing clinical features. If the onset is gradual, collateral circulation develops and can compensate for the obstruction of blood flow.[99] The onset is usually insidious, but when fully developed, it requires immediate attention. The most frequent symptom of SVCS is dyspnea, occurring in 63% of patients. Other common complaints include a feeling of fullness in the head with facial swelling (50%), cough (24%), and chest pain (15%).[160] The classic clinical picture of SVCS includes facial swelling, periorbital edema, and engorgement of veins across the upper torso. There is disagreement in the literature about the symptoms that occur early versus late in the course of SVCS. The onset and severity of signs and symptoms vary directly with the underlying disease and related pathophysiology. The presentation may be unilateral or bilateral. Because pressures in the head are higher in the supine than in the standing position, a person with early SVCS may initially have signs and symptoms only in the morning.[57] Most signs and

CLINICAL FEATURES

Superior Vena Cava Syndrome

Clinical Signs[57, 63, 143]

Edema of the face, neck, upper thorax, breasts, and upper extremities

Periorbital edema and/or edema of the conjunctivae, with or without protrusion of the eye

Horner's syndrome (sinking of eye with ptosis of eyelid)

Plethora (fullness) of the face

Increased pressure of the jugular veins

Dilation and prominence of collateral vessels in upper thorax and neck

Telangiectasia (capillary dilation)

Compensatory tachycardia

Symptoms

Respiratory compromise (dyspnea, shortness of breath, tachypnea, cough, orthopnea)

Feeling of facial fullness

Headache

Visual disturbances

Dizziness

Hoarseness

Chest pain

Stokes' sign (tightness of shirt collar)

Swelling of fingers (difficulty removing rings)

---

symptoms will be exacerbated by bending forward or the supine position.[57] Early detection of SVCS hinges on a careful in-depth history and physical assessment. The clinical features of SVCS are listed in the box.[39, 52, 65, 67, 72]

Progression of symptoms may lead to severe respiratory obstruction, paralyzed vocal cord, cyanosis of the upper torso, "wet brain syndrome" (manifested by drowsiness, stupor, unconsciousness, and seizures), and possible coma.[105]

DIAGNOSIS

The diagnostic evaluation of a patient with SVCS depends greatly on the patient's physical condition. If SVCS onset is insidious, the diagnostic work-up can proceed slowly, and treatment will not be initiated until a diagnosis is confirmed. If the onset is rapid and symptoms are acute, historically, a definitive diagnosis was deferred and treatment (usually radiation therapy) begun immediately. In the past SVCS was considered one of the rare occasions when treatment could be started even before a tissue diagnosis was confirmed. In this life-threatening situation, chest radiography, the results of which rarely appear normal, and clinical presentation

were considered diagnostic. A tissue biopsy to determine a primary lesion and further work-up for metastases proceeded during the course of treatment.

Current literature argues strongly for confirmation of tissue diagnosis prior to initiation of treatment whenever possible.* Present practice has been reported to obtain the diagnosis via bronchoalveolar lavage or thoracostomy as opposed to initiating immediate radiation therapy.[105] Emergency radiation therapy is considered appropriate without a tissue diagnosis when there is altered mental status and risk of brain damage from IICP, severe upper airway compression, or cardiovascular collapse.[108]

Chest films are abnormal in 80% of patients with SVCS.[108, 160] In 50% of patients, findings are a lung or mediastinal mass, most frequently on the right side because the SVC enters from the right. Also, 25% of patients may have mediastinal widening and pleural effusion.[57, 108] CT scan and MRI may further define the lesion and its location.[143] Important information obtained by radiographic findings includes more detailed information about the SVC and its tributaries as well as the source, size, and exact location of the mass in relation to the azygos vein. This information also provides anatomic detail necessary to establish the portals for radiation therapy. Accomplishing CT and MRI may be complicated by the patient's inability to tolerate the supine position. MRI has a 96% sensitivity rate for SVCS but requires longer scanning time and is more costly.[143]

Further diagnostic procedures must be evaluated for their risk versus benefit to the patient. Biopsy of palpable superficial lymph nodes, sputum for cytology, and bone marrow biopsy are associated with low risk and may provide information about the primary tumor. Invasive procedures such as bronchoscopy, mediastinoscopy, thoracoscopy, thoracotomy, or supraclavicular lymph node biopsy may be necessary but are associated with the risk of thrombosis or bleeding as a result of increased venous pressure. Improved techniques are decreasing the incidence of complications.[143] Immediate radiation therapy may impede later tissue biopsy because of radiation-induced tissue changes.

Bronchoscopy has established a diagnosis in approximately 70% of patients.[101] Percutaneous needle biopsy, mediastinoscopy, and thoracotomy are associated with increased risk of bleeding and, if possible, should be deferred until venous pressure is reduced. Superior venacavography is infrequently done. However, it can be most helpful in determining location and degree of obstruction, measuring venous pressure through the catheter, distinguishing between vascular and nonvascular lesions, evaluating collateral circulation, and assessing

---

*References 57, 72, 105, 108, 134, 143

operability.[143] Recently, CT-guided fine-needle biopsies have yielded diagnostic specimens from the lung mass with few complications.

TREATMENT MODALITIES

Four therapeutic modalities should be considered in the treatment of SVCS: radiation therapy, chemotherapy, surgery, and pharmacologic therapy. The goals are relief of symptoms and reduction of the obstructing lesion. Cure may be the goal when the primary diagnosis is SCLC, non-Hodgkin's lymphoma, or a germ cell tumor, which account for nearly half the malignant causes of SVCS.[160]

The choice of treatment depends on the rate of onset, the causative process (benign or malignant), and the type of mass (intraluminal or extraluminal). The goals of therapy for acute onset of symptoms related to SVCS are maintaining a patient airway and cardiac output.[99]

Radiation Therapy

Radiation therapy has been the treatment of choice for SVCS because of its local therapeutic response and minimal toxicities. Treatment is begun immediately in acute and life-threatening situations. The total dose, dose fractionation, and size and type of field depend on tumor histology, patient condition, radiologic response, and symptom relief. Delivery of radiation begins initially with high-dose fractionation at 3 to 4 Gy/d for the first 3 days, followed by a reduction of the daily dose to 1.5 to 2 Gy/d, for a total dose of 500 to 600 Gy in 5 to 7 weeks.[101, 143] The higher initial doses are favored because of an apparently more rapid tumor response. Patients with lymphoma require a lower total dose of 300 to 400 Gy, unless bulky masses are present, which may necessitate a total dose of 500 Gy.[39, 52, 134, 143, 160]

Tumor reduction usually occurs with radiation therapy, especially in patients with lymphoma and small (oat) cell lung cancer. Subjective improvement has been noted in 3 to 4 days in 75% of patients, regardless of tumor histology. Within 7 days, 91% obtain relief. Objective response, with decrease in facial swelling and plethora, reduction of venous engorgement, and shrinkage of tumor mass, is evident in 7 to 14 days.[72, 92]

Chemotherapy

The use of chemotherapy to treat SVCS has come to the forefront of the treatment regimen. It is an effective primary treatment when the cause of SVCS is SCLC, lymphoma, or a germ cell tumor.[160] Chemotherapy may be used alone if the mediastinal area has received a maximum of radiation or when reduction of tumor mass will provide a smaller radiation treatment field.

The choice of chemotherapeutic agents is based on the malignant cause of SVCS. More than 80% of patients with SCLC respond to platinum-based regimens. Relief of symptoms may be seen in 7 to 10 days with complete resolution of symptoms in about 2 weeks.[143] After the selection of agents, consideration must be given to intravneous administration. Edema and dilation of the veins in the upper extremities lead to impaired circulation. Limited venous access, poor drug distribution, and increased risk of venous irritation and extravasation of medications may contraindicate use of the upper extremities for therapy. In some situations the lower extremities may be used to administer chemotherapy by a central IV catheter placed in the femoral vein.[72]

Surgery

Specific surgical approaches to SVCS include stent placement or SVC bypass. The placement of a wire stent may open more than 90% of occluded SVC's and result in immediate and long-term palliation.[57] Use of a stent may be indicated when other treatments for SVCS are unusable or ineffective.[143] The most common situation is recurrence of SVCS after maximum-tolerance radiation or when the acuity of the symptoms contraindicates any delay in treatment related response. Stent placement is contraindicated when there is tumor invasion of the SVC.[143]

The stainless steel stent was designed by Gianturco and is usually referred to as the *Gianturco expandable wire stent* (GEWS) or *Gianturco Z stent.* Other products that are available are the balloon-expandable *Palmaz stent* and the self-expandable *Wallstent.* All the products are constructed of stainless steel wire in a cylindrical shape with similar function.[143] The stent is placed using a small balloon catheter inserted percutaneously with fluoroscopy with the patient under local anesthesia. The catheter is introduced into the vessel with the stent in a compressed form. When the stent is released, it expands and dilates the narrowed venous lumen. If the expansion is insufficient, the balloon is used to enlarge the stent to the desired diameter. Fibrinolytic therapy (with agents such as streptokinase, urokinase, or tissue-type plasminogen activator [TPA]) may be necessary prior to the procedure. Heparinization will be required during the procedure. The need for anticoagulants afterward is controversial, but may be recommended for 3 to 4 months for patients requiring pre-procedure thrombolysis or in whom there is significant post-procedural residual stenosis.[72] A period of about 4 weeks is necessary for the stent to become incorporated into the endothelium of the venous wall. The stent may remain patent for long periods because of its relatively low thrombo-genicity. Symptom relief may occur very quickly after stent placement (24–72 hours).[143]

One study has indicated some prognostic factors for longer-term palliation using the stent. It was found that patients with postirradiation fibrosis or slowly progressive pressure from a recurrent extrinsic tumor had longer relief of symptoms than patients whose symptoms resulted from direct tumor invasion. Complications from stent placement can include hematoma formation, SVC perforation, infection, and transient renal insufficiency.[99] Rarer adverse events may occur, such as stent migration into the right ventricle, stent fracture, and pulmonary edema from a rapid increase in blood flow to the lungs.[143]

Bypass of the SVC is used very judicially because postoperative morbidity is high. Bypass surgery is indicated when the tumor could be completely removed if the SVC were excised with it; when venous return is inadequate despite collateral circulation; and when the obstruction results from venous thrombosis, fibrosis, or a benign cause. This operative procedure is delicate and precise and depends on the same factors as in arterial grafts. The graft may be constructed using a synthetic Dacron prothesis or the patient's own saphenous vein. The graft creates a new vessel, which rechannels blood flow around the obstruction. One end of the graft is sutured to the right atrium, and the other is sutured to either the internal jugular or innominate vein.[160]

Patency of the bypass graft depends on the size of the anastomotic site, internal venous pressure, and blood flow. External rigidity of the graft is helpful to prevent collapse but is not required. Postoperatively, patients usually receive anticoagulation therapy and aspirin for an indefinite period to assist with graft patency.[52, 160] When patency is maintained for several weeks, it increases the likelihood of long-term function. Reports demonstrate patency beyond a year.

Pharmacologic Therapy

The increased use of indwelling central venous catheters has contributed to a rise in the incidence of SVCS.[52] Whatever the cause, irritation and inflammation of the SVC related to an intraluminal or extraluminal lesion produce platelet aggregation, leading to clot formation. Fibrinolytic therapy with streptokinase, urokinase, or TPA has been used to treat intraluminal thrombosis.[55, 76, 101, 160] Fibrinolytic therapy is contraindicated with brain or spinal cord metastases, bleeding disorders, or history of stroke.[57]

Fibrinolytic therapy is appropriate when initiated within 7 days of the SVCS symptoms. Anticoagulation is the preferred therapy if more than 7 days has elapsed. In-patient heparinization is followed by long-term oral warfarin (Coumadin).

Anticoagulation therapy is indicated for SVCS because of venous stasis. It may be used alone to resolve thrombus obstruction secondary to a central venous catheter or following initial fibrinolytic therapy. It is also used as a maintenance treatment to reduce the extent of the thrombus and prevent its progression. Removal of the central venous catheter should also be followed by anticoagulation to avoid embolization.[52, 160] Low-dose warfarin (Coumadin, 1 mg/d) may be used prophylactically in patients with central lines.[143]

During the administration of radiation therapy or chemotherapy, anticoagulants may be given concomitantly as a preventive treatment. Other medical interventions may be instituted as adjunctive therapy for SVCS. Diuretics may be given to reduce edema of the head and neck, which could improve cerebration and breathing. Caution should be used when giving diuretics because venous return to the heart is low and hypovolemia resulting from diuresis may induce decreased venous return, dehydration, thrombosis, and shock.[99] Corticosteroids may be administered during active treatment to reduce inflammation related to the obstruction, radiation, or chemotherapy and resulting tumor necrosis.[150] Their use remains controversial.[143] Oxygen therapy may be necessary for the management of respiratory complications and maintenance of oxygen saturation and patient comfort.

PROGNOSIS

Patients usually respond to treatment for SVCS, showing regression of the tumor. The signs and symptoms of SVCS are largely reversible and subside in 3 days to 2 weeks.[134] SVCS recurs in only 10% to 20% of patients.[108]

The prognosis of patients with SVCS strongly correlates with the prognosis of the underlying disease.[39, 105, 160] Some patients have not responded to treatment. This has been attributed to poor general condition, presence of thrombosis in the SVC, and metastatic disease. The best responses are seen in patients with lymphoma and SCLC. Other types of lung cancer have fewer long-term responses. Although a diagnosis of SVCS may not offer long-term survival, with prompt diagnosis and treatment, it can be managed and therefore improves the patient's quality of life.

Nursing management of the patient with SVCS is outlined in the accompanying box.

Nursing Management

SUPERIOR VENA CAVA SYNDROME

The nursing care of patients with superior vena cava syndrome (SVCS) begins with astute assessment skills. Identification should be made of those patients considered to be at risk, followed by close observation and baseline data collection. Documentation of vital signs, mental status, appearance, and level of activity are essential to facilitate detection of changes. Subtle changes in subjective complaints or objective parameters should be reported to the physician. Once a diagnosis of SVCS has been established, the role of the nurse continues to be important.

Nursing Diagnosis

- *Ineffective breathing pattern related to venous congestion in the upper torso*

Outcome Goals

Patient will be able to:

- Demonstrate knowledge related to ineffective breathing.
- Identify signs and symptoms of altered respiratory status.
- Identify factors that influence respiratory function.
- Exhibit effective breathing pattern, as evidenced by chest clear by auscultation, respirations regular and nonlabored, laboratory values and diagnostic tests approaching normal levels, and vital signs within patient's normal limits.

Interventions

- Determine current respiratory status:
    Observe for signs and symptoms of respiratory distress (dyspnea, shortness of breath, tachypnea, air hunger, stridor, orthopnea).
    Assess lungs. Observe ventilatory movements (rate and depth), patency of airway, use of accessory muscles, clubbing of fingernails, and discoloration of nail bed or mucous membranes.
    Palpate chest for fremitus, crepitance, deviation of the trachea, or nonsymmetric chest expansion.
    Percuss chest for density/consolidation and displacement of organs.
    Auscultate chest for breath sounds.
    Monitor laboratory and other respiratory function tests, CBC, electrolytes, ABGs, chest x-ray films, and scans.

- Assist with breathing and pulmonary toilet:
    Positioning for comfort and enhanced chest expansion
    Deep breathing and coughing every 2 hours
    Pursed-lip breathing
    Frequent mouth care
    Suctioning if necessary
- Provide oxygen and mechanical ventilation as indicated.
- Administer respiratory medications, steroids, and *analgesics* as prescribed.

Nursing Diagnoses

- *Decreased cardiac output related to decreased venous return caused by vena cava obstruction*
- *Impaired gas exchange related to venous congestion caused by vena cava obstruction*

Outcome Goals

Patient will be able to:

- Maintain optimal cardiac output, as evidenced by relief of chest pain, vital signs within patient's normal limits, cardiac rhythm without dysrhythmias, and adequate intake and output.
- Maintain adequate pulmonary function, as evidenced by laboratory values and diagnostic tests approaching patient's normal values and activity tolerance within patient's normal limits.
- Develop plan for behavioral and life-style changes.

Interventions

- Assess patient for changes in cardiac function:
    Obtain vital signs every 2 to 4 hours as indicated.
    Observe patient for signs of impedance of venous blood flow from the upper torso (plethora of the face; thoracic and neck vein distention; facial, trunk, and arm edema, especially in the morning; dyspnea, tachypnea, cough; cyanosis; mental status changes).
    Monitor laboratory values (CBC, ABGs, chest x-ray films, ECG, scans).
- Provide oxygen therapy as ordered.
- Position patient for comfort and enhancement of venous drainage from upper torso:
    Elevate and support upper extremities, especially if edematous.
    Avoid elevation of lower extremities.
    Avoid invasive or constrictive procedures involving upper extremities.

Avoid constrictive clothing.

Maintain a cool room temperature.

Avoid closed-in areas if possible.

- Prevent activities that increase intrathoracic or intracerebral pressure (Valsalva's maneuver, vomiting, bending over, stooping).
- Assist patient with physical activities as needed.
- Provide measures to decrease anxiety:

  Relaxation techniques

  Antianxiety medications

Nursing Diagnoses

- *Altered tissue perfusion, cerebral, related to upper torso venous stasis and decreased cardiac output*
- *Altered thought processes related to decreased cerebral tissue perfusion and impaired gas exchange*

Outcome Goal

Patient will be able to:

- Maintain adequate cardiac function, as evidenced by regular pulse, regular and nonlabored respirations, laboratory values within patient's normal limits, chest x-ray film showing no mediastinal mass, and ABGs within patient's normal limits.

Interventions

- Assess organ systems for malfunction related to ischemia.
- Note any changes in mental status.
- Monitor laboratory values closely.
- Administer vasoactive drugs as ordered.
- Provide oxygen as prescribed.
- Institute safety measures as indicated.

Nursing Diagnosis

- *Risk for impaired skin integrity in the chest/thorax area related to the effects of SVCS, radiation therapy*

Outcome Goal

Patient will be able to:

- Demonstrate strategies to promote optimal skin integrity.

Interventions

- Explain effects of SVCS and radiation on skin and prepare patient for temporary changes (edema, discoloration, pruritus).
- Outline proper skin hygiene:

  Use mild soap and tepid water and pat dry.

  Avoid use of lotions, creams, ointments, powders, and perfumes on skin in the treatment field.
- Wear loose cotton clothing on the chest.
- Protect chest from direct sunlight.
- Avoid application of heat to the area being treated.
- Report any discomfort to physician and nurse.

Nursing Diagnosis

- *Impaired swallowing related to inflammation of the esophagus caused by vena cava obstruction, effects of radiation therapy*

Outcome Goals

Patient will be able to:

- Identify signs and symptoms of difficulty swallowing and reports these to the health care team.
- Identify measures to improve swallowing ability.
- Exhibit stable nutritional status.

Interventions

- Assess patient's ability to swallow liquids and solids.
- Observe closely for aspiration.
- Provide analgesics as indicated.
- Change diet to avoid irritating foods (spicy or coarse).
- Avoid alcohol and tobacco use.
- Provide frequent mouth care.
- Alter medication schedule and form or rate (decrease pill size, liquids, etc.) as needed.
- Provide adequate hydration and nutrition.

As the acute phase of SVCS passes, the patient will be ready to become more involved in self-care, and anticipatory guidance can be given to facilitate continued therapy and detection of any changes in the patient's condition.

Data from references 57, 65, 67, 99, and 143.

Metabolic Oncologic Complications

Disseminated Intravascular Coagulation

DEFINITION

Disseminated intravascular coagulation (DIC) is considered to be a bleeding disorder. In the past it was referred to as a "consumptive coagulopathy." Bleeding disorders are classified as congenital or acquired. DIC is one of the acquired disorders. It is not a disease entity but rather an event that can accompany various disease processes. DIC is an alteration in the blood-clotting mechanism, with abnormal acceleration of the *coagulation cascade,* resulting in thrombosis. Hemorrhage occurs simultaneously as a result of the depletion of clotting factors.[99, 131, 120, 164]

ETIOLOGY AND RISK FACTORS

This disorder is not a primary independent disorder. An underlying pathology, benign or malignant, is responsible for DIC. The pathology creates the triggering mechanism or initiating event necessary for the activation of thrombin, which is responsible for the cascade of blood clot formation and clot dissolution, thus producing DIC.[54, 92, 125, 164] A variety of pathologies involve a triggering event, which can cause either endothelial tissue injury or blood vessel injury.

Endothelial injuries include[141, 164]:

Shock or trauma—head injury, burns
Infections—aspergillosis, gram-positive sepsis, or gram-negative sepsis
Obstetric complications—abruptio placentae, amniotic fluid embolism, eclampsia
Malignancies—acute promyelocytic myelogenous leukemia (APML), acute myelogenous leukemia (AML), mucin-producing GI adenocarcinomas (cancers of the lung, colon, breast, and prostate)

Blood vessel injuries include:

Infectious vasculitis—Rocky Mountain spotted fever, certain viral infections, severe glomerulonephritis
Vascular disorders—aortic aneurysm, giant hemangioma, angiography
Intravascular hemolysis—hemolytic transfusion reaction, multiple whole-blood transfusions, massive trauma, extracorporeal circulation devices (e.g., cardiopulmonary bypass machine, aortic balloon pump), heatstroke, peritoneovenous shunting
Miscellaneous—pancreatitis, liver disease (e.g., obstructive jaundice, acute hepatic failure), snakebite

In patients with cancer the incidence of DIC is less than 10% to 15%. It is usually related to the disease process or the treatment of the cancer and often occurs concomitantly with sepsis.[39, 43, 53]

Oncology-related DIC occurs with the most frequency in patients with APML. Approximately 85% of the patients with APML will develop DIC. The next most common cancers associated with DIC are the mucin-producing adenocarcinomas (lung, breast, stomach, pancreas, and prostate).[54] However, the most common cause of DIC is sepsis.[54] It is estimated that 10% to 20% of patients with gram-negative sepsis demonstrate the symptoms of DIC.[7]

PATHOPHYSIOLOGY

Body hemostasis depends on an intricate balance between blood clot formation and blood clot dissolution. The fibrin blood clot is the end-product of the blood-clotting mechanism. Normally this mechanism is initiated when tissues sustain an injury. Disruption of the vascular endothelium exposes collagen fibers to blood. Smooth muscle spasm then occurs, releasing serotonin. Vasoconstriction follows, which slows the flow of blood and causes circulating platelets to change shape and adhere to the rough surface of injured vessels within 1 to 2 seconds. More platelets aggregate and form a loose plug at the site of injury, creating a seal on the vessel wall to control bleeding. The injured vascular tissue also releases a phospholipid called *thromboplastin,* which initiates the clotting reaction.[8]

The fibrin blood clot is formed through a series of sequential reactions that are protein activated (Fig. 20–9). This protein activation occurs through two different cascades of reactions known as the intrinsic and extrinsic pathways, which operate jointly to form the blood clot. The *intrinsic pathway* is activated by injury to the blood vessel wall. The *extrinsic pathway* is activated after tissue injury. Central to each pathway is the conversion of prothrombin to thrombin through a series of reactions involving various blood factors (phospholipids, proteins, calcium). The thrombin then acts as a catalyst to convert fibrinogen (monomer) to fibrin (polymer). The fibrin polymers form a mesh of fibrin strands, which trap platelets, red blood cells (RBCs), and leukocytes, making an occlusive clot.

The series of reactions that forms the clot is balanced by a series of reactions that limits the size of the clot and later dissolves it. Therefore clot dissolution occurs in conjunction with clot formation. When the clot is no longer needed, it is converted from a polymer back to a monomer by *fibrinolysin* (*plasmin*). Fibrinolysin is formed in the presence of thrombin during coagulation when preactivators come in contact with a tissue enzyme known as *kinase.* Fibrinogen and fibrin are broken down

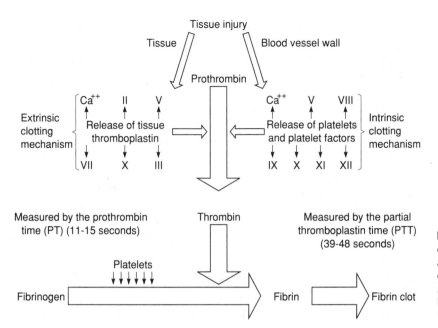

Formation of a blood clot. (From Yasko JM, Schafer SL: Disseminated intravascular coagulation. In Yasko JM, editor: *Guidelines for cancer care: symptom management,* Reston, VA, Reston, © 1983. Reprinted by permission of Prentice-Hall, Inc., Upper Saddle River, NJ.)

by fibrinolysis, resulting in *fibrin degradation products* (FDPs) or *fibrin split products* (FSPs). As these fragments circulate, they interfere with the formation of fibrin and coat the platelets, thus decreasing their adhesive ability. The result is anticoagulation along with the process of fibrinolysis; the body forms *antithrombins,* natural anticoagulants that also interfere with thrombin (clotting) activity. Hemostasis is therefore balanced between fibrin clot formation (*coagulation*) and clot dissolution by fibrinolysis (*anticoagulation*).

Disseminated intravascular coagulation is a disruption of body hemostasis. One of the triggering mechanisms from the underlying pathology initiates the process (Fig. 20–10), which results in the formation of

thrombin and fibrinolysin (plasmin). Thrombin acts to convert fibrinogen to fibrin to form clots. At the same time, fibrinolysin degrades some of the fibrin into a soluble monomer form; this initiates clot dissolution. The remaining portion of fibrin is an insoluble polymer, which continues to form clots. These clots may be deposited in the extremities or in organs such as the lungs, kidneys, and brain. Capillary clots slow the blood flow, resulting in tissue ischemia, hypoxia, and necrosis. The clots also trap circulating platelets in the microvasculature, which results in the thrombocytopenia. As the fibrinolysin continues to degrade fibrin, the by-products, FDPs are produced. These FDPs disrupt the conversion of fibrin to a polymer; coat platelets, decreasing their

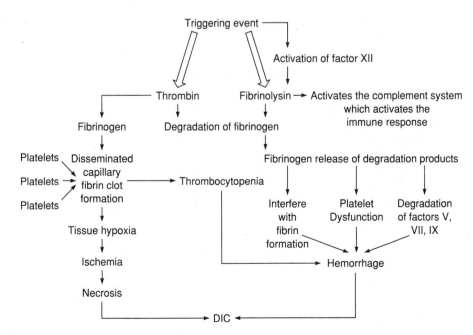

FIGURE 20–10
Pathophysiology of disseminated intravascular coagulation (*DIC*). (From Yasko JM, Schafer SL: Disseminated intravascular coagulation. In Yasko JM, editor: *Guidelines for cancer care: symptom management,* Reston, VA, Reston, © 1983. Reprinted by permission of Prentice-Hall, Inc., Upper Saddle River, NJ.)

adherence, and degrade factors V, VIII, and X, which leads to capillary hemorrhage.

Patients with hematalogic malignancies are at risk for DIC due to disseminated disease, risk for infection, and rapid cell turnover.[132] Patients with leukemia often have some of the characteristics of DIC without having the complete DIC syndrome. Occurrence of DIC in patients with leukemia is 1% to 2%. APML typically causes a low-grade or chronic form of DIC that is characterized by thrombotic complications such as deep vein thrombosis.[131] The blast cells in APML are hypergranular and release a procoagulant substance similar to thromboplastin (factor VIII) that stimulates the clotting cascade. This release may occur at any time, such as at diagnosis or after chemotherapy.

Solid tumors (mucin-producing adenocarcinomas) also tend to produce the more chronic form of DIC. They develop new blood vessels with abnormal endothelial linings that are thought to activate the procoagulant system. Necrotic tissue or tissue enzymes may also be released into circulation and stimulate coagulation.[53]

More acute forms of DIC are caused by extensive disease, tumor lysis syndrome, and sepsis.[132] Endotoxins associated with sepsis are thought to activate factor XII and initiate coagulation.[54] Gram-positive organisms, human immunodeficiency virus, varicella, hepatitis, and cytomegalovirus are also known to trigger the clotting cascade.[54]

If the underlying pathology with its triggering mechanism is not treated or otherwise eliminated, it will promote further coagulopathy. The term *consumptive coagulopathy* has been used to describe this increased use (consumption) of platelets and clotting factors, leading to a continuation of thrombocytopenia and a further decrease of clotting factors and resulting in bleeding. Thus the abnormal activation of thrombin in DIC results in a cyclic paradox of thrombosis or hemorrhage or both (see Fig. 20–10).

CLINICAL FEATURES

The onset of DIC may be acute, chronic, or somewhere in between. The clinical manifestations and laboratory findings depend on the triggering event and the body tissues involved. The presenting signs and symptoms result from disseminated clotting and bleeding, which may be overt or occult. Bleeding usually predominates.

Signs of bleeding are multiple and may be seen from any body orifice. Bleeding may range from oozing to frank bleeding or hemorrhage. Patients may have overt oozing from venipuncture sites, mucous membranes, needle puncture sites, or incisions. Petechiae, ecchymoses, purpura, or hematomas may be evident. Profound menstrual or GI bleeding may occur, as well as epistaxis or hemoptysis. The possibility of occult internal or intra-cerebral bleeding is equally critical. Abdominal distention, blood in stools, blood in urine or skin, and scleral changes may be observed. Other signs of occult bleeding may be mental status changes, orthopnea, and tachycardia.

Clotting resulting from fibrin deposits in the microcirculation will impede blood flow. Early signs of clotting may include oliguria, hypoxemia, and cool and mottled extremities.[131] Progression can cause severe tissue ischemia and lead to tissue necrosis. Multiple system changes may be observed. A major concern for a person experiencing DIC is the possibility of irreversible end-organ damage. The systems with the most risk of microvascular thrombosis include cardiac, pulmonary, renal, hepatic, and CNS.[16]

Observation of the skin may show acrocyanosis, also known as *Raynaud's sign* (generalized sweating with symmetric mottling of the nose, fingers, toes, and genitalia), and other ischemic changes, which can lead to superficial gangrene. Pulmonary signs, such as severe, sudden dyspnea at rest with tachypnea and progressive rales and rhonchi, are similar to those observed with adult respiratory distress syndrome (ARDS). The GI tract may have an ischemic insult appearing as an ulceration, and tubular necrosis of the kidney may lead to renal failure. If microcoagulation occurs in the brain, multifocal cerebrovascular accidents (CVAs, strokes), mental change, delirium, and coma may result. The associated symptoms of bleeding or clotting will vary depending on the system sustaining the ischemic insult or bleeding. Complaints include malaise, weakness, air hunger, altered sensorium, visual changes, and headaches. The presence and magnitude of these disturbances depend on the extent of the clotting and bleeding.

DIAGNOSIS

Laboratory findings substantiate a diagnosis of DIC (Table 20–6). No single blood test can confirm or exclude a diagnosis of DIC. Instead, screening has traditionally been accomplished by measuring the platelet count, prothrombin time (PT), partial thromboplastin time (PTT), and fibrinogen level. More recently, if abnormal results are obtained, the diagnosis is confirmed by the level of FDPs and D-dimer (a neoantigen formed when plasmin digests fibrin).[53, 79] D-dimer is abnormal in 93% of cases and FDP titer is abnormal in 75%.[16] Antithrombin III levels will be abnormal in 89%.

Platelet count is decreased. This indicates *thrombocytopenia*, which is the cardinal laboratory finding. More than 90% of patients with DIC have abnormal platelet count and PT. In about 50% of these patients, the platelet count is less than $50,000/mm^3$ (normal: 150,000–400,000/mm^3).

TABLE 20–6
DIC Lab Values

Test	Normal Value	DIC Value
PT	10–13 s	>15s, usually prolonged
PTT	39–48 s	Usually prolonged
Platelets	150,000–400,000 mm³	<150,000 mm³, decreased
Factor assay		Decreased factors VI, VIII, IX
Fibrinogen	150–350 mg/dL	<100–150 mg/dL, decreased
FDPs	10–40	>40, increased
D-dimer	<250 ng/mL	>500, increased
Antithrombin	85–125	<85, decreased

PT, prothrombin time; PTT, partial thromboplastin time; FDPs, fibrin degradation products.
Data from references 53, 120, 131, 141, and 162.

The PT is prolonged (normal: 10–13 seconds). This evaluates the extrinsic coagulation system, reflecting decreased levels of clotting factors II, V, and X and of fibrinogen.

Fibrinogen level is decreased (normal: 200–400 mg/dL). This results from the consumption of fibrinogen by thrombin-induced clotting and excessive fibrinolysis. Fibrinogen levels less than 150 mg/dL are found in 70% of patients with DIC.

The PTT is prolonged (normal: 39–48 seconds). This evaluates the intrinsic coagulation system.

The FDPs or FSPs are increased (normal: <10). They are 100% sensitive for DIC, but only 50% specific. The D-dimer level will be decreased. It is less sensitive than FDP but 100% specific. Together, the FDP and D-dimer have 100% specificity and sensitivity.[79]

Factor assays, especially V and VIII, are decreased.

Protamine sulfate precipitation test (thrombin activation test) is strongly positive (normal: negative).

Antithrombin III levels are decreased (normal: 89%–120%).[53, 120, 131, 141, 162]

Laboratory tests for DIC can be complicated by underlying conditions. Patients with liver disease have abnormal clotting studies and often thrombocytopenia. Laboratory findings in these patients show prolonged PT and decreased fibrinogen levels. Fibrinogen levels, usually elevated in the presence of sepsis, pregnancy, or malignancy, may fall within the normal range if DIC is present concurrently. Serum creatinine and liver transaminases are elevated with extensive clotting. Hemolysis will elevate reticulocytes and blood urea nitrogen (BUN) as the hemoglobin decreases.[131] Finally, multiple transfusions may cause alteration in the levels of clotting factors or platelets.

TREATMENT MODALITIES

The primary goal of therapy in DIC is to eliminate or alter the triggering event. Sepsis is treated with antibiotics. Surgery, chemotherapy, and radiation therapy are used to treat the underlying malignancy. If the DIC is chronic, only supportive measures may be necessary until the DIC is resolved. Depending on the progression of the DIC and the success of treating the triggering event and predominant signs and symptoms, therapy is directed at stopping the intravascular clotting process and controlling the bleeding. When bleeding is severe, blood component therapy is necessary to achieve hemostasis. It is used to correct the clotting deficiencies caused by the consumption of blood components during the DIC process. Common blood products used in treating DIC are as follows:

Platelets contain platelet factor III, which strengthens the endothelium, prevents petechial hemorrhage, facilitates the conversion of prothrombin to thrombin, and functions as a mechanical plug by adhering to the vessel wall. The amount and frequency of platelet replacement depend on the patient's platelet count and physical condition. Spontaneous hemorrhage is of concern especially when the platelet count falls below 15,000/mm³. Usually, 6 to 10 U is given and will raise the platelet count by 30,000 to 50,000/mm³.[21]

Fresh frozen plasma (FFP) is used for volume expansion. It contains clotting factors V, VIII, XIII, and antithrombin III. Usually, 2 to 4 U FFP is given once or twice a day. Each unit of infused FFP raises each clotting factor by 5%.

Packed red blood cells (PRBCs) are used to increase RBCs and clotting factors. PRBCs are used instead of whole blood to reduce the development of antibodies and fluid overload. Usually, 2 U is given when the hematocrit drops below 25%. Each unit of PRBCs should raise the hemoglobin count by 1.

Cryoprecipitate contains fibrinogen (approximately 200 mg/U) and factor VIII. It is used for patients with severe hypofibrinogenemia. Usually, 2 U cryoprecipitate is given every 6 hours when the fibrinogen level is below 50 mg/dL. A total of 10 U cryoprecipitate is administered. Each unit of cryoprecipitate increases the level of fibrinogen and factor VIII by 2%.

Heparin therapy, which inhibits thrombin formation, has met with controversy for the treatment of DIC. Research is lacking to support the risk/benefit ratio. The anticoagulation effects of heparin result from its prevention of the platelet aggregation that initiates the intrinsic pathway of the coagulation cascade. Heparin interferes with thrombin and stops the conversion of fibrinogen to fibrin, which prevents clot formation. It does not lyse those clots that are already formed; that requires thrombin to activate fibrinogen.

Doses of heparin have included 2500 to 5000 U subcutaneously every 8 to 12 hours, 50 U/kg of body weight by IV bolus every 4 to 6 hours, or 100 to 200 U/kg every 24 hours by IV infusion. Current recommendations are to use low-dose continuous infusion heparin for patients with the more chronic form of DIC (5–15 U/kg per hour).[7, 92, 164] Effective heparin therapy produces cessation of clot formation, a rise in platelet count and fibrinogen levels, and a decrease in the level of FDPs. PTT is monitored to assess the patient's response to heparin. A therapeutic level is reached when the patient's PTT is 1.5 to 2 times the normal level. Heparin is contraindicated in patients with any intracranial insult such as bleeding or CVA. It is also avoided in patients who have had recent surgery.[53, 54]

Failure to respond to heparin therapy has been attributed to a depletion of *antithrombin III* (AT-III). AT-III is a blood component factor that inhibits the competitive action of thrombin during heparin therapy.[107] Therefore, in patients with low AT-III levels and no response to heparin therapy, AT-III may be administered along with heparin; however, this form of therapy is not yet considered standard of care.[16, 131]

Finally, in addition to the control of clotting, medical attention is given to the control of bleeding. Usually, heparin therapy produces anticoagulation and at the same time controls fibrinolysis. In 5% of patients, however, fibrinolysis continues and uncontrolled bleeding results. In these patients, *antifibrinolytic therapy* may be administered, using a drug called *ε-aminocaproic acid* (EACA). EACA interferes with the intrinsic fibrinolytic process, which can lead to further clot formation. Therefore EACA is used only when intravascular clotting is effectively controlled.[54] The usual dose is 5 to 10 g given IV by slow bolus followed by 2 to 4 g every 1 to 2 hours for 24 hours or until bleeding stops. Patients receiving EACA must be closely monitored for hypotension, hypokalemia, cardiac dysrhythmias, and increased intravascular coagulation. A newer more potent fibrinolytic inhibitor, tranexamic acid, has less toxicity than EACA and is sometimes used with APML.[16, 127] Both EACA and tranexamic acid are controversial because they can cause widespread fibrin deposition that can lead to ischemia and organ failure.[54] Gabexate mesylate is a synthetic inhibitor of serine proteases that include both thrombin and plasmin. Hirudin is a synthetic thrombin inhibitor. The application of these agents requires further study.[7, 16]

PROGNOSIS

The prognosis of the patient with DIC depends on the underlying cause, the degree of disruption of the coagulation system, and the effects of bleeding and clotting. Most patients with cancer who develop DIC experience hemorrhage. A smaller number demonstrate thromboembolism. The estimated mortality rate for DIC is 54% to 68%. Mortality from DIC has decreased in the past decade. This is attributed to new antileukemia agents, combinations of anticancer therapies, and advances in blood component therapies. Prognostic factors including increasing age, severity of laboratory abnormalities, and number of clinical manifestations, increase the mortality from DIC. In the patient with DIC, a minor injury can have a fatal consequence. The most common cause of death in DIC is intracranial hemorrhage.[164]

Nursing management of DIC is outlined in the accompanying box.

Nursing Management

DISSEMINATED INTRAVASCULAR COAGULATION

The nursing management of patients with disseminated intravascular coagulation (DIC), as in the condition itself, is extremely complex. Depending on the onset and severity of DIC, the nurse's role may vary from watchful waiting to intensive participation in treatment. Nursing care focuses on minimizing the multitude of potentially life-threatening problems associated with DIC. Therefore care must be directed toward astute and ongoing assessment to detect bleeding (overt or occult) or thrombosis, provision of care for bleeding and thrombosis, prevention of further complications, and support of other needs.

Nursing Diagnosis

- *Risk for injury (bleeding, thrombosis) related to fibrous clot formation in the microcirculation, clotting factor consumption and decreased platelets, fibrinolysis or clot dissolution*

Outcome Goal

Patient will be able to:

- Exhibit resolution of signs and symptoms of DIC, as evidenced by cessation of bleeding, return of hematologic values to normal range, return of coagulation and fibrinogen levels to normal, and absence of cyanosis to extremities.

Interventions: *Observation for Signs of Bleeding and Thrombosis*

- Assess organ systems for evidence of bleeding and thrombosis:
    Integumentary: observe skin for evidence of bleeding (petechiae, ecchymosis, purpura, pallor, frank blood, oozing). Closely examine the mouth, including the mucous membranes of the palate and gums; sclera; nose; ears; urethra; vagina; and rectum. Check all venipuncture and puncture sites and wound sites.
    Pulmonary: auscultate lungs for crackles, wheezes, and stridor. Observe for dyspnea, tachypnea, cyanosis, hemoptysis, and chest pain.
    Cardiovascular: monitor for tachycardia, hypotension, and changes in peripheral pulses. Assess for palpitations and angina.
    Renal: measure intake and output. Observe for peripheral edema and oliguria.
    Gastrointestinal: palpate abdomen for pain. Measure abdominal girth daily.
    Neurologic: observe for irritability or changes in mental status. Assess frequently for headache, blurred vision, and vertigo.
- Monitor vital signs (temperature, pulse, blood pressure, respirations) every 4 hours.
- Test all excreta (urine, stool, sputum, vomitus) for blood.
- Assess for fatigue, lethargy, muscle weakness, and pain.
- Monitor laboratory values closely for abnormalities indicative of bleeding or infection, including complete blood count (CBC), platelet count, prothrombin time (PT), and fibrinogen level.

Interventions: *Measures to Prevent Further Tissue Trauma*

- Prevent further bleeding.
- Prevent skin breakdown.

- Institute safety measures:
    Keep bed rails up at night.
    Pad bed rails and any sharp objects.
    Instruct patient to ambulate with assistance.
- Perform activities that decrease risk of bleeding:
    Provide adequate hydration and soft diet.
    Avoid administration of aspirin or products that contain aspirin.
    Discourage activities that increase intracranial pressure (ICP) or intra-abdominal pressure (Valsalva's maneuver).
    Administer stool softeners as ordered.
- Prevent further clotting:
    Provide adequate hydration.
    Avoid constrictive clothing and devices.
    Use prescribed elastic support hose.
    Discourage dangling of legs, sitting for long periods, and crossing legs.
    Elevate legs at intermittent intervals to prevent venous stasis when sitting or lying.
    Perform range-of-motion (ROM) exercises for legs.
    Encourage deep breathing and coughing.
    Administer heparin therapy as ordered using an infusion-controlling device.

Nursing Diagnosis

- *Impaired skin integrity*

Outcome Goals

Patient/family/caregiver will be able to:

- Describe measures to prevent further trauma to damaged skin.
- State signs and symptoms that must be reported to health care team.
- Ensure patient's skin heals without development of infection.
- Perform necessary treatments and procedures to promote skin integrity.

Interventions

- Observe skin and mucous membranes for changes in integrity, color, and moisture.
- Provide meticulous skin care and lubrication.
- Maintain skin and mucosal integrity:
    Limit venipunctures, and when necessary, use small-gauge needles.
    Avoid subcutaneous (SC) and intramuscular (IM) injections.
    Apply pressure to puncture sites for 5 minutes.
    Administer medications orally (PO) or intravenously (IV).

Avoid rectal manipulation (rectal suppositories, thermometers, digital examinations).

Use electric razors instead of straight-edged razors.

Avoid indwelling catheters, and when necessary, keep them well lubricated and without tension.

Avoid vaginal manipulation (tampons, douches).

Use paper tape instead of adhesive tape and remove gently.

Use Montgomery straps on wound dressings.

Suction with care.

- Perform frequent gentle oral hygiene:

Use soft-bristled toothbrush or sponge toothettes.

Avoid mouthwashes with high alcohol content.

Lubricate mucous membranes and lips.

Nursing Diagnoses

- *Fluid volume deficit related to bleeding*
- *Risk for fluid volume deficit related to bleeding*

Outcome Goal

- Patient's fluid balance will be restored, as evidenced by blood pressure and pulse within patient's normal range, lungs clear to auscultation, absence of neck vein distention, absence of edema, normal sodium and serum osmolality, and urine output within patient's normal range.

Interventions

- Observe for signs of active bleeding, hypocalcemia, and hypoxia (decreased blood pressure, tachypnea, tachycardia, restlessness, irritability, confusion, dizziness, decreased urine output).

- Measure intake and output.
- Administer fluids, blood, and blood products as ordered.

Nursing Diagnosis

- *Altered tissue perfusion (periphera, renal, gastrointestinal, cerebral, cardiopulmonary) related to bleeding, thrombosis*

Outcome Goal

Patient will be able to:

- Maintain adequate perfusion through critical period, as evidenced by absent or diminished bleeding, adequate urine output, maintenance of circulation, and adequate respiratory function.

Interventions

- Assess organ systems for malfunctions resulting from ischemia.
- Monitor laboratory values closely.
- Measure intake and output.
- Provide oxygen therapy as prescribed.
- Administer vasoactive drugs as ordered.
- Administer pain medications as ordered.

The management of a patient with DIC is complex and difficult. The experience is often terrifying for the patient and family and frustrating for the nurse. The patient's condition can change rapidly. Everyone must be alert to and prepared for all possible sequelae of DIC.

Data from references 54, 99, 120, and 164.

Hypercalcemia

DEFINITION

Hypercalcemia is a metabolic condition that occurs when the serum calcium level rises above the normal level of 9 to 11 mg/dL.[83] Hypercalcemia is a frequent complication of certain types of malignancies and metastatic disease. It is a potentially life-threatening problem because the onset is variable and may go unnoticed until the problem becomes severe. Lack of intervention can lead to renal failure, coma, or cardiac arrest.[73] With prompt recognition and adequate treatment, this condition can be reversed.

ETIOLOGY AND RISK FACTORS

A variety of conditions can cause hypercalcemia (Table 20–7), with 90% of hypercalcemia caused by primary hyperparathyroidism (65%) or malignancy (35%).* Hypercalcemia is one of the most common oncologic emergencies, occurring in 10% to 20% of oncology patients.[11, 80, 73, 83] Malignancies associated with this condition include cancers of the breast and kidneys; squamous cell cancers of the lung, head, neck, or esophagus; lymphoma; leukemia; and multiple myeloma. Solid tumors, lung cancer, and breast cancer account

---

*References 11, 27, 80, 83, 102, 124

TABLE 20-7
Causes of Hypercalcemia

ENDOCRINE DISORDERS
Primary hyperparathyroidism
Multiple endocrine adenomatosis
Familial hyperparathyroidism
Familial hypocalciuric hypercalcemia
Hyperthyroidism
Hypoadrenalism
Pheochromocytoma

MALIGNANCY
Humoral hypercalcemia of malignancy (HHM)
   Parathyroid hormone-related protein (PTHRP)
   1,25-dihydroxyvitamin D
   Transforming growth factor (TGF-α)
   Interleukin-1 (IL-1)
   Granulocyte-macrophage colony-stimulating factor (GM-CSF)
   Tumor necrosis factor (TNF-α and β)
   Prostaglandin E_2 (PGE$_2$)
   Interferon
Local osteolytic hypercalcemia (LOH)

MEDICATIONS
Thiazide diuretics
Theophylline
Lithium
Estrogens and antiestrogens

GRANULOMATOUS DISORDERS
Sarcoidosis
Tuberculosis
Coccidioidomycosis
Histoplasmosis
Beryliosis
Candidiasis
Cryptococcosis
Leprosy

IMMOBILIZATION

RENAL DISEASE

DIET
Milk-alkali syndrome
Vitamin A or D intoxication

OTHER
Paget's disease
Adolescence
Parenteral nutrition

Data from references 37, 80, 83, and 102.

for 80% of malignancy-related hypercalcemia. The remaining 20% include causes from multiple myeloma, leukemia, and lymphoma. Patients with metastatic cancers being treated with estrogens or antiestrogens may experience progression of hypercalcemia, possibly from hormonal stimulation of the tumor.[11, 83] Bony metastasis from any malignant primary tumor may also be a causative condition. Nonmalignant conditions that can induce or worsen hypercalcemia include primary hyperparathyroidism, thyrotoxicosis, prolonged immobilization, vitamin A and D intoxication, renal failure, and diuretic therapy with thiazide preparations. Dehydration, volume depletion, and hypoalbuminemia may contribute to or aggravate hypercalcemia.

PATHOPHYSIOLOGY

Calcium is an essential inorganic element in the body. Most of it (99%) is found in skeletal tissue, providing strength and durability. The remaining 1% is in the serum. One half of the serum calcium (0.5%) is ionized and one half (0.5%) is bound to circulating albumin. Serum calcium levels include both the ionized portion and the protein-bound portion. Under normal conditions the ionized calcium is in equilibrium with the protein-bound calcium. Changes in serum albumin level directly affect serum calcium levels.

Serum calcium levels in the presence of hypoalbuminemia may not be representative of the true value for ionized calcium. Reduction of serum albumin, which is often seen in very ill patients or elderly patients, may result in a greater proportion of ionized calcium because of the unavailability of albumin for binding. Therefore the severity of hypercalcemia in a patient with hypoalbuminemia may be underestimated. Box 20–2 provides formulas to correct for decreased serum albumin. Only the ionized portion of calcium is capable of physiologic function. Calcium is responsible for bone and tooth formation, normal clotting mechanism, and cellular permeability. Calcium ion concentration regulates the contractility of the cardiac, smooth, and skeletal muscles and the excitability of nerve tissue.

Normal serum calcium levels are maintained in a state of equilibrium through a dynamic relationship among all three forms of calcium (stored, ionized, albu-

---

BOX 20-2

Calculation of Estimated Ionized Serum Calcium

Formulas to correct for changes in serum albumin concentrations (allow 0.8 mg/dL for each g/dL change in serum albumin):

1. Corrected serum calcium = measured total serum calcium value (mg/dL) + [4.0 − serum albumin value (g/dL)] × 0.8
2. Corrected serum calcium = measured total serum calcium value (mg/dL) − serum albumin value (g/dL) + 4.0

min bound), with a constant shifting from one form to another. Homeostasis is maintained through several body processes: GI calcium absorption, renal calcium reabsorption, and a balance of bone resorption of calcium and deposition of calcium through new bone formation. A balance is maintained between osteoclast (bone resorption) and osteoblast (bone formation) activity.[11] Metabolism of calcium is controlled by a negative feedback mechanism between calcium ion concentration and three hormones: parathyroid hormone (PTH, parathormone), activated vitamin D (1,25-dihydroxyvitamin D), and calcitonin.

A decrease in serum calcium stimulates an increase in PTH secretion (Fig. 20–11). PTH enhances calcium absorption from the GI tract and renal tubular reabsorption of calcium with increased excretion of phosphorus. Calcium ions and phosphorus ions have a directly inverse relationship: when the amount of one is increased, the amount of the other is decreased. PTH also promotes osteoclastic activity. *Osteoclasts* are multinucleated bone cells that function to remove damaged bone tissue. This results in the destruction of bones, releasing calcium into the bloodstream.

Vitamin D is activated by PTH and increases calcium absorption from the GI mucosa. Calcitonin is released by the thyroid gland in response to an increased serum calcium level and inhibits bone resorption of calcium. The effect of calcitonin is short lived. In general, hypercalcemia is the result of increased bone resorption of calcium, which exceeds renal ability to excrete the calcium overload. Hypercalcemia resulting from malignancies occurs through several different mechanisms, depending on the location and action of the cancer cells, as follows:

- Direct bony destruction by tumor cells, which causes osteoclastic activity, resulting in the release of calcium from bone into the serum

- Prolonged immobilization, which increases osteoclastic activity
- Ectopic PTH production by tumor cells, which enhances calcium resorption; secretion continues despite an elevated serum calcium level
- Metabolic substances produced by the tumor, such as osteoclast-activating factor (OAF), prostaglandin, or prostaglandin-like substances, all of which enhance osteoclastic activity
- Other contributing conditions include the following:

  Dehydration or volume depletion or both
  Hypervitaminosis of A and D (excessive use of vitamin A and D supplements)
  Excessive use of calcium supplements
  Hyperparathyroidism
  Prolonged use of thiazide diuretics

Historically, malignancy-related hypercalcemia has been closely associated with tumor invasion into the bone by direct tumor extension or metastasis. However, 15% of hypercalcemia in malignancy occurs in patients without bony metastases.[73] SCLC and prostate cancer, even though they commonly metastasize to the bone, are not frequently associated with hypercalcemia.[80] For these reasons, researchers continued investigating the pathophysiology of hypercalcemia in malignancy. The skeletal process, *local osteolytic hypercalcemia* (LOH), is no longer considered the most common mechanism of hypercalcemia. Approximately 80% of hypercalcemic malignancies have been found to be caused by humoral factors associated with the presence of malignant cells.[73] One of these, PTH-related peptide (PTHrP), is produced ectopically by malignant cells and is responsible for 80% to 90% of hypercalcemia of malignancy.[83] The humoral agents have a normal physiologic function in the body but can be induced by and released from malignant cells. They cause hypercalcemia by stimulating osteoclastic activity and bone resorption, inhibiting bone

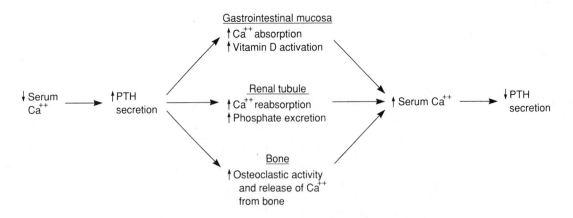

FIGURE 20–11 Effects of parathyroid hormone (*PTH*) on serum calcium levels.

formation, and increasing the renal tubular reabsorption of calcium. The various humoral factors are thought to act synergistically. In addition to PTH-rP, humoral factors associated with hypercalcemia include OAFs, transforming growth factors (TGFs), hematopoietic colony-stimulating factors (CSFs), prostaglandins (E series), and 1,25-dihydroxyvitamin D.[11, 73, 83]

CLINICAL FEATURES

Hypercalcemia disrupts normal cellular functions and adversely affects various organs. Clinical manifestations vary tremendously, depending on the level of serum calcium, the rate of onset, the underlying cause, and the patient's general condition. Patients may be asymptomatic, mildly symptomatic, or may have severe problems (Table 20–8). Onset may be insidious or acute. Diagnosis may be difficult because of multisystem involvement making it resemble other disorders, including side effect of chemotherapy and radiation therapy.

Signs and symptoms are directly related to cellular activity of the involved body system (see Table 20–8). Normal cell membranes are lined with calcium ions, which control the permeability of the cell. This gating mechanism allows sodium ions to enter the cell and depolarization to occur. Increased calcium ions decrease cellular permeability and subsequently alter cellular function. This decreases neuron permeability, resulting in a depressive effect on the CNS and peripheral nervous system (PNS).

CLINICAL FEATURES

Hypercalcemia

Clinical Signs[11, 27]

Lethargy
Change in mental status (restlessness, confusion, stupor, coma)
Vomiting
Dysrhythmias
Polyuria
ECG changes
Renal calculi
Renal failure

Symptoms

Anxiety
Fatigue and weakness
Anorexia
Nausea
Polydipsia
Constipation

Symptoms may include restlessness, agitation, lethargy, and confusion and may lead to coma. Skeletal muscles become hypotonic with decreased or absent deep tendon reflexes, ataxia, and fatigue. The smooth muscle action of the GI system slows, leading to decreased motility, anorexia, nausea, vomiting, constipa-

TABLE 20–8
Degrees of Hypercalcemia: Signs and Symptoms*

Body System Affected	Mild (<12 mg/dL)	Moderate (12–15 mg/dL)	Severe (>15 mg/dL)
Gastrointestinal	Anorexia, nausea, vomiting, vague abdominal pain	Constipation, increased abdominal pain, abdominal distention	Atonic ileus, obstipation
Neurologic	Restlessness, difficulty in concentrating, depression, apathy, lethargy, clouding of consciousness	Confusion, psychoses, somnolence	Coma, death
Muscular	Easily fatigued, muscle weakness (generalized or involving shoulders and hips), hyporeflexia	Increased muscular weakness, bone pain	Profound muscular weakness, ataxia, pathologic fractures
Renal	Nocturia, polyuria, polydipsia	Renal tubular acidosis, renal calculi	Oliguric renal failure, renal insufficiency, azotemia
Cardiovascular	Hypertension (may or may not be present)	Cardiac dysrhythmias, ECG abnormalities (shortening of QT interval on ECG, coving of ST-T wave, widening of T wave)	Cardiac arrest, death

Signs and symptoms regardless of serum calcium levels may vary from person to person.

From Poe CM, Radford AI: The challenges of hypercalcemia in cancer, *Oncol Nurs Forum* 12(6):29, 1985.

B O X   2 0 – 3

Definitions

Chvostek's sign—elicited by tapping the cheek below the temple near the facial nerve. Positive if lip or nose twitches.

Trousseau's sign—elicited by using a blood pressure cuff to occlude arterial flow in the arm for 1 to 5 minutes. Positive if the thumb adducts and the fingers extend.

Data from Stuckey LA: Acute tumor lysis syndrome: assessment and nursing implications, *Oncol Nurs Forum* 20:49, 1993.

tion, possible abdominal distention, and later, ileus. Impaired cardiac muscle conduction and contractility can result in dysrhythmias or even cardiac arrest.

Compensatory renal mechanisms increase urinary calcium reabsorption, leading to an inability to concentrate urine. This causes a syndrome similar to nephrogenic diabetes insipidus and is manifested by polyuria and polydipsia. The polyuria and hypercalciuria result in dehydration and a decrease in glomerular filtration rate (GFR). Dehydration from this event or from nausea and vomiting produces a further decline in the GFR of the kidney. The lowered GFR in turn increases reabsorption of sodium in the proximal tubules in an attempt to retain water. Because sodium and calcium work closely, calcium is also reabsorbed. This can further potentiate the hypercalcemia. Elevation of serum calcium levels produces a supersaturation of calcium and then precipitation. Precipitation in the kidneys can lead to calcium renal stones and possible renal failure, as evidenced by an elevated BUN and creatinine.

The clinical syndrome of hypercalcemia is complex because of the extreme variability in its manifestation of signs and symptoms. In addition, the symptomatology does not always correlate with serum calcium levels. These must be closely correlated with an in-depth history, physical examination, and laboratory profile. Because of its frequency in patients with cancer, hypercalcemia of malignancy should be one of the first differential diagnoses in patients who develop a change in mental status. Box 20–3 defines the Chvostek and Trousseau signs.

DIAGNOSIS

The diagnostic work-up for hypercalcemia begins with laboratory determination of the serum calcium level. Normal values are 9 to 11 mg/dL. Ionized serum calcium levels provide the most accurate values when albumin levels are below normal. If ionized levels are unavailable, the serum calcium and albumin levels can be used to calculate the ionized calcium (see Box 20–2).

Urinary calcium may also be measured. Hypercalciuria may be detected before an elevation in serum calcium. Other serum laboratory testing should include phosphorus, alkaline phosphatase, BUN, creatinine, electrolytes, and PTH. Patients with no bony involvement (e.g., squamous cell cancer of the head and neck) and whose tumor is producing PTH-like substances may have a normal serum phosphorus level. Hypercalcemia resulting from direct bony involvement (e.g., breast cancer, myeloma, renal cell carcinoma) often results in increased serum phosphorus levels.[9, 11] Furthermore, within this subset of patients, only those with breast cancer and bone metastasis usually have an elevated alkaline phosphatase.[9, 11] Serum albumin should be tested, because patients may be more hypercalcemic than serum levels indicate as a result of hypoalbuminemia, as discussed earlier.

Radiographic examinations can be helpful in differential diagnosis. A chest x-ray film may suggest tumor, sarcoidosis, or bony changes associated with hyperparathyroidism. Plain x-ray film or a radioisotope bone scan may demonstrate bone metastases or multiple myeloma. ECGs may show tachycardia, increased PR segment, shortened QT interval, and widening of the T wave. However, these changes may be subtle and difficult to detect.

TREATMENT MODALITIES

Decisions concerning whether and how to treat hypercalcemia caused by malignancy depend on the clinical situation. The degree of serum calcium elevation, the symptomatology, the patient's condition, and the ability to treat the underlying disease are determining factors in the decision-making process. Untreated cancer-induced hypercalcemia is typically progressive, and death is usually inevitable. Death from hypercalcemia may be a reasonable way to die for the patient with advanced cancer, because most people become comatose and do not experience pain. However, death may not be rapid, and unpleasant symptoms (anorexia, nausea, vomiting, sedation, confusion) may occur. Patients with advanced disease must be evaluated carefully. Although the only effective long-term treatment for hypercalcemia is antineoplastic therapy directed at the underlying malignancy, very potent, well-tolerated therapies now exist to readily correct hypercalcemia. If quality of life will not be improved, the decision may be to provide no treatment. When a decision is made to treat the hypercalcemia, the medical treatment is based on two principles: reduction of bone resorption of calcium and promotion of urinary excretion of calcium.[11]

Urgency of treatment is based on the degree of serum elevation and whether the patient is symptomatic. In general, a corrected serum calcium level greater than 13 to 14 mg/dL requires immediate intervention, regardless of symptoms. Asymptomatic patients with calcium levels between 12 and 13 mg/dL may be treated more conservatively. Symptomatic patients require intervention, regardless of the calcium level.

Hydration and Diuresis

Adequate hydration is usually the primary treatment for hypercalcemia and may be all that is needed for mild hypercalcemia. Increase fluids orally and intravenously rehydrate the patient and dilute the urine, which prevents supersaturation with calcium ions. Large volumes of isotonic saline restore plasma volume and promote urinary calcium excretion through sodium diuresis. Calcium loss follows sodium loss. Fluid volume in the range of about 5 to 8 liters daily is common for the first 24 hours, followed by 3 liters daily thereafter. Infusions of large volumes of fluids may necessitate CVP monitoring to avoid fluid overload. Accurate recordings of intake, output, and weight and laboratory studies should be done to prevent hyponatremia, hypomagnesemia, and hypokalemia.

Once the patient is rehydrated, loop diuretics (furosemide/Lasix and ethacrynic acid/Edecrin) are sometimes used to enhance the excretion of calcium. However, they must be used with caution and careful monitoring because extracellular fluid loss may exacerbate hypercalcemia by causing the reabsorption of calcium instead of the desired effect. Loop diuretics may also exacerbate serum depletion of magnesium and potassium.[83] During diuresis, serum levels of potassium and magnesium should be monitored closely and cardiac medication given cautiously. Thiazide diuretics are to be avoided because they decrease renal excretion of calcium.[73]

Pharmacologic Therapy

Biphosphonates are compounds that are selectively concentrated in bone and inhibit the action of osteoclasts. *Pamidronate,* a second-generation biphosphonate, has become first-line therapy for moderate to severe hypercalcemia.* Doses range from 60 to 90 mg and may be administered in 250 mL normal saline over 2 hours.[37] Reduction of serum calcium levels is seen in 24 to 48 hours with a peak effect in 7 days.[60] The infusion may be repeated weekly if needed to maintain normocalcemia until definitive treatment for the underlying malignancy is effective. The most common side effects include flu-like syndrome (managed with acetamenophen) and venous irritation (if peripheral IV route is used). Other side effects can include nausea, anorexia, taste alterations, and decreased serum phosphate, potassium, and magnesium.[83] Pamidronate may be used in combination with calcitonin.[106] Calcitonin has a more rapid onset of action (4–6 hours), but the inhibition of bone resorption is not long lasting. A usual dose is 4 IU/kg intramuscularly or subcutaneously every 12 hours.[112] As with pamidronate, one benefit of calcitonin is its safety in patients with renal failure. By using them together, there is a rapid initial drop in serum calcium levels from the calcitonin that is then maintained by the pamidronate.

Pamidronate has also demonstrated efficacy in the prevention of skeletal complication from bone metastases, including bone pain, pathologic fractures requiring radiation therapy or surgery, and spinal cord compression.[11, 15, 60, 80, 83, 102] For this indication, pamidronate is administered at 90 mg over 2 hours every 3 to 4 weeks.

Prior to the availability of pamidronate, *etidronate* (Didronel) had shown efficacy in more than 80% of patients with cancer-induced hypercalcemia. Lowered serum calcium was seen in 3 to 5 days after a regimen of 7.5 mg/kg per day IV for 4 to 5 days. The daily dose of etidronate is diluted in 250 mL normal saline and administered over at least 2 hours. IV administration can be followed with oral doses of 20 mg/kg per day for 7 to 10 days, which may be continued for up to 3 months.[112] Etidronate is contraindicated in patients with a serum creatinine level greater than 5 or those with renal failure. Hyperphosphatemia may result from etidronate therapy.[9]

Several third-generation biphosphonates are currently being investigated. Some of these include risedronate, ibandronate, and zoledronate. Early indications are that they may be more potent than the second-generation drugs.[119]

Gallium nitrate (gallium) is an antineoplastic agent noted to have hypocalcemic effects by directly inhibiting bone resorption without causing toxicity to bone cells. It is a very potent antihypercalcemic agent, but it must be administered over 24 hours daily for 5 days at a dose of 100 to 200 mg/m^2 mixed in 1 liter 0.9% normal saline or 5% dextrose in water. Adequate hydration must be maintained throughout the treatment period. Nephrotoxicity is the major side effect of gallium nitrate. The requirement of continuous infusion potentially limits its usefulness, especially in the outpatient setting.[9]

The use of *oral phosphates* is somewhat limited. It has been shown that patients with renal failure or serum phosphorus levels greater than 3.8 mg/L will not benefit from the use of phosphates. However, patients with low serum phosphorus levels may benefit from oral phosphorus administered in doses of 0.5 g four times a day. The mechanism of action, although uncertain, appears

---

*References 11, 36, 60, 80, 83, 102, 124

to be the reduction of bone resorption of calcium and impairment of the absorption of calcium from the intestine. Diarrhea, which can result at these high oral doses, may hamper the use of oral phosphorus. Large IV doses may cause precipitation of calcium in the heart, lung, or soft tissues, which can lead to renal failure; therefore, they are rarely indicated.

Glucocorticoids have been used to treat hypercalcemia associated with breast cancer, myeloma, and lymphoma. Prednisone, 40 to 60 mg/d, has been given. Glucocorticoids block bone resorption, increase calcium excretion, and decrease GI absorption.[73] Steroids may have some direct effect on the tumor itself, but the exact mechanism is unknown. Increasing the dose of the steroids does not increase their effectiveness. The effect of steroids may be delayed by a week. If used, they may be combined with calcitonin due to its more rapid effect on calcium levels. Chronic use of glucocorticoids enhances immunosuppression, which can result in osteolytic activity. Steroids are not recommended for long-term maintenance in view of the possible toxicities associated with chronic administration.[9]

Nonsteroidal anti-inflammatory drugs (NSAIDs) such as indomethacin (Indocin) or aspirin appear to inhibit prostaglandin synthesis and thus mediate bone resorption. Although their role in treating hypercalcemia is minor, they may be of value in patients with refractory hypercalcemia who are unable to tolerate other agents or if NSAIDs are part of a regimen for cancer pain control.[9] The usual dose of indomethacin is 75 to 100 mg/d in divided doses. Gastric upset is a frequent side effect of this drug. They are rarely used today.

Cisplatin, a widely used antineoplastic agent with a broad spectrum of antitumor activity, has demonstrated efficacy in reducing serum calcium levels. The calcium-lowering effect was delayed (10 days) and prolonged (mean duration: 38 days) and independent of antitumor activity because the decrease in calcium levels occurred in patients who experienced no tumor regression. The toxicities (GI, renal, neurologic) associated with cisplatin limit its consideration for antihypercalcemic therapy.[9]

Plicamycin (mithramycin) has calcium-lowering effects that may not appear for 24 to 48 hours. The usual dosage is a slow infusion of 15 to 25 μg/kg per day. Disadvantages of plicamycin are venous irritation, myelosuppressive effects, liver toxicity, and potential danger in patients with renal failure. The results are extremely unpredictable. It has been relegated to third-line therapy since the advent of pamidronate.[80]

Chemotherapy may be used to treat patients with underlying hematologic malignancies such as multiple myeloma or lymphoma. In patients with breast cancer, chemotherapy or hormonal therapy may produce a re-

mission. However, the initial use of hormonal therapy, especially tamoxifen (Nolvadex), may worsen the hypercalcemia. Some patients receiving hormonal therapy for breast cancer metastatic to the bone may experience episodes of increased serum calcium. This is often referred to as a "flare," which is indicative of tumor response to the hormone. These patients need to be monitored closely.

Part of the assessment in the treatment of increased serum calcium is to evaluate the other medications the patient is receiving. Many medications are known to precipitate hypercalcemia, such as estrogens, antiestrogens, thiazide diuretics, high doses of vitamin A and D, and calcium supplements. Whenever possible, these medications should be discontinued. However, it is not always necessary to stop antiestrogens in patients receiving them for treatment of cancer. Tumor flare, a temporary increase in tumor growth after initiating antiestrogens, is typically self-limiting. Temporary discontinuation of the antiestrogen and treatment with pamidronate is based on the degree of serum elevation and symptoms.[11, 83] Patients on digitalis must be carefully monitored because aggressive therapy for hypercalcemia can significantly lower potassium and magnesium levels, placing the digitalized patient at increased risk for dysrhytmias.[73] Table 20–9 outlines medications used to treat hypercalcemia.

Mobilization

Immobilization should be avoided because it will increase resorption of calcium from the bones. Activity should be appropriate for the patient's physical condition. Weight bearing through standing and ambulation produces physical stress at the ends of long bones, resulting in osteoblastic activity. Osteoblasts synthesize the collagen and glycoproteins to form a matrix and develop into osteocytes, which are mature bone cells. Muscle activity produces acid end-products needed to assist in the production of acid urine. Physical therapy may be helpful to establish a program of active exercises with resistance. A pain management program may be necessary to support activities.

Dietary Manipulation

Dietary intake of calcium has very little role in the hypercalcemia of malignancy. Patients with cancer typically have reduced GI absorption of calcium so dietary restriction is unfounded.[73] The only exception to this is in patients with elevated levels of 1,25-dihydroxyvitamin D (lymphoma), which enhances intestinal calcium absorption.

TABLE 20-9
Medications to Treat Hypercalcemia

Medication	Mode of Action	Dose	Toxicity	Comments
Furosemide	Blocks reabsorption of calcium at loop of Henle	80–100 mg q 1–2 h	Dehydration Electrolyte loss	May need CVP monitoring Only given after patient is rehydrated
Pamidronate	Biphosphonate inhibits osteoclast activity	60–90 mg in 250 mL over 2 h	Flulike syndrome Nausea Phlebitis	First-line therapy after hydration
Zoledronic acid (Zometa)	Biphosphonate inhibits osteoclast activity	4–8 mg in 30 mL over 15 min	Skeletal pain	First-line therapy after hydration
Etidronate	Biphosphonate	7.5 mg/kg/d in 250 mL or more over 2–3 h, then 20 mg/kg/d PO for 30 d	Nausea, vomiting Taste changes	Contraindicated in renal failure
Gallium nitrate	Inhibits bone resorption	100–200 mg/m^2/d × 5 d	Renal toxicity	Contraindicated in decreased renal function
Calcitonin	Inhibits bone resorption Increases urinary excretion	4 IU/kg q 12 h, may increase to 8 IU/kg	Nausea, vomiting Rash	Short-lived effectiveness Used in combination with pamidronate or glucocorticoids
Prednisone	Inhibits bone resorption Decreases GI absorption	40–100 mg/d IV	Hyperglycemia Na and H_2O retention	Used primarily for hematologic and breast cancers
Phosphates	Prevents GI absorption Inhibits bone resorption	0.5–3 g/d PO	Diarrhea	Used to correct hypophosphatemia
Plicamycin	Kills osteoclasts	15–25 μg/kg over 4–6 h × 3 d	Marrow suppression Hepatic toxicity Renal toxicity Nausea, vomiting	Unpredictable response Third-line agent, rarely used

Data from references 11, 60, 119, and 124.

Dialysis

Patients who are in renal failure secondary to hypercalcemia but who have a relatively good prognosis with their malignancy could benefit from renal dialysis. Saline diuresis is precluded in these patients so that dialysis will remove both excess calcium and phosphate. Serum phosphate levels should be measured and phosphates replaced as necessary.

PROGNOSIS

Cancer-induced hypercalcemia is a common complication of certain cancers and has the potential to be life-threatening. Clinical manifestations and onset vary greatly, but the course is usually progressive and can worsen quickly. Hypercalcemia is reversible in 80% of episodes if it is recognized and prompt aggressive therapy initiated. It has been shown that the more severe the hypercalcemia, the poorer the prognosis, and vice versa. Without prompt treatment, it is associated with a 50% mortality rate.[73] After the diagnosis of hypercalcemia, median survival is 3 months.[80] No treatment of hypercalcemia alone, with the possible exception of pamidronate has been demonstrated to improve the increased mortality rate associated with this complication.[80, 102, 119]

Nursing management of the patient with hypercalcemia is outlined in the accompanying box.

Nursing Management

HYPERCALCEMIA

Nursing care of the patient with hypercalcemia is directed at early detection and support through treatment. A thorough nursing assessment should include a history of the patient's cancer and cancer treatment and a review of all medications. Drugs that may cause or potentiate hypercalcemia, such as lithium carbonate, thiazide diuretics, vitamins A and D, and large doses of calcium supplements, should be reported and discontinued. Drugs whose action may be altered by high serum calcium, such as digitalis and some antihypertensive agents, should also be noted. Physical examination results should be correlated with potential symptomatology of hypercalcemia. This is often difficult because of the varying possibilities and degrees of clinical manifestations. However, the initial assessment will dictate the intensity of nursing care.

Nursing Diagnoses

- *Fluid volume deficit related to effects of the disease (impending renal failure with increased polyuria; fluid loss related to nausea and vomiting), effects of treatment (increased urine output secondary to diuretic therapy; fluid loss related to diarrhea)*
- *Fluid volume excess related to effects of treatment (hydration)*

Outcome Goals

Patient/family/caregiver will be able to:

- Demonstrate knowledge related to hypercalcemia.
- Identify signs and symptoms.
- Identify factors that influence serum calcium levels.
- Identify potential complications.
- Achieve serum calcium level within normal limits.
- Achieve fluid balance, as evidenced by adequate hydration and elimination status, diminished or absent nausea and vomiting, and vital signs and body weight within patient's normal range.

Interventions

- Assess for signs and symptoms of alterations in fluid volume:
    Excess: rales, shortness of breath, neck vein distention, weight gain, edema of sacrum and lower extremities
    Deficit: dry mucous membranes, poor skin turgor, weight loss, rapid thready pulse, orthostatic hypotension, restlessness
- Auscultate lungs for breath sounds every 4 hours.

- Monitor intake and output closely:
    Encourage oral fluids.
    Maintain IV fluids per physician orders (usually saline, 6–8 L/d).
    Monitor IV infusions carefully using flow regulator.
    Accurately measure urine output (maintain output at least at 50 mL/h).
- Obtain daily weight.
- Monitor laboratory values (serum BUN, creatinine, sodium, potassium).
- Administer diuretics as ordered. Thiazide diuretics are contraindicated because they inhibit urinary excretion of calcium and therefore may potentiate hypercalcemia.
- Obtain urine pH. An acidic urine should be maintained to prevent calcium precipitation, which can lead to renal calculi.

Nursing Diagnoses

- *Impaired physical mobility related to bone breakdown secondary to metastasis*
- *Risk for injury related to bone destruction*

Outcome Goals

Patient will be able to:

- Maintain activity and mobility appropriate to physical status.

Patient/family/caregiver will be able to:

- Identify/demonstrate measures to manage alteration in mobility.
- Demonstrate proper positioning and transfer techniques.
- Perform necessary treatments and procedures.
- Maintain good skin integrity and optimal level of physical activity.
- Identify signs and symptoms to report to health care team.

Interventions

- Assess patient for presence of spinal cord compression (signs and symptoms: pain, sensory loss or paresthesia, motor weakness or dysfunction, changes in patterns of elimination).
- Establish activity and exercise regimen according to patient's physical ability and physician orders:
    Change patient's position every 2 hours.
    Stand patient at bedside for short periods (several minutes) at least 4 to 6 times a day.

Use isometric exercises each hour while awake. Institute passive ROM exercises if patient is on bedrest.

- Provide a footboard for bedridden patients, and use a tilt table several times a day.
- Check for evidence of venous thrombosis in lower extremities caused by immobilization (redness, swelling, warmth, positive Homans' sign, pain, dorsiflexion).
- Monitor skin integrity and provide skin care.
- Promote and assist with regulation of elimination.
- Provide pain control as needed.
- Consult with physical therapy and occupational therapy for evaluation and assistance.
- Discuss and teach the use of assistive and supportive devices as needed.
- Use safety precautions:

    Move patients with care (use lift sheets and support joints).

    Assist patient with transfer and ambulation as needed.

    Place all articles within patient's reach.

    Pad bed rails.

    Modify bed surface with approved pressure-reducing mattress.

    Use bed rails at night.

    Closely monitor restless, anxious, or confused patients.

    Use restraints as necessary.

Nursing Diagnosis

- *Altered thought processes related to hypercalcemia*

Outcome Goals

Patient will be able to:

- Remain orientated to person, place, and time.
- Maintain mental and psychologic function at optimal level.

Interventions

- Assess level of consciousness and check for changes in mentation and behavior.
- Closely observe for restlessness or anxiety.
- Orient patient frequently to time and place.
- Allow time for verbalization of feelings regarding condition.
- Teach patient and family about changes caused by hypercalcemia, potential for its recurrence, and appropriate measures to be taken.

Nursing Diagnosis

- *Decreased cardiac output related to changes in serum calcium and electrolytes*

Outcome Goal

Patient will be able to:

- Maintain adequate fluid volume, as evidenced by serum electrolytes and serum calcium within patient's normal limits, vital signs and body weight within patient's normal limits, and return of cardiac function to patient's optimal level.

Interventions

- Assess for changes in cardiac function:

    Monitor for presence of dysrhythmias, bradycardia, and tachycardia.

    Observe ECG for shortened QT intervals or prolonged PR intervals.

    Obtain pulse and blood pressure every 4 hours.
- Monitor serum calcium and electrolytes.
- Administer oral potassium as ordered (hypokalemia frequently occurs in the presence of hypercalcemia).
- Monitor effects of digitalis and digoxin, if given to patient, because hypercalcemia potentiates their action. The dose is usually reduced in the presence of hypercalcemia.

Nursing Diagnosis

- *Diarrhea related to treatment for hypercalcemia*

Outcome Goal

Patient will be able to:

- Demonstrate regular and normal pattern of elimination, as evidenced by stools of normal frequency and consistency, normal bowel sounds, absence or minimal abdominal pain and cramping, and absence or minimal skin breakdown.

Interventions

- Monitor status of bowel elimination daily (color, texture, frequency of stools).
- Assess the abdomen daily:

    Observe for distention.

    Auscultate for the presence of bowel sounds.

    Palpate to determine any painful areas.
- Provide perianal hygiene and skin care, and use anesthesia and lubricants as ordered.
- Monitor perianal skin integrity.
- Avoid administration of antidiarrheal agents, because calcium is excreted via stool.
- Provide explanation of diarrhea to patient and family.

Hypercalcemia is one of the most common oncologic problems seen in patients with cancer. Therefore nurses practicing in all areas of cancer care should be educated regarding this problem. Nursing assessment of patients with cancer, especially those cancers typically associated with hypercalcemia (breast, lung, head and neck, lymphoma, myeloma, bony metastases), should focus on the potential manifestations of this problem.

Hypersensitivity Reaction to Antineoplastic Agents

DEFINITION

Severe hypersensitivity reactions (HSRs), or anaphylaxis, is defined as a life-threatening immunologic response to a foreign substance or antigen. Antineoplastic agents, like other drugs, may be recognized by the body's immune system as "not-self." This may initiate a type I reaction, characterized by the release of histamine and other inflammatory mediators that induce the symptoms of an anaphylactic reaction such as respiratory distress and cardiovascular failure.

ETIOLOGY AND RISK FACTORS

Risk factors associated with an increased incidence of HSR include age, gender, genetic makeup, nutritional status, stress level, and hormonal and environmental factors.[81, 86] Additional risk factors include the route of administration (IV versus oral, topical, or intramuscular), duration of administration (IV push versus slow infusion), and the immunologic characteristics of the drug.[33] The nitrosoureas (carmustine, lomustine) are the only class of antineoplastic agents that has never been documented to induce a HSR. One agent in the antitumor antibiotic class, dactinomycin, has yet to be noted in a HSR.[153] Increased risk of HSR is known to occur with drugs that are proteins, such as L-asparaginase (up to 33%); drugs prepared in antigenic diluents, as are the taxanes and podiphyllotoxins; as well as heavy metal compounds like cisplatin and carboplatin (Table 20–10).

PATHOPHYSIOLOGY

The Gell and Coombs classification includes four categories of immunologic reactions (Table 20–11). Most antineoplastic HSRs are thought to be type I reactions. However, there have been case reports of types II, III, and IV as well.[81]

Type I reactions occur in three phases. In the first phase, *sensitization,* the patient is exposed to the foreign substance or antigen, in this case the antineoplastic agent. This exposure causes the formation of specific IgE antibodies that attach to the receptors on basophils and mast cells. Once the patient receives the second exposure to the antigen, called the *activation phase,* the antigen attaches to the IgE molecules on the mast cell surfaces. An influx of calcium into the cells induces the mast cells to degranulate. This results in the release of pre-formed chemical mediators (histamine, heparin,

---

TABLE 20–10
Antineoplastic Agents Associated with HSR[33, 81, 154]

High Risk	Moderate Risk	Low Risk
L-Asparaginase	Anthracyclines	Cytosine arabinoside
Doxetaxel	Bleomycin	Cyclophosphamide
Paclitaxel	Carboplatin	Chlorambucil
Procarbazine	Cisplatin	Dacarbazine
Teniposide	Etoposide	5-Fluorouracil
Rituximab	Melphalan	Ifosfamide
	Methotrexate	Mitoxantrone
	Herceptin	Aldesleukin
		Gemcitabine
		Hydroxyurea
		Interferons
		Mechlorethamine
		6-Mercaptopurine
		Mitomycin
		Pentostatin
		Pegaspargase
		Vinca alkaloids

From Weiss RB: Miscellaneous toxicities. In DeVita VT Jr, Hellman S, Rosenberg SA, editors: Cancer: principles and practice of oncology, ed 5, Philadelphia, Lippincott-Raven, 1997:2804.

TABLE 20-11
Hypersensitivity Reaction Classifications

Type	Mechanisms	Sign/Symptoms	Examples
I. Anaphylactic or anaphylactoid	Antigen-antibody reaction. Mediator release from basophils and mast cells. Direct binding of antigen to mast cells. IgE antibody.	Urticaria, bronchospasm, hypotension, angioedema cramping, respiratory and cardiovascular collapse	Anaphylaxis to medication, bee stings, food
II. Cytotoxic	Antibody binding to cell surface. IgM and IgG antibodies.	Hemolysis	Hemolytic anemia, hemolysis from transfusion
III. Immune complex mediated	Immune complex formation by antigen–antibody interaction, or anaphylactoid reaction from complement activation	Tissue injury/manifestations depending on location of sickness, immune complex deposits	Systemic lupus, rheumatoid arthritis, horse serum Arthus reaction
IV. Cell-mediated (delayed hypersensitivity)	Sensitized T lymphocytes interact with antigen and release lymphokines	Mucositis, pneumonitis, contact dermatitis, granulomas, homograft rejection	Tuberculosis, poison ivy, granulomas, mechlorethamine sensitivity from topical application

Data from references 33, 51, and 81.

chondroitin sulfate, chemotactins) into the surrounding tissue and serum. Newly formed mediators are also released. These include prostaglandins and leukotrienes (also called SRSA—slow-reacting substances of anaphylaxis).[81]

Histamine release stimulates H1 and H2 receptors (located in the myocardium, vessel walls, and smooth muscle lining of the lung, ureters, bladder, and GI tract) that are responsible for many of the clinical features described below (Table 20–12). The final phase of the HSR, *effector,* involves the immediate neuromuscular and vascular responses seen in the organs targeted by the chemical mediators. Mast cells are concentrated in the skin, vasculature, connective tissue, and GI tract.

L-*Asparaginase* has been associated with the highest risk of HSR.[153] Incidence has been documented in up to 35% of cases with the overall risk of 5% to 8% per dose. Incidence may increase up to 33% after the fourth dose.[153] Reactions occur more frequently with significant time lapse between treatments (weekly or monthly versus daily during clinical trials).[153] L-Asparaginase is a polypeptide of bacterial origin. It is derived from *Escherichia coli.* Since the development of L-asparaginase, a substitute derived from *Erwinia chrysanthemia* (a plant pathogen) has been created. It has been the accepted substitute for L-asparaginase for more than 20 years.[153] Most recently, pegaspargase (Oncaspar, Enzon) has been made available and approved by the Food and Drug Administration. Pegaspargase is prepared from *E. coli* asparaginase, but is delivered in strands of polyethylene glycol (PEG) that allow it to escape detection by the immune system and a longer circulation time.[2, 3]

Cisplatin may be associated with an increased incidence of HSRs after prolonged use. Some studies indicated significant HSR occurrence with six or more doses. Incidence was more pronounced during early clinical trials prior to the advent of pre-medication with corticosteroids and antiemetics. The highest rate of reactions has been documented with multiple dose intravesicular administration for bladder cancer (10%–25%).[153] *Carboplatin* has rarely been associated with HSRs (reports of approximately 40 cases).[151] However, recent evidence indicates HSRs develop in patients treated repeatedly with the agent and may increase in frequency as carboplatin becomes more extensively used to treat malignancies.[93]

Bleomycin-related life-threatening events may actually be due to a massive release of endogenous human leukocyte pyrogens from the white blood cells as opposed to a true HSR. It has been customary to administer a small test dose of bleomycin and observe the patient for reactions, prior to administering the full prescribed dose.[33] However, practice patterns are now moving away from the test dose while maintaining close observation of the patient for signs of HSR. Risk may be increased for patients with lymphoma or those receiving IV administration.[33]

TABLE 20-12
Chemical Mediator Manifestations

Histamine	Heparin	Chondroitin Sulfate	Chemotactin	Prostaglandin	Leukotriene
H1 RECEPTOR	Coagulopathies	Edema	Eosinophilia	Vasodilatation	Vasodilatation
Pruritis		Pruritis	Neutrophilia	Smooth	Bronchoconstriction
Vasodilatation		Hypotension	Platelet aggregation	muscle	Mucus production
Smooth muscle		Bronchoconstriction		contraction	Hypotension
contraction		Vascular permeability		Viscous	Platelet
Vascular permeability		Smooth muscle		mucus	aggregation
Coronary artery		contraction		production	
vasospasm		Nerve fiber		Hypotension	
Vagal nerve irritation		stimulation		Platelet	
Increased mucus				aggregation	
viscosity					
Bronchospasm					
Edema					
Hypotension					
Tachycardia					
H2 RECEPTOR					
Increased heart					
contractility					
Increased heart rate					
Vasodilatation					
Goblet cell/bronchial					
gland mucus					
secretion					

Data from Craig JB, Capizzi RL: The prevention and treatment of immediate hypersensitivity reactions from cancer chemotherapy, Semin Oncol Nurs *1:285, 1985; and Gell PHG, Coombs RRA:* Clinical aspects of immunology, *Oxford, Blackwell Scientific Publications, 1975.*

Biologicals as an entire group are not commonly associated with HSRs. However the monoclonal antibodies (MoAbs) are conjugated from murine cells and are known to cause HSRs. Patients receiving interleukin (IL)-2 therapy may develop an increased sensitivity to radiologic contrast dye as well as to other antineoplastic agents, such as cisplatin.[156]

Procarbazine and *methotrexate* have induced interstitial pneumonitis and vasculitis, typical of a type III reaction.[154]

A significant number of HSRs related to antineoplastic agents are considered to be anaphylactoid instead of anaphylactic. *Anaphylactoid* reactions occur when the patient has not been previously exposed to the antigen. In these cases, the same mediators are released and the same clinical features are observed because the antigen binds directly to the mast cell surfaces inducing mediator release or triggers an uncontrolled activation of the complement cascade to produce inflammation and the immune response.[33, 81]

An example of an anaphylactoid HSR can occur with the administration of *paclitaxel* (Taxol). During clinical trials, up to 41% incidence of HSRs was seen.[115, 152] Further study indicated that paclitaxel was probably not the antigen. Taxol is prepared in a diluent made up of 50% dehydrated alcohol and 50% Cremaphor El.[115]

Cremaphor El is a polyoxyethylated castor oil vehicle that is known to induce HSRs (also seen in tenoposide, vitamin K, and cyclosporine).[122] Paclitaxel-related HSRs have been significantly reduced (1%-3%) with the advent of appropriate pre-medication.[122] Table 20-13 lists a standard regimen for paclitaxel premedication. Recent research has shown that IV dexamethasone 30 minutes before paclitaxel administration is just as efficacious as the oral regimen used previously (20 mg orally 12 hours and 6 hours prior to paclitaxel).[20, 93, 100]

Doxetaxel (Taxotere), an analogue to paclitaxel, has been associated with less incidence of HSRs; however, they do occur.[149] Doxetaxel is prepared in polysorbate

TABLE 20-13
Premedication Regimen for Paclitaxel Infusion

Coricosteroid	dexamethasone, 20 mg IV
H1 antagonist	diphenhydramine, 50 mg IV
H2 antagonist	cimetidine, 300 mg IV *or*
	ranitidine, 150 mg IV *or*
	famotidine, 20 mg IV

Data from references 20, 81, 93, and 110.

80 (Tween 80). Standard pre-medication consists of oral dexamethasone the day before, the day of, and the day following treatment. In this instance, premedication is given primarily to prevent fluid retention as opposed to prevention of HSR. Alterations in the premedication regime are made when the drug is given in low weekly doses.

CLINICAL FEATURES

The signs and symptoms from an antineoplastic-related HSR typically occur within minutes of initiating the agent IV and peak within 15 to 30 minutes.[6] Reactions to oral agents may take 2 hours. Reactions may be further delayed up to several hours depending on drug metabolism.[82] Once interventions wear off, recurrence of the HSR may be seen up to 8 to 24 hours later.

The most common effects include dyspnea, agitation, and hypotension. The patient may complain of a feeling of heat, chest or back pain, and trouble breathing. A more complete list of clinical features is listed in the Table 20–14.

The most common cause of death is asphyxiation secondary to laryngeal edema and spasm and can occur within minutes.[33, 81] Cardiovascular collapse and shock can occur without any cutaneous or respiratory symptoms.[81]

DIAGNOSIS

The diagnosis of antineoplastic-related HSR is made primarily by clinical assessment of the patient. Signs and symptoms of HSR typically occur within minutes of drug administration and are described above. Serum levels may be drawn to ascertain with certainty the evidence of a type I reaction, but are not commonly done. Plasma histamine levels may be detectable for 1 hour after

TABLE 20–14
Clinical Signs and Symptoms of HSR

Most Common	Less Common
Agitation	Nausea
Urticaria	Vomiting
Angioedema	Diarrhea
Upper airway edema	Abdominal cramping/bloating
Dyspnea	Rhinitis
Wheezing	Headache
Flushing	Substernal pain
Dizziness	Back pain
Hypotension	Seizure
	Sneezing
	Genital burning
	Metallic taste

Data from references 6, 33, 81, and 110.

symptoms occur. Urine histamine levels will remain elevated and can be detected in a 24-hour urine collection. Prostaglandin D_2 may also be measured in the urine and serum. Serum tryptase is also released from mast cells. These serum levels peak within 1 to 1.5 hours after the onset of symptoms and may remain elevated for up to 5 hours.[82, 86] Skin testing or the radioallergosorbent test (RAST) may also be used to evaluate hypersensitivity to a few specific drugs.[6, 81] Elevated cardiac enzymes and abnormal ECG readings may be seen from histamine-induced coronary artery vasospasm.[81]

A careful history must be taken to identify patients at high risk for HSR. History should include any prior exposure the agents to be administered, any prior antineoplastic-related or other HSRs and the specific agents involved, and any history of drug sensitivity or atopy (hereditary allergy).

TREATMENT MODALITIES

The primary treatment for HSR is prevention. By taking a careful history, the oncology nurse identifies patients who are high risk for HSR. Knowledge of the antineoplastic agents most likely to be associated with HSR and familiarity with appropriate pre-medication regimens are also valuable prevention tools. In addition, the oncology nurse carefully monitors the patient for signs of HSR, including blood pressure, pulse, and oxygen saturation. Emergency equipment and medications must be readily available, including oxygen supplies, cardiac monitor and defibrillator, intubation supplies, epinephrine 1 : 1000 or 1 : 10,000, diphenhydramine 50 mg, corticosteroids such as Solu-Medrol 125 mg, and other drugs such as aminophylline and dopamine sulfate. Antineoplastic agents likely to cause HSR are given in conjunction with patent IV access and compatible fluids.

In the event that the patient begins to experience symptoms compatible with HSR, administration of the antineoplastic agent is stopped immediately. IV fluids are continued at a rate consistent with maintaining adequate blood pressure. Administration of oxygen may be necessary to maintain a saturation above 92%. The patient should be continuously assessed for a patent airway.

It is recommended that standing orders be available for medication administration (Table 20–15). Many sources recommend the administration of *epinephrine* 1 : 1000, 0.3 to 0.5 mL every 5 to 20 minutes subcutaneously to slow the absorption of the antineoplastic agent as well as to counteract the effects of the HSR through bronchodilation, peripheral vasoconstriction, and increasing cardiac contractility and heart rate.[33, 81] Epinephrine also reduces mast cell degranulation.[81] In the event of airway compromise or shock, 0.1 mg/kg may be given IV over a minimum of 3 to 5 minutes.[89] *Diphen-*

T A B L E   2 0 – 1 5
Protocol for HSR Interventions

Stop the infusion
Call for help
Stay with the patient
Assess airway patency—prepare for possible intubation
Monitoring blood pressure, pulse, oxygenation and prepare
   for possible cardiopulmonary resuscitation
Administer epinephrine
   0.3–0.5 mg, 1:1000 SQ if no significant respiratory distress
   0.1 mg/kg, 1:10,000 IV if bronchospasm or stridor (over no
      less than 3–5 min)
Administer isotonic fluids (normal saline or Lactated Ringer's)
   to maintain blood pressure
Administer diphenhydramine 50 mg IV
Administer Solu-Medrol 125 mg IV

Data from references 20, 81, 100, and 110.

---

hydramine is an H1 antagonist that counteracts the dyspnea and wheezing caused by bronchospasm. H2 antagonists (cimetadine, ranitidine, or famotidine) may also be used, but are typically second-line therapy.[89] *Aminophylline* or nebulized β adrenergic agonists, such as *albuterol,* may be used when diphenhydramine is ineffective. Vasopressors, such as dopamine sulfate, may be needed if hypotension persists despite fluids. Corticosteroids, such as *Solu-Medrol,* may block the production of prostaglandins and leukotrienes and enhance the efficacy of epinephrine.[81] They may also prevent delayed or recurrent symptoms.[6] Patients taking β adrenergic blockers, angiotensin-converting enzyme inhibitors, monoamine oxidase inhibitors, or some tricyclic antidepressants may be difficult to treat for HSRs. These agents interfere with the effectiveness of epinephrine and the body's compensatory mechanisms.[81] IV glucagon (1–2 mg over 5 minutes or 1 mg in 1000 mL of D_5W at 5–15 mL/min) has been proven effective for people taking β blockers.[32, 89]

Many patients begin to have resolution of symptoms as soon as the antineoplastic administration is stopped. Others require some or all of the interventions described above. This author's experience with HSRs to paclitaxel have been successfully managed with the administration of Solu-Medrol 125 mg IV and diphenhydramine 50 mg IV, in addition to oxygen per nasal cannula.

There has always been controversy about the additional use of an antineoplastic agent for a patient who has experienced a serious HSR. This philosophy is changing in certain circumstances. One such instance is the use of paclitaxel to treat ovarian cancer. It is now considered to be first-line therapy that offers patients the best opportunity for cure. Recent research has shown that patients may be successfully rechallenged with paclitaxel by intensifying the pre-medication regimen and slowing the infusion time for the treatment.[110, 113] This success may be due in part to the fact that paclitaxel induces an anphylactoid response. Non-IgE-mediated reactions may be more amenable to desensitization and pre-medication. Successful re-challenge may be related to the specific agent involved, the mechanism of the HSR, the administration schedule, and the use of pre-medication.[113] There are some instances reported where re-challenge was not successful.[84]

PROGNOSIS

The outcome of a HSR reaction depends on a variety of factors. Immediate recognition and appropriate treatment are key factors to preventing a fatal event. Other variables include the amount of antigen absorbed and the degree of hypersensitivity manifested by the patient to the antineoplastic agent.[81]

Nursing management of HSR is described in the accompanying box.

Nursing Management

HYPERSENSITIVITY REACTIONS[148]

The importance of chemotherapy certification is clearly supported by the risk of chemotherapy-induced hypersensitivity reactions (HSR). Nurses administering chemotherapy must be knowledgeable about the agents most likely to cause HSR, and be skilled in recognizing and treating HSRs when they occur. The nursing history should include information about any previous allergies or reactions to medications. Baseline vital signs and mental status should be assessed and recorded. Emergency equipment and medications, as well as standing orders for HSR, should be readily available.

Nursing Diagnoses

- *Ineffective airway clearance related to airway edema and secretions*
- *Impaired gas exchange related to bronchospasm*

Outcome Goal

Patient will be able to:

- Demonstrate absence of respiratory distress within 10 minutes of treatment for HSR.

Interventions

- Stop infusion immediately.
- Maintain airway patency.
- Deliver high-flow oxygen at rate to maintain oxygen saturation.
- Administer emergency medications (see Table 20–15)
- Prepare to assist with intubation if required.

Nursing Diagnosis

- *Decreased cardiac output related to vasodilation and increased vasopermeability associated with histamine release*

Outcome Goal

- Exhibit baseline blood pressure and pulse within one hour of treatment.

Interventions

- Continuously monitor blood pressure and pulse if patient becomes symptomatic. Once stable, monitor every 15 minutes four times, then every hour four times, then every 4 hours.

- Deliver prescribed IV fluids at 200 mL/h or more to maintain blood pressure.
- Initiate vasopressors as prescribed if blood pressure does not respond to fluid challenge.
- Use Trendelenburg position if patient can tolerate due to respiratory symptoms.

Nursing Diagnosis

- *Anxiety related to the acute symptoms of HSR.*

Outcome Goal

- Verbalize understanding of the signs and symptoms of HSR to report immediately.
    Demonstrate effective coping strategies during and after the HSR.

Interventions

- Include education about the signs/symptoms and management of HSR when teaching the patient/family about chemotherapy.
    Review any premedication regimens.
    Discuss the rationale for vital sign monitoring.
    Describe the interventions that are used in the event an HSR occurs.
    Evaluate patient/family for level of anxiety and usual coping strategies.
    Carry out all interventions in a confident, efficient, and calm manner and explain each step to patient/family as it occurs.

Data from references 11, 27, and 73.

Malignant Pleural Effusion

DEFINITION

Pleural effusion, the abnormal accumulation of fluid in the pleural cavity, is a common complication of malignancy. Effusions in any body cavity are a potential problem with cancer, and the pleural space is the most frequent site, followed by the pericardial and the peritoneal spaces. Abnormal fluid accumulation results when the balance between secretion and reabsorption is altered.[49, 121] Malignant pleural effusion (MPE) is debilitating and life-threatening because the increased pleural fluid affects respiratory function by restricting lung expansion, decreasing lung volume, and altering gas exchange.

ETIOLOGY AND RISK FACTORS

Abnormal fluid accumulation in the pleural space may be the result of a benign or neoplastic process. Benign causes of pleural effusion include CHF, pericarditis, respiratory infections (pneumonia, tuberculosis), SVCS, mediastinal irradiation, ascites, hypoalbuminemia, and nephrosis.[42] Patients with cancer often develop pleural effusions in the course of their disease, especially if their disease involves primary or secondary intrathoracic malignancies. This may be the first sign of their cancer, a complication of existing disease, or a late manifestation in metastatic disease, or it may be related to a nonmalignant process.[17] Regardless of etiology, malignant pleural effusion causes alterations in ventilation and perfusion, hypoxia, and pain, and may lead to atelectasis, infection, and death.

Approximately 100,000 cases of malignant pleural effusion occur in the United States annually.[111, 121] MPE develops in about 50% of patients with cancer.[17, 111, 144] Lung and breast cancers are associated with about 75% of the cases.[121, 144] Other types of malignancy associated with MPE include ovarian, gastric, lymphoma, leukemia, melanoma, mesothelioma, uterine, cervical, sarcomas, and adeonocarcinomas of unknown origin.[17, 111, 121, 144] Gender incidence is primarily female (65%) due to the frequent occurrence in breast and gynecologic malignancies.[111, 121]

Malignant pleural effusion is the result of metastatic disease of the pleura or mediastinal lymph nodes. In the early 1980s, breast cancer was the leading malignancy associated with pleural effusion, but more recent studies report that lung cancer is the most common primary site to develop pulmonary metastases.[109] This probably reflects the increased incidence and death rate from lung cancer. The anatomic proximity and frequent invasion of the pulmonary vasculature with the embolization of the visceral pleural space from the lung cancer make it the most common cause of metastatic pleural malignancy.

PATHOPHYSIOLOGY

The pleura is a thin serosal membrane that envelops the lungs and lines the interior of the thoracic cavity (Fig. 20–12). There are two portions of the pleura, a visceral surface and a parietal surface lined by two thin layers of mesothelial cells. The *visceral pleura* adheres to the lung, encases each lobe, and extends within the interlobar fissures. Capillaries of the visceral pleura originate from the bronchial circulation. Lymphatic channels are present and coincide with the capillary bed. No nerve endings for pain are present. The *parietal pleura* lines the mediastinum, diaphragm, and chest wall. Capillaries of the parietal pleura are supplied by the intercostal arteries. Nerve endings for pain are present and, when stimulated, produce referred pain to the adjacent chest wall, shoulder, or abdomen. The right and left pleura have no communication.

A potential space exists between the two layers of pleural membrane, referred to as the *pleural space* or *pleural cavity*. Within the pleural space is a small amount of relatively protein-free transudative fluid produced by the mesothelial cells of the pleura, which flow across, from one pleura to the other, lubricating, moistening, and cushioning the pleural surfaces during respiration and providing lung movement without friction. Normally, 5 to 20 mL fluid is present in the pleural space.[17, 111, 121, 144] Fluid is continuously produced and shunted to the pleural space from the systemic capillaries of the parietal pleura. Approximately 80% to 90% of the fluid is then reabsorbed by the pulmonary capillaries of the visceral pleura. The remaining 10% to 20% of the pleural fluid, which contains large molecular substances, proteins, and erythrocytes, is reabsorbed through the lymphatic channels of the visceral pleura.[121]

Equilibrium of pleural fluid movement is regulated by five dynamic forces (see Fig. 20–12): capillary permeability, hydrostatic pressure (capillary and interstitial), colloidal osmotic pressure (plasma protein and interstitial protein), negative intrapleural pressure, and lymphatic drainage. The lymphatic channels regulate fluid

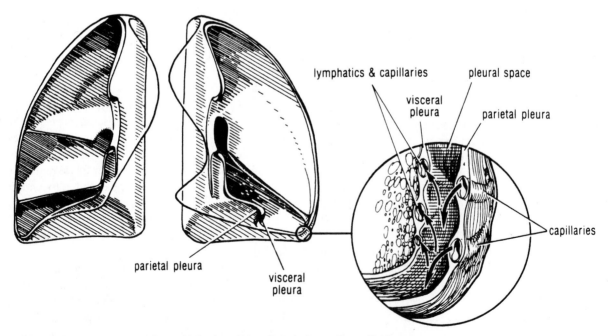

FIGURE 20–12 Right and left pleural membranes. Inset shows fluid movement from parietal pleura across pleural space to visceral pleura. (From Miller SE, Campbell DB: Pleural effusions in malignant disease. In Polomano RC, Miller SE, editors: *Understanding and managing oncologic emergencies,* Monograph, Columbus, OH, Adria Laboratories, 1987.)

and protein reabsorption. It is estimated that 5 to 10 liters fluid passes through the pleural space in 24 hours, but only 5 to 20 mL remains in the space at any given time.[111]

Abnormal fluid accumulation occurs when the regulating forces are disrupted, causing excessive fluid production or decreased fluid reabsorption. The two most common etiologies of MPE are pleural implants that cause irritation and inflammation leading to increased capillary permeability, and the obstruction of the pleural or pulmonary lymphatic systems by tumor.[17] Obstruction occurs by metastasis to mediastinal lymph nodes or tumor occluding the bronchus. Patients with ascites may also have spillover from the peritoneopleural channels.[121]

Malignant cells shed from the pleura and may grow freely in the pleural space, forming *tumor cell suspensions*. These collections of malignant cells are similar to pleural implants in origin and nature of growth. The difference between a tumor cell suspension and an implant is the greater number of cells found on cytologic examination. A tumor cell suspension may have cell counts higher than 4000 cells/mL, which is more than an implant. Ovarian cancer and lung cancer are often associated with tumor cell suspension.

Lymphatic blockage or venous obstruction interferes with drainage of fluid and large molecules from the pleural space, resulting in an overaccumulation of fluid. Lymphatic blockage is seen with lymphoma and metastasis from breast or lung cancer. Disruption of the capillary endothelium changes hydrostatic pressure gradients and allows fluid and protein to leak into the pleural space.

Necrotic malignant cells may shed into the pleural space, which raises its colloid osmotic pressure, thus reducing absorption of fluid by the visceral pleural capillaries. This occurs often in patients with lung or breast cancer. Obstruction and tearing of the thoracic duct may produce a true chylous (milky) pleural effusion, as seen with lymphoma.

Finally, other pathologies may contribute to the development of MPE effusion. These include SVCS, postobstructive pneumonitis, pericardial effusion, bronchial obstruction with atelectasis, hypoalbuminemia, and CHF. Any condition in which fluid formation in the pleural space exceeds fluid removal will lead to fluid accumulation. The space between the two pleural surfaces will then expand to accommodate the fluid (pleural effusion). Expansion of the pleural space leads to compression or collapse of the lung with decreased lung volume.

CLINICAL FEATURES

Alterations in pulmonary function by a pleural effusion produce clinical signs and symptoms related to impairment of lung expansion and hypoxia. The onset of a malignant pleural effusion may be slow or rapid. Insidiously developing effusions can produce a moderate to large amount of fluid overaccumulation before diagnosis. Thus, 25% of patients may be asymptomatic on presentation.[111, 144]

Symptoms expressed by a patient with MPE are related to alterations in pulmonary function, which result from impairment from the effusion, and baseline respiratory status. *Dyspnea* is the most common reported symptom and is typically accompanied by a dry, nonproductive cough and chest pain. Dyspnea is caused by pulmonary compression, decreased expansion, and alveolar collapse.[111, 121, 134] Pleural inflammation causes pleuritic chest wall pain. Parietal pleural metastases usually cause a dull continuous pain.[111] Cough is caused by compression of the bronchial walls by fluid.[111] The degree of symptomatology depends on the rapidity of

CLINICAL FEATURES
Malignant Pleural Effusion

Clinical Signs[35, 48, 111]

Labored breathing
Tachypnea
Restricted chest wall expansion
Decreased tactile fremitus on palpation
Dullness or flatness to percussion on affected side
Decreased diaphragmatic excursion with percussion
Diminished or absent breath sounds over affected area during auscultation
Pleuritic rub over affected area during auscultation
Egophony (change in transmitted sound) with auscultation just above level of effusion: the letter "e" spoken by the patient becomes higher pitched and sounds like an "a".
If the effusion is large, additional signs could include:
Bulging of intercostal spaces on affected side
Splinting of chest on affected side
Cyanosis
Chest tenderness
Shift in point of maximum intensity (PMI) to the left if effusion is on the right
Tracheal deviation to unaffected side

Symptoms

Dyspnea on exertion or at rest
Dry, nonproductive cough
Shortness of breath
Chest pain, often described as a "heaviness" or dull and aching rather than pleuritic
Desire to lie on the affected side
Malaise
Weight loss
Anxiety, fear of suffocation

fluid accumulation rather than the amount of fluid present.[49, 111]

Physical findings of a pleural effusion are often not enough to make a differential diagnosis from a pleural or pulmonary mass or to determine a malignant versus benign underlying process. Further work-up is necessary to confirm a diagnosis of MPE.

DIAGNOSIS

Pleural effusion is usually detected by chest x-ray films. The lateral and decubitus views are most helpful and reveal as little as 100 mL pleural fluid.[111] Accumulation must be about 300 mL to be seen in the upright antero-posterior position on chest x-ray film, where it appears as blunting of the costophrenic angle.[111] A more massive effusion (1500 mL) is seen as hemithorax opacification with mediastinal shift.[111] Additional radiographic studies could include an ultrasound of the chest or a CT scan of the thorax.[118, 134] These two tests, as well as serial chest x-ray films, are especially helpful in identifying a site for thoracentesis and demonstrating the mobility of fluid and absence of loculation that indicates the fluid is separated into cavities by adhesions. Confirmation of a pleural effusion in a patient with cancer does not necessarily indicate a malignant process. Aspiration and cytologic examination of the pleural fluid are required to identify the nature of the effusion. The mechanism of fluid accumulation should be ascertained, because it will guide treatment decisions.

Thoracentesis is a procedure in which a needle is introduced into the pleural space and fluid is aspirated. This procedure is indicated for diagnostic and therapeutic reasons. It is performed at the bedside. The patient is placed in the upright position with neck and dorsal spine flexed and arms extended and raised, usually over a bedside table. In this position, fluid will shift down into the dependent portion of the pleural space and the intercostal spaces will widen. A needle puncture is made, under local anesthesia, through the second intercostal space below the scapula on the affected side. The needle is directed inferiorly to avoid the neurovascular bundles located beneath and along the lower borders of the ribs. Fluid is removed by a syringe or vacuum drainage collection, depending on the amount present. A minimum of 25 to 50 mL fluid is needed for laboratory examination, but usually more than 250 mL is sent for analysis. Several puncture sites may be necessary if the fluid is loculated.

Initially, large volumes of fluid can be removed rapidly. However, this should not exceed 1500 mL because it could result in hypotension, circulatory collapse, or pulmonary edema.[111] The effusion should never be tapped dry. Leaving a small amount of fluid facilitates the placement of a chest tube. At an initial thoracentesis and when malignancy is suspected, 500 to 1000 mL of the fluid is usually aspirated. This amount will remove mesothelial cells, which may interfere with a definitive cytologic evaluation. The removal of amounts more than 1000 mL will encourage new fluid formation containing freshly shed malignant cells. Thoracentesis fluid is evaluated for cytology, Gram stain, culture, protein, lactic dehydrogenase (LDH), cell count and differential.[49, 121] Although thoracentesis is a relatively safe procedure, other potential complications include pneumothorax, if the lung is lacerated; hemorrhage, if a blood vessel is lacerated; vasovagal symptoms; and infection. To rule out complications, a chest x-ray film is done after the thoracentesis. Thoracentesis alone will not prevent fluid reaccumulation. Recurrence of pleural effusion is seen within a few days in as many as 87% of patients,[17, 121] and 97% of patients will have recurrence within 30 days.[111, 144] Repeated therapeutic thoracenteses for symptom relief may be warranted, but they are expensive and painful. In addition, they place the patient at risk for electrolyte imbalance, hypoproteinemia, pneumothorax, fluid loculation, and infection and may damage underlying lung parenchyma.

Pleural fluid analysis helps establish the underlying mechanism of fluid accumulation. Normal pleural fluid is straw colored. Fluid from an effusion is either a transudate or an exudate. A *transudate fluid* is a clear fluid usually attributed to an increased leakage of water. It is found in diseases characterized by sodium and water imbalances, such as CHF, cirrhosis, nephrotic syndrome, peritoneal dialysis hypoalbuminemia, and constrictive pericarditis.[35, 126] Although most diseases associated with transudate fluid are benign, 10% to 20% are malignant. An *exudate fluid* usually occurs with an excessive accumulation of protein in the pleural space. This is typically seen when the pleural surface is irritated or seeded with tumor. Although an exudate fluid does not specify neoplastic involvement in the pleural space, the most common cause is a malignancy.[35] Other causes of an exudative effusion are tuberculosis, pneumonia, SLE, pancreatitis, chylothorax, sarcoidosis, Meig's syndrome, prior radiation therapy, and mesothelioma. The color of the pleural fluid can further define the type of exudate, as follows[126]:

Purulent fluid—emphysema or infection (tuberculosis or pneumonia)

Chylous fluid (milky)—blockage of the thoracic duct with involvement of the mesenteric or retroperitoneal lymph nodes (lymphoma or benign disease process)

Bloody fluid (>100,000 erythrocytes/mm³)—usually indicates malignancy. A pleural fluid hematocrit higher than 50% than that of the blood characterizes hemothorax.

Malignant pleural effusions are always classified as an exudate. They usually have a bloody color and also must meet one of the following conditions: LDH level greater than 200 U, ratio of pleural fluid LDH level to serum LDH level greater than 0.6, or ratio of pleural fluid protein to serum protein greater than 0.5.[49]

Other less sensitive markers in the fluid that indicate a malignant effusion include the following:

White blood cell (WBC) count greater than $1000/mm^3$
RBC count greater than $100,000/mm^3$
Low pH
Low glucose
High specific gravity
High amylase
Carcinoembryonic antigen (CEA) level greater than 10 to 12 ng/mL[111]

Approximately one third of MPEs have a pleural fluid pH of less than 7.3. If there is also a low glucose level (<60 mg/dL), low oxygen tension, and a high LDH concentration, the prognosis is poorer.[111] These types of effusions are associated with large tumor burdens and fibrosis of the pleural space. The effusion tends to be chronic and may have been present for months.

Cytologic examination, which determines cell count and cell composition of fluid, is considered the most specific test for malignancy. Malignant cells tend to exfoliate more readily than normal cells. Approximately 60% to 80% of pleural specimens have been positive for malignant cells. A negative cytology does not exclude malignancy as the cause of the effusion. Repeated negative cytology is more common with lymphoma and warrants a pleural biopsy. In general, however, the patient with a malignant effusion will have other convincing evidence of cancer. Therefore a pleural biopsy may not be required.

In situations with a false-negative finding, however, other procedures can be done to make a differential diagnosis if necessary and if the patient can tolerate the work-up. Testing would include bronchoscopy, mediastinoscopy, thoracoscopy, transcutaneous needle biopsy, open-lung biopsy, or thoracotomy. Future techniques that may prove to be beneficial in identifying malignant cells are those involving MoAb and various types of chromosomal analysis.

TREATMENT MODALITIES

Once a diagnosis of malignant pleural effusion has been confirmed and the cause established, therapy is determined by the underlying cancer, the stage of disease, and the patient's life expectancy (Fig. 20–13).

Chemotherapy

If the underlying cancer is treatable, therapy is directed at the primary malignancy and not the effusion. After

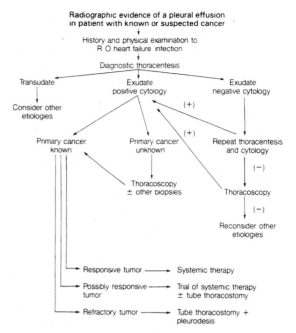

FIGURE 20–13 Clinical algorithm for prompt diagnosis and management of malignant pleural effusions. *RO,* Rule out; +, positive; −, negative. (From Ruckdeschel JC: Management of malignant pleural effusion: an overview, *Semin Oncol* 15[suppl 3]:27, 1988.)

diagnostic thoracentesis and lung reexpansion, systemic chemotherapy is initiated to prevent fluid reaccumulation in types of cancer that are sensitive to chemotherapy (SCLC, lymphoma, breast, and ovarian).[144] If the patient has a new diagnosis of lung cancer, a pleural effusion does not rule out surgery unless the cytology is positive. In that instance the tumor would be inoperable, and therapy would be determined by the responsiveness of the tumor. Treatment options (see Fig. 20–13) could be chest tube drainage with or without sclerosis, local radiation therapy, systemic chemotherapy, or any combination of these.

Radiation Therapy

Local radiation therapy may be used to treat malignant pleural effusions when the cause is a lymphoma or mediastinal lymphadenopathy from lung cancer.[121] Radiation therapy in these two diseases may be the primary treatment or may be combined with other types of treatment, such as chest tube drainage, pleurodesis, or systemic chemotherapy.

Chest tube drainage is considered a more appropriate means of controlling pleural effusion than repeated thoracenteses, which can lead to complications. A thoracostomy tube inserted into the pleural space will not prevent fluid recurrence but will facilitate drainage and then pleural sclerosing. The procedure can be performed at the patient's bedside. The patient should be premedicated with a systemic analgesic such as meperidine or morphine sulfate.

With the patient under local anesthesia the chest tube is inserted through the fifth intercostal space on the anterior or lateral chest wall. These sites are usually chosen for patient comfort when lying and to prevent occlusion or kinking of the tube. After insertion the tube is connected to a water-seal drainage system under suction. This restores negative pressure in the pleural space, removes the fluid, and allows the lung to reexpand. A chest x-ray film is done immediately after insertion of the chest tube to confirm its placement and to rule out a pneumothorax. Drainage usually requires 2 to 3 days, and subsequent chest films will be done, usually daily, to monitor fluid level and status of the lungs. Patients often complain of a cough as the lung reexpands.

Chest tube insertion may cause complications similar to those from thoracentesis, including pneumothorax, hemorrhage, infection, and damage to the lung parenchyma. An additional problem may be subcutaneous emphysema, or air under the subcutaneous tissues, although this is unusual unless the lung was injured. Fluid or air may leak around the insertion site, which would require future stitching at the insertion site and/or a more occlusive petroleum-based gauze dressing. Malfunctions of the drainage system are possible, so frequent monitoring of the drainage system for patency is required.

Pleurodesis (Chemical Sclerosing)

Needle thoracentesis and chest tube drainage can successfully remove fluid from the pleural cavity. However, neither procedure can consistently prevent recurrence of fluid accumulation.[144] Therefore, chest tube drainage is usually followed by pleurodesis (see Fig. 20–13), which is the chemical sclerosing of the two pleural membranes. The goal is to obliterate the pleural space by instilling an irritating chemical into the space, causing the formation of adhesions that prevent fluid accumulation around the lung.[42] These chemical agents damage the alveolar membrane and permeability, allowing clotting proteins such as fibrinogen to leak into the pleural space. Fibrinogen converts to fibrin, which accumulates and forms a lattice. Fibroblasts deposit collagen on the lattice and create the pleural adhesions. Pleurodesis can be done at the bedside after the effusion has been drained by the chest tube, producing less than 100 mL fluid in 24 hours.[144] Drainage of the effusion is confirmed by a chest x-ray film showing lung reexpansion. If larger quantities of fluid continue to drain, pleurodesis may be less effective and may require a repeat procedure.

Numerous agents have been used as sclerosants. The three most common have been tetracycline, bleomycin, and talc.[144] Other agents have included quinacrine, gold or phosphorous radioisotopes, antineoplastic agents, and antibiotics. The antineoplastic agents were used with the hope that there would be a cytotoxic effect, as well as sclerosing effect. Findings show that the effectiveness of neoplastic agents when used as sclerosants depends on the ability to cause irritation and not on their antineoplastic activity. Thiotepa, 5-FU, nitrogen mustard, doxorubicin (Adriamycin), and bleomycin were researched with varying results.[126] Bleomycin has been shown to have a success rate of 60% to 80%. Doses should not exceed 40 mg/m^2.[121] Tetracycline has been unavailable in the United States since 1991.[121] Both doxycycline and minocycline have been used; however, doxycycline has been associated with the need for multiple doses. Caution is required in patients with renal failure.[42] Sterile talc is the least expensive agent and is successful in 80% to 100% of patients.

Because the sclerosing agents work by irritation of the pleura, patient preparation for pleurodesis may involve sedation with an IV sedative (e.g., diazepam) or narcotic analgesic (e.g., meperidine, morphine sulfate). Even with intrapleural lidocaine, the pain may be quite severe. Success rates with sclerosing agents have been defined as no return of fluid after 30 and 90 days verified by a chest x-ray film.[144]

The chest tube is unclamped by the physician, who then slowly injects the prepared sclerosing mixture into the pleural cavity. The chest tube is clamped, and the patient may be asked or helped to turn from side to side to allow contact between the sclerosing agent and the entire surface of the pleura. Repositioning may be continued every 15 to 30 minutes for 2 to 6 hours. The chest tube is then opened to drainage and the amount of drainage monitored. Some feel that lung excursion allows for even distribution of the agent without the need for frequent position change.[48] The chest tube remains in place for approximately 24 hours. The drainage of pleural fluid usually decreases over a few days, and when the amount is less than 50 mL in an 8-hour period, the chest tube is removed. Expansion of the lung permits contact between the irritated vesical and parietal pleural surfaces. The inflammatory response of these membranes predicts total pleurodesis. A chest x-ray film is repeated to evaluate the success of the pleurodesis and to rule out a pneumothorax after chest tube removal.

Pleurodesis is contraindicated in patients with trapped lung (failure of lung to re-expand), and patients with comorbid CHF.[42, 144] Causes for failure of pleurodesis include irregularly scattered adhesions that prevent complete lung re-expansion, loculation of fluid in the pleural space by fibrin or adhesions, loss of pulmonary elasticity, extensive pleural metastases, or too much pleural fluid remaining in the pleural space at the time of pleurodesis.[42]

Surgery

Pleurectomy (Mechanical Pleurodesis). Surgical intervention for the management of pleural effusion is usually reserved for those situations when other treatment options fail to resolve the accumulation of fluid in the pleural cavity (see Fig. 20–13) and the patient has a life expectancy that makes the procedure worth the time and energy expenditure. Pleurectomy is the surgical removal of the parietal pleura with concomitant abrasion of the visceral pleura. Thus it is referred to as a mechanical pleurodesis. The goal of either type of pleurodesis is the same: obliteration of the pleural space. Both require adequate lung expansion to meet the chest wall. Therefore drainage of the pleural space by a chest tube is done preoperatively.

Removal of the parietal pleura involves the same considerations as for any other thoracotomy procedure. It is done in the operating room with the patient under general anesthesia. A thoracotomy incision is established, and the parietal pleura is separated and removed from the chest wall. The visceral pleura, on the lung, is then swabbed with dry gauze, which causes granulation and the formation of adhesions. Chest tubes are inserted and kept in place initially during the postoperative period to allow effective sclerosing. In certain cases of chylous effusions caused by neoplastic obstruction of the mediastinal lymphatics, the surgical procedure may include ligation of the thoracic duct at the level of the diaphragm.

Pleurectomy has produced excellent results; however, it has been accompanied by a morbidity rate of 20% or more and a 10% mortality rate.[111] Complications include air leaks, bleeding, and infection (pneumonia, empyema). Surgical removal of the pleura is a radical procedure usually reserved for patients in good physical condition and with a good life expectancy.

A less invasive approach to surgical pleurodesis is accomplished by video-assisted thoracostomy. It too is done under general anesthesia, but does not require the thoracotomy incision and is associated with less morbidity.[42] Mechanical or chemical pleurodesis may be accomplished. An aerosolized form of sterile talc has been approved for use with MPE since 1997 (Sclerosol).

Pleuroperitoneal Shunts. Another surgical treatment is available for intractable effusions when chemical pleurodesis is not feasible or has failed or when pleurectomy is not a viable option. The procedure involves the shunting of fluid from the pleural cavity into the abdominal cavity (Fig. 20–14).[111] With the patient under local anesthesia in the operating room, a commercially available device with one-way valve tubing is placed subcutaneously on the lateral chest wall. One end is inserted into the pleural cavity and the other into the abdominal cavity.

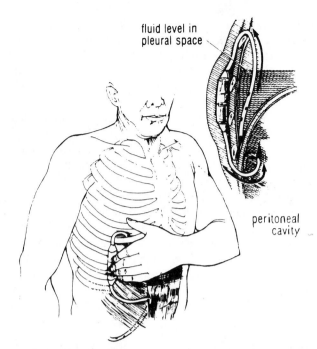

FIGURE 20–14 Pleuroperitoneal shunt procedure. Inset shows position of device on rib cage. Arrows indicate direction of flow. (From MIller SE, Campbell DB: Pleural effusions in malignant disease. In Polomano RC, Miller SE, editors: *Understanding and managing oncologic emergencies,* Monograph, Columbus, OH, Adria Laboratories, 1987.)

Early shunting devices were manually operated and required manual activation of the pump approximately 50 times a day. More recent devices are heparinized systems that drain spontaneously by positive pressure in the pleural cavity created by the effusion. This can be supplemented manually by applying pressure on the subcutaneous device (see Fig. 20–14). Patients are often taught to activate the device themselves. Success of the device depends on the amount and rate of fluid accumulation and proper pump function.

Long-Term Thoracotomy Access and Drainage. A final alternative for the control of pleural effusion is long-term thoracotomy access and drainage.[42] This approach is used for palliation. Patient selection is based on patient performance status and degree of disability, general health condition with attention to past and present pulmonary status, extent of underlying malignancy, and estimated life expectancy. Eligible patients include those with debilitating symptoms who have been unsuccessfully treated for pleural effusion by thoracentesis, chest tube drainage, pleurodesis, radiation therapy, or chemotherapy and those patients who are not candidates for surgery.

Access to the pleural cavity is accomplished by either a long-term access device, such as an implantable subcutaneous port, or by a chest tube. The subcutaneous port, with attached catheter or drainage tube, is placed into the pleural cavity by surgical implantation. The port is accessed through the usual subcutaneous method and fluid withdrawn intermittently. This can be done as often as deemed necessary but usually is done twice a week. Complications include infection, bleeding, occlusion, and device malfunctions.

Continuous long-term drainage can be accomplished by using either a standard chest tube or a small-bore catheter such as a Foley catheter placed into the pleural space. The smaller catheters are less traumatic to insert, may be sewn in place onto the skin, and will not cause splinting of the ribs, which is sometimes a complication with larger tubes. The principles and procedures of long-term drainage represent modifications of those for the standard short-term chest tube drainage system. The two necessary components of a long-term drainage system include the drainage tube and the collection equipment. Options are available, and choices depend on the patient's status. The following comparisons may help the decision process:

Standard Chest Tube	Small-Bore Catheter
Drainage Tube	
Large, allows view of fluid	Small, may or may not give view of fluid
Rigid, uncomfortable	Flexible, more comfortable
Anchored by sutures only	Inflatable bulb available in addition to sutures
Collection Equipment	
Drainage under water seal	Drainage without water seal (continuous urinary drainage bag or system may be used)
Large and cumbersome	Smaller and easier to handle
Expensive	Less expensive
May or may not be portable	Usually portable
Noisy, requires suction	Quiet, drains by gravity

A one-way valve (Heimlich valve) may or may not be used between the drainage tube and collection equipment. It is usually indicated when there is a risk of pneumothorax, because it allows the drainage of fluid and escape of air from the thorax but prevents their return. An advantage of the one-way valve is that the collection equipment can be kept at any level below or above the chest without adverse effects. However, if the one-way valve is not used, all collection equipment must be at or below the chest tube insertion site for adequate drainage and to prevent complications.

Long-term thoracotomy access drainage provides an important alternative method for managing intractable pleural effusions. It can reduce cost by decreasing the number of procedures and hospitalizations. Many patients can be managed at home using this method. This long-term treatment can provide comfort through relief of respiratory distress and control of associated symptoms. Most important, it can improve quality of life, the primary goal of any treatment.

PROGNOSIS

Patients with pleural effusion have a variable prognosis depending on the extent of the effusion and the success of treatment for the underlying disease. MPE is usually an indication of advanced disease. Survival rates vary from 3 months to 4 years, with the longest survival in patients with lymphoma.[121] Treatment efforts must be aimed at the underlying disease; however, they are always accompanied by measures to improve the patient's quality of life. Improving technology, earlier diagnosis and better interventions may increase survival rates.

Nursing management of the patient with MPE is outlined in the accompanying box.

Nursing Management

MALIGNANT PLEURAL EFFUSION[91]

Nursing care of a patient with pleural effusion depends on the extent of the effusion, the underlying disease, and the patient's overall condition. The problem is serious, and nursing care will be diverse, as with other oncologic complications. However, pleural effusions usually have a more gradual and detectable onset. This fact, coupled with a high recurrence rate, places great emphasis on the nurse's assessment skills.

Objective and subjective data must be collected systematically.

Nursing Diagnoses

- *Ineffective breathing pattern related to limited lung expansion secondary to pleural effusion*
- *Impaired gas exchange related to ineffective breathing patterns and pleural effusion*

Outcome Goals

Patient will be able to:

- Exhibit improved respiratory status, as evidenced by reduction in abnormal breath sounds, laboratory values and respiratory function tests approaching normal limits, ability to participate in self-care activities, and maintenance of normal respiratory rate and function.
- Identify/demonstrate emergency measures for acute respiratory distress.
- Maintain/return to activity tolerance levels.

Interventions

- Determine current respiratory status:
  - Observe for signs and symptoms of respiratory difficulty (dyspnea, shortness of breath, tachypnea, increased sputum production, change in color of sputum, hemoptysis, persistent cough, decreased activity tolerance, headache, chest, arm, or shoulder pain).
  - Assess lungs. Observe ventilatory movements (rate, depth), patency of the airway, use of accessory muscles, clubbing of fingernails, and discoloration of nailbeds or mucous membranes.
  - Palpate chest for fremitus, crepitance, deviation of trachea, or nonsymmetric chest expansion. Percuss chest for density or consolidation and displacement of organs. Auscultate chest for breath sounds.
  - Monitor laboratory and other respiratory function tests: complete blood count (CBC), electrolytes, arterial blood gases (ABGs), chest x-ray film, pulmonary function studies, and scans.
- Assist with breathing and pulmonary toilet:
  - Positioning for comfort and enhanced chest expansion
  - Deep breathing and coughing every 2 hours
  - Pursed-lip breathing
  - Postural drainage
  - Mouth care frequently with suctioning if necessary
- Provide oxygen therapy as indicated.
- Consult with physician regarding need for more aggressive pulmonary toilet measures (incentive spirometry, ultrasonic nebulizer, chest physical therapy).
- Administer respiratory medications as ordered.
- Provide mechanical ventilation if necessary.

- Teach measures to maintain optimal respiratory abilities:
  - Use of oxygen therapy
  - Pursed-lip breathing
  - Breathing exercises
  - Scheduled rest periods
  - Humidification
  - Adequate hydration and nutrition
  - Use of incentive spirometry and/or inhalers
  - Smoking cessation if indicated
  - Measures to decrease anxiety and stress (environmental manipulation, relaxation techniques, antianxiety medications)
- Make referrals to other health care professionals in the hospital and community as needed.
- Monitor chest tube drainage if indicated, as outlined in hospital procedure.
- Assist with pleurodesis if ordered, as outlined in hospital procedure.

Nursing Diagnosis

- *Altered tissue perfusion (peripheral, cerebral, cardiopulmonary) related to impaired gas exchange from pleural effusion*

Outcome Goals

Patient will be able to:

- Maintain adequate pulmonary function, as evidenced by vital signs and activity tolerance within patient's normal limits.
- Identify strategies for optimal pulmonary health.
- Develop plan for behavioral and life-style changes.

Interventions

- Assess organ systems for malfunction related to ischemia.
- Evaluate skin color of extremities.
- Note any change in mental status.
- Monitor laboratory values closely.
- Measure intake and output.
- Provide oxygen therapy as prescribed.
- Administer vasoactive drugs as ordered.

If the treatment used is surgery, the usual postoperative nursing care is implemented. The goal is to prevent or minimize complications. Patient assessment, pain management, oral hygiene, skin care, nutrition, and passive/active exercising are important aspects of surgical nursing care planning. When the patient is undergoing chemotherapy or radiation therapy, the nurse manages any side effects that may occur, such as fatigue, skin changes, alopecia, nausea, vomiting, diarrhea, and bone marrow suppression.

Discharge planning for patients treated for pleural effusion depends on their status after treatment. Some patients may be discharged symptom free and need only follow-up care to monitor for recurrence. Some patients may need support at home for intermittent or continuous pleural drainage. Other patients may require a hospice or extended care facility to continue management of the pleural effusion. The nurse is responsible for the transition from the hospital setting (see Chapter 28).

Septic Shock

DEFINITION

Shock comprises a group of diverse life-threatening syndromes that result from different pathophysiologic circumstances: decreased cardiac function, hemorrhage, trauma, antigen/antibody reaction, and sepsis. The three major classifications of shock are hypovolemic, cardiogenic, and distributive or vasogenic. *Hypovolemic shock* is a result of decreased intravascular volume. *Cardiogenic shock* results from the heart's impaired ability to pump blood adequately. *Distributive shock* or *vasogenic shock* is the result of an abnormality in the vascular system. Included under distributive shock are neurogenic, anaphylactic, and septic shock. The progression of septic shock produces a severe maldistribution of blood flow in the microcirculation. This leads to inadequate tissue perfusion, cellular ischemia, cellular hypoxia, and organ or system failure.

Sepsis and its sequelae are a complex compilation of related pathophysiologic processes. In 1991 the American College of Chest Physicians and the Society of Critical Care Medicine held a consensus conference to define the terms associated with sepsis and organ failure.[19] (Table 20–16). *Sepsis* was defined as the systemic inflammatory response to infection that is manifested by two or more of the following: temperature above 38°C or less than 36°C; heart rate greater than 90; respiratory rate greater than 20 or PaCO$_2$ less than 32 mm Hg; WBC above 12,000 mm^3, less than 4000 mm^3, or greater than 10% bands. Sepsis is classified as severe when it is associated with organ dysfunction, hypoperfusion, or hypotension. *Septic shock* is defined as sepsis-induced hypotension (despite fluid resuscitation) and organ perfusion abnormalities. Septic shock can lead to irreversible multiorgan dysfunction syndrome (MODS) and death.[19, 146, 147]

ETIOLOGY AND RISK FACTORS

Septic shock is the most common cause of noncoronary intensive care unit (ICU) deaths in the United States.[146, 147] The incidence of septic shock has increased steadily over the past 20 years.[147] Mortality rate ranges from 10% to 90%.[5, 103, 133] The incidence of sepsis in cancer patients is estimated at 45% with greater than 30% mortality.[133]

Patients with cancer are frequently immunosuppressed. Neutropenia is caused by most antineoplastic agents as well as radiation therapy to the long bones, pelvis, and sternum. Some antineoplastic drugs (asparaginase and vinca alkaloids) can alter the ability of neu-

---

TABLE 20–16
Definitions

Infection = microbial phenomenon characterized by an inflammatory response to the presence of microorganisms or the invasion of normally sterile host tissue by those organisms.

Bacteremia = the presence of viable bacteria in the blood.

Systemic inflammatory response syndrome (SIRS) = the systemic inflammatory response to a variety of severe clinical insults. The response is manifested by two or more of the following conditions: (1) temperature >38°C or <36°C; (2) heart rate >90 beats per minute; (3) respiratory rate >20 breaths per minute or PaCO$_2$ <32 mm Hg; and (4) white blood cell count >12,000/cu mm, <4,000/cu mm, or > 10% immature (band) forms

Sepsis = the systemic response to infection, manifested by two or more of the following conditions as a result of infection: (1) temperature >38°C or <36°C; (2) heart rate >90 beats per minute; (3) respiratory rate >20 breaths per minute or PaCO$_2$ <32 mm Hg; and white blood cell count >12,000/cu mm, <4,000/cu mm, or >10% immature (band) forms.

Severe sepsis = sepsis associated with organ dysfunction, hypoperfusion, or hypotension. Hypoperfusion and perfusion abnormalities may include, but are not limited to, lactic acidosis, oliguria, or an acute alteration in mental status.

Septic shock = sepsis-induced with hypotension despite adequate fluid resuscitation along with the presence of perfusion abnormalities that may include, but are not limited to, lactic acidosis, oliguria, or an acute alteration in mental status. Patients who are receiving inotropic or vasopressor agents may not be hypotensive at the time that perfusion abnormalities are measured.

Sepsis-induced hypotension = a systolic blood pressure <90 mm Hg or a reduction of ≥40 mm Hg from baseline in the absence of other causes for hypotension.

Multiple organ dysfunction syndrome (MODS) = presence of altered organ function in an acutely ill patient such that homeostasis cannot be maintained without intervention.

From Bone RG, Balk RA, Cerra FB, Dellinger RP: Definition for sepsis and organ failure and guidelines for the use of innovative therapy sepsis. Chest 101 (6): 1646, 1992.

trophil to migrate and phagocyytize bacteria. Patients with Hodgkin's disease may have impaired cellular immunity (macrophages and T lymphocytes). Patients with chronic lymphocytic leukemia (CLL) may have impaired antibody function that decreases the ability to attach to pathogens and enhance phagocytosis via the monocytes and macrophages. Macrophage function is also decreased in patients who have had a splenectomy.[96]

Septic shock can be caused by bacterial, fungal, viral, and protozoal organisms. Gram-negative bacteria (*E. coli, Klebsiella pneumoniae, Pseudomonas aeruginosa*) have historically been the primary organisms associated with septic shock. More recently there has been an increase in septic shock induced by gram-positive organisms (*Staphylococcus aureus, Staphylococcus epidermis*). This may be attributed to the increased use of long-term central venous access.[96] Another hypothesis is the prevalence of methicillin-resistant strains of staphylococcccus. Candida is the fungal organism most commonly associated with sepsis.[146] Due to the immunosupression in cancer patients, endogenous flora is frequently the source of infection.[65] The organism is not identified in 20% to 30% of cases due to previous exposure to antibiotics.[5] The most common sites of infection are the lung, abdomen, and urinary tract.[156]

A particular infectious life-threatening condition seen in patients with cancer is *neutropenic enterocolitis,* also called *typhilitis,* an inflammation of the small intestine or colon. The exact pathologic etiology is unclear. However, it is proposed to be initiated by direct cytotoxic damage from chemotherapy, radiation therapy, or neoplastic infiltration. Disruption of mucosal integrity, alteration of normal gut flora, and lack of neutrophil response lead to invasion of the GI tract by bacteria, viruses, and fungi. The implicated organisms include gram-negative bacilli such as *Klebsiella, Pseudomonas, E. coli, Candida,* and *Clostridium septicum.* Although *C. septicum* is not a flora, which is normally found in the gut, it may appear after the use of multiple antibiotics, which alter the normal gut flora. Neutropenic enterocolitis can lead to septic shock. Mortality rates have been estimated to be greater than 50%.

The factors that predispose a patient with cancer to infection and sepsis can be categorized according to the precipitating event, site of infection, and pathogen (Table 20–17). Each of the events that may initiate an infection leading to septic shock is a consequence of the underlying cancer or its treatment. All four treatment modalities (surgery, radiation therapy, chemotherapy, biotherapy) can result in profound suppression of host defense mechanisms. Monitoring the patient for effects of tumor growth and side effects of therapy is crucial to preventing septic shock.

PATHOPHYSIOLOGY

The presence of an invading pathogen (bacteria, fungus, virus, protozoa) should stimulate an immune response from the patient. In patients who are immunocompromised, infection may become established and the release of inflammatory mediators can lead to life-threatening complications that induce MODS. As bacterial pathogens are phagocytized, endotoxins (gram-negative bacteria) and exotoxins (gram-positive bacteria) are released into the blood stream (Fig. 20–15). The macrophages respond by releasing vasoactive mediators (histamine, kinins, interleukins, and tumor necrosis factor).[103] IL-1 and tumor necrosis factor-α alpha (TNF-α) are potent mediators of inflammation. Their release stimulates the release of additional inflammatory mediators such as IL-6, IL-8, thromboxanes, leukotrienes, platelet activating factor, prostaglandins, and complement.[5]

The inflammatory cascade leads to fever, chills, vasodilation, and hypotension. The vascular endothelium is altered by endotoxins and exotoxins. The endothelial alteration causes microthrombi to form and activates the complement, coagulation, and fibrinolytic systems. Bradykinin, histamine, and serotonin release increases capillary permeability. The patient in septic shock may exhibit hypovolemia, hypotension, hypoxia, tissue ischemia, DIC, ileus, oliguria, and liver failure (Fig. 20–16).

CLINICAL FEATURES

The first signs of progressive sepsis may be fever, shaking chills and mild hypotension.[41] The early phase of septic shock has been referred to as the warm, or hyperdynamic, phase. It is characterized by vasodilation, decreased peripheral vascular resistance, and increased cardiac output. The patient may present as warm and flushed. The respiratory rate is rapid, which leads to alkalosis. The patient may be nauseated, have diarrhea, and be mildly confused. As septic shock progresses, capillary leakage causes fluid to third-space, cardiac output decreases, and peripheral vascular resistance increases. The patient develops oliguria and metabolic acidosis. Peripheral vasoconstriction leads to ischemia and decreased blood flow to vital organs. Bleeding occurs in the patient with DIC. Peripheral edema becomes more severe. The patient becomes cold, clammy, and cyanotic. Confusion progresses to coma. Without successful intervention, symptoms progress to the cold phase, also known as late or refractory shock. At this point the condition is irreversible. Circulatory and respi-

Factors Predisposing Cancer Patients to Infection

Precipitating Event	Common Site of Infection	Common Organism
LOCAL EFFECTS OF TUMOR GROWTH OR TX		
Skin or mucous membrane breakdown	Cancer or TX of skin, head and neck, GI tract, female genital tract	Locally colonizing organisms
Obstruction of natural passages	Solid tumors or TX of cancer (especially pulmonary, biliary, and urinary tracts)	Locally colonizing organisms
Alterations in microbial flora	All cancer sites or TX of cancer (especially pulmonary, GI)	Locally colonizing organisms
Stasis of blood and body fluids secondary to obstruction or inactivity	All cancer sites or TX of cancer	Locally colonizing organisms
CNS dysfunction (brain or spinal cord tumors, metabolic abnormalities)	Pulmonary (aspiration pneumonia) Urinary tract	Locally colonizing organism
HYPOSPLENISM SECONDARY TO NEOPLASTIC INFILTRATION OR SPLENECTOMY	Disseminated	Bacteria: *Streptococcus pneumoniae*, *Neisseria meningitidis*, *Escherichia coli*, *Haemophilus influenzae*, *Clostridium difficile*, *Staphylococcus* species
GRANULOCYTOPENIA (neutropenia) prevalent with acute leukemia	Skin lesions, thrombophlebitis, pulmonary (pneumonia), sinuses pharynx, esophagus, colon, perianal	Gram-negative bacilli: *E. coli*, *Pseudomonas aeurginosa*, *Klebsiella pneumoniae*, *Staphylococcus aureus* Yeasts: *Candida* Filamentous fungi: *Aspergillus* species, agents of *mycosis*
CELLULAR IMMUNE DYSFUNCTION (T-cell immune alteration) prevalent with T-cell lymphoma	Disseminated	Bacteria: *Listeria monocytogenes*, *Salmonella* species, *Mycobacterium* species, *Nocardia steroides* Fungi: *Cryptococcus neoformans*, *Histoplasma capsulatum*, *Coccidioides immitis* Viruses: *Varicella zoster*, cytomegalovirus, herpes simplex Protozoa: *Pneumocystis carinii*, *Toxoplasma gondii*, *Cryptosporidium* Helminths: *Strongyloides stercoralis*
HUMORAL IMMUNE DYSFUNCTION (B-cell immune alteration) prevalent with multiple myeloma	Disseminated	*S. pneumoniae*, *H. influenzae*
IATROGENIC FACTORS (invasive procedures, devices equipment)	Skin Mucous membranes	*Staphylococcus epidermis* Locally colonizing organisms
Diagnostic procedures Genitourinary tract manipulations Bone marrow aspirations Biopsies Placement of shunts, stents, and tubes Venipuncture Long-term venous access devices Respiratory assist devices		
NOSOCOMIAL SOURCES		
Air	Pulmonary	*Aspergillus* species
Surface contact	Skin and mucous membranes	*S. aureus*
Food (fresh fruits/vegetables)		Bacteria, fungi
Water (stagnant sources)	Disseminated	*P. aeruginosa*, *Serratia marcescens*
Medical personnel (illness, organism transmission or cross-contamination, poor handwashing)	Various	Locally colonizing organisms
Extended prophylactic broad-spectrum antibiotics	Disseminated	Bacteria

Data from references 96, 103, 132, 146, and 155.

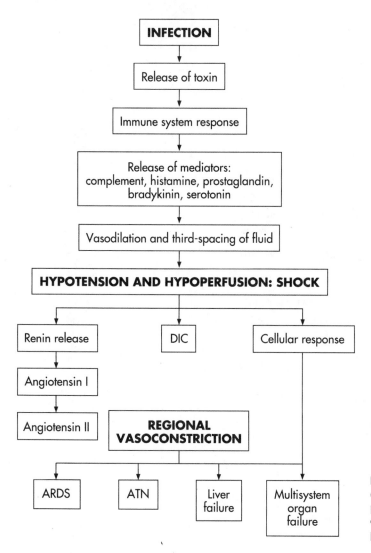

FIGURE 20-15 Pathophysiology of septic shock. (From McMorrow ME, Cooney-Daniello M: When to suspect septic shock, *RN* 54(10):32, 1991. [Published in *RN*; copyright © 1991, Medical Economics, Montvale, NJ. Reprinted by permission.])

ratory collapse ultimately occur.[41, 65] The Clinical Features box categorizes the clinical signs and symptoms into three stages of septic shock.[129]

Respiratory Features

Hyperventilation and respiratory alkalosis may occur both with and without fever.[146] Alveolar capillary leakage leads to pulmonary edema and hypoxemia.[146] ARDS occurs most frequently in patients with gram-negative infections.[146] The development of ARDS increases morbidity to 80% to 90%. Concomitant thrombocytopenia raises the morbidity rate even higher.[146]

Cardiovascular Features

Systemic vascular resistance drops dramatically due to vasodilation. Hypotension is associated with the release of complement, TNF-α, and IL-1. Metabolites of nitric oxide are also related to the decrease in vascular resis-

tance. Cardiac output increases to try and compensate. Systemic vascular resistance ultimately increases with vasoconstriction leading to ischemia and decreased organ perfusion. Elevated lactic acid levels occur with hypoperfusion of vital organs and hypoxemia. This is a poor prognostic sign.[146]

Hematologic Features

Gram-negative sepsis is also associated with the development of DIC. The release of bacterial toxins stimulates the clotting cascade that exhausts clotting factors and leads to simultaneous hemorrhage and thrombosis. (See previous discussion of DIC.) DIC is almost always associated with septic shock and may be one of the presenting signs.[133]

Other Features

Septic shock due to GI pathogens may also be accompanied by jaundice, stress ulcers, and bleeding. Renal

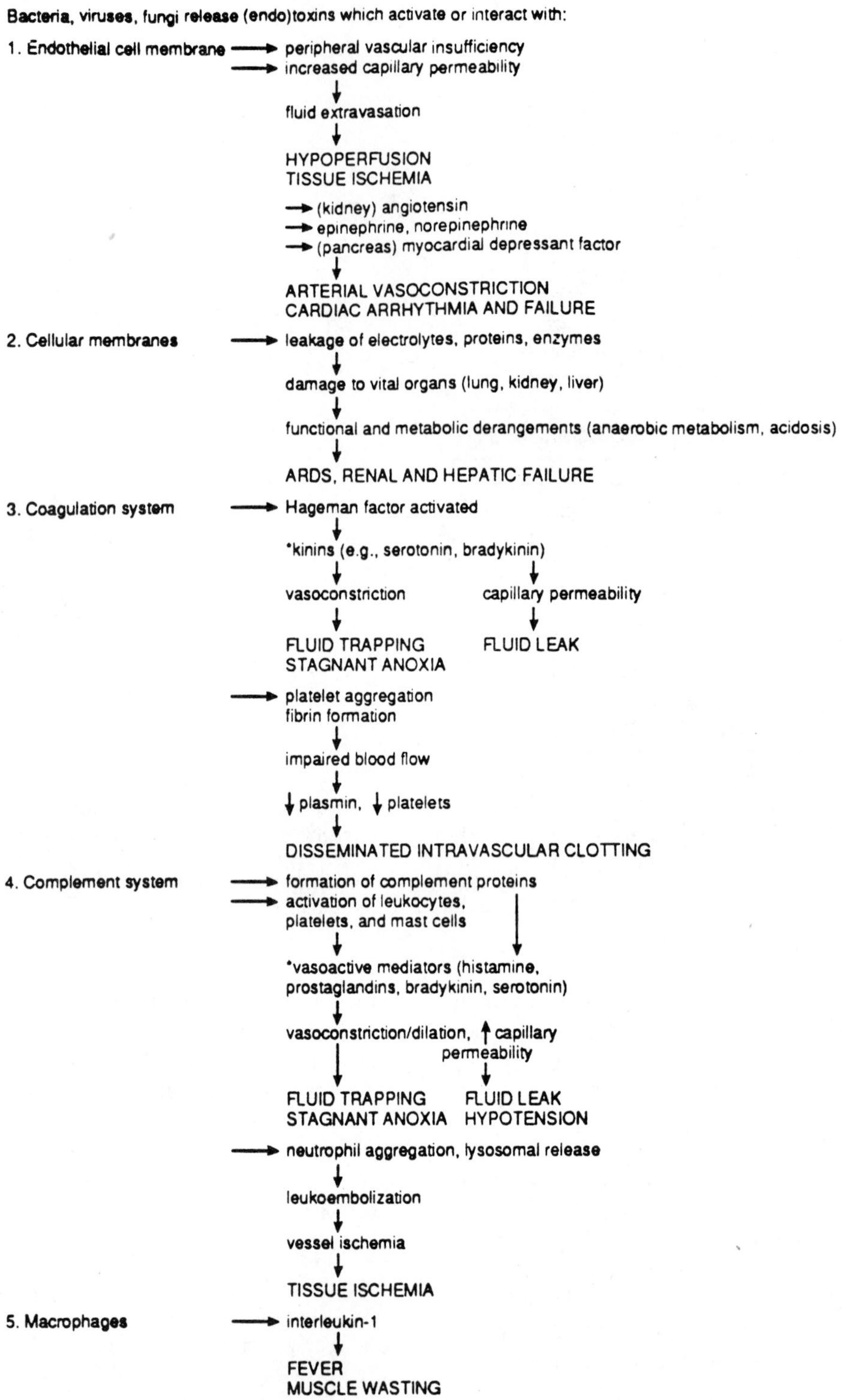

Bacteria, viruses, fungi release (endo)toxins which activate or interact with:

1. Endothelial cell membrane ⟶ peripheral vascular insufficiency
⟶ increased capillary permeability
↓
fluid extravasation
↓
HYPOPERFUSION
TISSUE ISCHEMIA

⟶ (kidney) angiotensin
⟶ epinephrine, norepinephrine
⟶ (pancreas) myocardial depressant factor

ARTERIAL VASOCONSTRICTION
CARDIAC ARRHYTHMIA AND FAILURE

2. Cellular membranes ⟶ leakage of electrolytes, proteins, enzymes
↓
damage to vital organs (lung, kidney, liver)
↓
functional and metabolic derangements (anaerobic metabolism, acidosis)
↓
ARDS, RENAL AND HEPATIC FAILURE

3. Coagulation system ⟶ Hageman factor activated
↓
*kinins (e.g., serotonin, bradykinin)
↓   ↓
vasoconstriction   capillary permeability
↓   ↓
FLUID TRAPPING   FLUID LEAK
STAGNANT ANOXIA

⟶ platelet aggregation
fibrin formation
↓
impaired blood flow
↓
↓ plasmin, ↓ platelets
↓
DISSEMINATED INTRAVASCULAR CLOTTING

4. Complement system ⟶ formation of complement proteins
⟶ activation of leukocytes,
platelets, and mast cells
↓
*vasoactive mediators (histamine,
prostaglandins, bradykinin, serotonin)
↓
vasoconstriction/dilation, ↑ capillary
permeability
↓   ↓
FLUID TRAPPING   FLUID LEAK
STAGNANT ANOXIA   HYPOTENSION

⟶ neutrophil aggregation, lysosomal release
↓
leukoembolization
↓
vessel ischemia
↓
TISSUE ISCHEMIA

5. Macrophages ⟶ interleukin-1
↓
FEVER
MUSCLE WASTING

*During a septic shock episode, shock mediators may be activated by more than one pathway.

FIGURE 20–16   Pathophysiology of septic shock. (From Harnett S: Septic shock in the oncology patient, *Cancer Nurs* 12(4):191, 1989.)

CLINICAL FEATURES
Stages of Shock

Stage One: Hyperdynamic Stage (early shock, warm shock)

Decreased tissue perfusion: 10% reduction in blood volume

Usually lasts less than 24 hours

Feelings of anxiety, apprehension, nervousness

Complaints of nausea

Altered mental status, restlessness, irritability, disorientation, inappropriate euphoria

Temperature normal, below normal, or above normal

Skin warm and flushed because of arteriole dilation

Peripheral cyanosis

Tachycardia and bounding peripheral pulses

Normal or slightly elevated blood pressure with a widening pulse pressure

Tachypnea, hyperventilation

Rales and decreased breath sounds

Respiratory alkalosis: decreased oxygen pressure

Renal output normal or elevated (polyuria)

BUN and creatinine may be slowly increasing

Hyperglycemia

Urine may test positive for sugar (glycosuria)

Urine specific gravity normal

No signs of bleeding

Coagulation profile normal

Stage Two: Normodynamic Stage (intermediate shock, cool shock)

Decreased tissue perfusion: 15% to 20% reduction in blood volume

Usually lasts a few hours

Complains of thirst

Altered mental status: lethargy, confusion

Skin pale, cool, and clammy because of peripheral vasoconstriction and diversion of blood to vital organs

Peripheral edema possible because of increased secretion of antidiuretic hormone and aldosterone leading to sodium and water retention

Temperature normal or subnormal

Tachycardia continues

Blood pressure decreases with a narrow pulse pressure because of decrease in cardiac output

Respirations slow and shallow

Respiratory acidosis

Renal output decreased (oliguria)

Urine specific gravity elevated

Abdominal distention because of air swallowing and decreased peristalsis

Hemorrhagic lesions may be apparent

Stage Three: Hypodynamic Stage (late shock, refractory shock, irreversible shock, cold shock, "classic" shock)

Decreased cardiac output, decrease in blood volume

Altered mental status, stupor, coma

Skin cold, possible cyanosis of digits and mottling

Temperature subnormal

Tachycardia

Weak or absent pulses because of decreased myocardial contractility: "pump failure"

Hypotension

Respiratory depression

Pulmonary edema, or "shock lung," because of decreased oxygen pressure and decreased pulmonary microcirculatory adult respiratory distress syndrome

Metabolic acidosis because of anaerobic metabolism and increased levels of lactic acid

Hypoglycemia

No renal output (anuria)

Renal failure: acute tubular necrosis

Hemorrhagic lesions

Data from references 5 and 133.

---

symptoms of oliguria and proteinuria may progress to acute tubular necrosis (ATN) and renal failure.[146]

DIAGNOSIS

The diagnosis of septic shock depends on astute observations of the patient. Sepsis may or may not have been confirmed. An initial finding could be as subtle a sign as the patient complaint of "just not feeling right." Physical assessment of all systems should be correlated with a brief recent history highlighting any changes and noting any possible sources of infection. Continuous assessment and monitoring of the patient is essential. This includes taking vital signs, observing tissue perfusion, watching for signs of bleeding, checking mental status, and assessing heart, lung, and kidney function.

In the neutropenic patient, fever may be the only sign of an infection. Elevated temperature is produced in the body by the monocytes, not the neutropihils. Some monocytes migrate into body tissue, where they become macrophages. The monocyte secretes an endogenous pyrogen that affects the thalamus, resulting in a rise in temperature. Fever in a neutropenic patient should be treated as an emergency. In a profoundly neutropenic patient, death can occur within 24 to 72 hours if appropriate antibiotic therapy is not initiated.[96]

Once fever is noted, cultures should be obtained from all potential sites of infection prior to the initiation of

TABLE 20-18
β-Lactam Antibiotics

penicillins
cephalosporins
carbapenems
monobactams

Data from Mann B, Sexton PA: Beta-lactam antibiotics, College of Health and Life Sciences, Fort Hays State University, http://www.fhsu.edu/nursing/otitis/b-lactam.html

antibiotics. Blood cultures are drawn peripherally, as well as centrally if the patient has a central line. Two sets of blood cultures are typically done 15 minutes apart to increase the chances of collecting the offending organism. Blood cultures may be repeated with each temperature spike until the organism is identified. When drawing blood from a central line for culture, the initial 5 to 6 mL should not be wasted, but used for the culture. Wasting the initial aspirate decreases the chances of collecting the pathogen. Sputum, urine, stool, central line exit sites, and any other areas where skin integrity is not intact, should be cultured.

A complete blood count is done to evaluate WBC and neutrophil levels. Chest x-ray is performed to evaluate lung status and rule out the lung as the site of infection. CT of the abdomen and pelvis or ultrasonograpy may be used to rule out intra-abdominal infections or abscesses.[146] Blood gases are done to evaluate any respiratory compromise. Coagulation panels are done to rule out or confirm DIC.[65] Additional lab results may include elevated serum glucose, cortisol, catecholamine, and lactate levels.

TREATMENT MODALITIES

The identified stage of septic shock will dictate the necessary medical interventions. Prompt medical treatment is essential to prevent progression of shock syndrome to the irreversible stage and subsequent death. Recognition of the signs and symptoms of shock and the determination of sepsis are the first medical interventions.

As with most oncologic emergencies, prevention is the ideal treatment for septic shock. Measures to protect immunocompromised patients from infection are critical. Some of these include meticulous handwashing, low bacterial diets, and avoidance of crowds. Patients in the acute care setting should have private rooms with limited visitors. Hematopoietic growth factors are used to promote neutrophil recovery after antineoplastic therapy.[133] Patients with prolonged neturopenia and candidates for bone marrow or stem cell transplant may benefit from antimicrobial prophylaxis.[133]

The patient in septic shock requires intervention in a critical care setting. Hemodynamic monitoring is nec-

essary, as is the vigilant nursing care that can be provided in the ICU. The goals of treatment are to maintain blood pressure and tissue perfusion while treating the underlying pathogen. Broad-spectrum antibiotics should be initiated within an hour of drawing blood cultures. The choice of empiric antibiotic treatment is based on the suspected site of infection and most likely pathogen.[103] High-risk patients currently receive two or more drugs to cover both gram-positive and gram-negative bacteria. Aminoglycosides (such as gentamycin or tobramycin) are included to cover gram-negative bacteria. If the skin is the suspected source of infection, penicillin or a first-generation cephalosporin may be used. Vancomycin is used when central venous access devices are the suspected source of infection and for methicillin-resistant strains.[103, 146] Some of the recommended combinations are listed below (Tables 20-18 and 20-19 for categories of β-lactams and generations of cephalosporins):

- A fourth-generation cephalosporin (Cefipime) or an antipseudomonal penicillin with an aminoglycoside[133]
- An antipseudomonal β-lactam and aminoglycoside[146]
- Ceftazidine and an aminoglycoside with or without vancomycin, *or* piperacillin/tazobactam, an aminoglycoside, and imipenem or meropenem.[146]
- An extended-spectrum penicillin (piperacillin, mezlocillin) or third-generation cephalosporin and aminoglycoside[103]
- For suspected anaerobes (GI/GU): extended-spectrum penicillin or third-generation cephalosporin and aminoglycoside combined with metronidazole *or* a penicillinase-inhibitor β-lactam combination such as piperacillin-tazobactam or ticarcillin-clavulante with an aminoglycoside *or* imipenem and an amiglycoside[103]

TABLE 20-19
Generations of Cephalosporins

FIRST GENERATION

cefadroxil	cephalexin	cephradine
cefazolin	cephapirin	

SECOND GENERATION

cefaclor	cefamandole	cefonicid
cefotetan*	cefoxitin*	cefprozil
cefuroxime		

THIRD GENERATION

cefdinir	cefixime	cefoperazone
cefotaxime	cefpodoxime	ceftazidime
ceftriaxone	ceftibuten	ceftizoxime

cephamycins (closely related β-lactam antibiotics)
Data from references 1 and 74.

Once culture and sensitivity results are obtained, the empiric therapy can be altered to include the most appropriate agents for the pathogens identified. If no pathogen is identified and the patient remains febrile despite broad-spectrum antibiotics, antifungal and/or antiviral agents, or both, must be added.[146]

Fluid replacement with crystalloids or colloids is done to correct hypovolemia. If the patient remains hypotensive, vasopressors such as dopamine or dobutamine are initiated to maintain perfusion of vital organs.[146] Norepinephrine may also be used.[156] Electrolyte imbalances should be corrected and urinary output maintained at 50 mL/h. Blood products may be needed for the patient with DIC or GI bleeding. Oxygen will be needed to help maintain oxygenation. Ventilatory assistance should be initiated early for patients with respiratory compromise.[146] Almost 85% of patients with septic shock will require ventilator support for 7 to 14 days.[156]

Any loculated sites of infection or drainable abscesses should be surgically drained.[146] Aggressive nutritional support is necessary for the patient with metabolic abnormalities and helps prevent tissue breakdown. TNF has been associated with cachexia. Glucose administration must be closely monitored because glucose uptake may be impaired due to insulin inhibition caused by hormones responding to the stress response. Protein and nutrient supplements are needed to meet the high energy demands of septic shock and to promote the healing process. Several studies have indicated that corticosteroids are not beneficial in the management of septic shock and may actually be detrimental to the outcome.[5, 34, 146, 147]

Much study is being done to identify interventions to counteract the inflammatory response to septic shock. Some agents under study include IL-1 receptor antagonists, anti-TNF antibodies, platelet-activating factor (PAF) receptor antagonists, bradykinin antagonists, ibuprofen, bactericidal permeablility-increasing protein, cationic antimicrobial protein, and *N*-acetylcysteine.[5, 103, 146, 147]

PROGNOSIS

Survival of patients with septic shock depends on preventing or reversing the process of shock and on the status of the underlying disease (nonfatal, ultimately fatal, rapidly fatal). Less than 5% of deaths are due to cardiac failure; 25% to 33% of patients die from hypotension that cannot be corrected with fluids and vasopressors.[5] The presence of ARDS raises morbidity to 80% to 90%.[146] Once the patient develops MODS, there is very little chance of reversal.[144] Prompt recognition and treatment of septic shock can mean the difference between life and death.

Nursing management of the patient in septic shock is outlined in the accompanying box.

Nursing Management

SEPSIS

The nursing care of a patient with sepsis varies with the identified stage of septic shock. Infection and sepsis have a high correlation with neutropenia. Patients at highest risk are those whose neutrophil count is less than 100/mm^3 for more than 3 weeks. Therefore the first nursing goal in the management of septic shock is prevention of infection. The following general measures outline the nursing care for the patient with neutropenia. Complete reverse isolation, although it reduces exogenous colonization, is no longer recommended for patients with neutropenia, because endogenous flora are the major source of infection. Thus current practice is to use protective isolation.

Nursing Diagnosis

• *Risk for infection (sepsis) related to neutropenia*

Outcome Goals

Patient will be able to:

• Remain infection free, as evidenced by temperature within normal limits, laboratory values within normal limits, and absence of inflammation.
• Demonstrate knowledge related to prevention of infection.
• Identify/demonstrate adequate nutrition and fluid intake.
• Identify/demonstrate appropriate hygenic measures.
• Alter environmental risk factors.
• Verbalize signs and symptoms to report to health care team.

Interventions

• Observe for signs and symptoms of infection:
   Monitor vital signs at least every shift. An elevated temperature and changes in blood pressure, pulse, and respiration may be the only sign of an impending infection, since neutropenic patients have a diminished inflammatory response.
   Observe for other general signs and symptoms of infection/sepsis: nausea, abdominal discom-

fort, changes in renal status, irritability, and changes in mental status.

Assess blood counts daily or every other day to determine the onset of infection, recovery of the bone marrow, status of renal function, and possible need to change antibiotic regimen. This should include CBC with differential, platelet count, and chemistry panel.

- Prevent cross-contamination:

    Place patient in a disinfected private room.

    Provide care first to patients with neutropenia before caring for other patients.

    Do not care for both patients with neutropenia and patients with infection.

    Wash hands consistently and thoroughly after each patient contact.

- Prevent disease transmission:

    Educate patient, staff, and visitors on all aspects of infection prophylaxis.

    Screen personnel and visitors. Patient should not be exposed to anyone with an infection, recent vaccination, or recent exposure to a communicable disease (e.g., bacterial infections, herpes, colds, influenza, chickenpox, measles).

    Limit the number of visitors.

- Eliminate possible sources of infection.

    Provide a neutropenic diet (microbiotic diet) that eliminates unpared fresh fruits and raw vegetables. All food items should be cooked.

    Avoid the placement of fresh fruits, flowers, or plants in patient's room.

    Change water to prevent stagnation (e.g., denture cups, water pitchers, humidifiers, respiratory equipment, irrigation containers).

- Maintain integrity of the skin and mucous membranes:

    Inspect patient's body daily with attention to the mouth, all orifices, all skin folds, and any site of an IV catheter insertion, a tube insertion, or a wound.

    Instruct patient and provide assistance in meticulous skin and mouth care. Provide lubrications to prevent dryness and cracking. Female patients should also keep the vaginal area clean and lubricated.

    Prevent trauma to the skin and mucous membranes by avoiding intramuscular or subcutaneous injections whenever possible; rectal manipulations, as with enemas, suppositories, or thermometers; urinary catheterization; and douching and using tampons with the female patient. If urinary catheterization is necessary, maintain a closed sterile drainage system.

    Avoid rectal trauma by preventing constipation with dietary measures or stool softeners.

- Assess respiratory status:

    Auscultate lungs at least every shift.

    Encourage mobility and frequent deep breathing and coughing.

- Provide nutritional support:

    Assess patient's food preferences.

    Administer nutrition (oral, tube feeding, or parenteral) to meet increased nutrition demands.

    Encourage and provide high-calorie, high-protein food items.

    Obtain dietitian consultation.

    Measure weight every day.

    Monitor laboratory values to assess for protein wasting, with particular attention to serum albumin level. Encourage fluid intake up to 3000 mL/d, *unless contraindicated.*

    Ensure patient conserves energy.

Nursing Diagnoses

- *Altered tissue perfusion (peripheral, cardiopulmonary, cerebral, renal, gastrointestinal) related to response to release of endotoxins*
- *Decreased cardiac output related to decreased cardiac function*

Outcome Goals

Patient will be able to:

- Maintain adequate tissue perfusion, as evidenced by vital signs within patient's normal limits, laboratory values and diagnostic tests approaching normal levels, and respiratory function within patient's normal limits.
- Maintain optimal cardiac output, as evidenced by relief of chest pain, vital signs within patient's normal limits, cardiac rhythm without dysrhythmias, central venous pressure (CVP) and pulmonary capillary wedge pressure (PCWP) within patient's normal limits, and adequate intake and output.

Interventions

- Monitor vital signs (temperature, pulse, blood pressure, respirations) every 4 hours.
- If hypotension is present, place patient flat in bed or in Trendelenburg position.
- Assess skin color, temperature, and moisture every 4 hours.
- Assess organ systems for malfunctions from ischemia.
- Monitor ECG for evidence of dysrhythmias.
- Monitor laboratory values closely.

- Obtain specimens for cultures and sensitivities as ordered:

    Blood samples are taken peripherally as well as from each port of central lines.

    Check urine, stool, throat, and sputum or any draining wound, IV catheter, or tube insertion site.
- Administer antibiotics as ordered. Observe patient closely for possible toxicities; nephrotoxicity and neurotoxicities are prevalent with the use of aminoglycosides (e.g., tobramycin, gentamicin).
- Provide oxygen therapy as prescribed.
- Administer vasopressive drugs as ordered.
- Administer pain medication as ordered.
- Control fever:

    Administer antipyretic medications such as acetaminophen.

    Lower room temperature.

    Use sponge bath with tepid water.

    Use hypothermia blanket.

    Monitor laboratory values with attention to K^+, BUN, and creatinine.

Nursing Diagnoses

- *Ineffective breathing pattern related to pulmonary edema and metabolic acidosis*
- *Impaired gas exchange related to circulatory collapse and pulmonary edema*

Outcome Goals

Patient will be able to:

- Maintain effective breathing pattern, as evidenced by chest clear to auscultation, laboratory values approaching patient's normal limits, respirations regular and nonlabored, and reduced signs and symptoms of respiratory impairment.

Patient/family/caregiver will be able to:

- Demonstrate measures to manage impaired ventilation.
- Perform necessary treatments and procedures.
- Demonstrate proper knowledge and administration of medication and oxygen.
- Identify/demonstrate emergency treatments for management of acute respiratory distress.
- Maintain vital signs within patient's normal limits.

Interventions

- Observe ventilatory function for difficulties: shallow respirations, tachypnea, dyspnea, frothy secretions, and jugular vein distention.
- Auscultate lungs for evidence of impairment: rales, chronic and diminished breath sounds.
- Monitor intake and output.
- Measure CVP.
- Obtain or assist with measurement of arterial blood gases (ABGs).
- Adjust position accordingly:

    High Fowler's position enhances lung expansion.

    Turn patient every 1 to 2 hours to mobilize secretions and prevent atelectasis, but keep most congested lung up to prevent further ventilation/perfusion problems.
- Administer humidified oxygen therapy by mask if ordered.
- Administer diuretics and decrease fluid intake as ordered.
- Suction nasopharynx and lungs as ordered.

Nursing Diagnosis

- *Fluid volume deficit related to capillary dilation or leakage leading to third spacing of fluid*

Outcome Goal

Patient will be able to:

- Maintain adequate fluid volume, as evidenced by laboratory values within normal limits; skin turgor, mucous membranes, and tongue hydration normal; daily intake and output balanced and adequate; absence of thirst or dry mouth; and vital signs within patient's normal limits.

Interventions

- Monitor intake and output every 30 to 60 minutes.
- Measure urine specific gravity.
- Insert indwelling urinary catheter as ordered.
- Measure CVP.
- Monitor blood pressure every 30 to 60 minutes.
- Administer crystalloids, colloids, and blood products as ordered to maintain circulating fluid volume.

The nursing management of a patient with septic shock is extremely complex and challenging. It requires astute assessment and often quick decision making. Because septicemia is the triggering event, infection prophylaxis is crucial.

Data from references 41, 46, 59, and 68.

Syndrome of Inappropriate Antidiuretic Hormone Secretion

DEFINITION

The syndrome of inappropriate antidiuretic hormone secretion (SIADH) is an endocrine paraneoplastic syndrome that causes a disorder of water balance.[74] Antidiuretic hormone (ADH), also called arginine vasopressin, regulates the body's water balance. SIADH is characterized by elevated serum blood levels of ADH, excessive water retention, hypo-osmolality, and hyponatremia.[74, 134]

ETIOLOGY AND RISK FACTORS

This syndrome develops in 1% to 2% of patients with cancer.[39, 134] Approximately two thirds of patients with documented SIADH have a neoplasm. The most common malignant disease associated with this syndrome is lung cancer, and about 80% of these cases are small (oat) cell carcinoma.[57] In fact, 50% of patients with SCLC have impaired water excretion. As many as 10% to 15% of these patients develop clinically evident SIADH.[39, 57, 69, 74] SIADH may be the presenting symptom in patients with SCLC.[39] Other cancers associated with SIADH include cancer of the esophagus, duodenum, pancreas, prostate, head and neck, and bladder; acute myelogenous leukemia; lymphoma; thymoma; mesothelioma; carcinoid tumors; CNS metastases; and non-SCLC.[39, 57, 74, 134] Several chemotherapeutic agents, including cisplatin, cyclophosphamide, melphalan, vinblastine, and vincristine, have been associated with the development of SIADH.[39, 57, 74, 135, 137] Other agents, such as antidepressants, antibiotics, opioids, chlorpropramide, nicotine, and ethanol have also been linked with SIADH.[39, 74, 135]

The incidence of SIADH is rising because of the increased incidence of SCLC and other cancers associated with the ectopic production of ADH.

Nonmalignant conditions that can account for SIADH are CNS disorders, pulmonary infections, asthma, the use of positive-pressure respirators.[74, 135]

PATHOPHYSIOLOGY

All body fluids are solutions containing various concentrations of solute (salt) and solvent (fluid or water). The concentration of salt in body fluid creates an osmotic pressure. Measurement of osmotic pressure (or concentration of a solution) is referred to as *osmolality* or *osmolarity*.[74] It is expressed in osmols (Osm) or milliosmols (mOsm) per kilogram of either water (osmolality) or solution (osmolarity). In a steady state, normal osmolality is maintained at a constant level of 280 to 300 mOsm/kg of body weight. The osmolality and volume of the extracellular fluid and the urine are maintained by a balance of fluid intake and urinary excretion.

Fluid intake is maintained by the thirst mechanism located in the hypothalamus (Fig. 20–17). Lack of water increases the osmolality of the extracellular fluid, which activates the sensation of thirst. Fluid intake is then increased to restore the fluid balance. If excess fluid is ingested, it is excreted to maintain the balance.

The second portion of the osmolality-regulating system is urinary excretion. The amount of urine excreted by the kidneys depends on how much fluid is reabsorbed and circulated throughout the body. This regulation of fluid intake and output through the kidneys is controlled by the presence of ADH in the kidneys.

Antidiuretic hormone is produced by the hypothalamus and transported to the posterior pituitary, where it is stored. Changes in ADH production and secretion (increase or decrease) are controlled by receptors in the kidneys, heart, and brain in response to extracellular or intravascular volume (see Fig. 20–17). ADH secretion is extremely sensitive and responds to a 1% to 2% change in osmolality.

When plasma osmolality is increased or plasma volume is decreased, ADH is secreted from the pituitary gland. Once in the kidneys, ADH increases the permeability of the distal tubule and the collection duct, which allows more water reabsorption. This enhanced amount of water enters the vascular system, diluting solutes, lowering plasma osmolality, and resulting in concentrated urine excretion. Decreased plasma or blood volume also stimulates ADH secretion. A moderate increase in ADH occurs with a 10% blood loss, and a 25% blood loss can produce 20 to 50 times the normal rate of ADH secretion. This response maintains arterial blood pressure.

If plasma osmolality is decreased, as in the presence of excessive water intake, ADH secretion is halted. This decreases the permeability to water of the renal distal tubule and the collecting duct, allowing more water to be excreted as dilute urine. An increase in plasma or blood volume also stops the release of ADH. Drinking alcohol inhibits ADH secretion. In summary, the thirst mechanism and the ADH feedback mechanisms (see Fig. 20–17) regulate body fluids and maintain a constant osmolality.

A variety of conditions can disrupt the body fluid regulating system and cause SIADH. The following three pathophysiologic mechanisms are responsible for SIADH:

- Inappropriate secretion of ADH from the supraoptic-hypophyseal system. This mechanism results from

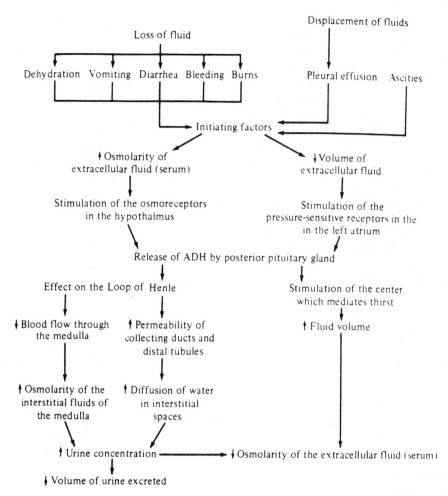

FIGURE 20–17 Feedback mechanism regulating the release of antidiuretic hormone (*ADH*). (From Yasko JM: Syndrome of inappropriate antidiuretic hormone secretion. In Yasko JM, editor: *Guidelines for cancer care: symptom management,* Reston, VA, Reston, © 1983. Reprinted by permission of Prentice-Hall, Inc., Upper Saddle River, NJ.)

CNS disorders such as head trauma, CVA (stroke), meningitis, brain abscess, CNS hemorrhage, CNS tumors (both primary and metastatic), encephalitis, and Guillain-Barre syndrome. Postoperative patients; patients in shock; patients experiencing status asthmaticus, pain, or high stress levels; and patients on positive-pressure breathing may also experience SIADH through this mechanism. These conditions increase intrathoracic pressure or decrease venous return to the heart. Cardiac output decreases, leading to decreased plasma volume, stimulating ADH secretion.

- ADH or an ADH-like substance is secreted by cells outside the supraoptic-hypophyseal system, referred to as *ectopic secretion.* Ectopic production of the endocrine peptide, ADH, has been demonstrated in a variety of malignancies and is the primary etiology for cancer-related SIADH. Cells in the atrium of the heart may also secrete a peptide, atrial natriuretic peptide, that can increase sodium excretion.[74] Infections within the pulmonary system such as those caused by bacteria or viruses may release ADH ec-

topically. This may also be one process leading to SIADH seen in patients with a malignancy.

- The action of ADH on the renal distal tubules is enhanced. Various drugs can stimulate or potentiate the release of ADH. These include narcotics such as morphine, nicotine, tranquilizers, barbiturates, general anesthetics, potassium supplements, thiazide diuretics, hypoglycemic agents such as chlorpropamide (Diabinese), clofibrate (Atromid-S), acetaminophen (paracetamol, Tylenol), isoproterenol, and five antineoplastic agents: cisplatin (Platinol), cyclophosphamide (Cytoxan), vinblastine (Velban), vincristine (Oncovin) and melphalan (Alkeran). Cyclophosphamide has a direct effect on the renal tubule and is also associated with vigorous hydration that can lead to SIADH.[57]

Patients with cancer may have SIADH resulting from any one of these three mechanisms. Intrathoracic or mediastinal tumors can increase intrathoracic pressure, resulting in a decreased venous return and decreased cardiac output, which stimulates the release of ADH. Patients with small (oat) cell lung cancer (50%), pancreatic cancer, lymphomas, and thymomas have demonstrated synthesis and secretion of ADH or an ADH-like substance from the neoplastic tissue. Patients receiving any of the chemotherapy agents listed above have the potential to develop SIADH.

The syndrome is associated with water excess and results from the ectopic production of ADH. ADH increases the permeability of the kidney to water, promoting water reabsorption and decreasing urine output. This may be associated with hyponatremia. Hyponatremia may be caused by excessive loss of sodium or excessive gain of water. It is always a result of a relatively greater water concentration than sodium concentration.

However, hyponatremia is not solely diagnostic of SIADH. Some other disorders may also stimulate SIADH. In hypothyroidism and hypoadrenocorticism, the hormone deficiency is responsible, but the exact mechanism is unknown.[46, 74, 105] SIADH can also be seen with hyponatremia secondary to sodium depletion (renal disease, vomiting, diarrhea, diabetic acidosis) hypokalemia, glucocorticoid deficiency, third-spacing, and dilutional hyponatremia related to CHF, renal failure, or ascites related to liver disease.

Two other particular situations will elicit hyponatremia. First, hyponatremia also occurs when nonsodium solutes accumulate in the extracellular space because they do not freely diffuse across cell membranes. This causes an osmotic gradient that allows water to move from the intracellular to the extracellular space. Two conditions can produce this phenomenon. Hyperglycemia is the most common cause of this disorder. The calculated and measured plasma osmolality will be the same, which is elevated because of hyperglycemia. IV mannitol therapy also demonstrates an elevated plasma osmolality, but the calculated level is lower than the measured value. In either situation, these are *not* true hypo-osmolar states.

Second, *pseudohyponatremia* may occur, also called *factitious hyponatremia*. These terms describe a low serum sodium concentration secondary to volume-displacing effects that can occur with hyperproteinemia and hyperlipidemia. Large macromolecules (proteins, lipids) are present and fictitiously lower plasma sodium levels, as measured in the clinical laboratory. However, measured plasma osmolality is normal.

These interesting situations must be evaluated in the presence of hyponatremia. Diagnostic work-up for any patient with hyponatremia requires determination of the existence of a hypo-osmolar state.

CLINICAL FEATURES

The clinical syndrome resulting from inappropriate secretion of ADH has the following features:

Hyponatremia (serum sodium less than normal level of 135–147 mEq/L)

Decreased osmolality of serum and extracellular fluid (less than normal level of 280–300 mOsm/kg)

Excessive water retention (water intoxication)

Urine osmolality greater than appropriate for plasma osmolality (>500 mmol/kg), producing less than maximally dilute urine (abnormally high urine specific gravity)

Continued urinary excretion of sodium (sodium in urine >20 mEq/L) (washing of sodium in urine)

Absence of fluid volume depletion (normal skin turgor and blood pressure)

Suppression of plasma renin

Normal renal, adrenal, and thyroid function

BUN possibly low because of volume expansion

Hypouricemia and hypophosphatemia may be present because of decreased proximal tubular reabsorption.

The symptomatology experienced by the patient with SIADH depends on the severity, rapidity, and duration of the hyponatremia and decreased plasma osmolality (Table 20–20).[39] Excessive water retention continues

TABLE 20–20
Signs and Symptoms of SIADH

MILD HYPONATREMIA: Serum Sodium 125–135 mEq/L

May be asymptomatic
Anorexia
Difficulty concentrating
Fatigue
Headache
Inappropriate behavior
Muscle cramps
Oliguria
Peripheral edema
Weakness
Weight gain

MODERATE HYPONATREMIA: Serum Sodium 115–125 mEq/L

Confusion
Decreased deep tendon reflexes
Hallucinations
Impaired taste
Incontinence
Lethargy
Nausea, vomiting, diarrhea
Oliguria
Personality changes
Thirst
Tremors
Weight gain

SEVERE HYPONATREMIA: Serum Sodium <115 mEq/L

Coma
Seizures
Inability to protect airway and mobilize secretions

Data from references 74 and 134.

despite a decrease in the osmolality of serum and extracellular fluid. Urine is concentrated and the extracellular fluid expands, and this results in hyponatremia. Patients complain of thirst, anorexia, nausea, and vomiting. Weight gain, lethargy, and muscle weakness occurs. Irritability, personality changes, and mental confusion may occur and lead to seizures and coma.

DIAGNOSIS

Asymptomatic SIADH is often found on routine serum chemistry.[57] SIADH is diagnosed from the combination of hyponatremia, decreased plasma osmolality, and increased urine osmality.[39, 57, 74] Associated lab values may include a decreased uric acid, albumin, BUN, and creatinine, and increased urine specific gravity.[74] It is possible to do radioimmunoassays of the urine and serum for elevated ADH levels. This is not commonly done due to cost and inconvenience. A water-loading test can also be performed. A calculated amount of water is administered, followed by monitoring intake, output, and specific gravity. This can only be done safely if the serum sodium is greater than 124 mEq/L and the patient is asymptomatic.[39]

TREATMENT MODALITIES

The primary treatment of choice for SIADH is to treat or eliminate the underlying cause; however, the sodium level and patient's neurologic status must be stabilized.[57] Treatment decisions are based on the severity of the hyponatremia and symptoms of water intoxication.

Mild hyponatremia is typically treated with fluid restriction (500–1000 mL/d). This promotes a negative water balance and will usually correct plasma sodium levels in 3 to 5 days.[57, 74] Mild to moderate hyponatremia that is chronic may be treated with demeclocycline, a derivative of tetracyline (600–1200 mg/d orally in divided doses). This drug inhibits the action of ADH on renal tubules so water can be excreted. Fluid restriction is not required with demeclocycline.[137] Side effects and toxicities may include nausea, photosensitivity, reversible diabetes insipidus, and azotemia (more common at higher doses).[39, 74, 137] Doses must be reduced for patients with decreased renal or hepatic function. Demeclocycline may be used for long-term therapy. Lithium carbonate (900–1200 mg/d) and urea (0.5 g/kg per day) are used less frequently.[74] Any drugs that can cause hyponatremia are discontinued (with the possible exception of certain chemotherapeutic agents).

Severe hyponatremia typically develops rapidly, over 1 to 2 days, and is a medical emergency. Un-treated, it will progress from seizures and coma to brain herniation and death. Increased intracellular fluid in brain cells (due to extracellular hypo-osmolality) increases ICP

and decreases cerebral blood flow.[74] Severe cases are treated with hypertonic saline infusions (3%) and Lasix diuresis.[57, 74] Care must be taken not to correct the hyponatremia too quickly, however, because this can lead to neurologic damage. Osmotic demyelination syndrome can occur within 2 to 6 days of too rapid correction of hyponatremia, particularly in patients with hypokalemia. Symptoms include rapidly progressive lower extremity weakness, dysarthria, and dysphagia. It is recommended to correct serum potassium levels prior to, or in conjunction with, initiating therapy for hyponatremia. One recommendation for hyponatremia is to begin sodium level correction at a rate not to exceed 0.5 to 1.0 mEq/L per hour.[74, 137, 138] Once mild hyponatremic levels are reached, therapy is changed to fluid restriction or pharmacologic agents such as demeclocycline.[74]

Using chemotherapy to treat the underlying malignancy in a patient with SIADH provides its own set of challenges. One drug used to treat SCLC is cisplatin, which requires the patient to be well hydrated to protect renal tissue from toxicity. Cisplatin can cause SIADH, as well as exacerbate existing SIADH. Administration of cyclophoshamide, used to treat many solid tumors, also requires hydration. Vigorous hydration may exacerbate SIADH. Patients with mild hyponatremia may be gently hydrated with normal saline prior to chemotherapy and then put on fluid restriction. Moderate SIADH may require saline hydration, electrolyte replacement, and diuresis prior to chemotherapy. Patients with severe hyponatremia will need to be neurologically stablized prior to the initiation of chemotherapy.[39]

Currently, no drugs are available that directly suppress the synthesis or release of ADH from malignant tissue; however, clinical trials are investigating agents that can block the action of ADH at the collecting duct system. These agents are called nonpeptide vasopressin V2 receptor antagonists.[70, 74]

PROGNOSIS

The syndrome can be successfully treated, as evidenced by a return to normal levels of serum and extracellular osmolality, serum sodium and urine osmolality, and specific gravity. The rapidity and duration of response depend greatly on the underlying cause. Neurologic impairment from water intoxication is usually reversible.

Usually, SIADH resolves with tumor regression, but it can persist despite control of the tumor. It may recur, suggesting tumor progression, but recurrence is sometimes seen with stable disease during the maintenance phase of therapy. If the underlying cause is not eliminated, the SIADH may be a chronic problem and require ongoing intermittent management.

Nursing management of the patient with SIADH is outlined in the accompanying box.

Nursing Management

SYNDROME OF INAPPROPRIATE DIURETIC HORMONE

The primary nursing intervention for a patient diagnosed with the syndrome of inappropriate secretion of antidiuretic hormone (SIADH) is patient education and emotional support to facilitate patient compliance.

Nursing Diagnoses

- *Fluid volume excess related to fluid retention (from SIADH) and hyponatremia*
- *Fluid volume deficit related to fluid restriction as treatment for SIADH*

Outcome Goal

Patient will be able to:

- Demonstrate resolution of SIADH, as evidenced by decreased or absent signs of SIADH, serum sodium range within normal limits, serum and urine osmolality within normal limits, normal urine output of at least 1500 mL/24 h, and normal body weight for patient.

Interventions

- Assess for signs or symptoms of alteration in fluid volume:
    - Excess: rales, shortness of breath, neck vein distention, weight gain, edema of sacrum and/or lower extremities
    - Deficit: dry mucous membranes, poor skin turgor, weight loss, rapid thready pulse, orthostatic hypotension, restlessness
- Auscultate lungs for breath sounds every 4 hours.
- Monitor cardiac function and tissue perfusion.
- Monitor intake and output closely:
    - Restrict fluids as ordered (500–1000 mL/24 h).
    - Allocate fluids per shift as per discussion with patient.
    - Give pills and medications with meals to allow flexibility with fluid rations.
    - Monitor IV infusions carefully using a flow regulator.
    - Accurately measure urine output. Intake and output should be almost equal until serum sodium is within normal limits.
- Obtain a daily weight.
- Monitor laboratory values (serum electrolytes, BUN, creatinine, calcium, magnesium) with special attention to the following:
    - Serum plasma osmolality: as SIADH progresses, plasma osmolality decreases, which causes the brain to swell and level of consciousness (LOC) to decrease. Therefore serum osmolality can predict LOC.
    - Serum sodium: hypernatremia may result from overcorrection of low serum levels. Accompanying signs and symptoms of hypernatremia include thirst, dry mucous membranes, irritability, lethargy, and seizures.
- Obtain urine osmolality and specific gravity.
- Monitor skin integrity and provide skin care.

Nursing Diagnosis

- *Altered oral mucous membrane related to fluid restriction*

Outcome Goal

Patient will be able to:

- Exhibit oral cavity, gums, and lips free of irritation, as evidenced by pink, moist mucosa and tongue; moist, soft lips with undisrupted integrity; pink, firm gingiva; watery saliva; and maintenance of adequate oral intake.

Interventions

- Thoroughly assess the oral cavity daily.
- Provide oral care every 2 to 4 hours as needed:
    - Use mouthwashes with little to no alcohol.
    - Discourage smoking and drinking alcohol.
    - Avoid spicy and mechanically harsh foods.
    - Use mouth moisturizers and artificial saliva as needed.

Nursing Diagnosis

- *Altered thought processes related to low serum sodium level*

Outcome Goals

Patient will be able to:

- Remain oriented to person, time, and place.
- Demonstrate safety-related behaviors.

Interventions

- Assess neurologic status:
    - Determine LOC, noting any changes in sensorium.

Check muscles and tendon reflexes for twitching.
Monitor for seizure activity if serum sodium level less than 120 mEq/L.
- Initiate safety precautions:
  Monitor patient activities.
  Assist patient with transfer and ambulation.
  Use bed rails at night.
- Increase safety measures if change in LOC or serum sodium level less than 120 mEq/L:
  Orient frequently to time and place.

Pad bed rails.
Use restraints as necessary.
Implement seizure precautions (e.g., padded tongue blade and airway at bedside, no oral thermometers).

Many patients with extreme hyponatremia cannot recollect much of their experience during the SIADH event. This points out the need to provide measures to ensure safety and to reduce anxiety.

Tumor Lysis Syndrome

DEFINITION

Tumor lysis syndrome (TLS) is an oncologic emergency that occurs with rapid lysis of malignant cells. The resultant metabolic imbalance can quickly lead to fatal renal, cardiac, and neurologic complications.

ETIOLOGY AND RISK FACTORS

Tumor lysis syndrome may occur spontaneously in patients with inordinately high tumor burdens. However, it is most commonly caused as a result of treatment-related malignant cell death. TLS has been reported to occur with surgery, biotherapy, hyperthermia, hormonal therapy, and radiation therapy, but it is most frequently associated with chemotherapy.[44, 88] It may occur anywhere from 24 hours to 7 days after antineoplastic therapy is initiated.[145] There are no published reports of incidence, but it is estimated to occur in 10% of lymphomas.[104] Patients most at risk are those who have large tumor cell burdens with high proliferative fractions (high-grade lymphomas), markedly elevated WBC counts (acute leukemias), elevated LDH (associated with bulky tumors) or uric acid levels, pre-existing renal dysfunction, splenomegaly, or lymphadeonopathy.[26, 44, 64, 145, 150] TLS is also seen in CLL in blast crisis, SCLC, metastatic breast cancer, and metastatic medulloblastoma.[39, 145]

PATHOPHYSIOLOGY

As malignant cells are lysed, intracelluar contents are rapidly released into the blood-stream. This results in high levels of potassium (hyperkalemia), phosphate (hyperphosphatemia), and uric acid (hyperuricemia). Because there is an inverse relationship between phosphate and calcium, a decrease in serum calcium (hypocalcemia) occurs. This metabolic imbalance may be even more pronounced in patients with certain types of cancers. Patients with lymphoblastic leukemia may have four times more intracellular phosphate.[39, 75] Leu-

kemic cells are also rich in purine nucleic acids that are metabolized into uric acid by the liver.[39, 44, 88] If the kidneys are unable to sufficiently excrete the by-products of malignant cell death, the clinical situation can rapidly become life-threatening. Hyperkalemia (K > 5.5 mEq/L) leads to bradycardia, heart block, ventricular fibrillation, and asystole.[45] Levels greater than 6.5 can cause ascending paralysis and respiratory failure.[45] Hypocalcemia can also cause arrhythmias and cardiac dysfunction. Hyperkalemia, hyperphosphatemia, and hyperuricemia all lead to renal failure. Uric acid is insoluble in acidic urine and can precipate in the kidneys. Elevated potassium and phosphate both cause renal insufficiency that can progress to renal failure. TLS can also stimulate the coagulation cascade that leads to DIC.

CLINICAL FEATURES

The clinical features of TLS are outlined in Table 20–21. Patients exhibit the signs and symptoms associated with each metabolic abnormality. Early signs may include nausea, vomiting, anorexia and diarrhea, and may be accompanied by muscle weakness and cramping. Later signs may progress to tetany, paresthesias, convulsions, anuria, and cardiac arrest.[120]

DIAGNOSIS

Tumor lysis syndrome is diagnosed by observation of the signs and symptoms outlined in Table 20–21 and by confirmation of abnormal laboratory values. Serum potassium, phosphate, calcium, and uric acid are diagnostic. Other important values include serum creatinine, BUN, and urine pH.[75]

TREATMENT MODALITIES

The best way to treat TLS is to *prevent* it by recognizing the patient population who is at risk and initiating prophylactic measures prior to initiation of antineoplastic therapy.[133] This includes pre-treatment *hydration* to maintain a urinary output of 100 mL/h. Hydration should begin 24 to 48 hours before treatment and con-

TABLE 20–21
Signs and Symptoms of Tumor Lysis Syndrome

	GI	Renal	Cardiac	Neuromuscular
Hyperkalemia	Nausea		BP/P changes	Twitching
			ECG changes	Cramping
	Vomiting		Arrhythmias	Weakness
	Diarrhea		Heart block	Paresthesias
	Anorexia		Asystole	Ascending flaccid paralysis
Hyperuricemia	Nausea	Edema		Lethargy
	Vomiting	Flank pain		Goutlike symptoms
	Diarrhea	Hematuria		
	Anorexia	Oliguria		
		Cloudy, sediment in urine		
		Anuria		
		Azotemia		
		Crystalluria		
Hyperphosphatemia		Oliguria		
		Anuria		
		Azotemia		
		Renal insufficiency		
Hypocalcemia			Hypotension	Twitching
			Heart block	Cramping
			Cardiac arrest	Tetany
				Chvostek's sign*
				Trousseau's sign*
				Laryngospasm
				Paresthesias
				Seizures
				Confusion

*See Box 20–3 for definitions.
Data from references 39, 44, 85, and 145.

tinue for at least 72 hours after treatment.[44] *Diuretics* may be used to promote the excretion of phosphate and uric acid.[145] *Allopurinol* is a xanthine oxidase inhibitor that prevents uric acid formation. It is begun a few days prior to treatment and should be continued for 3 to 5 days after treatment is completed. Dose recommendations range from 300 mg/d to a loading dose of 600 to 900 mg followed by 300 to 450 mg/d.[39, 75] Side effects of allopurinol may include a rash, eosinophilia, fever, hypersensitivity reaction, and exfoliative dermatitis.[44, 145] *Sodium bicarbonate* is used to maintain an alkaline urine (pH > 7) to prevent uric acid crystallization (50–100 mEq/L fluid or 50 mEq IV bolus).[145] Some controversy exists over whether alkalinization should be continued once treatment is started due to the risk of exacerbating hyperphosphatemia and hypocalcemia.[44, 75] Most references recommend continuing it until uric acid levels stablize.[88] Acetazolamide, a diuretic, may be used to decrease bicarbonate reabsorption in the kidney so that it is excreted in the urine where it enhances alkalinization.[44]

Electrolytes, urine pH, and accurate intake and output, must be assessed at least every 4 to 8 hours during treatment and for the following 3 to 5 days. 39 If TLS occurs, *diuretics* are used to prevent volume overload and promote the excretion of potassium in the urine. *Cation-exchange resins,* such as kaexylate, are used to bind with potassium so it can be excreted through the bowel (15–30 g with 50 mL 20% sorbitol orally 2–4 times a day; or 50 in 200 mL or 20% sorbitol as a retention enema for 30 to 60 minutes).[39] *Insulin-glucose* therapy may be added to enhance the shift of potassium back into the intracellular compartment. (1 U regular insulin is given for each 4 g glucose,[39] or 50 mL D50 and 10 U insulin over 1 hour.[88]) *Calcium gluconate* is used to correct hypocalcemia (1–3 amps of 10% IV push with cardiac monitoring).[145] Phosphate-binding gels, such as aluminum hydroxide, are given to form an insoluble complex that is excreted by the bowel.[145]

Medications containing phosphate should be discontinued (clindamycin, sodium-potassium phosphate). Phosphate-containing foods, such as milk, cheese, and carbonated beverages, may be restricted.[44] Other medications that can further elevate serum phosphate, and thus lower serum calcium, include furosemide, mithramycin, gallium nitrate, and anticonvulsants.[39, 44] Thiazide diuretics, aspirin, and probenecid can elevate uric acid levels.[145] Indomethacin and potassium-sparing diuretics (Aldactone/spironolactone, Dyrenium/triamterene, Midamor/amiloride HCL) are not recommended.[39, 145] Any nephrotoxic medications should be avoided as should radiographic contrast dyes.

When these measures are not successful, renal dialysis may be necessary. Critical laboratory values indicating a need for dialysis include potassium greater than 6.0 mEq/L, phosphate greater than 10 mg/dL, and uric acid greater than 10 mg/dL.[44, 65, 145]

PROGNOSIS

Successful treatment of TLS depends on preventing renal failure. TLS typically resolves within 7 days, once appropriate treatment is initiated.[85, 133]

Nursing Management of the patient with TLS is outlined in the accompanying box.

Nursing Management

TUMOR LYSIS SYNDROME

Oncology nurses should be aware of patients who are at high risk for tumor lysis syndrome (TLS). Nurses take an active role in the prevention of TLS by administering allopurinol and hydration prior to the initiation of treatment. Careful monitoring of lab values and observing the patient for early subtle changes allows prompt intervention and the prevention of cardiac abnormalities and renal failure.

Nursing Diagnoses

- *Altered tissue perfusion (renal) related to TLS induced hyperkalemia, hyperphosphatemia, hypocalcemia, and hyperuricemia.*
- *Altered urinary elimination related to uric acid nephropathy and acute renal failure*

Outcome Goals

Patient will be able to:

- Maintain normal levels of potassium, phosphorous, calcium, and uric acid.
- Maintain urinary elimination greater than 30 mL/h, balance intake and output, and BUN/creatinine/urine pH within normal limits

Interventions

- Identify patients at risk for TLS.
- Inititate hydration 24 to 48 hours prior to initiating chemotherapy in high-risk patients.
- Administer allopurinol before and during chemotherapy to maintain alkaline urine.
- Assess medications for those that contain phosphate or spare potassium and discuss discontinuation with physician.

- Monitor potassium, phosphorus, calcium, and uric acid levels.
- Assess patient for signs and symptoms of TLS (see Table 20–21)
    - Hyperkalemia—cardiac, GI, neuromuscular
    - Hyperphosphatemia—renal
    - Hypocalcemia—cardiac, neuromuscular
    - Hyperuricemia—GI, renal
- Administer diuretics, sodium bicarbonate, cation-exchange resins, insulin-glucose therapy, and phosphate-binding gels as appropriate.
- Monitor intake and output and notify physician if urinary output is less than 100 mL/h.
- Monitor urine pH and maintain at above 7.0 with sodium bicarbonate.
- Prepare the patient and family for dialysis if other measures are not effective.

Nursing Diagnosis

- *Decreased cardiac output*

Outcome Goal

Patient will be able to:

- Maintain optimal cardiac output, as evidenced by vital signs, cardiac rhythm and serum potassium and calcium within normal limits.

Interventions

- Monitor serum potassium and calcium.
- Obtain ECG for potassium greater than 6.0 mEq/L and calcium less than 8.0 mg/dL.
- Report ECG changes (peaked and narrow T-waves, shortened QT interval, widened QRS complex with decreased amplitude, loss of P-wave, ventricular tachycardia, ventricular fibrillation, blending of QRS into T-wave).

- Monitor blood pressure, pulse, and central venous pressure.
- Be prepared to transfer patient to ICU for hemodynamic monitoring.

Nursing Diagnosis

- *Fluid volume excess*

Outcome Goals

Patient will be able to:

- Maintain urinary output balanced with oral and IV fluid intake.

- Maintain stable blood pressure and pulse.
- Maintain lungs clear to auscultation.

Interventions

- Assess patient for jugular venous distention and peripheral edema.
- Auscultate lung sounds for signs of volume overload, assess rate and depth of respirations.
- Keep accurate intake and output.
- Weigh patient daily.
- Monitor blood pressure and pulse.
- Administer diuretics as ordered.

Data from references 117 and 145.

CONCLUSION

Successful management of patients with oncologic complications requires expertise from all members of the health care team. It requires in-depth knowledge in oncology but also in many related areas, such as immunology, pharmacology, cardiopulmonary care, and critical care. The nurse is in a pivotal role as coordinator of the care and as patient advocate to help the patient and family deal with the impact of the illness on their lives.

Chapter Questions

1. Two clinical findings that are classic features of cardiac tamponade are:
   a. Pulsus paradoxus, bradycardia
   b. Hepatojugular reflux, pitting edema
   c. Pulsus paradoxus, hepatojugular reflux
   d. Hepatojugular reflux, vasodilation
2. In which area of the spinal column are the majority of spinal metastases that cause spinal cord compression (SCC)?
   a. Cervical
   b. Lumbar
   c. Sacral
   d. Thoracic
3. Symptomatology is directly related to the location of the SCC. What is the *most* common presenting symptom of SCC?
   a. Motor weakness
   b. Pain
   c. Sexual dysfunction
   d. Sensory loss
4. The most common oncologic etiology for increased intracranial pressure (IICP) is:
   a. Syndrome of antidiuretic hormone (SIADH)
   b. Diabetes insipidus

   c. Brain metastases
   d. Intracranial bleeding
5. What is the first therapeutic measure after a confirmed diagnosis of superior vena cava syndrome (SVCS)?
   a. Surgery
   b. Radiation therapy
   c. Chemotherapy
   d. Biotherapy
6. Etiology and risk factors for disseminated intravascular coagulation (DIC) include:
   a. Shock, infection, acute leukemia, intravascular hemolysis
   b. Shock, infection, acute leukemia, breast cancer
   c. Shock, infection, lung cancer, intravascular hemolysis
   d. Shock, infection, testicular cancer, intravascular hemolysis
7. Components of the DIC laboratory test profile include:
   a. Complete blood count (CBC), serum aspartate aminotransferase (AST, SGOT), prothrombin times (PTs), fibrinogen levels
   b. PTs, fibrinogen levels, fibrin degradation products, D-dimer
   c. PTs, fibrinogen levels, CBC, type and crossmatch
   d. PTs, fibrinogen levels, platelet levels, HLA antigens
8. Clinical features for hypercalcemia include:
   a. Polyuria, polydipsia, change in mental status, absent deep tendon reflex
   b. Polyuria, polydipsia, change in mental status, increased deep tendon reflex
   c. Polydipsia, constipation, change in mental status, dyspnea
   d. Polyuria, constipation, change in mental status, dyspnea

9. Treatment modalities for hypercalcemia include:
   a. Hydration, dialysis, pharmacologic therapy, chemotherapy
   b. Hydration, dialysis, pharmacologic therapy, bed rest
   c. Hydration, pharmacologic therapy, radiation therapy, mobilization
   d. Hydration, dialysis, pharmacologic therapy, mobilization
10. Risk factors for hypersensitivity reaction (HSR) include:
    a. Specific agent, route of administration, gender
    b. Nutritional status, gender, alcoholism
    c. Specific agent, gender, weight
    d. Gender, age, nitrosurea drugs
11. Malignant pleural effusion is life-threatening because the:
    a. Decreased pleural fluid affects respiratory function.
    b. Increased pleural fluid affects respiratory function.
    c. Increased pericardial fluid affects respiratory function.
    d. Decreased pericardial fluid affects respiratory function.
12. The lymphatic channels regulate fluid and protein reabsorption. Normally how much fluid flows through the pleural space in 24 hours? How much fluid remains in the pleural space at any given time?
    a. 1 to 5 L; 5 to 10 mL
    b. 3 to 10 L; 10 to 20 mL
    c. 10 to 15 L; 5 to 10 mL
    d. 5 to 10 L; 5 to 20 mL
13. Septic shock may be classified by hyperdynamic stage (early), normodynamic stage (intermediate), and hypodynamic stage (late). Usual progression of the clinical features for these stages is:
    a. Tachycardia, increased respirations, hypertension, anuria
    b. Tachycardia, increased respirations, decreased urine output, altered mental status
    c. Tachycardia, decreased respirations, hypotension, anuria
    d. Tachycardia, respirations slow and shallow, hypertension, renal failure
14. Syndrome of inappropriate antidiuretic hormone secretion (SIADH) is *most* common in which type of cancer?
    a. Breast
    b. Leukemia
    c. Multiple myeloma
    d. Small cell lung cancer
15. The clinical manifestations of tumor lysis syndrome are due to:
    a. Hypercalcemia, hypokalemia, hypouricemia, hypophosphatemia
    b. Hyperkalemia, hyperphosphatemia, hyperuricemia, hypocalcemia
    c. Hypophosphatemia, hyperkalemia, hyperuricemia, hypercalcemia
    d. Hypokalemia, hyperuricemia, hyperphosphatemia, hypercalcemia

BIBLIOGRAPHY

1. *AHFS Drug Information 1999,* Bethesda, MD, American Society of Health System Pharmacists, Inc.
2. Alfieri DR: Pediatric drug information. Pegaspargase, *Pediatr Nurs* 21:471, 1995.
3. Anonymous: New drugs. Pegaspargase (Oncaspar): therapy for ALL evades immune reaction, *AJN* 95:56, 1995.
4. Arbour R: Aggressive management of intracranial dynamics, *Crit Care Nurse* 18:30, 1998.
5. Astiz ME, Rackow EC: Seminar. Septic shock, *Lancet* 351(9114):1501, 1998.
6. Atkinson TP, Kaliner MA: Anaphylaxis, *Med Clin North Am* 76:841, 1992.
7. Baglin T: Disseminated intravascular coagulation: diagnosis and treatment, *BMJ* 312:683, 1996.
8. Bailes BK: Disseminated intravascular coagulation: principles, treatment, nursing management, *AORN J* 55:517, 1992.
9. Bajournas DR: Clinical manifestations of cancer related hypercalcemia, *Semin Oncol* 17(suppl 5):16, 1990.
10. Barbiere CC: Are you listening? Cardiac tamponade: diagnosis and emergency intervention, *Crit Care Nurse* 10:7, 1990.
11. Barnett ML: Hypercalcemia, *Semin Oncol Nurs* 15:190, 1999.
12. Beattie S, Meinhardt SL: Transesophageal echocardiography: advanced technology for the cardiac patient, *Crit Care Nurse* 12:42, 1992.
13. Beauchamp KA: Pericardial tamponade: an oncologic emergency, *Clin J Oncol Nurs* 2:85, 1998.
14. Belford K: Central nervous system cancers. *In* Groenwald SL, Frogge MH, Goodman M, Yarbro CH, editors: *Cancer nursing: principles and practice,* ed 4, Boston, Jones & Bartlett, 1997:980.
15. Berenson JR, and others: Efficacy of pamidronate in reducing skeletal events in patients with advanced multiple myeloma, *N Engl J Med* 334:488, 1996.
16. Bick RL: Disseminated intravascular coagulation: objective criteria for diagnosis and management, *Med Clin North Am* 78:511, 1994.
17. Blendowski C, Haapoja IS: Pleural access port: a creative alternative to repeated thoracentesis, *Dev Supportive Cancer Care* 2:41-4, 1998.
18. Bohan EM: Neurosurgical management of patients with central nervous system malignancies, *Semin Oncol Nurs* 14:8, 1998.

19. Bone RC, and others: Definitions for sepsis and organ failure and guidelines for the use of innovative therapies in sepsis, *Chest* 101:1644, 1992.

20. Bookman MA, and others: Intravenous prophylaxis for paclitaxel-related hypersensitivity reactions, *Semin Oncol* 24(6 suppl 19):S19, 1997.

21. Borenstein MA: Best strategy for hematologic emergencies, *Emerg Med* 27:48, 1995.

22. Braunwald E: Pericaradial disease. In Braunwald E and others, editors: *Harrison's principles of internal medicine*, ed 11, New York, McGraw-Hill, 1987.

23. Bucholtz JD: Central nervous system metastases, *Semin Oncol Nurs* 14:61, 1998.

24. Bucholtz JD: Metastatic epidural spinal cord compression, *Semin Oncol Nurs* 15:150, 1999.

25. Campbell T, Farrell W: Radiotherapy. Palliative radiotherapy for advance cancer symptoms, *Int J Palliative Nurs* 4:292, 1998.

26. Camp-Sorrell D: Chemotherapy: toxicity management. In Groenwald SL, Frogge MH, Goodman M, Yarbro CH, editors: *Cancer nursing: principles and practice,* ed 4, Boston, Jones & Bartlett, 1997:385.

27. Camp-Sorrell D: Clinical focus. Hypercalcemia, *Clin J Oncol Nurs* 2:73, 1998.

28. Camp-Sorrell D: Clinical focus. Spinal cord compression, *Clin J Oncol Nurs* 2:12, 1998.

29. *Cancer Chemotherapy Guidelines and Recommendations for Practice*, ed 2, Fishman M, Mrozek-Orlowski M, editors. Pittsburgh, Oncology Nursing Press, 1999.

30. Cephalosporins. *AHFS Drug Information 1999,* Bethesda, MD, American Society of Health System Pharmacists, 1999.

31. Clayton K: Cancer-related hypercalcemia: how to spot it, how to manage it, *AJN* 97:43, 1997.

32. Compton J: Drug update: use of glucagon in intractable allergic reactions and as an alternative to epinephrine: an interesting case review, *J Emerg Nurs* 23:45, 1997.

33. Craig JB, Capizzi RL: The prevention and treatment of immediate hypersensitivity reactions from cancer chemotherapy, *Semin Oncol Nurs* 1:285, 1985.

34. Cronin L, and others: Corticosteroid treatment for sepsis: a critical appraisal and meta-analysis of the literature, *Crit Care Med* 23:1430, 1995.

35. Day MW: Caring for patients with pleural effusion, *Nursing* 28:56, 1998.

36. Deftos LJ: Hypercalcemia: mechanisms, differential diagnosis, and remedies, *Postgrad Med* 100:119, 1996.

37. Delaney TF, Oldfield EH: Spinal cord compression. In DeVita VT Jr, Hellman S, Rosenberg SA, editors: *Cancer: principles and practice of oncology,* ed 4, Philadelphia, Lippincott, 1993.

38. De Lalla F: Antibiotic treatment of febrile episodes in neutropenic cancer patients, clinical and economic considerations, *Drugs 1997* 53:789, 1997.

39. Dietz KA, Flaherty AM: Oncologic emergencies. In Groenwald SL, Frogge MH, Goodman M, Yarbro CH, editors: *Cancer nursing: principles and practice,* ed 3, Boston, Jones & Bartlett, 1993:821.

40. Dyck S: Surgical instrumentation as a palliative treatment for spinal cord compression, *Oncol Nurs Forum* 18:515, 1991.

41. Ellerhorst-Ryan JM: Infection. In Groenwald SL, Frogge MH, Goodman M, Yarbro CH, editors: *Cancer nursing: principles and practice,* ed 4, Boston, Jones & Bartlett, 1997:585.

42. Elpern EH and others: The technique of pleurodesis, *J Crit Illness* 9:1105, 1994.

43. Epstein C, Bakanauskas A: Clinical management of DIC: early nursing interventions, *Crit Care Nurse* 11:42, 1991.

44. Ezzone SA: Tumor lysis syndrome, *Semin Oncol Nurs* 15:202, 1999.

45. Fabius DB: How to recognize electrolyte imbalances on an ECG, *Nursing 98* 28(11):6, 1998.

46. Finley JP: Metabolic emergencies. In Itano JK, Taoka KN, editors: *Oncology Nursing Society core curriculum for oncology nursing,* ed 3, Philadelphia, Saunders, 1998:315.

47. Finley JP: Nursing care of patients with metabolic and physiological oncological emergencies. In Clark JC, McGee RF, editors: *Core curriculum for oncology nursing,* ed 2, Philadelphia, Saunders, 1991.

48. Fiocco M, Drasna MJ: The management of malignant pleural and pericardial effusions, *Hematol Oncol Clin North Am,* 99:253, 1997.

49. Fristoe B: Long-term cardiac and pulmonary complications in cancer care, *Nurse Practitioner Forum* 9:177, 1998.

50. Fuller BG, Heiss J, Oldfield EH: Spinal cord compression. In DeVita VT Jr, Hellman S, Rosenberg SA, editors: *Cancer: principles and practice of oncology,* ed. 5, Philadelphia, Lippincott-Raven, 1997:2476.

51. Gell PHG, Coombs RRA: *Clinical aspects of immunology, Oxford,* Blackwell Scientific Publications, 1995.

52. Glover DJ, Glick JH: Oncologic emergencies. In Holleb AI, Fink DJ, Murphy GP, editors: *American Cancer Society textbook of clinical oncology,* Atlanta, American Cancer Society, 1991.

53. Gobel BH: Bleeding disorders. In Groenwald SL, Frogge MH, Goodman M, Yarbro CH, editors: *Cancer nursing: principles and practice,* ed 4, Boston, Jones & Bartlett, 1997:604.

54. Gobel BH: Disseminated intravascular coagulation, *Semin Oncol Nurs* 15:174, 1999.

55. Gray BH and others: Safety and efficacy of thrombolytic therapy for superior vena cava syndrome, *Chest* 99:54, 1991.

56. Grossman SA, Lossignol D: Diagnosis and treatment of epidural metastases, *Oncology* 4:47, 1990.

57. Haapoja IS, Blendowski C: Superior vena cava syndrome, *Semin Oncol Nurs* 15:183, 1999.

58. Hardy J: Clinical management. Corticosteroids in palliative care, *Eur J Palliative Care* 5:46, 1998.

59. Harnett S: Septic shock in the oncology patient, *Cancer Nurs* 12:191, 1989.

60. Heatley S, Coleman R: Product focus. The use of bisphosphonates in the palliative care setting, *Int J Palliative Nurs* 5:74, 1999.

61. Hickman JL: Increased intracranial pressure. In Chernecky CG, Berger BJ, editors: *Advanced and critical care oncology nursing: managing primary complications,* Philadelphia, Saunders, 1998.

62. Hickey JV: *The clinical practice of neurological and neurosurgical nursing,* ed 3, Philadelphia, Lippincott, 1992.

63. Hillier R, Wee B: Clinical management. Palliative management of spinal cord compression, *Eur J Palliative Care* 4:189, 1997.

64. Hoffman V: Tumor lysis syndrome: implications for nursing, *Home Healthcare Nurse* 14:595, 1996.

65. Hogan DK, Rosenthal LD: Oncologic emergencies in the patient with lymphoma, *Semin Oncol Nurs* 14:312, 1998.

66. Hunter JC: Nursing care of patients with structural oncological emergencies. In Clark JC, McGee RF, editors: *Core curriculum for oncology nursing,* ed 2, Philadelphia, Saunders, 1992.

67. Hunter, JC: Structural emergencies. In Itano JK, Taoka KN, editors: *Oncology Nursing Society core curriculum for oncology nursing,* ed 3, Philadelphia, Saunders, 1998:340.

68. Hydzik CA: Alteration in cardiac output, decreased: related to cardiac tamponade. In McNally JC and others, editors: *Guidelines for oncology nursing practice,* ed 2, Philadelphia, Saunders, 1991.

69. Ingle RJ: Lung cancers. In Groenwald SL, Frogge MH, Goodman M, Yarbro CH, editors: *Cancer nursing: principles and practice,* ed 4, Boston, Jones & Bartlett, 1997:1260.

70. Ishikawa S, Toshikazu S: Therapeutic efficacy of vasopressin receptor antagonists, *Int Med* 37:217, 1998.

71. Joiner GA, Kolodychuk GR: Neoplastic cardiac tamponade, *Crit Care Nurse* 11:50, 1991.

72. Joyce M, Cunningham RS: Metastases that interfere with circulation, *Semin Oncol Nurs* 14:230, 1998.

73. Kaplan M: Hypercalcemia of malignancy: a review of advances in pathophysiology, *Oncol Nurs Forum* 21:1039, 1994.

74. Keenan AMM: Syndrome of inappropriate secretion of antidiuretic hormone in malignancy, *Semin Oncol Nurs* 15:160, 1999.

75. Kelly KM, Lange B: Oncologic emergencies. *Pediatr Clin North Am* 44:809, 1997.

76. Khandheria BK, Oh J: Transesophageal echocardiography: state-of-the-art and future directions, *Am J Cardiol* 69:61H, 1992.

77. King PA: Oncologic emergencies: assessment, identification, and interventions in the emergency department, *J Emerg Nurs* 21:213-8, 1995.

78. Knoop T, Willenberg K: Cardiac tamponade, *Semin Oncol Nurs* 15:168, 1999.

79. Koepke JA: Tips from the clinical experts. DIC workup, *Med Lab Observer* 29:18, 1997.

80. Kovacs CS and others: Hypercalcemia of malignancy in the palliative care patient: a treatment strategy, *J Pain Symptom Manage* 10:224, 1995.

81. Labovich TM: Acute hypersensitivity reactions to chemotherapy, *Semin Oncol Nurs* 15:222, 1999.

82. Labovich, TM: Selected complications in the patient with cancer: spinal cord compression, malignant bowel obstruction, malignant ascites, and gastrointestinal bleeding, *Semin Oncol Nurs* 10:189, 1994.

83. Lang-Kummer J: Hypercalcemia. In Groenwald SL, Frogge MH, Goodman M, Yarbro CH, editors, *Cancer nursing: principles and practice,* ed 4, Boston, Jones & Bartlett, 1997:684.

84. Laskin MS, Lucchesi KJ, Morgan M: Paclitaxel rechallenge failure after a major hypersensitivity reaction, *J Clin Oncol* 11:2456, 1993.

85. Lawrence J: Critical care issues in the patient with hematologic malignancy, *Semin Oncol Nurs* 14:198, 1998.

86. Lieberman P: Distinguishing anaphylaxis from other serious disorders, *J Respir Dis* 16:411, 1995.

87. Lokich J, Goodman R: Superior vena cava syndrome, *JAMA* 321:58, 1975.

88. Lorigan PC and others: Tumour lysis syndrome, case report and review of literature, *Ann Oncol* 7:631, 1996.

89. Mackan MM: Managing the patient with anaphylaxis part 2: therapeutic strategies, *Emerg Med* 27:20, 1995.

90. Maher DeLeon ME, Schnell S, Rozental JM: Tumors of the spine and spinal cord, *Semin Oncol Nurs* 14:43, 1998.

91. Mangan CM: Malignant pericardial effusions: pathophysiology and clinical correlates, *Oncol Nurs Forum* 19:215, 1991.

92. Mann B, Sexton PA: Beta-lactam antibiotics, College of Health and Life Sciences, Fort Hays State University, http://www.fhsu.edu/nursing/otitis/b-lactam.html.

93. Markman M and others: Clinical features of hypersensitivity reactions to carboplatin, *J Clin Oncol* 17:1141, 1999.

94. Maxwell MB: Malignant effusions and edemas. In Groenwald SL, Frogge MH, Goodman M, Yarbro CH, editors: *Cancer nursing: principles and practice,* ed 4, Boston, Jones & Bartlett, 1997:721.

95. McFadden ME, Sartorius SE: Multiple system organ failure in the patient with cancer. Part I. Pathophysiologic perspectives, *Oncol Nurs Forum* 19:719, 1992.

96. McIntyre WJ, Parr MD: Infections in the immunosuppressed patient. In Herfindal ET, Gourley DR, editors: *Textbook of therapeutics: drug and disease management,* Baltimore, Williams & Wilkins, 1996:1457.

97. McMorrow ME, Cooney-Daniello M: When to suspect septic shock, *RN* 54:32, 1991.

98. McNally JC and others, editors: *Guidelines for oncology nursing practice,* ed 2, Philadelphia, Saunders, 1991.

99. Miaskowski C: Oncologic emergencies. In Miaskowski CM, Buchsel P, editors: *Oncology nursing assessment and clinical care,* St. Louis, Mosby, 1999:221.

100. Micha JP and others: Single-dose dexamethasone paclitaxel premedication, *Gynecol Oncol* 69:122, 1998.

101. Miller SE, Campbell DB: Malignant pericardial effusions. In Polomano RC, Miller SE, editors: *Understanding and managing oncologic emergencies,* Monograph, Columbus, OH, Adria Laboratories, 1987.

102. Mundy GR, Guise TA: Hypercalcemia of malignancy, *Am J Med* 103:134, 1997.

103. Mutnick AH, Bergquist SC, Beltz E: Bacteremia and sepsis. In Herfindal ET, Gourley DR, editors: *Textbook of therapeutics: drug and disease management,* Baltimore, Williams & Wilkins, 1996:1471.

104. Moran TA: AIDS-related malignancies. In Groenwald SL, Frogge MH, Goodman M, Yarbro CH, editors: *Cancer nursing: principles and practice,* ed 4, Boston, Jones & Bartlett, 1997:845.

105. Nally AT: Critical care of the patient with lung cancer, *AACN Clinical Issues: Adv Pract Acute Crit Care* 7:79, 1996.

106. Neilan BA: Oncologic emergencies: treating acute problems resulting from cancer and chemotherapy, *Postgrad Med* 95:125, 1994.

107. O'Brien JF: The oncologic crisis, part 1: septic, hematologic, and metabolic emergencies, *Emerg Med* 28:24, 1996.

108. O'Brien JF: The oncologic crisis, part 2: cardiorespiratory and neurologic emergencies, *Emerg Med* 28:20, 1996.

109. Olopade OI, Ultmann JE: Malignant effusions, *CA Cancer J Clin* 41:167, 1991.

110. Olson JK and others: Taxol hypersensitivity: rapid retreatment is safe and cost effective. *Gynecol Oncol* 68:25, 1998.

111. Pass HI: Malignant pleural and pericardial effusions (in Chapter 50, Treatment of metastatic cancer). In DeVita VT Jr, Hellman S, Rosenberg SA, editors: *Cancer: principles and practice of oncology,* ed 5 Philadelphia, Lippincott-Raven, 1997:2586.

112. *PDR Nurse's Handbook,* 1999 edition, Albany, NY, Delmar Publishers and Medical Economics Company, 1999.

113. Peereboom DM and others: Successful re-treatment with taxol after major hypersensitivity reactions. *J Clin Oncol* 11:885, 1993.

114. Poe CM, Radford AI: The challenge of hypercalcemia in cancer, *Oncol Nurs Forum* 12:29, 1985.

115. Preston NJ: Chemotherapy. Paclitaxel (TAXOL)—a guide to administration, *Eur J Cancer Care* 5:147, 1996.

116. Rabbitt JE, Page MS: Selected complications in neurooncology patients, *Semin Oncol Nurs* 14:53, 1998.

117. Robison J: Tumor lysis syndrome. In Chernecky CG, Berger BJ, editors: *Advanced and critical care oncology nursing: managing primary complications,* Philadelphia, Saunders, 1998.

118. Rodriguez RM, Light RW: Pleural effusions: guidelines for identifying the cause: possible causes range from pulmonary embolism to intra-abdominal abscess, *J Crit Illness* 13:670, 1998.

119. Rogers MJ and others: Overview of bisphosphonates, *Cancer* 80(8 suppl):1652, 1997.

120. Rohaly-Davis J, Johnston K: Hematologic emergencies in the intensive care unit, *Crit Care Nurs Q* 18:35, 1996.

121. Rousseau P: Current concepts in pain management. Malignant pleural effusions: a brief synopsis, *Am J Hospice Palliative Care* 14:302, 1997.

122. Rowinsky EK, Donehower RC: Paclitaxel (Taxol), *N Engl J Med* 332:1004, 1995.

123. Ruckdeschel JC: Management of malignant pleural effusion: an overview, *Semin Oncol* 15(suppl 3):24, 1991.

124. Rutecki GW, Whittier FC: Recognizing hypercalcemia: the '3-hormone, 3-organ rule': uncovering clinically important abnormalities in calcium metabolism, *J Crit Illness* 13:59, 1998.

125. Rutherford IA: Haemostasis and disseminated intravascular coagulation, *Intensive Crit Care Nurs* 12:161, 1996.

126. Sahn SA: Diagnosis pleural effusion, *Hosp Med* 28:66, 1992.

127. Seto AH, Dunlap DS: Tranexamic acid in oncology, *Ann Pharmacother* 30:868, 1996.

128. Scott RC III: Evaluation and management of acute pericardial tamponade, *Topics Emerg Med* 20:95, 1998.

129. Schafer SL: Oncologic complications. In Otto SE, editor: *Oncology nursing,* ed 3, St. Louis, Mosby, 1997:447.

130. Schnell S, Maher De Leon ME: Anatomy of the central nervous system, *Semin Oncol Nurs* 14:2, 1998.

131. Shelton BK, Baker L, Stecker S: Critical care of the patient with hematologic malignancy, *AACN Clinical Issues: Adv Pract Acute Crit Care* 7:65, 1996.

132. Shelton BK: Disorders of hemostasis in sepsis, *Crit Care Nurs Clin North Am* 6:373, 1994.

133. Shelton BK: Sepsis, *Semin Oncol Nurs* 15:209, 1999.

134. Shivnan J, Shelton BK, Onners BK: Bone marrow transplantation: issues for critical care nurses, *AACN Clinical Issues* 7:95, 1996.

135. Shuey K: Heart, lung, and endocrine complications of solid tumors, *Semin Oncol Nurs* 10:177, 1994.

136. Sitton E: Central nervous system metastases, *Semin Oncol Nurs* 14:210, 1998.

137. Sorensen JB, Andersen MK, Hansen HH: Syndrome of inappropriate secretion of antidiuretic hormone (SIADH) in malignant disease, *J Int Med* 238:97, 1995.

138. Soupart A, Decaux G: Therapeutic recommendations for management of severe hyponatremia: current concepts on pathogenesis and prevention of neurologic complications, *Clin Nephrol* 46:149, 1996.

139. Spain RC, Wittlesey D: Respiratory emergencies in patients with cancer, *Semin Oncol* 16:471, 1989.

140. Spodick DH: Pathophysiology of cardiac tamponade, *Chest* 113:1372, 1998.

141. Statland BE: Tips from the clinical experts. Fibrin split products and DIC, *Med Lab Observer* 29:14, 1997.

142. Steffen S, Herringshaw M: Fulminate pneumococcal septicemia in the asplenic patient: a case study with urgent implications for recognition and prevention, *J Emerg Nurs* 25:102, 1999.

143. Stewart IE: Superior vena cava syndrome: an oncologic complication, *Semin Oncol Nurs* 12:312, 1996.

144. Stretton F, Edmons P, Marrdnan M: Clinical management. Malignant pleural effusions, *Eur J Palliative Care* 6:5, 1999.

145. Stucky LA: Acute tumor lysis syndrome: assessment and nursing implications. *Oncol Nurs Forum* 20:49, 1993.

146. Talan DA: Sepsis and septic shock, *Emerg Med* 29:54, 1997.

147. Toney JF, Parker MM: New perspectives on the management of septic shock in the cancer patient, *Infect Dis Clin North Am* 10:239, 1996.

148. Von Hohenleiten C, Webster JS: Anaphylaxis from chemotherapy. In Chernecky CG, Berger BJ, editors: *Advanced and critical care oncology nursing: managing primary complications,* Philadelphia, Saunders, 1998.

149. Wanders J and others: The EORTC-ECTG experience with acute hypersensitivity reactions (HSR) in taxotere studies, *Proceedings of ASCO* 12:73, abstract 94, March, 1993.

150. Warrell RP, Bockman RS: Metabolic emergencies. In DeVita VT Jr, Hellman S, Rosenberg SA, editors: *Cancer: principles and practice of oncology,* ed 4, Philadelphia, Lippincott, 1993.

151. Weidmann B and others: Hypersensitivity reactions to carboplatin, *Cancer* 73:2218, 1994.

152. Weiss RB and others: Hypersensitivity reactions from taxol, *J Clin Oncol* 8:1263, 1990.

153. Weiss RB: Hypersensitivity reactions. *Semin Oncol* 19:458, 1992.

154. Weiss RB: Miscellaneous toxicities. In DeVita VT Jr, Hellman S, Rosenberg SA, editors, *Cancer: principles and practice of oncology,* ed 5, Philadelphia, Lippincott-Raven, 1997:2796.

155. Wheeler AP, Bernard GR: Treating patients with severe sepsis, *N Engl J Med* 349:207, 1999.

156. Wheeler VS: Biotherapy. In Groenwald SL, Frogge MH, Goodman M, Yarbro CH, editors: *Cancer nursing: principles and practice,* ed 4, Boston, Jones & Bartlett, 1997:426.

157. Wilkes GM: Neurological disturbances. In Groenwald SL, others, editors: *Cancer symptom management,* Sudbury, MA, Jones & Bartlett, 1996.

158. Wilson JK, Masaryk TJ: Neurologic emergencies in cancer patients, *Semin Oncol* 16:490, 1989.

159. Woodard WL III, Hogan DK: Oncologic emergencies: implications for nurses, *J Intravenous Nurs* 19:256, 1996.

160. Yahalom J: Superior vena cava syndrome. In DeVita VT Jr, Hellman S, Rosenberg SA, editors: *Cancer: principles and practice of oncology,* ed 4, Philadelphia, Lippincott, 1993.

161. Yasko JM, editor: *Guidelines for cancer care: symptoms management,* Reston, VA, Reston, 1983.

162. Yasko JM, Schafer SL: Disseminated intravascular coagulation. In Yasko JM, editor: *Guidelines for cancer care: symptoms management,* Reston, VA, Reston, 1983.

163. Yasko JM, Schafer SL: Neoplastic pericardial tamponade. In Yasko JM, editor: *Guidelines for cancer care: symptoms management,* Reston, VA, Reston, 1983.

164. Zumsteg MM, Casperson DS: Paraneoplastic syndromes in metastatic disease, *Semin Oncol Nurs* 14:220, 1998.

Cancer Treatment Modalities

Surgery

Karen A. Pfeifer

Surgery is often the initial and preferred treatment of choice for many malignant tumors. Of the 40% of cancer patients treated by surgery alone, one third are cured. However, the key is finding the tumor while it is still localized. Surgical treatment failures are caused primarily by the presence of metastasis at the time of initial diagnosis. Metastasis has occurred in 50% of cancer patients by the time their tumor is of sufficient size to be clinically detected.*

The nurse may encounter the cancer patient anywhere along the surgical continuum, ranging from diagnosis to management of complications. It is imperative that the nurse have a strong fundamental knowledge of surgical oncology on which comprehensive plans of care can be designed and evaluated.

HISTORICAL PERSPECTIVE

Ephraim MacDowell is credited with describing modern surgical approaches to cancer in the United States. In 1809 he excised a 22-pound ovarian tumor from Mrs. Jane Todd Crawford, who lived 30 more years. This was the first of 13 ovarian resections performed by MacDowell, and it helped to advance the idea of elective surgery for cancer. Another important individual in the evolution of surgical oncology was Albert Theodore Billroth; between 1860 and 1890, he performed the first laryngectomy, gastrectomy, and esophagectomy. In the 1890s William Stewart Halsted clarified the principles of en bloc tumor resection.[14, 23, 27, 28, 30]

Building on the work of these early pioneers in surgical oncology, surgeons continued to remove the tumor and as much of the surrounding tissue as possible. Therefore, most surgical procedures were radical in nature. In the mid-1950s it was noted that despite the technical sophistication of these radical procedures, the mortality rates associated with certain cancer sites (e.g.,

breast cancer) were not improving. Many tumors thought to be local processes were discovered to be systemic diseases with metastatic lesions. It became evident that surgery alone, regardless of the magnitude of the procedure, was not effective for all tumors.[36]

APPLICATIONS FOR SURGICAL ONCOLOGY

Surgery has several applications in oncology, and these are described below.

Diagnosis of Disease

A histologic diagnosis is critical to planning treatment because it is the only definitive diagnostic method and different tumors respond differently to treatment. Surgical techniques used to obtain tissue samples for examination include incisional biopsy, excisional biopsy, needle biopsy, or endoscopy (Table 21–1). The technique used depends on the tumor's location, size, and growth characteristics. The current trend is a two-step process. The biopsy is done first, followed by a period of time (usually about 2 weeks), before any additional surgery is performed. This accomplishes two things: (1) it allows the patient and significant others to begin adjusting to the diagnosis, and (2) it allows the patient and significant others additional time to make decisions about treatment options.[24, 27, 30, 55]

Staging of Disease

Diagnosis includes determining the type and extent of cancer at one point in time, a process known as staging the disease. The tumor's stage provides information relating to the extent and location of disease and the prognosis. A staging laparotomy (or diagnostic laparotomy) may be performed before radical surgery to obtain tissue samples and determine disease sites.[24, 29]

Treatment of Disease

Surgical treatment of the cancer process focuses on five principal areas: primary treatment, adjuvant treatment,

---

*References 12, 14, 15, 23, 24, 46, 53.

TABLE 21-1
Biopsy Techniques

Type	Purpose	Technique	Advantages	Disadvantages
Incisional biopsy	Histologic study	Removal of a portion of tumor Secures a wedge of tumor tissue Usually performed at tumor margin Done on tumors > 3 cm in diameter	Usually requires only local anesthesia Simple method of obtaining diagnosis	Negative report does not eliminate possibility of cancer Specimen may not be large enough Tumor margins may not be defined Additional surgery is required to remove tumor
Excisional biopsy	Histologic study Cure/control	Removal of entire tumor mass with a margin of surrounding normal tissue Most common type of biopsy Performed on small (2–3 cm), accessible tumors	Usually requires only local anesthesia Can be definitive therapy (tumors of the lip, nose, ear, and breast) Quick, simple removal of tumor at time of biopsy Decreased costs	Cells may be implanted in tissue and incision, causing local recurrence
Needle biopsy	Histologic study	Aspiration of core tissue samples through special needle Either tissue or fluid samples can be obtained Performed during surgery or via percutaneous route	Simple to perform Reliable Inexpensive Causes little disturbance of surrounding tissue Done using local anesthesia Does not require hospitalization	Specimen may not be large enough Needle may miss tumor Improper handling may distort cells Technique poses risk of injury to adjacent structures; perforation/hemorrhage are additional risks
Endoscopy	Histologic study	Removal of small portions of tumor with forceps after visual examination Often used to diagnose tumors of the gastrointestinal, genitourinary, and pulmonary tracts	Allows access to tumors that might not otherwise be accessible except by laparotomy or thoracotomy Causes little disturbance of surrounding tissue Flexible instruments have made endoscopy more tolerable for patients and easier for surgeons	Tumor cells may be seeded along needle tract

Data from references 14, 24, 27, 30, 48, and 55.

salvage treatment, palliative treatment, and combination treatment.

Primary Treatment. Primary treatment involves removal of a malignant tumor and a margin of adjacent normal tissue. The goal is to achieve a cure by reducing the patient's total body tumor burden. Cure can be accomplished through several types of intervention. Local excision, for example, is the simple excision of a tumor and a small margin of normal tissue. This technique is often used to treat skin cancer. Wide excision or en bloc dissection involves removal of the primary tumor, regional lymph nodes, intervening lymphatic channels, and involved neighboring structures. Examples include radical mastectomy, radical neck dissection, and abdominal-perineal resection. Extended wide excision, another form of wide excision, involves removal of wide tumor infiltration in a particular region.[23, 30, 53, 55]

Adjuvant Treatment. Adjuvant treatment includes cytoreductive therapy, also known as debulking, which is surgery to remove a large tumor burden. If the quantity of cancer cells can be reduced to a very small number by surgical intervention, any remaining cancer cells are more likely to be destroyed by other systemic treatment. Cytoreductive therapy is commonly used in the treatment of ovarian cancer and for neuroblastomas and other childhood tumors. Adjuvant therapy also includes prophylactic surgery, or surgery performed on organs with underlying conditions marked by a high incidence of subsequent cancer. For example, ulcerative colitis carries with it a high incidence of cancer of the colon. Approximately 40% of patients with total involvement of the colon will ultimately die with colon cancer. Therefore, these lives could be prolonged by prophylactic colectomy. The decision to perform surgery is based on (1) the statistical risk of cancer based on the medical and family history, (2) the presence or absence of symptoms, (3) the degree of difficulty in diagnosing a cancer early should it develop, and (4) the patient's probable postoperative appearance and functioning.*

Salvage Treatment. Salvage treatment involves use of an extensive surgical approach to treat local recurrence after a less extensive primary approach has been implemented (e.g., mastectomy after lumpectomy and radiation therapy).[55]

Palliative Treatment. Palliative surgery is used to ameliorate disease- or treatment-related symptoms without trying to surgically cure the cancer. The goals of palliative surgery are to relieve distressing symptoms, to make the patient more comfortable, and to prevent symptoms that will occur if the patient goes untreated. The benefits of palliative treatment depend on the biologic pace of the cancer, the patient's projected life expectancy, and expected treatment outcomes.†

Examples of palliative surgical procedures include:

- Bone stabilization
- Relief of life-threatening obstruction or bleeding
- Removal of solitary metastasis (e.g., cerebral, hepatic)
- Treatment of oncologic emergencies (e.g., perforation, abscess, spinal cord compression, hypersplenism)
- Treatment of complications from chemotherapy and radiation therapy (e.g., skin breakdown, fistulas, perforation, radiation proctitis)
- Ablative surgery (removal of a hormone source) to alter the hormonal environment that encourages development and growth of a tumor (e.g., oophorectomy, orchiectomy, adrenalectomy)
- Management of cancer pain (e.g., nerve blocks, cordotomy, neurectomy, rhizotomy, sympathectomy, lobotomy, thalamotomy, tractotomy)

Combination Treatment. Combination treatment combines surgery with other treatment modalities to limit

the change in the patient's physical appearance and functional ability and improve tumor resectability and treatment outcomes. Examples include preoperative chemotherapy, radiation therapy, or biotherapy; intraoperative chemotherapy or radiation therapy; and postoperative chemotherapy, radiation therapy, or biotherapy.[5, 55]

Second-Look Procedures

Second-look procedures involve follow-up surgery after the original surgery or adjuvant treatment to check for the presence or absence of disease. These procedures usually are reserved for cancers that tend to recur locally (e.g., ovarian cancer). Second-look procedures are used less often than in the past because other laboratory tests, diagnostic procedures, and tumor markers are available to assess response to treatment.[55]

Reconstruction

Reconstructive surgery involves reconstruction of anatomic defects caused by extensive cancer surgery; its purpose is to improve function and cosmetic appearance. Cancer surgeries requiring the largest number of subsequent reconstructive surgeries are surgery of the head and neck (facial reconstruction), breasts (breast reconstruction after mastectomy), and superficial tissues (skin graft after resection for melanoma). The choice of method depends on several factors, including the site and extent of the tumor or tumors, loss of function and substance, chance of permanent cure, patient's age and psychological and general condition, availability of free skin grafts, and suitable internal prostheses.[24, 29, 55]

Prevention of Disease

Cancer prevention can entail preventive surgery. Surgery is the preferred treatment for precancerous and in situ lesions of all epithelial surfaces (e.g., skin, oral cavity, cervix). Benign polyps of the cervix, bladder, colon, and stomach often are removed surgically to reduce the risk of future cancer. Although rare, a second mastectomy sometimes is performed on women with a high potential for developing a second breast cancer.[23]

Insertion and Monitoring of Therapeutic/Supportive Hardware

Therapeutic/supportive hardware can be surgically implanted to improve the patient's comfort or ease delivery of treatment.[55] Several different types of hardware are discussed below.

Ventricular Reservoir (Ommaya Reservoir). A ventricular reservoir (Fig. 21–1) consists of a mushroom-

---

*References 12, 14, 23, 27, 29, 30, 53, 55, 60.
†References 2, 12, 21, 23, 27, 29, 30, 53, 55.

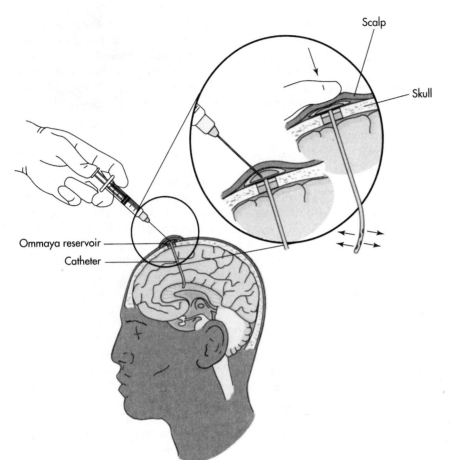

FIGURE 21–1 The Ommaya reservoir. (From Phipps WJ and others, editors, *Medical-surgical nursing: concepts and clinical practice,* ed 6, St. Louis, Mosby, 1999.)

shaped silicone dome that provides direct access to ventricular cerebrospinal fluid (CSF). The dome, which is approximately 3.4 cm in diameter, is attached to a silicone catheter. Ventricular reservoirs have three primary uses: (1) to more predictably and consistently deliver medication (e.g., chemotherapy drugs, pain medication) directly into the subarachnoid space and CSF (intrathecal administration); (2) to permit CSF to be sampled for pathologic examination; and (3) to permit measurement of CSF pressure.[33]

Central Venous Catheters. Central venous catheters are available for short- and long-term use. In short-term use, central venous catheters are used for brief intermittent or continuous administration of intravenous fluids, medications, parenteral hyperalimentation, or blood and blood products. They also may be used for obtaining blood samples. Most short-term central catheters are inserted via the subclavian or jugular vein and terminate in the superior vena cava near the right atrium. Most catheters have no cuff and do not pass through a subcutaneous tunnel.[33, 56]

Long-term central venous catheters (Fig. 21–2) are used when a prolonged course of parenteral therapy is expected. The silicone catheter is surgically placed percutaneously or by venous cutdown. The catheter is implanted via the subclavian or jugular vein, with the tip terminating in the superior vena cava near the right atrium. The catheter is then threaded subcutaneously to an exit site in the chest, usually to the right or left of midline. The procedure usually is done using local

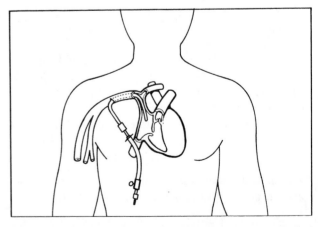

FIGURE 21–2 Anatomic location of long-term central venous catheter. (From Otto SE, editor: *Pocket guide to intravenous therapy,* ed 4, St. Louis, Mosby, 2001.)

anesthesia. A Dacron cuff forms a seal around the catheter; this cuff also stabilizes the catheter and reduces infection by preventing retrograde migration of organisms. The catheter may also be sutured in place to secure its placement.[33, 56]

Implantable Vascular Access Device (IVAD). The IVAD system (Fig. 21–3) consists of a self-sealing silicone rubber septum enclosed in a metal or plastic port that is attached to a silicone catheter. The port is surgically implanted beneath the skin, generally in the chest region. The catheter is then threaded subcutaneously and terminates in a body cavity, organ, epidural space, or blood vessel. Chemotherapy, intravenous fluids, pain medications and other drugs, and blood and blood products can be given intermittently or continuously via the port. The system is accessed by a needle puncture through the skin into the port's septum. Noncoring needles must be used when accessing the port to prevent damage to the silicone septum. Several commercially made ports are available in single or double lumens, lower profile ports for the smaller patient, and peripheral access ports for patients whose disease prevents the use of a traditional central venous access device.[33, 56]

Tenckhoff Catheter. The Tenckhoff catheter may be surgically placed for the treatment of malignant ascites, as often occurs with lymphomas and cancers of the ovary, colon, or stomach. In such cases the Tenckhoff catheter is used for administration of intraperitoneal chemotherapy.[6]

Implanted Infusion Pumps. Implanted infusion pumps (Fig. 21–4) are used for continuous regional infusion of chemotherapy or of pain medications or other drugs to specific body sites by way of an artery or vein or the CSF. Bolus injections also may be given by the pump's side port. These pumps have no external components and are accessed percutaneously. The pump is placed in a subcutaneous pocket of tissue. The silicone catheter most commonly terminates in the hepatic artery for treatment of liver cancer or liver metastasis, in the supe-

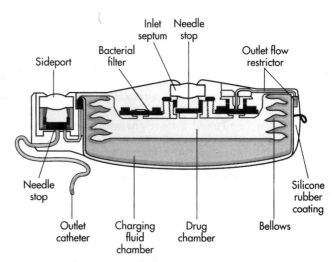

FIGURE 21–4 Implanted infusion pump. (From Phipps WJ and others, editors, *Medical-surgical nursing: concepts and clinical practice,* ed 6, St. Louis, Mosby, 1999.)

rior vena cava for systemic infusion of chemotherapy, or in the CSF for pain management.[56]

PRINCIPLES OF SURGICAL ONCOLOGY

When considering surgery for a patient with cancer, the surgeon critically evaluates three main elements: tumor factors, tumor cell kinetics, and patient variables.

Tumor Factors

Anatomic Location. The tumor's location can prevent or impede access for removal. Some tumors cannot be surgically treated because an adequate margin of normal tissue cannot be removed. Tumors that involve or are attached to vital structures usually do not benefit from surgical resection; superficial, well-encapsulated tumors are the type most easily removed by surgery.[23, 24, 27]

Histologic Type. Certain histologic types of cancer are not treated by surgery because they are disseminated at the outset of diagnosis. Examples of these are lymphomas, leukemias, and small-cell cancer of the lung.[27]

Tumor Size. Smaller tumors are less likely to have spread, and the patient is more likely to be cured by surgery. However, patients with large, localized tumors that have a poor blood supply respond more favorably to surgery than to other treatment modalities. This is because other treatment modalities (e.g., chemotherapy and radiation therapy) require tumors to have excellent blood supplies to cause cell destruction; surgery does not.[23, 27]

Tumor Cell Kinetics

Growth Rate or Biologic Aggressiveness. Well-differentiated, slow-growing tumors consisting of cells with long

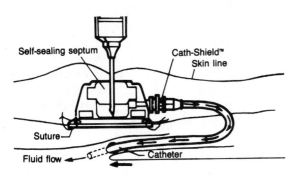

FIGURE 21–3 Cross-section of implantable port with needle. (Courtesy of SIMS Deltec, Inc., St. Paul, MN.)

cell cycles lend themselves best to surgical resection. These tumors are more likely to be confined locally. Poorly differentiated, rapid-growing tumors are less amenable to surgery.[23, 24]

Invasion. Any cell that remains after cancer therapy carries with it the potential for recurrence if that cell can reproduce. Therefore any surgery intended to be curative must include resection of normal tissue around the tumor to ensure removal of all cancer cells. Some cancers (e.g., melanomas) invade tissues deeply, thereby either requiring radical surgery or eliminating surgery as a treatment option.[23]

Metastatic Potential or Pattern and Extent of Metastatic Spread. Some tumors metastasize late or not at all. Even when advanced, these tumors may be cured by aggressive surgery. Other tumors are known to metastasize to certain regional lymph nodes, and cure may be achieved by removing the tumor-bearing organ and its nearby lymph nodes. Other tumors predictably metastasize early. Surgery may not be warranted for these tumor types, or, alternatively, it may be done to remove all visible tumor before the patient begins adjuvant treatment or to resect remaining diseased tissue after several courses of chemotherapy.[24, 50]

Patient Variables

General Health. The patient's general health plays a major role in determining the efficacy of surgery. As with any treatment, the surgical risk must be compared with the probability of long-term recovery. Cancer patients clearly are at greater risk of developing complications postoperatively or of succumbing to clinical problems.[23]

Host Resistance or Immune Competence. The patient's ability to initiate an immunologic response to the cancer cells that remain after surgery is critical. A person with cancer is less likely to be able to mount an effective immune response. However, the ability to resist infection has been shown to be closely related to total body tumor burden. Surgery can reduce the patient's tumor burden, thus improving the immune status.[23, 24]

Desire for Treatment. The surgeon must carefully assess the patient's desire for treatment. Even though surgery may be the most effective measure for tumor control, it is not appropriate for a patient who does not want an operation.[27, 39]

Quality of Life. Research has shown that some radical surgeries are not justified. Either they do not improve the end result, or they interfere with the patient's welfare. Selecting surgery as a treatment choice must include consideration of the quality of the patient's life when treatment is complete.[24]

SPECIAL SURGICAL TECHNIQUES

Several special surgical techniques are used in the treatment of cancer. These include electrosurgery, cryosurgery, chemosurgery, lasers, video-assisted thoracoscopy, intraoperative radiation therapy, and photodynamic therapy.

Electrosurgery

Electrosurgery eliminates cancer cells by using the cutting and coagulating effects of high-frequency electrical current applied by needles, blades, or electrodes. This technique may be an alternative treatment for certain cancers of the skin, oral cavity, and rectum.[23, 53]

Cryosurgery

Cryosurgery is the therapeutic destruction of tumors using subzero temperatures. The cryosurgical system produces temperatures below $-166.2°F$ $(-200°C)$. Freezing cells produces hypovolemia and a subsequent toxic level of electrolytes in the affected cells. As the freezing continues, cell membranes rupture. Indirect destruction of the microcirculation from the freezing of small blood vessels in the target area further contributes to hypoxic cellular death. The treated site then thaws naturally and becomes gelatinous, healing spontaneously. Most healing is complete within 6 to 8 weeks. Cells that are not frozen internally at the time of treatment become necrotic and subsequently die during the thawing process. Carbon dioxide, Freon, and nitrous oxide are the three common gaseous freezing agents used. Whereas original cryoprobes limited cryosurgery to the treatment of surface lesions (skin cancer and precancerous and cancerous gynecologic lesions), newer cryoprobe systems and innovative intraoperative radiology and ultrasound techniques allow detection and treatment of lesions deep within the body, most notably metastatic liver cancer and prostate cancer. Most patients require only one treatment; however, cryosurgery permits retreatment of recurrent lesions.[7, 8, 23, 30, 53, 55]

Chemosurgery

Chemosurgery, the combined use of layer-by-layer surgical resection of tissue and topical application of chemotherapeutic agents, was first described by Dr. Frederic Mohs in 1941. It involves mapping excised tissue in location to the wound; this allows the surgeon to remove mostly malignant tissue and little or no normal tissue, minimizing disfigurement.[30, 55]

Lasers

Coagulation and tissue ablation are two features of the laser, making it attractive to surgical oncologists. The term "laser" is derived from the process that creates laser light (*light amplification by stimulated emission of radiation*). In this process, photons are emitted and amplified by atoms and molecules. Safe, efficient use of lasers in surgical oncology requires an understanding of the various laser–tissue interactions. These interactions include photocoagulation, vaporization, photochemical ablation, and photochemical interactions.

In photocoagulation, proteins, enzymes, and other biologic molecules in tissue are heated to temperatures well above 932°F (500°C). The immediate result is denaturation of the treated tissues. Photocoagulation is used to prevent blood loss when heavily vascularized tissue is surgically incised.

Vaporization, or photothermal ablation, occurs at temperatures above 1832°F (1000°C), when tissue water boils. The production of steam results in removal of tissue in the form of microscopic particles. Vaporization is used for incision and removal of diseased tissue.

The term "photochemical ablation" was coined to specifically describe the unusually clean-cut incisions possible with short-wavelength, ultraviolet, pulsed excimer lasers. Short-wavelength photons have sufficient energy to break molecular bonds and have proved useful when extremely thin layers must be removed, as in skin cancer.

Photochemistry occurs when visible or ultraviolet radiation interacts with molecules. However, in most instances of laser use, the photochemical effects are dwarfed by temperature increases sufficient to cause thermal denaturation of tissue. With low dose rates, photochemistry may be the dominant mechanism, as occurs in photodynamic therapy (discussed later in this section).

Lasers have demonstrated their worth in removing tumors in difficult-to-access areas and in minimizing blood loss in highly vascular tissues. Established uses include local excision of head and neck cancer with the CO_2, argon, and KTP lasers. Nd:YAG has been used to debulk nasopharyngeal carcinomas. CO_2, argon, and Nd:YAG lasers also have been used in microsurgery with ultrasound to ablate or remove tumor tissue that is extremely close to critical neural tissue that must not be disturbed. Argon, CO_2, Nd:YAG, and KTP lasers have been used in urologic cancer surgery with both fiberoptic and cystoscopic delivery systems.*

Video-Assisted Thoracoscopy

Video-assisted thoracoscopy is revolutionizing a field once associated with long incisions and longer, painful recoveries. Until recently, thoracoscopy consisted of in-

---

*References 3, 4, 16, 30, 35, 51, 54, 55.

serting a small, lighted tube into the chest cavity, where, under direct vision, the surgeon performed pleural biopsies. Today, a multichip minicamera, accompanied by intense lighting, magnifies the image and transmits it to a video monitor. Video-assisted thoracoscopy has replaced approximately 70% of the thoracic procedures that previously required a standard thoracotomy; these include pulmonary wedge excisions, diagnosis and treatment of pleural effusions and pleural masses, biopsy or resection of mediastinal tumors, and, occasionally, sympathectomies, vagotomies, and thymectomies.

Video-assisted thoracoscopy is performed using general anesthesia with single-lung ventilation. Instead of the standard 20-cm thoracotomy incision, the surgeon makes three 1-cm incisions. A rigid telescope and camera are introduced through the first incision, and the endoscopic surgical instruments are introduced into the remaining incisions. Operating time ranges from 15 to 20 minutes to 2 to 3 hours, depending on the complexity of the surgery. Video-assisted thoracoscopy has opened treatment doors to patients previously ineligible for standard thoracotomy (e.g., severe emphysema). Contraindications include extensive pleural adhesions and bleeding disorders (which obstruct the camera lens) and recent myocardial infarction. Complications with video-assisted thoracoscopy are uncommon but include atelectasis, pneumonia, and postoperative air leaks that usually resolve within the first 24 hours postoperatively. Other reports have mentioned trocar injuries to the lung and other thoracic viscera, which usually are discovered and corrected during surgery.[1, 32, 40, 45]

Intraoperative Radiation Therapy

External-beam radiation therapy has been extensively used in patients with unresectable, locally advanced cancer and in patients with early stage cancer who, for medical reasons, cannot undergo surgery. Generally, the radiation field includes the primary tumor and lymph nodes that drain the area. However, the proximity of tumors to radiosensitive organs (lung, spinal cord, and heart) often limits the amount of radiation that can be delivered to the treatment site. Therefore, techniques are needed that allow delivery of high-dose radiation to the treatment site without exceeding the tolerance of radiosensitive organs.

One such technique is intraoperative electron-beam radiation therapy (IOEBRT). Using IOEBRT, tumoricidal doses of radiation can be delivered to tumors at the time of surgery while the dose to adjacent normal tissues is minimized. Dose-limiting normal tissues are protected by surgically placed lead shields or by physical displacement from the treatment field. IOEBRT, alone or in combination with preoperative or postoperative external-beam irradiation or neoadjuvant chemotherapy, has been used to treat various sites, including the stomach, bile duct, pancreas, retroperitoneum, and rectum.

For unresectable tumors inaccessible to the treatment cone of IOEBRT (e.g., sites deep in the inferior pelvis), intraoperative high-dose rate brachytherapy (IOHDRB) offers an alternative approach. In this approach, radioactive sealed sources are implanted surgically into the tumor or a cavity surrounding the tumor. For IOHDRB, treatment time depends on the total area to be treated and the activity of the source because a single source is used to treat the tumor. Because of the complex presentations of patients who are candidates for IOHDRB and the fact that most patients have received intensive multimodal therapy, it is difficult to differentiate surgical from radiation toxicities.

Lastly, stereotactic radiosurgery is worthy of mention. "Stereotaxy" refers to surgical techniques that rely on specialized instrumentation, including stereotactic frames, to perform procedures at precise locations. In stereotactic radiosurgery, surgical convention is replaced by multiple narrow radiation beams that are directed toward a common point to produce highly localized radiobiologic effects, such as blood vessel thrombosis.[10, 25, 26, 34, 43]

Photodynamic Therapy

Photodynamic therapy involves intravenous injection of a photosensitizing drug, followed by exposure to a laser light within 24 to 48 hours of injection. This results in fluorescence of cancer cells and cell death. It is important to note that, although photodynamic therapy involves use of a laser, the laser's mechanism of action does not involve cutting, cauterizing, or vaporizing (the more common uses associated with lasers). Photodynamic therapy has been used with varying success to treat basal and squamous cell cancers, malignant melanoma, Kaposi's sarcoma, recurrent breast cancer, head and neck cancer, bladder cancer, and endobronchial cancer. Bulky lesions and tumors that are inaccessible to light irradiation cannot be treated by photodynamic therapy.[20, 55, 58]

SPECIAL CONSIDERATIONS IN SURGICAL ONCOLOGY

Nutrition

Protein-calorie malnutrition is a common problem in cancer patients. Approximately 30% to 50% of cancer patients show moderate to severe degrees of malnutrition resulting from the primary tumor and from the diagnostic or treatment regimens used in the management of their disease. Protein-calorie malnutrition generally results from (1) a decrease in oral intake, (2) an increase in enteral losses as a result of malabsorption or development of intestinal fistulas, and (3) an increase in nutritional requirements caused by hypermetabolism or the presence of a tumor.[11, 12, 37, 59]

A nutritionally compromised cancer patient is a poor surgical risk. When subjected to the stress of surgery, the patient is unable to preserve lean body mass, and negative nitrogen balance ensues. The results are (1) poor wound healing, (2) anemia, (3) infection, (4) sepsis, (5) pneumonia, (6) further malnutrition, and (7) increased morbidity. Nutritional management is aimed first at reversing protein-calorie malnutrition and preventing weight loss. Once this has been accomplished, the nutrition plan can be as aggressive as the cancer treatment plan. The optimal duration of nutrition support varies with each cancer patient.[12, 24, 38, 49]

Blood Disorders

Anemia is common among cancer patients and should be corrected preoperatively with packed red blood cell transfusions to a hematocrit of 35% or above. In addition, some conditions (e.g., liver failure, uremia, leukemia) are associated with platelet dysfunction. It is generally accepted that 50,000 functionally active platelets per cubic millimeter are sufficient for surgery. An insufficient preoperative platelet count can result in postoperative bleeding and fatal hemorrhage, especially if the patient receives large volumes of blood products.[5]

The cancer patient is highly susceptible to changes in the hemostatic system, particularly hypercoagulability and thrombosis. Postoperative deep vein thrombosis is more likely to develop in cancer patients than in other surgery patients; therefore early postoperative ambulation is critical. Cancers commonly associated with recurring deep vein thrombosis are cancers of the brain, pancreas, stomach, and lung.[24, 31]

Complications of Multimodal Therapy

Tissue that has been irradiated is not biologically normal. Radiation causes fibrosis and obliterates lymphatic and vascular channels, interfering with postoperative wound healing. Patients who have received radiation therapy before surgery are candidates for postoperative infection, wound dehiscence, and necrosis.[24, 47, 61]

Certain chemotherapy drugs (methotrexate, cyclophosphamide, 5-fluorouracil, and doxorubicin) reduce the tensile strength of surgical wounds. Wound strength is significantly impaired when chemotherapy is administered within the first 4 days of surgery. This highlights the need for nonabsorbable sutures and for delaying chemotherapy when extensive surgical resection is required. Some chemotherapy drugs are toxic to specific organ systems, producing long-term side effects that can increase the cancer patient's risk of surgical complica-

T A B L E   2 1 – 2
Physiologic Changes Related to the Aging Process

Physiologic Changes	Effects	Potential Postoperative Complications
CARDIOVASCULAR SYSTEM		
Decreased elasticity of blood vessels Decreased cardiac output Decreased peripheral circulation	Decreased circulation to vital organs Slower blood flow	Shock (hypotension), thrombosis with pulmonary emboli, delayed wound healing, postoperative confusion, hypervolemia, decreased response to stress
RESPIRATORY SYSTEM		
Decreased elasticity of lungs and chest wall Increased residual lung volume Decreased ciliary action Fewer alveolar capillaries Decreased forced expiratory volume	Decreased vital capacity Decreased alveolar volume Decreased gas exchange Decreased cough reflex	Atelectasis, pneumonia, postoperative confusion
URINARY SYSTEM		
Decreased glomerular filtration rate Decreased bladder muscle tone Weakened perineal muscles	Decreased kidney function Stasis of urine in bladder Loss of urinary control	Prolonged response to anesthesia and drugs, overhydration with intravenous fluids, hyperkalemia, urinary tract infection, urinary incontinence
MUSCULOSKELETAL SYSTEM		
Decreased muscle strength Limitation of motion	Decreased activity	Atelectasis, pneumonia, thrombophlebitis, constipation or fecal impaction
GASTROINTESTINAL SYSTEM		
Decreased intestinal motility	Retention of feces	Constipation or fecal impaction
METABOLIC SYSTEM		
Decreased gamma globulin level	Decreased inflammatory response	Delayed wound healing, wound dehiscence, or evisceration
IMMUNE SYSTEM		
Fewer killer T cells Decreased response to foreign antigens	Decreased ability to protect against invasion by pathogenic microorganisms	Wound infection, wound dehiscence, pneumonia, urinary tract infection

Modified from Phipps WJ and others, editors: Medical-surgical nursing: concepts and clinical practice, *ed 6, St. Louis, Mosby, 1999.*

tions. For example, preoperative administration of bleomycin can predispose the patient to postoperative acute adult respiratory distress syndrome. Diuretics, aggressive pulmonary hygiene, and fluid restriction can prevent problems associated with preoperative bleomycin therapy. Preoperative administration of adriamycin or daunomycin (cumulative dose of 500 mg/m^2 or higher) increases the risk of intraoperative and postoperative congestive heart failure and pulmonary edema. Digitalis may be given preoperatively to increase ventricular contractility.[19, 24, 47, 52]

Surgical Risks in Older Patients

All surgical procedures must be considered high risk for the older cancer patient. However, if a careful baseline assessment permits preoperative correction of deficits and if the older patient is thoroughly instructed about

postoperative management, many complications can be avoided. Hypoxemia is the most common anesthesia-related problem in the older cancer patient. Age, obesity, and preexisting pulmonary disease all predispose the patient to hypoxemia, with the potential postoperative outcomes being pulmonary edema, myocardial infarction, decreased cardiac output, pulmonary thromboembolism, and aspiration pneumonia.[13] Table 21–2 presents additional information on physiologic changes related to the aging process that can affect surgical outcomes.

FUTURE DIRECTIONS AND ADVANCES IN SURGICAL ONCOLOGY

State-of-the-art surgical approaches of the future will reflect movement away from today's invasive procedures. The long incisions and visceral manipulation once considered necessary for adequate visualization, comprehensive resection, and anastomosis will be uncommon. Cancer surgery of the future will combine refined endoscopic equipment, videography, lasers, microscopes, and three-dimensional imaging devices, allowing surgeons to localize tumor tissue for ablation by microendoscopic resection or targeted intraluminal radiation. Current research with radiotagged antibodies, it is hoped, will lead to earlier detection of tumors, which will facilitate surgical cures for certain cancers. In the future, molecular surgery, the use of gene therapy for preoperative tumor debulking, may be used to treat localized head and neck cancer and ovarian cancer. The day may even come when organs damaged by chemotherapy or radiation, such as the heart, liver, and lungs, may be replaced in patients who demonstrate no evidence of disease after a period of time.[18, 24]

CONCLUSION

Current trends in tumor biology and interdisciplinary cancer management have changed our previous reliance on surgery as the only curative form of cancer therapy and precipitated changes in the extensiveness of surgical resections. By combining surgery, radiation therapy, chemotherapy, and biotherapy, disease-free intervals have been significantly expanded.[24]

Despite known limitations, surgery continues to be an important treatment modality for cancer. The nurse may encounter the cancer surgery patient at the time of initial diagnosis or when the patient returns for reconstructive surgery. This demands flexibility on the part of the nurse and a strong understanding of the foundations and principles of surgical oncology nursing.

Nursing Management

Nursing care of the surgical cancer patient is similar to the nursing care required for any surgery patient. However, the nurse must be aware of the problems that are unique to the cancer disease process. Unlike other surgery patients, the cancer patient's comprehensive plan of care must include nursing management of the psychosocial and existential aspects of and complications specific to the cancer.[24]

PREOPERATIVE CARE

Preoperative nursing care of the cancer patient focuses on assessment and intervention. To accomplish these tasks effectively, the nurse must know the answers to the following questions[30]:

What is the purpose of the surgery? Is it diagnosis, staging, cure, or palliation? Each purpose has a different meaning for the patient. By knowing the purpose of surgery, the nurse can better comprehend the patient's behavior. A patient who recently has been diagnosed as having cancer will exhibit different behaviors than will the patient with metastatic disease who undergoes palliative surgery for relief of intractable pain.

What kind of surgery will be performed? The nurse must know what preoperative preparation or care is required (e.g., bowel preparation, nutritional supplementation); where incisions will be made and how long they will be; and what devices will be attached to the patient (e.g., catheters, drains, chest tubes).

What has the patient or family been told about the surgery, diagnosis, and possibilities for future treatment? Patients often hear only the words "cancer"

and "surgery"; everything else is a blur. Therefore information needs to be repeated frequently.

Once answers to these questions have been obtained, preoperative nursing care of the cancer patient can focus on reducing anxiety, enhancing physical well-being, and teaching.[53]

Reducing Anxiety

Cancer has a profound psychological impact on patients and their significant others. Many patients with newly diagnosed cancer often feel hopeless, powerless, and depressed. Patients are often apprehensive about surgery and may be resentful, angry, anxious, and even panicky about the impending operation.[23, 41]

Some preoperative fear is normal, even positive, because it encourages the patient to take the surgery seriously and to make realistic plans for coping with it. For some, the question, "How do you think this surgery will change your life?" encourages the patient to explore fears, talk about related anxieties, and begin planning for change. This type of communication forms the basis for a supportive, trusting, and therapeutic relationship that will endure throughout subsequent readmissions to the hospital.[23, 41, 53]

Enhancing Physical Well-Being

The cancer patient may be debilitated as a result of advanced disease or because of the type of symptoms or length of time symptoms have been present. Enhancement of the patient's physical well-being in the preoperative period includes alleviating physical symptoms such as pain, diarrhea, nausea and vomiting, fatigue, bowel obstruction, and malnutrition. Stress-related symptoms, such as insomnia and headaches, also can be minimized. Proper preoperative treatment and management of physical symptoms will directly affect the patient's response postoperatively.[53] The table on pages 596 and 597 provides information specific to preoperative assessment of physiologic parameters in the surgical oncology patient.

Teaching

Anxiety appears to be more severe in patients who do not have accurate information about their impending surgery. During the preoperative period, concern about the diagnosis often is replaced by concern about the impending surgery. Nurses are in a primary position to correct misconceptions and fill in the gaps about surgical procedures. Honestly and clearly answering questions about the site, type, and extent of surgery, as well as probable pain, discomfort, or any body changes, often reduces rather than increases the patient's level of anxiety. Information should be provided and repeated as needed.[53]

PATIENT TEACHING PRIORITIES

Preoperative Instructions

Include information about:
Surgery to be performed
General preoperative activities and the reasons for them
General postoperative behaviors expected of the patient and the reasons for them
Techniques such as turning, coughing, and deep breathing (TCDB), incisional splinting, range-of-motion (ROM) exercises, and incentive spirometry
Types of equipment to be used before and after surgery
Plan of care and rationales for procedures
Anticipated care settings and equipment and experiences related to surgery
Self-care strategies to prevent and minimize complications of surgery

Outcomes of preoperative teaching:
Patient and/or significant other is able to:
State that anxiety about surgery has lessened
Demonstrate an understanding of preoperative procedures and routines through return demonstration, verbal feedback, and other means
Demonstrate an understanding of postoperative procedures and routines by return demonstration, verbal feedback, and other means
Participate in postoperative procedures and care

Preoperative patient teaching will be most successful if the nurse develops an individually tailored teaching plan based on a thorough assessment of the patient's knowledge deficits. These deficits must be handled as with any other nursing diagnosis, and the nursing process must serve as the basis for developing the teaching plan. Learning needs and goals or outcomes must be mutually identified and agreed on by the patient and/or family and the nurse. The Patient Teaching Priorities box lists preoperative teaching priorities and desired outcomes.[9, 53]

POSTOPERATIVE CARE

Postoperative nursing care of cancer patients depends on the type of cancer, the type of surgery performed, previous treatment, and preexisting physiologic deficits. Like preoperative care, postoperative care focuses on the patient's physical and psychological needs.[30]

Physical Needs

All surgery patients' immediate postoperative needs are primarily physical. From the moment the patient arrives in the recovery room or special care unit, certain definitive goals act as guides throughout the remaining postoperative course: to prevent postoperative complications and to promote cardiovascular function, tissue perfusion, respiratory function, nutrition and elimination, fluid and electrolyte balance, renal function, rest and comfort, wound healing, and early movement and ambulation.[6, 30] The reader is referred to any general surgical nursing text for a thorough discussion of these common postoperative goals.

Psychological Needs

As patients are roused from anesthesia, their first questions are often ones such as, "Do I have cancer? Did the doctor get all of it? Did the cancer spread? Did the doctor remove my (e.g., colon, leg, breast)?" The patient's questions should not be answered until recovery from the effects of anesthesia is complete and the surgeon or referring physician has had time to see the patient and offer an adequate explanation. However, the nurse must ensure that a supportive environment is provided when test results are shared with the patient and family.[30]

After surgery, cancer patients often grieve over real or imagined changes in body image and self-worth. Physical changes may be difficult for cancer patients to positively incorporate into their new self-image. Patients who attach great psychological sig-

Preoperative Assessment of Physiologic Parameters

Physiologic Parameters	Factors That Increase Surgical Risk	Assessment Factors	Laboratory Tests/Others
Nutritional status	Debilitation and malnourishment as a result of disease and/or previous therapy	Anorexia Eating habits Special diets Food restrictions Food preferences Availability of food Supplementation Nausea Vomiting Stomatitis Smell or taste changes Recent weight loss	Decreased serum albumin
Cardiovascular system	Congestive heart failure as a result of previous and prolonged chemotherapy	Dyspnea Fatigue Anorexia Nausea Vomiting Abdominal distention Right upper quadrant pain Tachycardia Weak, thready pulse Hypotension Rapid, labored respiration Frothy, blood-tinged sputum Moist rales Displaced apical pulse Weight gain Peripheral edema Dilation of peripheral veins	Increased pulmonary capillary pressure Decreased cardiac output Increased right atrial pressure
Pulmonary system	Pulmonary edema and/or fibrosis as a result of previous and prolonged chemotherapy	Nasal flaring Retractions Tachypnea Labored, noisy breathing Diaphoresis Rales Wheezing Persistent cough Frothy, blood-tinged sputum Restlessness Confusion Hypotension Tachycardia Lethargy Intake and output Sudden weight gain Swollen feet or ankles Chest pain	Decreased vital capacity Decreased minute volume Decreased cardiac output $Paco_2$ Pao_2 pH K^+ Na^+ Pulmonary capillary wedge pressure Pulmonary artery pressure Sputum specimens for culture and sensitivity Serial chest x-ray film reports
Genitourinary system	Renal insufficiency as a result of previous and prolonged chemotherapy	Frequency of voiding Dysuria Anuria Infection Urine (color, clarity)	Decreased creatinine clearance Increased blood urea nitrogen Increased uric acid levels Increased serum creatinine levels
Fluid and electrolyte status	Dehydration and electrolyte imbalance as a result of disease and/or previous therapy Hypovolemia as a result of disease	Intake and output Vomiting Diarrhea Bleeding	K^+ Mg^{++} Ca^{++} H^+

Preoperative Assessment of Physiologic Parameters *Continued*

Physiologic Parameters	Factors That Increase Surgical Risk	Assessment Factors	Laboratory Tests/Others
Liver function status	Metastatic liver disease	Jaundice Ascites Vague upper abdominal pain Anorexia Weight loss Splenomegaly Esophageal varices Fever of unknown origin Dependent edema	Total bilirubin
Hematologic factors	Platelet dysfunction as a result of disease and/or previous therapy Hypercoagulability as a result of disease Anemia as a result of disease	Easy bruising Excessive bleeding Dyspnea Fatigue Previous thrombophlebitis	Prothrombin time Partial thromboplastin Platelet count White blood cell (WBC) count Hemoglobin Hematocrit Red blood cell count
Potential for postoperative complications	Preoperative infection as a result of immunocompetence and/or previous therapy Previous radiation therapy	Sneezing Cough Sore throat Fever Skin lesions Rashes Radiation damage in relation to anticipated surgical incision	WBC count Throat culture Sputum culture

Data from references 6 and 57.

nificance to the physical changes associated with cancer surgery frequently restrict their physical and sexual activities unnecessarily, feeling they are now too frail and that their bodies are vulnerable. The nurse can assist these patients by acknowledging the painfulness of any physical changes and by ensuring that they grieve in a safe, nonjudgmental environment.[30, 41, 53]

It is important that the nurse assess the type and degree of support that significant others provide the patient. Postoperative anxiety often declines when the nurse includes family members in the care of the patient. However, the nurse must remember that cancer and surgery are crisis situations for the entire family. Initially the family may be emotionally and psychologically immobilized by the diagnosis. Often family members want to support the patient but do not know what to say or do. The nurse can guide them by aiding them in identifying what they can do to help.[30, 41]

Nurses must be aware of the psychological issues affecting cancer surgery patients to provide the most appropriate care and to encourage their patients to adapt positively to the demands of the disease and of therapy (see Chapter 32).

Nursing Diagnosis

- *Body image disturbance related to surgical removal of body part and to diagnosis of cancer*

Outcome Goal

Patient will be able to:

- Verbalize impact of surgery and diagnosis on self-image.

Interventions

- Encourage patient to discuss feelings and concerns with health care providers and significant others.
- Help patient identify, label, and express feelings about significance of lost body part, treatment modalities, and anticipated progress.
- Promote acceptance of a positive/realistic body image.

Nursing Diagnosis

- *Ineffective family coping: compromised related to diagnosis of cancer*

Outcome Goal

Family will be able to:

- Demonstrate effective coping strategies for living with cancer.

Interventions

- Provide opportunities for expression of feelings.
- Provide information to assist patients and their families in working through emotional reactions to the diagnosis, treatment, and prognosis.

Nursing Diagnosis

- *Ineffective individual coping related to diagnosis of cancer and to potential life-style changes*

Outcome Goal

Patient will be able to:

- Demonstrate effective coping strategies for living with cancer.

Interventions

- Provide opportunities for patient to express feelings about diagnosis and prognosis.
- Assist patient in meeting adaptations or changes in activities and relationships.

Nursing Diagnosis

- *Risk for fluid volume deficit related to surgical procedure, to excessive fluid loss from abnormal routes (indwelling tubes) and postoperative nausea/vomiting, and to inability to receive or absorb fluids*

Outcome Goal

Patient will be able to:

- Demonstrate no evidence of fluid volume deficit.

Interventions

- Monitor vital signs.
- Assess capillary refill time.
- Measure intake and output.
- Monitor electrolyte values.
- Measure urine specific gravity.
- Monitor hemoglobin and hematocrit.
- Assess oral mucous membranes.
- Assess skin turgor.
- Administer intravenous or oral fluids as ordered by physician.
- Administer antiemetics as ordered by physician.

Nursing Diagnosis

- *Fluid volume deficit related to surgical procedure (loss of 15%–20% of total blood volume during surgery)*

Outcome Goal

Patient will be able to:

- Demonstrate adequate fluid volume within 72 hours of surgery.

Interventions

- Maintain strict bed rest, with patient supine and head of bed elevated slightly.
- Limit all activities.
- Monitor vital signs every 5 to 15 minutes.
- Administer drugs as ordered to maintain blood pressure (BP) and increase cardiac output.
- Maintain patent intravenous line for administration of drugs.
- Administer fluids and volume expanders as ordered.
- Monitor urine output.
- Assess skin for color, temperature, and elasticity.
- Maintain accurate input and output records.
- Monitor arterial blood gases.
- Administer oxygen as ordered.
- Monitor respiratory rate and pattern.
- Monitor hemodynamic parameters as ordered.

Nursing Diagnosis

- *Impaired gas exchange related to embolization of thrombus*

Outcome Goal

Patient will be able to:

- Demonstrate no evidence of pulmonary embolus.

Intervention

- Observe for signs/symptoms of pulmonary embolus:
    Chest pain
    Dyspnea
    Tachypnea

Nursing Diagnosis

- *Risk for infection related to preoperative immunocompromised status stemming from disease and/or previous therapy*

Outcome Goal

Patient will be able to:

- Demonstrate no evidence of infection.

Interventions

- Assess for risk factors.
- Obtain cultures as ordered and report results.
- Monitor vital signs; check for increased pulse rate and signs of low-grade, intermittent fever.
- Inspect body secretions, excretions, and exudates for signs of infection; report abnormalities.
- Monitor hydration and electrolyte balance.
- Monitor changes in white blood cell (WBC) count.
- Wash hands before and after contact with patient.
- Make sure patient is not exposed to infected visitors or staff.
- Turn patient frequently; instruct in deep breathing.

Nursing Diagnosis

- Risk for infection related to break in skin's integrity (surgical incision)

Outcome Goal

Patient will be able to:

- Demonstrate no evidence of wound infection.

Intervention

- Monitor wound site for edema, redness, and undue pain.

Nursing Diagnosis

- Risk for infection related to urinary retention as a result of surgical procedure

Outcome Goal

Patient will be able to:

- Demonstrate no evidence of urinary tract infection.

Interventions

- Check urine output for amount, color, specific gravity, and odor.
- Administer antibiotics as ordered.
- Assess for abdominal pain.
- Force fluids.

Nursing Diagnosis

- Risk for injury related to peritonitis secondary to breakdown of anastomosis because of diminished tissue healing as a result of chemotherapy, radiation therapy, poor nutritional status, and/or tumor

Outcome Goal

Patient will be able to:

- Demonstrate no evidence of peritonitis.

Interventions

- Assess for signs/symptoms of peritonitis:
  Moderate to severe abdominal pain
  Burning ache aggravated by any motion, even respiration
  Anorexia
  Nausea
  Vomiting
  Fever within 48 hours after surgery
  Chills, thirst, scant urine output
  Inability to pass feces or flatus
  Abdominal distention
  Tachycardia with weak, thready pulses
  Rapid, shallow respirations
  Tachypnea

Nursing Diagnosis

- Risk for injury related to postoperative intestinal obstruction secondary to adhesions from radiation therapy

Outcome Goal

Patient will be able to:

- Demonstrate no evidence of intestinal obstruction.

Intervention

- Assess for signs/symptoms of intestinal obstruction:
  Vomiting
  Abdominal cramping
  Constipation

Nursing Diagnosis

- Risk for injury related to hypercoagulability and postoperative inactivity

Outcome Goal

Patient will be able to:

- Demonstrate no evidence of thrombophlebitis.

Interventions

- Assess calves daily.
- Observe for signs/symptoms of thrombophlebitis:
  Calf pain
  Calf tenderness
  Homans' sign
  Dilated superficial veins
  Edema of involved extremity
- Encourage early ambulation.

Nursing Diagnosis

* *Knowledge deficit related to such areas as self-care, activities related to health care regimen, and decision-making about health*

Outcome Goal

Patient will be able to:

* Express an understanding of and demonstrate important self-care and daily activities resulting from diagnosis and surgical procedure.

Interventions

* At every interaction, assess for knowledge deficits.
* Use patient's theories about illness as a starting point for teaching, and continually elicit patient's perception.
* During interactions, assess frequently to see if patient understands and accepts diagnosis.
* Simplify information to conform to patient's terms, thought patterns, and daily routines.
* Give explicit directions.
* Be available to patient for questions.
* Demonstrate to patient and family how to use information.
* Reinforce correct use of information.
* Teach patient how to mentally rehearse a necessary health action.
* Make sure patient is actively involved in decisions about care.
* Offer access to a peer support network and opportunities for patient to watch others successfully mastering similar health care problems.
* Provide instruction in several forms (visual, written, discussion), so that patient will remember it in various ways.
* Provide materials for patient to take home for review and to use what was learned (see box below).

Nursing Diagnosis

* *Impaired physical mobility related to surgical removal of limb*

Outcome Goal

Patient will be able to:

* Demonstrate activities that encourage adaptation to changes in physical mobility resulting from surgical procedure.

Interventions

* Help patient with ambulation; control distance.
* Have patient use walker, cane, or wheelchair as needed as assistive devices.
* Minimize environmental barriers.
* Encourage use of involved limb.
* Change patient's position slowly.
* Encourage moderate physical exercise, adequate rest, and ROM exercises.
* Balance nutritional intake; supplement protein.
* Discuss "phantom" pain with patient and family.

Nursing Diagnosis

* *Altered nutrition: less than body requirements related to surgical procedure for cancer that interferes with mechanical process of eating and with absorption of essential salts and nutrients*

Outcome Goal

Patient will be able to:

* Demonstrate no evidence of protein-calorie malnutrition.

Interventions

* Assess for signs/symptoms of protein-calorie malnutrition:
    Edema
    Hair dyspigmentation
    Easily pluckable hair
    Muscle wasting
    Dermatosis
* Review results of anthropometric test, dietary analysis, and clinical examination.
* Perform nutrition assessment:
    Assess problem area
    Food preferences
    Patterns and behaviors related to food intake
    Intake and output
    Calorie count
* Encourage good mouth care.
* Provide relaxed, pain-free environment.
* Observe presentation of food.
* Encourage family to bring in favorite foods when allowed.
* Confer with dietitian about diet and supplements that meet patient's needs.
* Provide proper care for and monitor intravenous total parenteral nutrition.
* Provide proper care for feeding tubes.
* Before discharge, provide nutrition teaching for patient and family.

Nursing Diagnosis

* *Pain related to surgical procedure and to complications at insertion sites of therapeutic hardware*

Outcome Goal

Patient will be able to:

- Express and demonstrate successful control of pain related to diagnosis and surgical procedure.

Interventions

- Incorporate the following when assessing patient's level of pain:
    Location and characteristics
    Onset
    Frequency
    Intensity (scale of 0–10)
    Quality
    Effective pain control measures
    Ineffective pain control measures
    Pain expression style
    Movement
    Muscle tone
    Emotional distress
    Effect of pain on postoperative activities
    Effect on sleep/wake pattern
- Identify strategies that eliminate or control pain.
- Explore strategies that have been successful in the past.
- Identify strategies that patient considers essential for reducing pain.
- Administer medication per physician's orders and protocols using appropriate delivery system:
    Monitor effect frequently.
    Graph pain assessment data.
    Provide physician with evidence of need to change medication.
- Intervene at onset of pain.
- Position for comfort.
- Provide distraction.
- Instruct patient in relaxation techniques; for acute pain, use short, simple techniques with nurse directing.
- Pace activities, and plan activities ahead of time.
- Provide supportive environment.
- Use several pain reduction strategies.

Nursing Diagnosis

- *Risk for impaired skin integrity related to tissue damage and/or poor tissue healing resulting from chemotherapy, radiation therapy, and/or poor nutritional status*

Outcome Goal

Patient will be able to:

- Demonstrate no evidence of tissue damage or poor tissue healing.

Interventions

- Inspect incision site for hematomas (swelling, discoloration).
- Assess patency of drains.
- Assess for signs/symptoms of dehiscence:
    Rapid onset of serosanguineous drainage
    Popping sensation
- Assess for signs of impending evisceration:
    Separation of incision
    Protrusion of abdominal contents
- Check use of abdominal binders for obese patients.

Nursing Diagnosis

- *Impaired skin integrity related to tissue damage and/or poor tissue healing resulting from chemotherapy, radiation therapy, and/or poor nutritional status*

Outcome Goal

Patient will be able to:

- Show adequate healing of affected tissues after appropriate medical and nursing intervention.

Interventions

- Assess for signs/symptoms of dehiscence:
    Monitor amount and color of drainage.
- If dehiscence occurs:
    Call physician immediately.
    Obtain vital signs.
    Prepare patient for surgery.
- Assess for signs of evisceration:
    Separation of incision
    Protrusion of abdominal contents
- If evisceration occurs:
    Apply sterile, moist towels over extruded intestine or omentum.
    Prepare patient for surgery.

Nursing Diagnosis

- *Altered tissue perfusion (peripheral) related to lymphedema secondary to dissection of lymph nodes*

Outcome Goal

Patient will be able to:

- Demonstrate no evidence of lymphedema.

Interventions

- Do not use affected limb to check BP, perform venipunctures, withdraw blood, or inject medications.

- Assess affected limb for signs/symptoms of lymph-edema:
    Redness
    Warmth
    Unusual hardness
    Swelling
- Use pillows to elevate affected limb above level of the heart.
- Observe for infection occurring secondary to lymphedema.
- Teach importance of good hygiene.
- Encourage progressive exercise of affected limb.

Nursing Diagnosis

- *Altered tissue perfusion (peripheral) related to hypercoagulability and postoperative inactivity*

Outcome Goal

Patient will be able to:

- Demonstrate no evidence of peripheral edema.

Interventions

- Keep patient on bed rest.
- Limit self-care activities.
- Raise affected limb above level of right atrium.
- Do not use knee gatch.
- If patient complains of pain, assess its quality and location.
- Administer analgesics as ordered.
- Measure calf or thigh (or both) daily and record findings.
- Assess circulation of affected extremity, and check pulses in all extremities. Use Doppler sensor if pulses seem to be absent.
- Use elastic stockings as ordered.
- Check vital signs every 4 to 8 hours.
- Administer anticoagulant therapy as ordered.
- Monitor results of prothrombin time and partial thromboplastin time studies.
- Initiate a progressive exercise program.
- Instruct patient to put on support stockings before ambulating and to avoid standing for long periods.

DISCHARGE PLANNING

The goal for the cancer patient is to develop or regain independence. This can be achieved by encouraging patients to participate in activities of daily living and to learn new self-care measures early in their hospitalization in preparation for discharge. However, in their eagerness to help patients, family members often try to do everything for them. This serves only to foster dependence in patients, contributing to feelings of helplessness. The nurse must guide the family in understanding the significance of the patient's early steps toward independence.[30]

Nurses sometimes mistakenly assume that, once the patient is discharged from the hospital, the patient will receive the care, attention, and support needed at home. However, some patients dread discharge from the hospital almost as much as admission to it. Some patients become very dependent on the hospital and their new sick role, particularly if their home life is unstable. An unstable home environment (e.g., poor communication, strained relationships) is likely to worsen after surgery. Whether the patient is able to adjust to changes in physical appearance or function is largely determined by the family's reaction to these same issues. If the patient feels rejected at home, the patient may fear rejection from society at large.[41]

Discharge planning therefore must begin when a patient is admitted to the hospital and continue throughout the hospital stay. The nurse's assessment must include information about the family and family situation; the patient's knowledge about the disease, its treatment, and available resources; the social setting; school and work; and diet. The health care team then can begin to make appropriate plans to ease the transition from hospital to home. Many times, prepar-

---

 PATIENT TEACHING PRIORITIES

Postoperative Instructions

Include information about:

Changes in self-care and other activities as a result of surgery

Progressive return to maximum activity level

Anticipated discharge medications

Wound management

Proper use of assistive or prosthetic devices

Symptoms to watch for: fever, pain, vomiting, diarrhea, bleeding, malnutrition

When and whom to call if problems arise

Where to get additional information about cancer or its treatment

How to contact support groups (e.g., Reach to Recovery, Make Today Count)

Resources or agencies that might be helpful to patient: physical therapy, occupational therapy, speech therapy, ostomy outpatient clinics, sources of prosthetic fitting devices, home care agencies

Sources of medical supplies

Possible follow-up care

Return to work

Any necessary job retraining

Resumption of driving

Resumption of sexual activity

ing the home to receive the patient takes longer than the hospitalization. Members of the health care team must be consulted for their evaluations of the family's ability to care for the patient. Evaluation may reveal that home care by private or visiting nurses or admission to an extended care facility may be needed when the patient leaves the hospital. If the family is experiencing communication problems and emotional difficulties, the health care team might consider referral to family therapy or a family support group.[30, 41] The postoperative instructions identified in the Patient Teaching Priorities box should be given to the patient in writing before discharge.

An astute nurse institutes and documents discharge planning based on a thorough admission assessment and history and makes every attempt to involve family members early in the process. If needed, referrals are made to appropriate members of the health care team so that all possible issues are addressed well before the patient's discharge from the hospital. Discharge planning allows patients and their families to prepare for living with cancer outside of the hospital. The nurse anticipates postoperative needs and concerns early, allowing the cancer patient and family to face the challenges that lie ahead.[30]

Chapter Questions

1. In stereotactic radiosurgery:
   a. External-beam radiation therapy is delivered to tumors.
   b. Photosensitizing drugs are injected intravenously.
   c. Multiple narrow radiation beams are directed toward tumors using specialized surgical instruments.
   d. Radioactive sealed sources are implanted surgically into tumors.
2. Local excision involves:
   a. Removal of a tumor, regional lymph nodes, lymphatic channels, and any involved neighboring structures
   b. Removal of a large tumor burden
   c. Excision of a tumor and a small margin of normal tissue
   d. Removal of a wedge of tumor tissue from a large tumor
3. Electrosurgery:
   a. Destroys precancerous or cancer cells by deep-freezing them
   b. Combines surgical resection of tissue with topical application of chemotherapy
   c. Destroys cancer cells by using the cutting and coagulating effects of high-frequency electrical current
   d. Uses a minicamera to transmit surgical images to a video monitor
4. Physiologic changes related to the aging process include all of the following except:
   a. Decreased cardiac output
   b. Decreased glomerular filtration rate
   c. Decreased residual lung volume
   d. Decreased muscle strength
5. Prophylactic surgery is considered what type of treatment?
   a. Salvage
   b. Adjuvant
   c. Palliative
   d. Primary
6. The disadvantages of needle biopsy include all of the following except:
   a. Improper handling may distort cells
   b. Needle may miss the tumor
   c. Requires general anesthesia
   d. Risk of injury to adjacent structures
7. Palliative surgery includes all of the following except:
   a. Management of cancer pain
   b. Treatment of chemotherapy-related complications
   c. Ablative surgery
   d. Second-look procedures
8. Surgery is recommended for:
   a. Cancers that are disseminated at the time of diagnosis
   b. Well-differentiated, slow-growing tumors
   c. Poorly differentiated, rapid-growing tumors
   d. Tumors that predictably metastasize early
9. Special surgical techniques for laser surgery requires knowledge and skill of laser-tissue interactions that include:
   a. Photocoagulation, vaporization, photochemical ablation, and photochemical interactions
   b. Photoanticoagulation, vaporization, photochemical ablation, and photochemical interactions
   c. Photocoagulation, cryoprobes, photochemical ablation, and photochemical interactions
   d. Photocoagulation, vaporization, stereotactic ablation, and photochemical interactions

10. Principles of surgical oncology require concepts of tumor cell kinetics and additional tumor factors that include:
  a. Tumor anatomic location, histologic type, response to surgical procedure, and growth rate
  b. Tumor anatomic location, histologic type, response to surgical procedure, and invasion
  c. Tumor anatomic location, histologic type, growth rate, and vertical spread
  d. Tumor anatomic location, histologic type, growth rate, and invasion

BIBLIOGRAPHY

1. Allen MS: Video-assisted thoracoscopy. In Morris PJ, Malt RA, editors: *Oxford textbook of surgery,* vol 2, New York, Oxford Medical Publications, 1994.
2. Anseline PF and others: Radiation injury of the rectum, *Ann Surg* 194:716, 1981.
3. Arbour R: Laser and ultrasound technology in aggressive management of central nervous system tumors, *J Neurosci Nurs* 26:30, 1994.
4. Aronoff BL: Lasers in surgical oncology. I, *Semin Surg Oncol* 11:281, 1995.
5. Baird RM, Rebbeck PA: Impact of preoperative chemotherapy for the surgeon, *Recent Results Cancer Res* 103:79, 1986.
6. Black JM, Matassarin-Jacobs E, editors: *Luckmann and Sorensen's medical-surgical nursing: a psychophysiologic approach,* ed 4, Philadelphia, Saunders, 1993.
7. Brandt BT and others: Hepatic cryosurgery for metastatic colorectal carcinoma, *Oncol Nurs Forum* 23:29, 1996.
8. Brenner ZR, Krenzer ME: Update on cryosurgical ablation for prostate cancer, *AJN* 95:44, 1995.
9. Brown MH and others: *Standards of oncology nursing practice,* New York, Wiley & Sons, 1986.
10. Bucholtz JD: Implications of radiation therapy for nursing. In Clark JC, McGee RF, editors: *Core curriculum for oncology nursing,* ed 2, Philadelphia, Saunders, 1992.
11. Butler J: Nutrition and cancer: a review of the literature, *Cancer Nurs* 3:131, 1980.
12. Calabresi P, Schein PS, Rosenberg SA, editors: *Medical oncology: basic principles and clinical management of cancer,* ed 2, New York, McGraw-Hill, 1993.
13. Derby SA: Cancer in the older patient. In Ashwander P and others, editors: *Oncology nursing: advances, treatments and trends into the 21st century,* Rockville, MD, 1990, Aspen, 1990.
14. DeVita VT Jr, Hellman S, Rosenberg SA, editors: *Cancer: principles and practice of oncology,* ed 5, Philadelphia, Lippincott-Raven, 1997.
15. DeVita VT Jr, Hellman S, Rosenberg SA, editors: *Important advances in oncology,* ed 12, Philadelphia, Lippincott-Raven, 1996.
16. Dixon J: Current laser applications in general surgery, *Ann Surg* 207:355, 1988.
17. Duke JH, Miller TA: Salt and water: fluid and electrolyte problems. In Condon R, DeCosse J, editors: *Surgical care,* Philadelphia, Lea & Febiger, 1980.
18. Engelking C: New approaches: innovations in cancer prevention, diagnosis, treatment, and support, *Oncol Nurs Forum* 21:62, 1994.
19. Falcone RE, Nappi JF: Chemotherapy and wound healing, *Surg Clin North Am* 64:779, 1984.
20. Fisher AMR, Murphree AL, Gomer CJ: Clinical and preclinical photodynamic therapy, *Lasers Surg Med* 17:2, 1995.
21. Forbes J: Principles and potential of palliative surgery in patients with advanced cancer, *Recent Results Cancer Res* 108:134, 1988.
22. Friel M: Concepts related to the nursing care of surgical oncology patients. In Vredevoe D, Derdiarian A, Sarna L, editors: *Concepts of oncology nursing,* Englewood Cliffs, NJ, Prentice Hall, 1981.
23. Griffiths MJ, Murray KH, Russo PC: *Oncology nursing: pathophysiology, assessment, and intervention,* New York, Macmillan, 1984.
24. Groenwald SL and others, editors: *Cancer nursing: principles and practice,* ed 3, Boston, Jones & Bartlett, 1993.
25. Haibeck S: Intraoperative radiation therapy, *Oncol Nurs Forum* 15:143, 1988.
26. Harrison LB, Enker WE, Anderson LL: High-dose-rate intraoperative radiation therapy for colorectal cancer, *Oncology* 9:737, 1995.
27. Haskel CM, editor: *Cancer treatment,* ed 4, Philadelphia, Saunders, 1995.
28. Hill G: Historic milestones in cancer surgery, *Semin Oncol* 6:409, 1979.
29. Holland JF, editor: *Cancer medicine,* ed 4, Philadelphia, Williams & Wilkins, 1997.
30. Howland WS: Preoperative evaluation of the cancer patient for emergency surgery. In Turnbull AD, editor: *Surgical emergencies in the cancer patient,* Chicago, Mosby, 1987.
31. Howland WS, Groeger JS, editors: *Critical care of the cancer patient,* ed 2, St. Louis, Mosby, 1991.
32. Landreneau RJ and others: The potential role of video-assisted thoracic surgery in the patient with lung cancer. In Pass HI and others, editors: *Lung cancer: principles and practice,* Philadelphia, Lippincott-Raven, 1996.
33. LaRocca JC, Otto SE: *Pocket guide to intravenous therapy,* ed 3, St. Louis, Mosby, 1997.
34. Larson DA, Flickinger JC, Loeffler JS: Stereotactic radiosurgery: techniques and results, *PPO Updates* 7:1, 1993.
35. Lehr P: Surgical lasers: how they work, current applications, *AORN J* 50:972, 1989.
36. Lewis SM, Collier IC, Heitkemper MM, editors: *Medical-surgical nursing: assessment and management of clinical problems,* ed 4, St. Louis, Mosby, 1996.
37. Lindsey A, Piper B, Stotts N: The phenomenon of cancer cachexia: a review, *Oncol Nurs Forum* 9:38, 1982.
38. Mullen J: Consequences of malnutrition in the surgical patient, *Surg Clin North Am* 61:465, 1981.
39. Murphy GP, Lenhard RE, Lawrence W Jr, editors: *American Cancer Society textbook of clinical oncology,* ed 2, Atlanta, American Cancer Society, 1995.
40. Nicholson C and others: Are you ready for video thoracoscopy? *AJN* 93:54, 1993.

41. Office of Cancer Communications: *Coping with cancer: a resource for the health professional,* Bethesda, MD, US Department of Health and Human Services, 1982.
42. Pack R, Lynds BG: Surgical intervention. In McIntire SN, Cioppa AL, editors: *Cancer nursing: a developmental approach,* New York, Wiley & Sons, 1984.
43. Pass HI and others, editors: *Lung cancer: principles and practice,* Philadelphia, Lippincott-Raven, 1996.
44. Patterson WB: Surgical issues in geriatric oncology, *Semin Oncol* 16:57, 1989.
45. Polomano R and others: Surgical critical care for cancer patients, *Semin Oncol Nurs* 10:165, 1994.
46. Schwartz SI, Shires GT, editors: *Principles of surgery,* ed 7, New York, McGraw-Hill, 1999.
47. Shamberger R: Effect of chemotherapy and radiotherapy on wound healing: experimental studies, *Recent Results Cancer Res* 98:17, 1985.
48. Sherman CD: Principles of surgical oncology. In Kahn SB and others, editors: *Concepts in cancer medicine,* New York, Grune & Stratton, 1983.
49. Shiplacoff TA: Concepts in surgical oncology. In Vredevoe D, Derdiarian A, Sarna L, editors: *Concepts of oncology nursing,* Englewood Cliffs, NJ, Prentice Hall, 1981.
50. Silberman AW: Surgical debulking of tumors, *Surg Gynecol Obstet* 155:577, 1982.
51. Sliney DH, Trokel SL: Medical lasers and their safe use, New York, Springer-Verlag, 1993.
52. Smith RW, Sampson MK, Lucas CE: Effects of vinblastine, etoposide, cisplatin and bleomycin in rodent wound healing, *Surg Gynecol Obstet* 161:323, 1985.
53. Snyder CC: *Oncology nursing,* Boston, Little, Brown, 1986.
54. Summers JL, Bollard GA: Visual laser-assisted prostatectomy, *J Urol Nurs* 13:861, 1994.
55. Szopa TJ: Implications of surgical treatment for nursing. In Clark JC, McGee RF, editors: *Core curriculum for oncology nursing,* ed 2, Philadelphia, Saunders, 1992.
56. Tenenbaum L, editor: *Cancer chemotherapy and biotherapy: a reference guide,* ed 2, Philadelphia, Saunders, 1994.
57. Thompson JM and others: *Mosby's clinical nursing,* ed 3, St. Louis, Mosby, 1993.
58. Tootla J, Easterling A: PDT: destroying malignant cells with laser beams—photodynamic therapy, *Nurs* 19:48, 1989.
59. Willard MP, Gilsdorf RB, Price RA: Protein-calorie malnutrition in a community hospital, *JAMA* 243:1720, 1980.
60. Wong RJ, DeCosse JJ: Cytoreductive surgery, *Surg Gynecol Obstet* 170:276, 1990.
61. Yasko J: *Care of the client receiving external radiation,* Reston, VA, Reston, 1982.

Radiation Therapy

Ryan Iwamoto

Radiation therapy is a localized treatment that is used alone or in conjunction with other treatments such as surgery or chemotherapy, or both. In certain situations, combining radiation therapy with other therapies maximizes cure rates because of the effect of the other therapies on radioresistant cells.[52] Radiation therapy may be administered before surgery to treat undisturbed tissues and to reduce the tumor's size to make resection feasible. Radiation therapy may also be delivered after surgery to treat cancer cells that may have been disseminated beyond the surgical margins or that may have remained in the tumor bed. In other instances, radiation is used before and after surgical resection. Chemotherapy may be combined with radiation therapy to control subclinical disease and enhance the local effect of radiation.[30, 51, 104] Table 22–1 lists the theoretical rationale for combining radiation therapy with chemotherapy.[104]

Radiation therapy is used for several purposes[115]: to cure by eradicating disease, allowing the person to live a normal life span; to control the growth and spread of the disease, allowing the person to live for a time without symptoms; to prevent microscopic disease, as with cranial irradiation for certain types of lung cancers; and to improve a person's quality of life by relieving or diminishing symptoms associated with advanced cancer. These symptoms include pain from bone metastasis; uncontrolled bleeding from the tumor; tumor obstruction around major blood vessels, gastrointestinal tract, kidneys, ureters, and trachea; spinal cord compression; and symptoms related to brain metastasis.[61, 115]

DEFINITION

Radiation therapy is the use of high-energy ionizing rays or particles to treat cancer. Approximately 60% of all persons with cancer will be treated with radiation therapy at some point during their illness.

HISTORICAL PERSPECTIVE

Radiation was one of the earliest ways cancer was treated. Since the late 19th century, when radium, radioactivity, and x-rays were discovered, radiation has been used to treat cancer. The first successful radiation treatment for cancer was reported in 1898. At that time, large doses were delivered in a single treatment, which resulted in many complications. Between 1920 and 1940, studies were conducted to evaluate the effects of radiation on tissues, and fractionation of the dose (dividing the total dose into several small doses) was started.

In 1952, the first patient was treated with radioactive cobalt. With the invention of the vacuum tube, treatment with higher energies to deeper tissues was possible. Linear accelerators were developed in the mid-1950s and provided treatment rays with deeper penetration and less scatter to normal tissues. Over the past 100 years, the specialty of radiation oncology has advanced with the use of computer technology, the refinement of treatment machines, and advancements in radiobiologic science.

PRINCIPLES OF RADIATION THERAPY

High-energy ionizing radiation destroys the ability of cancer cells to grow and multiply. Some cells are directly damaged by the ionizing rays or particles. However, more cells are indirectly affected when the ionizing rays or particles penetrate the cell's nucleus and interact with the water content of the nucleus to form hydroxyl (free) radicals. These unstable radicals then cause damage to the cell's DNA, with breakage of one or both chromosomal strands. Immediate cell death may occur if the chromosomal damage is irreparable. Some cells survive despite the chromosomal damage. However, these cells are unable to divide and die at the time of mitosis. As a result of radiation, some cells become giant cells, which continue to function but are unable to divide. These cells gradually degenerate and die.

The radiosensitivity of cancer cells depends on several factors:

Type of cell (Table 22–2)
Phase of cell life—cells in the resting stage are less sensitive to radiation than those in active cellular division

TABLE 22-1
Theoretic Rationale for Irradiation and Chemotherapy Interactions

Spatial cooperation
 Chemotherapy treats disease outside irradiation field
 Radiation therapy treats local disease and sanctuary sites
Toxicity independence
Tumor debulking by first modality leading to improved
  efficacy of second modality
 Improved chemotherapy delivery
 Improved oxygenation
 Smaller radiation therapy fields
Protection of normal tissues from irradiation damage
Prevention of emergence of resistant clones
Direct biochemical and molecular interactions
 Modification of slope of dose-response curve
 Synchronization of cells by chemotherapy into a more
  irradiation-sensitive phase of the cell cycle
 Improved sensitization of hypoxic cells to radiation therapy
  by chemotherapy
 Improved killing of hypoxic cells by chemotherapy
 Inhibition of repair of potentially lethal and sublethal x-ray
  damage
Inhibition of tumor repopulation during fractionated radiation
 therapy

From Rotman M, Aziz H, Wasserman TH: Chemotherapy and irradiation. In Perez CA, Brady LW, editors: Principles and practice of radiation oncology, *ed 3, Philadelphia, Lippincott-Raven, 1998:706.*

ADMINISTRATION OF RADIATION THERAPY

Radiation therapy can be delivered in many ways. External-beam radiation (teletherapy) uses a treatment machine placed at some distance from the body. Radiation can also be delivered by implanting a sealed radioactive source in or near the cancerous area to provide a localized treatment; this is called *brachytherapy*. The radioactive source may be placed in the body temporarily or permanently, depending on the radiation treatment plan. For brachytherapy patients receiving a temporary implant, isolation in a hospital room may be required while the implant is in place.

In other circumstances radioactive materials are injected intravenously or taken orally for a systemic effect (nonsealed sources). The radioactive substance travels to areas of the body requiring treatment. Thyroid cancer is frequently treated with radioactive iodine in this manner.

Coupling tumor-specific antibodies with radioactive isotopes combines the science of immunology with radiation therapy to maximize tumor treatment while minimizing normal tissue toxicity.[15, 123] These antibodies are designed to be attracted to specific antigens on certain tumor cells while sparing normal tissues. They are produced in animals and injected intravenously into the patient. When the radiolabeled antibodies are adminis-

Division rate of the cell—rapidly dividing cells are more sensitive to radiation than slowly dividing cells because more cells will be in the active cellular division stage

Degree of differentiation—poorly differentiated cells are more sensitive to radiation therapy than well-differentiated cells

Oxygenation—well-oxygenated tissues are more sensitive to radiation therapy because oxygen is needed to form the hydroxyl (free) radicals

Normal cells are also affected by the ionizing radiation. The sum total of the effects on each cell in the tissue accounts for the side effects of radiation therapy. However, normal cells are generally better able to repair the chromosomal damage done by the radiation. The treatments are delivered to kill as many cancer cells as possible while minimizing the damage to normal cells. Body tissues have limits to the amount of radiation that can be tolerated. Exceeding those limits can result in serious complications[6] (Table 22-3).

Radiation dose is recorded as the absorbed energy per unit mass.[52] The Systeme Internationale Unit for radiation dosage is the Gray. Dose of radiation may be reported as Gray (Gy) or centiGray (cGy = 1/100 Gray).

TABLE 22-2
Radiosensitivity of Various Tumors and Tissues

Tumors	Relative Radiosensitivity
Lymphoma, leukemia, seminoma, dysgerminoma	High
Squamous cell cancer of the oropharyngeal, glottis, bladder, skin, and cervical epithelia; adenocarcinomas of the alimentary tract	Fairly high
Vascular and connective tissue elements of all tumors, secondary neurovascularization, and astrocytomas	Medium
Salivary gland tumors, hepatomas, renal cancer, pancreatic cancer, chondrosarcoma, and osteogenic sarcoma	Fairly low
Rhabdomyosarcoma, leiomyosarcoma, and ganglioneurofibrosarcoma	Low

From Rubin P: Principles of radiation oncology and cancer radiotherapy. In Rubin P, editor: Clinical oncology for medical students and physicians, *New York, American Cancer Society, 1983.*

TABLE 22-3
Minimal and Maximal Tolerance Dose of Various Organs

Organ	Injury	Minimal Tolerance Dose TD$_{5/5}$* (cGy)	Maximal Tolerance Dose TD$_{50/5}$† (cGy)	Whole or Partial Organ (Field Size or Length)
Bone marrow	Aplasia, pancytopenia	250	450	Whole
		3000	4000	Segmental
Liver	Acute and chronic hepatitis	2500	4000	Whole
		1500	2000	Whole (strip)
Stomach	Perforation, ulcer, hemorrhage	4500	5500	100 cm
Intestine	Ulcer, perforation, hemorrhage	4500	5500	400 cm
		5000	6500	100 cm
Brain	Infarction, necrosis	5000	6000	Whole
Spinal cord	Infarction, necrosis	4500	5500	10 cm
Heart	Pericarditis, pancarditis	4500	5500	60%
		7000	8000	25%
Lung	Acute and chronic pneumonitis	3000	3500	100 cm
		1500	2500	Whole
Kidney	Acute and chronic nephrosclerosis	1500	2000	Whole (strip)
		2000	2500	Whole
Fetus	Death	200	400	Whole

*$TD_{5/5}$, minimal tolerance dose; the dose that, when given to a population of patients under a standard set of treatment conditions, results in a 5% rate of severe complications within 5 years of treatment.

†$TD_{50/5}$, maximal tolerance dose; the dose that, when given to a population of patients under a standard set of treatment conditions, results in a 50% rate of severe complications within 5 years of treatment.

From Rubin P, Cooper R, Phillips TL, editors: Radiation biology and radiation pathology syllabus. I. Radiation oncology, Chicago, American College of Radiology, 1975.

tered in the bloodstream, they seek out the tumor and the radioactivity attached to the antibody directly treats the cancer cells. Few acute side effects are associated with antibody administration. Allergic reactions may be noted during or soon after injection of the antibodies. Bone marrow suppression, particularly thrombocytopenia, may be noted 4 to 6 weeks after antibody administration.[15]

EXTERNAL RADIATION THERAPY

Treatment Planning

Before radiation treatments can begin, a plan is developed to determine the best way to deliver the treatments. A major part of the planning process is the localization procedure, which uses a simulator (Fig. 22–1). A *simulator* is a machine that simulates the treatment machine in its movement and positioning. Depending on the area being treated, a variety of radiographic studies, such as computed tomography (CT) scans, magnetic resonance imaging (MRI) studies, barium enemas, and intravenous pyelograms help define the exact area within the body that needs treatment as well as the normal organs to protect (Fig. 22–2). Marks or small tattoos placed on the body are used to position the patient for treatment. These marks ensure that treat-

ment delivery will be consistent. Special plastic or plaster forms or molds may be constructed to help support and assist the patient to maintain a precise position during each treatment (Fig. 22–3). The area of treatment is shaped with special shielding devices called blocks. These blocks, which are made of lead or high-

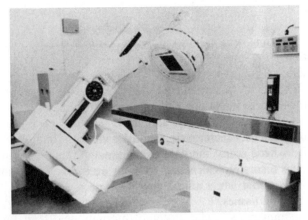

FIGURE 22-1 The simulator, which simulates the movement and positioning of the treatment machine, is used during the localization procedure. (Courtesy Virginia Mason Medical Center, Seattle, WA.)

tive treatments, such as for pain from bone metastasis, may be delivered at higher daily doses for fewer numbers of treatments. The actual treatment takes 2 to 5 minutes. More time is spent carefully positioning the patient on the treatment table.

A variety of machines are used in radiation therapy, depending on the type and extent of the tumor. These machines vary according to the energy produced and the ionizing particles delivered (Table 22–4). Linear accelerators are commonly used in cancer therapy (Fig. 22–4). The higher the energy produced by the machine, the greater the depth of penetration of the radiation beam. With higher energies, the maximum effect of the radiation occurs below the skin's surface and the dose to the skin is minimized; thus the term "skin-sparing effect." There is also less radiation scatter with higher energies (Fig. 22–5).

The number of treatments delivered during a course of radiation therapy depends on the type and extent of cancer, the area treated, and the dose. Because a single large dose of radiation is too toxic for normal tissues, the total radiation dose is divided into small daily doses or fractions to be given over a period of time. This

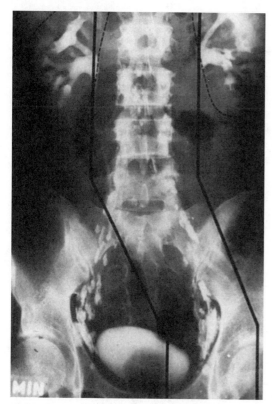

FIGURE 22–2 Simulation film. The radiation oncologist determines the treatment area using radiographic studies. The treatment area for this patient is the para-aortic and left inguinal lymph nodes. (Courtesy Virginia Mason Medical Center, Seattle, WA.)

density alloys, help minimize radiation exposure to normal tissues near the treatment area. Some treatment machines are equipped with a multileaf collimator to provide the blocking of the treatment rays to normal tissues. A compensating filter may also be used to differentially absorb the radiation beam to provide a uniform dose to the treatment volume. The treatment planning session usually lasts 1 to 2 hours. Patients who are in pain need to be appropriately medicated with analgesics prior to the localization procedure.

Advances in the planning of radiation therapy include the use of CT scans and MRI studies to three-dimensionally re-create the treatment volume. This process is sometimes referred to as a conformal treatment plan. With these specialized scans, the dose to the tumor volume can be more accurately calculated so as to maximize the dose to the tumor while minimizing the dose to normal surrounding tissues.[121]

Treatment Delivery

External radiation treatments are usually administered daily, Monday through Friday, for 2 to 8 weeks. Pallia-

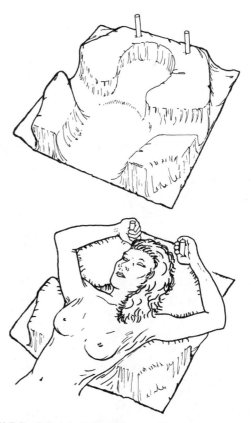

FIGURE 22–3 The Alpha-cradle helps a woman maintain the correct position for radiation therapy to the breast. Because the cradle is individually sized, the woman is able to conform to the exact position necessary for treatment.

Treatment Machines

Machine	Treatment Beam	
KILOVOLTAGE		
Mechanical	X-rays	Low-level energy; superficial treatment; scatter of radiation beam; intracavitary therapy
MEGAVOLTAGE		
Cobalt 60 radioactive source is in head of machine; replaced every 5–10 y because of decay of the isotope	γ-rays (1–4 MeV)	Deeper penetration than kilovoltage; below skin level; less scatter
SUPERVOLTAGE		
Linear accelerators	X-rays and electrons (4–35 MeV)	Less scatter; deep tumors
Betatron	Electrons	More DNA double-strand injury; less oxygen dependent; less cell-cycle specific
Cyclotron	Protons, neutrons, or electrons	

MeV, million electron volts; the energy of an electron accelerated across 1 million volts.

process is called *fractionation.* The dose is usually the same each day. Because fractionation allows normal cells to repair the sublethal damage after each treatment, more radiation can be delivered to the tumor while minimizing damage to normal tissues.[52] Fractionation also increases damage to the tumor because of reassortment of cells into radiosensitive phases of the cell cycle and an increased oxygenation in the tumor.[51] Large tumors usually contain cells that are far from a capillary network and as a result are hypoxic. As the tumor shrinks over time, oxygenation increases within the tumor as more cells have access to the capillary blood flow. As a result, the radiation's effectiveness is improved.

Some treatment schemes deliver treatments two to three times a day with at least 5 to 6 hours between each fraction. This is called *hyperfractionation.* Hyperfractionation may improve the treatment of large tumors, tumors with excessive bleeding, head and neck cancers, and brain tumors.[2, 54] The increased fractionation theoretically affects more mitotically active cells each day.

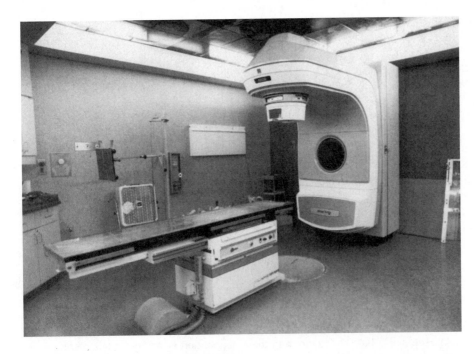

FIGURE 22–4 The linear accelerator delivers supervoltage treatment. (From Belcher AE: *Cancer nursing,* St. Louis, Mosby, 1992.)

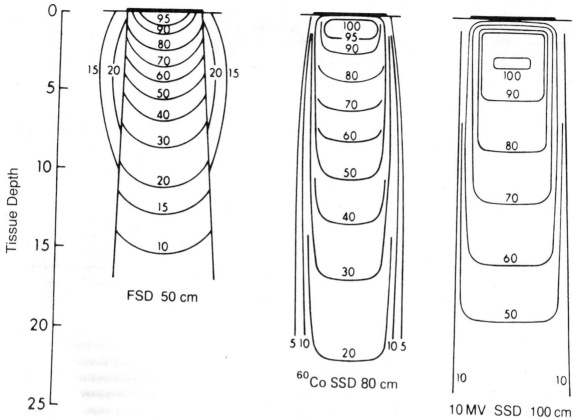

FIGURE 22–5 Isodose distributions (percentage of dose delivered) comparing increasing energies: kilovoltage (250 kVp), megavoltage (cobalt), and supervoltage (10 mV). *FSD* is the focal skin distance, or the distance from the focal spot in the x-ray tube to the patient's skin. *SSD* is the source-surface distance, or the distance from the front surface of the radiation source to the surface of the patient. As energy increases, the superficial tissues are spared, with the maximal radiation dose being delivered below the skin's surface; this results in fewer skin reactions and less sidescatter. (From Keller BE, Rubin P: Basic concepts of radiation physics. In Rubin P, editor: *Clinical oncology for medical students and physicians,* New York, American Cancer Society, 1983.)

The administration of radiation therapy depends on the reproducibility of the treatment setup. For most adults, teenagers and older children, this is easily accomplished. However, when working with young children and infants, special techniques are used to stabilize and sedate the patient to allow successful delivery of radiation therapy. "Body casts" can be created to immobilize the body or body part. However, these devices can cause even greater anxiety in a young child. Table 22–5 lists the medications commonly used for sedating young children for radiation therapy.[14] Chapter 19 further discusses issues in pediatric oncology nursing.

Total Body Irradiation

Leukemic cells are radiosensitive. In conjunction with bone marrow transplantation, supralethal radiation in the form of total body irradiation and chemotherapy are administered to reduce the tumor volume and provide immunosuppression to prevent the rejection of the marrow graft.[54] A variety of techniques provide a homogeneous dose of radiation to the entire body (Fig. 22–6). Doses range from 8 to 14 Gy, depending on fractionation. Acute side effects include nausea and vomiting, parotitis, anorexia, diarrhea, and fatigue. Effects such as stomatitis, pancytopenia, and interstitial pneumonitis occur during the weeks following total body irradiation. Delayed effects of total body irradiation include gonadal insufficiency and cataracts.[54]

INNOVATIONS IN RADIATION THERAPY

Intraoperative Radiation Therapy

Intraoperative radiation therapy (IORT) provides direct visualization and treatment of tumors to control

TABLE 22-5

Medications Commonly Used for Sedation during Radiation Therapy

Drug	Action	Dose Range	Route	Comments
Chloral hydrate	Sedative	50–100 mg/kg	Oral, rectal	Contraindicated with marked liver or kidney impairment May cause gastric irritation Bitter taste with oral preparation Minimal effect upon respiration No amnesic effect Maximum 2 g Especially useful with small infants Inexpensive
Pentobarbital	Sedative, hypnotic	2–6 mg/kg	Oral, rectal, IV	May cause cardiovascular depression and hypotension IM route not used because of local irritation IV administered as slow drip Not recommended for small infants
Fentanyl	Analgesic, amnesic	0.5 µg/kg every 2–3 min Max: 2 µg/kg	IM, IV	Rapid onset of action Short acting Administered as slow IV push May cause respiratory depression
Fentanyl	Analgesic, amnesic	1–2 µg/kg	IM, IV	Administered in combination with other drugs Respiratory effects may outlast amnesia
Midazolam	Sedative, tranquilizer	0.01 mg/kg every 3–5 min Max: 0.1 mg/kg	IM, IV	Severe, life-threatening cardiorespiratory effects can occur Partially reversible with naloxone
Meperidine*	Analgesic	2 mg/kg	IM, oral, rectal	Hypotension, respiratory depression and excessive sedation can occur
Promethazine*	Sedative	1 mg/kg	IM	No amnesic effect Administered as deep IM injection in single syringe
Chlorpromazine*	Sedative	1 mg/kg	IM	May titrate doses maintaining 2:1:1 ratio
Droperidol	Tranquilizer, sedative	0.12 mg/kg	IM, IV	Hypotension, orthostatic hypotension Fluids and measures to manage hypotension should be readily available Safe use in children under 2 years of age not established

IM, Intramuscular; IV, intravenous.

* Maximum doses: meperidine, 50 mg; promethazine, 25 mg; chlorpromazine, 25 mg

From Bucholtz JD: Issues concerning the sedation of children for radiation therapy, Oncol Nurs Forum 19:649, 1992.

local recurrence of cancer.[17] After surgical exposure, a targeting cone is placed directly on the tumor site. This cone helps to displace normal tissues and thus minimize toxicities. The treatment machine is carefully aligned with the cone. All persons leave the treatment room for the 15 to 25 minutes it takes to deliver the fairly large dose of electron irradiation (approximately 2000 cGy). Anesthesia personnel monitor the patient through a closed-circuit television.

Techniques using high-dose rate (HDR) remote afterloading equipment to deliver intraoperative radiation are also used.[48, 49] A dedicated and shielded surgical

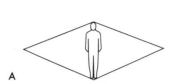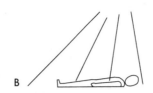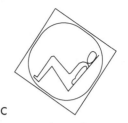

FIGURE 22–6 Methods of delivering total body irradiation. **A,** Lateral opposed beams. **B,** Supine and prone technique using three matching fields. **C,** Horizontal shrinking field technique: patient is in sitting position. (Adapted from Quast U: Total body irradiation, *Radiother Oncol* 9:95, 1987, with permission from Elsevier Science, and from Novack DH, Kiley JP: Total body irradiation, *Front Radiat Ther Oncol* 21:69, 1987, with permission from Karger, Basel.)

suite with HDR remote afterloading equipment is needed to perform the surgery and to deliver the HDR brachytherapy. This setup improves the convenience of providing IORT by avoiding the need to transport the patient from the surgical suite to the radiation therapy department, thus saving time, energy, and expense.

Intraoperative radiation is used to treat locally advanced abdominal cancers such as gastric, pancreatic, colorectal, bladder, cervical, and retroperitoneal sarcomas. Complications and side effects, no greater than with radiation therapy or surgery, may include nausea, vomiting, and anorexia.[44, 47] No increased risk for poor wound healing or postoperative infection has been reported, and severe complications, such as neuropathy, have been few.[22, 84, 107] Coordination between departments and disciplines is required to provide this complex therapy.[17, 47]

Radiosensitizers

Chemical radiosensitizing compounds are used to increase the lethal effects of radiation therapy in the treatment of gastrointestinal and bladder cancers.[83, 94] Nonhypoxic sensitizers such as iododeoxyuridine (IUdR) incorporate into the DNA and increase the susceptibility of the cell to radiation damage. Hypoxic cell sensitizers such as nitroimidazoles increase oxygen to hypoxic cells and promote damage of the DNA, preventing cell repair. Depending on the agent, side effects include peripheral neuropathy, nausea and vomiting, and skin rashes. The use of gadolinium texaphyrin is currently being investigated for its use with cancers in the thorax, brain, pelvis, bone, and soft tissues, and sites of lymph node metastases.[103] Certain chemotherapeutic agents, such as cyclophosphamide or cisplatin, are also being used not only for their cytotoxic effects but also as radiosensitizers and are given concurrently with radiation therapy.

Stereotactic External-Beam Irradiation

Stereotactic external-beam irradiation involves high-dose treatment of relatively small intracranial volumes with a three-dimensional distribution of the treatment beam.[70] This technique minimizes the radiation dose to normal tissues. Benign conditions, such as arteriovenous malformations, and malignancies, such as astrocytomas and brain metastases, are treated with stereotactic external-beam irradiation. Various machines are used, such as gamma units using cobalt ("gamma knife") and modified cobalt or linear accelerator units. Figure 22–7 depicts a gamma knife stereotactic radiation therapy unit. The treatment dose may be fractionated or given in a single fraction. Steroid medications are used to minimize cerebral edema. The concept of stereotactic radiation therapy is also being used for other applications where treatment of a small tissue volume within the body is desired.[9, 21, 78]

Radiopharmaceuticals

Strontium 89 and samarium 153 are radiopharmaceuticals with proven efficacy for treating pain from multiple osteoblastic bony metastases from prostate, lung, or breast cancer.[11, 97, 100] Pain relief may be noted within 1 to 2 weeks, or this relief may be delayed for up to 5 weeks; pain relief may last for several months. Repeated doses of radiopharmaceuticals may be given at the physician's discretion approximately every 2 to 3 months. However, toxicities such as myelosuppression increase. Radiopharmaceuticals may also be used in conjunction with external-beam radiation therapy.[5]

Strontium 89 (4 mCi) or samarium 153 (1 mCi/kg) is delivered intravenously to the patient in the outpatient setting. The radiopharmaceutical seeks out areas of bone metastases and provides radiation to the bony metastatic site. After administration of the radiopharmaceutical, assessment of pain and the use of analgesics are important. Consistently using a pain analog scale (e.g., asking the patient to rate the level of pain from 0 to 10) and reviewing the record of pharmacologic and nonpharmacologic methods of pain relief, the nurse monitors the efficacy of the radiopharmaceutical and teaches the patient and family ways to improve pain control.

Common side effects of radiopharmaceuticals include a temporary "flare" reaction of pain, which occurs

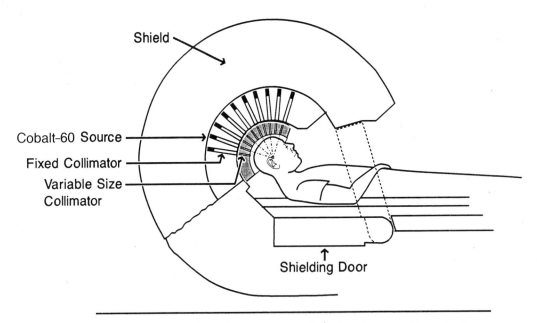

FIGURE 22–7 Gamma knife stereotactic radiation therapy unit. (From Alexander E: *Stereotactic radiosurgery,* New York, McGraw-Hill, 1993. Reproduced with permission of The McGraw-Hill Companies.)

approximately 3 to 5 days after administration of the radiopharmaceutical and lasts approximately 5 days, and myelosuppression. Because very little radiation is distributed outside of bone, the patient does not pose a risk of radiation exposure to others and contact with others is not limited. However, because radiopharmaceuticals are administered systemically, radioactive precautions for body fluids are necessary for approximately 7 days after administration. Patients and families must be taught these precautions (Box 22–1). Patients who are incontinent of urine may require a Foley catheter (or condom catheter for men) to control radioactive contamination of the household.

Patients should be advised that a flare reaction of pain may occur. They are instructed to continue taking pre-scribed analgesics and even increase the dose of medications as necessary during the time of the flare reaction. After administration of radiopharmaceuticals, complete blood counts are monitored every 2 to 3 weeks for approximately 8 to 12 weeks to monitor myelosuppression.

PHOTODYNAMIC THERAPY

Photodynamic therapy (PDT) involves the use of light-sensitive molecules, or photosensitizers, which are activated by light to form oxygen radicals, which in turn affect cell membranes, the cytoplasm, and the DNA, resulting in cell damage and death.[7, 72] Porfimer sodium is the most studied photosensitizer. Approximately 48 hours after administration of the photosensitizer, laser treatment with the appropriate wavelength is given. It takes approximately 48 hours for the tumor to reach the optimal concentration of porfimer sodium. Cutaneous photosensitivity can occur and can last for 6 to 8 weeks. PDT is used in the treatment of superficial bladder, skin, lung, esophageal, and superficial head and neck cancers; and for bone marrow purging for the treatment of leukemias and lymphomas. Patients and families are instructed on the extreme photosensitivity and the required precautions to prevent significant damage to the skin from sunlight and other sources of intense light such as examination lights.[7, 72, 77, 88]

INTERNAL RADIATION THERAPY

Brachytherapy

Radioactive implants deliver relatively large amounts of radiation to a specific site over a short time.[33] Tumors

---

BOX 22–1

Patient and Family Precautions with Radiopharmaceuticals

1. Flush toilet twice after use.
2. Wipe up spilled urine with a paper tissue and discard in the toilet before flushing.
3. Wash hands after using the toilet.
4. Immediately wash linen and clothes that become soiled with urine or blood. Wash these items separately from other laundry.
5. If an injury occurs and blood is spilled, wash away any spilled blood with water and a paper tissue and flush the paper tissue in the toilet.

TABLE 22-6
Cancers Treated with Brachytherapy

Cancer	Technique	Radioactive Source
Endometrial	Intracavitary	Radium, cesium
Cervical	Intracavitary	Radium, cesium
Prostate	Interstitial	Iodine, gold
Breast	Interstitial	Iridium
Ocular melanoma	Plaque therapy	Cobalt, iodine, palladium
Head and neck	Interstitial thermal	Iridium, cesium
Rectal	Interstitial	Cesium
Esophageal	Intraluminal	Cesium
Bronchogenic	Endobronchial	Iridium, iodine

From Dunne-Daly C: Principles of brachytherapy. In Dow KH and others, editors: Nursing care in radiation oncology, ed 2, Philadelphia, Saunders, 1997.

may be treated with an implant alone or after a course of radiation therapy to provide a boost of radiation to the tumor.[123] Cancers of the brain, tongue, lips, esophagus, lung, breast, vagina, cervix, endometrium, rectum, prostate, and bladder may be treated with brachytherapy. Table 22–6 lists the types of cancers treated with brachytherapy. Implants can be placed temporarily within the body cavity or structure with specifically designed applicators (Fig. 22–8). Because the radioactive material, ribbons, wires, seeds, capsules, needles, or tubes are encapsulated (sealed), body fluids are not contaminated. The radioactive isotopes are usually placed in the body with an afterloading technique of placing the applicators (needles, plastic or metal tubes) in the body in the operating room or under fluoroscopy. The applicators are sutured in or near the tumor. After the patient returns to the hospital room, the radioactive isotopes are then placed within the applicators. With this procedure, exposure of staff members to radiation is minimized. The implant then remains in the body for the prescribed length of time.

Intracavitary placement of implants within the vagina or uterus is performed using general or spinal anesthesia.[33] The vagina is packed with gauze to stabilize the applicator and separate the bladder and rectum from the radioactive source. Patients usually have a bowel cleansing before the applicator placement and are placed on a low-residue diet and diphenoxylate atropine to prevent a bowel movement while the implant is in place. Postoperative pain is managed with oral or parenteral medications.

With cervical and vaginal implants, the patient may experience fatigue and dysuria after implantation. Women may resume sexual intercourse within 2 to 3 weeks after implantation as tolerated.[33] Because a decrease in normal vaginal secretions may occur, use of a

water-based lubricant is recommended. Vaginal stenosis can also occur. Routine vaginal dilation is recommended to maintain the integrity of the vaginal walls.

Interstitial radioactive implants with needles, wires, seeds, or catheters are placed directly into the tissues. These implants may be temporary or permanent. Head and neck cancers are commonly treated with temporary interstitial implants. Goals of nursing care include minimizing airway obstruction and instructing the patient to perform oral care with saline irrigation every 3 to 4 hours. Nasogastric tube feedings are used to provide a high-protein, high-calorie liquid diet. Because talking is difficult and should be avoided, the patient communicates with a writing pad or specially created flash cards. With head and neck implants, the patient is permitted to get out of bed but must remain in the hospital room. Elevating the head of bed to 30 to 45 degrees will help minimize tissue swelling and aspiration of oral secretions.

Temporary interstitial implants of the breast are sometimes used. This implant is performed approximately 2 weeks after a course of external-beam radiation therapy to provide a higher dose of radiation to the site of tumor excision. Catheters are placed in the area where the tumor was excised using general anesthesia. The radioactive sources are then placed within the catheters once the woman returns to her hospital room.

In some instances permanent low-level radioactive implants may be placed percutaneously or intraoperatively in or near tumor masses such as in the head and neck region and chest. Because the level of radioactivity is low, radiation precautions are usually not required.

Permanent interstitial implants with radioactive iodine seeds are placed percutaneously with transrectal ultrasound guidance within the prostate gland to treat early stage prostate cancer.[43, 95] The radioactive source has a short half-life, and the patient's body tissues effectively shield any radiation. Patients are instructed to filter urine for radioactive seeds that may pass through the urine, to use condoms when having sexual intercourse, and to avoid close contact with pregnant women and children while the radioactive source decays. Patients are monitored for side effects such as cystitis, which is managed with the use of α-blocker medications, nonsteroidal medications, and analgesics.

Radioactive isotopes that deliver a high dose rate of radiation to a limited volume of tissue allow site-specific treatments over a shorter period.[33] Treatments can be delivered within a few hours and can be done in the outpatient setting. Use of a remote afterloading brachytherapy device reduces staff exposure to the high-dose isotopes used during therapy.[66] If the patient requires direct care, the sources can be momentarily removed

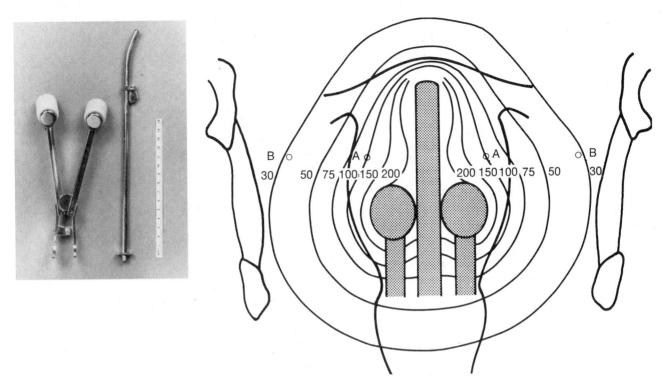

FIGURE 22–8 The Fletcher-Suit applicator is one of many kinds of applicators used to deliver intracavitary irradiation for carcinomas of the cervix and endometrium. The long central tandem is placed in the uterine cavity. (To the right is a section of tubing used to hold the radioactive sources and place them in the hollow tandem.) The movable sleeve on the tandem marks the cervical os, permitting localization of the os on x-ray film as a reference point for computerized dosimetry. The colpostats are placed in the lateral fornices. The entire apparatus is held in place with vaginal packing. After the applicator is in place, x-ray films are taken to confirm the accuracy of placement. Computerized dosimetry is then done to determine the best loading pattern and the time required for treatment. Finally, the radium or cesium sources are put into place. (Photograph courtesy Virginia Mason Medical Center, Seattle, WA; drawing from DiSaia P, Creasman W: *Clinical gynecological oncology,* ed 4, St. Louis, Mosby, 1993.)

through the applicators by remote control before nurses enter the room to assist the patient.

Educating patients about the implant, the process, its effects, and how to manage those effects is crucial.[10, 65] Brandt studied the informational needs of 22 patients receiving brachytherapy and found that most patients desired the maximum information about their illness.[10] Table 22–7 lists those items patients identified as important to know before implantation and following implantation.

Nonsealed Radioactive Therapy

When radioactive isotopes are injected intravenously or taken orally (nonsealed sources), the patient and the body secretions may be radioactive and nursing care must follow specific radiation safety precautions.[33] Depending on the isotope used, the patient usually must be isolated because of radioactivity for approximately

3 to 4 days. The amount of radioactivity emitted is carefully monitored during the patient's hospitalization. Table 22–8 lists the different radioactive isotopes used in cancer therapy.

TABLE 22–7

Important Information about Radioactive Implants as Identified by Patients

BEFORE IMPLANT

Symptom management
Activity restrictions while the implant is in place
Causes of their current symptoms
How the implant could affect those symptoms

AFTER IMPLANT

When to call the doctor
Potential side effects of treatment
How to manage those side effects

Data from reference 10.

T A B L E   2 2 – 8
Radioisotopes and Their Properties

Radioisotope	Symbols	Half-Life	Type
Cesium 137	^{137}Cs	30 y	Beta, gamma
Gold 198	^{198}Au	2.7 d	Beta, gamma
Iodine 125	^{125}I	60 d	Beta, gamma
Iodine 131	^{131}I	8 d	Beta, gamma
Iridium 192	^{192}Ir	74.4 d	Beta, gamma
Phosphorus 32	^{32}P	14.3 d	Beta
Radium 226	^{226}Ra	1620 y	Alpha, gamma
Strontium 90	^{90}Sr	28.1 y	Beta

From National Council on Radiation Protection and Measurements: Report #40, Protection against radiation from brachytherapy sources, Bethesda, MD, 1972.

Nursing Management

Understanding the principles of radiobiology is the key to understanding symptom management. The side effects associated with radiation therapy are localized and depend on the area treated, volume of tissue irradiated, fractionation, total dose, type of radiation, and individual differences. Variations of side effects will be observed among people receiving similar courses of treatment. A delay between the time of radiation exposure and the time the effects are seen can vary from days to weeks to months, depending on the cell's metabolic activity. Early reactions occur during or within weeks after treatment. Some symptoms do not subside until 2 or more weeks after treatment has ended. Delayed reactions occur months to years after therapy. Because radiation therapy has its greatest effect on rapidly dividing cells, the epithelial tissues, such as mucous membranes and the skin, are most susceptible to its effects. Selected nursing diagnoses related to radiation therapy include:

Nursing Diagnoses

- *Impaired skin integrity related to radiation therapy*
- *Risk for infection related to skin breakdown*
- *Activity intolerance related to radiation therapy*
- *Altered nutrition: less than body requirements, related to anorexia*
- *Altered oral mucous membrane related to head and neck irradiation*
- *Sensory/perceptual alterations: gustatory, related to head and neck irradiation*
- *Impaired swallowing related to pharyngitis or esophagitis*
- *Pain related to cough*
- *Altered nutrition: less than body requirements, related to nausea and vomiting*
- *Diarrhea related to pelvic irradiation*
- *Sexual dysfunction related to effects of pelvic irradiation*
- *Altered urinary elimination related to pelvic irradiation*
- *Ineffective individual coping related to alopecia*
- *Self-esteem disturbance related to alopecia*
- *Anxiety about radiation therapy*
- *Knowledge deficit about radiation therapy and self-care measures*

Outcome Goals

Patient or significant other will be able to:

- Maintain or restore skin integrity.
- Prevent skin breakdown and infection.
- Minimize fatigue and maintain activities of daily living.
- Maintain nutritional status and weight.
- Maintain integrity of oral mucous membranes.
- Control pain from pharyngitis/esophagitis and maintain nutritional intake.
- Minimize cough.
- Prevent or control nausea and vomiting and maintain nutritional status.
- Prevent or control diarrhea.
- Minimize cystitis.
- Maintain sexual functioning as desired.
- Successfully cope with alopecia.
- Control or minimize anxiety.

• Understand the use of radiation therapy for cancer and the self-care behaviors used to manage side effects of radiation therapy.

GENERAL SIDE EFFECTS

Skin

Certain skin reactions are normal and expected with radiation therapy.[114] The skin overlying the areas being treated may develop a reaction as soon as 2 weeks into the course of treatment.[114, 116, 122] Skin erythema may range from mild, light pink to deep and dusky red. Increased skin sensitivity and slight edema may also appear. As treatment continues, the skin reaction can progress, with the skin becoming slightly to moderately dry, itchy, and flaky (dry desquamation). In some cases the skin develops mild to severe moist desquamation, in which the epidermal layers of the skin slough, leaving a raw, painful area that may drain serous exudate. Areas of moist desquamation generally heal within several weeks.[114, 116]

Skin reactions vary but tend to be greater in those receiving large doses of radiation.[114] Also, treatments with electron beams usually produce more intense skin reactions because of the superficial concentration of the radiation dose. Some treatments involve the use of a bolus material placed on the skin to increase the surface dose. In addition, certain treatments are given from a tangential angle as opposed to perpendicular to the treatment site. These techniques can increase the skin reaction.[114] Certain areas of the skin, such as areas covering bony prominences or surgical wounds, tend to be more sensitive to the effects of radiation than others.[50] Areas having skin folds (e.g., the axillae, under the breasts, perineum, groin, gluteal folds) are also at increased risk for developing a skin reaction because of increased warmth and moisture and lack of aeration.[114, 116, 117] The skin on the face is particularly sensitive to the effects of radiation. Skin reactions may also occur where the radiation beams exit, that is, on the opposite side of the body from where the treatment is delivered. Evaluating the angle of the treatment beam will help determine where these reactions may occur. When chemotherapy is used in conjunction with radiation therapy, the patient is at higher risk of developing a skin reaction.[85]

Special consideration needs to be given to patients receiving pelvic irradiation after low anterior or anterior-posterior resection for rectal cancer. The surgical wound site is at increased risk for skin breakdown because the perineum is generally within the treatment field. The radiation oncologist may have the buttocks taped apart during the actual radiation treatment to minimize the skin reaction.[50] If a stoma (e.g., colostomy, ileostomy) is included in the treatment field, the stoma appliance and skin barrier can act as a bolus material and enhance the skin reaction. Daily assessments of the skin are necessary, and removal of the skin barrier and appliance may be required during the actual treatment to minimize peristomal skin breakdown.

Before beginning radiation therapy, instruct the patient to protect the skin and minimize sources of irritation and trauma. Nursing diagnoses related to skin care include *Actual or risk for impaired skin integrity* and *Risk for infection related to skin breakdown.* Assess the patient's usual skin care. Unintentional enhancement of skin reactions may occur if patients use skin lotions or ointments contraindicated during radiation therapy. Plan to educate the patient and family about skin care during radiation therapy. Cleanse the skin with lukewarm water as needed, and pat rather than rub the skin with a towel to dry. Avoid using soaps. When soap is necessary, use only nondeodorant, nonperfumed soaps. Powders, perfumes, and deodorants should not be applied to the irradiated skin, because they can dry and irritate the skin. Avoid the use of cornstarch in the axilla, groin, and gluteal folds.[114, 116, 117] Shaving with a razor blade within treatment areas should be avoided. An electric razor may be used if there is no skin irritation. Protect the treated skin from cold, heat, and sun. Only loose-fitting, cotton clothing should be worn close to the skin. Tight, restrictive clothing, such as bras and belts, over the treated area may chafe the skin and should not be worn. In addition, avoid placing adhesive tape over the irradiated skin, because this will further irritate the skin.

If the skin becomes dry, the patient may complain of tenderness and pruritus. A nonperfumed hydrophilic moisturizing lotion that contains no heavy metal ions may be applied to the skin on the recommendation of the radiation oncologist or radiation oncology nurse. Avoid having lotion on the skin during treatment because the lotion may increase the skin reaction. Remove excess lotion with a soft washcloth before treatment. Although topical steroids can help reduce pruritus and tenderness because of vasoconstriction, they must be used with extreme caution. Steroid creams and ointments can cause thinning of the skin and delay skin healing.[50] Fluorinated preparations are not recommended because they cause more vasoconstriction and thinning of the skin. Steroid preparations should not be used for moist skin reactions.[114, 116]

For moist desquamation, normal saline irrigations or cool compresses may be applied to the affected area three to four times a day to soothe the skin.

Cleansing with half-strength to third-strength hydrogen peroxide and saline followed by a rinse with saline may be used also.[114, 122] Caution with use of ointments and salves is important to avoid increasing the skin reaction. A thin layer of A&D ointment, lanolin, or Aquaphor may be applied to the moist desquamation. In some instances, treatment is stopped and zinc oxide or silver sulfadiazine cream is applied directly on the skin or onto a nonadherent dressing (Telfa pad or combine dressings), which is then applied to the moist reaction. Hydrogel and hydrocolloid dressings have been found effective to heal dermatitis and moist desquamation.[101] These dressings may be left on the skin reaction for up to 5 days to provide comfort. No increase in infection rates has been reported. Assess for signs of infection, and culture suspicious lesions and drainage. With painful skin reactions, systemic analgesics are sometimes necessary, especially at bedtime, to allow the patient to rest.

If moist desquamation occurs in the perineum, sitz baths, perineal compresses, and protective emollients may all be used. A hand-held blow dryer may be used on the cool setting to dry the perineum. These reactions are painful, and treatment is frequently stopped for a time to allow the tissues to heal. Use of analgesics is usually recommended.

Once radiation therapy is completed, the skin usually heals within a few weeks. Although the acute tenderness and erythema diminish within 2 weeks, the patient may be left with a tanned skin within the treatment field, which will usually subside. The irradiated skin may also remain more sensitive to heat or cold and damage more readily than untreated parts of the body.[114] The patient should continue to protect the irradiated skin by avoiding direct sun exposure by using clothing such as scarves and hats. A sunscreen with a high sun protection factor (SPF) should be used when sun exposure is unavoidable. Delayed effects to the skin from radiation include fibrosis and atrophy of the skin, telangiectasia, and lymphedema as a result of fibrosis of the lymph glands.[114] These delayed effects occur because of changes in the vascular component of the skin, which lead to tissue damage. Recall phenomenon occurs months to years after a course of radiation therapy. In this phenomenon, skin, mucous membrane, or pulmonary reactions occur within the treated area when certain chemotherapeutic agents, such as dactinomycin and doxorubicin, are given systemically. These reactions, which may be more severe than the skin reactions seen during radiation therapy, subside within 2 weeks.[3] Evaluate the patient's and family's understanding of potential and actual skin reactions and appropriate care and protection of the skin. The table below summarizes guidelines for skin care.

Fatigue

Fatigue, the subjective feeling of tiredness, is a significant symptom experienced by many people receiving radiation therapy.[86, 90, 114] The etiology of fatigue is

Nursing Care of Irradiated Skin

When treatment begins:	Assess skin integrity. Instruct patient to minimize trauma and protect skin within treatment field: Cleanse skin with lukewarm water as needed. Avoid use of soaps, powders, perfumes, and deodorants. Avoid shaving. Protect skin from cold, heat, and sun. Wear loose-fitting clothing over treatment site. Avoid adhesive tape on irradiated skin.
If dry desquamation occurs:	Use a hydrophilic moisturizing lotion or ointment two to three times a day (e.g., Aquaphor). Remove excess ointment from skin before daily treatment.
If moist desquamation occurs:	Saline irrigations or cool compresses may be used three to four times a day. Apply hydrogel dressing for comfort (e.g., Vigilon dressing). If treatment is withheld, zinc oxide or silver sulfadiazine may be applied to skin reaction and covered with a nonadherent dressing. Culture suspicious lesions and drainage. Use analgesics as necessary.
When treatment is completed and skin is healed:	Instruct patient to protect irradiated skin by avoiding exposure to sun, heat, or cold. Advise patient to use sunblock when sun exposure is unavoidable.

not well understood.[114] Fatigue may result from tumor breakdown, which releases by-products into the bloodstream. Another theory suggests an increased basal metabolic rate, which quickly uses the body's energy stores. Fatigue may occur after treatment each day and become chronic as treatment continues.[114, 123] In general, there is a gradual increase of fatigue over the period of radiation therapy, which then gradually decreases once treatment is completed. Variations, including less fatigue on Sundays because there is no treatment over the weekend, have been reported by patients. Fatigue is compounded by other symptoms such as pain, depression, anorexia, infection, anemia, and dyspnea. Although the level of fatigue varies among individuals, most people are able to continue their work and usual activities. Fatigue may persist weeks to months after completion of radiation therapy and disappear gradually.[114] In a study by Longman and colleagues,[75] fatigue was reported to be the most frequent and problematic side effect occurring over time in women receiving treatment for breast cancer. When radiation therapy is combined with other cancer therapies, the incidence of fatigue is increased. Woo and colleagues[130] found that women who received combination therapy for breast cancer experienced significantly more fatigue than women who received radiation therapy alone.

Nursing diagnoses of *Actual or risk for activity intolerance* can be made for the person receiving radiation therapy. Assess for the presence and pattern of fatigue. Evaluate factors that increase or decrease fatigue. Monitor blood counts for anemia, which can compound fatigue (see table below).

Assist patients and families to understand that fatigue can occur with radiation therapy. Help patients evaluate their activities so they can pace themselves throughout the day and plan for rest periods or naps as needed. Determining the times of the day when extra energy is needed can help a person plan rest periods through the day and evening. Taking a nap immediately after returning home from treatment helps some patients to have energy for the rest of the day. Plan for assistance with transportation, purchase and preparation of food, child care, and other activities of daily living. Evaluate the need for assistive devices, such as a cane or walker. These measures can help minimize exertion with certain activities and reduce fatigue. Regular mild aerobic exercises may actually be beneficial in improving well-being during radiation therapy. A walking exercise program during radiation therapy for women with breast cancer resulted in higher levels of physical functioning and lower levels of symptom intensity in the experimental group than in the women who did not participate in the program.[80] The walking exercise program consisted of an individualized, self-paced, home-based walking exercise program that the women participated in throughout the treatment period.

If the patient is experiencing pain, ensure adequate pain management with pharmacologic and nonpharmacologic measures. In addition, ensure that the person is maintaining an adequate nutritional intake. People with recent weight loss who are undergoing therapy will need additional nutritional supplementation. This supplementation will help the patient maintain or improve nutritional status and minimize fa-

Guidelines for Frequency of Blood Counts—Joint Center for Radiation Therapy

Site	No Prior Chemotherapy	Previous Chemotherapy <1 y	Previous Chemotherapy >1 y	Concomitant Chemotherapy
Breast	Baseline, 3 wk later if taking tamoxifen	Weekly—every other week	Every 3 wk	Biweekly—weekly
Head/neck	Every 3 wk	Every other week	Every 3 wk	Biweekly—weekly
Whole brain	Baseline only	Weekly	Every 3 wk	Weekly
Hodgkin's	Weekly	Weekly	Weekly	Biweekly
Lung/esophagus*	Weekly—every other week	Weekly—every other week	Weekly	Biweekly—weekly
Spine†	Weekly—every other week	Weekly	Weekly	Biweekly—weekly
Pelvis* Prostate	Every other week	Every other week	Weekly—every other week	Weekly
Colon	Every other week	Weekly	Weekly	Biweekly—weekly
GYN	Every other week	Weekly	Weekly	Biweekly—weekly

*Depends on field size, history of previous irradiation.

†Depends on the presence and extent of metastatic disease.

From Hirshfield-Bartek J and others: Monitoring the myelosuppressive effects of radiation therapy, Oncol Nurs Forum 15:547, 1988.

tigue. A dietitian is an excellent resource to help plan the patient's nutritional program. Evaluate the patient's and family's understanding of the causes of fatigue and their ability to modify activities to maintain or improve function (see Chapter 27).

Anorexia

Loss of appetite, or anorexia, sometimes is a result of cancer itself but also may be caused by cancer therapy. As with fatigue, the mechanisms that cause anorexia are unclear. Contributing factors include inactivity, medications, and inability to ingest and digest foods. The patient has a loss of appetite, which can result in weight loss and progressive fatigue.

Assess the loss of appetite in patients receiving radiation therapy. The nursing diagnosis *Altered nutrition: less than body requirements* is made for the person with anorexia. Discuss with the patient and family the fact that anorexia sometimes occurs in people undergoing radiation therapy, and suggest ways to overcome this problem. Assist the patient and family to plan ways to improve appetite to help the patient eat adequately and maintain body weight.

Frequent small meals rather than three large ones can help make eating less overwhelming and allow more food to be consumed throughout the day. Instruct the patient and family to have high-calorie, high-protein foods readily available at all times. Specially prepared nutritional supplements and carefully selected convenience foods can provide additional calories and protein. Because radiation treatments are given daily and considerable time is spent commuting to and from treatments, suggest that the patient carry snacks to consume during the commute. Some patients have found that having a meal at a restaurant each day is a special treat to look forward to. In addition, the use of an appetite stimulant such as megestrol acetate (400–800 mg/d) can be beneficial in improving appetite and nonfluid weight gain.[76, 87] Consult a dietitian to determine the nutritional needs of the patient, and plan additional ways to meet those needs. Help the patient and family understand the importance of nutrition during therapy. Evaluate their ability to use suggestions to enhance appetite and maintain optimal nutrition (see Chapter 29).

Bone Marrow Suppression

When large volumes of active bone marrow are treated with radiation, a decrease in bone marrow function occurs. These treatment areas include the pelvis, spine, sternum, ribs, metaphyses of long bones, and skull. Blood counts must be monitored routinely. The fall in blood counts usually develops slowly. However, if chemotherapy is combined with radiation therapy, the blood counts can fall precipitously and must be closely followed. See page 620 for guidelines for frequency of blood counts. Factors affecting the frequency of obtaining blood counts include the treatment site, use of other myelosuppressive therapies, the stage of disease, and the patient's age.

Assess for infections, bleeding, and fatigue. Plan and implement education for the patient and family about precautions for neutropenia, thrombocytopenia, and anemia. Transfusions of blood products are sometimes used and patients receiving combined modality therapy may receive colony-stimulating factors to minimize neutropenia. In some cases radiation therapy is withheld for a period of time to allow the blood counts to recover. Evaluate the patient's and family's understanding and use of self-care measures and precautions for bone marrow suppression (see Chapter 31).

SITE-SPECIFIC SIDE EFFECTS

Head and Neck

Treatment of head and neck cancers frequently involves combined modality therapy with surgery, radiation therapy, and chemotherapy.[30, 73] Significant toxicities can occur during treatment resulting in decreases in quality of life and functional ability. Although most acute side effects resolve following completion of therapy, chronic problems with xerostomia, taste changes, swallowing, hoarseness, and mouth pain may develop.[73] The potential need for enteral feeding by a feeding tube should be discussed with the patient and family. In some instances when patients are nutritionally compromised before the initiation of therapy, the feeding tube is placed before treatment starts to begin nutritional repletion. Radiation therapy is given to the head and neck regions for cancers of the mouth, tongue, and larynx. Some problems that develop are stomatitis, xerostomia, dental caries, taste changes, osteoradionecrosis, and hypopituitarism.[131]

Stomatitis. Stomatitis, or irritation of the mucosa in the mouth and oropharynx, can occur as the radiation affects the rapidly dividing cells of the oral mucosa. The patient may first note a tenderness in the mouth. This tenderness may be accompanied by mild to moderate erythema and edema of the mucosa. A whitish pseudomembrane may form on the surface of the mucosa; this membrane should be left undisturbed. Eventually this membrane pulls away from the underlying tissue, leaving a painful and friable ulcer. Bleeding often results when stomatitis is severe. Superimposed bacterial, fungal, and viral infections can also occur. The mucosal reaction may be enhanced by metallic tooth restorations in adjacent areas, which cause electron backscatter of radiation. During treatments, a material with a low atomic number, such as a piece of gauze or an oral stent made of dental acrylic, sometimes is placed between the tooth and mucosa to minimize this reaction.[64, 68]

Mouth care is crucial for the person receiving radiation therapy for head and neck cancer. Frequent cleansing of the mouth is important to protect the mucosa from irritants and prevent infections.[36] Tooth brushing and flossing, if tolerated, after meals and at bedtime will help remove debris from the teeth and gingiva. If tooth brushing becomes too painful, warm saline rinses and gentle swabbing with moistened gauze or a tooth sponge may be better tolerated. Instruct the patient and family in mouth care, including inspecting the oral cavity each day. Poorly fitting dental prostheses should not be worn until evaluated by a dentist; nor should the prosthesis be used when the mouth and gingiva become painful, because the prosthesis can cause more irritation and lead to mucosal breakdown. Oral pain is controlled with topical anesthetics or systemic analgesics. Mixtures containing viscous lidocaine, diphenhydramine, and Mylanta provide topical pain relief. Nonsteroidal anti-inflammatory drugs (NSAIDs) provide pain relief through anti-inflammatory action. In addition, sucralfate mouth rinses can coat ulcerations, reduce pain, and promote healing of oral tissues.[124] The use of biologic response modifiers such as recombinant human granulocyte-macrophage colony-stimulating factor to reduce radiation-induced mucositis by increasing the immune response in being investigated.[119, 127]

Instruct the patient to eat a soft, bland diet to make chewing and swallowing easier, allowing the patient to maintain nutritional intake.[82] For patients experiencing significant dysphagia, enteral feedings via a nasogastric or percutaneous endoscopic gastrostomy (PEG) tube should be implemented to maintain and improve the patient's nutritional status.[39] Topical thrombin can be applied to control minor areas of bleeding in the mouth and topical or systemic antibiotics are used to control oral infections.[93]

Xerostomia. Xerostomia, or dryness of the mouth, may occur 1 to 2 weeks into therapy and profoundly affects quality of life in patients.[60] When the treatment field includes the salivary glands, the saliva changes from a thin fluid to a thick, sticky, acidic one that is unable to cleanse the mouth. As a result, debris adheres more readily to the teeth and gingiva. The patient may note difficulty speaking, problems with retention of dentures, and difficulty eating certain foods such as crackers, breads, and peanut butter.[59]

With higher doses of radiation, xerostomia may remain a chronic problem. Older patients are at higher risk for xerostomia because of normally decreased levels of oral secretions.

Patient and family education is crucial to manage xerostomia and promote patient comfort.[60] Instruct the patient to perform mouth care before meals to help relieve xerostomia. Assist the patient and family to assess food choices and preparation to appropriately modify the patient's diet. Sauces, gravies, and other liquids taken with meals can moisten dry and thick foods. Frequent sips of fluids and atomizer mists are helpful. Sucking on sugarless sour candies can help stimulate salivation. Commercially available saliva substitutes such as Moi-Stir, Oralbalance, and Mouth Kote provide temporary relief of xerostomia. Two to three milliliters of solution is placed in the mouth and swished to coat the mucosal surfaces. Products containing lemon or glycerin should be avoided because these may cause further irritation and drying of the mucosa.[126, 129] Lemon juice also decalcifies teeth.[129] Commercial mouthwashes should be avoided because many contain alcohol and flavoring agents that further irritate the mucosa. Patients may find a room humidifier used at bedtime helps decrease mucosal dryness and minimize the frequency with which they awaken to drink fluids. In addition, some patients find that swishing a teaspoon of vegetable oil in the mouth at bedtime helps to provide lubrication and also prevents mouth dryness through the night.

At the completion of radiation therapy, oral pilocarpine, 5 mg three to four times a day may be used to help stimulate saliva production.[60, 99] The primary side effect associated with pilocarpine use is transient flushing and perspiration occurring within 30 minutes of taking the medication. The use of the radioprotectant amifostine has demonstrated protective benefits for salivary gland function with reduced chronic xerostomia without protecting the cancer.[18, 24, 109, 110] Amifostine is administered intravenously daily within 30 minutes prior to radiation therapy. The dose of 200 mg/m^2 is associated with minimal hypotension, but patients require hydration and antiemetics.

Tooth Decay and Caries. Tooth decay and caries become rampant as a result of xerostomia. Cariogenic bacteria adhere to the teeth and flourish in the acidic environment. Before treatment, a dentist evaluates the patient and provides prophylaxis, including extraction of teeth with extensive decay.[79] A daily program of fluoride application on debris-free teeth is important to prevent caries.[79] The fluoride is applied once or twice a day using specially constructed trays. These trays are filled with fluoride gel and placed over the teeth for approximately 5 to 10 minutes. The patient may expectorate the excess gel but should not rinse the mouth or drink fluids for at least 30 minutes. Because xerostomia can become a chronic problem, the use of fluoride must be continued even after radiation therapy is completed to prevent tooth decay.

Nursing Diagnoses: *Head and Neck Irradiation: Pretreatment Phase*

- *Anxiety related to radiation therapy*
- *Knowledge deficit related to radiation therapy and self-care measures*

Interventions: *Pretreatment Phase*

- Allow verbalization of fears, concerns, and questions.
- Provide education:
    Use of radiation therapy for head and neck cancer
    Potential side effects (stomatitis, taste changes, xerostomia, fatigue, and skin changes) and appropriate self-care measures.
- Consult dentist for evaluation and fluoride prophylaxis.
- Inspect mouth.

Nursing Diagnoses: *Treatment Phase*

- *Oral mucous membrane, altered, related to head and neck irradiation*
- *Sensory/perceptual alterations (gustatory) related to head and neck irradiation*
- *Skin integrity, impaired*
- *Activity intolerance*

Interventions: *Treatment Phase*

- Inspect mouth daily: assess for stomatitis and infections.
- Review mouth care:
    Brush and floss teeth if tolerated.
    As stomatitis progresses, use moistened gauze instead of tooth brushing and flossing to clean teeth.
    Rinse with normal saline at least four times a day.
- Provide soft, bland diet.
- Maintain hydration.
- Use saliva substitute and moisten foods when xerostomia occurs.
- Review use of radioprotectant with patient and family if prescribed:
    Assist with coordination of appointments for daily amifostine
    Manage symptoms such as nausea and vomiting associated with radioprotectant

- Offer topical anesthetics or analgesic medications before meals to relieve oral pain.
- Monitor weight.
- Instruct patient to perform mouth care before and after meals.
- Experiment with different foods and tastes, such as cold cooked chicken.
- Consider use of enteral feedings if significant dysphagia occurs
- Review skin care measures:
    Protect skin.
    Avoid using soap on the skin within treatment fields.
    Avoid constricting clothing or jewelry around the neck.
    Avoid shaving.
    Use moisturizing lotion if dryness occurs.
- If moist desquamation occurs:
    Burow's compresses four times a day.
    Hydrogel dressings applied to desquamated areas.
- Evaluate activities.
- Plan rest periods during the day.
- Assist in using community resources:
    Transportation to and from treatment center.
    Food purchasing and preparation.
    Social services referral.

Nursing Diagnosis: *Posttreatment Phase*

- *Oral mucous membrane, altered, related to head and neck irradiation*

Interventions: *Posttreatment Phase*

- Assess oral status (xerostomia, taste changes); inspect mouth.
- Review importance of oral hygiene and frequent visits to dentist.
- Instruct patient on use of pilocarpine if prescribed.
- To prevent osteoradionecrosis, continue prophylactic fluoride treatments.
- Continue dental evaluation and management of oral health.
- Review importance of minimizing alcohol and tobacco intake to reduce risk of oral complications.

Taste Change. Taste changes occur as the taste buds are affected by the radiation.[27] Occasionally patients report a bad or peculiar taste in the mouth. For instance, certain red meats may taste rancid or coffee may taste extremely bitter. In other cases there is a decrease in some or all taste sensations.[20] This can be very frustrating for patients who already have a loss of appetite and are trying to increase their nutritional intake. Although some recovery of taste may occur, alterations can persist 7 years or longer.[81] Therefore follow-up assessments of taste changes and their influence on nutrition should be ongoing.

Mouth care should be performed before and after each meal. Experimenting with different foods and using additional seasonings, if tolerated, can help make food more palatable.[41] If red meats are a problem, use other sources of protein such as fish, poultry, and vegetable protein. Marinating meats in wine or sweet and sour sauce before and during cooking can mask unpleasant tastes. Serving foods cold or at room temperature also blunts peculiar tastes.

Osteoradionecrosis. Osteoradionecrosis, a late and chronic effect of radiation therapy, can occur at anytime following radiation therapy and usually occurs in the mandible. Patients remain at risk for up to 20 years after treatment and probably indefinitely.[35] Trauma to the bone such as tooth decay and infections heals poorly because of compromised bone structure and can lead to necrosis of the bone. Patients who continue to use tobacco or drink alcohol are at a greater risk for developing this serious complication. Another risk factor is poorly fitting dentures, which abrade the mucosa. The mucosal breakdown can eventually reach the mandible. Treatment of osteoradionecrosis may include antibiotic therapy, surgical removal of the necrotic bone, and hyperbaric oxygen therapy (HBO) to promote healing of the bone and reduce pain.[23, 35, 74, 91] HBO therapy works by decreasing capillary filtration pressure to reduce edema, increasing oxygen diffusibility, improving collagen synthesis and neoangiogenesis, and enhancing antimicrobial defenses. After 30 HBO treatments, surgical management can be completed according to the extent of improvement achieved after HBO.[23]

Nursing care includes teaching and reinforcing the need to maintain good oral hygiene with frequent visits to the dentist for evaluation. Minimizing mouth irritants such as tobacco and alcohol and evaluating the fit and comfort of dentures will help decrease risk factors associated with osteoradionecrosis.

The nursing diagnoses *Altered oral mucous membrane related to head and neck irradiation* and *Sensory-perceptual alterations: gustatory, related to head and neck irradiation* are used when patients have alterations in the oral cavity as a result of radiation therapy. Assess mouth care practices and inspect the oral cavity for mouth changes. Evaluate the patient's ability to perform appropriate mouth care, minimize irritation, and prevent infections (see Chapter 12).

Hypopituitarism. The signs and symptoms of hypopituitarism are associated with decreased secretions of cortisol, thyroxine, and sex hormones[111] (see the accompanying table). The symptoms may develop

Signs and Symptoms of Hypopituitarism

Pituitary Deficiency	Target Organ Deficiency	Signs and Symptoms
ACTH	Cortisol	Fatigue, weakness, weight loss, anorexia, nausea, postural dizziness, muscle weakness, hypoglycemia
TSH	Thyroxine	Dry skin and hair, fatigue, edema, pallor, cold intolerance, hoarseness, weight gain, delayed deep tendon reflexes, alopecia, lethargy, mental and physical slowness, constipation
LH, FSH	Estrogen	Amenorrhea, decrease in sexual libido
	Testosterone	Decrease in sexual libido
GH		Short stature in children Asymptomatic in adults
PRL		Failure of lactation

ACTH, adrenocorticotropin; TSH, thyroid-stimulating hormone; LH, luteinizing hormone; FSH, follicle-stimulating hormone; GH, growth hormone; PRL, prolactin.

From Schultz PN: Hypopituitarism in patients with a history of irradiation to the head and neck area: diagnoses and implications for nursing, Oncol Nurs Forum *16:823, 1989.*

slowly within the first year after radiation therapy or up to 24 years after treatment. During times of stress, such as surgery or acute illness, the consequences of hypoadrenalism can be life-threatening.[111] Adrenal insufficiency is treated with adrenocorticosteroid replacement, and sex hormone deficits are replaced with appropriate hormone therapy.

Chest

Radiation therapy is given to the chest for lung cancer; lymphoma; cancers involving the mediastinum, including the esophagus; and breast cancer. Common side effects of radiation therapy to the chest are esophagitis and cough. Late effects include pneumonitis and, in rare cases, lung fibrosis. With current tissue-sparing techniques for treating breast cancer, the dose to the lung and esophagus is minimized and these patients have few if any of the just-mentioned effects.

With breast irradiation, breast edema can occur and cause discomfort. NSAIDs and manual lymph drainage can help decrease edema and inflammation of the breast tissue and provide pain relief. In some instances, the breast edema can become a chronic problem. A report of the use of HBO therapy to reduce breast edema and discomfort offers an innovative way to manage chronic breast edema.[19, 35]

Esophagitis. Esophagitis occurs if part of the esophagus is within the treatment field. Approximately 2 to 3 weeks from the start of therapy, the patient may note difficulty or pain with swallowing and may complain of a "lump in the throat." Esophagitis can become so severe that radiation treatments must be withheld for a short time. The nursing diagnosis of *Impaired swallowing related to esophagitis* is made when the patient experiences esophagitis. Assist the patient and family to plan a soft, bland, or liquid diet that provides a high-calorie, high-protein intake. Use of anesthetic and coating mouth rinses before meals can reduce the discomfort associated with eating and allow the patient to continue with therapy. Hilderley[55] described the beneficial use of a mouthwash containing viscous lidocaine, diphenhydramine elixir, and Mylanta taken 15 minutes before meals to relieve esophagitis. Other oral liquid pain medications may be used to numb the throat and relieve dysphagia.[32] Occasionally, systemic analgesics taken half an hour to an hour before meals are needed to obtain an acceptable level of pain relief. Evaluate the patient's and family's understanding and use of measures to relieve esophagitis and maintain an optimal nutritional intake.

Cough. A cough may develop or increase if lung tissue is within the treatment field, as with treatment for lung cancer. Initially the cough may be productive as trapped material is released by the previously blocked alveoli.[122] However, as treatment continues, the mucosa dries out and the cough becomes nonproductive. Assess the character, intensity, and frequency of cough, and monitor changes in lung sounds. The nursing diagnosis *Pain related to cough* is made if the patient develops a cough. Assist the patient to plan measures to relieve the cough. Make sure the patient has an adequate fluid intake. Humidification of the air and avoiding irritants such as smoke can reduce the cough. Use of cough preparations that contain codeine may be indicated for severe, dry, hacking coughing that results in fatigue or disrupts sleep. Monitor for signs and symptoms of respiratory infection, and instruct the patient to avoid sources of infection. Evaluate the patient's use of measures to minimize cough and risk of respiratory infections.

Radiation Pneumonitis. Radiation pneumonitis can occur approximately 1 to 3 months after radiation therapy to the lung. At first there may be an unproductive cough that eventually becomes productive. The symptoms include fever and dyspnea. The effect is similar to the adult respiratory distress syndrome (ARDS). Radiation pneumonitis is treated with steroids, bed rest, and antibiotics for any superimposed infections.[122]

Radiation Fibrosis. Radiation fibrosis may occur 6 to 12 months after treatment is completed. This consequence of radiation therapy is a restrictive disease of the lung. Lung fibrosis is seen primarily within the treated area of the lung and usually develops in areas of previous pneumonitis.[34] The primary symptom is shortness of breath. Treatment of radiation-induced lung fibrosis is limited to supportive care such as symptomatic control of dyspnea.

Abdomen

Gastritis may occur if part of the stomach is within the treatment field. A soft, bland diet is tolerated best. Antacids may be used if needed.

Altered nutrition: less than body requirements, related to nausea and vomiting is a likely nursing diagnosis if a large part of the abdomen, including the stomach, para-aortic area, or small bowel is within the treatment field. Nausea and vomiting usually occur within the first 6 hours after treatments and may last for 3 to 6 hours. In rare instances nausea may persist for longer periods. Assess patients for occurrence and pattern of nausea and vomiting. Prophylactic use of antiemetics before treatment each day and as needed after treatment can minimize and relieve nausea and vomiting from radiation therapy. For severe nausea and vomiting, around-the-clock antiemetics are recommended.[58] The table below provides guidelines for radiation-induced emesis.[42]

Guidelines for Radiation-Induced Emesis

RISK FACTORS FOR RADIATION-INDUCED EMESIS
A. High-Risk: Total body irradiation
   A serotonin receptor antagonist should be given with or without a corticosteroid before each fraction and for at least 24 h after.
B. Intermediate Risk: Hemibody irradiation, upper abdomen, abdominal-pelvic, mantle, cranial radiosurgery, and craniospinal radiotherapy
   A serotonin receptor antagonist or a dopamine receptor antagonist should be given before each fraction.
C. Low Risk: Radiation of the cranium only, breast, head and neck, extremities, pelvis, and thorax
   Treatment should be given on an as-needed basis only. Dopamine or serotonin receptor antagonists are advised. Antiemetics should be continued prophylactically for each remaining radiation treatment day.

From Gralla RJ and others: *Recommendations for the use of antiemetics: evidence-based, clinical practice guidelines,* J Clin Oncol 17:2971, 1999.

Relaxation techniques and distraction such as listening to soothing music and engaging in an enjoyable activity can help control nausea. Using relaxation techniques before and after treatments helps minimize the anxiety that can exacerbate nausea. Plan dietary modifications to minimize nausea and vomiting. A diet that is low in fat, low in sugar, and easily digested is best tolerated. Soups, broths, and other fluids should be consumed to maintain fluid intake and prevent dehydration (see Chapter 29). Evaluate the patient's and family's understanding of the potential and actual causes of nausea and vomiting. Also evaluate their ability to use appropriate measures to reduce or relieve nausea and vomiting and maintain the patient's nutritional status.

Pelvis

Diarrhea and cystitis commonly occur when the pelvis is being treated for gynecologic cancer, prostate cancer, testicular cancer, rectal cancer, or lymphomas. In addition, symptoms impacting sexual function also occur.[40, 113] When feasible, conformal radiation therapy limits the volume of treated tissue and results in fewer side effects than whole pelvis treatment.[4] Diagnoses include *Diarrhea related to pelvic irradiation, Altered patterns of urinary elimination related to pelvic irradiation* and *Sexual dysfunction related to effects of pelvic irradiation.*

Diarrhea. Diarrhea occurs as the bowel lining atrophies and resorption of fluids from the colon is decreased.[67] Malabsorption of bile salt may also cause diarrhea. Diarrhea can occur 2 to 3 weeks into treatment and may last throughout the course of therapy. Some patients produce an increased number of stools; others produce loose, watery stools with cramping. In certain instances treatment may be interrupted to allow the bowel to recover. Occasionally chronic enteritis develops.

Assess the patient's usual bowel pattern. If diarrhea occurs, help the patient and family plan measures to minimize diarrhea. Instruct the patient and family in the use of a low-residue diet. Reducing the amount of fat in the diet can also be helpful because fats are difficult to digest. If milk products are not tolerated, they should be avoided. If the diarrhea persists while the patient is on a low-residue diet, antidiarrheal medication such as diphenoxylate atropine or loperamide HCl may be indicated. If diarrhea tends to occur after meals as a result of the gastrocolic reflex, the antidiarrheal medication should be taken before meals. Tenesmus of the anal sphincter is controlled with antispasmodic and anticholinergic medications. Patients may also experience proctitis and hemorrhoidal discomfort. Frequent sitz baths, psyllium preparations (e.g., Metamucil) and hemorrhoidal preparations may be used to ease the discomfort. For chronic proctitis following radiation therapy, sucralfate enemas have been effective.[69] Evaluate the patient's and family's understanding and use of measures to minimize diarrhea, tenesmus and proctitis to maintain the patient's usual pattern of elimination.

Cystitis. Cystitis occurs if the bladder is within the treatment field. Symptoms include dysuria, decreased bladder capacity, urinary frequency and urgency, nocturia, and urinary hesitancy. In rare cases bleeding occurs. HBO therapy has shown therapeutic benefits in treating chronic radiation-induced cystitis that is refractory to conventional therapy.[25, 38, 89, 92, 125] HBO therapy increases tissue oxygenation and promotes vascularization and formation of granulation tissue. Patients sit in an HBO chamber and receive 100% oxygen for approximately 2 hours. One or two treatments a day are delivered for a total of as many as 60 treatments.

Assess and monitor symptoms of cystitis, including signs of hematuria. Instruct the patient to maintain an adequate fluid intake. As symptoms occur, bladder infections must be ruled out or treated. Obtain urine specimens for analysis and culture. Bladder analgesics such as phenazopyridine can relieve cystitis. Antispasmodic medications can provide some relief from bladder spasms. Evaluate the patient's understanding of the causes of cystitis and ways to relieve symptoms.

When the prostate is treated, the patient may experience bladder outlet irritation resulting in hesitancy, decreased force of urine stream, and urinary frequency from incomplete voiding. The use of an α-blocker medication such as terazocin or tamsulosin has demonstrated benefit for improving urinary flow for benign prostatic hypertrophy and can improve symptoms related to radiation therapy.[71]

Erectile Dysfunction. Erectile dysfunction after pelvic radiation may occur in men as a result of fibrosis of the pelvic vasculature and damage of pelvic nerves. A decline in the ability to attain and maintain an erection occurs gradually and may be permanent. Allow the patient and his partner to discuss concerns and feelings regarding changes in sexual functioning and body image. Consultation with a urologist may include a discussion of pharmacologic interventions and devices and prostheses that may be used.

Vaginal Stenosis. When the vaginal vault is included in the treatment field, vaginal stenosis may develop and cause dyspareunia and difficulties with pelvic examinations. Vaginal stenosis can be minimized or prevented by use of a vaginal dilator. With the patient lying supine with knees bent, the well-lubricated dilator is inserted into the vagina, withdrawn, and reinserted for 5 to 10 minutes.[98] Vaginal dilation needs to be performed three times a week for at least 1 year.

Ovarian Failure. Ovarian failure occurs with small amounts of radiation and produces symptoms associated with menopause: hot flashes, amenorrhea, decreased libido, and osteoporosis.[37] Older women are at a higher risk of ovarian failure than younger women. Replacement hormonal therapy with midcyclic estrogens and progesterone reverses the clinical effects of early menopause. In many circumstances the ovaries can be shielded from radiation. In one technique, oophoropexy, the ovaries are surgically placed outside the treatment field.

Testicles. The testicles are usually shielded from radiation. However, if exposure is needed or unavoidable, spermatogenesis will stop and usually results in permanent sterility.

Sexuality. Issues related to sexuality need to be explored with sensitivity. As physical changes occur, the patient and partner need to explore ways to satisfyingly express their sexuality and feelings (see Chapter 33).

Brain

Cerebral Edema. When the brain is treated for a primary brain tumor or brain metastasis, assessment for symptoms of cerebral edema is crucial. Cerebral edema occurs as tissues around the tumor become inflamed. These symptoms include headaches, nausea, vomiting, seizures, vision changes, motor function disabilities, slurred speech, and changes in mental status. Steroids are usually indicated during the course of treatment to minimize cerebral edema. If symptoms occur or increase, an evaluation is needed and may indicate a need to adjust the steroid dosage. Steroids may be needed on a continuing basis to control edema. Plan to ensure the patient's safety in the home and work place as well as during transportation to and from the treatment center. Evaluate the patient's and family's understanding of the cause of cerebral edema and the signs and symptoms they should monitor and report.

Alopecia. Alopecia, which occurs within the treatment area, depends on the dose and extent of radiation to the scalp. The hair loss may be regional or patchy, depending on the treatment technique. Alopecia starts when the dose to the scalp reaches 2500 to 3000 cGy, and the hair gradually thins over 2 to 3 weeks. With large doses of radiation (> 4000 cGy), as in the treatment for primary brain tumors, the hair loss is permanent. With small doses such as those given for palliative purposes, alopecia is more variable. Hair loss may also occur directly opposite the treatment site, where the x-rays exit. If regrowth of hair occurs, it may start 2 to 3 months after completion of therapy.[116]

Hair Texture and Color. Changes in hair texture and color may also occur. The scalp may develop pruritus and become very dry or peel. The scalp needs protection along guidelines for skin care outlined earlier in this chapter. Gentle brushing and combing of hair is recommended. Permanent waves and hair coloring during treatment and immediately following completion of therapy are contraindicated because they can irritate the scalp. Using a scarf, turban, hat, or cap to protect the scalp from the wind, cold, and sun is advisable. A wig may be worn. Make sure the wig lining is comfortable and does not further irritate the scalp. A mild shampoo may be used, but excessive shampooing should be avoided. The potential or actual loss of hair can be traumatic for the patient. Nursing diagnoses are *Ineffective individual coping related to alopecia* and *Self-esteem disturbance related to alopecia.* Help the patient cope with the psychological effects by recognizing the importance of alopecia, approaching the patient with gentleness, honesty, and caring, and allowing verbalization of fears, grief, and anger. Prepare the patient and family in advance for alopecia. Assess its significance. Provide information on what can be done to cover and care for the scalp. These activities communicate understanding of the loss and offer support to the patient as she adapts to the change in body image.

MINIMIZING THE NURSE'S EXPOSURE TO RADIATION

Nurses play a major role in dispelling the patient's and family's fears and misconceptions about radiation therapy. When working with patients with internal radiation therapy, nurses need to be aware of their own concerns so that care can be provided thoroughly and effectively while minimizing radiation exposure.[112] Nursing inservices about radiobiology and radiation safety principles, combined with discussions and practice laboratories, can help clarify how nurses can protect themselves and still provide comprehensive nursing care. Fear is highly contagious, and nurses need to develop awareness of their behavior and its impact on patients. National and state regulations keep individual exposure below levels that produce somatic or genetic damage.[33, 112]

When the nurse works with patients with a radioactive implant or systemic radiation, she should anticipate the patient's needs and use the principles of time, distance, and shielding to minimize radiation exposure.

Time—Minimize time spent in close proximity to the patient. Radiation exposure is directly related to the time spent within a specific distance of the source of radioactivity. Use time efficiently by organizing patient care activities and assembling necessary supplies before entering the patient's room. Before leaving the patient's room, place personal items within reach of the patient to avoid needing to reenter the room. Direct care is usually limited to one-half hour per person per shift. Encourage the patient to perform self-care activities.

Distance—Maximize the distance from the radioactive material. The amount of radiation decreases according to the inverse square law (Box 22–2). Visit frequently with the patient at the door to the patient's room.

Shielding—When appropriate, use shielding to decrease exposure to radiation. With radium or cesium implants, a 1-inch thick lead shield is positioned next to the bed to attenuate the radiation. Most nursing care is provided from behind the shields. The lead aprons used in diagnostic radiology can be cumbersome and actually result in the nurse requiring more time to perform essential bedside care. In addition, they are not sufficiently thick to stop gamma rays and therefore are not recommended.

Table 22–9 presents some general guidelines for working with patients receiving internal radiation therapy.

CONCLUSION

Nurses have always been involved in the development of radiation oncology as a specialty, whether being at

---

BOX 22-2

Inverse Square Law

Radioactive
Source

Meters	0 1 2 3 4 5 6 7 8
Exposure rate	$\frac{1}{1}$ $\frac{1}{4}$ $\frac{1}{16}$ $\frac{1}{64}$

If the exposure at 1 m from the radioactive source is x, the exposure at 2 m is one fourth of x, and at 4 m, one sixteenth.

According to the inverse square law, exposure decreases as the distance from the radioactive source increases.

$$\text{Exposure rate} = \frac{1}{(\text{distance})^2}$$

---

the bedside of the patient receiving radiation therapy, delivering the treatment, researching improved methods of symptom management, or helping to calm a confused or frightened patient on the treatment table. The fears and concerns of patients have changed very little, and the impact of the diagnosis of cancer remains profound.

The nurse provides leadership in the field of radiation oncology based on clinical expertise, education, and patient advocacy. In a collaborative role with the radiation oncology team, the nurse provides continuity and quality patient care.[11–13, 31] The nurse is in a prime position to assess, plan for, and evaluate interventions to prevent, minimize, or relieve side effects associated with radiation therapy. In working with colleagues in the hospital, home care, and ambulatory settings, and with patients and families, the nurse helps to advance the profession and improve the patient's quality of life throughout treatment and rehabilitation.

TABLE 22–9
Guidelines for Internal Radiation Therapy

	Sealed Sources	Unsealed Sources
Preparation of the patient	Instruct patient and family on procedure and visitation restrictions. Isolation is a temporary requirement and the nursing staff is available for all needs, but, by necessity, the nurse will work quickly and remain in the room for essential activities only. Preoperatively, patients may require bowel cleansing or placement of a Foley catheter, as with cervical/vaginal implants.	
Room assignment	Private room usually required.	Private room only.
Restrictions on staff and visitors	No one under 18 years of age and no one who is or may be pregnant. Time spent close to the patient must be limited as much as possible. Visits with the patient from the doorway are usually permitted for longer periods.	
Shielding	Stay behind lead shields. Lead aprons are not effective.	Lead aprons are not effective.
Level of patient's activity	Patient remains in room. Depending on location of implant, the patient's activities may be limited to bed rest. In some instances raising the head of the bed may also be limited. Diversional activities such as watching television or reading a book are recommended.	Patient remains in room. Bathroom privileges if tolerated. Patient should care for self.
Body fluid precautions	Body fluids and materials are not radioactive. No special precautions are necessary for handling these materials.	Secretions from the patient may be radioactive: • Prior to patient admission, cover the floor surfaces of the patient's room and bathroom with disposable waterproof liners (e.g., chux). Telephone handsets should also be covered with a waterproof liner. • Wear gloves when handling equipment or objects that may have come in contact with body fluids or materials (e.g., urinals, bedpans, and emesis basins). • Wash gloves before removing and place in designated waste container. • Wash hands thoroughly with soap and water after removing gloves. • Disposable shoe covers may be put on before entering the patient's room and removed before exiting. Shoe covers should be used if patient is incontinent. • Disposable items such as eating utensils, cups, and plates should be used. • Nondisposable items such as equipment and linens should not be removed from the patient's room until checked for radioactivity. Soiled items should be placed in a plastic bag, sealed, and left in the patient's room until checked for radioactivity. • Stool, urine, and emesis are usually discarded in the toilet in the patient's room. Instruct the patient to flush the toilet two or three times after each use. • Vomiting, stool or urinary incontinence, and excessive sweating may produce radioactive contamination of the room and linen. Use gloves to dispose of the material in the toilet, if appropriate, or in plastic bags, which are left in the patient's room for monitoring.

Table continued on following page

Guidelines for Internal Radiation Therapy *Continued*

	Sealed Sources	Unsealed Sources
		• If skin becomes contaminated, wash affected area immediately with soap and water.
		• If clothing becomes contaminated, have level of radioactivity evaluated before leaving the immediate area.
		• Take special room preparation and additional precautions according to specific institution's policies.
Special precautions	Check linens, clothing, and bedpans for signs of dislodged implant. If implant is dislodged, do not touch it; notify the physician immediately. If forceps are available, the radioactive source may be picked up with the forceps and placed in an available container, such as an emesis basin. The container should be placed in a corner of the room distant from the door. Immediately notify the physician. Dressings and packings should not be changed unless ordered by the physician.	
Discharge of patient from the hospital	The patient is no longer radioactive once the implant has been removed and placed in a lead-lined container.	The patient is discharged when total body retention of the radioactive isotope is at a safe level. After the patient is discharged, the patient's room and all items in it are surveyed for any residual radioactivity.

Nursing Management

HELPING PATIENTS AND FAMILIES COPE WITH RADIATION THERAPY

Radiation therapy can sound frightening, and many patients approach it with apprehension. The nurse is in a vital position to help the patient and family cope with this treatment and its sequelae.[56] Because most patients receive radiation therapy as an outpatient, self-care is supported by nurses through assessment, symptom management, and education.[31] Education can increase the patient's treatment-related knowledge while decreasing anxiety and general emotional distress during treatment.[96] The nursing diagnoses *Anxiety related to radiation therapy* and *Knowledge deficit related to radiation therapy and self-care measures* may be used. Support and counsel the patient and family who may need help to sort through their feelings about radiation therapy. Specifically assess the patient's expectations and concerns about therapy.

Patients are very interested in learning about their disease and treatment and ways to minimize symptoms and care for themselves. Dodd[28] studied the self-care behaviors of patients receiving radiation therapy and found that many patients used remedies for symptoms associated with radiation therapy, which were commonly known and used by the general public and presented in the media.

Patient education is challenging because of limited time to provide the education and because of patient and family variables such as anxiety, symptom distress, and lack of resources.[26] Identifying the major teaching needs and tailoring the education for the patients so that it is provided over a period of time helps make the information less overwhelming. For instance, a weekly patient newsletter or a series of cassette audio or videotapes can be used to give patients and families information throughout the treatment period.[45, 46, 120] A study conducted by Johnson and colleagues[62] evaluated the use of self-regulating, theory-based nursing interventions for patients receiving radiation therapy for breast or prostate cancer. Four 30-minute interventions were scheduled with patients. At each intervention, specific, concrete, and objective information was provided relevant to the point in the patient's treatment trajectory. The table below lists the content for each of the interventions.

Subjects who received the experimental interventions had less disruption in their usual activities during

Topic and Content of Each Experimental Intervention

FIRST INTERVENTION (BEFORE TREATMENT)
Topic: Description of the simulation and treatment
Content
- Purpose of the simulation
- Characteristics of the environment, including laser lights
- People involved and what they do
- Patient's positioning and what he or she will be asked to do
- Sensations from tubes, contours, tattoos, etc.
- Sounds of machines when moving
- Description of first treatment, including time required
- Description of room and patient preparation

SECOND INTERVENTION (FIRST WEEK OF TREATMENT)
Topic: Side effects
Content
- Side effects specific to site of treatment
- Cause of side effects
- When to expect side effects to start
- Time of day side effects will most likely occur
- Any sensations associated with side effects
- Suggestions for self-care activities (Written summaries of self-care activities were provided.)

THIRD INTERVENTION (LAST WEEK OF TREATMENT)
Topic: Side effects changes and end-of-treatment concerns
Content
- Pattern of subsidence of each side effect
- Reactions to treatment ending
- Return to usual life activities
- Individual concerns/expectations

FOURTH INTERVENTION (1 MONTH POSTTREATMENT)
Topic: Assessment of side effects and survivorship
Content
- Side effect status
- Return to usual life activities
- Prevention and detection activities for each cancer site
- Quality-of-life issues, including sexuality
- Resources available to patient
- Individualized content needs for each patient

From Johnson JE and others: The effects of nursing care guided by self-regulation theory on coping with radiation therapy. Oncol Nurs Forum 24:1041, 1997.

and following radiation therapy. In addition, a more positive mood was reported in identified pessimistic individuals who received the experimental interventions than similar individuals who did not receive the intervention.

Audiotapes can be helpful educational tools for patients receiving radiation therapy. Hagopian[46] described the use of six informational audiotapes for patients receiving radiation therapy. The audiotapes were between 7 to 10 minutes in length and covered topics such as radiation therapy, skin care, nutrition, fatigue, mouth care, diarrhea, and urinary frequency. The tapes described the side effects as well as suggested self-care measures to relieve the specific symptoms. Patients listened to the audiotapes of their choice at their convenience. The patients who used the audiotapes were more knowledgeable about radiation therapy and its side effects, used more self-care measures, and practiced more helpful self-care behaviors than the control group.

Concrete, objective information describing the common physical sensations experienced, the environmental surroundings, and information about timing of events helps to decrease the amount of disruption to the patient's usual activities during and after radiation therapy.[63] Educate the patient and family about the therapy and its side effects: what occurs, when it may occur, how long it lasts, and what they can do to manage the problem. Describe to the patient what he may experience.[122]

The patient may be in the treatment room for about 20 minutes, but the actual treatment lasts only 2 to 5 minutes.
The patient must lie on a hard table.
The patient must remain alone in the room for the actual treatment.
The patient may hear a buzzing, clicking, or whirring sound from the treatment machine.
The machine may rotate around the patient, depending on how the treatment is delivered.
The treatment itself is painless.

Many myths, fears, and anxieties surround radiation therapy. Many patients have heard from others about someone else's experience with radiation—the burns, disfigurement, and pain. Explain to the patient and family that not all treatments cause the same problems and that as technology advances, some side effects have become less common and less severe.

The treatment machines are large and can be intimidating as they hover closely over the patient. Some patients fear being crushed by the machine or parts of it. For some patients, being alone in the treatment room during the treatment reinforces the loneliness of having cancer.

A common misconception about external radiation therapy is the fear of radioactivity. Many people mistakenly believe that the patient is radioactive. Reassure the patient and family that with external radiation, the patient is *not* radioactive. There is no residue of radiation on the patient, and

---

PATIENT TEACHING PRIORITIES

External-Beam Radiation Therapy

Instruct Patient and Family About:

Use of radiation therapy to treat cancer.
Events that occur before, during, and after a course of radiation therapy: consultation, simulation, daily treatment, routine evaluations during course of therapy, and follow-up.
Time factors: length of simulation, length of daily treatment, length of course of radiation therapy.
Environmental information: description of surroundings, treatment room, and machine.

Effects and side effects of radiation therapy (general and site specific):

That radiation therapy is a localized treatment and expected side effects are site specific.
What happens, why it occurs.
When these effects are experienced.
How long these effects last and when they resolve.
That the patient is *not* radioactive; there is no need to isolate the patient from family and friends.

Measures That Patients and Families Can Use to Minimize or Prevent Side Effects:

General effects: skin care, nutrition, energy conservation.
Site-specific effects.
Delayed effects to monitor: skin care, fatigue, site-specific effects.
Follow-up care: routine follow-up with health care providers and adherence to recommendations for healthy living.

PATIENT TEACHING PRIORITIES

Internal Radiation Therapy—Sealed and Nonsealed Sources

Instruct the Patient and Family About:

Use of internal radiation therapy to treat cancer.
Patient preparation before therapy.
Procedures involved in the therapy.
Visitation restrictions: no one under 18 years of age, no one who is or may be pregnant.
Isolation requirements: temporary isolation, patient remains in room, nursing care for essential activities only, time spent in close proximity will be limited. If the patient with nonsealed radioactive source has bathroom privileges, the patient is instructed to flush the toilet two or three times after each use.
Patient activity may be restricted, depending on the procedure; diversional activities such as watching television or reading a book are recommended.
Discharge from the hospital: monitor for delayed effects such as fatigue; pelvic implants: diarrhea, urinary symptoms such as bladder infections, women are instructed to perform vaginal dilation three times a week for up to 1 year after implantation.[98]

---

therefore the patient should not be isolated from family or friends.

Community resources are available and can be gathered to assist the patient and family. These resources include a variety of services through the American Cancer Society, visiting nurses, home parenteral nutritional services, Meals on Wheels, accommodations for out-of-town patients, and transportation assistance for daily treatment.

Patient teaching priorities for external and internal beam radiation therapy and geriatric considerations are shown in the boxes.

Following a course of radiation therapy, follow-up with patients to assess and manage ongoing side effects is important in the rehabilitation period. These symptoms can be managed by nurses with telephone interviews.[102]

GERIATRIC CONSIDERATIONS
Radiation Therapy

Compromised body systems in the elderly place them at risk for developing side effects sooner and with greater severity:

Skin: Monitor for excessive dryness and early skin reactions.

Energy stores may be depleted and increase fatigue.

Medications prescribed for symptom management may need dosage adjustments to minimize adverse reactions.

Head and neck irradiation: Normally decreased oral secretions predispose the elderly for oral complications.

Check the fit and comfort of oral prostheses.

Taste acuity may be altered before start of irradiation.

Sexuality: Assess changes experienced. Provide education about the effects of radiation therapy. Because of the importance of preventing vaginal stenosis so that vaginal intercourse and pelvic examinations are feasible, instruct women who have received radiation therapy involving the vaginal vault to perform vaginal dilation three times a week for up to 1 year. Radiation therapy further decreases vaginal secretions. Women are instructed to use water-based lubricants for comfort. Some men experience erectile dysfunction with aging as a result of vascular changes. Pelvic irradiation may further damage the pelvic vasculature and cause nerve damage. Provide counseling or referral to specialist.

Social concerns:

Radiation therapy is usually delivered Monday through Friday for up to 7 weeks. The elderly may need to rely on public transportation or family and friends for daily transportation. In many situations, the patient is caring for a spouse or child and being away from home is difficult without a caretaker. Many elderly are on fixed incomes, and the added expense of therapy, transportation, out-of-town housing, and additional medications needed during therapy is a hardship.

Chapter Questions

1. The use of radiation therapy to treat cancer is based on the fact that radiation therapy:
   a. Is a systemic treatment
   b. Is rarely used with chemotherapy
   c. Uses heat to alter the cell's DNA
   d. Uses high-energy radiation

2. When educating a 70-year-old man about radiation therapy for prostate cancer, it will be most helpful if he receives information that:
   a. The treatment will last approximately 6 to 7 weeks.
   b. The actual treatment is very short.
   c. He may be alone in the treatment room for a long time.
   d. He may feel uncomfortable lying on the treatment table.

3. This gentleman should also receive information that during the course of treatment he should:
   a. Monitor for a cough
   b. Use a low-residue diet
   c. Limit fluid intake
   d. Avoid anticholinergic medications

4. When a patient has received a radiopharmaceutical to treat bone metastases, there:
   a. Is not contamination of body fluids
   b. Should be no contact with people in public areas
   c. May be a temporary increase in blood counts
   d. May be a temporary flare of bone pain

5. When caring for a hospitalized woman with a vaginal implant for cervical cancer:
   a. The patient may dangle her legs at the bedside.
   b. Monitor placement of the applicator and vaginal packing.
   c. A nasogastric tube is used for nutrition.
   d. Institute a bowel program to encourage bowel movements.

6. Recommendations for nursing care of the patient with a radioactive implant includes:
   a. Use of a lead apron when providing direct patient care
   b. Conversations with the patient at the bedside
   c. Use of a lead shield at the bedside
   d. Frequent Foley catheter care

7. When a moist desquamation of the skin occurs, use:
   a. Burow's compresses
   b. Fluorinated steroid creams
   c. Cornstarch powder
   d. Mentholated creams

8. Recommendations to manage fatigue during radiation therapy include all *except:*
   a. Walking in an exercise program
   b. Maintaining nutritional status
   c. Using community resources
   d. Avoiding naps during the day

9. When patients experience xerostomia due to salivary gland exposure to radiation therapy, it is recommended that they:
   a. Use commercial antibacterial mouthwashes
   b. Use lemon-glycerin swabs
   c. Perform frequent mouth rinses
   d. Consume high-protein foods such as peanut butter

10. Nausea and vomiting is associated with radiation therapy for:
   a. Breast cancer
   b. Rectal cancer
   c. Pancreatic cancer
   d. Brain cancer

BIBLIOGRAPHY

1. Anonymous: Samarium-153 lexidronam for painful bone metastases, *Med Lett Drugs Ther* 39:83, 1997.
2. Ang KK, Thames HD, Peters LJ: Altered fractionation schedules. In Perez CA, Brady LW editors, *Principles and practice of radiation oncology,* ed 3, Philadelphia, Lippincott-Raven, 1998.
3. Archambeau JO, Pezner R, Wasserman T: Pathophysiology of irradiated skin and breast, *Int J Radiat Oncol Biol Phys* 31:1171, 1995.
4. Beard CJ and others: Complications after treatment with external-beam irradiation in early-stage prostate cancer patients: a prospective multi-institutional outcomes study, *J Clin Oncol* 15:223, 1997.
5. Ben-Josef E and others: Radiotherapeutic management of osseous metastases: a survey of current patterns of care, *Int J Rad Oncol Biol Phys* 40:915, 1998.
6. Bentel GC, Nelson CE, Noell KT: Elements of clinical radiation oncology. In Bentel GC, Nelson CE, Noell KT, editors: *Treatment planning and dose calculation in radiation oncology,* ed 4, New York, Pergamon, 1989.
7. Biel MA: Photodynamic therapy and the treatment of head and neck neoplasia. *Laryngoscope* 108:1259, 1998.
8. Blanke CD and others: Concurrent paclitaxel and thoracic irradiation for locally advanced esophageal cancer, *Semin Radiat Oncol* 9(2 suppl 1):43, 1999.
9. Blomgren H and others: Radiosurgery for tumors in the body: clinical experience using a new method, *J Radiosurg* 1:63, 1998.
10. Brandt B: Informational needs and selected variables in patients receiving brachytherapy, *Oncol Nurs Forum* 18:1221, 1991.
11. Bruner DW: Report on the radiation oncology nursing subcommittee of the American College of Radiology task force on standards development, *Oncology* 4:80, 1990.
12. Bruner DW and others, editors: *Manual for radiation oncology nursing practice and education,* Pittsburgh, Oncology Nursing Society, 1992.
13. Bruner DW and others, editors: *Manual for radiation oncology nursing practice and education,* Pittsburgh, Oncology Nursing Press, 1998.
14. Bucholtz JD: Issues concerning the sedation of children for radiation therapy, *Oncol Nurs Forum* 19:649, 1992.
15. Bucholtz JD: Radiolabeled antibody therapy, *Semin Oncol Nurs* 3:67, 1987.
16. Campbell J, Lane C: Developing a skin-care protocol in radiotherapy, *Professional Nurse* 12:105, 1996.
17. Campbell C, Iwamoto R: Intraoperative radiation therapy, *Todays OR Nurse* 14:1, 1992.
18. Capizzi RL: Clinical status and optimal use of amifostine, *Oncology* 13:47, 1999.
19. Carl UM, Hartmann KA: Hyperbaric oxygen treatment for symptomatic breast edema after radiation therapy, *Undersea Hyperb Med* 25:233, 1998.
20. Conger A: Loss and recovery of taste acuity in patients irradiated to the oral cavity, *Radiat Res* 53:338, 1973.
21. Corn BW and others: Stereotactic radiosurgery and radiotherapy: new developments and new directions, *Semin Oncol* 24:707, 1997.
22. Cromack DT and others: Are complications in intraoperative radiation therapy more frequent than in conventional treatment? *Arch Surg* 124:229, 1989.
23. Cronje FJ: A review of the Marx protocols: prevention and management of osteoradionecrosis by combining surgery and hyperbaric oxygen therapy. *SADJ.* 53:469, 1998.
24. Curran WJ: Radiation-induced toxicities: the role of radioprotectants, *Semin Radiat Oncol* 8(4 suppl 1):2, 1998.
25. Del Pizzo JJ and others: Treatment of radiation induced hemorrhagic cystitis with hyperbaric oxygen: long-term follow-up. *J Urol* 160(3 Pt1):731, 1998.
26. DeMuth JS: Patient teaching in the ambulatory setting, *Nurs Clin North Am* 24:645, 1989.
27. DeWys W, Walters K: Abnormalities of taste sensation in cancer patients, *Cancer* 36:1888, 1975.
28. Dodd MJ: Patterns of self care in cancer patients receiving radiation therapy, *Oncol Nurs Forum* 11:23, 1984.
29. Dorr RT: Radioprotectants: pharmacology and clinical applications of amifostine, *Semin Radiat Oncol* 8(4 suppl 1):10, 1998.
30. Dowell JE and others: Seven-week continuous-infusion paclitaxel concurrent with radiation therapy for locally advanced non-small cell lung and head and neck cancer, *Semin Radiat Oncol* 9(2 suppl 1):97, 1999.
31. Downing J: Radiotherapy nursing: understanding the nurse's role, *Nurs Standard* 12:42, 1998.
32. Dunne CF: Oral analgesics to relieve radiation-induced esophagitis, *Oncol Nurs Forum* 18:785, 1991.
33. Dunne-Daly C: Principles of brachytherapy. In Dow KH and others, editors: *Nursing care in radiation oncology,* ed 2, Philadelphia, Saunders, 1997.
34. Emami B, Graham MV: Lung. In Perez CA, Brady LW editors, *Principles and practice of radiation oncology,* ed 3, Philadelphia, Lippincott-Raven, 1998.

35. Epstein J and others: Postradiation osteonecrosis of the mandible: a long-term follow-up study, *Oral Surg Oral Med Oral Pathol Oral Radiol Endod* 83:657, 1997.

36. Feber T: Management of mucositis in oral irradiation, *Clin Oncol (R C Radiol)* 8:106, 1996.

37. Feldman JE: Ovarian failure and cancer treatment: incidence and interventions for the premenopausal woman, *Oncol Nurs Forum* 16:651, 1989.

38. Feldmeier JJ and others: Hyperbaric oxygen an adjunctive treatment for delayed radiation injuries of the abdomen and pelvis, *Undersea Hyperb Med* 23:205, 1996.

39. Fiekau R: Principles of feeding cancer patients via enteral or parenteral nutrition during radiotherapy, *Strahlenther Onkol* 174(suppl 3):47, 1998.

40. Franklin CI, Parker CA, Morton KM: Late effects of radiation therapy for prostate carcinoma: the patient's perspective of bladder, bowel and sexual morbidity, *Australas Radiol* 42:58, 1998.

41. Gallucci BB, Iwamoto RR: Taste alterations in patients with cancer: nursing care of the cancer patient with nutritional problems, *Report of the Ross Oncology Nursing Roundtable* 40, 1981.

42. Gralla RJ and others: Recommendations for the use of antiemetics: evidence-bases, clinical practice guidelines, *J Clin Oncol* 17:2971, 1999.

43. Greenburg S and others: Interstitially implanted I-125 for prostate cancer using transrectal ultrasound, *Oncol Nurs Forum* 17:849, 1990.

44. Gunderson LL: Past, present, and future of intraoperative irradiation for colorectal cancer, *Int J Radiat Oncol Biol Phys* 34:741, 1996.

45. Hagopian GA: The effects of informational audiotapes on knowledge and self care behaviors of patients undergoing radiation therapy, *Oncol Nursg Forum* 23:697, 1996.

46. Hagopian GA: The effects of a weekly radiation therapy newsletter on patients, *Oncol Nurs Forum* 18:1199, 1991.

47. Haibeck SV: Intraoperative radiation therapy, *Oncol Nurs Forum* 15:143, 1988.

48. Harrison LB, Enker WE, Anderson LL: High-dose-rate intraoperative radiation therapy for colorectal cancer: part I, *Oncology* 9:679, 1995a.

49. Harrison LB, Enker WE, Anderson LL: High-dose-rate intraoperative radiation therapy for colorectal cancer: part II, *Oncology* 9:679, 1995b.

50. Hassey KM: Skin care for patients receiving radiation therapy for rectal cancer, *J Enterostom Ther* 14:197, 1987.

51. Hellman S: Principles of cancer management: radiation therapy. In DeVita VT Jr, Hellman S, Rosenberg SA, editors: *Cancer: principles and practice of oncology,* ed 5, Philadelphia, Lippincott-Raven, 1997.

52. Hendrickson FR, Withers HR: Principles of radiation oncology. In Holleb AI, Fink DJ, Murphy GP, editors: *American Cancer Society textbook of clinical oncology,* Atlanta, American Cancer Society, 1991.

53. Herscher LL, Cook J: Taxanes as radiosensitizers for head and neck cancer, *Curr Opin Oncol* 11:183, 1999.

54. Hilderley LJ: Principles of teletherapy. In Dow KH and others, editors: *Nursing care in radiation oncology,* ed 2, Philadelphia, Saunders, 1997.

55. Hilderley L: Relieving radiation esophagitis, *Oncol Nurs Forum* 13:71, 1986.

56. Hilderley LJ: The role of the nurse in radiation oncology, *Semin Oncol* 7:39, 1980.

57. Hirshfield-Bartek J and others: Monitoring the myelosuppressive effects of radiation therapy, *Oncol Nurs Forum* 15:547, 1988.

58. Hogan CM, Grant M: Physiologic mechanisms of nausea and vomiting in patients with cancer, *Oncol Nurs Forum* 24(7 suppl):8, 1997

59. Iwamoto RR: Xerostomia. In Yarbro CH, Frogge MH, Goodman M, editors: *Cancer symptom management,* ed 2, Boston, Jones & Bartlett, 1999.

60. Iwamoto RR: A nursing perspective on radiation-induced xerostomia, *Oncology* 10(3 suppl):12, 1996.

61. Janjan NA: Radiation for bone metastases: conventional techniques and the role of systemic radiopharmaceuticals, *Cancer* 80(8 suppl):1628, 1997.

62. Johnson JE and others: The effects of nursing care guided by self-regulation theory on coping with radiation therapy, *Oncol Nurs Forum* 24:1041, 1997.

63. Johnson JE and others: Reducing the negative impact of radiation therapy on functional status, *Cancer* 61:46, 1988.

64. Jones D, Hafermann MD: A radiolucent bite-block apparatus, *Int J Radiat Oncol Biol Phys* 13:129, 1986.

65. Jordan LN, Buck SS: A teaching booklet for patients receiving high dose rate brachytherapy, *Oncol Nurs Forum* 18:1235, 1991.

66. Jordan LN, Mantravadi RVP: Nursing care of the patient receiving high dose rate brachytherapy, *Oncol Nurs Forum* 18:1167, 1991.

67. Kelvin JF: Gastrointestinal cancers. In Dow KH and others, editors: *Nursing care in radiation oncology,* ed 2, Philadelphia, Saunders, 1997.

68. Klevenhagen SC, Lambert GD, Arbabi A: Backscattering in electron beam therapy for energies between 3 and 35 MeV, *Phys Med Biol* 27:363, 1982.

69. Kochlar R and others: Sucralfate enema in ulcerative rectosigmoid lesions, *Dis Colon Rectum* 33:49, 1990.

70. Larson DA and others: Stereotactic external-beam irradiation. In Perez CA, Brady LW, editors: *Principles and practice of radiation oncology,* ed 2, Philadelphia, Lippincott, 1992.

71. Lepor H: Phase III multicenter placebo-controlled study of tamsulosin in benign prostatic hyperplasia, *Urology* 51:892, 1998.

72. Levy JG: Photosensitizers in photodynamic therapy, *Semin Oncol* 21:4, 1994.

73. List MA and others: Quality of life and performance in advanced head and neck cancer patients on concurrent chemoradiotherapy: prospective examination, *J Clin Oncol* 17:1020, 1999.

74. London SD and others: Hyperbaric oxygen for the management of radionecrosis of bone and cartilage, *Laryngoscope* 108:1291, 1998.

75. Longman AJ, Braden CJ, Mishel MH: Pattern of association over time of side-effects burden, self-help and self-care in women with breast cancer, *Oncol Nurs Forum* 24:1555, 1997.

76. Loprinzi CL and others: Phase III evaluation of four doses of megestrol acetate as therapy for patients with cancer anorexia and/or cachexia. *J Clin Oncol* 11:762, 1993.

77. McCaughan JS Jr, Williams TE: Photodynamic therapy for endobronchial malignant disease: a prospective fourteen-year study, *J Thorac Cardiovasc Surg* 114:940, 1997.

78. McGinn CJ and others: Treatment of intrahepatic cancers with radiation doses based on a normal tissue complication probability model, *J Clin Oncol* 16:2246, 1998.

79. Meraw SJ, Reeve CM: Dental considerations and treatment of the oncology patient receiving radiation therapy, *J Am Dent Assoc* 129:201, 1998.

80. Mock V and others: Effects of exercise on fatigue, physical functioning and emotional distress during radiation therapy for breast cancer, *Oncol Nurs Forum* 24:991, 1997.

81. Mossman K, Shatzman A, Chencharick J: Long term effects of radiotherapy on taste and salivary function in man, *Int J Radiat Oncol Biol Phys* 8:991, 1982.

82. Murray T and others: Acute and chronic changes in swallowing and quality of life following intraarterial chemoradiation for organ preservation in patients with advanced head and neck cancer, *Head Neck* 20:31, 1998.

83. Noll L, Riese N: Chemical modifiers of radiation therapy. In Dow KH and others, editors: *Nursing care in radiation oncology*, ed 2, Philadelphia, Saunders, 1997.

84. Noyes RD and others: Surgical complications of intraoperative radiation therapy: the Radiation Therapy Oncology Group experience, *J Surg Oncol* 50:209, 1992.

85. O'Rourke ME: Enhanced cutaneous effects in combined modality therapy, *Oncol Nurs Forum* 14:31, 1987.

86. O'Rourke ME, Lee C: Radiation and chemotherapy-associated fatigue, *Clin J Oncol Nurs* 2:151, 1998.

87. Ottery FD, Walsh D, Strawford A: Pharmacologic management of anorexia/cachexia, *Semin Oncol* 25(2 suppl 6):35, 1998.

88. Overholt BF, Panjehpour M, Haydek JM: Photodynamic therapy for Barrett's esophagus: follow-up in 100 patients, *Gastrointest Endosc* 49:1, 1999.

89. Peusch-Dreyer D and others: Management of postoperative radiation injury of the urinary bladder by hyperbaric oxygen (HBO), *Strahlenther Onkol* 174(suppl 3):99, 1998.

90. Piper BF, Lindsey AM, Dodd MJ: Fatigue mechanisms in cancer patients: developing nursing theory, *Oncol Nurs Forum* 14:17, 1987.

91. Plafki C and others: The treatment of late radiation effects with hyperbaric oxygenation (HBO). *Strahlenther Onkol* 174(suppl 3):66, 1998.

92. Pomeroy BD, Keim LW, Taylor RJ: Preoperative hyperbaric oxygen therapy for radiation induced injuries, *J Urol* 159:1630, 1998.

93. Preston FA: Management of oral bleeding caused by thrombocytopenia, *Oncol Nurs Forum* 10:59, 1983.

94. Pu AT, Robertson JM, Lawrence TS: Current status of radiation sensitization by fluoropyrimidines, *Oncology* 9:707, 1995.

95. Ragde H and others: Ten-year disease free survival after transperineal sonography-guided iodine-125 brachyther-apy with or without 45-Gray external beam irradiation in the treatment of patients with clinically localized, low to high Gleason grade prostate carcinoma, *Cancer* 83:989, 1998.

96. Rainey L: Effects of preparatory patient education for radiation oncology patients, *Cancer* 56:1056, 1985.

97. Resche I and others: A dose-controlled study of 153 Am-ethylenediaminetetramethyleneposphonate (EDTMP) in the treatment of patients with painful bone metastases, *Eur J Cancer* 33:1583, 1997.

98. Richards S, Hiratzka S: Vaginal dilatation post pelvic irradiation: a patient education tool, *Oncol Nurs Forum* 13:89, 1986.

99. Rieke JW and others: Oral pilocarpine for radiation-induced xerostomia: integrated efficacy and safety results from two prospective randomized clinical trials, *Int J Radiat Oncol Biol Phys* 31:661, 1995.

100. Robinson RG and others: Strontium 89 therapy for the palliation of pain due to osseous metastases, *JAMA* 274:420, 1995.

101. Roof LM: The use of Vigilon primary wound dressing in the treatment of radiation dermatitis, *Oncol Nurs Forum* 18:133, 1991.

102. Rose MA and others: Identifying patient symptoms after radiotherapy using a nurse-managed telephone interview, *Oncol Nurs Forum* 23:99, 1996.

103. Rosenthal DI and others: A phase I single-dose trial of gadolinium texaphyrin (Gd-Tex), a tumor selective radiation sensitizer detectable by magnetic resonance imaging, *Clin Cancer Res* 5:739, 1999.

104. Rotman M, Aziz H, Wasserman TH: Chemotherapy and irradiation. In Perez CA, Brady LW, editors: *Principles and practice of radiation oncology*, ed 3, Philadelphia, Lippincott-Raven, 1998.

105. Rubin P: Principles of radiation oncology and cancer radiotherapy. In Rubin P, editor: *Clinical oncology for medical students and physicians*, New York, American Cancer Society, 1983.

106. Rubin P, Cooper R, Phillips T, editors: *Radiation biology and radiation pathology syllabus. I, radiation oncology*, Chicago, American College of Radiology, 1975.

107. Saclarides TJ: Radiation injuries of the gastrointestinal tract, *Surg Clin North Am* 77:261, 1997.

108. Safran H and others: Paclitaxel and concurrent radiation therapy for locally advanced adenocarcinomas of the pancreas, stomach, and gastroesophageal junction, *Semin Rad Oncol* 9(2 suppl 1):53, 1999.

109. Schuchter LM: Guidelines for the administration of amifostine, *Semin Oncol* 23:40, 1996.

110. Schuchter LM: Current role of protective agents in cancer treatment, *Oncology* 11:505, 1997.

111. Schultz PN: Hypopituitarism in patients with a history of irradiation to the head and neck area: diagnoses and implications for nursing, *Oncol Nurs Forum* 16:823, 1989.

112. Sedhom LN, Yanni MIY: Radiation therapy and nurses' fears of radiation exposure, *Cancer Nurs* 8:129, 1985.

113. Shrader-Bogen CL and others: Quality of life and treatment outcomes: prostate carcinoma patients' perspectives after prostatectomy or radiation therapy, *Cancer* 79:1977, 1997.

114. Sitton E: Managing side effects of skin changes and fatigue. In Dow KH and others, editors: *Nursing care in radiation oncology,* ed 2, Philadelphia, Saunders, 1997.

115. Sitton E: Nursing implications of radiation therapy. In Itano JK, Taoka KN, editors: *Core curriculum for oncology nursing,* ed 3, Philadelphia, Saunders, 1998.

116. Sitton E: Early and late radiation-induced skin alterations. I, mechanisms of skin changes, *Oncol Nurs Forum* 19:801, 1992.

117. Sitton E: Early and late radiation-induced skin alterations. II, nursing care of irradiated skin, *Oncol Nurs Forum* 19:907, 1992.

118. Smets EM and others: Fatigue and radiotherapy: an experience in patients undergoing treatment, *Br J Cancer* 78:899, 1998.

119. Sonis S, Edwards L, Lucey C: The biological basis for the attenuation of mucositis: the example of interleukin-11, *Leukemia* 13:831, 1999.

120. Sporkin E: A newsletter for radiation therapy patients, *Oncol Nurs Forum* 14(suppl):149, 1987 (abstract).

121. Stephenson JA, Wiley AL: Current techniques in three-dimensional CT simulation and radiation treatment planning, *Oncology* 9:1225, 1995.

122. Strohl RA: The nursing role in radiation oncology: symptom management of acute and chronic reactions, *Oncol Nurs Forum* 15:429, 1988.

123. Strohl RA: Radiation therapy: recent advances and nursing implications, *Nurs Clin North Am* 25:309, 1990.

124. Sur RK: Sucralfate in radiation-induced mucositis, *South Afr Med J* 87:337, 1997.

125. Suzuki K and others: Successful treatment of radiation cystitis with hyperbaric oxygen therapy: resolution of bleeding event and changes of histopathological findings of the bladder mucosa, *Int J Urol Nephrol* 30:267, 1998.

126. Van Drimmelen J, Rollins HF: Evaluation of a commonly used oral hygiene agent, *Nurs Res* 18:327, 1969.

127. Wagner W and others: Treatment of irradiation-induced mucositis with growth factors (rhGM-CSF) in patients with head and neck cancer, *Anticancer Res* 19(1B):799, 1999.

128. Wasserman TH, Rich KM, Drzymala RE: Stereotactic irradiation. In Perez CA, Brady LW editors, *Principles and practice of radiation oncology,* ed 3, Philadelphia, Lippincott-Raven, 1998.

129. Wiley SB: Why glycerol and lemon juice? *Am J Nurs* 69:342, 1969.

130. Woo B and others: Differences in fatigue by treatment methods in women with breast cancer, *Oncol Nurs Forum* 25:915:1998.

131. Woodtli MA, Van Ort S: Nursing diagnoses and functional health patterns in patients receiving external radiation therapy: cancer of the head and neck, *Nurs Diagn* 2:171, 1991.

Chemotherapy

Shirley E. Otto

It is estimated that 1,220,100 people in the United States were newly diagnosed as having cancer in 2000. More than half of these people will receive systemic chemotherapy as a form of treatment because of disease recurrence, as secondary therapy after a local treatment, or for treatment of hematologic disease. The primary focus of chemotherapy is to prevent cancer cells from multiplying, invading adjacent tissue, or developing metastasis.[37, 39]

DEFINITION

Chemotherapy is the use of cytotoxic drugs in the treatment of cancer. It is one of the four treatment modalities (the others being surgery, radiation therapy, and biotherapy) that provide cure, control, or palliation. Chemotherapy is a systemic treatment, rather than localized therapy, such as surgery and radiation therapy. Chemotherapy may be used in five ways:

Adjuvant therapy—a course of chemotherapy used in conjunction with another treatment modality (surgery, radiation therapy, or biotherapy) and aimed at treating micrometastases

Neoadjuvant chemotherapy—administration of chemotherapy to shrink a tumor before it is removed surgically

Primary therapy—the treatment of patients who have localized cancer for which an alternative but less than completely effective treatment is available

Induction chemotherapy—drug therapy given as the primary treatment for patients who have cancer for which no alternative treatment exists

Combination chemotherapy—administration of two or more chemotherapeutic agents to treat cancer; this allows each medication to enhance the action of the other or to act synergistically with it (an example of combination chemotherapy is the widely known MOPP regimen of nitrogen mustard, vincristine [Oncovin], procarbazine, and prednisone, which is used to treat patients with Hodgkin's disease[23])

HISTORICAL PERSPECTIVE

Systemic therapy, in the form of metallic salts (arsenic, copper, lead), began with the Egyptian and Greek civilizations. This practice continued for centuries with limited success. Each generation had its own specific remedy for various illnesses. In the late 1880s some bacterial compounds were developed. However, none of these methods proved reliable and effective in treating these varied illnesses.

Research for chemotherapy began in the early 1900s, when Paul Ehrlich used rodent models of infectious diseases to develop antibiotics. Further developments led to the use of rodents to test potential cancer chemotherapeutic agents. An additional discovery in drug development was made as the result of servicemen's exposure to mustard gas during World War I and World War II. This exposure led to the observation that alkylating agents caused marrow and lymphoid suppression in humans. This experience resulted in the use of these agents to treat Hodgkin's and other lymphomas; the therapy was first attempted at Yale's New Haven Medical Center in 1940. Because of the secret nature of the gas warfare program, the work was not published until 1946. Chemotherapy as a treatment modality was introduced in the late 1950s and became established in medical practice in the 1970s.[23, 39, 90]

Since the start of cytotoxic drug research, thousands of chemical agents have been tested for their ability to destroy cancer cells. More than 200 cytotoxic agents are available for commercial or experimental use with approval by the federal Food and Drug Administration. Research continues to contribute discoveries in the area of chemotherapy as a cancer treatment modality, and as a result of this intensive investigation, new areas have been tapped for further study, such as the use of chemotherapeutic agents as radiosensitizers, chemoprotectants, and compounds to reduce multidrug resistance.[23, 39, 76, 90]

PRINCIPLES OF CHEMOTHERAPY

Cell Generation Cycle

The cell cycle is the sequence of events that results in replication of DNA and equal distribution into daughter cells, a process called *mitosis.* Normal cells and cancer cells go through the same division cycle, which is characterized by the following phases: G_0—resting or dormant phase; G_1—phase in which protein synthesis takes place in preparation for the S-phase–DNA synthesis; and G_2—phase for further protein synthesis in preparation for the M phase—mitosis and cell division. The generation time, or the time it takes a cell to complete the phase or cycle, varies from hours to days. Chemotherapeutic drugs are most active against frequently dividing cells, or in all the phases of the cell cycle except G_0. Normal cells with rapid growth changes that are most commonly affected by chemotherapeutic agents include bone marrow (platelets and red and white blood cells), hair follicles, the mucosal lining of the gastrointestinal (GI) tract, and skin and germinal cells (sperm and ova). Chemotherapy is given according to schedules that have proved most effective for tumor kill and that are planned to allow normal cells to recover.[23, 39, 77, 87]

Tumor Growth

The regulatory mechanism that controls the growth of cancer cells differs from that of normal cells. Unlike normal cells, cancer cells grow by means of a pyramid effect; however, they grow at the same rate as the tissue from which they originated (e.g., breast cancer develops at the same rate of growth as normal breast tissue development). The time required for a tumor mass to reach a certain size is called *doubling time.* Tumors probably have undergone approximately 30 doublings from a single cell before they are clinically detected. Between the seventh and tenth doubling time, the possibility arises for the tumor to shed cells, a process called *micrometastasis.* During the early stages of tumor growth, doubling time is more rapid than at later stages; this pattern of growth is called *gompertzian function.* Tumor cells are more sensitive than normal cells to chemotherapy agents that are toxic to rapidly dividing cells.[50, 76, 90]

Curative treatment for cancer focuses on killing the stem cells responsible for the neoplastic disease clone. In their attempts to understand the growth of tumor cells, investigators are trying to identify tumor-specific stem cells and then determine which cytotoxic drug is most effective against the tumor. Many investigators have tried to increase the efficiency of chemotherapy by using assays to evaluate the tumor clone's response to specific chemotherapy agents.[23]

The roles of tumor growth and cell kinetics are important in understanding the action of cytotoxic therapy. Hematologic diseases, such as leukemia and lymphoma, have many rapidly dividing cells. When chemotherapy is initiated, there is the potential for rapid, extensive cellular destruction because of the nature of the bone marrow stem cells and the rapidly dividing cancer cells.[5, 6, 30] The treatment implications for these diseases and others are discussed later in the chapter. (See Chapter 1 for a detailed discussion of the cell generation cycle and properties of tumor growth.)

FACTORS INFLUENCING CHEMOTHERAPY SELECTION AND ADMINISTRATION

Blood–Brain Barrier

An understanding of the blood–brain barrier (BBB) is essential in comprehending the effects of some chemotherapeutic agents on brain and central nervous system (CNS) tumors. Brain tumors create greater obstacles for treatment by chemotherapy than do other tumors. This is partly because of the existence of the BBB, the tumor's location inside the skull, and the lack of an adequate lymphatic drainage system. Certain metabolites, electrolytes, and chemicals have varying abilities to cross the barrier into the brain. This can have serious implications because certain chemotherapeutic agents (e.g., nitrosureas) have a greater propensity than others for crossing the barrier.[4]

The BBB is made up of cellular structures that can inhibit certain substances from entering the brain or cerebrospinal fluid (CSF). The barrier is formed by continuous supporting cells, particularly astrocytes, and the endothelial cells of brain capillaries, which form intertwining junctions. The passage of substances across the lipid membranes of endothelial cells depends on molecular weight, lipid solubility, and ionization state. Large, water-soluble (e.g., glucose) charged particles and compounds bound to plasma proteins are unable to penetrate the BBB; conversely, small water-soluble chemotherapeutic drugs (carmustine, lomustine, cytarabine), normally excluded from the brain by the BBB, may reach enhancing areas of the tumor. In many cases the BBB acts as a screening device, protecting the brain and CSF from harmful particles or agents, although the exact nature of this mechanism is unknown. The permeability of the BBB can be inconsistent throughout the tumor; it tends to be greater in or near the center of the tumor, where the blood supply usually is diminished. In addition, there frequently is a slowly dividing tumor core containing tumor cells that are not identical and therefore are prone to drug resistance (Fig. 23–1).[4, 83, 87, 90]

Chemotherapy drug administration via the intrathecal route (Ommaya reservoir) effectively bypasses the BBB and permits delivery of drugs directly into the CSF. This intrathecal method (Ommaya reservoir or lumbar puncture) allows access to the CNS for drug (analgesia and chemotherapy) administration and permits sampling of the CSF. Intrathecal drug administration provides more consistent drug levels in the CSF, thereby increasing cell kill in primary or metastatic tumors located in the brain.[4, 59, 83, 106]

Chemoprevention

Chemoprevention is the study of prevention in the development of cancer in humans. Currently there are four major approaches to cancer prevention. *Primary prevention* involves reducing the risk of cancer by eliminating or limiting exposure to agents that cause cancer, such as chemicals, radiation exposure, or viruses. Addi-

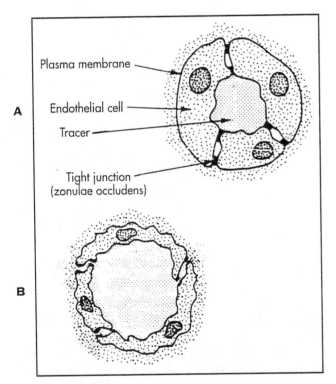

FIGURE 23-1 Schematic representation of the blood–brain barrier. **A,** Normal cerebral capillary showing tight junctions. **B,** Blood–brain barrier opening created by widening of the interendothelial tight junctions. When the endothelial cells shrink in a hypertonic environment, the permeability of the junctions increases. (From Groenwald SL and others: *Cancer nursing: principles and practice,* ed 4, Jones & Bartlett Publishers, Sudbury, MA. Reprinted with permission. 1997.)

In the figure, the labels read: Plasma membrane, Endothelial cell, Tracer, Tight junction (zonulae occludens), with panels marked **A** and **B**.

tionally the individual needs to participate in health promotion activities that *decreases* the individual's cancer risk: healthy diet, scheduled exercise, and avoiding tobacco products. *Secondary prevention* is the screening of individuals who are at increased risk for a particular malignancy in hopes of increasing their chances of survival with early detection and treatment. The American Cancer Society recommendations for health-wellness practices for certain individuals include monthly self-breast examination, annual clinical breast examination, mammogram, gynecologic examination, annual digital rectal examination with prostate-specific antigen, and colorectal tests. Recent advances in genetic testing have made it possible to determine an individual's inherited cancer susceptibility, and this information is valuable in determining the populations that would benefit from early preventive interventions. *Tertiary prevention* is targeted to individuals who have survived a cancer disease and assists them to retain an optimal level of functioning regardless of their potential disabling condition.[33, 34, 58, 97]

Chemoprevention via a pharmacologic intervention refers to the concept of reducing cancer risk in individuals who are highly susceptible to certain cancers by prescribing certain natural or chemical synthetic products or chemotherapy drugs that may reduce or suppress the process of carcinogenesis. The development of cancer can be the result of a chemical, physical, or genetic insult to a cell. Carcinogenesis is a stepwise process that begins at the genetic level and progresses with cellular changes that initiate and promote the development of a malignancy. Chemoprevention seeks to arrest the process of carcinogenesis before the tumor develops.[23, 33, 58]

Early work in the area of chemoprevention focused on the results of epidemiologic studies, which indicated that some substances that occur naturally in the diet were related to a decreased cancer incidence (vitamin A, vitamin E, aspirin, calcium, and selenium). This area of work in chemoprevention began in the 1980s, examining selective compounds. Originally the number of compounds thought to have an inhibitory effect on cancer was believed to be very large. The majority of the early prevention studies focused on the cancer-chemopreventive effect on epithelial tissue sites such as oral cavity, skin, bladder, lung, breast, and prostate.[33, 34, 58, 65]

Chemoprevention trials generally are conducted in noncancer populations more than in populations at high risk for the development of cancer. The phases of chemoprevention drug trials follow the same pattern of investigation and progression as other chemotherapy drug trials: phase Ia, single drug dose; phase Ib, continuing drug dose; phase IIa, dose deescalation and fixed-dose single-arm trials, surrogate end-point biomarkers; IIb, randomized, placebo-controlled, double-blind trials; III, definitive, cancer incidence end-point. Each phase of the trial may vary from weeks, to months, and or years to complete before clinical efficacy is determined.[33, 34, 58]

Today, under the National Cancer Institute's Chemoprevention Program, more than 400 possible chemoprevention agents are being studied, including 50 compounds in more than 100 clinical trials. Important points being reviewed are the drug's efficacy and safety and the overall potential of its chemoprevention properties. The population of trial subjects includes those at high risk for specific cancers (breast, prostate, colorectal, melanoma) as well as subjects from the general population. "Designer estrogens" appear to be the new focused attention of the clinical researchers. These selective estrogen-receptor modulators appear to act as potent estrogen agonists in some tissues but as estrogen antagonists in other tissues. "Aromatase inhibitors" are the second group of drugs gaining research attention via their selectivity in depriving the "breast cancer tumor" of estrogen, thereby exhibiting cell kill. These new compounds are undergoing clinical trials in the prevention of breast cancer for certain individuals. Finasteride (inhibits the conversion of testosterone to its active metabolite dihydrotestosterone) has been used in the largest phase III trial (Prostate Cancer Prevention) ever conducted in the United States.[23, 26, 28, 31, 42, 47, 97] (Refer to Chapters 7 and 10 for detailed information regarding cancer prevention trials for breast and prostate cancers).

The role of chemoprevention in cancer care of the future is both exhilarating and challenging. There is now a significant interest in the biochemical and biologic mechanisms of cancer development. A concerted effort continues to develop new methods of identifying those individuals who are at greatest risk and in turn to counsel those individuals in the areas of genetics, adjustment of life-styles, and avoidance of environmental factors. Chemoprevention as an area of study holds the promise of reducing cancer morbidity and mortality through early intervention, before carcinogenesis occurs or progresses to invasive disease.[40, 58, 97]

Chronotherapy/Circadian Rhythm

Circadian rhythm is a term used to describe a regular, repeated fluctuation in biologic functions during a 24-hour period. The term often is used in conjunction with the term *diurnal*, which refers to "events happening in the daytime." In the many ongoing physiologic mechanisms that occur in the human body, many variables are affected by circadian rhythms. These *circadian variables* can influence drug absorption, metabolism, distribution, and elimination.[51, 52, 74]

One of several possible examples is hepatic blood flow, which can be a major factor in the clearance of lipophilic, rapidly metabolized drugs. Age-related changes occur in hepatic function, such as a decrease in liver size, a decline in the number of functioning hepatocytes, less hepatic blood flow, and less ability to metabolize drugs. Today, chronotherapy using antineoplastic agents is a relatively new strategy. Its purpose is to allow both dose intensification of the drug and reduction of cytotoxic side effects. Previous studies have revealed "time-dependent variations for both toxic side effects and therapeutic drug efficacy." Circadian variations are evident in several human parameters, such as DNA synthesis in the intestinal mucosal tissue, skin, bone marrow, spleen, testis, and thymus tissue. The numbers of circulating leukocytes, lymphocytes, erythrocytes, and platelets are not constant but are subject to diurnal fluctuations. Likewise, high-amplitude circadian rhythms in the epithelium of the human gut show the greatest DNA synthetic activity occurring each day at approximately 7 AM, fasting or nonfasting.[19, 51, 52, 66]

Clinical trials conducted in this country and abroad thus far have sought to determine the benefit/risk ratio and efficacy of chemotherapeutic chronotherapy versus continuous infusion. Chronotherapy allows a subject to receive scheduled drug delivery at specific, predetermined time slots during a 24-hour period: short-term infusion for 30 minutes at 4 AM, or 6 AM, or 4 PM, or 6 PM; continuous infusion times included variations: 6 PM to 3 AM, or 3 AM to 6 PM. Prior investigations determined that the therapeutic indices of these drugs can be affected by varying the timing of drug delivery, whereas a continuous, steady-rate infusion of antineoplastic agents can be a means of increasing antitumor activity with reduced toxicity. This is because a constant supply of the drug provides continuous exposure to the cancer cells and thus increases the probability of cytotoxic damage. An additional benefit is the avoidance of peak drug concentrations, which should minimize host cell injury.[19, 51, 52, 66]

Drugs, such as fluorouracil, doxorubicin, cisplatin, and interferon, have been used in multiple circadian rhythm clinical trials for solid tumor diseases such as breast, colorectal, endometrial, and renal cell cancers. The circadian scheduling of drug administration allowed an increase in dose intensity while reducing toxicities (e.g., anemia, diarrhea, nausea, neutropenia, and stomatitis). Further clinical trials in the area of chronotherapy should investigate efficacy, toxicities, and drug dosing limits. This therapy's role in the treatment of cancer could allow maximum dosing for antitumor effect while limiting harmful toxicities.[19, 28, 50, 62, 74, 80]

Cytoprotectants

This new category of drugs has emerged in the past decade. Cytoprotectants are used to prevent or decrease specific system (e.g., cardiotoxicity, nephrotoxicity, bladder toxicity, and hemopoietic toxicity) related to certain drug therapies. These drugs selectively protect normal tissues from the cytotoxic effects of drugs or irradiation while preserving their antitumor effects. *Usual* administration and monitoring guidelines for cytoprotectants include:*

1. Follow the specific manufacturer's guidelines related to preparation, reconstitution, and timed infusion administration components.
2. Administer the cytoprotectant *30 to 60 minutes prior* to the chemotherapy and radiation therapy treatment. The optimal time to administer some of the chemoprotectants remains to be defined.
3. Refer to the manufacturer's product literature regarding drug specificity side effects such as nausea, vomiting, transient hypotension, warm flushed feeling, diarrhea, and joint pain.

The current cytoprotectant drugs and their respective system toxicity include[102, 104, 108]:

- Dexrazoxane (Zinecard) used to prevent or decrease doxorubicin-associated cardiotoxicity
- Mesna (Mesnex) used to prevent or decrease hemorrhagic cystitis induced by ifosfamide (Ifex) and cyclophosphamide (Cytoxan).
- Amifostine (Ethyol) is used as a pancytoprotectant and to decrease cumulative renal toxicity associated with repeated administration of cisplatin in patients with ovarian and non–small-cell lung cancer.

Cytoprotectants offer many patients with cancers such as breast, non–small-cell lung, or ovarian, or those patients requiring chemotherapy dose-intensification therapy for peripheral blood stem cell or marrow transplantation, an improved quality of life. Multiple clinical drug trials are currently in process and future trials will continue to explore new drugs, different drug combinations, and dosing guidelines related to drug infusion, initiation, duration, and frequency of dosing schedule. As chemotherapy-dose intensification therapy options increase and become available to more patients, chemoprotectants offers a much-desired multisystem toxicity protection.†

Liposomes

Liposomes, microscopic spherical structures that are formed when phospholipids are placed in water, were initially discovered in the early 1960s by the British scientist, Alec Bangham. Following the discovery, this new concept received extensive investigation by biophysicists, biochemists, and the pharmaceutical and medical industries. The Greek roots of the word liposome mean *fat body,* yet a more precise definition describes them as hollow structures made of phospholipids—the same molecule that form the membrane of *all* animal cells. A number of skin care products that describe the benefits of liposomes in reducing the signs of the aging process can be found in varied cosmetic, lotion, and cream skin care products.[5, 63, 70, 78]

Advances in liposome technology used for drug delivery purposes are that the drugs can be manipulated and tailored to penetrate specific target tissues. Some of the specific designed technology (antifungal and antitumor antibiotic drugs) has been labeled as STEALTH technology for the "drug package" and "drug delivery" system. This novel system allows more drug to penetrate the targeted tissue (cancer cells) with an increased dose delivery specificity, while minimizing drug side effects at or near the adjacent tissue.[63, 70, 78]

Chemotherapy drugs currently being investigated or approved (Doxil—doxorubicin HCL liposome, DaunoXome—daunorubicin liposome, Evacet—doxorubicin) are used for patients with AIDS-related Kaposi's sarcoma and breast and ovarian cancers. Mucositis, nausea, vomiting, lumbar pain, skin rash, and headache were the most frequent reported side effects. Drug-related myelosuppression and vesicant extravasation that are usually associated with antitumor antibiotics (daunorubicin, doxorubicin) were not as evident or cumulative with the above-mentioned drugs. Administration guidelines include: *DO NOT* mix with other drugs or use an in-line filter, follow manufacturer's preparation and infusion time guidelines, premedications are not necessary, and if an untoward clinical event occurs during drug infusion, stop the infusion immediately.[63, 69, 70, 77–79]

The other category of new liposome drugs are the antifungal agents. Traditionally amphotericin-B has been a long-standing drug used for treatment of fungal infections for the immunosuppressed patient. This drug has been very effective regarding organism treatment specificity, but the accompanying side effects related to nephrotoxicity, neurotoxicity, fever, chills, and bone pain have limited its use in some patients. Current liposomal antifungal agents in use include Abelcet, AmBisome, and Amphotec. These drugs have specificities regarding diluent (e.g., D_5W only), test dose requirements, infusion initiation, and time duration; *NOT* mixing with other drugs, solutions, or products; and ongoing system monitoring requirements. The drug-related side effects include moderate fever and chills, transient hypotension, skin rash, nausea, and a dose-dependent renal toxicity.[63, 69, 70, 78, 79]

Radiosensitizers

The use of concomitant continuous infusion chemotherapy (CCIC) and radiation therapy in the treatment of

---

* References 65, 73, 78, 96, 102, 108.
† References 57, 61, 73, 79, 96, 102, 106, 108.

a variety of tumors has produced substantial improvement in complete response and survival rates. The emphasis in chemotherapeutics has been directed toward treatment of systemic metastases, with seemingly less interest shown in improving the cure of local and local/regional disease. The goal of radiotherapy is to achieve maximum tumor cell kill while minimizing injury to normal tissues; this is called the *therapeutic ratio*. Efforts to improve the therapeutic ratio have led to the development of certain compounds called *radiosensitizers*.[20, 35, 48]

Radiosensitizers are compounds that enhance the sensitivity of tumors to the effects of radiation, but not normal tissue. This concept includes administering concomitant chemotherapy at cytotoxic doses followed by radiotherapy that allows better control on micrometastases and better local control on the tumor due to radiosensitization by the chemotherapy drugs. Initially, in 1930s radiosensitization was attempted with oxygen and progressed to using hyperbaric oxygen in 1950s. Well-oxygenated tumors are more responsive to radiation and more radiosensitive than poorly oxygenated tumors. The 1950s and 1960s brought systemic chemicals that changed the DNA structure and enhanced radiation response. The first hypoxic cell sensitizers were used in the 1970s and 1980s. It was thought that if irradiation and chemotherapy were administered concurrently, treatment could be enhanced by the biochemical or molecular interactions that occur between them. This led to clinical use of the halogenated pyrimidines: iododeoxyuridine, bromodeoxyuridine, and fluorodeoxyuridine. The toxicities caused by combining these early drugs with irradiation were so severe that interest turned to the use of chemotherapeutic agents as radiosensitizers.[20, 23, 35]

Today patients often receive combination treatment with radiation therapy and chemotherapy at some point in their management. The combination of radiation therapy and chemotherapy has potential benefit for patients. It may be part of a planned protocol, may be used when patients who have not responded to one modality are rescued by treatment with another, or may be used to reduce radioresistance. Clinical trials are under way for various malignancies using concomitant chemotherapy and radiation therapy.[2, 43, 48, 73, 89, 91]

Important principles and definitions in chemotherapy include:

1. *Spatial cooperation* is the ability of one agent to control disease spatially missed by the other, such as the practice of administering chemotherapy to eradicate micrometastases that are outside the radiation field.
2. *Radiosensitizers* are compounds that apparently promote fixation of the free radicals produced by radiation damage at the molecular level.
3. *Radioprotection* involves using drugs that may protect against radiation damage to normal tissue.

4. It has been postulated that the drug and irradiation have a direct interaction within the tumor, producing greater cell kill than would be expected with either modality used alone.

When a drug is selected to be used with radiation therapy, the drug's pharmacokinetics and the tumor cell kinetics are important considerations. Many chemotherapeutic agents are active in the cell during the phase of DNA synthesis. In some tumors this phase of the cell cycle is relatively short, and these chemotherapeutic agents usually have short half-lives; therefore bolus administration of the drug, with its rapid clearance, does not usually provide adequate exposure of the drug during this critical time in the cell cycle. The response to any chemotherapy is proportional to the serum concentration of the drug and the duration of exposure.[38, 43, 48, 73, 89, 91]

If the tumor is one in which the DNA synthesis phase can vary from minutes to hours, prolonged drug exposure ensures that adequate amounts of the drug are present during the critical period. To achieve this, a continuous infusion is the route of choice, especially if the chemotherapeutic agent has a short half-life or is characterized by low cellular uptake or rapid cellular excretion. In addition, continuous infusion usually has low hematologic potential because no peak drug concentrations occur, as happens with a bolus administration.[38]

The mechanism of action that occurs with chemotherapy and irradiation is not well known. One school of thought is that the separate effect of each modality may have an added therapeutic impact on the tumor. Several studies support radiosensitizers as repair inhibitors; that is, they have the potential to increase the amount of residual DNA and chromosome damage after irradiation thus targeting the S-phase cell component. Induction of DNA damage in all phases of the cell cycle by irradiation could create DNA sites for drug incorporation possibly inducing cell kill in cells outside the S phase.[38, 43, 48, 89, 91]

Many classes of drugs have been found to interact with irradiation. Amifostine, 5-fluorouracil (5-FU), cisplatin, doxorubicin, docetaxel, fludarabine, gemcitabine, hydroxyurea, and paclitaxel have been documented and evaluated as radiosensitizers. Initially, 5-FU was developed in 1957 and since has been widely used in the treatment of breast and GI cancers. Various clinical studies have demonstrated that doses of radiotherapy that were growth inhibitory but not curative in rodents could be made curative by adding 5-FU. The exact mechanism of 5-FU and radiation therapy interaction is unknown. 5-FU is a pyrimidine analog that inhibits the synthesis of DNA. It also is taken up into the cell and combines with RNA, which leads to defective RNA synthesis.[38, 89, 94]

Cisplatin is used as a radiation sensitizer, but its mechanism of action is also elusive. Covalent links are formed between cisplatin, DNA, and RNA. In the presence of irradiation, these links break down. Doxorubicin inhibits mitochondria and enzymatic repair of breaks in the DNA strands. The combination of doxorubicin and irradiation is synergistic at low doses. Despite many reports that the radiation-doxorubicin combination is well tolerated, its use has been avoided. Many believed that it was cardiotoxic and was associated with increased enteritis, esophagitis, and a recall reaction.[10, 20, 38, 94]

Several studies have been done to evaluate the efficacy of other chemotherapeutic agents as radiosensitizers, including amifostine, docetaxel, fludarabine, gemcitabine, hydroxyurea, and paclitaxel. The increasing use of CCIC with radiotherapy has provided clinicians with a wealth of information on the ability of radiosensitizers to improve the response rate in treating all but the most advanced carcinomas of the anus, bladder, esophagus, non–small-cell lung, and rectum. Gains also have been demonstrated with dose enhancement using CCIC in soft-tissue sarcomas and multiple solid tumors. In certain gynecologic and colon malignancies, when liver metastasis is anticipated, it is not unreasonable to suggest the use of 5-FU infusion and radiation therapy not only for the primary tumor and lymph nodes, but also for the liver.[38, 43, 89, 91]

Radiation therapy and CCIC used in the treatment of a variety of tumors has produced substantial improvement in the complete response and survival rates. Current research is aimed at defining the required total dosing, fractionation of irradiation, optimal concentration of drugs, and proper scheduling of the infusion. Randomized trials are needed to answer these and other questions about long-term toxicity. This form of therapy has had a major positive impact on survival and organ preservation and in reducing the need for radical surgery.[38, 43, 89, 91]

CHEMOTHERAPY DRUG CLASSIFICATION

Chemotherapeutic agents are classified according to their pharmacologic action and their interference with cellular reproduction. Following are the basic groups and their potential action.[32, 45, 85]

Cell cycle phase-specific drugs are active on cells undergoing division in the cell cycle; examples include antimetabolites, vinca plant alkaloids, and miscellaneous agents such as asparaginase and dacarbazine. These drugs are most effective against actively growing tumors that have a greater proportion of cells cycling through the phase in which the drug attacks the cancer cell. Cell cycle phase-specific drugs are given in minimal concentration via continuous dosing methods.

Cell cycle phase-nonspecific drugs are active on cells in either a dividing or resting state; examples include alkylating agents, antitumor antibiotics, nitrosureas, hormone and steroid drugs, and miscellaneous agents such as procarbazine. These agents are active in all phases of the cell cycle and may be effective in large tumors that have few active cells dividing at the time of administration. Drugs of this nature are often given as single bolus injections.

The mechanism of most chemotherapeutic drugs is targeting of the cell DNA in some manner. This action may result in direct interference with the DNA, inhibition of enzymes related to RNA or DNA synthesis or both, or destruction of the cells' necessary proteins.[23, 40, 90]

A general description of each drug classification follows, and detailed information about the specific drugs in each class can be found in Appendix 23-A at the end of this chapter.

Alkylating agents are cell cycle phase-nonspecific. They act primarily to form a molecular bond with the nucleic acids, which interferes with nucleic acid duplication, preventing mitosis. This category of drugs has a phase activity similar to that observed in radiation therapy, with two peaks of maximum lethal activity, one in G_2 to M phase and one near the G_1 to S phase boundary.

Antibiotics (*antitumor agents*) are cell cycle phase-nonspecific. These drugs disrupt DNA transcription and inhibit DNA and RNA synthesis.

Antimetabolites are cell cycle phase-specific. They exhibit their action by blocking essential enzymes necessary for DNA synthesis or by becoming incorporated into the DNA and RNA, so that a false message is transmitted.

Hormones are cell cycle phase-nonspecific. These chemicals, which are secreted by the endocrine glands, alter the environment of the cell by affecting the cell membrane's permeability. By manipulating hormone levels, tumor growth can be suppressed. Hormone therapies are not cytotoxic and therefore not curative. Their purpose is to prevent cell division and further growth of hormone-dependent tumors.

Antihormonal agents derive their antineoplastic effect from their ability to neutralize the effect of or inhibit the production of natural hormones used by hormone-dependent tumors.

Nitrosureas are cell cycle phase-nonspecific. They have the ability to cross the BBB. Their action is similar to that of the alkylating agents; synthesis of both DNA and RNA is inhibited.

Corticosteroids exert an anti-inflammatory effect on body tissues (e.g., they reduce intracranial or spinal cord compression and suppress lymphocytes). They may also promote a feeling of well-being and increase the appetite.

Vinca plant alkaloids are cell cycle phase-specific. They exert a cytotoxic effect by binding to microtubular proteins during metaphase, causing mitotic arrest. The cell loses its ability to divide and so dies.

Miscellaneous agents may be cell cycle phase-specific or nonspecific or both. These drugs act by a variety of mechanisms. For example, L-asparaginase is unique because it is an enzyme product that acts primarily by inhibiting protein synthesis.

Cell Kill Hypothesis

A single cancer cell is capable of multiplying and eventually killing the host. Every tumor cell must be killed to cure cancer. With each course of the drug therapy, a given dose of chemotherapeutic drug kills only a fraction, not all, of the cancer cells present (Fig. 23–2). Repeated courses of chemotherapy must be used to reduce the total number of cancer cells. This cardinal rule of chemotherapy—the inverse relationship between cell number and curability—was established by Skipper and colleagues in the early 1960s.[23, 40, 90]

Factors Considered in Drug Selection

Patient's eligibility for chemotherapy (confirmed diagnosis; age; bone marrow, nutritional, cardiac, hepatic, respiratory, and renal status; expectation of longevity; history of chemotherapy and radiation therapy)[23, 81]

Cancer cell type (e.g., squamous cell, adenocarcinoma)

Rate of drug absorption (e.g., treatment interval and routes—oral, intravenous, intraperitoneal)[14, 30]

Tumor location (many drugs do not cross the BBB)[4, 64, 83]

Tumor load (larger tumors are generally less responsive to chemotherapy)[49]

Tumor resistance to chemotherapy (tumor cells can mutate and produce variant cells distinct from the tumor stem cell of origin)[2, 5, 6]

Combination Chemotherapy

Chemotherapeutic drugs are most often given in combination because this enhances the effect of the drugs on the tumor cell kill. Considerations for drugs used in combination include verified effectiveness as a single agent, results in increased tumor cell kill, increased patient survival, presence of a synergistic action, varied toxicities, different mechanisms of action, and administration in repeated courses to minimize the immunosuppressive effects that might otherwise occur. Combination chemotherapy provides additional benefits that are not possible with single-drug treatment, such as maximal cell kill within the range of toxicity tolerated by the host for each drug, a broader range of coverage of resistant cell lines in a heterogeneous tumor population, and prevention or slowing of the development of new resistant lines.[2, 49, 60, 61, 64]

Because numerous cellular variants exist within a metastasis by the time it is detected, therapy for metastatic disease often is directed toward characteristics of the secondary tumor rather than those of the primary tumor. Using combination chemotherapy rather than single sequential therapy maximizes the therapeutic response by addressing the diversity of cellular response.

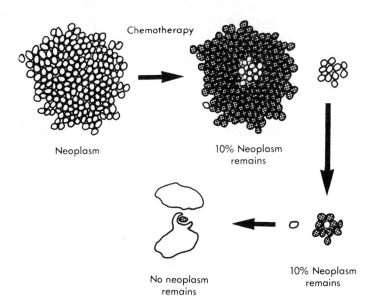

Neoplasm

10% Neoplasm remains

10% Neoplasm remains

No neoplasm remains

FIGURE 23–2 Cell kill hypothesis. (From Goodman MS: *Cancer: chemotherapy and care,* Evansville, IN, Bristol Laboratories, Bristol-Myers Co.)

BOX 23-1

Combination Chemotherapy Regimens

Breast Cancer

CMF—cyclophosphamide, methotrexate, 5-fluoro-
  uracil
FUVAC—5-fluorouracil, vinblastine, Adriamycin, cyclophosphamide

Lung Cancer

CAV—cisplatin, Adriamycin, vinblastine
CAMP—cyclophosphamide, Adriamycin, methotrexate, procarbazine

Hodgkin's Disease

ABVD—Adriamycin, bleomycin, vinblastine, dacarbazine
MOPP—nitrogen mustard, Oncovin, prednisone, procarbazine

Lymphoma

CHOP-BLEO—cyclophosphamide, Adriamycin, Oncovin, prednisone, bleomycin
Transplantation: BEAC—BCNU, etoposide, cytosine
  arabinoside, cyclophosphamide

Testicular Cancer

VBP—vinblastine, bleomycin, cisplatin
VPV—VP-16 (etoposide), cisplatin, vinblastine

See examples of commonly used combination therapies in Box 23–1.

CHEMOTHERAPY ADMINISTRATION

Calculation of Drug Dosage

The drug dosage for cancer chemotherapy is based on body surface area (BSA) in both adults and children. The dosages of some drugs are calculated proportionally to the patient's BSA. BSA is calculated in square meters (m^2). A nomogram is used to correlate height with weight to determine the BSA. Ensure that an accurate patient height and weight is obtained on a scheduled frequency. Fluctuations in weight may occur because of side effects of chemotherapy drugs from anorexia, nausea, and vomiting. The drug dose is ordered in milligrams per square meter. All drug calculations should be verified by a second person to ensure accuracy of the dose. The dosage range of a drug may vary with different drug regimens.[15, 16, 22, 36, 95]

Drug Reconstitution

Pharmacy staff should reconstitute all drugs and pre-prime the intravenous (IV) tubings under a class II biologic safety cabinet. In certain conditions (the drug has short-term stability after mixing and the required administration time is unknown, as is the case with intrathecal injection of methotrexate using preservative-free diluent), nurses may be required to reconstitute medications. When the drugs are prepared and reconstituted, aseptic technique must be used in accordance with manufacturer's current recommendations. All syringes of reconstituted drugs are immediately labeled with the name of the drug. Many chemotherapeutic agents are colorless and cannot be distinguished from one another after reconstitution (see Safe Handling of Chemotherapeutic Agents, page 653).[3, 85, 101]

Administration Guidelines

Routes[29, 36, 72]

Oral route. Emphasize the importance of the patient's complying with the prescribed schedule. Plan for drugs with emetic potential to be taken with meals; drugs that require hydration (e.g., Cytoxan) need to be taken early in the day.

Subcutaneous and intramuscular route. Demonstration with a return demonstration may be needed if the patient is giving self-injections. Encourage patient to rotate injection sites for each dose and to keep a log of drug dosing schedule.

Topical administration. Cover surface area with a thin film of medication; instruct the patient to wear loose-fitting cotton clothing. Wear gloves and be sure to wash hands thoroughly after procedure. Caution the patient not to touch ointment.

Intra-arterial route. This method requires catheter placement in an artery near the tumor; because of arterial pressure, administer the drug in a heparinized solution through an infusion pump. Throughout the infusion, monitor vital signs, color and temperature of extremity, and potential for bleeding at site. Instruct the patient and family in the care of the catheter and infusion pumps (e.g., routine filling and maintenance of the infusion pump) if chemotherapy is to be given at home.

Intracavity route. Instill the drug into the bladder through a catheter or chest tube (or both) into the pleural cavity. Follow prescribed premedication dosage to minimize local irritation.

Intraperitoneal route. Deliver the drug into the abdominal cavity through the implantable port or external suprapubic catheter (e.g., Tenckhoff catheter). Use dry heat to warm the infusate solution to body temperature before administration. Monitor the patient for abdominal pressure, pain, fever, and electrolyte imbalance after the infusion; measure abdominal girth.

Intrathecal route. Reconstitute all intrathecal medications with preservative-free sterile normal saline or sterile water. Medication may be infused through an Ommaya reservoir or implantable pump, if available, or through lumbar puncture. Usually the volume of medication given via an Ommaya reservoir or lumbar puncture is 15 mL or less. Maintain sterile technique throughout the procedure. The medication should be injected slowly. If chemotherapeutic drugs (cytarabine or methotrexate or both) are given in high doses, monitor the patient closely for potential neurotoxicity. *Usually a physician administers intrathecal drugs via an Ommaya reservoir or lumbar puncture.*

Intravenous route. Drugs administered IV may be given through central venous catheters or peripheral venous access. Methods of administration include:

- Push (bolus)—medication is administered through syringe directly into the vein.
- Piggyback (secondary setup)—drug is administered using a secondary bag (bottle) and tubing; primary infusion is concurrently maintained throughout drug administration.
- Side arm—drug is administered through a syringe and needle into the side port of a running (free-flowing) IV infusion.
- Infusion—drug is added to the prescribed volume of fluid in IV bag or bottle. Check for blood return before, during, and after infusion of chemotherapeutic drugs. Follow the agency's guidelines on how often continuous chemotherapeutic infusions are to be monitored. For continuous infusion of a vesicant drug, suggestions include validating blood return every 2 hours; for continuous infusion of a nonvesicant drug, validate blood return every 4 hours.[13, 85]

Vein Selection and Venipuncture. Many chemotherapeutic agents irritate the veins and surrounding tissues. Venipuncture sites must be changed on a planned basis every 48 hours to reduce the possibility of phlebitis and infiltration. Peripheral sites should be changed daily before administration of vesicants. Veins suitable for venipuncture feel smooth and pliable, not hard or sclerotic. Select a vein that is large enough to allow adequate blood flow around the IV device.[3, 17, 32, 53, 84]

Selection of the appropriate site and equipment is determined by the patient's age and vein status, the drugs to be infused, and the expected period of infusion. Observe and palpate the extremity. Use distal veins first, and choose a vein above areas of flexion. The distal veins of the hands and arms should be used first, and subsequent venipuncture should be done proximal to previous sites. Select the shortest catheter with the smallest gauge appropriate for the type and duration of the infusion. Veins commonly used include the basilic, cephalic, and metacarpal veins (Fig. 23–3).

Large veins on the forearm are the preferred site. If a drug extravasates in this area, maximum soft-tissue

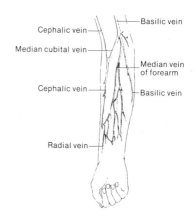

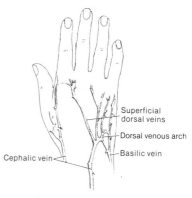

FIGURE 23–3 Venous anatomy. (From Perry AG, Potter PA: *Clinical nursing skills and techniques,* ed 4, St. Louis, Mosby, 1998.)

coverage is present to prevent functional impairment. Do not use the antecubital fossa and the wrist because extravasation in these areas can destroy nerves and tendons, resulting in loss of function.[84, 88, 89]

Procedure for Administering Chemotherapeutic Drugs*

Verify the patient's identification, drug, dose, route, and time of administration with the physician's order.

Review drug allergy history with the patient.

Anticipate and plan for possible side effects or major system toxicity (Tables 23–1 and 23–2).

Review appropriate laboratory data and other tests.

Verify informed consent for treatment.

Select appropriate equipment and supplies.

Calculate the dose and reconstitute the drug using aseptic technique; follow safe handling guidelines.

Explain the procedure to the patient and family.

Administer antiemetics or other prescribed medications.

---

* References 36, 41, 84, 85, 99, 101, 106, 107.

Text continued on page 652

TABLE 23-1

Patient Teaching for Self-Management of Most Common Side Effects from Chemotherapeutic Drugs

Side Effects	Points to Cover
ACHES AND PAINS *Nursing Intervention* Assess location, intensity, quality, and duration of pain.	Pain medication should be taken on a regular and duration of pain schedule. Side effects of pain medicine are constipation, dry mouth, and drowsiness. Rest and relaxation strategies include music, progressive relaxation exercise, distraction, and positive imaging.
ALOPECIA *Hair Loss* Bleomycin, cyclophosphamide, dacarbazine, dactinomycin, daunorubicin, doxorubicin, idarubicin, ifosfamide, irinotecan, mechlorethamine, mitomycin, paclitaxel, teniposide, topotecan, vinblastine, and vinorelbine *Hair Thinning* Bleomycin, etoposide, 5-fluorouracil, floxuridine, and vincristine	Hair loss occurs 10–21 d after drug administration. Hair loss is temporary, and hair will regrow when drug is stopped. Hair loss may occur suddenly and in large amounts; select wig, cap, scarf, or turban before hair loss occurs. Avoid use of hair dryers, curling irons, and harsh or frequent shampoos. Keep the head covered in summer to prevent a severe sunburn and in winter to prevent heat loss.
ANOREXIA *Nursing Intervention* Assess dietary history, monitor serum transferrin levels and weight loss.	Eating is a social event; eat with others in a pleasant area with soft music and attractive settings. Freshen up before meals, with mouth care and exercise, for example. Small, frequent meals (five to six meals daily); avoid drinking fluids with meals to prevent feeling of fullness. Concentrate on eating foods high in protein, such as eggs, milk products, peanut butter, tuna, beans, peas. Breakfast may be the most tolerable meal of the day; try to include one third of daily calories at this time. Monitor and record weight weekly; report weight loss.
CONSTIPATION Drugs associated with potential for: vinblastine, vincristine, vindesine, vinorelbine, and opioids *Nursing Interventions* Determine normal bowel habits; advise the patient not to strain with bowel evacuation, and to respond immediately to the urge to defecate.	Increase intake of high-fiber foods, such as whole-grain products, bran, fresh fruit, raw vegetables, popcorn. Increase fluid intake to 2–3 qt of liquids daily; encourage fresh fruit juices, prunes, hot liquids on waking. Follow prescribed schedule for use of stool softener; follow prescribed physician orders if no bowel movement for 3 d or more.
CYSTITIS Drug associated with potential for: cyclophosphamide and ifosfamide *Nursing Interventions* Observe urine for color and amount, and assess frequency of voiding; advise patient to take oral cyclophosphamide early in the day. Verify physician order for administration of mesna.	Increase fluid intake to 3 qt daily Empty bladder at least every 4 h, especially at bedtime and at least once during the night. Promptly report to the physician increasing symptoms and frequency of bleeding, burning, pain, fever, and chills.
DEPRESSION *Nursing Intervention* Assess for changes in mood or affect	Set small goals that are achievable daily. Participate in enjoyable and diversionary activities, such as music, meditations, reading, outings. Share feelings and concerns with someone.
DIARRHEA Drugs with potential for: 5-fluorouracil, irinotecan, methotrexate *Nursing Intervention* Monitor serum electrolytes and fluid intake and number, color, frequency, and consistency of diarrhea stools.	Avoid eating high-roughage, greasy, and spicy foods. Avoid using milk products or use boiled skim milk. Avoid caffeine and alcoholic products. Eat a bland diet. Increase fluid intake to 3 qt of liquids daily (weak, tepid tea, bouillon, grape juice).

TABLE 23-1

Patient Teaching for Self-Management of Most Common Side Effects from Chemotherapeutic Drugs *Continued*

Side Effects	Points to Cover
	Record number and consistency of daily bowel movements; report information to the physician. Follow prescribed medication schedule if problem persists beyond 1 d. Cleanse rectal area after each bowel movement.
FATIGUE *Nursing Intervention* Assess for possible causes (anemia, chronic pain, stress, depression, and insufficient rest or nutritional intake).	Conserve energy; rest when tired; plan rest periods. Plan for gradual accommodation of activities into life-style. Monitor dietary and fluid intake daily.
HEMATOPOIETIC CHANGES: LEUKOPENIA Most myelosuppressive agents produce white blood cell (WBC) nadir 7–14 d after drug administration; myelosuppression will be severe and prolonged with increased dosages: for example, with cytarabine 3–6 g; busulfex 2–6 g; cyclophosphamide 2–3 g; methotrexate 6–8 g; etoposide 2–3 g. *Nursing Intervention* Monitor WBC and differential; change equipment as indicated—for example, O₂ setup, denture cups, IV supplies; teach sexual hygiene.	Avoid sources of infection, such as people with bacterial infections, colds, sore throats, flu, chickenpox, measles, or cold sores or people recently vaccinated with live vaccines such as measles-mumps-rubella (MMR) or diphtheria-pertussis-tetanus (DPT). Avoid having fresh fruit, live plants, and flowers at or near bedside. Avoid eating raw vegetables, fruits, and eggs. Avoid cleaning animal litter boxes because feces contain high levels of bacteria and fungi. Maintain good personal hygiene—for example, bathe daily, wash hands before eating and preparing food, clean carefully after bowel movements, and keep nails clean and clipped short and straight across; maintain adequate fluid intake. Conserve energy; get adequate rest and exercise. Prevent trauma to the skin and mucous membranes. Avoid elective dental work or surgery. Avoid enemas, rectal suppositories and temperatures, and catheterizations. Use toothettes or nonabrasive dental cleaning devices. Report signs and symptoms of infection immediately to the physician; for example, report fever of 38°C or greater, cough, sore throat, a shaking chill, painful or frequent urination, or vaginal discharge.
HEMATOPOIETIC CHANGES: THROMBOCYTOPENIA Drugs associated with a delayed cumulative effect: mitomycin and all nitrosureas *Nursing Intervention* Monitor platelet counts; observe bleeding precautions; apply firm pressure to venipuncture site for 3–5 min; monitor pad count on menstruating females; monitor environment for sharp objects.	Avoid use of straight-edge razor, power tools, and physical activity that could cause injury. Avoid use of drugs containing aspirin. Humidify the air; use lotion and lubricants on skin and lips; use a soft bristle toothbrush. Avoid invasive procedures; no intramuscular injections, rectal or vaginal exams, enemas, suppositories, or the use of rectal thermometers. Discourage bare feet when ambulatory. Use sanitary pads instead of tampons. Immediately report the following signs and symptoms to the physician: bleeding gums, increased bruising, petechiae, purpura, hypermenorrhea, tarry-colored stools, blood in urine, or coffee-ground emesis. Check with the physician before any dental work.
HEMATOPOIETIC CHANGES: ANEMIA *Nursing Intervention* Monitor hematocrit and hemoglobin, especially during drug nadir.	Adjust physical activity to accommodate periods of rest. Report the following signs and symptoms promptly to the physician: fatigue, dizziness, shortness of breath, and palpitations.

Table continued on following page

TABLE 23-1

Patient Teaching for Self-Management of Most Common Side Effects from Chemotherapeutic Drugs *Continued*

Side Effects	Points to Cover
MUCOSITIS, RECTAL Symptoms occur 3–5 d after chemotherapy *Nursing Intervention* Monitor for electrolyte imbalance and granulocyte count; monitor number, consistency, and amount of bowel movements and urine output; assess for rectal bleeding.	Report weight loss to physician. Eat low-residue and easily digestible foods. Increase intake of liquids to replace fluid loss. Follow prescribed medication schedule, such as antidiarrheal and pain control drugs. Wash rectal area with soap and water following each bowel movement; pat or air dry.
MUCOSITIS VAGINAL Symptoms occur 3–5 d after chemotherapy and subside in 7–10 d after therapy.	Report pain, ulceration, or bleeding of mucous membranes lining the perineum and vagina to physician. Sitz bath with warm salt water may provide relief of vaginal itching and odor. Use hydrogen peroxide (one-quarter strength) with warm water after voiding to rinse perineal area. Avoid commercial douches, tampons, and vaginal pads or liners containing deodorants.
NAUSEAS AND VOMITING Drugs with high emetic potential: asparaginase, carmustine, cisplatin, dacarbazine, dactinomycin, daunorubicin, doxorubicin, idarubicin, ifosfamide, mechlorethamine, methotrexate, mitoxantrone, procarbazine, streptozocin, teniposide, and high-dose cytarabine, cyclophosphamide, and methotrexate *Nursing Intervention* Premedicate with antiemetic before nausea begins, for example, 30 min before meals; patient may require routine antiemetics for 3–5 d following some chemotherapy protocols; monitor fluid and electrolyte status.	Eat frequent, small meals. Avoid greasy or fatty foods and very sweet foods or candies. Avoid unpleasant sights, odors, and tastes. Cold foods, salty foods, dry crackers, and dry toast may be more tolerable. If vomiting is severe, restrict diet to clear liquids and notify the physician. Consider diversionary activities, such as music therapy and relaxation techniques. Recall strategies that were successful during pregnancy, illness, or other times of stress, for example, sipping on a flat cola drink.
PHARYNGITIS AND ESOPHAGITIS Symptoms are often first noted by difficult or painful swallowing.	Eat a soft pureed or liquid diet. Follow prescribed scheduled medication to relieve discomfort. Report to the physician symptoms that persist more than 3 d.
SKIN CHANGES	Maintain good personal hygiene. Use topical preparations to minimize itching, such as creams or lotions containing vitamins A, D, or E. Avoid use of perfume and perfumed lotion, wearing fabrics such as wool or corduroy, and wearing tight-fitting clothes such as jeans or pantyhose.
STOMATITIS (ORAL) Symptoms occur 5–7 d after chemotherapy and persist up to 10 d.	Continue brushing regularly; use soft toothbrush. Use nonirritant mouthwash, such as salt, soda, and water solution (¼ tsp salt, pinch of soda, 8 oz water) at least four times daily. Avoid irritants to the mouth, such as tobacco, alcoholic beverages, spices, and commercial mouthwashes. Avoid wearing dentures until mouth soreness heals. Maintain good nutritional intake; eat soft or liquid foods high in protein; add sauces or gravies in foods to make food soupier. Follow prescribed medication schedule, such as scheduled drugs for oral candidiasis. Report persistent symptoms promptly to physician, and report if white patches occur on tongue, back of throat, or gums.

From Otto SE, editor: Pocket guide to intravenous therapy, ed 4, St. Louis, Mosby, 2001.

TABLE 23-2

Major System Toxicity or Dysfunction and Nursing Management

Toxicity/Dysfunction	Nursing Management
CARDIAC TOXICITY Drugs associated with potential for: chlorambucil, cyclophosphamide, dactinomycin, daunorubicin, doxorubicin, mitoxantrone, and high-dose ifosfamide, paclitaxel	Verify baseline cardiac studies (e.g., ECG, ejection fraction, cardiac enzymes) before drug administration. Monitor cardiac status and report symptoms regarding tachycardia, shortness of breath, distended neck veins, gallop heart rhythm, and ankle edema. Monitor and record total cumulative dose of drug in the patient's medical record; doxorubicin approximate maximum lifetime dose is 500 mg/m^2.
HEMATOPOIETIC TOXICITY (see Table 23–1) **HEPATIC TOXICITY** Drugs associated with potential for: asparaginase, busulfan, carmustine, chlorambucil, cytarabine, doxorubicin, 5-fluorouracil, lomustine, mercaptopurine, methotrexate, mitoxantrone, mithramycin, mitomycin, paclitaxel, and streptozocin	Verify physician order for administration of Zinecard. Monitor liver function studies, such as lactic dehydrogenase (LDH), bilirubin, prothrombin time, and live function tests (SGOT, SGPT) Report to the physician signs of jaundice, tenderness over the liver, and urine and stool color changes.
HYPERSENSITIVITY REACTION Drugs associated with potential for: asparaginase, bleomycin, docetaxel, doxorubicin (local erythema), etoposide, paclitaxel, and teniposide	Review the patient's allergy history. Monitor for symptoms of hypersensitivity and anaphylaxis, such as agitation, urticaria, rash, chills, cyanosis, bronchospasm, abdominal cramping, and hypotension; onset may be rapid or delayed; advise the patient to report subjective symptoms promptly. Ensure proper medical equipment is nearby and in good working condition. Drugs for emergency intervention should be readily available. When administering a drug with potential for a reaction, give a test dose, monitor vital signs, and observe for allergic response. If allergic response occurs, stop drug administration and notify the physician immediately.
METABOLIC ALTERATIONS *Hypercalcemia*	Monitor serum level; observe for anorexia, constipation, nausea, vomiting, polyuria, and mental status change.
Hyperglycemia	Monitor serum and urine levels; observe for symptoms of thirst, hunger, glucosuria, and weight loss.
Hyperkalemia	Monitor serum level: observe for symptoms of confusion, complaints of numbness or tingling, weakness, and cardiac arrhythmias.
Hypernatremia	Monitor serum level and weight loss; observe for symptoms of thirst, dry mucous membranes, poor skin turgor, rapid thready pulse, restlessness, lethargy.
Hyperuricemia Potential with treatment of highly proliferative tumors, such as leukemia and lymphoma	Monitor serum and urine levels; daily intake and output. Initiate prescribed drug therapy (e.g., allopurinol) to inhibit the formation of uric acid before administration of chemotherapy drug. Provide vigorous hydration, such as oral and IV fluid intake (2000–3000 mL), beginning 12–24 h after initiation of chemotherapy. Alkalize urine to pH > 7.0 by administration of IV NaHCO$_3$ (sodium bicarbonate). Report symptoms of pain, chills, fever, and diminished urinary output.
Hypocalcemia	Monitor serum level; observe for symptoms of muscle cramping, tingling of extremities, depression, and tetany.
Hypomagnesemia	Monitor serum level; observe for symptoms of personality changes, anorexia, nausea, vomiting, lethargy, weakness, and tetany.

Table continued on following page

TABLE 23-2
Major System Toxicity or Dysfunction and Nursing Management *Continued*

Toxicity/Dysfunction	Nursing Management
Hyponatremia	Monitor serum level; observe for symptoms of rales, shortness of breath, distended neck vein, weight gain, edema of sacrum or lower extremity, increasing mental status changes.
NEUROTOXICITY Drugs associated with potential for: ifosfamide, vinblastine, vincristine, high peak plasma levels of etoposide, 5-fluorouracil; high-dose and/or intrathecal administration of cytarabine, carboplatin, cisplatin, and methotrexate	Monitor and report symptoms of weakness, numbness, and tingling sensation of hands, arms, and feet; also monitor and report symptoms of hoarseness, jaw pain, hallucinations, mental depression, decreased or absent deep tendon reflexes, slapping gait or footdrop, severe constipation, and paralytic ileus.
OTOTOXICITY Drug associated with potential for: cisplatin	Verify physician order for administration of amifostine (Ethyol). Verify baseline audiogram. Monitor and report symptoms of tinnitus, hearing loss, and vertigo.
PULMONARY TOXICITY Drugs associated with potential for: bleomycin, busulfan, carmustine	Verify baseline respiratory function. Individuals older than age 70 years have increased risk. Monitor respiratory status and report symptoms of dyspnea, dry cough, rales, tachypnea, and fever.
RENAL SYSTEM TOXICITY Drugs associated with potential for: carmustine, cisplatin, cyclophosphamide, ifosfamide, methotrexate, mitomycin C, streptozocin, and thiotepa	Assess 24-h urine creatinine clearance before treatment, 2–3 liters for 24 h before and after therapy. Verify baseline renal function. Encourage adequate fluid intake, such as 2–3 liters for 24 h before and after therapy. Monitor intake and output, weight changes. Report diminished output to physician, e.g., > 500 mL in 24 h. Administer drug mesna concomitant with ifosfamide, high-dose cyclophosphamide, and thiotepa.
REPRODUCTIVE SYSTEM DYSFUNCTION Drugs associated with potential for: busulfan, chlorambucil, cyclophosphamide, mechlorethamine, melphalan, thalidomide, thiotepa, vinblastine, and vincristine Antihormonal agents: fenretinide, finasteride, flutamide, goserelin, letrozole, leuprolide, tamoxifen	Assess for nature and frequency of sexual dysfunction. Counsel patients regarding avoidance of pregnancy and sperm banking before chemotherapy administration; provide information on contraceptives. Birth control practices are recommended by most practitioners for 2 y following chemotherapy to provide for evaluation of disease response, avoidance of possible teratogenic drug effects, and in male patients, recovery of spermatogenesis. Inform the patients of potential for temporary or permanent infertility and loss of libido. Women may experience symptoms including amenorrhea, "hot flashes," insomnia, dyspareunia, and vaginal dryness; estrogen therapy may be helpful in management of these symptoms.

From Otto SE, editor: *Pocket guide to intravenous therapy, ed 4,* St. Louis, Mosby, 2001.

Initiate peripheral IV site or prepare central venous access site.

Administer chemotherapeutic agents.

Monitor the patient at scheduled intervals throughout the course of drug administration.

Dispose of all used supplies and unused drugs in approved, puncture-proof, leak-proof containers outside of patient area.

Document procedure according to agency policy and procedure.

Documentation Recommendations[16, 29, 68, 80, 85]

Site assessment before and after infusion or injection of chemotherapeutic drug

Establishment of blood return before, during, and after IV and intra-arterial infusion of chemotherapy

Establishment of catheter or device patency before, during, and after infusion of chemotherapy (e.g., intraperitoneal, intrathecal administration)

Patient and family education about chemotherapy protocol: potential side effects and toxicities, self-management of side effects, and schedule of follow-up blood counts, tests, and procedures

Chemotherapeutic drug, dose, and route and time administered

Premedications, postmedications, other infusions, and supplies used for chemotherapeutic regimen

Any complaints by the patient of discomfort and symptoms experienced before, during, and after chemotherapeutic infusion

SAFE HANDLING OF CHEMOTHERAPEUTIC AGENTS

The number of chemotherapeutic agents available and their use have increased considerably in recent years. Consequently, concern has emerged among health care workers about potential occupational hazards associated with the handling of these drugs. Clinical studies have indicated that many agents are carcinogenic, mutagenic, and teratogenic, or any combination of the three. Exposure to these chemotherapeutic agents can occur by inhalation, absorption, or digestion. Safe handling guidelines should be followed when implementing policy and procedure within each agency that prepares, administers, stores, or disposes of supplies or unused chemotherapeutic agents.*

Safe handling guidelines cover the following[55, 98, 100, 101].

Drug preparation
Drug administration
Disposal of supplies and unused drugs
Management of spills
Care of patients receiving chemotherapy (e.g., linen contamination, patient's excreta)
Staff education
Employment practice regarding reproductive health

Drug Preparation

To ensure safe handling, all chemotherapeutic drugs should be prepared according to the package insert in a class II biologic safety cabinet (BSC). Venting to the outside is desirable where feasible. Personal protective equipment includes disposable surgical latex gloves and

---

* Recommendations for safe handling of chemotherapeutic drugs are available from the Occupational Safety and Health Administration (OSHA), the National Cytotoxic Study Commission, and the American Society of Hospital Pharmacists.

a gown made of lint-free, low-permeability fabric with a closed front, long sleeves, and elastic or knit cuffs. Eye-protective splash goggles or a face shield must be worn when these drugs are prepared if BSC is not used. Consider the use of multiple latex-free products for personnel who experience latex allergies.[55, 84, 85, 86, 101]

Gloves should be changed between preparation and administration of the drug and at least every 30 minutes during preparation and administration. Suggestions to minimize exposure include:

Wash hands before and after drug handling.
Limit access to drug preparation area.
Keep labeled drug spill kit near preparation area.
Put on gloves before handling drugs.
Use aseptic technique when preparing drugs.
Avoid eating, drinking, chewing gum, applying cosmetics, or storing food in or near drug preparation area.
Place absorbent pad on work surface.
Use Luer-Lok equipment.
Open drug vials and ampules away from body.
Vent vials with a hydrophobic filter needle or pin to prevent spraying of drug.
Wrap alcohol wipe around neck of ampule before opening.
Prime lines containing drugs inside BSC using original drug vial or a zip-close plastic bag.
Cover tip of needle with sterile gauze or alcohol wipe when expelling air from syringe.
Label all chemotherapeutic drugs.
Clean up any spills immediately.
Transport drugs to delivery area in a leak-proof, puncture-proof container.

Drug Administration

Wear protective equipment (gloves, gown, eyewear, Fig. 23–4).
Explain to the patient that chemotherapeutic drugs are harmful to normal cells and that protective measures used by personnel minimize their exposure to these drugs.
Administer drugs in a safe, unhurried environment.
Place a plastic-backed absorbent pad under the tubing during administration to catch any leakage.
Do not dispose of any supplies or unused drugs in patient care areas (see next section).

Disposal of Supplies and Unused Drugs

Do not clip or recap needles or break syringes.
Place all used supplies intact in a leak-proof, puncture-proof, appropriately labeled container.
Place all unused drugs in containers in a leak-proof, closeable, puncture-proof, appropriately labeled con-

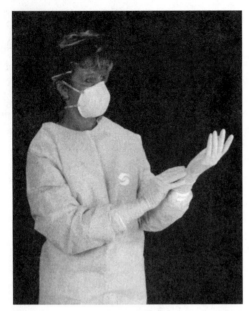

FIGURE 23–4 Woman wearing gloves, gown, eyewear, and mask. (Courtesy Biosafety Systems, Inc., San Diego, CA.)

tainer; keep these containers in every area where drugs are prepared or administered so that waste materials need not be moved from one area to another.

Dispose of containers filled with chemotherapeutic supplies and unused drugs in accordance with regulations of hazardous wastes (e.g., in a licensed sanitary landfill, or incinerate at 1832°F (1000°C).

Management of Chemotherapy Spills

Chemotherapy spills should be cleaned up immediately by properly protected personnel trained in the appropriate procedures. A spill should be identified with a warning sign so that other people will not be contaminated. The following are recommended supplies and procedures for managing a chemotherapy spill on hard surfaces, linens, personnel, and patients.[86, 98, 100, 101]

Supplies

Chemotherapy spill kit (Fig. 23–5)
    Respirator mask for airborne powder spills
    Plastic safety glasses or goggles
    Heavy-duty rubber gloves
    Absorbent pads to contain liquid spills
    Absorbent towels for cleanup after spill
    Small scoop to collect glass fragments
    Two large waste disposal bags
Protective disposable gown
Containers of detergent solution and clear tapwater for cleaning up after the spill

Puncture-proof, leak-proof closeable container approved for chemotherapy waste disposal
Approved, specially labeled, impervious laundry bag.
Eyewash faucet adapters or fountain in or near work area

Procedure for Spill on Hard Surface

Restrict area of spill.
Obtain drug spill kit.
Put on protective gown, gloves, and goggles and, if powder spill is involved, a respirator mask.
Open waste disposal bags (double bag).
Place absorbent pads gently on spill, being careful not to touch it.
Place saturated absorbent pads in waste bag.
Clean surface with absorbent towels using detergent solution and rinse clean with clean tapwater. Wipe dry.
Place all contaminated materials (e.g., gown, gloves, saturated absorbent pads, towels) in double-bagged waste disposal bags.
Discard waste bag and contents in approved container.
Wash hands thoroughly with soap and water.

Procedure for Spill on Linen

Restrict area of spill.
Obtain drug spill kit.
Obtain specially marked, approved laundry bag and labeled, impervious bag.
Put on protective gown, gloves, and goggles.
Remove soiled, contaminated linen from patient's bedside.
Place linen in approved, specially marked, impervious laundry bag.
Contaminated linen should be washed two times in the laundry; laundry personnel should wear surgical latex gloves and gown when handling this material.

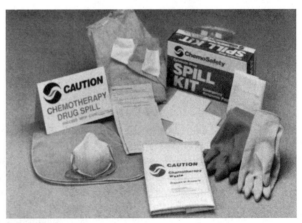

FIGURE 23–5 Chemotherapy spill kit. (Courtesy Biosafety Systems, Inc., San Diego, CA.)

Clean contaminated area with absorbent towels and detergent solution.

Place all contaminated supplies used for management of spill in waste disposal bag and discard in approved waste disposal container.

Wash hands thoroughly with soap and water.

Procedure for Spill on Personnel or Patient

Restrict area of spill.

Obtain drug spill kit.

Immediately remove contaminated protective garments or linen.

Wash affected area of skin with soap and water.

Eye exposure: immediately flood affected eye with water for at least 5 minutes; obtain medical attention promptly.

Follow procedures for contaminated linen.

Notify physician if drug spills on patient.

Documentation

Document in patient's medical record the management of the drug spill and notification of the patient's physician.

Document on the agency's approved forms the management of the spill and whether it occurred on a hard surface, linen, or individual.

Caring for Patients Receiving Chemotherapeutic Drugs

Personnel handling blood, vomitus, or excreta from patients who have received chemotherapy within the previous 48 hours should wear disposable surgical latex gloves and gowns, which are discarded appropriately after use. Linen contaminated with chemotherapeutic drugs, blood, vomitus, or excreta from a patient who has received these drugs within 48 hours before should be placed in a specially marked, impervious laundry bag according to procedures for drug spills on linen.[55, 84, 85, 98, 101]

Staff Education

All personnel involved in any aspect of the handling of chemotherapeutic agents should receive an orientation to chemotherapeutic drugs, including their known risks, relevant techniques and procedures for handling, proper use of protective equipment and materials, spill procedures, and medical policies covering personnel handling chemotherapeutic agents who are pregnant or actively trying to conceive children (per Occupational Safety and Health Administration [OSHA] requirements). Staff compliance can be evaluated through monitoring clinical performance monitoring on a scheduled frequency.

Employment Practices Regarding Reproductive Issues

The handling of chemotherapeutic agents by women who either are pregnant or are actively trying to conceive and by those who are breastfeeding remains a sensitive and unsettled issue. Some suggest offering these employees the opportunity to transfer to areas that do not involve chemotherapeutic agents. All safe handling guidelines should be practiced with utmost care by all pregnant personnel.[100, 101]

Extravasation Management

Vesicant extravasation is the accidental leakage of a drug that causes pain, necrosis, or sloughing of tissue into the subcutaneous tissue. A *vesicant* is an agent that can produce a blister or tissue destruction, or both. An *irritant* is an agent that can cause aching, tightness, and phlebitis at the injection site or along the vein line with or without an inflammatory reaction. A *flare* is a local allergic reaction without pain that usually is accompanied by red blotches along the vein line. Local allergic symptoms subside within 30 minutes with or without treatment.[13, 84, 85]

Injuries that may occur as the result of extravasation include tissue sloughing, infection, pain, and loss of mobility in an extremity. The degree of tissue damage is related to several factors, including drug vesicant potential, drug concentration, amount of drug extravasated, duration of tissue exposure, veinpuncture site/device, and needle insertion technique and individual tissue responses (Fig. 23–6). *Delayed extravasation* is an extravasation in which symptoms occur 48 hours after the drug is administered.[84, 85]

Because of the harmful effect of vesicants on tissues, studies in human subjects are limited; thus controlled clinical trials demonstrating the effectiveness of treatment have been difficult to achieve. Most extravasation interventions have been based on preclinical studies using animal models, including mice, pigs, rabbits, and dogs. Other clinical data regarding extravasation management has been collected from isolated drug clinical events. Treatment strategies for managing extravasation involve using specific antidotes and guidelines for immediate intervention to minimize tissue damage. Preventing extravasation and instituting prompt intervention are the key elements for successful management. Tissue destruction from drug extravasation may be subtle and progressive. Initial symptoms include pain or burning at the IV site, progressing to erythema, edema, and superficial skin loss (Figs. 23–7 and 23–8). Tissue necrosis may not develop for 1 to 4 weeks after extravasation. A list of nonvesicant chemotherapeutic drugs follows[15, 32, 84, 85]:

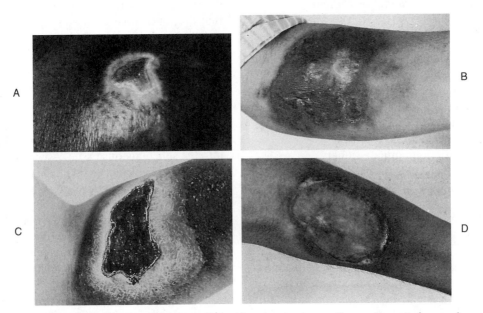

FIGURE 23-6 A, Cutaneous effects of vesicant extravasation; note central necrosis and surrounding erythema and induration. **B,** Lateral progression of initial cutaneous effects, which occurs over a period of weeks. **C,** Eschar requiring surgical debridement eventually develops. **D,** Wide surgical excision of involved area on forearm. (Courtesy Robert Dorr, University of Arizona, *Progressions* 2(4):4, 1990; Mosby.)

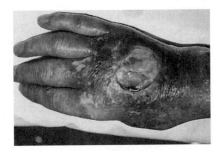

FIGURE 23-7 Doxorubicin extravasation in dorsum of right hand; note depth of wound. (From *Progressions* 2(4):4, 1990; Mosby.)

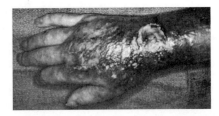

FIGURE 23-8 One month after doxorubicin extravasation in dorsum of right hand. (Courtesy Robert Dorr, University of Arizona, *Progressions* 2(4):4, 1990; Mosby.)

Chemotherapeutic Drugs, Nonvesicants*

Generic Name	Trade Name
Asparaginase	Elspar
Bleomycin	Blenoxane
Busulfan	Busulfex
Carboplatin	Paraplatin
Cisplatin	Platinol
Cladribine	Leustatin
Cyclophosphamide	Cytoxan
Cytarabine (ara-C)	Cytosar-U
Docetaxel	Taxotere
Floxuridine	FUDR
Fludarabine	Fludara
Fluorouracil	Efudex
Gemcitabine	Gemzar
Irinotecan	Camptosar
Methotrexate	Methotrexate
Mitoxantrone	Novantrone
Oxaliplatin	Eloxatin
Pentostatin	Deoxycoformycin
Thalidomide	Thalomid
Thiotepa	Thioplex
Topotecan	Hycamtin

Chemotherapeutic Drugs with Vesicant Potential†

Generic Name	Trade Name
Dactinomycin	Actinomycin D, Cosmegen
Daunorubicin	Cerubidine, Daunomycin
Doxorubicin	Adriamycin
Epirubicin	Pharmorubicin
Esorubicin	4-Deoxydrorubicin
Idarubicin	Idamycin
Mechlorethamine	Nitrogen Mustard, Mustargen
Mitomycin C	Mutamycin
Menogaril	Tomosar
Paclitaxel	Taxol
Oxantrazole	Piroxantrone
Plicamycin	Mithracin
Vinblastine	Velban
Vincristine	Oncovin
Vindesine	Eldisine
Vinorelbine	Navelbine

Chemotherapeutic Drugs with Irritant Potential*

Generic Name	Trade Name
Carmustine (BCNU)	BiCNU
Dacarbazine	DTIC-Dome
Etoposide	VePesid
Ifosfamide	Ifex
Mitoguazone	Methyl-GAG, MGBG
Streptozocin	Zanosar
Teniposide	Vumon

Controversial Topics

Management of extravasation of chemotherapeutic drugs involves some controversial issues.[84, 85, 101]

Use of Antecubital Fossa for Drug Administration

Favor Antecubital Fossa Access

Larger veins permit faster infusion of drug.
Larger veins permit potentially irritating drugs to reach the general circulation sooner with less irritation.

Oppose Antecubital Fossa Access

Arm mobility is restricted.
Infiltration may require extensive reconstructive efforts.
Early infiltration may be difficult to assess.
Potential for venous fibrosis; blood drawing from antecubital fossa may be more difficult.

Methods of Drug Sequencing

Favor Administering Vesicants First

Vascular integrity declines over time.
Initial assessment of vein patency is most accurate.
Possibility of diminishing patient awareness of symptoms related to drug infiltration.

Favor Administering Vesicants Last

Vesicants are irritating and may increase fragility of veins.
Venous spasm may occur at onset of drug administration and alter assessment of venous access.

Needle or Catheter Size

Favor Large Gauge (18–19)

Irritating chemotherapeutic agents can reach circulation sooner with less irritating effect on peripheral veins.

---

*From Otto SE, editor: Pocket guide to intravenous therapy, *ed 4, St. Louis, Mosby, 2001.*

† From Otto SE, editor: Pocket guide to intravenous therapy, *ed 4, St. Louis, Mosby, 2001.*

---

*Adapted from Oncology Nursing Society Task Force: Cancer chemotherapy guidelines and recommendations for nursing education and practice: 1999 guidelines, *Pittsburgh, The Society, 1999.*

Favor Small Gauge (20–23)

Smaller-gauge devices are less likely to puncture the wall of a small vein.

Increased blood flow around a smaller gauge device increases dilution of chemotherapeutic agents.

Phlebitis may be minimized with smaller gauge device.

Prevention of Extravasation

Nursing staff responsibilities for preventing extravasation include the following:

Acquiring a knowledge of drugs with vesicant potential (see list on page 657).

Explaining the vesicant potential to the patient before administering the drug, to obtain true informed consent for this treatment. This practice can significantly aid in identifying an early extravasation if one should occur.

Developing skill in drug administration.

Identifying risk factors (e.g., history of drug allergy, multiple venipunctures, previous treatment).

Anticipating extravasation and being knowledgeable about the approved management protocol.

Obtaining a new venipuncture site daily if peripheral access is used.

Considering central venous access if peripheral access is difficult.

Being aware that most sources recommend 24–hour vesicant infusion via central venous access only.

Administering the drug in a quiet, unhurried environment.

Testing vein patency without using chemotherapeutic agents.

Providing adequate drug dilution (e.g., side port infusion via free-flowing IV infusion)

Carefully observing the access site and extremity throughout the procedure.

Validating blood return from the IV site before, during, and after infusion of the vesicant drug.

Educating patients about the symptoms of drug infiltration (e.g., pain, burning and stinging sensations at IV site).

Protocol for Extravasation Management at a Peripheral Site

Agency policy and procedure for management of extravasation with the responsible physician's prescription should be easily accessible to the staff. The approved antidotes should be readily available, and the following procedure should be initiated with a physician's prescription as soon as extravasation of a vesicant or irritant agent is suspected or occurs.[13, 84, 85]

Stop the chemotherapeutic drug infusion.
Leave the needle or catheter in place.

Aspirate any residual drug and blood in the IV tubing, needle, or catheter and suspected infiltration site.

Instill the IV antidote (Table 23–3).

Remove the needle.

If unable to aspirate the residual drug from the IV tubing, remove the needle or catheter.

Inject the antidote subcutaneously (SQ) clockwise into the infiltrated site using a 25-gauge needle; change the needle with each new infection.

Avoid applying pressure to the suspected infiltration site.

Photograph the suspected area of extravasation according to the agency's policy and procedure for documentation and follow-up.

Apply a topical ointment if ordered.

Cover lightly with an occlusive sterile dressing.

Apply cold or warm compresses as indicated (see Table 23–3).

Elevate the extremity.

Observe regularly for pain, erythema, induration, and necrosis.

Documentation of extravasation management:
    Date
    Time
    Needle or catheter size and type
    Insertion site
    Drug sequence
    Approximate amount of drug extravasated
    Nursing management of extravasation
    Photographic documentation
    Patient's complaints and statements
    Appearance of site
    Notification of physician
    Follow-up measures
    Nurse's signature

Anaphylaxis

Nursing personnel administering chemotherapy in all settings should follow the listed guidelines for drug preparation, administration and disposal, vein selection, documentation of drug infusion, selection of venous access device and possible side effects, teaching of the patient about self-management of most common side effects, and management of chemotherapy spills and drug extravasation. In addition to these guidelines, all nursing personnel should be alert and prepared for the possible complications of anaphylaxis. The drugs and supplies needed to manage these complications must be readily available. The nurse must be informed about and prepared for the specific drugs known to pose a risk of anaphylaxis. Test dosing before infusing the drug and following infusion precautions reduces the occurrence of anaphylaxis (Table 23–4). Emergency medications and supplies for managing anaphylaxis include:

TABLE 23–3
Chemotherapeutic Vesicant Drugs with Recommended Antidotes

Drug	Antidote
ALKYLATING AGENTS Mechlorethamine (Mustargen, Nitrogen Mustard), mitomycin C (Mutamycin)	Isotonic sodium thiosulfate 1/6 molar, 4.4 g/10 mL Dilute 1.6 mL sodium thiosulfate 25% with 8.4 mL sterile water for injection; apply cold compresses
ANTIBIOTICS Daunorubicin (daunomycin) Doxorubicin (Adriamycin), mitomycin-C (Mutamycin)	Apply *ice cold* compresses immediately for 30–60 min Alternate protocol: topical dimethyl sulfoxide (DMSO) 1–2 mL of 1 mmol DMSO 50%–100%; apply topically one time at site; apply *cold* compresses
BISANTRENE	Sodium bicarbonate 1 mEq/mL Mix equal parts of sodium bicarbonate with sterile normal saline (1:1 solution); resulting solution is 0.5 mEq/mL Inject 2–6 mL (1–3 mEq) IV through existing IV line and SQ into extravasated site; apply cold compresses
VINCA ALKALOIDS Teniposide, vinblastine, vincristine, vindesine, vinorelbine	Hyaluronidase (Wydase) 150 U/mL Add 1 mL sterile sodium chloride Inject 1–6 mL (150–900 U) SQ into extravasated site with multiple injections; apply warm compresses; *do not* inject corticosteroids
DRUGS WITH NO KNOWN SPECIFIC ANTIDOTES Dactinomycin, epirubicin, esorubicin, idarubicin, menogaril, mitoxantrone, piroxantrone	Specific treatment for extravasation unknown at this time
TAXANES Docetaxel (Taxotere) Paclitaxel (Taxol)	Specific treatment for extravasation unknown at this time

From Otto SE, editor: Pocket guide to intravenous therapy, *ed 4, St. Louis, Mosby, 2001.*

Injectable aminophylline, diphenhydramine hydrochloride (Benadryl), dopamine, epinephrine, heparin, hydrocortisone
Oxygen setup, tubing cannula, or mask and airway device
Suction equipment
IV fluids (isotonic solutions)
IV tubings and supplies for venous access

Prompt, effective nursing intervention for anaphylaxis reduces complications. The nurse must be alert to the signs and symptoms of an anaphylactic response to a chemotherapeutic drug. All or some of these symptoms may be present: anxiety, hypotension, urticaria, cyanosis, respiratory distress, abdominal cramping, flushed appearance, and chills. The calm, reassuring presence of the nurse facilitates management of these symptoms, which proceeds as follows[15, 22, 36, 54, 75, 85]:

Immediately stop the drug infusion.
Maintain an IV line with isotonic saline.
Position the patient for comfort and to promote perfusion of the vital organs.
Notify the physician, nursing agency, or emergency medical services.
Maintain the airway and anticipate the need for cardiopulmonary resuscitation.
Monitor the vital signs according to agency policy.
Administer the appropriate medications with an approved physician's order.
Follow the nursing agency's protocol for follow-up care (e.g., evaluation of the patient by a physician).
Document the incident in the patient's medical record.

An anaphylactic episode is upsetting to the patient and family. Follow-up care is required to diminish their anxiety and to monitor for delayed side effects. Instruct the patient and family in the pertinent drug side effects, when and where to call for assistance, and what symptoms require immediate health care intervention (shortness of breath, rash on the body that increases in size and intensity, flushed appearance, fever, chills, abdominal cramping, feeling of anxiousness).

ALTERNATIVE CARE SETTINGS

Improved drug delivery, cost containment, and consideration of the quality of life have affected trends in chemotherapy administration. Management of symp-

T A B L E 2 3 – 4
Chemotherapeutic Drugs with Potential for Anaphylaxis

Drugs	Signs and Symptoms	Precautions
Asparaginase (Elspar) *Test Dose Procedure:* Prepare 10,000 IU asparaginase with 5 mL NS; inject 0.1 mL of this solution (200 IU) into 9.9 mL NS; inject 0.1 mL of this concentration (2 IU) intradermally to make a wheal in inner aspect of arm; observe wheal for 60 minutes for erythema, swelling, and itching before doing infusion.	Respiratory distress, increased pulse, respirations, hypotension, facial edema, anxiety, flushed appearance, hives, itching; risk for anaphylaxis increases with each dose	Test dose before initial IV/IM dosing; monitor 30 min IM or 60 min IV after drug administration; keep vein open with IV normal saline before, during, and 30/60 min after IV administration of asparaginase. Initiate drug infusion slowly (mg/m²/titrate infusion). Emergency Care; O₂ suction, drugs for anaphylaxis at or near patient's bedside
Bleomycin (Blenoxane) *Test Dose Procedure:* Inject 2 U of bleomycin intradermally to make a wheal in inner aspect of arm; observe for erythema or edema and itching before first 2 doses of bleomycin are infused.	Dyspnea, hypotension, increased pulse and respiration, rash	Test dose before initial IV dosing; initiate drug infusion slowly (10–20 mL/15 min); monitor vital signs and auscultate breath sounds every 4 h during infusion and for 24 h afterward, and/or on scheduled basis in outpatient setting.
Etoposide (VePesid, VP-16)	Hypotension, bronchospasm, chest pain, increased pulse and respirations, facial flush, fever, chills, diaphoresis	Initiate drug infusion slowly (10–20 mL/15 min). Infuse total volume over at least 60 min. Monitor vital signs every 15 min × 4; every 30 min × 2; and every 4 h during and for 24 h after infusion.
Teniposide (Vumon, VM-26)	Severe hypotension, anxiety, increased pulse and respirations, fever	Initiate drug infusion *slowly* (10–20 mL/30 min). Total infusion time 60–120 min. Monitor vital signs every 15 min × 4; every 30 min × 2 during and after infusion; then monitor every 4 h × 24 h.
Paclitaxel (Taxol) Docetaxel (Taxotere)	Increased or decreased BP, increased temperature and pulse, restlessness, dyspnea, bronchospasm, facial flushing, hives *If any of these symptoms occur, stop drug infusion and notify physician immediately.*	Premedicate with the following before Taxol or Taxotere infusion: dexamethasone 10–20 mg PO/IV 12 and 6 h, diphenhydramine 50 mg IV push 30–60 min; cimetidine 300 mg IV over 30 min; infuse Taxol/Taxotere in a glass bottle with non-PVC tubing and a 0.22-μm filter, obtain baseline VS, then monitor every 15 min × 4, every 1 hr × 4, and every 4 h × 4 during infusion. Ensure that emergency medications (Benadryl 50 mg, hydrocortisone 100 mg, adrenaline [epinephrine] 1:1000—all IV bolus), as well as O₂ and suction equipment are assembled and ready for use.

BP, blood pressure; IM, intramuscular; NS, normal saline; PO, oral; PVC, polyvinyl chloride; VS, vital signs.
From Otto SE, editor: Pocket guide to intravenous therapy, *ed 4, St. Louis, Mosby, 2001.*

toms, such as controlling nausea and vomiting and innovative pain management, have reduced the need for hospitalization. Options for giving chemotherapy in outpatient settings include ambulatory care centers, physicians' offices, extended care facilities, and home health agencies. Certain principles of chemotherapy administration and standards of care for patients must be maintained by the staff regardless of the setting.[3, 12, 59, 101]

Home health care has extensively expanded in the past decade to include more varied care options for oncology patients. Criteria specific to home administration of chemotherapy include:

1. A caregiver is available who is able and willing to assist.
2. The patient's physical condition is stable and within the range of home care capabilities.
3. Living conditions are stable and suitable (cleanliness, plumbing, refrigeration, telephone).
4. The patient has access to emergency assistance.

Patients and family members involved in the infusion of chemotherapeutic drugs or the management of side effects, or both, require verbal, written, demonstration, and return demonstration procedural information. Following are suggested nursing interventions to facilitate education of the patient and family in drug administration in the home.[3]

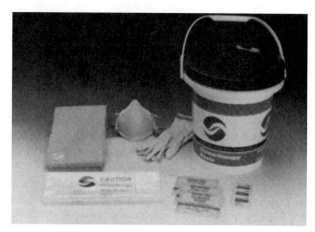

FIGURE 23 – 9 Home health care kit. (Courtesy Biosafety Systems, Inc., San Diego, CA.)

Interventions

- Assess the patient's ability and willingness to learn, the availability of a caregiver, the home environment, the patient's ability to assume self-care, and compliance with the treatment regimen.
- Describe the purpose, schedule, and procedure of the chemotherapeutic regimen.
- Explain to the patient the possible side effects of chemotherapeutic drugs (nausea and vomiting, anorexia, stomatitis, constipation, diarrhea, alopecia, skin and hematopoietic changes).
- Instruct the patient or caregiver in dealing with specific side effects.
- Review symptoms, such as temperature elevation over 100.4°F (38°C), severe constipation or diarrhea, persistent bleeding from any site, sudden weight gain or loss, shortness of breath, pain that is not relieved by prescribed medications, and severe nausea and vomiting more than 24 hours after treatment. *Emphasize* the importance of promptly reporting these symptoms to the physician.
- Instruct the patient or caregiver in the management of infusion devices.
- Validate the aseptic technique and skills of the patient or caregiver for prescribed self-administration and discontinuation of chemotherapeutic drugs.
- Explain the safe handling precautions for administration and disposal of chemotherapeutic drugs.
- Provide information and a list of resources for obtaining, storing, and disposing of drugs and supplies. Also provide a schedule of follow-up tests and care.
- Record the drug, dose, route, and time given in the home and provide this information to the agency responsible for care management.
- Discard all unused drugs and used supplies in a recommended puncture-proof, leak-proof, closeable container. Return this container to the appropriate agency for disposal (Fig. 23–9).

- Use plastic sheeting to protect bedding or furniture if incontinence is possible.
- Carefully handle linen contaminated by chemotherapeutic drugs and excreta, and wash twice, separately from all other linen.

It is recommended that the patient receive the first chemotherapy dose in an acute care or outpatient setting.

CANCER CARE FOR THE ELDERLY

A combination of factors, such as the increasing number of older people in the population and the increasing number of older people with cancer, has brought to the forefront the need to understand the special problems involved in treating older cancer patients. It is estimated that the number of Americans over age 85 will increase fourfold between 1980 and 2030. As the United States has entered the year 2000, the population of those turning age 50 years was at the rate of 8 people per minute. This increasing number of people older than 50 years is coupled with an increased incidence of cancer associated with an aged person; the risk for a person over age 65 of developing cancer is 10 times that of a younger person. Even though more than half of all cancers are diagnosed in people over age 67, studies rarely consistently enroll patients over age 70.[12, 14, 37, 42, 80, 81]

The physiologic changes that occur with biologic aging are an important consideration in the treatment of cancer and chemotherapy pharmacokinetics. The hematopoietic system's inability to respond as readily as in a younger person partly determines the selection of chemotherapeutic agents and dose intensities and imposes an increased risk of infection. A gradual wasting of body muscle mass and an increase in fat can influence drug distribution, and decreased liver function and renal excretion affect drug metabolism and excretion. Cardiovascular changes must be considered when cardiotoxic chemotherapeutic agents or surgery are the possible cancer treatment modalities.[14, 80, 81]

In the older age group, perhaps more than any other, we have concern for the quality of life we are providing as well as the rate of cure. In caring for these individuals, any treatment of the tumor affects and is affected by the patient's previous experiences, behavior, and coping mechanisms and any support systems available.

Likewise, it is important to remember that there can be wide degree of variability among older adults. Although many individuals in their seventies and eighties are physiologically challenged, others in the same age group are running relays. Therefore, though we recognize older adults as a group that has a greater vulnerability to cancer and the effects of treatment modalities, we also recognize a wide range of variability among individuals. Treatments should be selected based on the individual patient information, not age. Research should be conducted to determine the most appropriate use of current treatments and the efficacy of new treatments for this age group, so that regimens are developed that address their needs.*

FUTURE DIRECTIONS AND ADVANCES IN CHEMOTHERAPY

Future directions in chemotherapy offer many exciting opportunities. The use of effective adjuvant, neoadjuvant, and combination chemotherapies, as well as the use of chemotherapy in combination with other treatment modalities, will continue to increase. Ongoing clinical research will focus on new drug development and dose intensity schedules for most of the major cancer diseases, regarding uses of circadian chronotherapy, chemoprevention, liposomal agents, and radiosensitizers. The emergence and ground swell of managed care packages, along with changes in insurance coverage, will increase the demand for ambulatory/short-stay program for most chemotherapy administration. The "graying" of our population will create a larger population of oncology patients, whether for screening and detection, treatment, or palliative care. This will evolve into the need for drugs that have greater efficacy, are administered in a timely fashion, and have limited side effects.*

CONCLUSION

Nurses have major responsibilities in caring for patients who receive chemotherapeutic agents. It is important that nurses know the treatment goals, drug classifications and modes of action, principles of tumor growth and cell kill, and administration protocols. Chemotherapeutic agents should be administered only by nurses who have been taught and are skilled in the various procedures. Patient and family education on the many aspects of chemotherapy (e.g., procedure, potential side effects and toxicities, follow-up care) requires competent nursing assessment and intervention. The nurse should encourage the patient and family to become an integral part of planning and implementing care. Keeping abreast of all the new drugs and their implications, along with the responsibilities just mentioned, offers many challenges for the nurse in the varied settings of oncology practice.†

---

* References 14, 24, 44, 48, 57, 66, 81.

---

* References 5, 37, 38, 43, 58, 60, 66, 76, 79.

† References 24, 28, 35, 44, 48, 49, 58, 60, 61, 66, 78, 89.

Nursing Management

Nursing management of the patient receiving chemotherapy requires multiple assessment and intervention strategies. Nursing care begins with a thorough understanding of five primary elements: the patient's condition; the goal of therapy; the treating drug's dosage, route, and schedule; the principles of administration; and the potential side effects. Additional nursing management includes monitoring responses to therapy, reassessing and documenting signs and symptoms, and communicating pertinent information to other members of the health care team. Continual psychosocial evaluation and patient teaching components require astute nursing interventions. Many resources are available, both locally and nationally. The Oncology Nursing Society, the American Cancer Society, the National Cancer Institute, and the Leukemia Society all provide lay and professional educational materials.

NURSING ASSESSMENT AND INTERVENTION

Chemotherapeutic drugs may cause adverse side effects and major system toxicity and dysfunction. Side effects and toxicity vary in severity according to the patient's individual response to the drug therapy. The most frequent side effects are myelosuppression, nausea, and vomiting. Myelosuppression can be a dose-limiting toxicity. Myelosuppression, stomatitis, mucositis, and skin integrity are discussed extensively in Chapter 31. The chemotherapeutic drugs work by destroying or suppressing new leukocytes, platelets, and erythrocytes. These effects are monitored by evaluating the blood count at scheduled intervals. The time or level at which a blood count reaches its lowest point is the nadir. The nadir varies with individual drugs but usually occurs between 7 and 21 days after administration.[12, 15]

Nausea and vomiting often are the most distressing side effects of chemotherapy; they may be acute, anticipatory, delayed, or persistent. Acute nausea and vomiting occur within 1 to 2 hours of treatment and last approximately 24 to 48 hours. Anticipatory nausea and vomiting occur before the treatment. Nausea and vomiting after the initial 24 hours of treatment may be referred to as *delayed* or *persistent*. Cisplatin in particular is associated with this symptom. An estimated 60% of patients experience delayed emesis after receiving cisplatin, even if emesis is adequately controlled during the first 24 hours. Assessing and reporting the frequency, severity, and pattern of nausea and vomiting are critical to the patient's recovery process.

In the past 10 to 15 years, antiemetic research has had a profound effect on the treatment of chemotherapy-induced nausea and vomiting. The incidence of these side effects is related to the emetic potential of the chemotherapy drug (see the table below); the dose; the route, schedule, and duration; and combinations of drug administration. The combination of antiemetic drugs with different mechanisms, round-the-clock administration, and higher dosages have proved more effective than single-agent dosing and as-needed (PRN) schedules. Several agents now used as single agents or in combination are metoclopramide, haloperidol, dexamethasone, lorazepam, and prochlorperazine (see the tables on page 664). Many of these drugs act on the chemoreceptor trigger zone in the brain by blocking dopamine receptors. Although these antiemetics have demonstrated their effectiveness, they are associated with undesirable side effects: sedation, extrapyramidal reactions, anxiety, mood changes, and diarrhea. Another major drawback is that most of these drugs are administered intravenously and thus have limited use in the outpatient setting.[24, 27, 44]

Emetic Potential of Common Chemotherapeutic Drugs

Mild Potential	Moderate Potential	Severe Potential
Bleomycin	Carboplatin	Carmustine
Busulfan	Cytarabine	Cisplatin
Chlorambucil	Daunorubicin	Cyclophosamide
5-Fluorouracil	Doxorubicin	Dacarbazine
Hydroxyurea	Ifosfamide	Dactinomycin
Mercaptopurine	Mitomycin C	Etoposide
Methotrexate (low dose)	Procarbazine	Mechlorethamine
Paclitaxel	Mitoxantrone	Streptozotocin
Vinblastine		

Selected Parenteral Antiemetic Regimens (Adult)

Drug	Dosage	Schedule
Metoclopramide (Reglan)	1–3 mg/kg IV	30 min before and 90 min after chemotherapy, then every 4 h PRN
Dexamethasone (Decadron)	20 mg IV	30–40 min before chemotherapy
Lorazepam (Ativan) or	1.5 mg/m^2 IV	30 min before chemotherapy
Diphenhydramine (Benadryl)	50 mg IV	30 min before chemotherapy
(The above drugs are used in varying doses and schedules depending upon severity of emetic episode.)		
Dolasetron (Anzemet)	1.8 mg/kg IV 100 mg PO	30 min before chemotherapy 60 min before chemotherapy
Granisetron (Kytril)	10 μg IV 2 mg PO	30 min before chemotherapy 60 min before chemotherapy
Ondansetron (Zofran)	0.15 mg/kg IV in 30–50 mL; infused over 15–30 min	30 min before chemotherapy, then at 4 and 8 h after initial dose
	(IV dose 16–32 mg/d) 4–8 mg PO TID	

Data from American Society of Hospital Pharmacists, Bethesda, MD, 1999.

Selected Oral Antiemetic Regimens (Adult)

Drugs	Dosage	Schedule
Chlorpromazine hydrochloride (Thorazine)	10, 25, 50, 100, 200 mg tablets; 75, 150, 200, 300 mg slow-release (SR) capsules	Give 30–75 mg in 2–4 h in divided doses; give 1 h before chemotherapy administration, then every 4–6 h PRN.
Dolasetron (Anzemet)	100 mg	Give 100 mg 30–60 min before chemotherapy administration
Dronabinol (Marinol)	2.5, 5, 10 mg SR capsules	Give 1–3 h before chemotherapy administration; then 4–6 doses per day every 2–4 h (maximum 15 mg/m^2 per dose).
Granisetron (Kytril)	1 mg	Give initial 1 mg dose 1 h before chemotherapy administration and next dose 12 h after first.
Ondansetron (Zofran)	8 mg (12 y of age or older)	Give initial 8 mg dose 30 min before chemotherapy (maximum dose 3 times per day for 2–3 d).
	4 mg (4–11 y of age)	Give initial 4 mg dose 30 min before chemotherapy (maximum dose 3 times per day for 2–3 days).
Prochlorperazine (Compazine)	5, 10, 25 mg tablets; 10, 15, 30 mg SR capsules	Give 10–25 mg 1 h before chemotherapy administration, then 15–30 mg SR capsules every 12 h; repeat one of above doses every 3–4 1/2 h.
Promethazine (Phenergan)	12.5, 25, 50 mg tablets	Give 25–50 mg 1 h before chemotherapy administration, then 12.5–25 mg 4 times per day.
Trimethobenzamide hydrochloride (Tigan)	100, 250 mg capsules	Give 250 mg 1 h before chemotherapy administration, then 250 mg 4 times per day.
Perphenazine (Trilafon)	16 mg/5 mL solution 2,4,8,16 mg tablets	Give 4–8 mg PO 1 h before chemotherapy administration, then 4 mg every 4–6 h.

Data from Physician drug reference, Montvale, NJ, Medical Economics Data, Medical Economic Co, 1999, and American Hospital Formulary Service, Bethesda, MD, 1999.

With the development and use of the serotonin (5-HT3) antagonists (e.g., dolasetron [Anzemet], granisetron [Kytril], and ondansetron [Zofran]), new strides have been made in effective antiemetic therapy. Although more costly than previous antiemetic drugs, the dosing schedule is less frequent (30 minutes before chemotherapy, and thereafter the dose frequency varies after the initial dose). Side effects thus far are mild: headache, constipation, and transient elevation of liver enzymes. All three of these agents have demonstrated effectiveness as oral agents and may be suitable for outpatient therapy and for children.[24, 27, 44, 92]

The remaining side effects listed in Table 23–1 (e.g, aches and pains, alopecia, anorexia, constipation, cystitis, diarrhea, depression, fatigue, mucositis, pharyngitis, stomatitis) have listed nursing actions and points to cover for patient and family teaching. The nurse's responsibilities include evaluating the patient's response to the drugs, teaching the patient or caregiver self-management interventions, and monitoring laboratory data, as well as signs, and symptoms reported by the patient. This information is useful in developing the plan of care for the patient receiving chemotherapy.*

Pertinent information related to the major system toxicities (cardiac, hematopoietic, hepatic, hypersensitivity, neurologic, ototoxicity, pulmonary, reproductive, renal) and to metabolic alterations (see Table 23–2) imposes dose-limiting restrictions on many of the drugs. If symptoms occur and the chemotherapeutic drug dose or schedule (or both) is not altered or evaluated, the potential for irreversible side effects grows. All the toxicities listed in Table 23–2 require astute observation and prompt intervention by all members of the health care team. Additional circumstances that may affect the patient's response to a drug include the setting in which the drug is administered (acute care or home care), the needs posed by activities of daily living, and life-style changes.*

Selected nursing diagnoses and interventions appropriate for the patient receiving chemotherapy are listed below. Additional nursing diagnoses may be determined by assessing the patient's health and psychosocial issues and the specific side effects of the chemotherapeutic drugs.

Nursing Diagnosis

- *Knowledge deficit related to chemotherapeutic side effects*

---

* References 9, 12, 21, 25, 28, 46, 59, 82, 93, 99.

Outcome Goal

Patient will be able to:

- State drug side effects.

Interventions

- Assess educational level, ability, desire to learn, and barriers to learning.
- Assess knowledge level relative to cancer, previous experience with diagnosis, and treatment of cancer.
- Evaluate understanding relative to the specific diagnosis, disease process, and potential treatment planned.
- Assess previous experience with chemotherapy.
- Determine availability of caregiver to participate in patient's care and treatment.
- Assess patient's and family's needs for consultation with various resources (e.g., I Can Cope Support Group, Reach to Recovery, Look Good–Feel Better, and ostomy, and laryngectomy support groups)

Nursing Diagnosis

- *Oral mucous membrane, altered, related to side effects of drugs*

Outcome Goals

Patient will be able to:

- Exhibit signs of a healthy oral mucosa.
- Identify/demonstrate measures that promote good oral hygiene.

Interventions

- Assess history of alcohol and tobacco use or other risk factors.
- Obtain history of current treatment: radiation therapy, chemotherapy, surgery, and biotherapy.
- Query patient about usual regimen for oral hygiene and date of last dental examination.
- Assess oral mucosa: palate, tongue, gums, teeth, lips, floor of mouth, and inner aspects of cheeks. Note redness, ulcerations, bleeding, and white patches, as well as color, amount, and consistency of saliva.

Nursing Diagnosis

- *Injury, risk for, related to alteration in immune system; clotting factors*

Outcome Goals

Patient will be able to:

- Identify/report signs and symptoms of infection.
- Identify/demonstrate infection potential precautions.

Interventions

- Monitor complete blood count (CBC), hemoglobin, prothrombin time (PT), partial thromboplastin time (PTT), and platelet count.
- Assess type of therapy (chemotherapy, radiation therapy) and current drugs (aspirin, anticoagulants) that may alter bleeding and clotting times.
- Assess factors (fever, sepsis, altered hepatic function, bone marrow function) that may alter clotting process.
- Observe for and report symptoms: bruising; bleeding from venous access sites, nose, gums, vagina, rectum; hemoptysis, hematemesis; black, tarry, or gross blood in stools; increase in usual menstrual flow; change in vital signs; spontaneous petechiae or hematomas.

Nursing Diagnosis

- *Nutrition, altered: less than body requirements, related to nausea and vomiting*

Outcome Goals

Patient will be able to:

- Maintain laboratory values within normal limits.
- Identify/demonstrate measures to minimize nausea and vomiting episodes.
- Consume sufficient calories to maintain weight goal.

Interventions

- Assess nauseous episodes, including amount, color, consistency, and frequency of emesis.
- Determine what factors facilitate or prevent nausea and vomiting.
- Query patient about past strategies that were helpful in managing nausea and vomiting.
- Assess baseline weight before illness, onset of illness, changes since onset of treatment, and weight 1 month ago; note weight gains/losses.
- Monitor laboratory values: serum albumin, serum transferrin, CBC, electrolytes.
- Assess dietary history: food habits, food likes/dislikes, amount and type of food eaten at breakfast, lunch, supper, and snacks.

- Note altered bowel habits and presence of other related gastrointestinal (GI) distress (heartburn, feeling of fullness, cramping).
- Consult dietary services and/or plan with patient recommendations for nutritional intake that will stimulate appetite and facilitate calorie intake (e.g., cold foods, salads, cheeses, fruits, salty foods, colas).

Nursing Diagnosis

- *Sensory/perceptual alterations, visual, related to photosensitivity and auditory related to ototoxicity*

Interventions

- Determine chemotherapy or other treatment-related protocol that may affect sensory alterations.
- Assess severity of symptoms regarding compromises in activities in daily living.
- Assess environmental conditions (light, noise, room temperature).
- Assess sensory alteration: onset, severity, changes in duration, other discomforting symptoms.
- Instruct patient in precautions to follow: photosensitivity (wear sunglasses when outside, dim room lights, observe driving and/or work-related restrictions), ototoxicity (limit or restrict environmental noise).
- Inform health care team about symptoms and restrictions affecting work, driving, and activities of daily living.

Nursing Diagnosis

- *Body image disturbance related to alopecia*

Outcome Goals

Patient will be able to:

- Identify measures to protect/minimize scalp and hair damage.
- Use resources regarding changes in body image.

Interventions

- Inform patient that hair loss is temporary and hair will regrow after treatment stops (hair growth usually returns in 2–6 months).
- Provide resources for purchase or loan of wigs, scarves, and caps.
- Inform patient about health care measures to protect scalp: use gentle shampoos, avoid hair dryers, curling irons, permanents, and hair drying; protect scalp in winter and summer (cold/heat loss); wear protective head covering when outdoors.

PATIENT TEACHING PRIORITIES

Chemotherapy

Assess willingness, readiness to learn, and barriers to learning (acuity of illness, sensory deficits, pain, and/or fear and anxiety regarding diagnosis/treatment).

Inform patient/family about schedule of activities for chemotherapy administration and monitoring of laboratory and diagnostic tests.

Encourage practice and repetition of newly learned skill to enhance learner's performance for at-risk procedures.

Validate aseptic technique and skills of patient or caregiver for prescribed self-administration and discontinuation of chemotherapeutic drugs.

Provide written materials (e.g., those from the National Cancer Institute, "Chemotherapy and You." "What Are Clinical Trials All About"), 1-800-4-CANCER telephone number, and other materials as needed.

Teach and review specific drugs and related side effects patient may experience, and when, where, how, and whom to call if problems arise.

Provide information and list of resources for obtaining, storing, and disposing of drugs and supplies.

- Encourage sharing of feelings regarding body image changes. Inform patient about American Cancer Society support groups (e.g., I Can Cope, Look Good–Feel Better).

Nursing Diagnosis

- *Pain related to bone metastasis*
- *Oral mucous membrane, altered (mucositis)*

Outcome Goals

Patient will be able to:

- Achieve adequate control of pain.
- Identify/demonstrate measures to control or minimize pain episodes.

Interventions

- Determine onset, location, duration, severity, intensity, and radiation of symptoms.
- Assess symptoms with patient's and family's suggestions: What makes the symptoms/discomfort better?
- What makes the symptoms/discomfort worse? For example: types and frequency of interventions; treatment-related interventions affecting hygiene, nutrition, and pain; time of intervention regarding food intake and mobility.

- Provide physician-prescribed medications and treatment interventions.
- Encourage relaxation/meditation/distraction strategies to facilitate coping with discomfort and enhance effects of medications and treatment interventions.
- Monitor electrolyte balance and granulocyte count.
- Assess skin, especially hidden areas (between toes, skin folds of breasts, buttocks, perineal area) on a scheduled basis; report changes and findings promptly.

Nursing Diagnosis

- *Infection, risk for, resulting from immunosuppression, break in skin, or contamination of supplies*

GERIATRIC CONSIDERATIONS

Chemotherapy

Consider potential for cardiac, renal, respiratory, and hepatic systems compromise: medication dosage or schedule of administration may be altered.

High-dose drug regimens have been associated with increased toxicity (e.g., neurotoxicity with high-dose cytarabine—patients over 50 years of age are particularly susceptible to this toxicity).

Consider neuromuscular and sensory deficits that may be present, such as visual and hearing losses and arthritic joints; plan individualized teaching sessions; use printed materials with large print for reading ease; return demonstration techniques may require more simplistic steps to facilitate patient/family ease in learning required technique.

Consider age-related changes in body function accommodations: bowel and bladder tonicity (unable to hold large-volume hydration, unable to retain large-volume bowel cleansing preparations); provide prompt and frequent elimination needs.

Premedications may cause drowsiness; encourage patient/family to use transportation resources (family, public, American Cancer Society) if receiving chemotherapy or undergoing required laboratory test monitoring.

Query patient/caregiver regarding over-the-counter or previous physician-prescribed medications; some of these medications may alter bleeding and clotting times or interfere with prescribed chemotherapy medications.

Assess abilities of patient and caregiver, and determine if additional resources are needed, such as a home care agency, Meals on Wheels, and social services for financial assistance.

Outcome Goals

Patient/caregiver will be able to:

- Identify and report signs and symptoms of infection.
- Identify/demonstrate appropriate hygiene measures.

Interventions

- Monitor CBC and acute granulocyte count.
- Monitor expectation of nadir related to chemotherapy.
- Teach and monitor prudent handwashing technique: before any nursing intervention, before and after meals, after bathroom use, before any treatment-related activity for self-care.

- Restrict visitors with potential infections or those recently immunized with attenuated live vaccines, such as diphtheria-pertussis-tetanus (DPT) or measles-mumps-rubella (MMR).
- Monitor food intake: explain restrictions (no fresh vegetables or fruits) and emphasize that the nurse must be consulted before patient eats food brought into hospital.
- Ensure cleanliness of room and supplies used in routine care; change all supplies on a scheduled basis.
- Examine all sterile supplies before use; note expiration date for sterility, observe for any defect or interruption of product's integrity, and use sterile technique when opening and using product.
- See Patient Teaching Priorities and Geriatric Considerations.

Chapter Questions

1. Factors considered in chemotherapy drug selection for cancer treatment include:
   a. Cancer cell type, bone marrow status, tumor burden, tumor resistance
   b. Cardiac, hepatic, renal, and sexuality status
   c. Patient's age, diagnosis, pain status, tumor burden
   d. Rate of drug absorption, nausea potential, renal status, tumor burden

2. Chemotherapy drugs that have potential for cardiac toxicity include:
   a. Carmustine, cisplatin, dactinomycin, daunorubicin
   b. Chlorambucil, cyclophosphamide, daunorubicin, doxorubicin
   c. Dactinomycin, daunorubicin, doxorubicin, deoxycoformycin
   d. Dactinomycin, daunorubicin, docetaxel, dexamethasone

3. Chemotherapy vesicant drugs with extravasation potential include:
   a. Antitumor antibiotics, alkylating agents, antiestrogens
   b. Antitumor antibiotics, alkylating agents, vinca alkaloids
   c. Antitumor antibiotics, antimetabolites, vinca alkaloids
   d. Antitumor antibiotics, alkylating agents, antihormonal agents

4. Clinical features that may occur during a hypersensitivity or anaphylaxis event are
   a. Anxiety, cyanosis, dyspnea, urticara
   b. Anxiety, chills, fever, hives
   c. Anxiety, facial edema, hoarseness, weakness
   d. Cyanosis, dyspnea, hives, vertigo

5. Chemotherapy drugs that cause neurotoxicity symptoms such as numbness, jaw pain, absent deep tendon reflexes and/or severe constipation include:
   a. Alkeran, busulfan, cisplatin, dactinomycin
   b. Bleomycin, carboplatin, cytarabine, doxorubicin
   c. Cisplatin, dactinomycin, etoposide, fludarabine
   d. Etoposide, ifosfamide, vinblastine, vincristine

6. Interventions for nausea and vomiting associated with chemotherapy drugs include:
   a. Offer antiemetics at least every 12 hours, avoid greasy or cold foods, eat large meals
   b. Offer antiemetics at least every 24 hours, avoid fatty foods, eat small meals, dry toast
   c. Offer antiemetics before chemotherapy, avoid greasy or fatty foods, eat small meals
   d. Offer antiemetics after chemotherapy, eat cold or salty foods, dry crackers or toast

7. Nursing interventions for chemotherapy drug extravasation include:
   a. Knowing drugs with vesicant potential, test vein with normal saline, carefully observe drug administration, validate blood return before, during and after
   b. Knowing drugs with irritant potential, test vein with distilled water, carefully observe drug ad-

ministration, validate blood return before, during, and after

c. Knowing drugs with nonvesicant potential, test vein with normal saline, carefully observe drug administration, validate blood return before and after

d. Knowing drugs with vesicant potential, test vein with normal saline, carefully observe drug administration, validate blood return during and after

8. "Circadian variables" in the concept of circadian rhythm include:

a. Drug absorption, distribution, dose modification, metabolism

b. Drug absorption, metabolism, drug administration, elimination

c. Drug absorption, metabolism, distribution, elimination

d. Drug absorption, distribution, dose intensification, elimination

9. Critical elements of chemotherapy documentation include:

a. Drug dose, route, site assessment, physician order for drug(s)

b. Drug dose, route, IV access, blood return status

c. Drug dose, route, IV access, pharmacy preparation of drug

d. Drug dose, route, IV access, safe handling preparation

10. Factors related to blood–brain barrier drug administration include:

a. Abundant lymphatic drainage, permeability consistency for drug delivery

b. Adequate lymphatic drainage, permeability inconsistency for drug delivery

c. Inadequate lymphatic drainage, permeability consistency for drug delivery

d. Inadequate lymphatic drainage, permeability inconsistency for drug delivery

BIBLIOGRAPHY

1. Abbokinase Open-Cath (urokinase for catheter clearance) prescribing information. Abbott Laboratories, North Chicago, IL, revised 1999.

2. Akpek G and others: Chemotherapy with etoposide, vincristine, doxorubicin, bolus cyclophosphamide, and oral prednisone in patients with refractory cutaneous T-cell lymphoma, *Cancer* 86:1368, 1999.

3. Bean CA and others: High-tech homecare infusion therapies, *Crit Care Nurs Clin North Am* 10:287, 1998.

4. Belford K: Central nervous systems cancers. In Groenwald SL, Frogge MH, Goodman M, Yarbro CH, editors: *Cancer nursing: principles and practice,* ed 4, Boston, Jones & Bartlett, 1997.

5. Berg D and others: Overcoming multidrug resistance: valspodar as a paradigm for nursing care, *Oncol Nurs Forum* 26:711, 1999.

6. Berg D: Irinotecan hydrochloride: drug profile and nursing implications of a topoisomerase I inhibitor in patients with advanced colorectal cancer, *Oncol Nurs Forum* 25:535, 1998.

7. Berenson JR, Lipton A: Use of bisphosphonates in patients with metastatic bone disease, *Oncology* 12:1573, 1998.

8. Biffi R and others: Totally implantable central venous access ports for high-dose chemotherapy administration and autologous stem cell transplantation: analysis of overall and septic complications in 68 cases using a single type of device, *Bone Marrow Transplant* 24:89, 1999.

9. Body JJ and others: A dose-finding study of zoledronate in hypercalcemic cancer patients, *J Bone Miner Res* 14:1557, 1999.

10. Brown MC: An adverse interaction between warfarin and 5-fluorouracil: a case report and review of the literature, *Chemotherapy* 45:392, 1999.

11. Calia KA, Herbst SL, Sidawy EN: Management of central venous catheter occlusions: the emerging role of altephase, Gardiner-Caldwell SynerMed, San Francisco, 1999.

12. Camp-Sorrell D: Surviving the cancer, surviving the treatment: acute cardiac and pulmonary toxicity, *Oncol Nurs Forum* 26:983, 1999.

13. Camp-Sorrell D: Developing extravasation protocols and monitoring outcomes, *INS* 21:232, 1998.

14. Cohen JH: Geriatric principles of treatment applied to medical oncology: an overview, *Semin Oncol* 22(1 suppl):1, 1995.

15. Cohen MR: IV *Drug safety,* Institute for Safe Medication Practice, Huntington Valley, PA, 1999.

16. Cohen MR, editor: *Medication errors,* American Pharmaceutical Association, Washington, DC, The Association, 1999.

17. Cole D: Selection and management of central venous access devices in the home setting, *INS* 22:315, 1999.

18. Comley AL and others: Effect of subcutaneous granulocyte colony-stimulating factor injectate volume on drug efficacy, site complications, and client comfort, *Oncol Nurs Forum* 26:87, 1999.

19. Corneliasen G and others: Chronomedical aspects of oncology and geriatrics, *IN-Vivo* 13:77, 1999.

20. Curran WJ: Radiation-induced toxicities: the role of radioprotectants, *Semin Radiat Oncol* 8(4 Suppl 1):2, 1998.

21. Dalakas MC: *Autoimmune peripheral neuropathies, pathogenesis and treatment,* Nebraska Health Science Center, Clinical Communications Inc., Omaha, 1998.

22. Davis L, Drogasch M: Triple check procedure prevents chemotherapy errors, *Oncol Nurs Forum* 24:641, 1997.

23. DeVita VT Jr: Principles of cancer management: chemotherapy. In DeVita VT Jr, Hellman S, Roseman SA, editors: *Cancer: principles and practice of oncology,* ed 5, Philadelphia, Lippincott-Raven, 1997.

24. Doherty KM: Closing the gap in prophylactic antiemetic therapy: patient factors in calculating for emetogenic potential of chemotherapy, *Clin J Oncol Nurs* 3:113, 1999.

25. Dorr VJ: A practitioner's guide to cancer-related alopecia, *Semin Oncol* 25:562, 1998.

26. Dowsett M: Theoretical considerations for the ideal aromatase inhibitor, *Breast Cancer Res Treat* 49(suppl 1):S39, 1998.

27. Engstrom C and others: The efficacy and cost effectiveness of new antiemetic guidelines, *Oncol Nurs Forum* 26:1453, 1999.

28. Fall-Dickson JM, Rose L: Caring for patients who experience chemotherapy-induced side effects: the meaning for oncology nurses, *Oncol Nurs Forum* 26:901, 1999.

29. Fiesta J: Legal aspects of medication administration, *Nurs Manage* 29:22, 1998.

30. Finiewicz KJ, Larson RA: Dose-intensive therapy for adult acute lymphoblastic leukemia, *Semin Oncol* 26:6, 1999.

31. Fisher B: Highlights from recent National Surgical Adjunct Breast and Bowel Project studies in the treatment and prevention of breast cancer, *CA J Clin* 49:159, 1999.

32. Gahart BL, Nazareno AR: *Intravenous medications,* ed 16, St. Louis, Mosby, 2000.

33. Garay CA, Engstrom PF: Chemoprevention of colorectal cancer: dietary and pharmacologic approaches, *Oncology* 13:89, 1999.

34. Giovannucci E: The prevention of colorectal cancer by aspirin use, *Biomed Pharmacother* 53:303, 1999.

35. Gordon GS, Vokes EE: Chemoradiation for locally advanced, unresectable NSCLC. New standard of care, emerging strategies, *Oncology* 13:1075, 1999.

36. Gotaskie G, Robinson KD: Routes of administration and error precautions, administration of chemotherapy. In Yasko JM: Nursing management of symptoms associated with chemotherapy, Bala Cynwyd, PA, Pharmacia & Upjohn, Meniscus Health Care Communications, 1998.

37. Greenlee RT and others: Cancer statistics, 2000, *CA Cancer J Clin* 50:7, 2000.

38. Greqoire V and others: Chemo-radiotherapy: radiosensitizing nucleoside analogues, *Oncol Rep* 6:949, 1999.

39. Grever MR, Chabner BA: Cancer drug discovery and development. In DeVita VT Jr, Hellman S, Roseman SA editors: *Cancer: principles and practice of oncology,* ed 5, Philadelphia, Lippincott-Raven, 1997.

40. Guyton AC, Hall J: *Textbook of medical physiology,* ed 9, Philadelphia, Saunders, 1996.

41. Hadaway LC: Vascular access devices: meeting patients' needs, *Medsurg Nurs* 8:296, 1999.

42. Heerdt AS, Borgen PI: Current status of tamoxifen use: an update for the surgical oncologist, *J Surg Oncol* 72:42, 1999.

43. Herscher LL, Cook J: Taxanes as radiosensitizers for head and neck cancer, *Curr Opin Oncol* 11:183, 1999.

44. Hineman L, editor: *Clinical management of chemotherapy-induced nausea and vomiting: focus on oral 5-HT3-receptor antagonists,* Springfield, NJ, Scientific Therapeutics Information, 1999.

45. Hodgson BB, Kizior RJ: *Saunders nursing drug handbook,* Philadelphia, Saunders, 2000.

46. Hogan CM: The nurse's role in diarrhea management, *Oncol Nurs Forum* 25:879, 1998.

47. Hortobagyi GN, Hung MC, Buzdar AU: Recent developments in breast cancer therapy, *Semin Oncol* 26(4 suppl 12):11, 1999.

48. Hoskin PJ, Saunders MI, Dische S: Hypoxic radiosensitizers in radical radiotherapy for patients with bladder carcinoma: hyperbartic oxygen, misonidazole, and accelerated radiotherapy, carbogen and nicotinamide, *Cancer* 86:1322, 1999.

49. Hudis CA, Münster PN: High-dose therapy for breast cancer, *Semin Oncol* 26:35, 1999.

50. Hudson MM, Donaldson SS: Treatment of pediatric Hodgkin's lymphoma, *Semin Hematol* 36:313, 1999.

51. Hrushesky W, Bjarnason G: Circadian cancer therapy, *J Clin Oncol* 11:1403, 1993.

52. Iacobelli S and others: A phase I study of recombinant interferon-α administered as a seven-day continuous venous infusion at circadian rhythm-modulated rate in patients with cancer, *Am J Clin Oncol* 18:27, 1995.

53. Infusion management update: needlestick safety legislation steadily moving forward, *Infusion Manage* 9:4, 1999.

54. Itano JK, Taoka KN, editors: *Core curriculum for oncology nursing,* ed 3, Philadelphia, Saunders, 1998.

55. Jagger J, Perry J: Shield staff from occupational exposure, *Nurs Manage* 30:53, 1999.

56. Johnson BL, Gross J: *Handbook of oncology nursing,* ed 3, Boston, Jones & Bartlett, 1998.

57. Karius D, Marriott MA: Immunologic advances in monoclonal antibody therapy: implications for oncology nursing, *Oncol Nurs Forum* 24:483, 1997.

58. Khuri FR: Chemoprevention of cancer, *Highlights Oncol Pract* 16:100, 1999.

59. Kosier MB, Minkler P: Nursing management of patients with an implanted ommaya reservoir, *Clin J Oncol Nurs* 3:63, 1999.

60. Kositis C, Callaghan M: Rituximab: a new monoclonal antibody therapy for non-Hodgkin's lymphoma, *Oncol Nurs Forum* 27:51, 2000.

61. Krishna R, St. Louis M, Mayer LD: Increased intracellular drug accumulation and complete chemosensitization achieved in multidrug-resistant solid tumors by co-administering valspodar (PSC 833), *Int J Cancer* 85:131, 2000.

62. Labovich TM: Acute hypersensitivity reactions to chemotherapy, *Semin Oncol Nurs* 15:222, 1999.

63. Lasic D: Liposomes, *Am Sci* 80:20, 1992.

64. Laurence AD, Goldstone AH: High-dose therapy with hematopoietic transplantation for Hodgkin's lymphoma, *Semin Hematol* 36:303, 1999.

65. Lehnert M, de Giuli R, Twentyman PR: Sensitive and rapid bioassy for analysis of P-glycoprotein-inhibiting activity of chemosensitizers in patient serum, *Clin Cancer Res* 2:403, 1996.

66. Levi F: Cancer chronotherapy, *J Pharm Pharmacol* 51:891, 1999.

67. Levin B: An overview of preventive strategies for pancreatic cancer, *Ann Oncol* 10(suppl 4):193, 1999.

68. Lipson JE, Dibble SL, Minarik PA, editors: *Culture and nursing care: a pocket guide,* U of California, San Francisco, USCF Nursing Press, 1996.

69. Lopez AM and others: Topical DMSO treatments for pegylated liposomal doxorubicin-induced palmar-planta erythrodysesthesia, *Cancer Chemother Pharmacol* 44: 303, 1999.

70. Martin FJ: STEALTH Liposome Technology: an overview, *DOXIL Clinical Series,* 1(1), 1997.

71. Marsee V: Ethical perspectives. In Chernecky C, Berger B, editors: *Advanced and critical care oncology nursing,* Philadelphia, Saunders, 1998.

72. Mayer DK: Cancer patient empowerment, *Oncol Nurs Updates* 6:1, 1999.

73. Mehta MP: Protection of normal tissues from the cytotoxic effects of radiation: focus on amifostine, *Semin Radiat Oncol* 8(4 suppl 1):14, 1998.

74. Metzger G and others: Spontaneous or imposed circadian changes in plasma concentrations of 5-fluorouracil coadministered with folinic acid and oxaliplatin: relationship with mucousal toxicity in patients with cancer, *Clin Pharmacol Ther* 56:190, 1994.

75. Mohler M and others: The reliability of blood sampling from peripheral intravenous infusion lines: complete blood counts, electrolyte panels, and survey panels, *INS* 21:209, 1999.

76. Moran P: Cellular effects of cancer chemotherapy administration, *INS* 23:44, 2000.

77. Murray V: A survey of the sequence-specific interaction of damaging agents with DNA: emphasis on antitumor agents, *Prog Nucleic Acid Res Mol Biol* 63:367, 1999.

78. Myers JS: Supportive care in preventing and reducing cancer therapy-induced toxicities, *New Therapies Symposia Highlights,* 10, Bala Cynwyd, PA, Meniscus, 1999.

79. Myers JS: Integrating today's and anticipating tomorrow's therapeutic advances, *New Therapies Symposia Highlights,* 10, Bala Cynwyd, PA, Meniscus, 1999.

80. National Cancer Institute. *Common toxicity criteria,* Bethesda, MD, National Cancer Institute, 1998.

81. Nitsu N: Non-Hodgkin's lymphoma in the elderly: a guide to drug treatment, *Drugs Aging* 14:447, 1999.

82. Northwestern University, Robert H. Lurie Comprehensive Cancer Center: *evaluation and management guidelines for the treatment of chemotherapy-induced diarrhea: a primer,* 1999.

83. Oinonen R, Franssila K, Elonen E: Central nervous system involvement in patients with mantle cell lymphoma, *Ann Hematol* 78:145, 1999.

84. Oncology Nursing Society: *Access device guidelines,* Pittsburgh, Oncology Nursing Press, 1996.

85. Oncology Nursing Society: *Cancer chemotherapy guidelines and recommendations for practice,* Pittsburgh, Oncology Nursing Press, 1999.

86. Orenstein R: The benefits and limitations of needle protectors and needleless intravenous systems, *INS* 22: 122, 1999.

87. Ozols R: Ovarian cancer: current treatment and controversies. In *Negotiating optimal ovarian cancer care,* 10, Bala Cynwyd, PA, Meniscus, 1999.

88. Perry AG, Potter PA: *Clinical nursing skills & techniques,* ed 4, St. Louis, Mosby, 1998.

89. Pisters PW: Chemoradiation treatment strategies for localized sarcoma: conventional and investigational approaches, *Semin Surg Oncol* 17:66, 1999.

90. Restifo NP, Wunderlich JR: Essentials of immunology. In DeVita VT Jr, Hellman S, Roseman SA, editors: *Cancer: principles and practice of oncology,* ed 5, Philadelphia, Lippincott-Raven, 1997.

91. Rich TA: Chemoradiation for pancreatic and biliary cancer: current status of RTOG studies, *Ann Oncol* 10(suppl 4):231, 1999.

92. Rhodes VA, McDaniel: The index of nausea, vomiting, and retching: a new format of the index of nausea and vomiting, *Oncol Nurs Forum* 26:889, 1999.

93. Rutledge DN, Engelking C: Cancer-related diarrhea: selected findings of a national survey on oncology nurse experiences, *Oncol Nurs Forum* 25:861, 1998.

94. Schmoll HJ and others: Where do we stand with 5-fluorouracil? *Semin Oncol* 26:589, 1999.

95. Schulmeister L: Chemotherapy medication errors: descriptions, severity, and contributing factors, *Oncol Nurs Forum* 26:1033, 1999.

96. Schuchter LM: Current role of protective agents in cancer treatment, *Oncology* 11:505, 1997.

97. Singh DK, Lippman SM: Cancer chemoprevention, part 2: hormones nonclassic antioxidant natural agents, NSAIDs, and other agents, *Oncology* 12:1787, 1999.

98. Singleton LC, Connor TH: An evaluation of the permeability of chemotherapy gloves to three cancer chemotherapy drugs, *Oncol Nurs Forum* 26:1491, 1999.

99. Steele CA: Access devices, administration of chemotherapy. In Yasko JM: *Nursing management of symptoms associated with chemotherapy,* Pharmacia & Upjohn, Meniscus Health Care Communications, Bala Cynwyd, PA, 1998.

100. Thomas CS: Management of infectious waste in the home care setting, *INS* 20:188, 1997.

101. US Department of Labor, Office of Occupational Medicine, OSHA: Controlling occupational exposure to hazardous, CPL 2-2.20B CH-4, Washington, DC, US Government Printing Office, 1995.

102. Viele CS, Holmes BC: Amifostine: drug profile and nursing implications of the first pancytoprotectant, *Oncol Nurs Forum* 25:515, 1998.

103. Viale PH, Yamamoto DS, Geyton JE: Extravasation of infusate via implanted ports: two case studies, *Clin J Oncol Nurs* 3:145, 1999.

104. Von Hoff DD: Phase I trials of dexazoxane and other potential applications for the agent, *Semin Oncol* 25(4 suppl 10):31, 1998.

105. Weiss RB: Introduction: dose-intensive therapy for adult malignancies, *Semin Oncol* 26:1, 1999.

106. Wickham RS and others: Taste changes experienced by patients receiving chemotherapy, *Oncol Nurs Forum* 26:697, 1999.

107. Williams J, Wood C, Cunningham-Warburton P: A narrative study of chemotherapy-induced alopecia, *Oncol Nurs Forum* 26:1463, 1999.

108. Winston DJ, Schiller GJ, Territo MC: Liposomal amphotericin B for fever and neutropenia, *N Engl J Med* 341:1154, 1999.

Most Commonly Used Chemotherapy Drugs (Adult)

Drug Class	Disease	Route	Dose (mg/m²)	Nadir	Major Side Effects/Toxicities	Nursing Action
ALKYLATING AGENTS						
Busulfan (Myleran) Busulfex (Busulfan injection)	CML, BMT preparation Allogeneic BMT preparation	PO IV	2–6 g 360–400 Varies mg/kg and ablative therapy goal	12–30 d q 4 wk	Myelosuppression, N&V, pulmonary fibrosis, alopecia, VOD; neurotoxicity with high dose or IV	Increased toxicity with high dose. Ensure total dose is given as scheduled. Premedicate for N&V
Carboplatin (Paraplatin)	Ovarian, leukemia, SCLC	IV, IP	250–600	21 d	Myelosuppression, N&V, mild nephrotoxicity and neurotoxicity	Hydration, premedicate with antiemetics. Drug decomposes if mixed with NS
Chlorambucil (Leukeran)	Lymphoma, CLL	PO, IV	0.1–0.3 mg/kg 50–100	7–14 d	Myelosuppression, sterility, stomatitis, pulmonary infiltrates, hepatotoxicity	Promote compliance, inform patient about sexuality changes
Cisplatin (Platinol)	Testicular, ovarian, lung, H&N, cervical, neuroblastoma, osteogenic sarcoma	IV, IP, IA	50–150	21 d	Nephrotoxicity, neurotoxicity, N&V, ototoxicity, electrolyte imbalance (K, Ca⁺⁺, Mg, P), hypersensitivity reaction	Hydration, monitor I&O, premedicate with antiemetics, obtain 12–24 h creatinine clearance
Cyclophosphamide (Cytoxan)	Leukemia, breast, pre-BMT, lymphoma, lung, ovarian, myeloma, neuroblastoma, Wilms', Ewing's sarcoma	IV, PO	50–200 High-dose 2–6 g	7–14 d	Myelosuppression, alopecia, hemorrhagic cystitis, N&V, cardiotoxicity, pulmonary fibrosis, temporary sterility, hypersensitivity reaction	Hydration, monitor I&O, encourage to void every 2–4 h, ECG/MUGA scan with high doses. Ensure hydration/bladder irrigation with HD BMT preparation; mesna
Dacarbazine (DTIC)	Hodgkin's, soft-tissue sarcoma, melanoma	IV	75–1500	7–21 d	Myelosuppression, N&V, alopecia, diarrhea, anaphylaxis, extravasation, flulike syndrome, hepatotoxic and renal impairment	VESICANT. Administer drug via free-flowing IV, premedicate with antiemetic
Ifosfamide (Ifex)	Breast, lung, sarcoma, ovarian, lymphoma, testicular	IV	700 mg to 2 g High dose	7–21 d	Cardiotoxicity (HD), alopecia, nephrotoxicity, N&V, hemorrhagic cystitis, myelosuppression	Concurrent administration with mesna, hydration, monitor I&O, premedicate with antiemetics
Melphalan (Alkeran)	Myeloma, ovarian, breast, multiple myeloma	PO	Varies	7–14 d	Myelosuppression (HD), N&V, hypersensitivity reaction	Premedicate with antiemetics

ALKYLATING AGENTS—continued

Drug	Uses	Route	Dose	Nadir	Side effects	Nursing considerations
Mechlorethamine HCL (Nitrogen mustard)	Hodgkin's, lymphoma, leukemia	IV, topical	Dose varies with protocol	7–21 d	Severe N&V, stomatitis, myelosuppression, alopecia, diarrhea, extravasation, hypersensitivity reactions	VESICANT, premedicate with antiemetics; administer drug within 60 min after drug reconstitution
Temozolomide (Temodal)	Refractory anaplastic astrocytoma	PO	100–250 mg	14–21 d	Myelosuppression, N&V, headache, fatigue. Avoid if hepatic or renal impaired.	Capsules supplied in amber container; take on empty stomach q 5 d × 28 d
Thiotepa (Thioplex)	Preparation BMT, breast, lymphoma, leukemia, bladder	PO, IV, Instill bladder	6–10	7–28 d	Myelosuppression, N&V, menstrual & spermatogenesis dysfunction	Myelosuppression increases with HD, monitor side effects

ANTITUMOR ANTIBIOTICS

Drug	Uses	Route	Dose	Nadir	Side effects	Nursing considerations
Bleomycin (Blenoxane)	Testicular, cervical, lung, Hodgkin's, lymphoma,	IV, IM, SC	10–20 U/m²	7 d	Anaphylaxis, N&V, rash, pneumonitis, pulmonary fibrosis, alopecia, stomatitis, hyper-pigmentation, cystitis	Test dose prior to initial administration, auscultate breath sounds on a scheduled frequency
Dactinomycin (Actinomycin D Cosmegen)	Choriocarcinoma, Ewing's and soft tissue sarcoma, Wilms' rhabdomyosarcoma	IV	1–2	7–14 d	Myelosuppression, extravasation, hepatotoxic, allergic reaction, alopecia, radiation recall, stomatitis	VESICANT, monitor skin irritation
Daunorubicin HCL (Cerubidine Daunomycin)	Leukemia (ALL, AML)	IV	30–60	7–14 d	Myelosuppression, cardiotoxic, ECG changes, extravasation, N&V, alopecia, stomatitis, anorexia, allergic reaction, dermatitis in previous irradiated areas	VESICANT, cumulative dose ~500 mg/m², monitor skin desquamation changes, inform patient re red urine 24/48 h status
Doxorubicin HCL (Adriamycin)	Breast, endometrial, H&N Ewing's, and osteogenic sarcomas, hepatic, leukemia (ALL, AML), myeloma, NHL, Wilms' neuro-retinoblastomas	IV	Varies with protocol	7–14 d	Myelosuppression, cardiotoxic, ECG changes, extravasation, N&V, alopecia, stomatitis, anorexia, allergic reaction, red urine (24–48 h), dermatitis in previously irradiated areas	VESICANT, cumulative dose ~550 mg/m², monitor skin desquamation changes, inform patient re red urine status. Doxorubicin is incompatible with many drugs. Use Zinecard/ chemoprotectant
Epirubicin HCL (Ellence)	Breast cancer	IV	100–120	7–14 d	Myelosuppression, alopecia, N&V, stomatitis, diarrhea, cardiotoxicity, chromo-somal sperm/ovarian changes	VESICANT, red urine 24–48 h. Amenorrhea in premenopausal female. Use contraceptive methods

Table continued on following page

673

Drug Class	Disease	Route	Dose (mg/m²)	Nadir	Major Side Effects/ Toxicities	Nursing Action
ANTITUMOR ANTIBIOTICS—*continued*						
Idarubicin HCL (Idamycin)	Breast, leukemia	IV	18–25	7–14 d	Myelosuppression, myocardial toxicity, extravasation, N&V, alopecia, stomatitis, diarrhea	VESICANT
Mitomycin C (Mutamycin)	Colorectal, gastric, esophageal, Ewing's and soft-tissue sarcomas	IV	10–20	21 d	Myelosuppression, pulmonary toxicity, hepatotoxicity, renal toxicity, N&V, extravasation, alopecia, urine color changes, stomatitis	VESICANT, inform patient re urine color changes
ANTIMETABOLITES						
Capecitabine (Xeloda)	Metastatic breast cancer	PO	250 mg × 14	14–21 d	Diarrhea, N&V, stomatitis, dermatitis, hyperbilirubinemia, fever, neutropenia	Administer with food; monitor altered coagulation if taken with coumarin derivatives
Cytarabine (Cytosar Ara-C)	Leukemia (ALL, AML), lymphoma, myelodysplastic syndrome	IV, IT, IP, SC	Varies with protocol	7–10 d	Myelosuppression, neurotoxicity, sudden respiratory distress with HD, rash, N&V, stomatitis, diarrhea, alopecia conjunctivitis, hepatotoxic, anaphylaxis	Monitor neurotoxicity via scheduled neuro assessments, premedicate with antiemetic. Use decadron eye drops as prophylaxis for conjunctivitis; preservative-free diluent IT administration
Cytarabine (DepoCyt)	Intrathecal liposome cytarabine to eradicate cancer cells in the cerebrospinal axis and systemic chemotherapy	IT	50 mg	5 days	Headache, fever, nausea, vomiting, neck rigidity, limb numbness	Monitor for neurotoxicity, potential to develop within 5 days of drug administration
Floxuridine (FUDR)	Colorectal, hepatic metastasis, liver	IA	5–20	7–14 d	Myelosuppression, N&V, oral and GI ulceration, alopecia, dermatitis, hepatic dysfunction	Requires placement of temporary arterial catheter and/or implantable pump for drug infusion; monitor catheter and extremity on a scheduled basis
Fludarabine phosphate (Fludara O)	Leukemia (CLL, hairy cell), low-grade NHL, B-cell CLL alt with Cytoxan	IV	30	7–14 d	Myelosuppression, CNS toxicity, visual disturbance, N&V, renal damage with HD, tumor lysis syndrome	Hydration, premedicate with antiemetics, monitor CNS toxicities on a scheduled frequency.

ANTIMETABOLITES—continued

Drug	Indications	Route	Dosage	Toxicities	Comments
5-Fluorouracil (5-FU)	Breast, colorectal, liver, endometrial, esophageal, pancreatic, bladder	IV	400–600	Myelosuppression, diarrhea, oral and GI ulcerations, alopecia, hyperpigmentation, N&V	Diarrhea and ulcerations are more severe when 5-FU is given in combination with leucovorin; incompatible with anthracyclines
Gemcitabine (Gemzar)	Pancreatic, lung cancer, breast, ovarian	IV	1 g over 30 min/wk	Myelosuppression, N&V, fatigue, fever, alopecia, rash; transient elevations of liver and renal serum levels	Premedicate with antiemetics; monitor side effects; serum transaminases; proteinuria and hematuria; dyspnea
Hydroxyurea (Hydrea)	CML chronic phase	IV, PO	1000–1500, 1000	Myelosuppression, N&V, stomatitis, dysuria, alopecia, allergic reaction	Premedicate with antiemetics, administer in divided doses, monitor allergic reaction
Irinotecan (CPT-11) (Camptosar) (Camptothecin)	Metastatic: colorectal, breast, pancreatic, gastric, glioma, gallbladder, bile duct, (topoisomerase I inhibitor)	IV	125 over 90 min × 4 wk	Myelosuppression, severe diarrhea, N&V, abdominal cramping, diaphoresis, flushing, alopecia, dyspnea	Administer antiemetic; antidiarrheal meds and IV fluids 30 min prior to drug infusion, 48 h post; DW/solution
6-Mercaptopurine (6-MP)	Leukemia (ALL, CML)	PO	100	Myelosuppression, N&V, diarrhea, oral and GI ulcerations, pancreatitis	Monitor oral dosing compliance
Methotrexate (MTX, Folex)	Breast, lymphoma, leukemia (ALL), bladder, choriocarcinoma, H&N, esophageal, mycosis fungoides	IV, IT, PO, IM	Varies with protocol	Myelosuppression, diarrhea, oral and GI ulcerations, pulmonary infiltrates and fibrosis, N&V, stomatitis, renal toxicity, hepatotoxic, CNS toxicity with IT infusion, alopecia; hypersensitivity reactions	Dosage 1 g/m² or greater requires hydration and alkalization of urine and leucovorin rescue; diarrhea and ulcerations are more severe when drug is given in HD, preservative-free diluent with IT administration.
Oxaliplatin (Eloxatin)	Metastatic colorectal cancer	IV	25 mg/m² via 6 h inf	Myelosuppression, oesthenia (fatigue) neuropathy	Drug usually administered in combination with 5-FU/Leucovorin
6-Thioguanine (6-TG)	Leukemia (ALL)	PO	100	Myelosuppression, diarrhea, stomatitis, hepatic damage	Monitor oral dosing compliance
Trimetrexate (Neutrexin)	Pneumocystis carinii, H&N, SCLC, urothelial cancer	IV	8–12 for 5 d	Myelosuppression, mucositis, fever, chills, N&V, rash, pruritus, hyperpigmentation, nephrotoxicity, diarrhea	Monitor toxicities; administer antiemetic and antidiarrheal drugs

Table continued on following page

Most Commonly Used Chemotherapy Drugs (Adult) *Continued*

Drug Class	Disease	Route	Dose (mg/m²)	Nadir	Major Side Effects/ Toxicities	Nursing Action
HORMONAL AGENTS		**Varied**	**NOT IN mg/m²**			
Aminoglutethimide (Cytadren)	Breast, prostate	PO	500–1000 mg	None	Nausea, hypotension, fever, rash, masculinization, hypo- and/or hyper-glycemia	Produces medical adrenalectomy, drug interactions with Warfarin, digoxin, theophylline
Anastrozole (Arimidex)	Metastatic breast cancer	PO	1 mg/d	None	Nausea, headache, hot flashes, pain, back pain, diarrhea	Inform patient about side effects
Bicalutamide (Casodex)	Metastatic prostate cancer	PO	50 mg daily	None	Pain, hypertension, hot flashes, nausea	Inform patient about sexuality changes; drug not indicated in women
Corticosteriods (Dexamethasone, Decadron, Solu-Cortef, Solu-Medrol, Prednisone)	Used in many chemo-therapy disease protocols	PO, IV, IM	Varies with protocol	None	Fluid and electrolyte disturbances, neuro-muscular imbalances, changes in appetite and energy, requires glucose/insulin adjustments, potential weight gain	Decadron IV rapid bolus will result in severe rectal itching. Corticosteriods long-term use requires dose tapering principles.
Diethylstilbesterol (DES)	Breast, prostate	PO	Varies	None	N&V, gynecomastia in males, breast tenderness, loss of libido, hyper-tension, changes in menstrual flow	Inform patient about sexuality changes
Fenretinide (Raloxifene)	Antiestrogen, chemo-prevention breast cancer	PO	200 mg	None	Headache, rash, hair loss, vertigo, diarrhea, N&V, joint pain	Inform patient about sexuality changes
Finasteride (Proscar)	Prostate	PO	5 mg	None	Impotence, decreased libido, teratogenic	Inform patient about sexuality changes. Monitor liver enzymes; triglycerides
Flutamide (Eulexin)	Prostate	PO	250–750 mg	None	Nausea, diarrhea, gyneco-mastia, hepatotoxicity	Inform patient about sexuality changes
Goserelin acetate (Zoladex)	Breast, prostate	IM, SC	Varies	None	Postmenopausal symptoms, impotence, testicular atrophy, gynecomastia, hot flashes, transient increased bone pain	Inform patient about sexuality changes

HORMONAL AGENTS—continued

Drug	Uses	Route	Dose NOT IN mg/m²	Nadir	Side Effects	Nursing Considerations
Leuprolide (Lupron)	Prostate	Varied IM, SC	Varies	None	Impotence, testicular atrophy, hot flashes, gynecomastia, CNS effects, peripheral edema, transient increase in bone pain	Inform patient about sexuality changes
Letrozole (Femara)	Antiestrogen, metastatic breast cancer	PO	0.5–2.5 mg	None	Mild hot flashes, vaginal dryness, weight gain	Inform patient about sexuality changes
Megestrol (Megace)	Breast, prostate	PO	Varies	None	Menstrual changes, hot flashes, N&V, headache, fluid retention, weight gain	Inform patient about sexuality changes (appetite stimulant for anorexia)
Nilutamide (Nilandron)	Antiandrogen; metastatic prostate cancer	PO	50 mg	None	Pain, hot flashes, nausea, constipation, dizziness, insomnia	Sexuality changes; monitor liver function studies
Tamoxifen (Nolvadex)	Breast	PO	Varies	None	Vaginal bleeding and discharge, hot flashes, rash, N&V, hypercalcemia, bone pain, peripheral edema, weight gain	Inform patient about sexuality changes
Toremifene citrate (Fareston)	Metastatic breast cancer	PO	60 mg	NA	Hot flashes, nausea, vaginal discharge, bone pain, hypercalcemia	Inform patient about sexuality changes
NITROSOUREA						
Carmustine (BCNU)	Glioblastoma myeloma, lymphoma, pre-BMT	IV	200–225	3–4 wk	Myelosuppression, N&V, pulmonary fibrosis, renal and liver damage, seizures, myocardial ischemia, leukemia, phlebitis	Irritant, administer slowly, contains alcohol, patient may feel inebriated; myelosuppression is increased with HD administration
Carmustine (Gliadel wafer)	Implant for glioblastoma	Cranial implant	7.7 mg each wafer (may implant up to 8 wafers)	Varies	Seizure, brain edema, intracranial infection	Monitor for neurotoxicity by recommended postoperative protocol
Lomustine (CCNU)	Brain, leukemia, Hodgkin's lymphoma, melanoma, myeloma, bladder	PO	100–150	4–6 wk	Myelosuppression, N&V, pulmonary fibrosis, neurologic reactions, renal damage, leukemia, elevated liver enzymes	Administer at bedtime with antiemetics
Semustine (Methyl-CCNU)	Brain, colorectal, gastric	PO	150–200	4–6 wk	Myelosuppression, N&V, renal and hepatic toxicities	Administer on an empty stomach with antiemetics
Streptozocin (Zanosar)	Colorectal, liver, pancreas	IV	Varies	2–4 wk	Myelosuppression, CNS effects, renal/liver damage, hypo/hyperglycemia, N&V	Irritant, monitor for phlebitis and glucose/insulin levels

Table continued on following page

APPENDIX
Most Commonly Used Chemotherapy Drugs (Adult) *Continued*

Drug Class	Disease	Route	Dose (mg/m²)	Nadir	Major Side Effects/Toxicities	Nursing Action
VINCA ALKALOIDS Etoposide (VePesid, VP-16)	Lung, testicular, Kaposi's and osteogenic sarcomas, leukemia, neuroblastoma, preparation BMT, lymphoma	IV, PO	50–100, 200	7–10 d	Myelosuppression, N&V, diarrhea, fever, hypotension, phlebitis, anaphylaxis, rash, alopecia, peripheral neuropathy, mucositis, and hepatic damage with high dose	Administer drug slowly IV; increased severity of side effects with HD
Teniposide (Vumon, VM-26)	Leukemia (childhood ALL), SCLC	IV	165	7–14 d	Myelosuppression, extravasation, alopecia, constipation, neuropathy	VESICANT, monitor neurotoxicities and bowel function, promote hydration
Vinblastine sulfate (Velban)	Testicular, Hodgkin's, lung, lymphoma, bladder, Kaposi's sarcoma, renal	IV	2–6	5–10 d	Myelosuppression, extravasation, N&V, alopecia, stomatitis, loss of deep tendon reflexes, jaw pain, paralytic ileus	VESICANT, monitor neurotoxicity and promote hydration and high-fiber diet, administer oral stool softener
Vincristine sulfate (Oncovin)	Leukemia (ALL, CML), lymphoma, myeloma, retinoblastoma, Wilms', brain, Ewing's & Kaposi's sarcoma, rhabdomyosarcoma, SCLC	IV	0.5–2 mg	5–7 d	Extravasation, alopecia, stomatitis, constipation, paralytic ileus, peripheral neuropathy, jaw pain, inappropriate ADH secretion, mild myelosuppression, optic atrophy	VESICANT, monitor bowel function, promote hydration and high-fiber diet, administer oral stool softener, monitor neurotoxicity changes
Vindesine (Eldesine VDS)	Squamous cell-esophagus	IV	2–4	7–14 d	Myelosuppression, peripheral neuropathy, constipation, extravasation, skin changes	VESICANT, monitor neuropathy and constipation, promote hydration
Vinorelbine tartrate (Navelbine)	Breast, non-SCLC, Hodgkin's, H&N	IV	30 dilute conc. > 3 mL	7–10 d	Myelosuppression, bronchospasm, alopecia, injection site reactions (erythema, discoloration, phlebitis, pain), N&V, anorexia, stomatitis, peripheral neuropathy, constipation, weakness, fatigue	VESICANT, IRRITANT, monitor neurotoxicity and bowel function; follow manufacturer's reconstitution guidelines; pre- and posthydration 100 mL to flush the vein; administer drug over 10 min via free-flow IV

MISCELLANEOUS CHEMOTHERAPY DRUGS

Drug	Indications	Route	Dose	Nadir	Toxicities	Nursing considerations
L-Asparaginase (El-spar)	Leukemia (ALL)	IV, IM	1000–6000 IU/kg	None	Anaphylaxis, N&V, chills, headache, CNS depression, abdominal pain, coagulation defects, hyperglycemia, hepatic and renal damage, fever	Maintain IV access, follow anaphylaxis protocol, monitor for 2–4 h after drug infusion
Cladribine (Leustatin 2-CdA)	Hairy cell leukemia, low-grade lymphoma	IV CI × 7 d	0.09 mg/kg amb. pump	7–14 d	Myelosuppression, peripheral neuropathy with HD, fever, fatigue	Incompatible with D_5W; calculate dose by multiplying patient's weight in kg by 0.09 mg
2-Deoxycoformycin (Pentostatin)	Hairy cell leukemia, chronic lymphocytic leukemia, lymphoma	IV, SC	2–4	7–14 d	Myelosuppression, nephrotoxicity, CNS depression, N&V, myalgia, rash, photophobia, conjunctivitis	Monitor toxicities; teach patient to recognize and report symptoms
Docetaxel (Taxotere)	Breast, non-SCLC, ovarian	IV	100	7–14 d	Anaphylaxis, myelosuppression, fluid retention, skin desquamation, mucositis, phlebitis, localized erythema, vomiting, & diarrhea, fluid retention	Premedicate; maintain IV access, follow anaphylaxis protocol; use non-PVC tubing/glass bottle for drug administration. VESICANT
Hexamethyl-melamine (Altretamine)	Lymphoma, lung, H&N, breast, ovarian	PO	150–400 in 4 divided doses	21 d	Myelosuppression, N&V, CNS depression, peripheral neuropathy, ataxia, tremors, alopecia, rash	Premedicate with antiemetics, ensure medication is taken QID (PC & HS)
Leucovorin (Folic Acid)	Used in multiple chemotherapy regimens, e.g., 5-FU	PO, IV	Varies	7–14 d	Hypersensitivity, pruritus, erythema, urticaria, wheezing	Promote hydration and compliance in self-administration regimens
Levamisole (Ergamisol)	Used in multiple chemotherapy regimens	PO	1–5 mg/kg	None	Mild GI complaints	Observe
Lysodren (Mitotane)	Adrenocortical carcinoma	PO	9–10 g/d divided doses	None	CNS depression, N&V, diarrhea, visual disturbance, rash, pulmonary infiltrates, hypertension	Provide hydration, monitor CNS effects
Mitoxantrone (Novantrone)	Leukemia, breast, lymphoma, childhood T-cell ALL and lymphoma	IV	15	7–14 d	Myelosuppression, cardiotoxicity, alopecia, N&V, stomatitis, phlebitis, hepatic and renal damage	Inform patient re urine and sclera blue-green pigment changes 24–48 h postdrug infusion
Octreotide (Sandostatin)	Antidiarrhea 50 μg IV TID; carcinoid cancers; NHL	IV SC	100–600 μg	None	Abdominal pain and cramps; headache, nausea; insomnia; USE with caution in CNS disease	Culture and sensitivity for diarrhea; monitor for dehydration/hydration

Table continued on following page

APPENDIX
Most Commonly Used Chemotherapy Drugs (Adult) *Continued*

Drug Class	Disease	Route	Dose (mg/m²)	Nadir	Major Side Effects/ Toxicities	Nursing Action
MISCELLANEOUS CHEMOTHERAPY DRUGS—*continued*						
Paclitaxel (Taxol)	Breast, non-SCLC melanoma, H&N, ovarian	IV	175–200	7–14 d	Anaphylaxis, myelosuppression, angioedema, dyspnea, hypotension, alopecia, urticaria, cardiotoxic, peripheral neuropathy	Premedicate; maintain IV access, follow anaphylaxis protocol; use non-PVC tubing/glass bottle for drug administration. VESICANT
Procarbazine (Matulane)	Lymphoma, lung, brain, Hodgkin's	PO	100–150	3–5 wk	Myelosuppression, CNS depression, N&V, stomatitis, avoid alcohol, foods rich in tyramine (yeast)	Teach patient diet (e.g., bananas, yogurt, and ethanol restrictions); antidepressants/ antihistamines
Thalidomide (Thalomid)	Multiple myeloma, melanoma, H*N, brain, Kaposi's sarcoma	IV, PO	50–200 mg/d	7–14 d	Myelosuppression, nausea and vomiting, skin rash, impairment of fertility	Life-threatening human birth defects. Female patients require effective contraception for at least 1 mo before beginning drug, during thalidomide therapy, and for 1 mo after discontinuation of thalidomide. Two reliable forms of contraception must be used simultaneously.
Topotecan HCL (Hycamtin)	Lung, breast, esophagus, ovarian, leukemia, myelodysplastic syndrome	IV	2 mg CI over 5 d	7–14 d	Myelosuppression, N&V, diarrhea, fever, fatigue, alopecia, mucositis, rash, fever/flu-like syndrome; elevated liver enzymes	DₗW preferred solution, reconstitute and use within 24 hours, Administer antiemetics and antipyretics.
Tretinoin (Vesanoid ATRA)	Acute promyelocytic leukemia; may be given in combination with CTY	Oral	45 mg/m² daily	None	Fever, skin mucous membrane dryness, bone pain, N&V, alopecia, pruritus, HA, retinoic acid-APL syndrome—leukocytosis; CNS, respiratory, hypercholesterolemia	Monitor drug side effects and progression of clinical symptoms. Provide scheduled CNS, respiratory, and myelosuppression assessment and interventions
INVESTIGATIONAL CHEMOTHERAPY DRUGS						
Azacitidine (5-Azacytidine)	Leukemia (refractory AML)	IV	200	7–14 d	Myelosuppression, fever, rash, diarrhea, N&V, drowsiness, hepatic and cardiotoxicity	Premedicate with antiemetics

INVESTIGATIONAL CHEMOTHERAPY DRUGS—*continued*

Drug	Indication	Route	Dose	Nadir	Side effects	Nursing considerations
Chlorozotocin (DCNU)	GI and pancreatic clinical trials	IV	Varies	2–4 wk	Myelosuppression, N&V, phlebitis, renal and liver damage, diarrhea, hyperglycemia, fever	IRRITANT, monitor glucose/insulin levels
Didemnin B	Lung, breast, ovarian, sarcoma, kidney	IV	5	7–14 d	Anaphylaxis, N&V, diarrhea, elevated liver enzymes	Follow anaphylaxis protocol, premedicate with antiemetics
Dolastatin (DOLA-10)	Metastatic advanced breast	IV	Varies	7–14 d	Neutropenia, thrombocytopenia, diarrhea, paresthesia, neuropathy	Administer IV bolus via NS-D$_5$W IV-Y-site
Edatrexate (10-Edam)	H&N, colorectal, breast, lymphoma, lung, soft-tissue sarcomas	IV	350	7–14 d	Myelosuppression, mucositis, fatigue, diarrhea, alopecia, N&V	Premedicate with antiemetics
Fazarabine	Lung, pancreas	IV	2	7–14 d	Myelosuppression, elevated liver enzymes, N&V	Reconstitute with D$_5$W or lactated Ringer's solution
Iressa	NSC lung, pancreatic	PO	250–500 mg	7–14 d	Diarrhea, acne, elevated liver enzymes	Increased toxicities may occur when combined with radiation therapy
Isotretinoin (Accutane)	Cervical	PO	1 mg/kg	7–14 d	Fatigue, headache, N&V, xerostomia, rash, conjunctivitis, anorexia, pruritus, bone and joint pain, nosebleeds	Provide prudent mouth care and offer medications for dry eyes/conjunctivitis
Merberone	Pancreatic, gastric, melanoma	IV	1 g CI 5 d	7–14 d	Alopecia, elevated liver enzymes, N&V, diarrhea, phlebitis, anorexia	IRRITANT, premedicate with antiemetics, monitor liver enzymes
Pala	Colorectal	IV	250	7–14 d	N&V, diarrhea, stomatitis	Premedicate with antiemetics
Piroxantrone (Oxantrazole)	Breast, prostate, H&N, melanoma	IV	150	7–14 d	Myelosuppression, N&V, alopecia, mucositis, diarrhea, lethargy, extravasation	VESICANT, premedicate with antiemetics
Pirtrexin	Melanoma, urothelial cancers, H&N	PO	75–150 mg, bid	7–14 d	Myelosuppression, mucositis, stomatitis, N&V, anorexia, skin rash	Premedicate with antiemetics
STI 571	Chronic myelogenous leukemia	PO	25–600 mg	7 d	Myelosuppression, nausea, vomiting	Avoid coadministration of hydroxyurea
Suramin	Prostate, breast, multiple myeloma	IV	350–1400	7–14 d	Myelosuppression, proteinuria, photophobia, elevated liver enzymes and serum creatinine	Inform patient of side effects and visual changes

MISCELLANEOUS DRUGS

Prophylactic Drugs

Drug	Indication	Route	Dose	Nadir	Side effects	Nursing considerations
Allopurinol (Zyloprim)	Leukemia, Hodgkin's, lymphoma	PO	200–600 mg/QD	None	Myelosuppression, headache, drowsiness, anorexia, N&V, alopecia	Promote hydration, administer prior to chemotherapy drug initiation

Table continued on following page

APPENDIX
Most Commonly Used Chemotherapy Drugs (Adult) *Continued*

Drug Class	Disease	Route	Dose (mg/m²)	Nadir	Major Side Effects/Toxicities	Nursing Action
MISCELLANEOUS DRUGS—continued						
Prophylactic Drugs—continued						
Allopurinol (Aloprim)	Leukemia, lymphoma, and solid tumor malignancies	IV	200–600 mg/QD	None	Myelosuppression, headache, drowsiness, anorexia, N&V, alopecia	Promote hydration, administer prior to chemotherapy drug initiation
Pamidronate (Aredia)	Hypercalcemia, related to bone metastasis in breast, prostate, multiple myeloma	IV	90 mg over 2–4 h q 3–4 wk	None	Soft tissue symptoms (redness, edema, pain on palpation); hypertension, mild fever, N&V, anorexia, constipation, bone pain	Assess and provide comfort measures, e.g., pain, nausea, fever
Zoledronic acid (Zometa)	Hypercalcemia, related to bone metastasis in breast, prostate, multiple myeloma	IV	4–8 mg over 15 min	NA	Mild skeletal pain, nausea	Promote hydration
Cytoprotectant Drugs						
Amifostine (Ethyol)	Ovarian, NSC lung; minimizes potential cumulative nephrotoxicity	IV	700/900 mg over 15 min	7–14 d	Hypotension (transient), N&V, chills, skin rash, somnolence, flushed sensation	Premedicate (hydration and antiemetics). Monitor VS on a scheduled frequency during infusion
Amifostine (Ethyol)	Reduce the incidence of moderate to severe xerostomia in patients undergoing radiation treatment for H&N cancer	IV	200 mg/m² daily as 3-min IV infusion	None	Hypotension (transient), N&V, sensations of warmth, chills, fever, dizziness, somnolence, hiccups, and sneezing	Administer 15–30 min prior to scheduled radiation therapy treatments; ensure hydration
Dexrazoxane (Zinecard)	Breast cancer; diminishes the potential maximum dose of doxorubicin (cardiac toxicity)	IV	1 g IV over 15 min	NA	N&V, transient hypotension (blocks cardiotoxic effects)	Administer Zinecard 30 min prior to doxorubicin administration
Mesna (Mesnex)	Prophylaxis to reduce incidence of ifosfamide and cyclophosfamide and induced hemorrhagic cystitis	IV bolus	240 mg	None	N&V, diarrhea, altered taste, rash, headache, fatigue, joint pain, hypotension	Always administer with each dose of ifosfamide and/or high-dose cyclosphosphamide
Liposomal Agents						
Amphotericin B (Abelcet)	Treatment of aspergillosis	IV	Dose varies with protocol	NA	Hypotension, N&V, diarrhea, electrolyte imbalance, dyspnea, skin rash, fever, and chills	Monitor side effects; follow physician prescribed administration protocol
Amphotericin B (Am-Bisome)	Empiric therapy for presumed fungal infection in febrile, neutropenic patients	IV	Dose varies with protocol	NA	Abdominal and back pain, chills, N&V, blood product transfusion reaction, hypotension and	Monitor side effects; follow physician prescribed administration protocol

Liposomal Agents—continued

Drug	Description/Indication	Route	Dose	Nadir	Toxicities	Nursing considerations
Depocyt	Sustained-released cytarabine encapsulated with depofoam particles; neoplastic meningitis	IT	50 mg	NA	hypertension, electrolyte imbalance, arthralgia, facial edema; Headache, fever, nausea, vomiting, neck rigidity, asthma	
Doxorubicin HCL (Doxil)	Kaposi's sarcoma, AIDS, metastatic carcinoma of the ovary refractory to paclitaxel and platinum-based chemotherapy regimens	IV	36 mg/kg	7–14 d	Myelosuppression, dyspnea, headache, chills, back pain, tightness in chest and throat, hypotension, stomatitis, hand-foot syndrome	IRRITANT; do not administer IM or SC; irritant; monitor CBC levels, and complications related to myelosuppression
Multidrug Resistant (MDR) Valspodar (PSC 833)	Acute myelogenous leukemia, lymphoma, multiple myeloma, ovarian and gastric cancers, and thymus gland	IV	2 mg/kg over 2 h	None	Inflammation and mild skin reactions at injection site, mild dizziness, numbness, ataxia. Abstain from alcohol products and sedatives during drug administration	Initiate the infusion ONE day before the scheduled chemotherapy drug; infusion stable only 24 h after diluted
MONOCLONAL ANTIBODIES Gemtuzumabozogamicin (Myelotarg)	$CD33^+$ antigen acute myeloid leukemia	IV	9 mg/m^2	7–14 d	Myelosuppression, nausea, fever, chills, transient changes in bilirubin and liver enzymes	Premedicate with acetaminophen PO and diphenhydramine IV
Rituximab (Rituxan)	B-cell NHL (low-grade follicular), drug targets the CD20 antigen found on the surface of B cells	IV	375–400 mg/m^2	7–14 d	Fever and chills (rigors), N&V, urticaria, fatigue, dyspnea, hypotension, bronchospasm, flushing and pain at disease sites	Do not administer as an IV push or bolus; initial infusion rate 50 mg/h; may increase rate to 100 mg/h q 30 min; MAX 400 mg/h if no clinical event occurs; incompatible with other drugs; premedicate with acetaminophen PO and diphenhydramine IV
Trastuzumab (Herceptin)	Anti-HER2 antibody treatment for metastatic breast cancer with an overexpression of HER-2 protein	IV	2–4 mg weekly	7–14 d	Cardiac toxicity (CHF), leukopenia, anemia, diarrhea, abdominal pain, headache, rhinitis, pruritus, chills, fever, N&V	Do not administer as an IV push or bolus; incompatible with other drugs and D$_5$W solution.

ABMT, autologous bone marrow transplantation; ALL, acute lymphocytic leukemia; ADH, antidiuretic hormone; bid, twice a day; BMT, bone marrow transplantation; Ca^{++}, calcium; CHF, congestive heart failure; CI, continuous infusion; CLL, chronic lymphocytic leukemia; CML, chronic myelogenous leukemia; CNS, central nervous system; D$_5$W, dextrose water 5%; ECG, electrocardiogram; GI, gastrointestinal; HD, high dose; HIV, human immunodeficiency virus; H&N, head and neck; I&O, intake and output; IA, intra-arterial; IM, intramuscular; IP, intraperitoneal; IT, intrathecal; IV, intravenous; SC, subcutaneous; K$^+$, potassium; Mg, magnesium; P, phosphorus; PO, oral; qd, daily; VOD, veno-occlusive disease; SCLC, small-cell lung carcinoma; N&V, nausea and vomiting; NHL, non-Hodgkin's lymphoma; CTY, chemotherapy; HER2, human epidermal growth factor 2

Biotherapy

Carol Pappas Appel

The rapid introduction of novel agents and approaches and an improved understanding of the biology of cancer have opened an exciting era in cancer therapy. Traditionally, surgery, radiation therapy, and chemotherapy, either singly or in combination, have been the mainstays of cancer therapy. Since the 1980s, biotherapy, or biologic therapy, has emerged as an important fourth modality for treating cancer, and in recent years provided multiple options for patients receiving high-dose chemotherapy regimens and bone marrow or stem cell transplantations.[65, 83, 96, 131, 195]

Oncology nurses whose patients receive biotherapy need a basic understanding of the immune system, the rationale for this therapy, and its primary clinical agents (see Chapter 31 for a review of the immune system). This chapter reviews the history of immunotherapy and other biotherapy approaches, scientific advances that led to clinical trials with biologic agents, the rationale for the use of these agents, their clinical indications, and the associated nursing care for patients receiving them.

THEORY OF IMMUNE SURVEILLANCE

Host defense mechanisms protect the body by detecting and eliminating substances recognized as "foreign" or "nonself." The theory of immune surveillance, refined and expanded by McFarlane Burnet,[38, 117, 142] states that certain cells undergo neoplastic transformation but are recognized by the immune system as foreign and subsequently destroyed. At first, T cells were thought to be primarily responsible for this reaction, but it is now known that other immune cells such as natural killer (NK) cells and macrophages are also involved.[142] If an atypical cell somehow escapes detection or destruction, a clinically detectable tumor eventually develops.

Although this theory remains controversial, many clinical phenomena and laboratory observations support it. Spontaneous tumor regression has been observed in patients with solid tumors such as melanoma and renal cancer and with acute leukemia[233]; that is, tumors shrank or patients entered remission without treatment. Some of these regressions have been associated with infectious complications, which may suggest an immunologic mechanism.[117, 192, 233]

Immunologic defense mechanisms are relatively weak in the young and the aged, and the incidence of malignancy in humans peaks correspondingly during early childhood and old age. In these periods, impaired or immature defense mechanisms may allow abnormal cells to escape immune surveillance and proliferate. An increased incidence of cancer is also seen in patients with immune deficiencies resulting from immunosuppressive therapy or other causes, for example, individuals undergoing chronic immunosuppressive therapy for the maintenance of organ and marrow allografts. Patients with immunodeficiencies exhibit a higher incidence of malignancies, especially of the lymphoid type, than does the general population.[142, 203]

The fact that immune cells infiltrate tumors also supports this theory. Pathologic examination of surgical specimens shows infiltration by lymphocytes, macrophages, and plasma cells, and it has been suggested that immune mechanisms may be responsible for reducing the growth rate of tumors.[210] A variety of experiments lend further support to the theory of immune surveillance. Neonatal thymectomy causes mice to accept tumor transplants, whereas mice possessing normal thymic function reject the transplants.[3] The use of antilymphocyte serum and immunosuppressive therapy in animals can increase the incidence and development of both spontaneous tumors and those induced by viruses and chemical carcinogens. Lymphocytes appear to be essential to the recognition and destruction of aberrant cells.[117]

If, as this evidence suggests, immune surveillance is an important part of antitumor host defense, how do transformed cells escape detection by the immune system? Krueger[142] proposes four basic mechanisms: (1) a basic defect in function of effector cells responsible for immune surveillance; (2) an imbalance of the immune response to the tumor; (3) malignant cells not sufficiently immunogenic to elicit an immune response; and (4) production of blocking factors that interfere with the immune response to tumors. Although skepticism remains regarding the theory of immune surveillance, it is an attractive explanation for the occurrence of cancer. Further experimentation will continue to clarify the relationship between the immune system and malignant cells.[83]

HISTORICAL PERSPECTIVE

The observation of interactions between the immune system and malignant cells led to the development of therapies that could manipulate this natural process. Traditionally, this field has been known as *immunotherapy.*[117, 233] The immunotherapy of cancer can be divided into two approaches, active and passive. *Active immunotherapy* consists of giving a tumor-bearing host agents that are designed to elicit an immune response capable of retarding or eliminating tumor growth. The two types of active immunotherapy are specific and nonspecific. *Active specific* immunotherapy is immunization with tumor cells or tumor cell extracts, either alone or in vaccines. The use of monoclonal antibodies as vaccines is an area of active investigation. *Active nonspecific immunotherapy* is an attempt to boost overall immunity through the use of adjuvants such as bacterial extracts. The latter approach was based on the observation that adjuvants administered in animal systems could cause tumor regression. It was also based on the idea that those with tumors have diminished defense mechanisms.[117, 233]

Passive immunotherapy is the administration or transfer of previously sensitized immunologic reagents such as antisera (which contain sensitized antibodies) or immune-reactive cells to a tumor-bearing host. These reagents directly or indirectly mediate antitumor responses. The term *adoptive immunotherapy* is still used to refer to the passive transfer of sensitized cells such as lymphocytes or macrophages.[117, 231, 233]

Principles for immunotherapy of human cancer are based mainly on knowledge gained from animal experiments. *First,* immunotherapeutic approaches appeared most successful for small tumor burdens. Therefore tumor burden was to be reduced by conventional treatment, followed by immunotherapy. *Second,* the host had to be immunocompetent, or immunocompetence had to be restored, for immunotherapy to be maximally effective. *Third,* the timing of immunotherapy was crucial. How long after conventional treatment immunotherapy should be started to allow for restoration of immunosup-

pressive effects was a concern. *Fourth,* the site of immunization for active immunotherapy, especially active specific immunotherapy, was extremely important. Active specific immunotherapy was often given in tumor-free lymphatic drainage areas.[117]

Initial attempts at boosting the immune systems of cancer patients to destroy tumors used a variety of microorganisms, fractions of microbial products, or other immunomodulators. Since the 1960s many clinical studies have attempted nonspecific stimulation of the immune system by using such products as bacille Calmette-Guerin (BCG) or its methanol extraction residue (MER), *Corynebacterium parvum,* and levamisole. Although initial trials seemed positive, well-controlled, prospective, randomized trials did not show significant overall survival gains in the arm using immunotherapy.[195] These early trials failed to establish immunotherapy as a major modality most likely for a variety of reasons, such as the lack of purity and definition of immunotherapeutic agents, lack of analogy between animal model systems and humans, variability of experimental procedures, and inadequate administration of immunotherapeutic agents.[195, 233]

TECHNOLOGIC ADVANCES

During the 1970s and 1980s, several scientific and technologic developments led biologic therapy to emerge as a major modality in the treatment of cancer. Our overall understanding of the relationship between host defense mechanisms and cancer and of the basic biology of cancer has improved. Recombinant DNA technology (Fig. 24-1) has allowed the production of large quantities of highly purified products from the human genome, as hybridoma technology has done for highly purified, highly specific immunoglobulin reagents. Methods of growing large volumes of effector cells in culture have been developed, and advances in computer hardware and software have led to the isolation and purification of biologic molecules.[95, 195]

These discoveries have led to the modern era of biotherapy. The use of this term is more appropriate than heretofore because this field encompasses a much broader basis than only the immune system. Although the use of agents affecting the immune system remains a subcategory, biotherapy includes treatments affecting other biologic responses such as growth and differentiation factors, chimeric molecules (genetically engineered molecules that may have some parts added or removed to tailor them for a particular use, as when a chimeric monoclonal antibody [MoAb] has part human and part murine fragments), and agents that may affect the ability of tumor cells to metastasize.

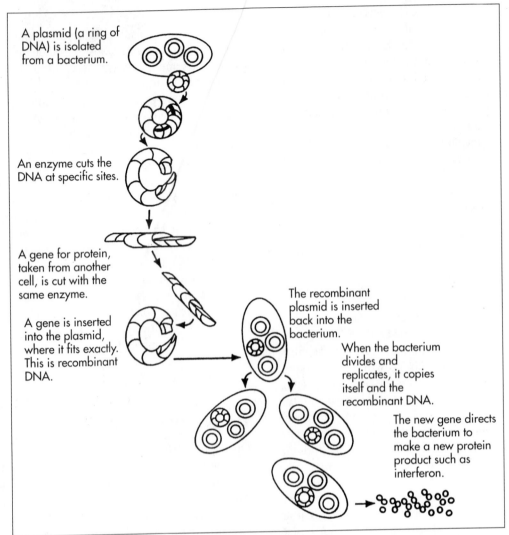

A plasmid (a ring of DNA) is isolated from a bacterium.

An enzyme cuts the DNA at specific sites.

A gene for protein, taken from another cell, is cut with the same enzyme.

A gene is inserted into the plasmid, where it fits exactly. This is recombinant DNA.

The recombinant plasmid is inserted back into the bacterium.

When the bacterium divides and replicates, it copies itself and the recombinant DNA.

The new gene directs the bacterium to make a new protein product such as interferon.

FIGURE 24–1 Recombinant DNA technology. Genetic engineering, known as recombinant DNA technology, allows scientists to pluck genes from one type of organism and combine them with genes of a second organism, inducing cells to make large quantities of human protein, such as interferon and interleukins. Microorganisms also can be made to manufacture proteins from infectious agents, such as the hepatitis virus and the AIDS virus, for use in vaccines. (From Schindler LW: *Understanding the immune system,* NIH Publication No. 88-529, Bethesda, MD, US Department of Health and Human Services, 1988.)

BIOTHERAPY DEFINED

Biotherapy may be defined as treatment with agents derived from biologic sources and/or affecting biologic responses. Most of its agents are derived from the mammalian genome.[195] The Subcommittee on Biologic Response Modifiers (BRMs) of the National Cancer Institute (NCI) Division of Cancer Treatment defines BRMs as "agents or approaches that modify the relationship between tumor and host by modifying the host's biologic response to tumor cells, with a resultant therapeutic effect."[174]

The explosion of biotherapy research, coupled with the technologic advances, has led to the use of numerous agents, both commercially and in clinical trials. These include nonspecific immunomodulating agents such as BCG and *C. parvum,* and newer agents, such as interferons (IFNs), interleukins, MoAbs, and hematopoietic growth factors (Tables 24–1 and 24–2). Many of these are naturally occurring body substances that act as messengers between cells. A generic term for these messengers is *cytokine,* which refers to protein products from cells that serve as cell regulators. More

TABLE 24–1
Biologic Activity of Cytokines

Cytokine	Abbreviation	Primary Cellular Source	Biologic Activity
INTERFERONS			
Interferon-α	IFN-α	Leukocytes	Antiviral activity.
Interferon-β	IFN-β	Fibroblasts	Antiproliferative effects; augments NK cell activity; induces MHC class I antigens.
Interferon-γ	IFN-γ	T cells, NK cells, monocytes/macrophages	Antiviral activity; induces MHC class I, II antigens; potent immunomodulatory effects; interacts with other cytokines; enhances tumor-associated antigen expression; regulates differentiation.
HEMATOPOIETIC GROWTH FACTORS			
Granulocyte colony-stimulating factor	G-CSF	Stromal cells, endothelial cells, monocytes/ macrophages	Stimulates growth of granulocyte colonies; activates mature granulocytes; augments ADCC; stimulates proliferation and differentiation of leukemic cells.
Granulocyte/macrophage colony-stimulating factor	GM-CSF	Fibroblasts, endothelial cells, T cells, stromal cells	Stimulates growth of monocyte, granulocyte, and early erythroid progenitors; activates mature granulocytes and monocytes; enhances ADCC and cell-mediated cytotoxicity.
Macrophage colony-stimulating factor	M-CSF	Fibroblasts, stromal cells, monocytes/macrophages	Stimulates growth of monocyte colonies; activates mature monocytes.
Erythropoietin	Epo	Peritubular cells in the kidney	Stimulates erythrocyte progenitors; primary regulator of erythropoiesis.
Thrombopoietin	Tpo	Hepatic cells, endothelial cells, fibroblasts	Primary regulator of platelet production.
Stem cell factor	SCF	Stromal-derived cells	Stimulates multiple and committed stem cells, mast cells, megakaryocytes; potent costimulatory factor.
INTERLEUKINS			
Interleukin-1	IL-1	Monocytes/macrophages; B, T, and NK cells; fibroblasts; endothelial cells	Hematopoietic effects; induces acute-phase responses (e.g., fever, sleep, ACTH release); mediates inflammation; activates resting T cells.
Interleukin-2	IL-2	T cells	Primary T-cell growth factor; cofactor for growth and differentiation of B cells; induction/release of cytokines.
Interleukin-3	IL-3	T cells	Stimulates early progenitor cell growth; supports mast cell growth; supports growth of pre-B cell lines.
Interleukin-4	IL-4	T cells, mast cells, macrophages	Growth factor for activated B cells; growth factor for resting T cells; supports mast cell growth; enhances cytolytic activity of cytotoxic T cells.
Interleukin-5	IL-5	T cells, mast cells	Induces differentiation and proliferation of eosinophil progenitors; cofactor for induction of cytotoxic T cells; increases proliferation of IgG and IgL immunoglobulins.
Interleukin-6	IL-6	T cells, monocytes/ macrophages, fibroblasts, endothelial cells	Costimulates T cells; induces IL-2 production; induces acute phase response; hematopoietic effects; augments NK and LAK cytotoxicity; synergizes with other growth factors to promote colony growth; enhances IgG secretion by B cells; induces B-cell differentiation.
Interleukin-7	IL-7	Bone marrow stromal cells	Induces LAK activity; supports growth of B-cell precursors; induces cytokine secretion by monocytes.

Table continued on following page

TABLE 24-1
Biologic Activity of Cytokines *Continued*

Cytokine	Abbreviation	Primary Cellular Source	Biologic Activity
Interleukin-8	IL-8	Monocytes/macrophages	Strongly chemotactic for neutrophils, T and B cells, and monocytes; depending on cofactor, enhances or inhibits growth of hematopoietic progenitors.
Interleukin-9	IL-9	T-helper cells	Stimulates antigen-specific T-helper cell clones; stimulates mast cell growth; supports erythroid colony formation; potentiates IL-4-induced IgE synthesis by B cells.
Interleukin-10	IL-10	T cells, B cells, macrophages	Costimulator to enhance growth of mast-cell lines; costimulator for proliferation of activated T cells; inhibits macrophage activity; stimulates B-cell proliferation; cytokine synthesis inhibitory factor T helper-1 cells.
Interleukin-11	IL-11	Stromal fibroblasts	Synergizes with IL-3 to support megakaryocyte colonies; stimulates proliferation of CD34$^+$ cells.
Interleukin-12	IL-12	B lymphoblastoid cell lines	Enhances NK activity; stimulates antigen-activated CD4$^+$ and CD8$^+$ cells; induces production of IFN-γ; hematopoietic effects; stimulates IFN-γ secretion by resting and activated human PBLs.
Interleukin-13	IL-13	T cells	Induces IgE synthesis; enhances class II MHC antigen expression on resting B cells.
Interleukin-14	IL-14	T cells	Induces B-cell proliferation; inhibits immunoglobulin secretion and selectively expands certain B cells.
Interleukin-15	IL-15	Activated monocytes/macrophages	T-cell growth factor (some functions overlap with those of IL-2); stimulates NK cells.
Interleukin-16	IL-16	Mast cells, CD8$^+$ T cells	CD4$^+$ T-cell chemoattractant
Interleukin-17	IL-17	T cells, particularly activated CD4$^+$ cells	Proinflammatory cytokine, activates fibroblasts, stromal cells, epithelial cells, and endothelial cells to secrete proinflammatory cytokines, autocrine function on murine T cells.
Interleukin-18	IL-18	Osteoblasts	Regulates IFN-γ production by T cells and NK cells, inhibits osteoclast formation via GM-CSF.

ACTH, adrenocorticotropic hormone; ADCC, antibody-dependent cellular cytotoxicity; LAK, lymphokine-activated killer; MHC, major histocompatibility complex; NK, natural killer; PBL, peripheral blood lymphocyte.

Data from Tushinski RJ, Mulé JJ: Biology of cytokines: the interleukins. In DeVita VT, Hellman S, Rosenberg SA, editors: The biologic therapy of cancer, ed 3, Philadelphia, Lippincott, 1998; and Rosenberg SA: Principles of cancer management. In DeVita VT, Hellman S, Rosenberg SA, editors: Cancer: principles and practice of oncology, ed 5, Philadelphia, Lippincott, 1997.

specifically, lymphokines are products of lymphocytes, and monokines are products of monocytes. The name *interleukin* refers to proteins that act as messengers between cells.[60, 210, 233]

A system of classification is often useful for looking at the agents' mechanisms of action. However, the way many BRMs work against tumors is not fully understood. Many agents may have more than one antitumor mode of action, and with certain agents it is often difficult to determine which mode of action is most important to the antitumor effect. It may be one action or the combination of several. In addition,

many agents have both immunologic actions and other biologic effects.

Although several classification schemes exist, in general, BRMs can be classified into three major divisions: agents that augment, modulate, or restore the host's immunologic mechanisms; agents that have direct antitumor activity (cytotoxic or antiproliferative mechanisms); and agents that exert other biologic effects (those that affect differentiation or maturation of cells, that interfere with the ability of a tumor cell to metastasize, or that affect initiation or maintenance of neoplastic transformation).[50, 141]

TABLE 24-2
Clinical Status of Major Biologic Response Modifiers

Agent	Status/Indication
INTERFERONS	
Interferon-α	
Interferon alfa-2a (Roferon-A)	FDA approved for hairy cell leukemia, AIDS-related Kaposi's sarcoma, chronic myelogenous leukemia
Interferon alfa-2b (Intron-A)	FDA approved for hairy cell leukemia, AIDS-related Kaposi's sarcoma, adjuvant therapy for high-risk melanoma, condyloma acuminata, chronic hepatitis non-A, non-B/C, chronic hepatitis
Interferon-α leukocyte (Alferon)	Condyloma acuminata
Interferon-β	
Interferon-β (Betaseron)	FDA approved for multiple sclerosis
Interferon-γ	
Interferon γ-1b (Actimmune)	FDA approved for chronic granulomatous disease
INTERLEUKINS	
IL-1-α	In clinical trials
IL-1-β	In clinical trials
IL-2 (Proleukin, Chiron)	FDA approved for renal cell cancer, malignant melanoma
IL-4	In clinical trials
IL-6	In clinical trials
IL-12	In clinical trials
HEMATOPOIETIC GROWTH FACTORS	
GM-CSF	
Sargramostim	
(Leukine, Prokine, Granulocyte-macrophage colony-stimulating factor [GM-CSF])	FDA approved for acceleration of myeloid recovery in patients with non-Hodgkin's lymphoma, acute lymphoblastic leukemia, and Hodgkin's disease undergoing autologous BMT, treatment of delayed engraftment, support of elderly patients with acute myelogenous leukemia (AML) receiving high-dose chemotherapy
G-CSF	
Filgrastim	
(Neupogen, Granulocyte colony-stimulating factor [G-CSF])	FDA approved to reduce incidence of infection in patients with nonmyeloid malignancies receiving myelosuppressive anticancer drugs, autologous bone marrow transplantation, cyclic neutropenias, mobilization of peripheral blood stem cells
Erythropoietin	
(Procrit, Epogen, Epoetin alfa)	FDA approved for treatment of anemia in cancer patients undergoing chemotherapy or radiation therapy. Indicated for treatment of anemia in patients with chronic renal failure and anemia related to therapy with zidovudine (AZT) in patients infected with HIV.
Oprelvekin (Neumega)	FDA approved for prevention of severe thrombocytopenia and the reduction of the need for platelet transfusion following myelosuppressive chemotherapy in patients with nonmyeloid malignancies
Multicolony-stimulating factor (M-CSF)	In clinical trials
PIXY 321 (GM-CS and IL-3 fused together with a linker protein, stem cell factor)	In clinical trials
Erythropoietin	
(Epoetin alfa)	
(Epogen Amgen)	Indicated for treatment of anemia in patients with chronic renal failure
(Procrit (Ortho Biotech))	Indicated for treatment of: anemia in patients with chronic renal failure; anemia related to therapy with zidovudine (AZT) in patients infected with the human immunodeficiency virus (HIV); and anemia in cancer patients undergoing chemotherapy
IL-11	
Thrombopoietin	
Stem cell factor	In clinical trials
MONOKINES	
Tumor necrosis factor (TNF)	In clinical trials
MONOCLONAL ANTIBODIES (MOABS)	
Capromab (Prostascint)	FDA approved for imaging of prostate cancers
Fumomab (CEA-scan)	FDA approved for imaging of colorectal and hepatic metastasis
Muromonab-CD3 (Orthoclone OKT3)	FDA approved for acute allograft rejection
Nofetumomab (Verluma)	FDA approved for imaging of small-cell and non–small-cell lung cancer

Table continued on following page

TABLE 24–2
Clinical Status of Major Biologic Response Modifiers *Continued*

Agent	Status/Indication
Rituximab (Rituxan)	FDA approved for the treatment of patients with relapsed or refractory low-grade or follicular CD20-positive B-cell non-Hodgkin's lymphoma
Satumomab (Oncoscint)	FDA approved for diagnostic imaging of colon and ovarian cancer
Trastuzumab (Herceptin)	FDA approved for the treatment of mesastatic breast cancer in patients who have tumors that overexpress the HER2 protein
RETINOIDS	
all-*trans*-retinoic acid (ATRA)	
Tretinoin (Vesanoid)	FDA approved for the induction of remission in patients with acute promyelocytic leukemia
13-*cis*-retinoic acid (13-cRA)	In clinical trials
(cRA, Isotretinoin)	
Etretinate	In clinical trials
Fenretinide	In clinical trials
EFFECTOR CELLS	
Gene-altered tumor-infiltrating lymphocytes (TILs)	In clinical trials
Lymphokine-activated killer cells (LAK)	In clinical trials
Tumor-infiltrating lymphocytes (TILs)	In clinical trials

Major Agents in Use

Interferons

Interferon (IFN) was first characterized in 1957 by virologists Isaacs and Lindemann.[125] They found that this newly discovered protein was produced by virally infected cells and was capable of protecting other cells from viral infection. A great deal has been learned since about the IFN system and its biologic effects. IFN has proved effective in the treatment of several malignancies and viral diseases. IFNs are divided into three major classes, according to antigenic type: alpha, beta, and gamma. IFN-α and IFN-β are produced primarily by leukocytes and fibroblasts respectively; IFN-γ is made primarily by T lymphocytes. The IFNs may be called a family of glycoprotein hormones possessing pleiotropic biologic effects.[16, 80]

BIOLOGIC EFFECTS

All IFNs mediate their cellular effects after binding to a specific receptor. IFN-α and IFN-β share a receptor, whereas IFN-γ uses a different one. The IFNs have a wide range of biologic effects, including antiviral, antiproliferative, and immunomodulatory. Exactly how they exert their antitumor effects is unknown. It is unclear which of their many biologic effects may be most important in obtaining tumor responses (e.g., direct effects versus immune stimulation). This is further complicated by the likely diversity of patients' responses to the agents and the differing effects of IFN on different diseases. In addition, there are differences in biologic effects between different classes of IFN.[16, 80]

The antiviral activity of IFN renders uninfected cells resistant to attack by the offending virus as well as by a variety of other viruses. Internalization of the IFN-receptor complex causes a sequence of events that results in the production of antiviral proteins and enzymes. Both in vitro and in vivo experimentation have demonstrated the antiproliferative effects of IFN. Although the exact mechanism is unknown, IFN extends all phases of the cell cycle and lengthens overall cell generation time. The proteins also may inhibit DNA and protein synthesis to block the growth of tumor cells. Cellular protooncogenes play an important role in the regulation of cell growth, and IFNs are known to inhibit expression of protooncogenes.

A variety of immunomodulatory effects have been described for the IFNs; these differ for the different classes of IFN. In vitro, IFN increases the killing potential of NK cells by recruiting pre-NK cells and enhancing the cytotoxic activity of activated cells. Low doses of IFN appear to stimulate antibody production, but higher doses have a suppressive effect. IFN-γ appears to be a more potent activator of macrophage function than IFN-α or IFN-β; however, all three are capable of inducing tumoricidal activity and increasing phagocytosis. IFNs also are capable of affecting the production of other lymphokines that regulate immune responses. Little is known about the positive and negative feedback regulation between IFNs and other lymphokines. Current investigations will continue to define the immunomodulatory effects on IFNs and their interactions with other cytokines.[16, 80]

PHENOTYPIC EFFECTS

Interferon is also capable of affecting the phenotypic properties of neoplastic cells. In vitro studies have shown that IFN can enhance differentiation of certain cell lines. IFN can also induce or enhance expression of human leukocyte antigens (HLAs) and increases tumor-associated antigens in melanoma and other cell lines. This may improve endogenous host antitumor activity.[16, 80]

CLINICAL INDICATIONS

Initial clinical trials with IFN were carried out in the early 1970s using the Cantell preparation of leukocyte IFN (IFN-α), which was manufactured by Kari Cantell and coworkers at the Finnish blood bank.[42] Although supplies of leukocyte IFN were scarce, expensive, and very impure, a few important pharmacologic studies were done. The NCI in 1975 and the American Cancer Society in 1978 expanded this work. Although initial trials showed responses in patients with breast cancer and lymphoma, large-scale clinical trials have not supported widespread efficacy in these two diseases. Large-scale clinical trials with IFN became possible during the 1980s with the advent of recombinant DNA technology. Large quantities of very pure IFNs of all types are now available because of these industrial-scale production methods.[204]

The U.S. Food and Drug Administration (FDA) approved two recombinant IFN-α products for the treatment of hairy-cell leukemia (HCL) in 1986: IFN alfa-2b (Intron A) and IFN alfa-2a (Roferon A). Use of these IFNs in high doses has also been approved for the treatment of Kaposi's sarcoma related to acquired immunodeficiency syndrome (AIDS).[228, 239] Since then, Intron A has received additional approval for the treatment of condyloma acuminata, chronic hepatitis C, and chronic hepatitis B, and as adjuvant therapy in patients with melanoma at high risk for recurrence.[239] In late 1995, Roferon A received regulatory approval for the treatment of patients with chronic myelogenous leukemia (CML) in the chronic phase.[228]

The treatment of HCL with IFN-α has shown dramatic antitumor effects. Doses as low as 3 million U/m^2 per day have been of benefit in as many as 95% of patients.[212, 213] The median time to response is 4 to 6 months, with most patients achieving normalization of peripheral blood values, resulting in a decrease in transfusion requirements and incidence of infection. Once therapy is stopped, patients ultimately relapse. Today, newer therapies, such as cladribine, have replaced IFN-α as frontline therapy for HCL. CML, a more common leukemia, is characterized by the presence of the Philadelphia chromosome in most patients. The use of IFN in this population, at doses of 2 to 5 million U/m^2 per day results in normalization of peripheral blood counts. In approximately 15% of patients with chronic phase CML, IFN therapy has been shown to eliminate the malignant clone of cells (those bearing the Philadelphia chromosome).[99, 263, 264, 265] Other hematologic diseases against which IFN-α has shown efficacy include low-grade lymphomas[251, 272] and multiple myeloma.[161] In these diseases several studies have shown the use of IFN as maintenance therapy after chemotherapy to result in an improved rate of failure-free survival and median survival. In solid tumors, such as melanoma, renal cell cancer, ovarian carcinoma (using the intraperitoneal route), and superficial bladder carcinoma, IFN has also demonstrated efficacy[2] (Tables 24-3 and 24-4). In patients with melanoma, no adjuvant therapy has traditionally been effective in extending relapse-free or overall survival. In late 1995, based on a study by the Eastern Cooperative Oncology Group, Intron A was approved as an adjuvant to surgical treatment of melanoma in patients who are free of disease but at a high risk for recurrence. These are patients with a deep primary lesion (>4 mm thickness) or any patient with primary or recurrent nodal involvement. Median disease-free survival was extended from 1 to 1.7 years, overall survival from 2.8 to 3.8 years, and 5-year survival from 37%

TABLE 24-3

Response of Various Hematologic Malignancies to IFN-α

Tumor Type	Response Rate*
Hairy-cell leukemia	80–90%
Chronic myelogenous leukemia	
Newly diagnosed	70–80%
Advanced	10–25%
Philadelphia-negative myeloproliferative disorders	
Essential thrombocythemia and polycythemia vera	75%
Cutaneous T-cell lymphomas	
No prior therapy	80%
Previously treated	55%
Non-Hodgkin's lymphomas (relapsed)	
Low grade	40–50%
Intermediate and high grade	15%
Hodgkin's disease (relapsed)	20%
Multiple myeloma	
No previous therapy	50%
Previously treated	15–25%
Chronic lymphocytic leukemia	10–15%
Acute leukemia	10–20%

Responses signify a partial or complete regression of tumor.

From Kurzrock R, Talpaz M, Gutterman JU: Other tumors. In DeVita VT, Hellman S, Rosenberg SA, editors: The biologic therapy of cancer, ed 2, Philadelphia, Lippincott, 1995.

T A B L E   2 4 – 4
Response of Various Solid Tumors to IFN-α

Tumor Type	Response Rate*
Cervical intraepithelial neoplasia	80–90%
Basal cell cancer	90%
Superficial bladder cancer	60–70%
Malignant neuroendocrine tumors	30–80%
Kaposi's sarcoma (AIDS related)	35%
Ovarian cancer	
Parenteral administration	10–15%
Intraperitoneal administration	40%
Gliomas	30%
Renal cell cancer	15–20%
Nasopharyngeal cancer	20%
Melanoma	10–15%
Colorectal cancer	<10%
Osteogenic sarcoma	<10%
Lung (small and non-small cell)	<10%
Breast cancer	<10%

* Responses signify partial or complete tumor regression.

From Kurzrock R, Talpaz M, Gutterman JU: Other tumors. In DeVita VT, Hellman S, Rosenberg SA, editors: The biologic therapy of cancer, ed 2, Philadelphia, Lippincott, 1995.

to 46%.[48, 76, 136] (For a comprehensive review of IFN therapy, see references 65, 80, 200, 225, 233, 247, and 295.) In patients with metastatic renal cell carcinoma, IFN-α demonstrated a 12% improvement in 1-year survival and a 2.5-month improvement in overall survival over patients treated with medroxyprogesterone acetate.[41, 247]

Interferon-β1a and 1b remain under clinical investigation in patients with cancer but have received regulatory approval for the treatment of multiple sclerosis.[26] IFN-γ was found to significantly increase the severity of graft-versus-host disease (GVHD) in patients undergoing autologous bone marrow transplantation for breast cancer. Clinical trials comparing it with placebo in patients with metastatic renal cell carcinoma showed no benefit. IFN-γ is still under investigation in cancer,[215] though it is commercially available for the treatment of chronic granulomatous disease.[94, 97]

Interferon continues to be explored as a single agent and in combination with other BRMs and chemotherapeutic agents.[185, 221–223] Initial clinical trials evaluating the combination of IFN and fluorouracil (5-FU) for the treatment of colon cancer yielded exciting results. A pilot study conducted by Wadler and others[284] reported a response rate of 81% with 13 of 16 previously untreated patients with advanced colon carcinoma. These results led other investigators to attempt to duplicate Wadler's regimen and to evaluate this combination in other cancers. However, several recent large-scale randomized studies have not demonstrated any clear superiority for the combination, compared with 5-FU alone.[56] The investigation of IFN-α in combination with DTIC in the treatment of metastatic melanoma showed initial promise in a single institution study involving 61 patients. However, subsequent trials of the same regimen failed to show statistical benefit over chemotherapy alone. Clinical trials involving combination chemotherapeutic agents, such as the Dartmouth regimen (DTIC, BCNU, cisplatin, tamoxifen), the BOLD regimen (bleomycin, vincristine, CCNU, DTIC), and CVD (cisplatin, vinblastine, DTIC) have been undertaken. Response rates were encouraging, ranging from 26% to 68%, with the highest responses occurring in the BOLD/IFN-α trial. Unfortunately, these response rates were not statistically significant and the addition of IFN did not appear to improve overall survival when compared to combination chemotherapy alone.[48] An additional area of investigation is the combination of IFN-α and 13-*cis*-retinoic acid (13-cRA) for the treatment of squamous cell carcinomas of the skin and cervix.[153] Although responses have been demonstrated, randomized trials are required to clarify the ultimate role of the combination in these diseases. Phase I trials of IFN-α, cRA, and paclitaxel for hormone-refractory prostate cancer and other advanced cancers identified that IFN and cRA act synergistically to inhibit tumor growth and appeared to have some activity in advanced cancers.[74] Randomized trials have demonstrated no additional benefit for the addition of IFN-α to high-dose therapy with interleukin-2 (IL-2) in patients with melanoma or renal cell carcinoma.[70]

An occasional problem in patients receiving chronic treatment with IFN-α is development of neutralizing antibodies. Although the clinical significance of this phenomenon is uncertain, in a number of clinical trials the development of neutralizing antibodies has been associated with resistance to therapy. Factors that may contribute to formation of antibodies are immunogenicity, underlying disease, routes of administration, dosing regimens, and duration of treatment. It has been difficult to determine the true incidence of antibody formation. Additional factors that may be important are blood sampling time and assay methodology. Until comparative studies are well controlled for these variables, the formation of antibodies and their effect will remain controversial.[12]

ADMINISTRATION

Although numerous clinical trials have been conducted, the optimal dose, route, and frequency of administration for IFN have yet to be determined. The most common routes of administration are intramuscular (IM) and subcutaneous (SC), although IFN is also given intravenously (IV), intralesionally, intraperitoneally, intravesically, intraarterially, and intrathecally.[55, 233] Pharmacokinetics differ by types of IFN and route of administration. IV administration results in rapid clearance with a half-life of 4 to 8 hours. With Sc or IM administration, peak serum levels occur at about 6 to 8 hours and complete clearance occurs by 16 to 24 hours.[107] IFN is metabolized in the kidneys, and most metabolites are completely reabsorbed. Although at first IFN was given by a predetermined standard dosage, it is now more commonly prescribed by body surface area (million U/m^2). Dosage requirements for IFN-α vary among patients and diseases. High-dose IFN is usually prescribed at doses over 10 million U/m^2, whereas low-dose therapy is given in 0 to 3 million U/m^2 (Table 24–5). In general, the higher the dose, the more severe the side effects and the inhibition of the patient's performance status.

Interferon-α is supplied commercially as a sterile, lyophilized powder with accompanying diluent or as a sterile solution. It must be stored in a refrigerator at 35.6° to 46.4°F (2°–8°C). The vial should not be shaken when the powder is reconstituted because this will make the medication foam. For further information, such as the availability of differing vial strengths and shelf-life stability, see the manufacturer's product literature.[228, 239]

Handling issues are a concern to all oncology nurses. To date there has been no formal research on the safest way to handle IFNs or other BRMs. Many institutions place BRMs in the same classification as chemotherapy, instructing staff to follow institutional policy on the handling and disposal of cytotoxic drugs. Patients taught to self-administer IFN are advised to dispose of vials, needles, and syringes in a puncture-resistant container. Guidelines for disposal of used equipment in the home setting are available from the U.S. Environmental Protection Agency. In some clinical trials, patients are requested to return unused vials to the dispensing institution.[55, 110, 221–223]

SIDE EFFECTS

The toxicity of IFN has been well established. In general, side effects are similar for all classes of IFN, with slight variations according to dosage, schedule, and type. High-dose IFN therapy can be very debilitating. Nearly all patients receiving it report fatigue (with almost 25%

reporting grade III fatigue). Coupled with flulike symptoms and gastrointestinal symptoms, these side effects are most frequently cited as reasons to discontinue therapy.[76] Side effects are generally reversible on cessation of therapy. Because IFN is generally given as long-term therapy, side effects can be divided into those occurring early (acute) and those occurring as therapy progresses (late or chronic). Some side effects occur only occasionally or rarely.

Nearly all patients beginning therapy with IFN have flulike symptoms. Although the symptoms may be severe at first, tachyphylaxis (adjustment to symptoms over time) prevents them from becoming dose limiting. Symptoms include chills 2 to 4 hours after injection followed by fever spikes up to 104°F (40°C). Patients may have headaches, myalgia, arthralgia, and malaise. High-risk patients (e.g., those with a history of cardiac problems, debilitated patients) should be premedicated, monitored closely, and kept well hydrated.[108]

Chronic side effects tend to increase in intensity and maintain their level of intensity after patients have been undergoing therapy for several weeks. Of prime concern are fatigue and anorexia with resultant weight loss; these can become dose limiting. The patient's IFN therapy may have to be halted or the dosage reduced if these side effects become too severe. Patients also experience lethargy, lack of concentration,[173] neutropenia, mild thrombocytopenia, elevated transaminase levels, proteinuria, and asymptomatic hypotension.

A number of side effects are less widespread; they vary in frequency between individual patients and in intensity depending on the dose. These include gastrointestinal effects such as nausea, vomiting, diarrhea, and altered taste (patients complain of foods tasting metallic or bitter). Nausea, in particular, is more commonly seen in patients with malignant melanoma who are receiving higher doses of IFN-α by the IV route during the induction phase. Patients may exhibit central nervous system (CNS) or neurologic changes such as depression, mood alterations, decreased libido, memory problems, electroencephalographic (EEG) abnormalities, and peripheral neuropathies.[173] In a study of patients receiving IFN and low-dose cytarabine for CML, Hensley and others[116] found 24% of the 91 patients experienced grade III or IV neurotoxicity (all but 2 patients returned to their baseline status on discontinuation of therapy).

Inflammation at the injection site, reactivation of herpes simplex, rash, exacerbation of psoriasis, and mild alopecia (thinning of hair as opposed to full-scale hair loss) have all been reported. Laboratory values should be watched for changes indicating anemia, hypercalcemia, hyperkalemia, elevated blood urea nitrogen (BUN), and elevated lactate dehydrogenase.[213, 233, 281] In general, patients receiving low doses tolerate side effects well. Although not proved by research, a fre-

TABLE 24–5
Interferon Dosage

Interferon Protocol	Dose (million U/m^2)
Low dose	0–3
Intermediate dose	3–10
High dose	> 10

quent recommendation is that IFN be given at bedtime so that patients will sleep through the worst of the side effects. The most common life-threatening toxicity is acute cardiac failure,[41] which is extremely rare. It is generally recommended that patients with a strong history of cardiovascular disease should not undergo IFN therapy.

Interleukins

The term *interleukin* literally means "between leukocytes." Traditionally, when biologic proteins were characterized, they were given acronyms based on their functional properties (e.g., T-cell growth factor). When genes for these cytokines were ultimately cloned, it was found that a number of these substances were in fact the same molecule. At international symposia, the terminology interleukins was agreed on to name these biologic proteins. Hence, as more of these cytokines are discovered and their amino acid sequences established, they are named numerically (e.g., IL-5, IL-6) (see Table 24–1). Research has progressed through the discovery of IL-15.[149] This section will concentrate on interleukin-2 (IL-2), which received FDA approval in 1992, and will briefly cover other interleukins that are currently in clinical trials. Interleukin-3 will be covered under the discussion of hematopoietic growth factors.

INTERLEUKIN-1

Interleukin-1 (IL-1) was originally described as an endogenous pyrogen and lymphocyte-activating factor.[72] It is a complex and heterogeneous molecule now known to be produced by a variety of cells. Its biologic activities include serving as an endogenous pyrogen; inducing the release of lymphokines from activated T cells and fibroblasts; enhancing antibody responsiveness through synergism with other lymphokines that affect B-cell function; inducing the proliferation of fibroblasts; serving as a chemotactic factor for neutrophils, macrophages, and lymphocytes; and serving as a mediator of the inflammatory response.[72, 256] Two genes coding for proteins with IL-1 properties have been discovered. These have been called *interleukin-1-alpha* (*IL-1-α*) and *interleukin-1-beta* (*IL-1-β*). They share the same cell surface receptor and various biologic activities.[62]

Several phase I trials have evaluated IL-1 in patients.[133, 256, 278] In general, these studies demonstrated a delayed increase in leukocytes and platelets. In patients receiving IL-1-β after treatment with 5-FU, it appeared to exert a myeloprotective effect (fewer days of neutropenia).[58] However, the difference between those patients receiving IL-1-β and those receiving 5-FU alone was not statistically significant. A study by Vadhan-

Raj and others,[278] demonstrated that IL-1-α increased circulating platelet counts and enhanced platelet recovery after treatment with carboplatin (CBDCA) in patients with ovarian cancer. Common toxicities experienced in these phase I trials were chills and fever, constitutional symptoms (headache, myalgia, arthralgia, fatigue, nausea), hypotension at higher doses, tachycardia, and inflammation at injection sites. Occasional toxicities, especially at doses above 300 ng/kg, were cardiac dysrhythmias, reversible renal insufficiency, abdominal pain, and transient CNS changes. Further studies evaluating IL-1 in a variety of settings, as well as IL-1 in combination with IL-2, are in progress. Future trials will continue to evaluate the role of IL-1 in the pathology of septic shock, inflammatory bowel disease, and autoimmune diseases such as rheumatoid arthritis.[242, 256] Clinical studies are now investigating the role of IL-1 receptor antagonist (IL-1RA), a molecule capable of blocking the biologic effects of IL-1. This agent may have efficacy in the treatment of septic shock or as a means of selectively suppressing the toxic effects of other cytokines such as IL-2.

INTERLEUKIN-2

Interleukin-2 is a glycoprotein mainly produced by activated T-helper cells. First discovered in 1976 by Morgan and others,[179] it was originally named T-cell growth factor. Since then, intensive research has proved IL-2 to be a potent modulator of immune responses. The release of IL-2 in vivo occurs in response to two signals presented to T lymphocytes. The first is activation of T cells by antigen or mitogen, and the second is through interactions with IL-1. Like many polypeptide hormones, IL-2 exerts its biologic effects by binding to membrane-bound receptors on certain immune cells. It is now known that the IL-2 receptor has low-, intermediate-, and high-affinity forms. Hence, a resting cell may display very few IL-2 receptors. Once activated, it may display thousands of receptors and respond to activation by IL-2.[9, 16, 60, 248, 285]

Biologic Effects

The biologic effects of IL-2 are numerous and have been well documented.[9, 16, 60, 248, 285] IL-2 supports the growth and maturation of subpopulations of T cells both in vitro and in vivo, stimulates cytotoxic T cells, stimulates the proliferation and activity of NK cells, and develops the capacity in lymphoid cells incubated with IL-2 to lyse fresh tumor cells. These cells, known as lymphokine-activated killer (LAK) cells, have served as the basis for adoptive immunotherapy regimens. IL-2 also enhances antibody responses by activating other lymphocytes to produce lymphokines important to B-cell function

(IL-4 and IL-6), stimulates the expression of its own cell surface receptor, and induces the release of other lymphokines, such as IFN-γ and granulocyte/macrophage colony-stimulating factor (GM-CSF), that can mediate physiologic effects. Both in vitro and in vivo studies have demonstrated that IL-2 can reverse immune deficiencies in mice and humans. It appears that there are no differences in activity between naturally occurring IL-2 and the recombinant forms available.

Clinical Indications

In 1992, IL-2 (aldesleukin) was approved by the FDA for the treatment of renal cell cancer[46] and in 1998, it was approved for the treatment of metastatic melanoma. The approved regimen uses high doses of IL-2: 600,000 or 720,000 IU/kg by IV bolus every 8 hours, up to 14 doses. (For a complete chronology on the clinical investigation of IL-2, see references 8, 9, 70, 87, 140, 201, 231, 233, 234, 242, 260, 285, and 288.) The first phase I clinical evaluations of IL-2 began in 1983 with IL-2 obtained from a human lymphoma tumor cell line. Although production methods limited supplies, a few clinical trials were conducted for patients with malignant tumors or AIDS. Therapy was given IV and produced minimal side effects. However, no therapeutic responses were seen.[155, 156]

When the DNA sequence coding for IL-2 was elucidated, recombinant DNA technology made possible the production of large quantities of purified IL-2. As a result, phase I trials using recombinant IL-2 (rIL-2) were initiated in 1984.[155] Concurrently, studies conducted by Rosenberg[233] showed that adoptive immunotherapy with LAK cells was well tolerated by patients. These LAK cells were generated from fresh peripheral blood lymphocytes obtained through lymphocytapheresis and then incubated with IL-2.

In 1984, studies of the combination of IL-2 and LAK cells began. Results reported by Rosenberg and associates[233] in December 1985 showed that of 25 patients, 11 exhibited tumor responses. These responses were seen in patients with melanoma, renal cancer, and colorectal and pulmonary adenocarcinoma. The excitement over these results generated an explosion of clinical trials with IL-2. Numerous clinical trials have evaluated a variety of doses, routes of administration, and schedules for IL-2. Trials have been conducted using IL-2 alone and in combination with LAK cells. Although patients with a variety of cancers have been treated, most trials have focused on patients with renal cell cancer and melanoma because of the successes seen in these solid tumors. Randomized trials have now demonstrated that the addition of LAK cells does not offer an advantage over the use of high-dose IL-2 alone.[8, 70, 71, 87]

Research efforts continued to find cells with more potent antitumor activity. A different subpopulation of lymphocytes, denoted *tumor-infiltrating lymphocytes (TILs)*, appeared to have greater efficacy in the treatment of experimental tumors than did LAK cells. TILs are obtained by removing tumor specimens from the host. Human TILs are T cells and can be isolated by growth in single-cell suspensions. They appear to be less dependent on adjunctive systemically administered IL-2 than are LAK cells. Early clinical trials using IL-2 plus TILs by Rosenberg and coworkers reported remissions in 11 of 20 patients with metastatic melanoma treated with this combination. A report on their 5-year experience with this combination showed an overall response rate of 34% in patients with advanced melanoma. Work continues on how to achieve the optimal therapeutic benefit and to find predictors of response.[233]

The combination of IL-2 with other cytokines, MoAbs, and chemotherapy is another active area of focus. Preclinical studies in animal models have shown antitumor activity to be enhanced by use of the combinations just mentioned.* Phase I and II trials evaluating the efficacy of these combinations continue. One promising area appears to be the use of IL-2 in combination with chemotherapy in patients with melanoma. Several clinical trials across the country are evaluating multidrug chemotherapy, using cisplatin, dacarbazine, carmustine, and tamoxifen (Dartmouth regimen) or cisplatin, vinblastine, and dacarbazine (CVD), in combination with IL-2 and IFN-α.[191] Reported response rates to these combinations have been 53% or higher, although toxic effects are severe. In an attempt to maximize response, minimize toxicity, and provide cost effective chemobiotherapy on an outpatient basis, the Cytokine Working Group (CWG) began a randomized, phase II clinical trial. This two-arm trial combines DTIC and cisplatin IV, days 1 to 3, followed by IFN-α2b SC, days 6, 8, 10, 13, and 15. IL-2 is given in both arms on days 6 to 10 and 13 to 15, but in different doses and different routes. One arm consists of an IV bolus IL-2 at 18.0 MU/m^2 and the other arm consists of SC IL-2 at 5.0 MU/m^2. Eighty patients were randomized to each arm. Results of this trial are forthcoming. Randomized studies are in progress to determine whether biochemotherapy is truly superior to chemotherapy alone.[39, 87] Also of important consideration in these regimens is whether biotherapy is given before, during, or after chemotherapy.

Evaluation of chimeric molecules is an active area of pursuit. One such example is the use of an IL-2 molecule with diphtheria toxin attached that is administered to patients whose malignancies express the IL-2 receptor. Phase I and II trials with this molecule continue,[199] as

---

*References 9, 10, 70, 71, 86, 87, 158, 185, 186, 201.

does its evaluation for the treatment of rheumatoid arthritis. In patients who have received both autologous and allogeneic bone marrow transplantation (BMT),[88] administration of low-dose IL-2 to reduce the incidence of relapse by stimulating a graft-versus-leukemia effect and to restore immune function is under investigation. A current area of focus, especially in patients with renal cell cancer, is the use of low-dose regimens administered in the ambulatory setting that maintain efficacy yet reduce toxicity.[255] Preliminary studies of low-dose, SC IL-2 in combination with IFN-α, with or without 5-FU, appear to be well-tolerated. However, they do not appear to have the same response rates as have been achieved with high dose IL-2 alone. Over the next several years, increased use of IL-2 will be seen in the clinical setting as research defines optimal dosing and schedules and its concomitant use with effector cells and other biologic or chemotherapeutic agents.[87, 242, 288]

Administration

As with other BRMs, the optimal therapeutic dosage, route, and schedule for IL-2 have yet to be determined. The most common route of administration is IV, using either bolus or continuous infusion.[47] Investigations continue to evaluate other routes such as SC, intraperitoneal, and intra-arterial, with most ambulatory regimens using the SC route. A study investigating the use of inhalation IL-2 versus low-dose IV IL-2 revealed a reduction in side effects sufficient enough to restore quality of life in the inhalation arm of the study.[114] Bernsen and others[27] propose treating patients with IL-2 by local injection of IL-2 instead of systemic therapy. They believe this is the key to getting a response, as is keeping the tumor in place instead of excising as much as possible.

The recommended dose for aldesleukin (Proleukin) is 600,000 IU/kg every 8 hours by a 15-minute IV infusion, for a total of 15 doses.[47] Pharmacokinetic studies show rapid initial plasma clearance (6–7 minutes) after bolus administration. With longer infusions, however, a more prolonged clearance is seen (half-life of approximately 30 minutes). These observations suggest a multicompartmental model of pharmacokinetics.[7, 155, 156] Inactivation appears to occur in the kidneys, with inactive metabolites excreted in the urine.

Other concerns about drug administration that are important to nurses include handling procedures, which are determined by hospital policy; manufacturer's instructions for administration; how long the drug is stable in solution; whether the drug can pass through a micropore filter; and evaluation of compatibility with concomitant medications such as antiemetics and vasopressors.[55, 221–223]

Side Effects

Although responses to therapy with IL-2 are seen, severe systemic toxicities associated with high-dose IL-2 therapy make it difficult to tolerate. The range and severity of toxicity seen with IL-2 are related to and influenced by dose, schedule, and concomitant use of adoptive immunotherapy, other BRMs, and chemotherapy.[244]

How many side effects arise from IL-2 remains a mystery. Although IL-2 may directly cause some side effects, the induction of other cytokines by IL-2 may also play a role. One encouraging note is that most IL-2-related side effects disappear once therapy is completed. IL-2 is often administered on a cyclic basis similar to that of chemotherapy. This gives patients an opportunity to recuperate between cycles or courses, although cumulative toxicity does occur with repeated cycles. Patients have exhibited a marked decline in performance status over time, and more severe toxicity and impairment have been observed as the dose increases. Because the toxicity of existing IL-2 regimens can be severe enough to require hospitalization, ongoing trials continue to search for dosage schedules that can maximize therapeutic responses with a more acceptable level of toxicity.[87, 242, 288] Box 24–1 summarizes the side effects of IL-2 by system.

As with other BRMs, patients receiving IL-2 have constitutional or flulike symptoms, including chills followed by fever of up to 104°F (40°C), headache, myalgia, arthralgia, and general malaise. Pretreatment with acetaminophen and indomethacin or another nonsteroidal anti-inflammatory drug (NSAID) helps control these side effects. With continuous infusions of IL-2, the medications just mentioned are often necessary around the clock to control fevers. The major cardiovascular and pulmonary toxicity associated with IL-2 administration stems from cumulative, dose-related fluid imbalances caused by a capillary leak syndrome. Shortly after administration, a rapid decrease in systemic vascular resistance occurs and fluids shift from the vascular bed to the interstitium. This causes a drop in mean arterial blood pressure, increased cardiac output, and increased heart rate.[41, 233]

Weight gains of as much as 10% of baseline weight have been observed in high-dose trials.[233] Fluid retention is usually manifested as peripheral edema and abdominal ascites. These effects may progress to interstitial pulmonary edema, with subsequent dyspnea and decreased partial oxygen pressure (Po_2) in some patients. In extreme cases of respiratory distress, patients require intubation.[41, 82] Although clinically patients appear fluid overloaded, in reality they are hypovolemic. This hypovolemia leads to hypotension, decreased central venous pressure (CVP), and renal hypoperfusion.

BOX 24–1

Interleukin-2 Toxicities

Constitutional Symptoms

Chills, fever
Headaches
Malaise
Myalgia, arthralgia
Fatigue
Nasal congestion

Cardiovascular System

Hypotension
Decreased systemic vascular resistance
Tachycardia
Atrial arrhythmias
Edema
Weight gain
Ascites

Pulmonary System

Pulmonary edema
Dyspnea
Decreased Po_2

Renal Function

Oliguria
Increased BUN, creatinine
Proteinuria
Azotemia

Gastrointestinal System

Nausea, vomiting
Diarrhea
Decreased appetite
Mucositis
Glossitis
Xerostomia

Endocrine System

Hypothyroidism

Integumentary System

Erythema
Erythematous rash
Dry skin
Pruritus
Dry desquamation

Central Nervous System

Confusion, disorientation
Somnolence
Lethargy
Combativeness
Psychoses
Anxiety
Depression

Hematologic Function

Anemia
Thrombocytopenia
Eosinophilia
Lymphopenia

Hepatic Function

Increased bilirubin
Elevated aspartate aminotransferase (AST,
    formerly SGOT), alanine aminotransferase
    (ALT, formerly SGPT), and lactate
    dehydrogenase (LDH)

Related Laboratory Values

Hypophosphatemia
Hypocalcemia
Hypomagnesemia
Decreased serum albumin

Other

Potential for catheter-related sepsis

From Rieger PT, Weatherly B: Can your nursing skills meet the challenge of a patient receiving IL-27? *Dimens Oncol Nurs* 3(3):9, 1989. Additional data from references 8, 27, and 88.

These physiologic changes increase the demand on the heart, and transient dysrhythmias may be observed. Because of this, patients usually undergo rigorous pretherapy screening for underlying cardiac problems before beginning treatment with IL-2. Medical treatment includes administration of colloid solutions (5% albumin), judicious use of fluids to avoid pulmonary edema, and the use of vasopressors.[222, 223, 225, 293]

The multiple hemodynamic abnormalities associated with IL-2 therapy often lead to the development of renal hypoperfusion and prerenal azotemia. Renal toxicity is evidenced by oliguria, proteinuria, azotemia, and increases in BUN and creatinine levels. These effects, seen at various doses, usually return to baseline after therapy. Medical treatment includes fluids, diuretics (if blood pressure and CVP are within normal limits), and pressors such as low-dose dopamine to stimulate renal blood flow.[41]

Acute gastrointestinal effects are common with IL-2. Nausea and vomiting closely parallel chemotherapy-associated nausea and vomiting. Patients often complain that food odors increase nausea. Unfortunately, for some patients, IL-2-associated nausea and vomiting have proved resistant to pharmacologic treatment. Often, aggressive use of multiple antiemetics around the clock is required. In addition, patients lose their appetite; therefore, weight loss over time becomes a major concern. Diarrhea may be acute or chronic and is often watery and profuse. Mucositis, glossitis, and xerostomia can further damage nutritional status.

Baseline assessment of mental status is important in patients receiving IL-2. CNS toxicity may be manifested as confusion, lethargy, decreased concentration, extreme somnolence, depression, hallucination, paranoia, agitation, combativeness, and nightmares.[23, 64, 127, 173, 253] Occasionally these toxicities are severe enough to cause the delay or discontinuation of therapy.

Skin changes occurring with IL-2 therapy are profound and cumulative; they are a major source of discomfort for patients. Varying degrees of erythema, erythematous rash, pruritus, dryness, and occasionally dry desquamation all may be seen, either alone or in combination. Skin biopsies have not elucidated the etiology of these skin changes. Aggravation of underlying dermatologic conditions, as well as recall phenomena, may also be seen.[93]

Patients may develop neutropenia, thrombocytopenia, or anemia. In programs using lymphocytapheresis, anemia is often exacerbated. With prolonged IL-2 administration, marked eosinophilia often occurs. The clinical significance of this is uncertain, although it may be responsible for the fluid shifts observed.[219] Significant lymphopenia occurs within minutes of IL-2 administration. However, rebound lymphocytosis occurs within 24 hours after discontinuation of a treatment. As with other IL-2 side effects, these changes are usually reversible on cessation of therapy.

Patients receiving IL-2 often have several abnormal laboratory values. Patients should be monitored for increased bilirubin, elevated hepatic enzymes (aspartate

---

BOX 24-2

Medications Commonly Used in the Management of IL-2 Toxicity

Antipyretic Analgesic Agents

Acetaminophen

Antiinflammatory Agents

Indomethacin
Naproxen
Sulindac

Histamine H$_2$-Antagonist Agents

Cimetidine
Ranitidine

Antiemetic Agents

Lorazepam
Prochlorperazine maleate
Promethazine HCl
Droperidol
Ondansetron
ABH (lorazepam, diphenhydramine, haloperidol)
Scopolamine patches

Antidiarrheal Agents

Codeine phosphate
Kaolin and pectin
Opium tincture
Diphenoxylate HCl with atropine SO$_4$

Antianxiety, Antihallucinogen, and Hypnotic Agents

Diphenhydramine
Diazepam
Fentanyl
Flurazepam
Haloperidol

Diuretic Agents

Furosemide
Metolazone

Agents to Control Chills

Meperidine HCl
Indomethacin
Dilaudid SL

Vasopressors and Antiarrhythmic Agents

Dopamine HCl
Verapamil HCl
Atropine So$_4$

Antihypotensive Measures

0.9% sodium chloride boluses
5% N serum albumin

Antipruritic Agents

Hydroxyzine hydrochloride
Diphenhydramine
Colloidal oatmeal

From Rieger PT: Patient management. In Rieger PT, editor: *Biotherapy: a comprehensive overview* (ed 2), Boston, Jones & Bartlett, 1999. Adapted and revised from original source: Padavic-Shaller K: *Semin Oncol Nurs* 4(2):142, 1988.

aminotransaminase [AST], alanine aminotransaminase [ALT], lactic dehydrogenase [LDH]), hypomagnesemia, hypophosphatemia, hypocalcemia, decreased serum albumin, and respiratory alkalosis. Replacement therapy should be instituted as appropriate.

The incidence of catheter-related sepsis appears higher in patients receiving high doses of IL-2. Trials have evaluated the use of prophylactic antibiotics in this patient population. In patients with indwelling catheters, antibiotics are often administered prophylactically. It is often difficult to differentiate signs of infection from those associated with IL-2; therefore patients must be monitored closely.[293] In patients receiving adoptive immunotherapy with either LAK or TILs, most side effects are attributable to IL-2. Chills and fever are the major side effects noted with cell infusions. These are readily treatable with meperidine. A further risk is that of infection, because lymphocytes incubated in culture medium for 3 to 4 days may be contaminated with viruses or bacteria.[233] Box 24–2 lists medications commonly used during IL-2 therapy.

INTERLEUKIN-4

Primarily produced by activated T cells and mast cells, IL-4 has a number of biologic effects. It stimulates the growth and differentiation of B cells; it increases production of IgG and IgE immunoglobulins; it may stimulate certain T-cell lines; it enhances the expansion of activated CD4 cells and the killing potential of NK, LAK and TIL cells[62]; and it may stimulate growth and maturation of mast cells. These effects depend on the type of cell, the presence of other cytokines such as IL-2, and the state of activation of the cytotoxic cells.*

Several phase I trials have evaluated tolerance of IL-4 in patients, using several routes of administration: IV bolus, short-term IV infusion, and SC injection. Toxicities experienced were low-grade delayed fevers, nausea, reversible elevation in liver enzymes, and nasal congestion. Occasional toxicities, especially at higher doses, were chills, hypotension, and edema with weight gain. Rare instances of therapy complicated by gastroduodenal erosion or ulceration have been reported.[235] A phase II outpatient dose and schedule have been established at 5 μg/kg per day by the SC route. Clinical trials are in progress in hematologic malignancies (multiple myeloma, indolent lymphoma, B-cell chronic lymphocytic leukemia [BCLL], intermediate-grade lymphoma, Hodgkin's disease, and CML). Several clinical trials have evaluated the combination of IL-2 and IL-4, with both high-dose and low-dose regimens for each of these agents. As yet the few responses documented have

been in patients with either renal cell cancer or melanoma.[242, 269, 288]

INTERLEUKIN-6

Interleukin-6 (IL-6) is a cytokine produced by many cells in the body and induced by other cytokines such as tumor necrosis factor (TNF) and IL-1. As with other cytokines, it has pleiotropic effects and plays an important role in coordinating systemic host defense responses to injury. Its expression has been noted in several disease states, and it may be involved in certain aspects of the pathogenesis of infection, autoimmunity, and malignancy. Multiple myeloma has been linked to autocrine growth stimulation by IL-6. IL-6 has an important role in promoting differentiation of B lymphocytes into antibody-secreting cells, is involved in the activation of T cells and promotion of T-cell differentiation, induces production of acute phase proteins by the liver, increases the proliferation of multilineage progenitor cells and increases the number of megakaryocytes, and serves as a messenger between the nervous and immune systems. It works synergistically with many other cytokines in vivo.[30, 60, 144, 145, 269]

Phase I/II trials are in progress evaluating the use of IL-6 in patients with cancer as both an antitumor and as a myeloprotective agent. In a study published by Weber and colleagues[286] at the NCI, IL-6 given by the SC route resulted in no clinical responses. Elevations in platelet counts were seen at higher doses. The most common toxic effects included constitutional symptoms, transient anemia, and hyperglycemia. Other investigators have administered IL-6 by the IV route in patients with melanoma or renal cell cancer; minor clinical responses were documented. Further study is necessary to determine this agent's utility as an anticancer agent, as well as its optimal dose, route, and schedule. Dose-limiting toxicities include neurotoxicity, hepatotoxicity, and cardiac dysrhythmias.[41, 62] Its value as a marker of disease activity is also under investigation.[144, 145, 288]

Hematopoietic Growth Factors

Hematopoietic growth factors (HGFs) are a family of glycoprotein hormones responsible for the proliferation, differentiation, and maturation of hematopoietic cells in vitro. They also stimulate functions of certain mature leukocytes.[51] The four classic growth factors, known as colony-stimulating factors (CSFs), are GM-CSF, granulocyte colony-stimulating factor (G-CSF), macrophage colony-stimulating factor (M-CSF), and IL-3 (multi-CSF). All are now produced in recombinant form. GM-CSF (sargramostim) and G-CSF (filgrastim) have both received regulatory approval, whereas clinical trials with

---

* References 60, 128, 144, 211, 242, 269.

Pluripotent stem cell

CFU-Blast

flk-2/flt-3 ligand
SCF

flk-2/flt-3 ligand

flk-2/flt-3 ligand
SCF

flk-2/flt-3 ligand
SCF

CFU-GEMM

Stimulate proliferation
of CFU-Blast

Lymphoid
stem cell

NK
precursor

SCF
IL-3

MGDF/TPO
SCF
IL-3

SCF
IL-3
flk-2/flt-3
ligand

SCF
IL-3

SCF
IL-3

SCF
IL-3

SCF
IL-7
flk-2/flt-3
ligand

SCF
IL-7
flk-2/flt-3
ligand

BFU-E

CFU-Meg

CFU-GM

CFU-Eo

CFU-Ba

CFU-Mast

Pre-B cell

Pre-T cell

SCF
IL-3
GM-CSF
EPO

SCF
IL-3
GM-CSF
IL-11
IL-6
MGDF/TPO

IL-3
GM-CSF

IL-3
G-CSF
GM-CSF

IL-7

CFU-E

CFU-M

CFU-G

IL-3
GM-CSF
EPO

IL-3
GM-CSF
M-CSF

IL-3
GM-CSF
G-CSF

IL-3
CM-CSF

IL-3

IL-3
SCF

IL-6

Reticulocyte

Megakaryocyte

Monocyte

GM-CSF
M-CSF

B lymphocyte

IL-2
IL-7

SCF
IL-2

Proplatelet

Red blood cell

Platelets

Macrophage

Neutrophil

Eosinophil

Basophil

Tissue mast cell

Plasma cell

T lymphocyte

NK cell

F I G U R E   2 4 – 2   Hematopoietic tree. All hematopoietic cells are derived from a common stem cell under the influence of various growth factors or combinations of growth factors. *BFU-E,* erythrocyte burst-forming units; *CFU,* colony-forming units; *CFU-Ba,* basophil CFU; *CFU-Eo,* eosinophil CFU; *CFU-g,* granulocyte CFU; *CFU-GEMM,* granulocyte/erythroid/macrophage/megakaryocyte CFU; *CFU-GM,* granulocyte/macrophage CFU; *CFU-M,* macrophage CFU; *CFU-mast,* mast cell CFU; *CFU-Meg,* megakaryocyte CFU; *NK,* natural killer; *SCF,* stem cell factor; *IL-3,* interleukin-3; *GM-CSF,* granulocyte-macrophage colony-stimulating factor; *Epo,* erythropoietin; *IL-11,* interleukin-11; *IL-6,* interleukin-6; *MGDF,* megakaryocyte growth and development factor; *Tpo,* thrombopoietin; *M-CSF,* macrophage colony-stimulating factor; *G-CSF,* granulocyte colony-stimulating factor; *IL-7,* interleukin-7; *IL-2,* interleukin-2. (Reprinted from Hunt P, Foote MA: *Curr Opin Biotech* 6:692, © 1995, with permission from Elsevier Science.)

IL-3 and M-CSF continue. The characterization of other HGFs is also being pursued. After in vitro studies elucidate their biology, the next step will be assessment of their clinical efficacy in vivo.[92] For the four classic CSFs, current investigations attempt to further define appropriate dosages, schedules, and routes of administration, as well as the diseases and conditions for which these agents are best used.[169–171, 282]

The HGFs were discovered through research into the process and regulation of hematopoiesis. These glycoproteins were detected because of their mandatory and unique role in stimulating hematopoietic cells to proliferate[75] (Fig. 24–2). The use of semisolid colony assay systems to culture hematopoietic cells revealed that specific regulatory molecules (CSFs) were necessary to sustain progenitor cells and to form colonies. The ability to clone these agents greatly enhanced the ability to study them. There appear to be overlapping functions, as well as synergism, between different HGFs. Because these are all receptor-mediated molecules, differences in effects on different hematopoietic lineages may be related to the distribution of receptors.[169–171]

To understand the HGFs, one needs a basic understanding of hematopoiesis, or the production and development of blood cells. This process normally occurs in the bone marrow, where cells of various lineages proliferate, differentiate, and mature. Most blood cells have a relatively short life span; therefore, they must be constantly produced to offset continual turnover. For example, baseline levels of granulocytes and macrophages are maintained within a narrow range. However, the body has a remarkable ability to increase production in response to stresses such as infection and inflammation. Factors thought to be important in the control of hematopoiesis are the bone marrow microenvironment, cell-to-cell interaction, and humoral substances.[154]

The process starts with a multipotent or pluripotent stem cell. These cells have the capacity for self-renewal and the ability to form multilineage colonies, although they are relatively quiescent under normal circumstances. Cells become successively more proliferative during differentiation, and their capacities to renew themselves and to form multilineage colonies become more restricted. The factors controlling hematopoiesis have not been entirely delineated. Constitutive substances that may affect the lineage commitment status of a cell are being investigated. CSFs appear more important in the stress response, and they seem to help control the number of effector cells in the immune response.[109, 154]

BIOLOGY AND CLINICAL APPLICATIONS

The biologic activity of the HGFs is summarized in Table 24–1. In vitro studies suggested that the CSFs may have clinical value in a variety of settings. CSF clinical trials continue to evaluate (1) reducing cancer treatment morbidity by decreasing myelosuppression (both intensity and duration) and the incidence of febrile neutropenia; (2) improving survival by allowing patients to receive chemotherapy treatments on schedule; (3) speeding marrow recovery after bone marrow transplantation; (4) supporting the harvest of peripheral blood stem cells; (5) restoring bone marrow function in aplastic anemia, myelodysplastic syndrome, myelomas, leukemias, and acquired and congenital neutropenias; (6) combining CSFs with other BRMs to further enhance effector cell functions; (7) treating leukemia by promoting terminal cell maturation; and (8) treating burns, overwhelming sepsis-related infections, and parasitic infections.[92, 169, 183, 282, 292] Although the use of HGFs has had a significant impact as supportive therapy in patients receiving chemotherapy and after bone marrow transplantation,[190] issues of cost effectiveness are a continuing concern. Because a major issue in the changing health care environment is controlling cost, the American Society of Clinical Oncology published guidelines and recommendations for the use of these factors in 1995.[175]

GRANULOCYTE/MACROPHAGE COLONY-STIMULATING FACTOR

Of the multilineage CSFs, GM-CSF has received the most extensive clinical evaluation. Early clinical trials evaluated its application in patients with AIDS,[106] myelodysplastic syndromes, and aplastic anemia,[274, 275] and in cancer patients after chemotherapy[11] and autologous BMT.[31] All studies showed dose-dependent increases in leukocytes, especially neutrophils, eosinophils, and monocytes. The duration of neutropenia appeared shorter after chemotherapy, and leukocyte recovery was enhanced after transplantation, compared with controls. Overall, no significant effects on platelet recovery were seen. Counts rose during therapy in a dose-dependent manner but fell rapidly once therapy was discontinued. In general, courses were well tolerated, and side effects were dose dependent. Recombinant human GM-CSF, sargramostim (Leukine), received regulatory approval in 1991 for the acceleration of myeloid recovery in patients with non-Hodgkin's lymphoma (NHL), acute lymphoblastic leukemia (ALL), and those with Hodgkin's disease who were undergoing autologous BMT.[123] Patients receiving GM-CSF had neutrophil recovery 7 days earlier than the group receiving placebo, fewer infections, fewer days taking antibiotics, and fewer days of hospitalization. Subsequent approvals include use in BMT graft failure and engraftment delay and as supportive therapy for elderly patients with acute myelogenous leukemia (AML) receiving high-dose chemotherapy.[250] Current trials have focused on whether GM-CSF given before chemotherapy could protect hematopoietic cells from cytotoxic effects. Kobrinsky and others[138] found that this approach in adjuvant breast cancer treatment resulted in earlier nadir and more rapid recovery of neutrophila and platelet counts. Also, the duration and severity of thrombocytopenia was reduced with GM-CSF given prior to adjuvant chemotherapy. Issues to be addressed in future trials include evaluation of the effects of GM-CSF on the incidence and seriousness of neutropenic infections after chemotherapy or transplantation, the timing of therapy in relation to administration of chemotherapy, long-term toxicity, its antitumor effect in both solid tumors and leukemias, and its use in infectious disease.[169, 178, 209, 276, 292]

Administration

Several pharmaceutical companies manufacture GM-CSF; however, only one brand is commercially available in the United States. Nurses should consult pharmacy resource personnel or the package insert about issues related to reconstitution, filterability, and stability. Pharmacology studies show GM-CSF has a relatively short half-life, with the second phase lasting 1 to 3 hours.[43] In early trials GM-CSF was given by IV infusion (continuous infusion, bolus); however, SC administration is also used.

In general, doses of 125 to 250 $\mu g/m^2$ (3–5 $\mu g/kg$) are fairly well tolerated. The recommended dose for sargramostim is 250 $\mu g/m^2$ per day for 21 days as a 2-hour IV infusion beginning 2 to 4 hours after the autologous bone marrow infusion.[123] Toxicity is dose related, and the dose-limiting side effects are myalgia, arthralgia, capillary leak syndrome with edema, and pericardial and pleural effusions, which develop at doses above 16 to 32 $\mu g/kg$.[11, 41]

Side Effects

Side effects are affected by the dosage, route of administration, patient population, and setting used (postchemotherapy, post-BMT). Common side effects are constitutional symptoms (low-grade fever), bone pain, fatigue, and anorexia. Other reported side effects, generally seen at higher doses, are rashes, flushing, phlebitis,[106] gastrointestinal disturbances, erythema at the injection site, hypotension, fluid retention, pericarditis, pleural and pericardial effusion, thrombocytopenia, and

thrombus formation at the catheter tip. These effects are generally reversible when therapy stops.*

GRANULOCYTE COLONY-STIMULATING FACTOR

The early clinical trials investigating G-CSF focused on its use after chemotherapy.[183] Trials with combination chemotherapy for urothelial carcinoma[91] and high-dose chemotherapy for small-cell lung cancer[33] demonstrated a shorter duration of severe neutropenia after G-CSF therapy. Gabrilove's study showed that patients who received G-CSF had fewer days of antibiotic therapy and a reduced incidence and severity of mucositis and were more likely to be able to stay on their chemotherapy schedules than other patients. Patients exhibited a dose-dependent increase in leukocyte counts, mainly because of an increase in the absolute number of neutrophils. Counts fell rapidly once therapy was stopped. G-CSF has also been investigated in neutropenia arising from other causes.[84] In patients with HCL, for example, G-CSF dramatically increased the absolute neutrophil count.[100] In patients with myelodysplastic syndrome, patients have increased their neutrophil counts over baseline levels 5- to 40-fold.[183]

Recombinant human G-CSF, filgrastim (Neupogen), received FDA approval in 1991. Its initial indication was to reduce the incidence of infection in patients with nonmyeloid malignancies receiving myelosuppressive anticancer drugs associated with a significant incidence of severe neutropenia with fever. In 1994, filgrastim received regulatory approval for use in BMT in nonmyeloid malignancies. An additional indication is the use of filgrastim to treat patients with severe chronic neutropenia.[4] Current clinical trials continue to study its use in a variety of bone marrow failure states, infections, in dose-intensified chemotherapy, mobilization of peripheral blood stem cells, radiotherapy, and in combination with other HGFs.[112, 159, 183, 209, 292]

Administration and Side Effects

The recommended starting dose of filgrastim is 5 $\mu g/kg$ per day, administered SC or IV as a single daily injection[4] 24 hours after chemotherapy (for complete dosing instructions, consult the package insert). Nurses should consult pharmacy resource personnel or the package insert about issues related to reconstitution, filterability, and stability. Therapy is generally well tolerated, with medullary bone pain as the only consistent toxicity reported. This pain is usually mild to moderate in severity and is generally well controlled with nonnarcotic analge-

---

* References 11, 31, 42, 109, 158, 274, 275.

BOX 24-3

Clinical Potential of GM-CSF and G-CSF

Adjunct to standard chemotherapy
- Reduce morbidity
- Allow full doses to be delivered on time

Permit dose intensification of chemotherapy
- Reduce the morbidity of autologous or allogeneic marrow or peripheral stem-cell transplantation
- Allow larger doses of drugs to be administered
- Increase the frequency of chemotherapy cycles

Reversal of marrow failure
- Malignancies with marrow infiltration, chronic lymphatic leukemia, hairy cell leukemia, lymphoma

Differentiation-inducing agents
- Myelodysplastic syndromes
- Myeloid leukemia

Recruitment of malignant cells before chemotherapy
- Myeloid leukemia

Direct anticancer effects

From Metcalf D, Morstyn G: Colony-stimulating factors: general biology. In DeVita VT, Hellman S, Rosenberg SA, editors: *Biologic therapy of cancer*, ed 2, Philadelphia, Lippincott, 1995.

---

sics. Erythema is occasionally seen at the site of subcutaneous injections. Box 24–3 reviews potential clinical uses of GM-CSF and G-CSF.

ERYTHROPOIETIN

Physiologically, erythropoietin is a natural body glycoprotein essential for the growth of erythroid progenitor cells. Erythropoiesis is regulated by erythropoietin in response to changes in tissue oxygenation. Secreted primarily by the kidneys, erythropoietin acts on specific target cells in the bone marrow to increase the rate of production and release of red blood cells.[254] Recombinant human erythropoietin, epoetin alfa (Epogen and Procrit), was approved by the FDA in 1989 as a treatment for chronic anemia in end-stage renal disease after phase I and II trials demonstrated clinical efficacy.[79] The recombinant form is produced in cultured mammalian cells. When receiving it IV three times a week, virtually all patients achieved normalization of hematocrit and were transfusion independent. Therapy is well tolerated in general, and most side effects (hypertension, seizures, increased clotting of venous access grafts) appear to be related to increased hematocrit.[6] Patients are generally started at a dosage of 50 to 100 U/kg three times a week IV or SC. Maintenance doses are generally titrated in 25-U increments to keep the hematocrit in a chosen target range (e.g., 36–38%).

Anemia is one of the major side effects of treatment with zidovudine, an antiviral drug used in the treatment of patients infected with the human immunodeficiency virus (HIV). Double-blind, placebo-controlled trials led to regulatory approval of epoetin alfa in this population for patients with an endogenous serum erythropoietin level below 500 U/L. Doses of epoetin alfa at 100 U/kg by IV infusion three times a week resulted in an increase in hematocrit and a decrease in transfusion requirements. In 1993, Procrit received regulatory approval for the treatment of anemia in cancer patients undergoing chemotherapy.[1, 197, 224, 296] At doses of 150 U/kg given by SC injection three times weekly, patients experienced an increase in hematocrit values from baseline and a decrease in transfusion requirements. Quality of life indices in responding patients showed improvement in energy levels, ability to engage in daily activities, and improvement in overall quality of life.[63, 101] Epoetin alfa is being studied for its use in autologous blood donation, acute blood loss and surgery, and treatment of myelodysplastic syndrome, as well as in combination with other HGFs.

MACROPHAGE COLONY-STIMULATING FACTOR

The inherent biologic activity of M-CSF has aroused considerable interest in its use, alone or in combination with other biologic agents, in the treatment of malignancy.[15, 187, 189] Early phase I/II trials are in the process of evaluating dosage and toxicity for both the SC and IV routes. In trials evaluating SC administration, doses up to 12,800 μg/m^2 have been administered. In general, toxicity has been mild, consisting of local reaction, arthralgia, and fatigue. At the highest dose levels, thrombocytopenia and monocytosis have been observed.[38] A dose-dependent decrease in cholesterol and lipoproteins has also been observed. Future trials will further define dosage and evaluate the efficacy of M-CSF in treating cancer. It is also being studied as a treatment for fungal infections in patients undergoing BMT.[282]

INTERLEUKIN-3

The ability of IL-3 to target multipotential-committed progenitor cells provides a strong rationale for its evaluation in the treatment of bone marrow failure states. IL-3 is produced by activated T lymphocytes. Phase I/II clinical trials continue to evaluate the use of IL-3 alone and in combination with other HGFs for patients with bone marrow failure, normal hematopoiesis but advanced malignancy, or prolonged cytopenia after radiotherapy or chemotherapy.[115, 142] In trials with IL-3 alone, all studies showed a delayed increase in leukocytes (granulocytes, eosinophils, and basophils), and occasional increases in platelets and reticulocytes. Effective doses range from 60 to 500 μg/m^2 per day for 15 days, though clinical trials with doses up to 1000 μg/m^2 per day have been fairly well tolerated.[98, 143, 282] There appears to be no difference between the IV and SC routes, though the SC route has less toxicity associated with it. The most common toxicities experienced include flulike symptoms, such as low-grade fever, headaches, and stiff neck. Facial flushing, erythema at injection sites, bone pain, lethargy, and nausea and vomiting can also occur. Future trials will further refine dosage and the application of IL-3 in bone marrow failure states and its ability to provide a myeloprotective effect after chemotherapy or radiotherapy.[209, 282, 292] In studies with IL-3 and GM-CSF, there is marked production of immature neutrophils when IL-3 is given after GM-CSF.[75] Preliminary clinical results suggest that this combination may have a synergistic effect on hematopoietic progenitor cells and may be of value in reducing chemotherapy-induced neutropenia.

PIXY321

PIXY321 is a recombinantly engineered fusion molecule. It consists of GM-CSF and IL-3, fused together with a linker protein. It has demonstrated biologic effects consistent with both of these growth factors and is thought to have a greater multilineage effect than either alone. PIXY321 is being evaluated both (1) alone in a variety of bone marrow failure states or after chemotherapy and (2) in combination with other HGFs. Doses range from 750 to 1000 μg/m^2 per day as an IV or SC injection 24 hours after chemotherapy (per protocol) for up to 14 days. Studies have shown a dose-dependent increase in white blood cell counts (mainly neutrophils) and platelets. Common toxic effects include erythema at the injection site, flulike symptoms, bone pain, and fatigue. Phase III confirmatory trials of PIXY321 are in progress at several centers, evaluating its use in the areas of chemotherapy-induced cytopenias and high-dose chemotherapy and BMT.[209, 282, 292]

INTERLEUKIN-11

Interleukin-11 is a thrombopoietic growth factor that stimulates the proliferation of hematopoietic stem cells and megakaryocyte progenitor cells. IL-11 also induces the maturation of megakaryocytes, thereby increasing platelet production. IL-11 (oprelvekin) was approved by the FDA in 1998 for the prevention of severe thrombocytopenia and reduction in need for platelet transfusions following myelosuppressive chemotherapy for nonmyeloid cancers. In randomized, double-blinded, placebo-controlled trials evaluating patients receiving myelosuppressive chemotherapy, the oprelvekin arm had fewer patients requiring platelet transfusions (72% versus 93% in the placebo arm). This was true among patients who had previously been treated with chemotherapy, as well as those who had not undergone prior treatment.[104, 126, 266] Oprelvekin is given SC in doses of 50 μg/kg daily, beginning 6 to 24 hours after chemotherapy. Doses continue on a daily basis until the postnadir platelet count is 50,000 cells/μL or greater. Side effects are usually mild to moderate in intensity and include nausea, vomiting, edema, mucositis, diarrhea, pain, chills, and dyspnea.[126]

MEGAKARYOCYTE GROWTH AND DEVELOPMENT FACTOR

Investigators over the past 40 years have suggested the existence of a growth factor (or factors) that regulates megakaryocytopoiesis and thrombopoiesis. This factor, which was thought to be a group of cytokines was termed thrombopoietin (TPO). The oncogene c-Mpl was isolated from a human erythroleukemia cell line and was found to have the characteristics of a hematopoietic growth factor. In 1994, the ligand for the c-Mpl cytokine receptor was cloned and was renamed megakaryocyte growth and development factor (MGDF). Recombinant human megakaryocyte growth and development factor (rHuMGDF) is a truncated form of Mpl ligand with the identical biologic activity. A pegylated form of MGDF (PEGrHuMGDF) was developed and is 10 times more potent than nonpegylated MGDF in vivo.[119, 135] In clinical trials using PEGrHuMGDF alone, in doses ranging from 0.3 to 1.0 μg/kg, patients experienced increases in platelet counts ranging from 51% to 584%. Doses were given either once before chemotherapy or daily for 10 days. There were no effects on neutrophil counts or hematocrits.[22, 273] In studies using PEGrHuMGDF after chemotherapy and G-CSF, the platelet nadir count occurred earlier and lasted for a shorter period of time.[21] The same effect did not occur when PEGrHuMGDF was given without G-CSF after chemotherapy. Fanucchi and colleagues[81] found a higher platelet nadir and time to recovery of platelets shorter when PEGrHuMGDF was given in this manner. Several ongoing trials are investigating the use of PEGrHuMGDF in the high-dose chemotherapy with peripheral blood stem cell (PBSC) support, and its use in the treatment of platelet donors or patients suffering from chronic thrombocytopenia disorders.

Tumor Necrosis Factor

Discovered in 1975 in the serum of animals treated with injections of BCG or *C. parvum* followed by endotoxins, tumor necrosis factor (TNF) is a protein that selectively targets transformed cells.[16] Normal human fibroblasts appeared insensitive to TNF. These findings generated considerable interest in the use of TNF in the treatment of cancer. The gene for TNF has been isolated, identified, and cloned to produce recombinant TNF (rTNF). Further investigations have analyzed the relationships of TNF with other cytotoxic factors produced by immune effector cells. Cachectin was isolated by Beutler and colleagues,[28] who believed it to be important in the pathogenesis of cachexia. Amino acid sequencing and cloning techniques proved human cachectin and TNF to be the same molecule.[28, 268] This TNF, primarily produced by activated macrophages, is called *TNF-α*. Another cytokine, lymphotoxin, which shares biologic activity with TNF-α, has been called TNF-β. It is produced primarily by lymphocytes. This section focuses on TNF-α.

BIOLOGIC EFFECTS

Although primarily synthesized in vivo by activated macrophages, TNF is also produced by lymphocytes, NK cells, astrocytes, and microglial cells of the brain. This polypeptide hormone, pivotal in the pathogenesis of infection, inflammation, and injury, participates in the beneficial processes of host defense and tissue homeostasis. TNF interacts with high-affinity receptors on normal tissue cells, with resultant internalization of the receptor-ligand complex. Details of this process remain unclear. Several biologic activities of TNF may be responsible for its antitumor effects: it is cytotoxic or cytostatic to some human tumor cells; it promotes the induction of other mediators (IL-2 and GM-CSF)[90, 268]; it enhances chemotactic, phagocytic, and cytotoxic activity of macrophages and neutrophils; and it causes the induction of several cell-surface antigens. It also serves as the primary mediator of endotoxic shock[162] and as a growth factor by stimulating fibroblasts and mesenchymal cell proliferation.[16, 36, 268]

CLINICAL INDICATIONS

Both preclinical studies in animal models and human clinical trials have evaluated the effectiveness of TNF as an antitumor agent. An overview of phase I experience with TNF in the United States indicates that more than 200 patients with a variety of malignancies have undergone therapy with TNF. However, to date, therapeutic responses are unimpressive.[29, 45, 90, 245] An editorial by Frei[90] concludes that until the cellular mechanisms of TNF cytotoxicity and tumor cell resistance are understood, clinical trials will not be able to exploit the full potential of this agent. Current efforts are focused on phase II investigations and on evaluating combination therapy of TNF with other cytokines,[185, 186] isolated limb perfusions in combination with IFN-γ and in the transfer of the gene coding for TNF into TIL (a form of gene therapy).[231]

ADMINISTRATION

Tumor necrosis factor has been administered by IM, SC, IV[29, 245] (via both bolus and continuous infusion), and intraperitoneal routes. The maximum tolerated dose as defined in phase I trials varies with route and schedule. TNF has not received FDA approval and therefore is administered only in investigational settings.

Pharmacy resource personnel should be consulted about stability, filterability, and other administration concerns (e.g., IV lines are often preprimed with albumin and normal saline before TNF administration). Handling procedures should follow agency policy.

SIDE EFFECTS

Toxicity associated with TNF has been well documented in early clinical trials.[36] The side effects are similar to those seen with other biologic agents, are dose dependent, and in general resolve on discontinuation of therapy. Dose-limiting toxicities with IV administration have been constitutional symptoms and shocklike manifestations, including fever and hypotension.[36, 41] As with IFN, patients may exhibit tachyphylaxis to many of the side effects.

Common side effects include fever, severe chills or rigors, fatigue, myalgia, headache, soreness at the injection site (erythema and tenderness), nausea or vomiting, diarrhea, and loss of appetite, with resultant weight loss. Pretreatment with meperidine is often helpful in controlling chills and rigors. Depending on the dose and schedule, these side effects may lessen or disappear with subsequent doses.

Occasional side effects include hematologic changes (leukopenia, thrombocytopenia), cardiovascular changes (hypotension, dizziness), hepatic changes (elevated transaminases, hyperbilirubinemia), elevated triglycerides, and decreased serum cholesterol. These changes are usually reversible with cessation of therapy. Hypotension can generally be managed with fluid administration, with prehydration used at higher IV doses of TNF ($\geq 100 \ \mu g/m^2$).[41]

Although rare, more severe toxicity associated with changes in the central nervous or respiratory systems has occurred.[173] Neurologic deficits observed include transient ischemic attacks and strokelike symptoms. Patients who develop these symptoms should be removed from the study and evaluated to determine the etiology of the symptoms. Respiratory insufficiency, evidenced primarily by dyspnea, has also been observed. Morice and associates[180] monitored 19 patients receiving SC or

IV TNF. All but two demonstrated impairment of gas exchange as measured by diffusion lung capacity (DLCO), a measurement of alveolar gas exchange. This toxicity appeared to be dose related but resolved in most patients with the cessation of therapy.

Monoclonal Antibodies

Monoclonal antibodies (MoAbs), produced by the fusion of antibody-producing cells and myeloma tumor cells (hybridomas), are highly specific for a single target antigen. With the development of hybridoma technology in 1975,[139] large amounts of pure antibodies with a predetermined specificity could be produced. This rekindled interest in the use of antibodies for the diagnosis and treatment of cancer. Their potential was implicated in the early 1900s, when Paul Ehrlich observed that antiserum from tumor-bearing mice, when injected into tumor-bearing animals of the same strain, was capable of causing tumor rejection. He called these antibodies magic bullets and proposed using them as carriers to deliver drugs and toxins to tumor cells.[77]

An antigen is any substance that the body recognizes as foreign and attacks with an immune response. The humoral immune response produces immunoglobulins against the invading antigen from B cell-derived plasma cells. These immunoglobulins, or antibodies, react specifically with the antigenic determinants or epitopes of the inducing antigen. The antigenic determinants are parts of the antigen recognized by the antibodies. Each antigen has any number of epitopes, depending on the complexity of its structure. Individual B cells produce an antibody specific for a single antigenic determinant; therefore, when an antigen invades the body, a variety of antibodies against it are produced.[134, 210]

Hybridoma technology begins with immunizing a mouse with a chosen antigen (Fig. 24–3). After the mouse mounts an immune response, its spleen is removed to obtain B lymphocyte-producing antibodies. Because lymphocytes cannot grow indefinitely in culture, they are fused with mouse myeloma cells (plasma cells) to immortalize the antibody-producing B lymphocytes. These new cells, *hybridomas,* can grow indefinitely in culture and produce antibodies with predetermined specificity—MoAbs. The next step is to select and clone for the desired antibody. Once the desired hybridoma is obtained, it can be frozen for future use, grown in culture to produce continuous quantities of MoAbs, or reinjected into mice and grown as tumors to produce MoAbs in ascites fluid.[66]

When the body encounters a foreign substance, an immune response is mounted. It has long been hypothesized that tumor cells express cell-surface molecules (antigens) different from those expressed on normal

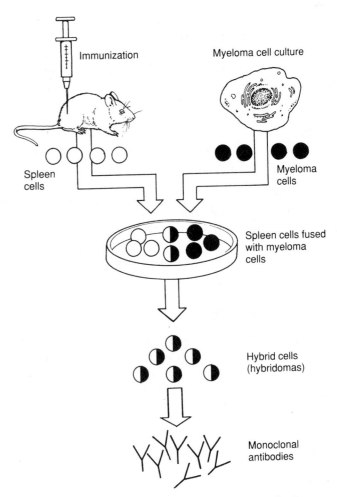

FIGURE 24–3 Monoclonal antibody production.

cells. Antigens found only on malignant cells are called *tumor-specific antigens (TSAs),* whereas antigens found also on normal tissues but to a greater degree in malignant cells are called *tumor-associated antigens (TAAs).*[17, 66, 70, 134, 240] Most malignant cells express TAA. One example is oncofetal antigens, which are normally expressed on embryonic cells and later reexpressed on malignant cells. Whereas most current therapies are toxic for both malignant and normal cells, MoAbs can be used to attack the tumor cell directly. Theoretically, antibody therapy is the most tumor-specific approach to cancer treatment.[66, 70]

UNCONJUGATED ANTIBODY

Biology and Clinical Applications

Numerous clinical trials have been conducted with native MoAbs—those not bound to drugs, toxins, or isotopes—for a large number of malignancies. An unconjugated antibody may demonstrate an anticancer effect in several ways. One is to mediate an antitumor cytotoxic effect through complement-dependent cytotoxicity or antibody-dependent cellular cytotoxicity. The constant region (F_c) of the immunoglobulin reacts with either the first component of the complement system or with immune effector cells; the end result is tumor cell lysis.[17] Tumor cells express a variety of receptors important for growth and proliferation advantages. A second approach uses MoAbs directed against cell surface receptors involved in proliferation, such as the epidermal growth factor (EGF) receptor. The intent is to block or downgrade the number of available receptors, thereby inducing an antiproliferative effect.[17, 19, 70, 240] An extensively studied approach is the use of anti-idiotype antibodies. Idiotypes are the variable regions of the immunoglobulin molecule that contain the antigen-combining region. A malignant B-cell clone produces cells that express and occasionally secrete a specific antibody. Infusions of antibodies directed against a B-cell lymphoma idiotype may suppress that clone back to its baseline.[66, 70, 134, 240]

Another approach, actually a method of passive immunization, uses antibodies as surrogate tumor antigens to stimulate an immune response against the tumor. For example, suppose a murine antibody (AB1) is selected to recognize a certain TAA. A second antibody (AB2) is raised against the idiotype of AB1. This second antibody, AB2, is an anti-idiotype antibody. The patient is immunized with this antibody. An anti-idiotype response to AB2 produces a third antibody, AB3. This third antibody has the same capacity to react with the desired TAA as AB1 because its idiotype is the mirror image of this antigen. In essence, by receiving AB2, the patient becomes self-immunized, developing his own human antibodies against the tumor. This technique is also used to immunize against invading organisms such as viruses because it avoids vaccination with whole virus or viral antigens (Fig. 24–4).

In 1997, the first MoAb was approved by the FDA specifically for the treatment of human malignancy. Rituxan (mouse/human chimeric anti-CD20 MoAb rituximab) received approval for demonstrating activity in B-cell lymphoma.[241, 283] In clinical trials, objective response rates of 60% for patients with follicular lymphomas and 30% for large-cell or mantle-zone lymphomas were achieved. The response rates increase to 95% to 100% when rituximab is combined with chemotherapy regimens, such as CHOP (cyclophosphamide, doxorubicin, vincristine, and prednisone).[52, 68, 160, 167] Current trials explore rituximab in the high-dose chemotherapy with autologous stem cell rescue setting to purge the CD20+ cells before stem cell collection, and after marrow recovery, use as consolidation therapy. The use of rituximab in consolidation therapy for CLL and myeloma is also being explored.

In 1998, the FDA approved a second MoAb, trastuzumab (Herceptin), the first for use in solid tumors. This agent has a specific use in a group of metastatic breast cancer patients whose tumors overexpress the HER2/neu receptor. HER2/neu is a member of the EGF tyrosine kinase receptor family. Overexpression of the *erb*B-2 proto-oncogene, results in overexpression of the HER2/neu receptor on the cell surface. This causes increased cell proliferation. In clinical trials, weekly

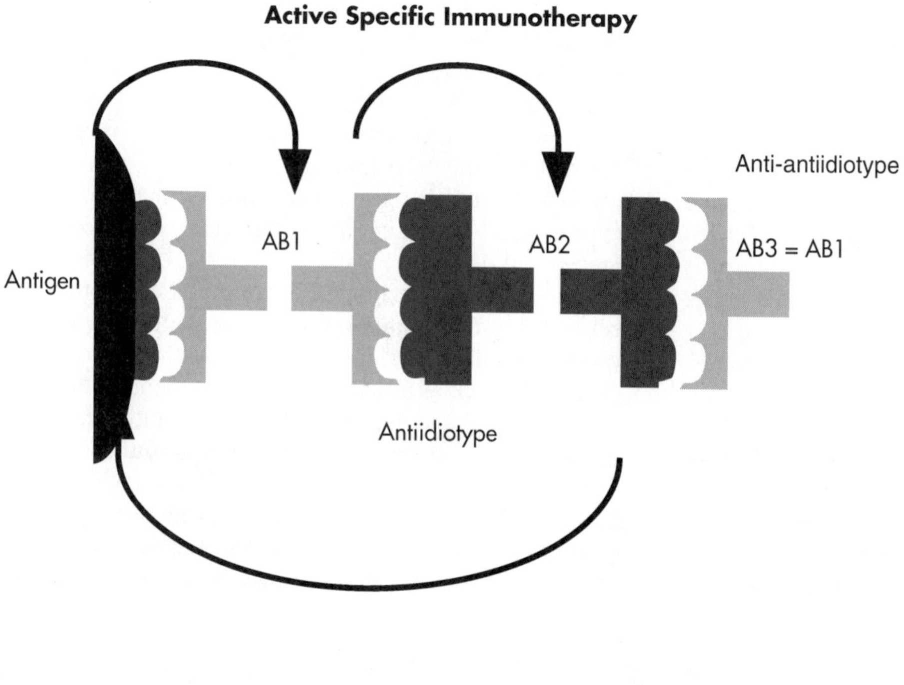

Active Specific Immunotherapy

FIGURE 24–4 Production of MoAbs to be used as vaccines. A murine antibody (AB1) is chosen to recognize a certain tumor-associated antigen, such as a melanoma-associated antigen. A second antibody (AB2) is made to recognize the idiotype of AB1; this second antibody is an anti-idiotype antibody, which is used as the vaccine. The patient is immunized with AB2 and responds by producing an anti-idiotype antibody against AB2; this third antibody, designated AB3, has the same ability to react with the desired tumor-associated antigen as AB1, because its idiotype is the mirror image of AB1. Thus the patient becomes self-immunized, developing his own human antibodies against the tumor.

administration of trastuzumab alone over 10 weeks resulted in objective tumor responses of 12%.[20] Subsequent trials of trastuzumab in combination with chemotherapy yielded response rates of 21% to 53%.[18, 202]

Several problems can affect the therapeutic efficacy or toxicity (or both) of MoAbs. A major concern is the development of human antimouse antibodies (HAMA) after murine MoAbs are administered.[17, 66, 216] HAMA may trigger immune complex formation, which mediates tissue damage, neutralization of MoAbs (preventing them from binding to tumor cells), and alteration of MoAb clearance and organ distribution. Strategies being evaluated to abrogate the development of HAMA include infusion of antibody fragments, infusion of large doses of MoAb to induce tolerance, immunosuppressive therapy, and use of human or chimeric[17, 66] antibodies.

Another concern is antigenic modulation. Surface antigens decline during this process, being either internalized and later reexpressed or shed from the cell surface. Antigenic modulation is especially problematic in hematologic malignancies. Within minutes of exposure to MoAbs, modulation can occur. Once circulating levels of MoAb decrease, antigen is reexpressed. Obviously, once modulation occurs, MoAbs cannot effectively bind to malignant cells. Strategies for circumventing this problem include administration of mixed MoAbs (a cocktail) to recognize different antigens and choosing MoAbs specific for nonmodulating antigens. The 17-1A MoAb, edrecolomab, is a mouse IgG2 MoAb that reacts with glycoproteins found on various adenocarcinomas and normal epithelial tissue. The antigen is not shed into the circulation and it appears to be involved in cell adhesion.[66, 70, 240]

Other problems include poor tumor vascularity (poor circulation inhibits delivery of MoAbs to the tumor site), cross-reactivity of MoAbs with normal tissues, tumor heterogeneity (expression of more than one TAA), lack of sufficient antigen expression on the tumor cell surface, and lack of in vivo cytotoxicity of the antibody alone. Clinical trials are evaluating strategies to overcome these obstacles so that the full therapeutic benefit of MoAbs can be realized.[17, 66, 216] For example, one area of focus is the combination of native MoAbs and other BRMs. An example is the use of an HGF such as GM-CSF to increase the number of immune cells capable of interacting with MoAbs to destroy tumor cells.[17]

Immunoconjugates

An active area of investigation is the conjugation of MoAbs to toxins (immunotoxins),[199] chemotherapy (chemoimmunotoxins),[205] radioisotopes (radioimmunotherapy),[103, 291] and BRMs (immunobiologics).[17] The ricin A chain, a toxin, has been conjugated to several antitumor murine MoAbs, and clinical trials are progressing.[199, 253] Although most responses are transient, patients with hematopoietic tumors tend to respond better than those with solid tumors. The most significant complications have included a capillary leak type of syndrome exhibited clinically by hypoalbuminemia, proteinuria, weight gain, and pulmonary edema. Clinical trials are investigating immunoconjugates of chemotherapeutic agents such as methotrexate, doxorubicin, and cisplatin, to MoAbs.[195] By selectively delivering these drugs to the tumor, investigators hope to increase tumor cell kill while avoiding systemic toxicity. Problems include acquired drug resistance and the need to deliver large amounts of drug (as opposed to small amounts with toxins) to the tumor.

Another exciting area is conjugation of radioisotopes to MoAbs. Two important advantages to this approach are the ability to kill antigen-negative bystander cells and elimination of the need for internalization by the tumor cell to exhibit their cytotoxic effect. Clinical trials are in progress in this area, with most successes seen in the hematologic malignancies.[66, 103, 168] Major problems with all types of conjugates include damage to normal tissue as a result of cross-reactivity and systemic toxicity should the MoAb and the conjugate dissociate. Toxicity is related primarily to the effects of the radioisotope on the bone marrow, with platelets being the most sensitive.

Diagnostic Imaging with Radiolabeled Antibodies

The use of radiolabeled MoAbs in diagnostic imaging has received intense study.[147, 233] When low doses of radioisotopes such as indium-111 and iodine-131 are conjugated with MoAbs that react to specific tumor antigens, MoAbs can be used to locate both primary and metastatic tumors. The ability of radiolabeled MoAbs to detect tumors is being compared with conventional x-rays and isotope scans. In some instances, antibodies are more sensitive than conventional scans.[168] Currently, there are four radiolabeled antibodies that have been approved by the FDA for radioimmunodetection of cancer. These include satumonab (OncoScint), capromab (ProstaScint), nofetumomab (Verluma), and arcitumomab (CEA-Scan).

OncoScint was the first FDA-approved MoAb for cancer radioimmunoimaging. It is reactive with 83% of colorectal adenocarcinomas and 97% of epitheleial ovarian cancers, as well as a majority of breast, pancreatic, gastric and esophageal cancers.[267] ProstaScint is reactive with over 95% of prostate cancers. It was studied in men with localized prostate cancer who were at high risk for metastatic disease and in men with suspicious recurrent or residual disease.[150] Verluma reacts with most small-cell and non–small-cell lung cancers, as well as breast, ovary, colorectal, and prostate adenocarcinomas.[32] CEA-Scan is a MoAb that targets carcinoembryonic antigen (CEA). This allows for early imaging of hepatic metastases, potentially when surgically resectable. Trials were conducted to increase the sensitivity of computed tomography (CT) scanning and, with the addition of CEA-Scan, sensitivity of CT scan improved from 86% to 97% in the ability to detect metastatic disease.[177] Problems that are associated with radioimmunoimaging include tumor size (lesions < 1 cm in size do not image well), tumor heterogeneity, nonspecific uptake of MoAbs by other organs (especially the liver and spleen), tumor vascularity, toxicities, and the HAMA response, which may limit administration to a single course. A current area of investigation is the use of a handheld probe during surgery to detect radiolabeled areas of tumor foci within the abdomen. This approach might be used to rule out metastasis in the lymph nodes and to determine tumor-free margins for resection.[17]

Other Clinical Applications

For diagnosis, MoAbs may be used in serologic detection of clinically unapparent tumors or to aid in the differential diagnosis of tumors that look alike on routinely processed light microscopy specimens. The latter field, *immunohistochemistry,* has been used increasingly over the past several years. MoAbs have been used extensively to classify leukemias and lymphomas.[240]

The MoAbs have also been used in BMT. One of the more severe complications of allogeneic transplantation is the development of GVHD. In an attempt to prevent the development of GVHD, MoAbs reactive with immunocompetent T cells are incubated in vitro with donor marrow before the marrow is infused into the recipient. An attractive therapeutic option in this area is the use of MoAbs to purge autologous marrow of lingering malignant cells before transplantation. The future holds further exploration and refinement in this area and investigation into the use of human monoclonal antibodies, chimeric monoclonal antibodies, and bifunctional antibodies (Box 24–4). Also, a considerable number of clinical trials are investigating the use of MoAb-based therapies in other disease states.

Administration

Administration of MoAbs involves IV, intra-arterial, intraperitoneal, and intralymphatic routes.[66, 233] Dosage depends on investigational protocols and whether the MoAb is being used for diagnostic or therapeutic purposes. Antibodies are generally diluted in normal saline and administered over several hours via an infusion pump to prevent accidental bolus infusion.[55, 225, 236] Handling procedures may vary among agencies; however,

---

BOX 24–4

Antibodies in Cancer Therapy

Antibodies
  Cytotoxic
  Regulatory
  Immunization
Immunoconjugates
  Radiolabeled antibodies
  Chemoimmunoconjugates
  Immunotoxins
  Immunobiologics
Bone marrow transplantation
  Allogeneic
  Autologous

From Dillman RO: Antibody therapy. In Oldham RK, editor: *Principles of cancer biotherapy,* ed 2, New York, Marcel Dekker, 1991. Additional data from references 70 and 233.

---

appropriate cytotoxic handling procedures should be used with chemoimmunoconjugates and immunotoxins. Radiation safety procedures should be used whenever radiolabeled MoAbs are used. Pharmacy resource personnel should be consulted about filterability, solution compatibility, stability, and other pertinent issues.[225, 232]

Side Effects

Allergic reaction to mouse protein is a major concern for patients receiving murine MoAbs. The major acute toxicity is anaphylaxis, manifested as generalized flushing or urticaria, followed by pallor or cyanosis. Respiratory distress may also occur. If left untreated, anaphylaxis can progress to systemic vascular collapse, unconsciousness, and death. Fortunately, its occurrence is rare. Treatment involves immediately stopping the antibody infusion and administering fluids and emergency drugs such as epinephrine, diphenhydramine, and hydrocortisone sodium succinate.

Subacute toxicity includes fever, chills, and rigors, diaphoresis, malaise, urticaria, pruritus, nausea, vomiting, dyspnea, and hypotension. Fevers, chills, diaphoresis, and shaking rigors are often seen when MoAbs bind to circulating leukemic cells.[67, 69] These toxicities can occur in the first 24 hours to 1 week after the infusion. They are usually easily treated before or during the infusion with acetaminophen, antihistamines, meperidine, or antiemetics.*

Serum sickness, the major delayed toxicity seen with MoAb therapy, can occur 2 to 4 weeks after infusion.

---

* References 66, 67, 69, 221–223.

It results when circulating immune complexes are deposited in the tissues and produces symptoms such as urticaria, pruritus, arthralgia, generalized adenopathy, and flulike symptoms. Treatment includes aspirin, acetaminophen, and occasionally corticosteroids. Symptoms usually resolve as the complexes are cleared from the body.[66, 67, 69]

On occasion, when MoAbs cross-react with normal tissues, other types of toxic effects may be seen. For example, antibodies targeted against the GD$_2$ ganglioside in melanoma cause intense pain during infusion. This is hypothesized to be a result of cross-reactivity with nerve tissue.[17]

Retinoids

The retinoids are a class of agents consisting of vitamin A (retinol) and related derivatives (all-*trans*-retinoic acid [ATRA; tretinoin] and 13-*cis*-retinoic acid [13-cRA] isotretinoin) that are involved in growth, reproduction, epithelial cell differentiation, and immune function. Specific effects of the retinoids on the immune system include enhancement of humoral antibody responses and certain cell-mediated immune responses, and improved phagocytosis by macrophages. The biologic effects of retinoids appear to occur from changes in gene expression that occur via specific nuclear receptors. Retinol and retinoic acid (RA) are known to bind to cellular retinol or RA-binding proteins. These proteins facilitate the transfer of RA and retinol from the cytoplasm to the nucleus, where they bind to one of several nuclear RA receptors. This ultimately leads to the transcription of appropriate target genes through binding to specific DNA sequences.[120, 153, 249]

Preclinical studies with RA have demonstrated several potentially beneficial effects: induction of cell differentiation in both normal epithelial cells and certain tumor cell lines, and direct growth inhibition with or without differentiation. Because of the unique biology of the retinoids, a number of clinical trials are evaluating their use in the treatment of cancer patients. Toxicity in these trials can be classified according to mucocutaneous, visual, skeletal, lipid, liver, and teratogenic side effects. Mucocutaneous toxicities are generally the most troublesome and include dryness of the mucosal tissues, erythema and desquamation of the skin, and cheilitis. Because of the strong teratogenic effect of the retinoids, extreme caution should be exercised to avoid their use during pregnancy.[120, 153, 249]

A series of clinical studies with oral RA has demonstrated high complete remission rates (CR) in patients with acute promyelocytic leukemia (APL).[262] Recent studies revealed that patients with APL that expressed CD56 resulted in short duration of response to combined chemotherapy and ATRA.[85] In November 1995, tretinoin (Vesanoid) received regulatory approval for the treatment of APL for induction of remission in patients who are refractory to or who have relapsed from anthracycline chemotherapy, or for whom anthracycline-based therapy is contraindicated. Because optimal consolidation or maintenance regimens have not been determined, all patients should receive a standard consolidation or maintenance chemotherapy regimen for APL after induction therapy with Vesanoid unless otherwise contraindicated.[229] Additional clinical trials, both phase I and phase II, are evaluating the use of RA alone and in combination with other agents such as IFN in myelodysplastic syndrome, other hematologic malignancies (multiple myeloma, mycosis fungoides), and solid tumors (cervical, squamous cell cancer of the head and neck, breast, and prostate carcinoma).[120, 153, 249]

Another exciting area is the use of retinoids in the chemoprevention of lung and upper aerodigestive tract carcinomas.[14, 24, 151, 152] Clinical trials have evaluated the effectiveness of both natural agents and synthetic retinoids in reversing oral premalignant lesions. A randomized, placebo-controlled trial of 13-cRA has been reported by Hong and associates.[120] Reversal of dysplasia occurred in 54% of the retinoid group and in only 10% of the placebo group. Two significant problems were encountered in this study: toxicity from 13-cRA and a relapse rate of over 50% within 3 months of stopping therapy. A second trial evaluated an induction phase with higher doses (1.5 mg/kg per day) followed by a 9-month maintenance program with either low-dose 13-cRA (0.5 mg/kg per day) or β-carotene (30 mg/d). Preliminary data demonstrate that the relapse rate after 9 months is 8% in the low-dose 13-cRA group and 55% in the β-carotene group. Other trials include evaluation of high-dose 13-cRA to prevent second primary tumors (SPT) in patients with squamous cell cancer of the head and neck. With a median follow-up of 42 months, only 6% of the 13-cRA group developed SPT compared with 28% of the placebo group. Two important directions for future chemoprevention trials will be establishing effective doses that reduce toxicity and evaluating other retinoids, such as fenretinide[271] or etretinate.[57] A phase III trial comparing tretinoin with β-carotene in the treatment of oral premalignant lesions is in progress.

Other Immunomodulators

This section briefly reviews agents that either boost immunologic responses (specifically or nonspecifically) or cause the induction of cytokines. Although many of these agents were more actively investigated in the 1960s and 1970s, they may still be encountered today. For example, they may now be used alone via different routes (intraperitoneal, intrapleural), or smaller subunits may be used in an attempt to elicit an immune response. Further possible uses include combining these agents with newer BRMs.

BACILLUS CALMETTE-GUERIN

Bacillus Calmette-Guerin (BCG) was used in first-generation immunotherapy trials.[117] Developed in the early 1900s, it is an attenuated form of the living bovine tubercle bacillus. It is believed to have a nonspecific immunostimulating effect. The initial work with BCG in animal models was done by Old and coworkers,[194] who demonstrated that BCG could stimulate the reticuloendothelial system and the immune response. Clinical trials reported by Mathe and others[163] demonstrated positive therapeutic results of BCG therapy for children with ALL. Although early trials with BCG in a multitude of settings appeared promising, further investigations did not support these results.[117, 233] Trials with BCG continue. When comparing the results of different clinical trials of BCG, it is of prime importance to note the variability in the strains of BCG used (Pasteur, Glaxo, Phipps, and so on), as well as the route of administration, dosage, and schedule. BCG is approved for the treatment of bladder cancer by intravesical instillation.[238]

Bacillus Calmette-Guerin can be administered intralesionally; intradermally by scarification, the tine technique, or the Heafgun; or intracavitarily (to the pleura, peritoneum, or bladder). Side effects can include local inflammatory reactions, flulike symptoms, hypersensitivity, and the serious complication of disseminated BCG infection.

LEVAMISOLE

Levamisole is an orally active synthetic agent that is an isomer of tetramisole, a broad-spectrum antihelminthic agent. Ergamisol[129] has been approved by the FDA for use with 5-FU as an adjuvant treatment for colon cancer (Duke's stage C). A randomized study showed that patients in Duke's stage C disease who were treated with levamisole and 5-FU had a higher 5-year survival rate than untreated patients.[148] Toxicity has been minimal with levamisole alone, and no more severe than expected for 5-FU alone, when the two drugs were combined.

TUMOR ANTIGENS

This form of therapy rests on the premise that tumor cells express immunogenic determinants that are not associated, or are associated to a lesser degree, with normal cells. The immune system will theoretically recognize these cells as foreign and mount an immunologic response. Tumor vaccines use tumor cells or purified components of tumor cell membrane. To increase the immunogenicity of the cells, the surface is often treated with viruses, irradiation, or neuramidase. Tumor vaccines are also given in combination with other immunostimulants such as BCG or *C. parvum*.[261] Clinical trials treating stage II melanomas and metastatic melanomas with tumor vaccines, with or without low doses of chemotherapy, are ongoing. There are response rates of 12% to 15% in patients with metastatic disease and 26% in patients who were surgically resected free of disease.[25, 40, 176] Vaccines are usually administered by multiple intradermal injections, with patients receiving vaccines prepared from their own tumor cells. One hindrance has been the technical limitations of such individualized vaccines. The process is technologically complex, labor intensive, and expensive. Research with MoAbs may lead to characterization and purification of reactive antigenic molecules that could be mass produced as a generic vaccine.[17, 111, 261]

Gene Therapy

An exciting but controversial area of current focus is gene therapy, defined as the insertion of a functioning gene into the cells of a patient to correct an inborn genetic error or to provide a new function to the cell. Somatic cell gene therapy, which does not have the potential of passing changes on to future generations, is currently the only technique approved for use in humans.[132, 227] The recent death of a patient undergoing gene therapy on an approved clinical trial heightened the awareness of the substantial risks to patient's safety when any part of the lengthy and rigorous process necessary for institutional, FDA, and National Institutes of Health authorization is circumvented.

Research in the area of gene therapy has been pioneered by Rosenberg and associates at the NCI. Trials evaluating the insertion of the gene for TNF into TIL cells have not been as effective as was originally expected. Theoretically, TILs would secrete large amounts of TNF locally at the tumor site.[230, 231] Other studies include administration of fibroblasts, transduced with the gene coding for IL-4, and tumor vaccines in patients with advanced melanoma or renal cell, breast, or colon cancer. Another approach under investigation is insertion of the multidrug resistance gene into bone marrow progenitor cells in an attempt to prevent dose-limiting myelosuppression while using higher doses of chemotherapy.[122]

To date, the most common approach for insertion of genes into somatic cells is through the use of a retroviral vector. A retrovirus, incapable of replicating, is used as a carrier to enter the cell and insert the desired gene into the cell's genome.[222, 235] Safety concerns include the fear of replication-competent viruses arising from vector cell lines or the disruption of normal cell growth when the retroviral vector randomly inserts the gene into the target cell. To address these issues, alternative delivery systems such as the use of the gene gun or antibody-coated liposomes are under evaluation. At this point, minimal toxic effects have been noted with gene therapy. However, it is important to remember that this therapy is still in its infancy and much remains to be learned. Ethical concerns over the manipulation of genes remain an ongoing area of importance. As genetic tests are developed to identify patients at risk for developing certain types of cancer, the use of gene therapy to inactivate or replace defective genes will become more prevalent.[227]

FUTURE DIRECTIONS AND ADVANCES IN BIOTHERAPY

Treatment with biologic agents is becoming more and more widespread, and new agents and novel combinations of agents will continue to make their way into the clinical setting.* It is imperative that oncology nurses be knowledgeable about biotherapy to be able to care for patients receiving it. In their roles as educator, advocate, and caregiver, nurses are key figures in facilitating management of patients receiving biologic agents. Over the next few years, BRMs will continue to receive FDA approval, which will increase their availability. Clinical trials will continue to define appropriate dosage, route, and clinical indications for many agents and combinations.[7, 185, 186] In addition, research efforts are now focusing on delineating the pathophysiology of BRM-associated side effects. It is hoped that these efforts will lead to improved tolerance of the more severe side effects.[219, 241]

For years, determination of the maximum tolerated dose has been the standard in chemotherapy trials. However, this approach may not be appropriate for biotherapy. Recent attention has focused on determining the optimal immunomodulatory dose. Lower doses may be more effective than the maximum tolerated dose in boosting an immune response. In addition, determining the full range of biologic effects in vivo will assist in determining dosage. Investigators are also faced with the challenge of developing therapeutic regimens that maximize response yet are tolerable to patients, cost effective, and realistically managed.[221–223, 233]

Clinical investigations evaluating combinations of cytokines and of cytokines and chemotherapy continue to

be an area of active focus. The availability of recombinant cytokines has led to evaluation of their efficacy in vivo as single-modality cancer therapy. Although clinical benefits have been achieved, few patients have been cured. An additional problem is the toxicity of cytokines when given at high doses. Is there a way to maximize response while achieving acceptable toxicity? Studies in animal models using combinations of cytokines have demonstrated synergism and a resultant increase in antitumor effect. Combining agents may make it possible to use smaller doses while maintaining therapeutic benefit. This has provided a rationale for the use of combinations of cytokines such as IFN-α and IL-2, TNF, and IL-2, and MoAbs and IL-2. It is hoped that effective combinations of BRMs with or without chemotherapy will result in improved therapeutic benefits and decreased toxicity.[10, 185, 186] Randomized trials will ultimately be necessary to prove any benefit for combination therapies.[71]

Progress in the basic sciences will continue to explore the mystery of cancer on a cellular level. This new understanding will serve as the foundation for future cancer therapies.[144, 145, 226, 294] Key regulatory molecules and signaling pathways in the cells will provide important targets for future diagnostic, therapeutic, and preventive strategies. Therapies will become increasingly selective and targeted toward repairing or blocking the negative effects of the underlying cellular defect. Depending on the existing mutation, strategies might be designed either to block or to stimulate transcription of a gene. Examples of this approach currently under clinical investigation include the use of "antisense" therapy, synthetic strands of DNA that bind to specific sites on the nucleic acids and inhibit the synthesis of disease-related proteins.[257] Numerous current and future clinical trials are aimed at restoring normal function to the mutated p53 gene.[44] This gene, classified as a tumor suppressor gene, is important in controlling abnormal cell growth.[287] As basic research begins to describe the metastatic process, new avenues for therapeutic intervention will be opened. One example under clinical investigation is the use of antiangiogenesis factors that ultimately would deprive a tumor of its blood supply.[113]

A final area of concern is reimbursement. Because of recent economic trends in health care, funding agencies and third-party payers often are unwilling to underwrite the cost of phase I and II investigations for drugs not approved by the FDA.[53] In the case of approved agents, they may be unwilling to pay for indications not included in the original FDA approval. Treatment with many BRMs can be costly in both the inpatient and ambulatory care setting; therefore, this problem is of major importance to both patients and health care professionals.[165, 297] Patients who receive investigational drugs as part of an approved clinical trial receive the drug at no cost; however,

---

* References 37, 54, 78, 115, 144, 145, 195, 226, 232, 270.

they are responsible for all other associated costs. In the case of an FDA-approved drug, patients must pay for the drug. Because extended therapy can be quite expensive, some pharmaceutical companies have programs to assist patients in receiving drugs if they are no longer able to pay or have reached a yearly maximum (cost assistance programs).[5, 46, 124, 197] In addition, most pharmaceutical companies sponsor reimbursement hotlines that will assist patients and health care professionals with reimbursement concerns.

CONCLUSION

Oncology nurses who care for patients receiving biotherapy are on the cutting edge of cancer therapy. They must stay abreast of continual changes, be knowledgeable about therapeutic agents and modalities, and develop standards of care and nursing interventions to manage toxicity. The possibilities for nurses to participate in this exciting new therapeutic modality are limitless.

Nursing Management

Caring for patients receiving biotherapy is both challenging and exciting. Because many biologic response modifiers (BRMs) are now available for commercial use, many oncology nurses have become more familiar with this once new form of therapy. As research continues, biotherapy advances over the next few years will be exponential. Nurses working in this area will be compelled to remain up-to-date and will have an opportunity to be on the cutting edge in developing standards of care for patients receiving biotherapy.[83, 131] Although the mode of action and pattern of toxicity for biotherapy differ from those for chemotherapy, nurses can draw on their expertise in managing chemotherapy-related side effects to meet the challenge of dealing with side effects unique to biotherapy.

Nursing Diagnoses: *Neurologic Function*

- *Sensory/perceptual alterations (visual, auditory)*
- *Sleep pattern disturbance*
- *Social interaction, impaired*
- *Thought processes, altered*

Nursing Diagnosis: *Renal Function*

- *Urinary elimination, altered*

Nursing Diagnoses: *Hematologic Function*

- *Injury, risk for, related to weakness or bleeding*
- *Infection, risk for, related to decreased WBC*
- *Activity intolerance related to anemia*

Nursing Diagnosis: *Skin*

- *Skin integrity, impaired*

Nursing Diagnoses: *Gastrointestinal System*

- *Nutrition, altered: less than body requirements*
- *Diarrhea*
- *Oral mucous membrane, altered*
- *Skin integrity, impaired, risk for, related to diarrhea*

Nursing Diagnoses: *Cardiovascular System*

- *Tissue perfusion, altered cardiopulmonary, peripheral*
- *Fluid volume deficit*

Nursing Diagnoses: *Pulmonary System*

- *Gas exchange, impaired*
- *Anxiety related to respiratory distress*

Nursing Diagnoses: *Miscellaneous*

- *Fatigue*
- *Activity intolerance*
- *Body temperature, altered, risk for*
- *Pain*
- *Self-care deficit (hygiene, grooming, feeding)*
- *Knowledge deficit (biotherapy treatment side effects)*

Nursing Diagnoses: *Psychosocial Adjustment*

- *Coping, ineffective, individual or family*
- *Decisional conflict (treatment regimen)*
- *Hopelessness*
- *Sexuality patterns, altered*

Outcome Goals

Patient/significant other/caregiver will be able to:

- Discuss their disease and the rationale for the use

of biotherapy in their disease (e.g., as treatment, for detection or diagnosis, as a supportive measure).

- Describe their treatment regimen and associated laboratory and diagnostic tests, clinic visits, hospitalizations, and other special requirements.
- State the side effects common to the agent they are receiving and specific management strategies.
- Verbalize reportable signs and symptoms.
- Demonstrate proper skills for self-administration of medications.
- List resources available to assist them in coping with their disease and treatment (e.g., financial and reimbursement issues, community resources).

Assessment and Planning

From the first encounter, nurses play a key role in managing patients undergoing biotherapy. (For the purposes of this chapter, the word *patient* includes the patient and family or significant other as applicable.) The physician generally obtains a detailed history and physical examination before starting a patient on therapy. The physician explains the purpose of therapy, the treatment schedule, associated side effects, and financial concerns as appropriate. The physician also obtains informed consent for patients in a clinical trial. It is important that nurses understand the ethical and legal foundations of informed consent, for they serve as both educator and advocate for the patient.* The nurse may have to answer many questions that the patient is either afraid or embarrassed to ask the physician. Within the scope of independent nursing practice, the nurse can do much to reinforce information and clarify misconceptions. Assessing whether patients understand their therapeutic plan is crucial, and this information should be relayed to other members of the health care team as appropriate.

The nurse should perform a baseline assessment using a body systems approach, including psychosocial concerns, before the patient starts therapy. This should include current symptoms related to disease or previous treatment, level of functional status, and hopes, fears, and expectations related to therapy. Documentation of other intercurrent medical illnesses (e.g., cardiovascular disease) that may place the patient at risk for more severe toxic effects is essential. A medication profile should also be obtained, because many medications are contraindicated with certain biologic agents or can contribute to side effects. The initial assessment should also include evaluation of the patient's support systems. When biotherapy trials are investigational, the patient often receives therapy away from home and her usual support systems. Patients may be concerned about finances; appropriate housing; family, friends, and job while they are away loneliness; and fear of the unknown. It is especially helpful to allow patients to voice their concerns and resolve problems through appropriate referrals.

The nurse plays a crucial role in assessing and facilitating the patient's tolerance of side effects while undergoing therapy. A basic understanding of the biology, mode of action, and side effects (acute and chronic) of the agent administered is a must. This knowledge can be applied through regular, systematic assessment of the patient. It is necessary to evaluate symptoms for duration, frequency, and severity to plan the appropriate care. Information and care plans should be documented in the patient's medical record.

The nurse must also assess the therapeutic plan to develop a plan of care and intervene appropriately. Questions would include the following:

Will the therapy be given in the hospital, an ambulatory care setting, or both? In the ambulatory care setting, assessment of the patient's compliance with the therapeutic plan is especially important.

What types of laboratory tests (routine laboratory work, special laboratory work, and pharmacology) and diagnostic procedures will be required?

What agent or agents will the patient receive, and what are the associated side effects?

Is the agent under investigation or FDA approved?

If under investigation, has informed consent been secured?

What is the nature of the agent? Are there special handling precautions or storage requirements? Is any special equipment or are any emergency supplies needed?

What type of teaching will the patient need (e.g., self-administration techniques, side effects, and management)?

What type of monitoring will be required? Are special vital signs necessary (e.g., orthostatic blood pressures)?

A thorough assessment both before and during therapy helps in formulating and updating the patient's plan of care.*

HANDLING ISSUES

Handling issues are a matter of concern to all oncology nurses. Policies and procedures governing safe han-

---

* References 129, 149, 209, 228, 229, 264, 280, 290.

* References 34, 35, 55, 121, 130, 164, 225.

dling of cytotoxic agents during preparation, administration, and disposal have been well established nationwide. However, there has been no formal research to date regarding the safest way to handle biologic agents. The nurse is advised to check institutional policy regarding handling of BRMs at the place of employment. Most BRMs do not directly affect DNA and are therefore not considered genotoxic substances; however, many institutions place them in the category of cytotoxic products requiring special handling. In the future, new generations of BRMs may require special handling. The addition of chemotherapeutic agents or toxins to BRMs would necessitate special handling, and the addition of radioisotopes would require appropriate radiation safety procedures.[55, 233]

MANAGEMENT OF SIDE EFFECTS

The oncology nurse plays a key role in the management of side effects associated with biologic therapy. This is especially true because many of these effects are not "life-threatening" but have a tremendous impact on the patient's quality of life. A sound foundation in symptom management can guide the nurse in developing strategies to manage biotherapy-related side effects.[217]

Neurologic Side Effects

To ensure prompt recognition of CNS toxicity, patients should be assessed before therapy for baseline data and regularly during therapy for changes in level of consciousness, orientation, and mental status. Changes should be reported to the physician. The nurse should also evaluate the patient's medication profile for other drugs that can contribute to CNS toxicity. The patient should be taught which signs and symptoms to report. Family members are often the first to recognize subtle changes and should be encouraged to report them to the health care team. Often the nurse and the patient together can creatively deal with minor CNS changes, such as slowed thinking, decreased concentration, and memory problems.[23, 49, 127, 173]

For more serious problems, such as confusion, disorientation, and somnolence, safety concerns arise. Patients should be protected from injury when appropriate with fall precautions or bed sensors and should be reoriented as needed. Especially in the intensive care unit, the nurse should allow normal periods of sleep and rest. Patients receiving BRMs may experience depression. Allowing patients to verbalize their feelings is often helpful. However, a psychiatric consultation should be sought when appropriate.

For a review of BRM-related side effects and their frequency of occurrence, see pages 716 and 717.

Renal Side Effects

In all treatment settings, patients should be evaluated for renal toxicity through assessment of blood urea nitrogen (BUN) and creatinine levels, and change should be reported to the physician. With IL-2 therapy, renal toxicity is more problematic. Patients should be placed on strict intake and output and weighed regularly. Because urine output is often decreased, intake and output usually will not balance. The physician usually sets a minimum output per shift that can be used as a guideline for reporting changes. Nursing includes administration of fluids, diuretics, and pressors as ordered.[55, 218, 221–223, 293]

Hematologic Side Effects

Patients are monitored for changes in complete blood count, including differential and platelet counts. When ordered, the coagulation profile should also be assessed. The patient should be taught signs and symptoms to report, along with appropriate precautions (e.g., bleeding precautions for thrombocytopenia, measures to guard against infection should white cell counts decrease, conservation of energy for anemia), in case a problem develops. Replacement therapy with blood and platelets should be administered as ordered. With biologic therapy, counts generally recover very quickly after therapy stops.

Hepatic Side Effects

Nursing includes assessing the patient for changes in serum transaminases and bilirubin and for jaundice or hepatomegaly. Nursing diagnoses should be formulated as appropriate. If significant changes occur in laboratory values, therapy may need to be withheld and reinstituted at a lower dose after laboratory measurements recovery and the patient's status improves.

Skin Changes

Skin changes are most commonly seen with IL-2 and retinoid therapy, although rashes have been reported with IFN and GM-CSF. The baseline assessment of skin condition should include a history of underlying

Side Effects of Biologic Response Modifiers

System	Interferons	Interleukin-2	Hematopoietic Growth Factors	Monoclonal Antibodies	Tumor Necrosis Factor	Retinoids
Central nervous system	Impaired concentration, headache, lethargy, confusion, depression	Impaired concentration, headache, lethargy, confusion, anxiety, psychoses, depression	Rare	Rare	Confusion, seizures (rare)	Headache,* visual disturbances, changed visual acuity, anxiety, insomnia, depression
General	Constitutional symptoms,* fatigue*	Constitutional symptoms,* fatigue,* weight gain during therapy, followed by weight loss*	Mild constitutional symptoms, fatigue (mostly with GM-CSF)	Constitutional symptoms, allergic reactions, anaphylaxis (rare)	Constitutional symptoms,* rigors,* fatigue*	Fever,* malaise
Cardiovascular system	Hypotension, tachycardia, arrhythmias, myocardial ischemia (rare)	Hypotension,* edema,* ascites, arrhythmias, decreased systemic vascular resistance*	Hypertension (rare) with epoetin alfa	Hypotension, chest pain	Hypotension,* arrhythmias	Hypotension, hypertension, flushing
Pulmonary system	Rare	Dyspnea, pulmonary edema	Rare occurrence of dyspnea with first dose of GM-CSF	Dyspnea, wheezing	Dyspnea	Dyspnea, pleural effusion in patients with APL experiencing RA-APL syndrome
Renal/hepatic systems	Proteinuria, elevated liver enzymes*	Oliguria,* increased BUN, creatinine* proteinuria, azotemia, increased bilirubin, SGOT, SGPT, LDH	Elevation of LDH (rare), alkaline phosphatase with G-CSF	Rare	Increased bilirubin, liver enzymes	Elevation of triglycerides and cholesterol*; elevation of liver function tests*

System						
Gastrointestinal system	Nausea, vomiting, diarrhea, anorexia*	Nausea, vomiting,* diarrhea,* anorexia,* mucositis	Rare	Nausea, vomiting	Nausea, vomiting, anorexia, diarrhea	Nausea, vomiting, mucositis,* diarrhea
Genitourinary system	Impotence, decreased libido	Decreased libido	Rare	Rare	Decreased libido	Rare
Integument	Alopecia, rash	Rash,* dry desquamation,* erythema,* pruritus,* inflammatory reaction at injection sites*	GM-CSF/G-CSF: inflammation at injection site; rash (rare)	Urticaria, rash, pruritus	Inflammatory reaction at injection sites	Dryness of skin and mucous membranes,* pruritis, increased sweating
Hematologic system	Leukopenia,* anemia, thrombocytopenia	Anemia,* thrombocytopenia, lymphopenia,* eosinophilia*	Leukocytosis (expected biologic effect of HGF use); eosinophilia (GM-CSF)	Leukopenia in hematologic malignancies	Thrombocytopenia, granulocytopenia	Leukocytosis in patients with APL
Musculoskeletal system	Myalgia,* arthralgias*	Myalgia, arthralgia	Bone pain* with GM-CSF and G-CSF	Arthralgia (rare)	Myalgia, arthralgia	Bone pain,* myalgias,* arthralgia*

* Common side effect.

APL, Acute premyelocytic anemia; BUN, blood urea nitrogen; G-CSF, granulocyte colony-stimulating factor; GM-CSF, granulocyte/macrophage colony-stimulating factor; LDH, lactate dehydrogenase; SGOT, aspartate aminotransferase (AST); SGPT, alanine aminotransferase (ALT).

Modified from Rieger PT: Biotherapy: the fourth modality of therapy. In Barton-Burke M, editor: Cancer chemotherapy: a nursing process approach, Boston, Jones & Bartlett, 1996.

skin conditions such as psoriasis. Patients should be taught signs and symptoms to be expected as well as an appropriate skin care routine. Skin should be observed daily for signs of infection and breakdown. Therapeutic measures for dry skin include gentle cleansing (avoid scrubbing the skin), tepid rather than hot baths, frequent use of water-based lotions and creams, soft cotton clothing, and bath oils.* Patients should be taught to avoid the use of perfumed lotion, because it can further irritate already sensitive skin. Pruritus can also be a major problem. Helpful measures include antipruritic medications (often with around-the-clock administration), soft clothing, and the use of colloidal oatmeal baths. In some cases a room humidifier is helpful.[218] It is important to cautionpatients against the use of topical steroids, because this is contraindicated in many IL-2 protocols.

Irritation, with resultant erythema and swelling, may occur at subcutaneous injection sites. Patients should be reassured that this inflammatory reaction usually resolves within several days. In patients receiving IL-2 by SC injection, "knots" may persist under the skin for several months. Although not generally painful, they reduce the number of sites available for subsequent injections.[288] For inflammatory reactions, no treatment is generally necessary; however, if applications of cold or heat are considered, they should be verified with the physician.

Gastrointestinal Side Effects

Teaching the patient to maintain nutritional status is of prime importance because anorexia and weight loss over time are common side effects of many BRMs. Baseline nutritional status and dietary intake should be assessed and documented. Measures commonly used with other oncology patients (e.g., small, frequent meals and calorie supplements) are appropriate here. A dietary consultant should be used as necessary. If weight loss becomes significant, tube feedings or hyperalimentation may have to be considered. Antiemetics usually abate nausea and vomiting; however, with IL-2, more aggressive around-the-clock therapy is usually necessary. Prophylactic antiemetic administration and an odor-free environment are often necessary with IL-2. Diarrhea is controlled through the use of antidiarrheal medications. Special consideration should also be given to the skin integrity in the perianal area through assessment, hygienic measures, and use of barrier creams as indicated.†

Mucositis may also occur, especially with IL-2 therapy. The oral cavity should be assessed and its condition documented. A pretreatment oral assessment by a dental oncologist to identify and treat preexisting oral disease may be recommended. Patients should be taught meticulous oral hygiene using saline and baking soda mouth rinses, soft toothbrushes, alterations in diet for comfort, and avoidance of solutions such as commercial mouthwashes, which can exacerbate oral dryness. If dryness of oral mucous membranes is extreme, artificial saliva may be helpful.[218]

Cardiovascular/Pulmonary Side Effects

A thorough assessment of cardiopulmonary parameters is important with all biologic agents, but it is extremely important with IL-2 therapy or in patients receiving ricin-based immunotoxins, because of capillary leak syndrome. Nursing specific for this syndrome includes evaluation of cardiovascular status by monitoring heart rate, blood pressure (including orthostatic checks), central venous pressure as indicated, and other cardiac indices. Accurate daily weight and strict intake and output measures are necessary to evaluate fluid imbalances.*

Patients should be assessed for edema and abdominal ascites. They should be taught signs and symptoms to report, as well as to rise from a lying to a sitting position slowly to prevent dizziness that may result from sudden drops in blood pressure. Because of edema, the use of tight clothing or restrictive jewelry should be avoided. Bed rest may be indicated if the systolic blood pressure consistently runs below 80 mm Hg and the patient is symptomatic. Nursing assessment of pulmonary status includes monitoring the respiratory rate, ausculating breath sounds, monitoring laboratory values of oxygenation, and heeding complaints of shortness of breath or altered breathing patterns. Patients should be taught which signs and symptoms to report and should be reassured that toxicity is dose related and reversible. Nurses should position patients for maximum respiratory effort.

Constitutional Symptoms

Chills followed by fever are seen with almost all biologic agents.[108] Patients should be told to expect this reaction and that tachyphylaxis will occur. Because chills are usually transient and self-limiting, nursing focuses primarily on comfort measures. Patients are often premedicated with acetaminophen or other NSAIDs. They should be kept warm with blankets and warm clothing during chills and should be instructed to avoid cold beverages. For severe chills, IV meperidine or sublingual morphine may be necessary.

---

* References 55, 59, 93, 130, 221–223.
† References 55, 59, 93, 130, 217, 221–223, 236.

---

* References 41, 55, 82, 121, 130, 221–223, 231, 241, 293.

Fevers are usually controlled with regular administration of acetaminophen. However, for prolonged or extreme temperature elevations, cool sponging or hypothermia blankets may be necessary. When therapy is initiated, vital signs, including temperature, are usually monitored for the first day or so; patients with cardiovascular or pulmonary problems require more intensive monitoring. Patients should monitor their temperature several times a day so that fever patterns can be established. It should never be assumed that all fevers in a patient receiving a BRM are related to the therapy. Variables such as length of time the patient has been receiving the agent, comparison of the fever with the patient's usual fever patterns, spiking fevers despite administration of antipyretics, and other signs and symptoms of infection should all be considered. Appropriate interventions can then be instituted. An adequate fluid intake should be encouraged during high fevers to prevent dehydration. Acetaminophen, massage, and heating pads can be used as appropriate to control headache, myalgia, arthralgia, and bone pain.

Fatigue

Fatigue is common with many biologic agents, is usually chronic, and in some instances can be the dose-limiting side effect.[246] Because its etiology is unknown, nursing interventions are aimed at helping patients cope with this often distressing side effect. Although few tools can objectively measure fatigue, nurses can document the patient's fatigue by gathering data on contributing factors (e.g., anemia, stressors, depression, other treatment regimens); diagnosis, disease stage, and prognosis; degree of immobility; manifestations of fatigue; and patterns of fatigue. Which factors alleviate fatigue and which exacerbate it? When is fatigue the greatest? How long does it persist? Interventions focus on four areas: conservation of energy, nutritional management, stress management, and management of contributing factors.* When teaching patients about this side effect and its management, nurses should stress that this fatigue is chronic, not acute, and that more sleep often exacerbates the problem instead of alleviating it. Many patients fear that increased fatigue signals progression of disease. The nurse should reassure such patients that fatigue is an expected side effect of the medication. If fatigue becomes so severe that the patient's functional status is acutely impaired, therapy may have to be stopped or the dosage reduced. Nursing research is beginning to evaluate the use of exercise programs as an intervention for managing cancer-related fatigue.

* References 23, 49, 61, 83, 105, 188, 206, 207, 208, 246, 289, 292.

Allergic Reactions

Allergic reactions are most commonly associated with MoAb infusions.[68, 69, 221–223] The patient's vital signs should be monitored regularly, in many cases as often as every 15 minutes, and observed closely. Emergency drugs must be kept at the bedside, and a crash cart must be on hand. Nursing may include medication of the patient before or during therapy to prevent chills, fever, and urticaria. Fever is common with certain MoAbs, and should be evaluated for its relationship to the course of therapy (early versus late).

Psychosocial Difficulties

When investigational biotherapy is used, patients often are extremely optimistic that therapy is going to help them, especially if there is no effective therapy for their particular disease or if they have failed several courses of therapy. Although hope is important, expectations should be realistic. The nurse can be instrumental in helping patients voice their hopes and fears, answering questions, and discussing the patient's expectations. Depression is common, either as a side effect of BRMs, related to fatigue, or as a result of failing therapy. The failure of therapy can be extremely difficult for patients, and the nurse's most effective tool is often her presence. Even when a cure is not possible, the nurse can foster hope that something can be done for the patient and can reassure the patient that he will not be abandoned. Patients are often away from their usual support systems. Family dynamics are often disrupted, and therapy may be more difficult to tolerate than anticipated. Support groups, individual counseling, and simple ventilation of feelings to the nurse all can be helpful. Serving as an advocate for the patient, the nurse can make appropriate referrals to help resolve problems.[23, 49, 118]

Patient Instructions

The nurse is responsible for teaching patients about the particular biologic agent or agents they are to receive, for preparing them for participation in experimental trials, for describing side effects and how to cope with them, and for teaching self-administration of the medication.[181, 220, 237, 243, 259] The keys are early assessment of the patient for learning needs and barriers (physical, psychological, and verbal deficiencies and dysfunctions) and use of appropriate written and audiovisual materials that reinforce teaching. Patient education resources available from the various pharmaceutical companies are listed on page 720. A teaching plan specific for the patient can be formulated and documented in the medical record.

Sufficient time should be allotted to teach patients to administer their medication. This should always be

Educational Resources Available from Pharmaceutical Companies

Amgen, Inc.[4, 5, 6]
Analogy Book
Calendar with Laboratory Data
Chemotherapy and Neupogen
Neupogen (Filgrastim) Patient Fact Sheet
Neupogen Reimbursement Guide for the Patient
Patient Guide to Therapy with Neupogen (video, handout)
Pediatric Package (includes Sammy Syringe, Marvin's Marvelous Medicine, Your Body and G-CSF–pamphlets)
Questions and Answers About Therapy with Neupogen (Filgrastim)
Self-Injection Chart (step-by-step guide)
Self-Injection Video (English and Spanish)
Your Personal Daily Journal

Chiron Therapeutics[46, 47]
Proleukin Therapy: Information for Patients and Their Families (video)

Immunex Corp.[123, 124]
The Cells of the Hematopoietic Cascade (video, monograph)
Hematopoiesis Chart
A Patient Guide to Self-Injection (video)
A Patient Guide to Self-Injection (instruction and site recording chart)
Understanding Your Bone Marrow Transplant: A Videotape for Patients Understanding Your Bone Marrow Transplant: A Patient Guide (written accompanying BMT videotape)

Ortho Biotech, Inc.[197, 198]
Anemia in Cancer: Getting Your Energy Back
Coping with Fatigue Videotape

Dimensions of Caring: Understanding and Overcoming Fatigue
Patient Diary
Resource Catalogue
r-HuEpo and the Anemia of Cancer and Chemotherapy: Two Sides of an Inpatient Story (book and audio-cassette)
Self-Injection Starter Kit
Subcutaneous Injection: A Patient Guide to Correct Injection Technique (video, flipchart)
Understanding and Overcoming Fatigue (audiotape)
Understanding and Overcoming Fatigue (brochure)

Roche Laboratories[228, 229]
Complete home administration kit
Medication travel cooler
Patient Guide
Refrigerator magnet for expiration date
Self-Administration (video)
Syringe disposal container

Schering-Plough Corp.[239]
Patient Information Card
Patient kit: home supplies plus brochures on self-administration and side effect management
Self-Injection (video)
Taking Control of Your Therapy (booklet)
An A-B-C Approach to Managing Your Therapy: Intron A (teaching card)
Intron A Therapy—Making it Work for You (videotape)

Modified from Rumsey KA: Patient education. In Rieger PT, editor: *Biotherapy: a comprehensive overview* (ed 2), Boston, Jones & Bartlett, 1999.

---

anticipated with interferon therapy and CSFs. Patients need to learn how to reconstitute the medications (if applicable), how to draw up the proper dose, the proper technique for intramuscular or SC injection, the proper technique for site selection and rotation, storage requirements for the medication, and proper disposal of needles and syringes at home. A variety of vital concentrations are available for IFN. The nurse can exercise considerable latitude in selecting a concentration that is cost effective and easy for the patient to use. The nurse also should accommodate dose escalations if applicable without the need to reteach the patient continually. Because many biologic agents require refrigeration or freezing, special arrangements for transport must be made. Patients are also instructed in reportable signs and symptoms. With CNS side effects, changes are often subtle. Family members are usually the first to recognize changes and can report them to the health care team. Many patients are asked to keep a daily log or diary of associated side effects, time and location of injections, and other medications used. If the patient is not self-sufficient, appropriate referrals should be made before discharge. Priorities for patient teaching in biotherapy and geriatric considerations are given in the appropriate boxes.[165]

PATIENT TEACHING PRIORITIES
Biotherapy

Assessment

Time available
Learning needs
People available to teach
Barriers to learning
Resources needed
Teaching content

Treatment Plan

Goals of therapy
Commercial versus investigational agent
Treatment regimen
Associated laboratory and diagnostic tests
Special requirements

Side Effects

Expected side effects
Management of symptoms experienced
Reportable signs and symptoms

Self-Administration of BRMs

Aseptic technique
Reconstitution of powdered medications
Drawing up the proper dose
Proper site selection and rotation
Administration of the injection
Storage of the drug
Proper disposal of equipment at home

Psychosocial/Economic Concerns

Coping skills/resources
Reimbursement resources

Documentation

Time frame for teaching
Patient/significant others taught
Tasks/information disseminated
Resources utilized
Evaluation/need for referrals

GERIATRIC CONSIDERATIONS
Biotherapy

Factors Affecting Medication Dosage and Administration

Alterations in hepatic and renal function may necessitate adjustment of dosage and/or schedule.
Decreases in cardiovascular function may require lower doses of BRMs such as IFN and IL-2, which have side effects that may stress the cardiovascular system.
Alterations in neurosensory/perceptual protective mechanisms may place elderly patients at higher risk for problems with CNS-associated side effects of BRMs such as confusion, depression, memory loss, or slowed thinking.
Decreased functional status may place patients at a higher risk for intolerance of fatigue associated with many BRMs.
Altered nutritional intake (less than body requirements) may be increased due to anorexia associated with some BRMs.
Decreased tissue, skin, and mucous membrane integrity may place patients at higher risk for IL-2–related skin toxicity.
The patient's current medication profile should be evaluated to detect drugs that may be contraindicated with BRMs and may cause additive toxicity.

Factors Affecting Patient Teaching

Assess for neuromuscular and sensory deficits (e.g., vision problems, hearing losses, arthritic joints) that may inhibit teaching/learning. Use appropriate teaching tools for deficits present (e.g., large print, minimal illustrations for patient with vision problems).
Assess for reading level and comprehension, because many people 65 or older have completed 8 or fewer years of formal schooling. Use reading materials targeted for the appropriate reading level and audiovisual aids. Frequently reinforce information presented.

Factors Affecting Social Support Systems

Approximately 30% of patients 65 or older live alone, the majority being women. The difficulties of living alone are often intensified by poverty, having few relatives or other social supports, and decreased functional status.
Many BRMs are given on an outpatient basis; hence patients are required to learn self-care. Evaluation of formal and informal support networks, functional capacity, and economic status should be incorporated into the nursing assessment and referrals made to community resources as needed.
Spouses should be evaluated for early indicators of caregiver role strain and appropriate interventions initiated.

Modified from Boyle DM and others: *Oncol Nurs Forum* 19:913, 1992. Additional data from references 41, 221.

NURSING RESEARCH

Biotherapy follows a pattern different from that of standard chemotherapy, often lasting months to years. The associated toxicities are complex, chronic, usually subjective, and prone to having a major effect on the quality of life.[41, 114, 159] The etiology of many side effects is unknown, which makes treating them difficult or empirical. A clearer understanding of the nature of these side effects is essential to the development of effective strategies for dealing with them.

Biologic therapy is ripe with opportunities for research, including nursing research in conjunction with clinical trials.[55, 76, 258]

One difficulty with research in this area is accurately measuring symptoms.[89, 166] Although observer-rated toxicity scales used in clinical trials have been adapted to accommodate symptoms associated with BRMs, often they are not sensitive enough for research purposes.[193] The subjective nature of most BRM-associated symptoms makes their measurement a challenge. Nursing research efforts require a means to quantify side effects before interventions to pre-

vent and control them can be studied.[221-223] These research efforts might be focused on the development of tools to measure side effects, determination of the most effective time of drug administration to alleviate side effects, interventions to control or prevent toxicity, evaluation of teaching methods, evaluation of quality of life and symptom distress, and drug handling issues. Such studies have begun; however, a great deal of work remains to be completed.*

---

* See references 61, 127, 221–223, 261, 271, 283.

Chapter Questions

1. All the following are biologic response modifiers *except:*
   a. G-CSF
   b. IL-2
   c. Taxotere
   d. Rituximab
2. A naturally occurring body substance that acts as a messenger between cells is known as a:
   a. Protein
   b. Toxin
   c. Protokine
   d. Cytokine
3. All of the following are true about biotherapy *except:*
   a. Biologic response modifiers must be FDA approved before they can be used in a clinical trial.
   b. Biologic response modifiers cause patients to experience flulike symptoms.
   c. Biotherapy encompasses tumor vaccine therapy, interferons, and interleukins.
   d. Biotherapy is a major treatment modality.
4. Interferon therapy is:
   a. Only effective in adjuvant treatment therapies
   b. Only approved for use with high-risk melanoma
   c. Usually given intramuscularly for renal cell cancer
   d. Usually the higher the dose, the more severe the side effects
5. In patients receiving high-dose IL-2 for metastatic melanoma:
   a. They must receive all 14 planned doses of therapy before discharge
   b. Premedicate before each dose with Decadron to reduce nausea and vomiting
   c. The nurse monitors for signs of capillary leak syndrome

   d. Administer IV fluids at 200 mL/h to maintain blood pressure
6. All the following are known toxicities of IL-2 therapy *except:*
   a. Oliguria
   b. Combativeness
   c. Diarrhea
   d. Pulmonary embolus
7. Biologic response modifiers that are highly specific for a single target antigen are:
   a. TNF
   b. MoAbs
   c. NK
   d. G-CSF
8. Which of the following biotherapeutic agents can be given alone or in combination with chemotherapy?
   a. IL-2
   b. IFN
   c. GM-CSF
   d. All of the above
   e. None of the above
9. A significant clinical application for retinoids is used in:
   a. Chemoprevention of breast cancer
   b. Chemoprevention of lung cancer
   c. Chemoprotection of breast cancer
   d. Chemoprotection of lung cancer
10. Which of the following is a platelet growth factor?
    a. IL-2
    b. IL-11
    c. M-CSF
    d. MoAb
11. Radiolabeled MoAbs use in diagnostic imaging has been related to their ability to:
    a. Detect, locate, and measure the exact tumor size
    b. Detect, locate, primary tumors less than 1 cm in size
    c. Detect, locate, primary and metastatic tumors
    d. Detect, locate, react to multiple tumor antigens

12. Controversial issues and concerns in gene therapy include:
   a. Safety, ethics
   b. Safety, financial
   c. Ethics, financial
   d. Ethics, MTD

BIBLIOGRAPHY

1. Abels RI: Use of recombinant human erythropoietin in the treatment of anemia in patients who have cancer, *Semin Oncol* 19(suppl 8):29, 1992.
2. Aggarwala SS, Kirkwood JM: Interferons in the therapy of solid tumors, *Oncology* 51:129, 1994.
3. Allison AC, Taylor RB: Observations on thymectomy and carcinogenesis, *Cancer Res* 27:703, 1967.
4. Amgen, Inc: Neupogen (filgrastim) (package insert), Thousand Oaks, CA, Amgen, 1998.
5. Amgen, Inc: Neupogen reimbursement hotline: (1-800-272-9376), Thousand Oaks, CA, Amgen, 1998.
6. Amgen: Epogen (epoetin alfa) (package insert), Thousand Oaks, CA, Amgen, 1999.
7. Atkins MB and others: Phase I evaluation of recombinant interleukin-2 in patients with advanced malignant disease, *J Clin Oncol* 4:1380, 1986.
8. Atkins MB and others: Recombinant interleukin 2 therapy for patients with metastatic melanoma: analysis of 270 patients treated between 1985 and 1993, *J Clin Oncol* 17:2105, 1999.
9. Atkins M, Mier JW, editors: *Therapeutic applications of interleukin-2*, New York, Marcel Dekker, 1993.
10. Atkins MB, Mier JW, Trehu EG: Combination cytokine therapy. In DeVita VT Jr, Hellman S, Rosenberg SA, editors: *Biologic therapy of cancer,* ed 2, Philadelphia, Lippincott, 1995.
11. Antman KS and others: Effect of recombinant human granulocyte-macrophage colony-stimulating factor on chemotherapy-induced myelosuppression, *N Engl J Med* 319:593, 1988.
12. Antonelli G: Development of neutralizing and binding antibodies to interferon (IFN) in patients undergoing IFN therapy, *Antiviral Res* 24:235, 1994.
13. Aulitzky WE and others: Interleukins: clinical pharmacology and therapeutic use, *Drugs* 48:667, 1994.
14. Ayoub J and others: Placebo-controlled trial of 13-*cis*-retinoic acid activity on retinoic acid receptor-beta expression in a population at high risk: implications for chemoprevention of lung cancer, *J Clin Oncol* 17:3546, 1999.
15. Bajorin DF, Cheung NV, Houghton AN: Macrophage colony-stimulating factor: biological effects and potential applications for cancer therapy, *Semin Hematol* 28(suppl 2):42, 1991.
16. Balkwill FR, editor: *Cytokines in cancer therapy,* Oxford, Oxford University, 1989.
17. Baquiran DC, Dantis L, McKerrow J: Monoclonal antibodies: innovations in diagnosis and therapy, *Semin Oncol Nurs* 12:130, 1996.
18. Baselga JU and others: Recombinant humanized anti-HER2 antibody (Herceptin) enhances the antitumor activity of paclitaxel and doxorubicin against HER2/neu-overexpressing human breast cancer xenografts, *Cancer Res* 58:2825, 1998.
19. Baselga J and others: Phase I studies of anti-epidermal growth factor receptor chimeric antibody c225 alone and in combination with cisplatin, *J Clin Oncol* 18:904, 2000.
20. Baselga J and others: Phase II study of weekly intravenous recombinant humanized anti-p185HER2 monoclonal antibody in patients with HER2/neu-overexpressing metastatic breast cancer, *J Clin Oncol* 14:737, 1996.
21. Basser RL and others: Randomized, blinded, placebo-controlled phase I trial of pegylated recombinant human megakaryocyte growth and development factor with filgrastim after dose-intensive chemotherapy in patients with advanced cancer, *Blood* 89:3118, 1997.
22. Basser RL and others: Thrombopoietic effects of pegylated recombinant human megakaryocyte growth and development factor (PEGrHuMGDF) in patients with advanced cancer, *Lancet* 348:1279, 1996.
23. Bender CM: Cognitive dysfunction associated with biological response modifier therapy, *Oncol Nurs Forum* 21:515, 1995.
24. Benner SE, Lippman SM, Hong WK: Chemoprevention strategies for a lung and upper aerodigestive tract cancer, *Cancer Res* 52(suppl):2758, 1992.
25. Berd D and others: Treatment of metastatic melanoma with an autologous tumor-cell vaccine: clinical and immunologic results in 64 patients, *J Clin Oncol* 8:1858, 1990.
26. Berlex Laboratories: Betaseron (interferon-beta 1B) package insert, Richmond, CA, Berlex Laboratories, 1997.
27. Bernsen MR and others: Interleukin 2 (IL-2) therapy: potential advantages of locoregional versus systemic administration, *Cancer Treat Rev* 25:73, 1999.
28. Beutler B, Cerami A: Cachectin: more than a tumor necrosis factor, *N Engl J Med* 316:379, 1987.
29. Blick M and others: Phase I study of recombinant tumor necrosis factor in cancer patients, *Cancer Res* 47:2986, 1987.
30. Borden EC, Chin P: Interleukin-6: a cytokine with potential diagnostic and therapeutic roles, *J Lab Clin Med* 123:824, 1994.
31. Brandt SJ and others: Effects of recombinant human granulocyte-macrophage colony-stimulating factor on hematopoietic reconstitution after high-dose chemotherapy and autologous bone marrow transplantation, *N Engl J Med* 318:869, 1988.
32. Breitz HB, Sullivan K, Nelp WB: Imaging lung cancer with radiolabeled antibodies, *Semin Nuclear Med* 23:127, 1993.
33. Bronchud MH and others: Phase I/II study of recombinant human granulocyte colony-stimulating factor in patients receiving intensive chemotherapy for small cell lung cancer, *Br J Cancer* 56:809, 1987.
34. Brophy LR, Rieger PT: Biotherapy. In Clark JC, McGee RF, editors: *Core curriculum for oncology nursing,* ed 2, Philadelphia, Saunders, 1992.

35. Brophy LR, Sharp EJ: Physical symptoms of combination biotherapy: a quality-of-life issue, *Oncol Nurs Forum* 18(suppl):25, 1991.

36. Brophy LR: Tumor necrosis factor. In Rieger PT, editor: *Biotherapy: a comprehensive overview,* Boston, Jones & Bartlett, 1995.

37. Brunda MJ, Gately MK: Interleukin-12: potential role in cancer therapy. In DeVita VT Jr, Hellman S, Rosenberg SA, editors: *Important advances in oncology,* Philadelphia, Lippincott, 1995.

38. Burnet FM: The concept of immunological surveillance, *Prog Exp Tumor Res* 13:1, 1970.

39. Buzaid AC, Legha SS: Combination of chemotherapy with interleukin-2 and interferon-alfa for the treatment of advanced melanoma, *Semin Oncol* 6:23, 1994.

40. Bystryn JC and others: Relationship between immune response to melanoma vaccine immunization and clinical outcome in stage II malignant melanoma, *Cancer* 69:1157, 1992.

41. Camp-Sorrell D: Surviving the cancer, surviving the treatment: acute cardiac and pulmonary toxicity, *Oncol Nurs Forum* 26:983, 1999.

42. Cantell K, Hirvonen S: Preparation of human leukocyte interferon for clinical use, *Tex Rep Biol Med* 35:138, 1977.

43. Cebon J and others: Pharmacokinetics of human granulocyte-macrophage colony-stimulating factor using a sensitive immunoassay, *Blood* 72:1093, 1988.

44. Chang F, Syrjanen S, Syrjanen K: Implications of the p53 tumor-suppressor gene in clinical oncology, *J Clin Oncol* 13:1009, 1995.

45. Chapman P and others: Clinical pharmacology of recombinant human tumor necrosis factor in patients with advanced cancer, *J Clin Oncol* 5:1942, 1987.

46. Chiron Corp: Proleukin reimbursement line (1-800-775-7533), San Francisco, CA, Chiron, 1999.

47. Chiron Therapeutics: Proleukin (aldesleukin) for injection (package insert), Emeryville, CA, Chiron Corp., 1999.

48. Chowdhury S, Vaughn MM, Gore ME: New approaches to the systemic treatment of melanoma, *Cancer Treat Rev* 25:259, 1999.

49. Cimprich B: Symptom management: loss of concentration, *Semin Oncol Nurs* 11:279, 1995.

50. Clark J, Longo D: Biological response modifiers, *Mediguide Oncol* 6:1, 1986.

51. Clark SC, Kamen R: The human hematopoietic colony-stimulating factors, *Science* 236:1229, 1987.

52. Coiffier B and others: Rituximab (anti-CD20 monoclonal antibody) for the treatment of patients with relapsing or refractory aggressive lymphoma: a multicenter phase II study, *Blood* 92:1927, 1998.

53. Coleman T: Health system reform and clinical research, *Oncology* 9:118, 1995.

54. Cohen JS, Hogan ME: The new genetic medicines, *Sci Am* 271:76, 1994.

55. Conrad KJ, Horrell CJ, editors: *Biotherapy: recommendations for nursing course content and clinical practicum,* Pittsburgh, Oncology Nursing Press, 1995.

56. Corfu-A Study Group: Phase III randomized study of two fluorouracil combinations with either interferon alfa-2a or leucovorin for advanced colorectal cancer, *J Clin Oncol* 13:921, 1995.

57. Costa A and others: Prospects of chemoprevention of human cancers with the synthetic retinoid fenretinide, *Cancer Res* 54(suppl 7):2032, 1994.

58. Crown J and others: A phase I trial of recombinant human interleukin-1 alone and in combination with myelosuppressive doses of 5-fluorouracil in patients with gastrointestinal cancer, *Blood* 78:1420, 1991.

59. Dangel RB: Pruritus and cancer, *Oncol Nurs Forum* 13:17, 1986.

60. Dawson MM, editor: *Lymphokines and interleukins,* Boca Raton, FL, CRC Press, 1991.

61. Dean GE and others: Fatigue in patients with cancer receiving interferon-alpha, *Cancer Pract* 3:164, 1995.

62. DeLaPena L and others: Programmed instruction: biotherapy, module IV. Interleukins, *Cancer Nurs* 19:60, 1996.

63. Demetri GD and others: Quality of life benefit in chemotherapy patients treated with epotin alpha is independent of disease response or tumor type: results from a prospective community oncology study, *J Clin Oncol* 16:3412, 1998.

64. Denicoff KD and others: The neuropsychiatric effects of interleukin-2/lymphokine-activated killer cell therapy, *Ann Intern Med* 107:293, 1987.

65. DeVita VT Jr, Hellman S, Rosenberg SA, editors: *Biologic therapy of cancer,* ed 2, Philadelphia, Lippincott, 1995.

66. DiJulio JE, Liles TM: Monoclonal antibodies. In Rieger PT, editor: *Biotherapy: a comprehensive overview,* Boston, Jones & Bartlett, 1995.

67. Dillman JB: Toxicity of monoclonal antibodies in the treatment of cancer, *Semin Oncol Nurs* 4:107, 1988.

68. Dillman RO and others: Toxicities associated with monoclonal antibody infusions in cancer patients, *Mol Biother* 1:81, 1988.

69. Dillman RO and others: Toxicities and side effects associated with intravenous infusions of monoclonal antibodies, *J Biol Response Mod* 5:73, 1986.

70. Dillman RO: Antibodies as cytotoxic therapy, *J Clin Oncol* 12:1497, 1994.

71. Dillman RO: The clinical experience with interleukin-2 in cancer therapy, *Cancer Biother* 9:183, 1994.

72. Dinarello CA: Interleukin-1 and interleukin-1 antagonism, *Blood* 77:1627, 1991.

73. Dinarello CA, Mier JW: Lymphokines, *N Engl J Med* 317:940, 1987.

74. DiPaola RS and others: Phase I clinical and pharmacologic study of 13-*cis*-retinoic acid, interferon alfa, and paclitaxel in patients with prostate cancer and other advanced malignancies, *J Clin Oncol* 17:2213, 1999.

75. Donahue RE and others: Stimulation of hematopoiesis in primates by continuous infusion of recombinant human GM-CSF, *Nature* 321:872, 1986.

76. Donnelly S: Patient management strategies for interferon alfa-2b as adjuvant therapy of high-risk melanoma, *Oncol Nurs Forum* 25:921, 1998.

77. Ehrlich P: *Studies in immunity,* ed 2, New York, Wiley & Sons, 1910.

78. Engelking C: New approaches: innovations in cancer prevention, diagnosis, treatment and support, *Oncol Nurs Forum* 21:62, 1994.

79. Eschbach JW and others: Correction of the anemia of end-stage renal disease with recombinant human erythropoietin, *N Engl J Med* 316:73, 1987.

80. Estrov Z, Kurzrock R, Talpaz M, editors: *Interferons: basic principles and clinical applications,* Austin, TX, Landis, 1993.

81. Fanucchi M and others: Effects of polyethylene glycol-conjugated recombinant human megakaryoctye growth and development factor on platelet counts after chemotherapy for lung cancer, *N Engl J Med* 336:404, 1997.

82. Farrell MM: The challenge of adult respiratory distress syndrome during interleukin-2 therapy, *Oncol Nurs Forum* 19:475, 1992.

83. Farrell MM: Biotherapy and the oncology nurse, *Semin Oncol Nurs* 12:82, 1996.

84. Fazio MT, Glaspy JA: The impact of granulocyte colony-stimulating factor on quality of life in patients with severe chronic neutropenia, *Oncol Nurs Forum* 18:1411, 1991.

85. Ferrara F and others: CD56 expression is an indicator of poor clinical outcome in patients with acute promyelocytic leukemia treated with simultaneous all-*trans*-retinoic acid and chemotherapy, *J Clin Oncol* 18:1295, 2000.

86. Figlin RA and others: Concomitant administration of recombinant human interleukin-2 and recombinant interferon alfa-2a: an active outpatient regimen in metastatic renal cell carcinoma, *J Clin Oncol* 10:414, 1992.

87. Fisher R, editor: Interleukin-2: advances in clinical research and treatment, *Semin Oncol* 20(suppl 9):1, 1993.

88. Foelber R: Autologous stem cell transplant plus interleukin-2 for breast cancer: review and nursing management, *Oncol Nurs Forum* 25:563, 1998.

89. Frank-Stromborg M, editor: *Instruments for clinical nursing research,* Boston, Jones & Bartlett, 1992.

90. Frei E, Spriggs D: Tumor necrosis factor: still a promising agent, *J Clin Oncol* 7:291, 1989.

91. Gabrilove JL and others: Effect of granulocyte colony-stimulating factor on neutropenia and associated morbidity due to chemotherapy for transitional-cell carcinoma of the urothelium, *N Engl J Med* 318:1414, 1988.

92. Gabrilove JL, Golde D: Hematopoietic growth factors. In DeVita VT Jr, Hellman S, Rosenberg SA, editors: *Cancer: principles and practice of oncology,* ed 5, Philadelphia, Lippincott, 1997.

93. Gallagher J: Management of cutaneous symptoms, *Semin Oncol Nurs* 11:239, 1995.

94. Gallin JI and others: Interferon-gamma in the management of infectious diseases, *Ann Intern Med* 123:216, 1995.

95. Gallucci B: The immune system and cancer, *Oncol Nurs Forum* 14(suppl 6):3, 1987.

96. Galvani DW, Cawley JC, editors: *Cytokine therapy,* New York, Cambridge University Press, 1992.

97. Genentech, Inc: Actimmune (Interferon gamma 1 b) (package insert), San Francisco, CA, Genentech, Inc., 1996

98. Gianella-Borradori A: Present and future clinical relevance of interleukin-3, *Stem Cells* 12(suppl 1):21, 1994.

99. Giralt S and others: The natural history of chronic myelogenous leukemia in the interferon era, *Semin Hematol* 32:152, 1995.

100. Glaspy JA and others: Therapy for neutropenia in hairy cell leukemia with recombinant granulocyte colony-stimulating factor, *Ann Intern Med* 109:789, 1988.

101. Glaspy J and others: Impact of therapy with epoetin alfa on clinical outcomes in patients with nonmyeloid malignancies during cancer chemotherapy in community oncology practices, *J Clin Oncol* 15:1218, 1997.

102. Goldenberg D: New developments in monoclonal antibody for cancer detection and therapy, *CA Cancer J Clin* 44:43, 1994.

103. Goldenberg DM, editor: *Cancer therapy with radiolabeled antibodies,* Boca Raton, FL, CRC Press, 1995.

104. Gordon MS and others: A phase I trial of recombinant human interleukin-11 (Neumega rhIL-11 growth factor) in women with breast cancer receiving chemotherapy, *Blood* 87:3615, 1996.

105. Graydon JE and others: Fatigue-reducing strategies used by patients receiving treatment for cancer, *Cancer Nurs* 18:23, 1995.

106. Groopman JE and others: Effect of recombinant human granulocyte-macrophage colony-stimulating factor on myelopoiesis in the acquired immunodeficiency syndrome, *N Engl J Med* 317:593, 1987.

107. Gutterman JU and others: Recombinant leukocyte α-IFN: pharmacokinetics, single-dose tolerance, and biologic effects in cancer patients, *Ann Intern Med* 96:549, 1982.

108. Haeuber D: The flu-like syndrome. In Rieger PT, editor: *Biotherapy: a comprehensive overview,* Boston, Jones & Bartlett, 1995.

109. Haeuber D, DiJulio JE: Hematopoietic colony-stimulating factors: an overview, *Oncol Nurs Forum* 16:247, 1989.

110. Hahn MB, Jassak PF: Nursing management of patients receiving interferon, *Semin Oncol Nurs* 4:95, 1988.

111. Hanna MG and others: Fundamental and applied aspects of successful active specific immunotherapy of cancer. In Oldham RK, editor: *Principles of cancer biotherapy,* New York, Marcel Dekker, 1991.

112. Harousseau JL and others; Granulocyte colony-stimulating factor after intensive consolidation chemotherapy in acute myeloid leukemia: results of a randomized trial of the Groupe Ouest-Est Leucemies Aigues Myeloblastiques, *J Clin Oncol* 18:780, 2000.

113. Hawkins MJ: Clinical trials of antiangiogenic agents, *Curr Opin Oncol* 7:90, 1995.

114. Heinzer H and others: Subjective and objective prospective, long-term analysis of quality of life during inhaled interleukin-2 immunotherapy, *J Clin Oncol* 17:3612, 1999.

115. Hendrzak JA, Brunda MJ: Interleukin-12: biologic activity, therapeutic utility, and role in disease, *Lab Invest* 72:619, 1995.

116. Hensley ML and others: Risk factors for severe neuropsychiatric toxicity in patients receiving interferon alfa-2b and low dose cytarabine for chronic myelogenous leu-

kemia: analysis of Cancer and Leukemia Group B 9013, *J Clin Oncol* 18:1301, 2000.

117. Hersh EM, Gutterman JU, Mavligit G, editors: *Immunotherapy of cancer in man: scientific basis and current status,* Springfield, IL, Thomas, 1973.

118. Hogan CM: Coping with biotherapy: physiological and psychosocial concerns, *Oncol Nurs Forum* 18(suppl 1): 19, 1991.

119. Hokom MM and others: Pegylated megakaryocyte growth and development factor abrogated the lethal thrombocytopenia associated with carboplatin and irradiation in mice, *Blood* 86:4486, 1995.

120. Hong WK, Lotan R, editors: *Retinoids in oncology,* New York, Marcel Dekker, 1993.

121. Hood LE, Abemathy E: Biological response modifiers. In McCorckle R, Baird SB, Grant M, editors: *Cancer nursing: comprehensive textbook,* ed 2, Philadelphia, Saunders, 1996.

122. Hwu P: Gene therapy of cancer. *Principles and practice of oncology updates,* Philadelphia, Lippincott, 1995.

123. Immunex Corp: Leukine (sargramostim) (package insert), Seattle, Immunex, 1999.

124. Immunex Corp: A reimbursement support program for Leukine (1-800-321-4669), Seattle, Immunex, 1999.

125. Isaacs A, Lindemann J: Virus interference, *Proc Soc Biol* 147:257, 1957.

126. Isaacs C and others: Randomized placebo-controlled study of recombinant human interleukin-11 to prevent chemotherapy-induced thrombocytopenia in patients with breast cancer receiving dose-intensive cyclophosphamide and doxorubicin, *J Clin Oncol* 15:3368, 1997.

127. Jackson BS and others: Long-term biopsychosocial effects of interleukin-2 therapy, *Oncol Nurs Forum* 18: 683, 1991.

128. Jansen JH and others: Interleukin-4: a regulatory protein, *Blut* 60:269, 1990.

129. Janssen Pharmaceutica: Ergamisol (levamisole hydrochloride) (package insert), Piscataway, NJ, Janssen Pharmaceutica, 1998.

130. Jassak PF: Biotherapy. In Groenwald SL and others, editors: *Cancer nursing: principles and practice,* ed 4, Boston, Jones & Bartlett, 1997.

131. Jassak P: An overview of biotherapy. In Rieger PT, editor: *Biotherapy: a comprehensive overview,* Boston, Jones & Bartlett, 1995.

132. Jenkins J, Wheeler V, Albright L: Gene therapy for cancer, *Cancer Nurs* 17:447, 1994.

133. Johnson C: Interleukin-1: therapeutic potential for solid tumors, *Cancer Invest* 11:600, 1993.

134. Karius D, Marriott MA: Immunologic advances in monoclonal antibody therapy: implications for oncology nursing, *Oncol Nurs Forum* 24:483, 1997.

135. Kaushansky K: Thrombopoietin: primary regulator of platelet function, *Blood* 86:419, 1995.

136. Kirkwood JM and others: Interferon alfa-2b adjuvant therapy of high-risk resected cutaneous melanoma: the Eastern Cooperative Oncology Group Trial EST 1684, *J Clin Oncol* 14:7, 1996.

137. Kobayashi S and others: Interleukin-11, *Leuk Lymphoma* 15:45, 1994.

138. Kobrinsky NL and others: Granulocyte-macrophage colony-stimulating factor treatment before doxorubicin and cyclophosphamide chemotherapy priming in women with early-stage breast cancer, *J Clin Oncol* 17:3426, 1999.

139. Kohler G, Milstein C: Continuous cultures of fused cells secreting antibody of predefined specificity, *Nature* 256:495, 1975.

140. Kolitz JE, Mertelsmann R: The immunotherapy of human cancer with interleukin-2: present status and future directions, *Cancer Invest* 9:529, 1991.

141. Krown SE, Jacubowski A, Houghton A: Biologic response modifiers. In Wittes RE, editor: *Manual of oncologic therapeutics 1991/1992,* Philadelphia, Lippincott, 1991.

142. Krueger GRF: Abnormal variation of the immune system as related to cancer. In Herberman RB, editor: *Influence of the host on tumor development,* Dordrecht, Kluwer, 1989.

143. Kurzrock R and others: Phase I study of recombinant human interleukin-3 in patients with bone marrow failure, *J Clin Oncol* 9:1241, 1991.

144. Kurzrock R, Talpaz M, editors: *Cytokines: interleukins and their receptors,* Boston, Kluwer, 1995.

145. Kurzrock R, Talpaz M, editors: *Molecular biology in cancer medicine,* New York, Oxford University Press, 1995.

146. Kuzel TM, Rosen ST: Antibodies in the treatment of human cancer, *Curr Opin Oncol* 6:622, 1994.

147. Larson SM and others: Overview of clinical radioimmunodetection of human tumors, *Cancer* 73(suppl 3):832, 1994.

148. Laurie JA and others: Surgical adjuvant therapy of large-bowel carcinoma: an evaluation of levamisole and the combination of levamisole and fluorouracil, *J Clin Oncol* 7:1447, 1989.

149. Leuko WM and others: Interleukin-15 and the growth of tumor-derived activated cells, *Cancer Biother* 10:13, 1995.

150. Levesque PE and others: Radiolabeled monoclonal antibody indium 111-labeled CYT-356 localizes extraprostatic recurrent carcinoma after prostatectomy, *Urology* 15:978, 1998.

151. Lippman SM, Benner SE, Hong WK: Cancer chemoprevention, *J Clin Oncol* 12:851, 1994.

152. Lippman SM and others: Strategies for chemoprevention study of premalignancy and second primary tumors in the head and neck, *Curr Opin Oncol* 7:234, 1995.

153. Livera MA, Vidali G, editors: *Retinoids: from basic science to clinical application,* Boston, Birkhausen Verlag, 1994.

154. Long MW, Wicha MS, editors: *The hematopoietic microenvironment: the functional and structural basis of blood cell development,* Baltimore, Johns Hopkins University Press, 1993.

155. Lotze MT and others: In vivo administration of purified human interleukin-2. I. Half-life and immunologic effects of the Jurkat cell line-n-derived IL-2, *J Immunol* 134:157, 1985.

156. Lotze MT and others: In vivo administration of purified human interleukin-2. II. Half-life, immunologic effects and expansion of peripheral lymphoid cells in vivo with recombinant IL-2, *J Immunol* 135:2865, 1985.

157. Lyman AD, Williams DE: Biological activities and potential therapeutic uses of steel factor, *Am J Pediatr Hematol Oncol* 14:1, 1992.

158. Lynch M, Yanes L, Todd R: Nursing care of AIDS patients participating in a phase I/II trial of recombinant human granulocyte-macrophage colony-stimulating factor, *Oncol Nurs Forum* 15:463, 1988.

159. Macquart-Moulin G and others: High-dose sequential chemotherapy with recombinant granulocyte colony-stimulating factor and repeated stem-cell support for inflammatory breast cancer patients: does impact on quality of life jeopardize feasibility and acceptability of treatment?, *J Clin Oncol* 18:754, 2000.

160. Maloney DG and others: IDEC-C2B8: results of a phase I multiple-dose trial in patients with relapsed non-Hodgkin's lymphoma, *J Clin Oncol* 15:3266, 1997.

161. Mandelli F and others: Maintenance treatment with recombinant interferon alfa-2b in patients with multiple myeloma responding to conventional induction chemotherapy, *N Engl J Med* 322:1430, 1990.

162. Marincola FM and others: Combination therapy with interferon alfa-2a and interleukin-2 for the treatment of metastatic cancer, *J Clin Oncol* 13:1110, 1995.

163. Mathe G and others: Active immunotherapy for acute lymphoblastic leukemia, *Lancet* 1:697, 1969.

164. Mayer DK: Biotherapy: recent advances and nursing implications, *Nurs Clin North Am* 25:291, 1990.

165. McCabe MS: Reimbursement for biotherapy. In Rieger PT, editor: *Biotherapy: a comprehensive overview*, ed 2, Boston, Jones & Bartlett, 1999.

166. McCorkle R, Young K: Development of a symptom distress scale, *Cancer Nurs* 1:373, 1978.

167. McLaughlin P and others: Rituximab chimeric anti-CD20 monoclonal antibody therapy for relapsed indolent lymphoma: half of patients responded to a four-dose treatment program, *J Clin Oncol* 16:2825, 1998.

168. Meredith RF, LoBuglio AF: Recent progress in radioimmunotherapy for cancer, *Oncology* 11:979, 1997.

169. Mertelsmann R, Herrmann F, editors: *Hematopoietic growth factors in clinical applications*, ed 2, New York, Marcel Dekker, 1995.

170. Metcalf D: The granulocyte-macrophage colony-stimulating factors, *Science* 229:16, 1985.

171. Metcalf D: The colony-stimulating factors: discovery, development and clinical applications, *Cancer* 65:2185, 1990.

172. Metcalf D: Thrombopoietin: at last, *Nature* 369:519, 1994.

173. Meyers C: Mental status changes. In Rieger PT, editor: *Biotherapy: a comprehensive overview*, Boston, Jones & Bartlett, 1995.

174. Mihich E, Fefer A, editors: *Biological response modifiers: subcommittee report*, National Cancer Institute Monograph, p. 63, 1983.

175. Miller L, editor: American Society of Clinical Oncology recommendations for the use of hematopoietic colony-stimulating factors: evidence-based, clinical practice guidelines, *J Clin Oncol* 12:2471, 1994.

176. Mitchell MS and others Active-specific immunotherapy for melanoma, *J Clin Oncol* 8:856, 1990.

177. Moffat FL Jr and others: Clinical utility of external immunoscintigraphy with the IMMU-4 technetium-99m Fab' antibody fragment in patients undergoing surgery for carcinoma of the colon and rectum: results of a pivotal, phase III trial—the Immunomedics Study Group, *J Clin Oncol* 14:2295, 1996.

178. Moore MAS: Does stem cell exhaustion result from combining hematopoietic growth factors with chemotherapy? If so, how do we prevent it? *Blood* 80:3, 1992.

179. Morgan DA, Ruscetti FW, Gallo RC: Selective in vitro growth of T lymphocytes from normal human bone marrows, *Science* 193:1007, 1976.

180. Morice RC and others: Pulmonary toxicity of recombinant tumor necrosis factor (rTNF), *Proc Am Soc Clin Oncol* 6:29, 1987 (abstract).

181. Morra ME, Grant M, editors: Cancer patient education, *Semin Oncol Nurs* 7:79, 1991.

182. Morstyn G and others: Treatment of chemotherapy-induced neutropenia by subcutaneously administered granulocyte colony-stimulating factor with optimization of dose and duration of therapy, *J Clin Oncol* 1:1554, 1989.

183. Morstyn G, Dexter TM, editors: *Filgrastim (r-metHuG-Csf) in clinical practice*, New York, Marcel Dekker, 1994.

184. Morstyn G and others: Stem cell factor is a potent synergistic factor in hematopoiesis, *Oncology* 51:205, 1994.

185. Mule JJ, Rosenberg SA: Combination cytokine therapy: experimental and clinical trials. In DeVita VT Jr, Hellman S, Rosenberg SA, editors: *Biologic therapy of cancer*, ed 2, Philadelphia, Lippincott, 1995.

186. Mule JJ, Rosenberg SA: Immunotherapy with lymphokine combinations. In DeVita VT, Hellman S, Rosenberg SA, editors: *Important advances in oncology*, Philadelphia, Lippincott, 1991.

187. Munn DH, Cheung N-KV: Preclinical and clinical studies of macrophage colony-stimulating factor, *Semin Oncol* 19:395, 1992.

188. Nail LM, Winningham ML: Fatigue and weakness in cancer patients: the symptom experience, *Semin Oncol Nurs* 11:272, 1995.

189. Nemunaitis J: Macrophage function-activating cytokines: potential clinical application, *Crit Rev Oncol Hematol* 14:153, 1993.

190. Nemunaitis J: Overview of the role of hematopoietic growth factors in bone marrow transplant recovery and bone marrow transplant failure, *Support Care Cancer* 2:374, 1994.

191. O'Day SJ and others: Advantages of concurrent biochemotherapy modified by decrescendo interleukin-2, granulocyte colony-stimulating factor, and tamoxifen for patients with metastatic melanoma, *J Clin Oncol* 17:2752, 1999.

192. Oettgen HF, Old LJ: The history of cancer immunotherapy. In DeVita VT Jr, Hellman S, Rosenberg SA, editors:

Biologic therapy of cancer, ed 2, Philadelphia, Lippincott, 1995.

193. Oken MM and others: Toxicity and response criteria of the Eastern Cooperative Oncology Group, *Am J Clin Oncol* 5:649, 1982.

194. Old LJ and others: The role of the reticuloendothelial system in the host reaction to neoplasia, *Cancer Res* 21:1281, 1961.

195. Oldham RK: Biotherapy: general principles. In Oldham RK, editor: *Principles of cancer biotherapy,* ed 2, New York, Marcel Dekker, 1991.

196. Oratz R and others: Antimelanoma monoclonal antibody—ricin A chain immunoconjugate (XMMME-001-RTA) plus cyclophosphamide in the treatment of metastatic malignant melanoma: results of a phase II trial, *J Biol Response Mod* 9:345, 1990.

197. Ortho Biotech: Procrit (epoetin alfa) (package insert), Raritan, NJ, Ortho Pharmaceutical, 1999.

198. Ortho Biotech: PROCRIT line (reimbursement hotline 1-800-553-3851), Raritan, NJ, Ortho Pharmaceutical, 1999.

199. Pai LH: Immunotoxins and recombinant toxins. In DeVita VT Jr, Hellman S, Rosenberg S, editors: *Biologic therapy of cancer,* ed 2, Philadelphia, Lippincott, 1995.

200. Parkinson DR (guest editor): The expanding role of interferon-alfa in the treatment of cancer, *Semin Oncol* 21(6 suppl 14):1, 1994.

201. Parkinson DR, Sznol M: High-dose interleukin-2 in the therapy of metastatic renal cell carcinoma, *Semin Oncol* 22:61, 1995.

202. Pegram MD and others: Phase II study of receptor-enhanced chemosensitivity using recombinant humanized anti-p185HER2/neu monoclonal antibody plus cisplatin in patients with HER2/neu-overexpressing metastatic breast cancer refractory to chemotherapy treatment, *J Clin Oncol* 16:2659, 1998.

203. Penn I: Principles of tumor immunity: immunocompetence and cancer. In DeVita VT Jr, Hellman S, Rosenberg SA, editors: *Biologic therapy of cancer,* ed 2, Philadelphia, Lippincott, 1995.

204. Pestka S: The purification and manufacture of human interferons, *Sci Am* 249:37, 1983.

205. Pietersz GA and others: Chemoimmunoconjugates for the treatment of cancer, *Adv Immunol* 56:301, 1994.

206. Piper BF, Lindsey AM, Dodd MJ: Fatigue mechanisms in cancer patients: developing a nursing theory, *Oncol Nurs Forum* 14:17, 1987.

207. Piper BF and others: Recent advances in the management of biotherapy-related side effects: fatigue, *Oncol Nurs Forum* 16(suppl6):27, 1989.

208. Piper BF: Alteration in comfort: fatigue. In McNally JC and others, editors: *Guidelines for oncology nursing practice,* ed 2, Philadelphia, Saunders, 1991.

209. Pitler LR: Hematopoietic growth factors, *Semin Oncol Nurs* 12:115, 1996.

210. Post-White J: The immune system, *Semin Oncol Nurs* 12:89, 1996.

211. Puri R, Siegel J: Interleukin-4 and cancer therapy, *Cancer Invest* 11:473, 1993.

212. Quesada JR and others: Interferon for induction of remission in hairy cell leukemia, *N Engl J Med* 310:15, 1984.

213. Quesada JR, Gutterman JU, Hersh EV: Treatment of hairy cell leukemia with alpha interferons, *Cancer* 57:1678, 1986.

214. Quesada JR and others: Clinical toxicity of interferons in cancer patients: a review, *J Clin Oncol* 4:234, 1986.

215. Quesada JR: Biologic therapy with interferon-gamma. In DeVita VT, Hellman S, Rosenberg SA, editors: *Biologic therapy of cancer,* ed 2, Philadelphia, Lippincott, 1995.

216. Reilly RM and others: Problems of delivery of monoclonal antibodies: pharmaceutical and pharmacokinetic solutions, *Clin Pharmacol Ther* 28:126, 1995.

217. Rhodes VA, McDaniel RW, editors: Cancer symptom management, *Semin Oncol Nurs* 11:231, 1995.

218. Rieger PT, Weatherly B: Can your nursing skills meet the challenge of a patient receiving IL-27? *Dimens Oncol Nurs* 3:9, 1989.

219. Rieger PT: The pathophysiology of selected symptoms associated with BRM therapy (monograph), Emeryville, CA, Cetus Corp., 1992.

220. Rieger PT, Rumsey KA: Responding to the educational needs of patients receiving biotherapy. In Carroll-Johnson RM, editor: *The biotherapy of cancer.* V (monograph), Pittsburgh, Oncology Nursing Press, 1992.

221. Rieger PT: Dosing and scheduling of biological response modifiers. In Rieger PT, editor: *Biotherapy: a comprehensive overview,* ed 2, Boston, Jones & Bartlett, 1999.

222. Rieger PT, editor: *Biotherapy: a comprehensive overview,* ed 2, Boston, Jones & Bartlett, 1999.

223. Rieger PT: Patient management. In Rieger PT, editor: *Biotherapy: a comprehensive overview,* ed 2, Boston, Jones & Bartlett, 1995.

224. Rieger PT, Haeuber D: A new approach to managing chemotherapy-related anemia: nursing implications of epoetin alfa, *Oncol Nurs Forum* 22:71, 1995.

225. Rieger PT: Interferon-alpha: a clinical update, *Cancer Practice* 3:356, 1995.

226. Rieger PT: Future projections in biotherapy, *Semin Oncol Nurs* 12:163, 1996.

227. Robinson KD, Abernathy E, Conrad KJ: Gene therapy of cancer, *Semin Oncol Nurs* 12:142, 1996.

228. Roche Laboratories: Roferon-A (package insert), Nutley, NJ, Hoffman-LaRoche, 1999.

229. Roche Laboratories: Vesanoid (package insert), Nutley, NJ, Hoffman-LaRoche, 1998.

230. Rosenberg SA: Gene therapy of cancer. In DeVita VT Jr, Hellman S, Rosenberg SA, editors: *Important advances in oncology,* Philadelphia, Lippincott, 1991.

231. Rosenberg SA: The immunotherapy and gene therapy of cancer, *J Clin Oncol* 10:180, 1992.

232. Rosenberg SA, Barry JM, editors: *The transformed cell: unlocking the mysteries of cancer,* New York, Putnam, 1992.

233. Rosenberg SA: Principles and applications of biologic therapy. In DeVita VT, Hellman S, Rosenberg SA, editors: *Cancer: principles and practice of oncology,* ed 5, Philadelphia, Lippincott, 1997.

234. Rosenberg SA and others: Treatment of 283 consecutive patients with metastatic melanoma or renal cell cancer using high-dose bolus interleukin-2, *JAMA* 271:907, 1994.

235. Roth JA, Molldrem J, Smythe WR: The current status of cancer gene therapy trials, *Principles and Practice of Oncology Updates* 13:1, 1999.

236. Rubin JT, Lotze MT: Acute gastric mucosal injury associated with the systemic administration of interleukin-4, *Surgery* 111:274, 1992.

237. Rumsey KA: Patient education. In Rieger PT, editor: *Biotherapy: a comprehensive overview,* Boston, Jones & Bartlett, 1995.

238. Schellhammer PF, Ladaga LE, Fillion MB: Bacillus Calmette-Guerin for superficial transitional cell carcinoma of the bladder, *J Urol* 135:261, 1986.

239. Schering Corp: Intron A: interferon alfa-2b recombinant for injection, Kenilworth, NJ, Schering, 1999.

240. Schlom J: Monoclonal antibodies in cancer therapy. In DeVita VT Jr, Hellman S, Rosenberg SA, editors: *Biologic therapy of cancer,* ed 2, Philadelphia, Lippincott, 1995.

241. Scott SD: Rituximab: a new therapeutic monoclonal antibody for non-Hodgkin's lymphoma, *Cancer Pract* 6:195, 1998.

242. Sharp E: The interleukins. In Rieger PT, editor: *Biotherapy: a comprehensive overview,* Boston, Jones & Bartlett, 1995.

243. Sharp E and others: A teaching tool for patients receiving continuous IV infusion recombinant interleukin-2 therapy, *Oncol Nurs Forum* 21:911, 1994.

244. Siegel JP, Puri RK: Interleukin-2 toxicity, *J Clin Oncol* 9:694, 1991.

245. Silverman P, Berger NA: Recent clinical experience with tumor necrosis factor and advances in understanding its physiologic function and cellular activities, *Curr Opinion Oncol* 2:1133, 1990.

246. Skalla KA, Rieger PT: Fatigue. In Rieger PT, editor: *Biotherapy: a comprehensive overview,* Boston, Jones & Bartlett, 1995.

247. Skalla KA: The interferons, *Semin Oncol Nurs* 12:97, 1996.

248. Smith KA: Interleukin-2, *Sci Am* 262:50, 1990.

249. Smith MA and others: Retinoids in cancer therapy, *J Clin Oncol* 10:839, 1992.

250. Smith TJ: Role of granulocyte-and granulocyte-Macrophage colony-stimulating factors in clinical practice: Balancing clinical and economic concerns, *American Society of Clincal Oncology Educational Book,* p 275, 1999.

251. Solal-Celigny P and others: Recombinant interferon alfa-2b combined with a regimen containing doxorubicin in patient with advanced follicular lymphoma, *N Engl J Med* 329:1608, 1993.

252. Sparber A, Biller-Sparber K: Immunotherapy and neuropsychiatric toxicity, *Cancer Nurs* 16:188, 1993.

253. Spitler LE: Immunotoxins. In Oldham RK, editor: *Principles of cancer biotherapy,* ed 3, Norwell, MA, Kluwer Academic Publishers, 1997.

254. Spivak JL, editor: Erythropoietin: basic and clinical aspects, *Hematol Oncol Clin North Am* 8:863, 1994.

255. Stadler WM, Vogelzang NJ: Low-dose interleukin-2 in the treatment of metastatic renal cell carcinoma, *Semin Oncol* 22:67, 1995.

256. Stames HF: Biological effects and possible clinical applications of interleukin 1, *Semin Hematol* 28(suppl 2):34, 1991.

257. Stein CA, Narayanan R: Antisense oligodeoxynucleotides, *Curr Opin Oncol* 6:587, 1994.

258. Stetz KM and others: 1994 Oncology Nursing Society research priorities survey, *Oncol Nurs Forum* 22:785, 1995.

259. Straw LJ, Conrad KJ: Patient education resources related to biotherapy and the immune system, *Oncol Nurs Forum* 212:1223, 1994.

260. Sznol M, Parkinson DR: Clinical applications of IL-2, *Oncology* 8:61, 1994.

261. Sznol M: Emerging concepts in cancer vaccine development, *Principles and Practice of Oncology Updates* 13:1, 1999.

262. Tallman MS: All-*trans*-retinoic acid in acute promyelocytic leukemia and its potential in other hematologic malignancies, *Semin Hematol* 31(4 suppl 5):38, 1994.

263. Talpaz M and others: Hematologic remissions and cytogenic improvement induced by recombinant human interferon A in chronic myelogenous leukemia, *N Engl J Med* 314:1065, 1986.

264. Talpaz M and others: Interferon alpha in the therapy of CML, *Br J Haematol* 79(suppl)1:38, 1991.

265. Talpaz M: Use of interferon in the treatment of chronic myelogenous leukemia, *Semin Oncol* 6:3, 1994.

266. Tepler I and others: A randomized placebo-controlled trial of recombinant human interleukin-11 in cancer patients with severe thrombocytopenia due to chemotherapy, *Blood* 87:3607, 1996.

267. Thor A and others: Distribution of oncofetal antigen tumor-associated glycoprotein-72 defined by monoclonal antibody B72.3, *Cancer Res* 46:3118, 1986.

268. Tracey KJ, Vlassara H, Cerami A: Cachectin tumor necrosis factor, *Lancet* 1:1122, 1989.

269. Truitt RL and others: Role of IL-4, IL-6 and IL-12 in cancer therapy. In DeVita VT Jr Hellman S, Rosenberg SA, editors: *Biologic therapy of cancer,* ed 2, Philadelphia, Lippincott, 1995.

270. Tushinski RJ, Mule JJ: Biology of cytokines: the interleukins. In DeVita VT Jr Hellman S, Rosenberg SA, editors: *Biologic therapy of cancer,* ed 2, Philadelphia, Lippincott, 1995.

271. Ulukaya E, Wood EJ: Fenretinide and its relation to cancer, *Cancer Treat Rev* 25:229, 1999.

272. Urabe A: Interferons for the treatment of hematological malignancies, *Oncology* 51:137, 1994.

273. Vadhan-Raj S and others: Stimulation of megakaryocyte and platelet production by a single dose of recombinant human thrombopoietin in patients with cancer, *Ann Intern Med* 126:673, 1997.

274. Vadhan-Raj S and others: Effects of recombinant human granulocyte-macrophage colony-stimulating factor in patients with myelodysplastic syndromes, *N Engl J Med* 317:1545, 1987.

275. Vadhan-Raj S and others: Stimulation of myelopoiesis in patients with aplastic anemia by recombinant human granulocyte-macrophage colony-stimulating factor, *N Engl J Med* 319:1628, 1988.

276. Vadhan-Raj S and others: Abrogating chemotherapy-induced myelosuppression by recombinant granulocyte-macrophage colony-stimulating factor in patients with sarcoma: protection at the progenitor cell level, *J Clin Oncol* 10:1266, 1992.

277. Vadhan-Raj S and others: Effects of PIXY321, a granulocyte-macrophage colony-stimulating factor/interleukin-3 fusion protein, on chemotherapy-induced multilineage myelosuppression in patient with sarcoma, *J Clin Oncol* 12:715, 1994.

278. Vadhan-Raj S and others: Effects of interleukin-1α on carboplatin-induced thrombocytopenia in patients with recurrent ovarian cancer, *J Clin Oncol* 12:707, 1994.

279. Vadhan-Raj S: PIXY321 (GM-CSF/IL-3 fusion protein): biology and early clinical development, *Stem Cells (Dayt)* 12:253, 1994.

280. Varrichio CG, Jassak PF: Informed consent: an overview, *Semin Oncol Nurs* 5:95, 1989.

281. Vial T, Descotes J: Clinical toxicity of the interferons, *Drug Safety* 10:115, 1994.

282. Vose JM, Armitage JO: Clinical applications of hematopoietic growth factors, *J Clin Oncol* 4:1023, 1995.

283. Vose JM and others: Multicenter phase II study of iodine-131 tositumomab for chemotherapy-relapsed/refractory low-grade and transformed low-grade B-cell non-Hodgkin's lymphomas, *J Clin Oncol* 18:1316, 2000.

284. Wadler S and others: Fluorouracil and recombinant alfa-2a-interferon: an active regimen against advanced colorectal carcinoma, *J Clin Oncol* 7:1769, 1989.

285. Wagstaff J, editor: *The role of interleukin-2 in the treatment of cancer patients,* Boston, Kluwer, 1993.

286. Weber J and others: Phase I trial of subcutaneous interleukin-6 in patients with advanced malignancies, *J Clin Oncol* 11:499, 1993.

287. Weinberg R: Oncogenes and cancer suppressor genes, CA *Cancer J Clin* 44:160, 1994.

288. Wheeler V: Interleukins: the search for an anticancer therapy, *Semin Oncol Nurs* 12:106, 1996.

289. Winningham ML and others: Fatigue and the cancer experience: the state of the knowledge, *Oncol Nurs Forum* 21:23, 1994.

290. Winters W, Glass E, Sakurai C: Ethical issues in oncology nursing practice: an overview of topics and strategies, *Oncol Nurs Forum* 20(suppl):21, 1993.

291. Witzig TE and others: Phase I/II trial of IDEC-Y2B8 radioimmunotherapy for treatment of relapsed or refractory CD20+ B-cell non-Hodgkin's lymphoma, *J Clin Oncol* 17:3793, 1999.

292. Wujcik D: Hematopoietic growth factors. In Rieger PT, editor: *Biotherapy: a comprehensive overview,* ed 2, Boston, Jones & Bartlett, 1999.

293. Yarbro CH, editor: Management of patients receiving interleukin-2 therapy, *Semin Oncol Nurs* 9(suppl 3):1, 1993.

294. Yarbro JW: The new biology of cancer: future clinical applications, *Semin Oncol* 16:254, 1989.

295. Yarbro JW, Bornstein RS, Mastrangelo MJ: Interferon: advances in biotherapy, *Semin Oncol* 18(suppl 7):1, 1991.

296. Yarbro JW, Bornstein RS, Mastrangelo MJ: Management of anemia in oncology, *Semin Oncol* 19(suppl 8):1, 1992.

297. Yasko JM, Ver Furth M: Closing comments: economic trends, *Semin Oncol Nurs* 8:156, 1992.

Bone Marrow and Stem Cell Transplantation

Claire Keller

Stem cells are found in the bone marrow, the spongy tissue found in the inner cavities of bone and in the peripheral blood. Stem cells eventually proliferate into mature erythrocytes, leukocytes, and platelets (see Chapters 14 and 31 for further information). Historically bone marrow transplantation (BMT) has been the process of replacing diseased or damaged bone marrow with normal-functioning bone marrow. BMT has been used in the treatment of a variety of diseases. More recently peripheral blood stem cell (PBSC) transplantation has become widely used. In both cases the treatment offers a chance for long-term survival.

HISTORICAL PERSPECTIVE

The first known documented cases of human BMT occurred as early as the 19th century. Medical practitioners experimented with bone marrow as a treatment modality for poorly understood diseases for which there was no existing treatment. Bone marrow was injected into or sometimes even fed to patients. Some positive results occurred; however, these benefits were sporadic, and the reasons for improvement were poorly understood. These primitive attempts were for the most part abandoned.

Later in the 20th century an interest in BMT again arose as an experimental approach for the treatment of some hematologic diseases. A variety of approaches were used, and many important discoveries were made. Developments in antibacterial, fungal, and viral therapies; blood-banking techniques; chemotherapeutic regimens; growth factors; graft-versus-host disease (GVHD) prophylaxis and treatment; and tissue typing have made BMT a more effective, viable treatment option. Table 25–1 summarizes the highlights of these significant developments.

TYPES OF BONE MARROW AND STEM CELL TRANSPLANTATION

There are two major types of transplant: autologous and allogeneic. The type of transplant is identified by the recipient's relationship to the donor. An *autologous transplant* is a transplant in which the patient's own bone marrow or stem cells are collected (harvested), placed in frozen storage (cryopreserved), and reinfused into the patient after the conditioning regimen. Therefore, the patient is his own donor. An *allogeneic transplant* is a transplant in which the patient receives someone else's bone marrow or stem cells. There are several types of allogeneic transplant, with each type named according to the donor: *syngeneic*—the donor is the patient's identical twin; *related*—the donor is related to the recipient and is usually a sibling; *unrelated*—the donor is no relation to the recipient.

SOURCES OF STEM CELLS

Autologous Peripheral Blood Stem Cells

Although stem cells have been traditionally harvested from bone marrow cavities, functional hematopoietic stem cells can also be found circulating in peripheral blood. PBSCs can be effectively transplanted, as evidenced in 1986 when the first successful PBSC transplants were reported.[8, 87] Today the collection of PBSCs for hematopoietic support after high-dose chemotherapy (HDCT) has become standard practice in the treatment of a variety of diseases (Table 25–2). Advocates of PBSC transplant cite early engraftment as a cost-saving measure because of shortened length of stay and the need for fewer blood products and antibiotics.[22] It appears that bone marrow harvest has become a thing of the past. Few centers collect bone marrow except

TABLE 25–1
Significant Historical Events in Bone Marrow Transplantation (BMT)

Year	Researcher	Significant Finding
1896	Quine	Attempted BMT by injecting or feeding bone marrow to patients; poor results.
1939	Osgood et al.	Attempted to cure aplastic anemia by massive intravenous (IV) injections of marrow cells.
1950	Relders et al.	Attempted BMT in dogs. Adequate doses of bone marrow, but inadequate radiation exposure did not allow for sufficient immunosuppression for engraftment.
1951	Lorenzo et al.	Demonstrated that guinea pigs and mice exposed to lethal radiation could be protected by infusion of bone marrow.
1955	Lindsley et al.	Radiation protection described earlier was result of growth of donor bone marrow.
1956	Ford et al.	Cytogenetic techniques used to show that radiation protection resulted from transfer and survival of donor marrow cells.
1957	Thomas et al.	Large quantities of bone marrow could be safely infused IV; one patient showed transient engraftment. Estimated necessary dose of marrow cells and warned against graft-versus-host disease reactions.
1959	Thomas et al.	Demonstrated that IV infusion of marrow from identical twin could protect against lethal radiation doses in patients with refractory leukemia.
1964	Mathe	First to achieve enduring bone marrow graft in patient with leukemia.
1968	Epstein et al.	Detected DL-A antigen in dogs and showed that marrow grafts between litter mates were almost always successful.
1968	Gatti et al.	Performed first marrow transplant from a matched sibling for an infant with immunodeficiency.
1975	Thomas et al.	Performed series of successful transplants using HLA-A identical siblings.

TABLE 25–2
Diseases Treated with Bone Marrow and Stem Cell Transplant

Type	Disease
Malignant	Acute myelogenous leukemia
	Acute lymphocytic leukemia
	Chronic myelogenous leukemia
	Myelodysplastic syndrome
	Hodgkin's disease
	Non-Hodgkin's lymphoma
	Multiple myeloma*
	Breast cancer*
	Neuroblastoma
	Testicular cancer*
	Ewing's sarcoma*
	Rhabdomyosarcoma*
	Wilms' tumor*
	Malignant melanoma*
	Lung cancer*
	Brain tumors*
	Ovarian cancer*
Nonmalignant	Aplastic anemia
	Myelofibrosis
	Wiskott-Aldrich syndrome
	Severe combined immunodeficiency syndrome
	Mucopolysacharoidosis
	Osteopetrosis
	Lipid storage diseases*
	Thalassemia*
	Paroxysmal nocturnal hemoglobinuria*

Role of transplantation is still under investigation.

when unable to obtain an adequate cell dose during apheresis. However, there is still some debate over the advantages and disadvantages of PBSC collection versus bone marrow harvest (Table 25–3).

The process of PBSC collection consists of two phases: mobilization, apheresis.

Mobilization. Peripheral blood in its steady state does not contain adequate numbers of stem cells to allow for efficient collection. Bone marrow contains up to 100 times the number of stem cells found in peripheral blood.[48, 91] To collect an adequate number of stem cells in the least number of apheresis sessions, it is necessary to stimulate the production of PBSCs through a process called *mobilization*. There are two techniques typically used to mobilize PBSCs, using hematopoietic growth factors (granulocyte colony-stimulating factor [G-CSF] or granulocyte/macrophage CSF [GM-CSF]) alone or in combination with chemotherapy.

When growth factors are used alone, they are generally given for a set number of days and followed by a preset number of apheresis sessions. The main advantage to this approach is that the apheresis sessions can be scheduled in advance.[44] Cyclophosphamide is the most frequently used chemotherapeutic agent in PBSC mobilization, although other agents have been used. Chemotherapy is used to treat the disease and to take advantage of the accelerated hematopoiesis that occurs during the recovery period that follows myelosuppressive treatment.[45] When chemotherapy and growth factors are used together, there is an increase in the number of stem cells in the blood and a lengthening in the time

TABLE 25-3

Advantages and Disadvantages of Peripheral Blood Stem Cell (PBSC) Transplant and Autologous Bone Marrow Transplant (ABMT)

Advantages	Disadvantages
PBSC TRANSPLANT	
Outpatient procedure	Processing and cryopreservation of PBSCs labor intensive
No general anesthesia needed for PBSC collection	Low cell yield requires multiple pheresis sessions
No harvest-related pain	Malignant cells may be present
Can be done when bone marrow is fibrotic, hypocellular, or diseased	Requires large-bore double-lumen central venous catheter
Possibility of less tumor contamination than in bone marrow	
Tumor cells in peripheral blood may have less ability to proliferate	
More rapid hematopoietic recovery; may result in lower costs from increased need for blood products and antibiotics, increased risk of infection, and shorter length of stay	
Faster reconstitution of immune function from increase in number of committed lymphocytes	
Potential for serial transplants	
ABMT	
Offers treatment options for older adults	Longer period of neutropenia
	Harvest requires general anesthesia and hospitalization
	Pain from multiple aspirations

they are present.[91] There are two primary disadvantages to chemotherapy-induced mobilization: it can result in neutropenic fever and infection, and it is difficult to predict when the patient will be ready to begin apheresis. However, the most significant mobilization seems to occur when chemotherapy and growth factors are used together rather than when either is used alone.[91] It has been reported that the combined use of chemotherapy and growth factors for mobilization also enhances engraftment.[91]

Apheresis. The PBSCs are collected by a process called *apheresis,* using standard commercially available cell separators. The cell separators are programmed to collect either lymphocytes or low-density leukocytes.[45, 48] The remaining blood components are returned to the patient. Apheresis is performed for 1 to 10 days. In recent years the process has become more efficient and an adequate number of cells can usually be collected in one to three sessions. Each session is 3 to 4 hours long, but the duration is based on the rate of blood flow through the central venous catheter. A flow rate of 50 to 70 mL/min is considered optimal.[91] A single large volume collection can decrease collection time while providing a safe cost-effective harvest method.[51]

To collect PBSCs, a large-bore, double-lumen central venous catheter is required. This is necessary to provide adequate blood flow through the cell separator. A variety of catheters are in use; generally at least a 12 French is needed to maintain blood flow. Catheters that have narrower lumens or those constructed of soft material

such as silicone may not be able to provide adequate flow rates.[17, 94] Complications related to the central venous catheters have been reported, including thrombosis, occlusion, malpositioning, and infection. These complications contribute to the morbidity and cost of the procedure. The "ideal" apheresis catheter has not yet been found. Current technology does not allow one to identify the circulating stem cells. Several techniques are in development to help determine if an adequate number of stem cells have been collected to ensure engraftment. The easiest and most accessible is to measure the number of mononuclear cells in the apheresis product. Mononuclear cell counts of 4 to 5×10^8/kg patient body weight routinely contain adequate stem cells for engraftment. Another method is to measure the population of cells that express CD34$^+$ using flow cytometry. It is believed that stem cells are found within the group of cells carrying the CD34$^+$ antigen. Currently this is one of the most widely used methods to estimate the number of stem cells in the apheresis product.[45]

Side effects of apheresis are minimal but include transient hypocalcemia from the anticoagulant used in the apheresis process, fatigue, anemia, and thrombocytopenia. After each collection the stem cells are placed in a blood bag and cryopreserved using dimethylsulfide (DMSO) as a cryoprotectant. The cells are kept frozen at $-196°C$.

Allogeneic Peripheral Blood Stem Cells

In recent years many centers have turned to PBSCs as the source of stem cells for allogeneic transplants. The advantages of using allogeneic PBSCs include: faster engraftment and decreased transplant related mortality, the ability to obtain a larger number of stem cells, the possibility of faster reconstitution of the immune system and comparable rates of GVHD.[1]

Allogeneic PBSC collection consists of two phases, mobilization and apheresis.

Mobilization. Mobilization of PBSCs is necessary in the normal donor as there is not an adequate number available in the peripheral circulation in its steady state.[48] With normal donors only the use of growth factors specifically G-CSF is considered safe for mobilization. An adequate number of CD34$^+$ cells are available in the circulation after 4 to 5 days of G-CSF administration.[1] Side effects reported include bone pain, headache, fatigue, nausea and insomnia.[85] These side effects can be managed with oral analgesics in most cases and resolve on their own after the G-CSF is discontinued. Long-term effects of normal donors receiving G-CSF are not known, but it has been speculated that the risk for leukemia may increase by as much as 10-fold.[1]

Apheresis. As with autologous PBSCs, allogeneic PBSCs are collected by a process called *apheresis,* using standard commercially available cell separators. The cell separators are programmed to collect either lymphocytes or low-density leukocytes.[48] In normal donors most commonly peripheral lines in the antecubital veins are used for venous access; in some cases a temporary central may be needed. An adequate number of CD34$^+$ cells can collected in one or two sessions in most cases.[1] The most significant side effect is a 30% to 50% drop in platelet count. The platelet count may take a week or more to recover and donor follow-up is important.[3]

Bone Marrow Harvest

Harvesting is the process of obtaining bone marrow for transplantation. Bone marrow harvests are becoming less frequent because many centers have turned to PBSCs for autologous and allogeneic transplants. This procedure occurs in the operating room, typically with the patient under general anesthesia. Bone marrow is obtained by performing multiple punctures with a large-bore needle into the patient's posterior and occasionally anterior iliac crests. Usually two physicians work simultaneously, one on either side of the patient. Multiple punctures are necessary because each aspiration obtains only 2 to 5 mL bone marrow.

The amount of bone marrow collected depends on the size of the recipient and donor as well as the type of BMT (autologous or allogeneic). Usually, 10 to 15 mL/kg body weight will yield the amount of needed stem cells. Therefore, a 50-kg patient would contribute approximately 500 to 750 mL bone marrow, and if ob-

taining about 5 mL/aspiration, approximately 100 to 150 aspirations are required to obtain the desired 500 to 750 mL marrow. This is only about 5% of the body's total marrow volume. Ideally, this amount of marrow should contain 1 to 4 $\times$ 10^8 nucleated cells.[2]

Once collected, the marrow is mixed with a heparinized solution, filtered to remove bone fragments and fat, and placed in a blood bag. At this point the marrow can be treated or purged. *Purging* is the process of removing residual malignant cells from the marrow for autologous transplant. It is performed using monoclonal antibodies or chemotherapeutic agents. Marrow collected for allogeneic BMT may also be treated. One such treatment is that of T-cell depletion, which is the process of removing T lymphocytes from the marrow to prevent acute GVHD. If an ABO incompatibility exists, the red blood cells (RBCs) may also be removed from the allogeneic marrow.

When an allogeneic BMT is to be done, the marrow is immediately transfused into the recipient. The marrow is usually brought directly to the recipient's room from the operating room. For an autologous BMT, the collected marrow is mixed with the preservative DMSO, placed in a blood bag, and cryopreserved. It is thawed and transplanted at a later date.

After bone marrow harvest, postoperative recovery time is minimal. A large pressure dressing will have been applied to the iliac crests. Nursing responsibilities after bone marrow harvest include routine postoperative care such as maintaining comfort and mobility, providing care of the dressing, and monitoring vital signs and blood counts. Postoperatively, patients can expect discomfort at the sites for approximately 1 week. This discomfort can typically be relieved with acetaminophen. With an allogeneic BMT, the donor's psychological and emotional needs must not be overlooked. Many donors experience anxiety over whether the BMT will be a success or a failure. Nursing must allow for the ventilation of donor feelings and offer support.

Unrelated Donors

Another option for donor availability is the attainment of an unrelated donor. The National Marrow Donor Program (NMDP) was established in 1987 for this purpose. The registry contains more than 4 million available bone marrow donors, all of whom have had tissue typing completed and have expressed a desire to donate bone marrow. In 1999, the NMDP developed a central registry of cord blood banks to enable transplant centers to search cord blood banks more efficiently. Ethnic minorities remain underrepresented in the registry. The NMDP continues to place major emphasis on the recruitment of minority donors. The registry search determines which listed donors have compatible typing with the recipient patient. There are several other donor registries that contain approximately 1 million donors located throughout the world who are available for searches. It is not inconceivable that a patient in the United States could receive bone marrow from a donor located somewhere in Europe, Asia, Africa, or anywhere else in the world. The system is an anonymous one. When chosen, the donor does not know who is receiving the marrow, and the recipient does not know from which donor the marrow came or where that donor is located. More than 9000 unrelated BMTs have been made possible as a result of efforts of the NMDP.

Cord Blood Transplantation

As with bone marrow, umbilical cord blood (UCB) is rich in stem cells. It is now possible to collect and store cord blood for use in place of bone marrow or PBSCs. The first successful UCB transplant was performed in 1988 on a child with Fanconi's anemia.[40] Cord blood transplants have been successfully performed in patients with leukemia, aplastic anemia, Fanconi's anemia, immunodeficiency, and genetic and metabolic disorders.

Most early cord blood transplants were from siblings, but cord blood transplants from unrelated donors have increased dramatically in recent years.[71] The New York Blood Bank Center has banked more than 8000 cord blood samples.[71] In addition there are many smaller cord blood banks across the country and around the world. So far, cord blood has been used primarily in children because of the relatively low number of stem cells in the cord blood. It is not yet known how many stem cells are required to ensure engraftment, but at least four patients weighing more than 70 kg have been successfully transplanted.[14] Because the uses of UCB for transplantation is a relatively new approach and long term follow-up short, some questions cannot yet be answered. Is UCB transplant associated with a different relapse rate than other sources of stem cells? Will targeted collection of UCB increase the transplant opportunities for ethnic and racial minorities? Only time will answer these questions.

Collecting UCB is a simple procedure and poses no risk to the donor. After delivery, the umbilical cord is clamped and the blood withdrawn from the umbilical vein using a needle and syringe. It is then cryopreserved in much the same way as PBSCs or bone marrow.[36, 70]

Cord blood banking for transplant has several advantages and some disadvantages; these are outlined in Table 25–4. In addition to the clinical issues related to UCB transplantation, ethical issues will need to be addressed. These include the process and timing of the consent process; many cord blood banks obtain consent while the mother is in labor. Another key issue is whether identifiers linking the mother and the baby should be maintained or if all identifying links should be severed at the time of donation. UCB transplant will likely be the focus of much clinical, regulatory and ethical scrutiny for the foreseeable future.

Human Leukocyte Antigen Typing

Tissue typing of the patient and potential donors is the first step in identifying whether a patient has a compatible donor. To determine a person's tissue type, a small amount of peripheral blood is drawn, and antigens on the surface of the leukocytes are analyzed. These antigens make up the human leukocyte antigen (HLA) system, which plays a role in immune surveillance by constantly identifying "self" from "nonself."[34] There are a pair of antigens at several sites on the white blood cells (WBCs) called *loci*. Three of these loci, the HLA-A, HLA-B, and HLA-DR, are important in determining whether a patient and potential donor are compatible. The best match is one in which the antigens of the patient and potential donor match at all three loci. Matching at the A, B, and DR loci minimizes the risk of GVHD and graft rejection.

The antigens that make up the HLA system are inherited from one's parents. Each offspring receives a set

T A B L E   2 5 – 4
Advantages and Disadvantages of Cord Blood

Advantages	Disadvantages
1. Shorter interval to transplant, readily available	1. Slightly increased risk of graft failure
2. Rarely contaminated with latent viruses	2. Genetic/developmental abnormalities may go undetected
3. Collection poses no risk to the donor	3. Donor unavailable if additional cells needed
4. Decreased risk of GVHD, fewer activated T cells, graft is immunologically tolerant	4. Minimum number of nucleated cells needed for engraftment unknown
5. Able to transplant up to 3 antigen mismatch	
6. Eliminates risk of donor attrition	

Data from Wagner J: Umbilical cord transplantation, Leukemia *12(suppl 1):530, 1998.*

of antigens, referred to as a *haplotype,* from each parent (Fig. 25–1). Thus the best chance of finding a matched donor occurs among full siblings. Statistically, each sibling has a one in four (25%) chance of receiving the same haplotypes from the same parents. It is possible but unlikely that parents or children of a patient will match, because they are usually only a one-haplotype (half) match. In general, relatives outside the immediate family have approximately the same chance of matching as someone from the general population. Overall, the chances of matching someone in the general population are approximately 1 in 20,000, depending on how common the individual's haplotypes are.

HLA-A and HLA-B (class I) antigens are identified by serologic testing using a small blood sample and a typing tray containing known antisera.[95] HLA-DR antigens are identified using DNA technology. DNA technology identifies genes that specify the DR and DQ antigens; this allows for more accurate DR typing and therefore the identification of better matches. DNA technology has become the standard method used by many transplant centers and is now required by the NMDP.[95]

Mixed lymphocyte culture (MLC) testing, in which donor and recipient lymphocytes are grown in culture together to assess their reaction, was considered important in determining HLA-DR antigen compatibility, but the results are often difficult to analyze or reproduce. The advent of DNA technology has caused many centers to consider MLC testing obsolete.[95]

Mismatched donors are used in allogeneic transplants, for which no true match exists. Mismatches currently considered for transplant are either one or two antigen mismatches. The mismatch can occur at either the A, B, or DR loci. The higher the number of mismatches, the higher the incidence is of GVHD or graft rejection and the poorer the chances are of the patient's survival.[4]

Mismatching does not refer to ABO incompatibility. Corrections can be made to overcome ABO incompati-

bility so that, for example, a patient with blood type O can receive a transplant from a donor with blood type A. When ABO incompatibility occurs, the donor's erythrocytes can be removed from the bone marrow before transplant. Therefore the donor's erythrocytes are not infused and side effects from the ABO incompatibility are minimized. The recipient will eventually seroconvert to the donor's blood type.

INDICATIONS FOR BONE MARROW AND STEM CELL TRANSPLANTATION

Bone marrow transplantation is a treatment modality for a variety of malignant and nonmalignant diseases (see Table 25–2). Most BMTs are performed for malignancies. The type and stage of the disease, the patient's age and performance status, and donor availability determine the type of transplant that can be done and the chances of survival. Table 25–5 identifies approximate 5-year disease-free survival (DFS) for autologous and allogeneic transplants. Allogeneic transplant is used for the treatment of patients with hematologic malignancies, marrow failure, severe combined immunodefi-

TABLE 25–5

Survival Rates: Approximate 5-Year Disease-Free Survival (DFS) of Patients Receiving Autologous or Matched-Sibling Transplant

Disease	DFS
AUTOLOGOUS TRANSPLANTS	
AML (1st CR)	40–50%
AML (2nd CR)	30–40%
ALL (1st CR)	40–50%
ALL (2nd CR)	30%
CML (chronic)*	10%
Hodgkin's disease	20–60%
Non-Hodgkin's	40–60%
Breast cancer	Stage II and III: 75%
	Stage IV: 20%
ALLOGENEIC TRANSPLANTS	
AML (1st CR)	50–65%
AML (>1st CR)	25–35%
ALL (1st CR)	40–60%
ALL (2nd CR)	30–60%
CML (chronic)	65%
CML (accelerated)	30–45%
CML (blastic)	15%
Hodgkin's disease	25–55%
Non-Hodgkin's	20–65%
Multiple myeloma*	30%
Aplastic anemia	60–80%
MDS	30–60%

See text for abbreviations.

* Limited number of patients and follow-up.

	Mother			Father	
	M-1	M-2		F-1	F-2
A	1	2		3	9
B	5	7		12	13
DR	1	2		4	5

	Child #1		Child #2		Child #3		Child #4	
	M-1	F-1	M-1	F-2	M-2	F-1	M-2	F-2
A	1	3	1	9	2	3	2	9
B	5	12	5	13	7	12	7	13
DR	1	4	1	5	2	4	2	5

FIGURE 25–1 Human leukocyte antigen (HLA) inheritance.

ciency syndrome (SCIDS), and some inherited metabolic disorders. Currently, most allogeneic transplants are performed for acute myelocytic leukemia (AML), acute lymphocytic leukemia (ALL), and chronic myelogenous leukemia (CML).[39] Autologous BMT is used primarily for the treatment of diseases in which the patient's own bone marrow contains adequate PBSCs that can eventually generate functioning erythrocytes, leukocytes, and platelets. For example, autologous BMT is not a viable option for the treatment of aplastic anemia because the patient's own bone marrow is lacking PBSCs; however, it can be a treatment option for patients with limited disease in their bone marrow.

Autologous BMT is being used increasingly for the treatment of hematologic malignancies. Since 1990 the number of autologous BMTs has outpaced the number of allogeneic BMTs.[88]

A variety of approaches are being used to improve the efficacy of autologous transplant. The most promising is the use of dose-intensity therapy. BMT allows for the use of much higher doses of chemotherapy or radiation than would otherwise be possible. By increasing the dose intensity of the treatment, one can increase the likelihood of curing patients of their disease.[20, 79, 88] A second approach is the use of sequential autologous BMTs. Often, using PBSCs this approach allows for several courses of dose-intensive therapy with PBSC rescue in the hope of curing the patient's disease.

A concern associated with autologous transplant and PBSC transplant is the potential for contamination with tumor cells. A variety of purging techniques have been developed. A lack of prospective clinical trials, a lack of sensitive and specific assays to measure residual tumor, and the concern that stem cells can be damaged during the purging process have kept marrow purging controversial.[28]

Hematologic Malignancies

Leukemia

Acute Lymphocytic Leukemia. Allogeneic BMT has been performed on patients with ALL in remission and in relapse. Survival for patients transplanted in first remission is comparable to survival with conventional chemotherapy.[39] However, performing an allogeneic BMT in first remission is beneficial for patients who present with a high WBC count at diagnosis, the Philadelphia chromosome, or other chromosomal abnormalities. Allogeneic BMT for ALL in second or subsequent remission has shown a survival advantage over conventional chemotherapy.

Autologous BMT and PBSC transplant may also be done if no suitable donor is available. ALL is the most common leukemia among children; 60% to 70% of these children are cured with conventional chemotherapy. For most children with ALL, BMT is not considered unless the child relapses while in treatment. BMT in first remission is indicated only if the Philadelphia chromosome or other chromosomal abnormality is present.[67, 74] For patients who do not have a suitable donor, autologous BMT has been done, but these patients have a relapse rate of 70% to 75%.[74]

Acute Myelocytic Leukemia. Survival rates of AML patients with allogeneic BMT are 35% to 60%, compared with conventional chemotherapy survival rates of 20% to 50%. Timing of transplant remains controversial, but survival is best when the patient is transplanted in first remission. For patients without suitable donors, autologous and PBSC transplants done during first remission offer survival rates of 40% to 50%. The relapse rate is higher after autologous BMT, but complications of allogeneic BMT (e.g., GVHD) result in similar DFS rates.

Chronic Myelogenous Leukemia. For patients with CML, allogeneic BMT is the only treatment option that is curative.[10, 55, 57] The disease phase at the time of transplantation is the factor most strongly associated with treatment success.[56] Patients who have a BMT in the chronic phase have higher rates of success. The best results are seen in young patients, transplanted in chronic phase within a year of the diagnosis.[2]

For patients without a suitable donor, autologous BMTs for CML are under investigation. In some studies PBSCs are collected while the patient is in chronic phase. Patients undergo transplant when they progress to accelerated phase. Although this treatment is not curative, chronic phase CML has been successfully restored for 4 months to 1 year.[88] Other investigators are looking at transplantation earlier in the course of the disease and purging techniques.[10, 15]

Five percent of the leukemias in children are chronic. There are two types, adult-type CML and juvenile chronic myelogenous leukemia (JCML). Adult-type CML is more common and is characterized by high WBC count and the presence of the Philadelphia chromosome. Allogeneic BMT is the only hope of cure and should be performed early after diagnosis. JCML occurs in very young children, usually less than 5 years of age. JCML frequently presents like acute leukemia but cannot be effectively treated with chemotherapy. Allogeneic BMT provides a 30% to 50% chance of survival and the only hope of cure.[67, 74]

Lymphoma. BMT in the malignant lymphomas, Hodgkin's and non-Hodgkin's, is widely used as a salvage treatment. Because of the high chemotherapy and radiation sensitivity of these tumors, patients with lymphoma are optimal candidates for BMT.[82]

Autologous, allogeneic, and recent PBSC transplants are used, although autologous BMTs are done most frequently because of better donor availability and decreased complications. Autologous BMT also allows for treatment of older patients, which is especially important in non-Hodgkin's lymphoma.

The best results have been seen in lymphoma patients treated in second remission or in relapse with disease that is still responsive to chemotherapy.[88] In Hodgkin's disease, BMT is usually indicated for patients who fail to achieve a complete response to three or four courses of chemotherapy or who are in early relapse after initial complete response.[23] In non-Hodgkin's lymphoma, BMT is usually indicated for patients who have relapsed after an initial complete response or who remain responsive to chemotherapy but have residual disease.[11] For patients with residual disease or highly aggressive non-Hodgkin's lymphoma, BMT should be carried out as a consolidation procedure.[12]

Other Hematologic Malignancies

Myelodysplastic Syndrome (MDS). MDS consists of a number of disorders characterized by peripheral cytopenias. Allogeneic BMT is the only curative treatment for patients with MDS. Results are better in patients without excess blasts; cure rates of 60% to 70% have been reported in this population. Patients with excess blasts have a survival rate of 25% to 40%.[4]

Multiple Myeloma. Allogeneic BMT is being more closely scrutinized as studies have shown a higher rate of treatment related mortality over autologous transplants.[9] Overall survival rates for patients undergoing allogeneic transplant who fail first-line chemotherapy average 30% to 35%.[4] Allogeneic BMT is not an option for many patients with multiple myeloma because of their advanced age and lack of suitable donors. Autologous BMT can be tolerated by patients up to age 65. Favorable results reported with autologous BMT showed that patients most likely to benefit have primary resistant or responding disease with low β-microglobulin and lactate dehydrogenase (LDH) levels.[90]

Solid Tumors

Autologous BMT is most often done for patients with solid tumors. Solid tumors are the malignancies most frequently treated with dose-intensive strategies. For BMT to be effective, the disease must be responsive to treatment. Although BMTs are currently being performed on a variety of solid tumors, many are still considered investigational. The diseases currently receiving the most attention and study are breast cancer and neuroblastoma. Other tumors for which BMT has shown some positive responses are Ewing's sarcoma, malignant melanoma, rhabdomyosarcoma, testicular cancer, Wilms' tumor, ovarian cancer, and small-cell lung cancer.

Breast Cancer. Breast cancer now represents the most common disease treated by autologous BMT.[88] Conventional chemotherapy shows a dose-response effect, providing the rationale for the use of HDCT.[11] Studies show that HDCT with PBSC or marrow transplant in patients with chemotherapy-responsive metastatic disease has a 50% rate of complete remission, with a 5-year DFS rate of 20%. For patients with high-risk stage II (10 nodes or more) and stage III disease, the 5-year DFS rate with conventional treatment is 25% to 57%. With HDCT and PBSC transplant, this increases to 70%. Indicators of favorable prognosis for these patients are chemotherapy-responsive disease, limited tumor bulk, limited number of disease sites, absence of liver involvement, and good performance status. HDCT and autologous transplant alone are not curative; dose-intensive therapies must be integrated with other treatment modalities into the overall treatment of breast cancer.[11, 85]

The role for HDCT and stem cell transplantation in breast cancer remains controversial. No definitive randomized clinical trials have been completed. Ongoing study is needed in this area.

Neuroblastoma. Neuroblastoma is the most frequent pediatric solid tumor treated with BMT. Approximately 60% of patients have advanced disease and only a 10% chance of cure with conventional therapy.[54] Studies of autologous BMT in these patients suggests an overall 5-year DFS of 20% to 40%. Again, the small number of patients and the brief follow-up make these results encouraging but inconclusive. Further clinical trials are needed to determine if autologous BMT provides optimal treatment.[75]

Nonmalignant Diseases

Aplastic Anemia. Allogeneic BMT is responsible for approximately an 80% overall survival rate in patients with aplastic anemia.[2] Patients who have had blood product transfusions before BMT have a higher rate of graft rejection. Therefore, at the time of diagnosis, HLA typing is done on the entire family. All patients younger than age 45 should be considered for BMT. Although patients are immunosuppressed because of the disease, a conditioning regimen is usually administered. This is especially important for patients who have received transfusions because of the increased possibility of rejection.[2]

Severe Combined Immunodeficiency Syndrome. The earliest successful BMTs were in patients with SCIDS.[20] Most patients with SCIDS die within 1 year of diagnosis, and because this disease occurs so early in life, a matched sibling donor may be unavailable. Therefore, the use of a haplo-identical parent and, in some patients, matched unrelated donors is considered.[20] Approximately 70% of patients receiving a matched BMT will be cured.[66] The survival rate is slightly lower for patients receiving a haplo-identical parent match because of the increased incidence of graft rejection and GVHD.[66] Because the disease has already immunosuppressed the patient, no conditioning regimen is usually given.

BONE MARROW AND STEM CELL TRANSPLANTATION PROCESS

Pretreatment Work-up

An extensive evaluation is performed on the BMT recipient before transplant. This is done to establish the recipient's physical and psychosocial status. For allogeneic transplants, the donor is also thoroughly assessed. The assessment is done on an outpatient basis and includes a variety of tests, procedures, and consultations (Box 25–1). A team approach is usually used and typically includes psychology, social work, surgery, chaplaincy, and radiology in addition to nursing and medicine.

The patient's family and significant others are also included in this process. These evaluations alert the BMT team to potential problems that can occur, such as physical hindrances, negative coping mechanisms, or financial difficulties. This assessment also ensures that the patient has adequate support systems to help him throughout the rigorous BMT process.

Conditioning Regimens

The conditioning regimen is the process of preparing the patient to receive bone marrow or stem cells. It accomplishes three vital functions: obliterate the malignant disease, destroy the patient's preexisting immunologic state, and create space in the marrow cavity for the proliferation of the transplanted stem cells.[67] In effect, conditioning regimens destroy the patient's own bone marrow. The proliferation of new erythrocytes, leukocytes, and platelets cannot occur unless new functioning bone marrow or stem cells are given to the patient. On completion of the conditioning regimen, the patient must receive a transplant or die. The conditioning regimen consists of HDCT with or without total-body irradiation (TBI). There are several regimens using various combinations of chemotherapy or radiation or both that last 4 to 10 days (Table 25–6). Cyclophosphamide, carmustine, etoposide, busulfan, and cytarabine are all common chemotherapeutic agents used in conditioning regimens. The regimen chosen depends on the type of disease and the amount and response to previous radiation or chemotherapy.

In addition to severe myelosuppression, the patient may experience many other side effects (Table 25–7). Most of these are immediate responses to the chemo-

---

BOX 25-1

Pretransplantation Evaluation

Bone Marrow/Stem Cell Recipient

History and physical examination
Bone marrow biopsy and aspiration with cytogenetics
Chemistry profile
Complete blood count, platelets, reticulocyte count
ABO and Rh typing
Coagulation profile
Serum immunoelectrophoresis
Quantitative immunoglobulins
Hepatitis screen
Cytomegalovirus, human immunodeficiency virus (HIV), and herpes simplex virus titers
Urinalysis, creatinine clearance, and protein quantification
Chest x-ray film
Electrocardiogram, echocardiogram, or radionucleotide ventriculogram
Pulmonary function testing
Sinus x-ray film
Allergy testing
Audiology consult
Physical therapy consult
Dental consult
Dietary consult
Social work consult
Psychology/psychiatry consult
Ophthalmology consult
Surgery consult, insertion of multilumen catheter

Bone Marrow/Stem Cell Donor

History and physical examination
Chemistry profile
Complete blood count, platelet count
ABO and Rh typing
Hepatitis screen
Cytomegalovirus, HIV, and herpes simplex virus titers
Chest x-ray film
Electrocardiogram
Urinalysis

---

therapy and radiation and can continue for several weeks after transplantation. Management of these side effects focuses on control of the symptoms, prevention of further complications, and maintenance of patient comfort. Long-term effects, such as cataracts and gonadal dysfunction, also can occur and are discussed in the section on complications.

Nonmyeloablative Conditioning Regimens

In recent years transplanters have begun to look at nonmyeloablative conditioning regimens. This may pro-

TABLE 25–6
Common Conditioning Regimens for Transplant

Regimen	Description

BUSULFAN/CYCLOPHOSPHAMIDE

	−7	−6	−5	−4	−3	−2	−1	0
Day								
Busulfan 1 mg/kg every 6 h	×	×	×	×				
Cyclophosphamide 60 mg/kg/d					×	×		
Rest day							×	
Transplant day								×

BUSULFAN/CYTARABINE/CYCLOPHOSPHAMIDE

	−9	−8	−7	−6	−5	−4	−3	−2	−1	0
Day										
Busulfan 1 mg/kg every 6 h	×	×	×	×						
Cytarabine 2 g/m² every 12 h					×	×				
Cyclophosphamide 60 mg/kg/d							×	×		
Rest day									×	
Transplant day										×

CYCLOPHOSPHAMIDE/TOTAL-BODY IRRADIATION (TBI)

	−6	−5	−4	−3	−2	−1	0
Day							
Cyclophosphamide 60 mg/kg/d	×	×					
Rest day			×				
TBI 200 Gy twice daily				×	×	×	
Transplant day							×

CYCLOPHOSPHAMIDE/ETOPOSIDE/CARMUSTINE

	−7	−6	−5	−4	−3	−2	−1	0
Day								
Cyclophosphamide 1.8 g/m²/d	×	×	×	×				
Etoposide 200 mg/m² every 12 h	×	×	×	×				
Carmustine 600 mg/m²/day					×			
Rest day						×	×	
Transplant day								×

CYCLOPHOSPHAMIDE/TBI

	−8	−7	−6	−5	−4	−3	−2	−1	0
Day									
Cyclophosphamide 50 mg/kg/d	×	×	×	×					
TBI 300 Gy every day					×	×	×*	×	
Transplant day									×

CYCLOPHOSPHAMIDE

	−5	−4	−3	−2	−1	0
Day						
Cyclophosphamide 50 mg/kg/d	×	×	×	×		
Rest day					×	
Transplant day						×

CYCLOPHOSPHAMIDE/CISPLATIN/CARMUSTINE

	−6	−5	−4	−3	−2	−1	0
Day							
Cyclophosphamide 1875 mg/m²/d	×	×	×				
Cisplatin 55 mg/m²	×	×	×				
Carmustine 600 mg/m²				×			
Rest					×	×	
Transplant day							×

Lungs shielded for this dose.

vide an alternative for patients for whom a traditional allogeneic transplant may be too toxic. Appropriate patients are over the age of 55 with some preexisting organ damage. Nonmyeloablative transplants have also been called mini-transplants, low-intensity transplants, or transplant lite. The theory behind nonmyeloablative transplants is based on the belief that it is the immune-mediated graft-versus-tumor effect that provides the

TABLE 25–7

Side Effects of Conditioning Regimens for Transplant

Regimen	Major Side Effects	Management
Busulfan	Nausea, vomiting, diarrhea, seizures (possible during administration and up to 48 h after last dose)	Administer antiemetic at scheduled intervals. Check emesis for busulfan tablets and replace 1 for 1. Establish seizure precautions and monitor for seizure activity. Administer anticonvulsant at scheduled intervals as ordered.
Carmustine (BCNU)	Nausea, vomiting, diarrhea Hypotension Alcohol intoxication (drug is reconstituted in an alcohol base) Stomatitis Veno-occlusive disease (hepatic failure occurs in first 4 weeks)	Administer antiemetic at scheduled intervals. Monitor blood pressure (BP) throughout administration. Maintain adequate hydration. Monitor for possible intoxication, maintain safe environment, and keep patient in bed during administration and several hours afterward. Monitor for ascites, edema, and elevated liver function. Administer diuretics, lactulose, and albumin and restrict fluids as ordered.
Cyclophosphamide (Cytoxan)	Nausea, vomiting, diarrhea Hemorrhagic cystitis Alopecia Cardiac toxicity	Administer antiemetic at scheduled intervals. Maintain adequate hydration. Monitor for blood in urine. Maintain continuous bladder irrigation as ordered and provide catheter care. Administer mesna and pain medications as ordered. Ensure that electrocardiogram is done and verified before administration of each dose.
Cytarabine (ARA-C)	Nausea, vomiting, diarrhea Erythema Neurotoxicity Hemorrhagic conjunctivitis Alopecia	Administer antiemetics at scheduled intervals. Monitor palms and soles for erythema, provide creams and assistance with activities of daily living as needed. Monitor for cerebellar toxicity (ataxia). Administer steroid eye drops at scheduled intervals up to 48 h after last dose.
Etoposide (VP-16)	Nausea, vomiting, diarrhea Hypotension Alopecia	Administer antiemetics at scheduled intervals. Monitor BP throughout administration. Maintain adequate hydration. See Chapter 23 for additional chemotherapy drug information.
Total-body irradiation (TBI)	Nausea, vomiting, diarrhea Stomatitis Alopecia Veno-occlusive disease Fever Parotitis Erythema	Administer antiemetics 30 min before and immediately after treatment. Monitor for ascites, edema, and elevated liver function. Administer diuretics, lactulose, albumin, and fluid restriction as ordered. Monitor temperature every 2 to 4 hours and observe fever pattern. Assess for signs and symptoms of infection. Administer antipyretics as ordered. Apply hot/cold packs to affected areas. Administer pain medications as ordered. Monitor skin integrity and keep skin clean and dry. Avoid harsh soaps and irritants. If desquamation occurs, use dressings, ointments only as ordered. See Chapter 22 for additional radiation therapy information.

cure of the disease not the conditioning regimen itself.[42] Specific regimens remain under investigation; fludarabine, single-dose TBI or a combination have been used.

Transplantation of Marrow and Stem Cells

After completion of the conditioning regimen, the bone marrow or stem cells must be infused. If the regimen was one in which chemotherapy was the last treatment given, there is a rest period of 24 to 72 hours before transplant. This rest period is necessary because of the drug's half-life. Compared with the donor search, extensive pretransplant work-up, and toxic conditioning regimen, most patients describe the actual transplantation of marrow as quite anticlimactic.

For autologous BMT, the frozen marrow or stem cells are brought to the recipient's room for transplant. The bag of cells is thawed in a normal saline bath, drawn up in large syringes, and given through a rapid intravenous (IV) push via central venous catheter. The

TABLE 25-8
Common Antibiotics, Antifungals, and Antivirals Administered after Transplant

Medication	Route/Dose	Indications/Precautions
ANTIBIOTICS		
Cefoperazone	IV 2 g every 8 h	Suspected gram-negative sepsis. Infuse over 30 min. Not approved for pediatric patients. Monitor prothrombin time and for diarrhea. Administer vitamin K as ordered.
Ceftazidime	IV 150 mg/kg/d every 8 h	Suspected gram-negative sepsis. Infuse over 30 min. Maximum dose 2 g every 8 h. Monotherapy for pediatric patients, second-line therapy for adults. Monitor for diarrhea and development of drug resistance.
Norfloxacin	PO 400 mg BID	Reduction of bowel flora, anaerobes. Administer on empty stomach. Do not administer with antacids or carafate. Monitor for rash, nausea, vomiting, and diarrhea. Discontinue when granulocyte recovery is maintained.
Penicillin VK	PO 250 mg BID	Prophylaxis of gram-positive infections after BMT. Check for allergy to penicillin. Monitor for rash.
Tobramycin	IV 5 mg/kg/d	Suspected gram-negative sepsis. Infuse over 20-30 min. Do not administer at same time as ceftazidime or cefoperozone. Monitor peak and trough blood levels. Monitor for nephrotoxicity (elevated BUN and creatinine) and ototoxicity (ataxia, diminished hearing).
Trimethoprim-sulfamethoxazole	PO 1 DS tablet BID IV 15-20 mg/kg/d	Prophylaxis of *Pneumocystis carinii* pneumonia after BMT. Avoid with sulfa allergy. Administer per transplant center protocol. Monitor for rash, decreasing WBC, and increasing BUN and creatinine.
Vancomycin	IV 1 g every 12 h (adult patients) IV 40 mg/kg/d (pediatric patients) PO 125 mg every 6 h	Suspected or proven gram-positive infections. Infuse over 60 min. PO is used for *Clostridium difficile* enterocolitis only (not absorbed orally). Monitor peak and trough blood levels. Monitor for nephrotoxicity (elevated BUN and creatinine) and ototoxicity (ataxia, diminished hearing).
ANTIFUNGALS		
Amphotericin B	IV 0.5-1 mg/kg/d	Treatment of fungal infections resistant to fluconazole. Infuse through D_5W only over 3-6 h. Administer test dose at initiation of therapy (1 mg in 100 mL D_5W). Monitor for increased temperature and chilling rigor during infusion. Premedicate with diphenhydramine, acetaminophen, or hydrocortisone as ordered. Monitor electrolytes and for nephrotoxicity.
Fluconazole	PO 500 mg BID IV 100-200 mg/d	PO for reduction of bowel flora (used with norfloxacin). IV for treatment of fungemia. Monitor for overgrowth of resistant strains of fungus—surveillance cultures. Monitor for elevated liver function tests and nephrotoxicity. Discontinue PO when granulocyte recovery is maintained.
ANTIVIRALS		
Acyclovir	PO or IV 250-500 mg/m² every 8 h	Prophylaxis and treatment of herpes simplex virus (HSV) or cytomegalovirus (CMV). Infuse over 2 h (doses > 500 mg must be diluted in 500 mL fluid). Monitor for increased BUN and creatinine.

TABLE 25-8

Common Antibiotics, Antifungals, and Antivirals Administered after Transplant *Continued*

Medication	Route/Dose	Indications/Precautions
Ganciclovir	IV 2.5 mg/kg every 8 h IV 5 mg/kg every 12 h	Prophylaxis and treatment of CMV. Infuse over 1 h; handle administration and disposal using chemotherapy precautions. Administer with immunoglobulin for cases of CMV pneumonitis. Monitor for decreased WBC and increased BUN and creatinine. Colony-stimulating factors may be given to maintain WBC.
Foscarnet	IV 40–60 mg/kg every 8 h	Second-line therapy for HSV or CMV infections. Monitor for electrolyte distrubances, nephrotoxicity, and decreased WBC. Monitor for seizure activity.
Immunoglobulin	IV 0.4 g/kg every week for 6 wk PO 50 mg/kg/d every 6 h	IV prophylaxis for HSV and CMV. IV treatment for CMV pneumonitis in conjunction with ganciclovir. PO treatment of rotavirus. Administer IV slowly 20–30 mL/h. Monitor for chills, hypotension, and increased temperature during infusion.

bag of cells can also be hung and transfused. The entire process takes approximately 20 to 30 minutes depending on the volume of cells being transplanted. Patients often experience minimal shortness of breath, because of the rapid infusion of the bone marrow or stem cells, and nausea and vomiting from the preservative DMSO. DMSO also gives off a strange garlic-like odor as it is excreted through the patient's respiratory system for 24 to 48 hours after autologous transplant.

For allogeneic BMT, the marrow or stem cells are infused on the same day as they are collected. This procedure resembles an RBC transfusion in that the bag of marrow is hung and transfused via the patient's central venous catheter. Unfiltered tubing must be used to prevent precious stem cells from becoming trapped and not being infused. The total time of infusion depends on the amount of marrow or stem cells but usually lasts between 1 and 5 hours. Possible side effects from an allogeneic transplant are similar to those that can occur with a blood transfusion: shortness of breath, chills, fever, rash, chest pain, and hypotension. These reactions are more likely to occur if the marrow is ABO incompatible. If reactions do occur, the patient is treated with diphenhydramine, hydrocortisone, epinephrine, and oxygen therapy as necessary.

Patients may be premedicated with diphenhydramine or hydrocortisone or both to prevent or minimize these reactions. In both transplant procedures, emergency equipment is always available at the patient's bedside. The physician is also available throughout the entire transplant. The nursing staff is responsible for closely monitoring vital signs and for signs and symptoms of reaction. Teaching is also an important aspect of nursing care. The patient and family/significant others will have been exposed to much information about this procedure before its occurrence; however, several questions always arise, along with patient and family anxiety, on this eventful day. Some patients view their transplant day as a "birthday" of sorts, because in their eyes they are given a new chance at life.

Engraftment Period

The engraftment period is the time immediately after transplant when the transfused stem cells migrate, by some unknown phenomenon, to the recipient's bone marrow space and begin to regenerate. The time to engraftment varies with the source of the stem cells. Engraftment of bone marrow typically takes 2 to 3 weeks. Patients receiving PBSCs engraft as early as 5 days and on average 11 to 16 days after stem cell reinfusion. Cord blood takes an average of 26 days but as long as 42 days to engraft. During this period the patient experiences severe pancytopenia and immunosuppression. Immediate complications that can occur include infection and bleeding. The patient's care during this time focuses on prevention of and early treatment of infection and bleeding. Patients typically receive antibiotics and blood components during this time (Tables 25–8 and 25–9).

Because infections and bleeding can be major complications immediately after transplant, one goal is to shorten the length of the pancytopenic period. Hematopoietic growth factors aid in this process (see Chapter 24). These include, but are not limited to, GM-CSF and G-CSF. These factors affect the function of mature myeloid cells and the ability to stimulate the proliferation of myeloid precursor cells at various stages of differentiation.[100]

TABLE 25-9
Blood Component Therapy

Component	Indications	Special Considerations
PACKED RED BLOOD CELLS (PRBCs)	Hemoglobin is < 8.0 g. Patient is symptomatic. Active bleeding occurs.	Type and cross-match procedure is necessary. Infuse over 2–4 h. Monitor for transfusion reaction (fever, chills, urticaria).
Leukocyte-poor PRBCs: leukocytes are removed during transfusion.	Patient has experienced febrile transfusion reactions. Patient is at risk for alloimmunization.	Infuse through a special filter (Pall).
Washed PRBCs: blood is washed with 1000 mL normal saline and repacked before transfusion.	Patient has known severe allergic reaction to plasma and leukocytes.	Infuse at 20–30 gt/min until completion of unit. Unit expires within 24 h of washing.
PLATELET CONCENTRATES	Platelet count is < 20,000 Active bleeding occurs. Platelets are given before minor procedures or surgery.	ABO compatibility is preferred but not necessary. 1-h or 24-h posttransfusion increments are monitored to determine effectiveness. Splenomegaly, disseminated intravascular coagulation, fever, and sepsis may increase demand. Monitor for transfusion reactions. Prophylaxis is done with diphenhydramine, acetaminophen, and hydrocortisone.
Random-donor platelets (RDPs): several units (6–10) harvested from whole blood are pooled into one bag.	Patient has had no prior transfusions. Patient has had no reactions or alloimmunization.	Units expire about 4 h after pooling.
Leukocyte-poor RDPs: leukocytes are removed before or during transfusion.	Patient is at risk for alloimmunization. Patient has experienced febrile transfusion reactions.	Unit is either centrifuged and leukocytes mechanically trapped (Leukotrap) or a special filter (Pall) is used for infusion.
Single-donor platelets (SDPs): platelets are collected by pheresis from one donor.	Patient is refractory to RDPs Patient is at risk for alloimmunization	Try to match ABO/Rh of patient. Usually transfuse with special filter (Pall). Unit expires within 24 h of collection.
HLA-matched platelets: platelets are collected by pheresis from a donor whose HLA typing closely matches patient's type.	Patient is refractory to RDPs and SDPs Patient is at risk for alloimmunization.	Patient must have been HLA typed. Unit expires within 24 h of collection.
Resuspended platelets: plasma is removed from pooled units, and an equivalent amount of normal saline is added.	Patient has experienced severe reaction to platelet concentrates despite prophylaxis.	Prophylaxis is usually needed.
FRESH FROZEN PLASMA	Patient has had multiple PRBC transfusions. Abnormal coagulation factors are evident.	Provide ABO-compatible component. Transfuse immediately after thawing.
IRRADIATED COMPONENTS	Severely immunocompromised patients are at risk for GVHD.	Component is not radioactive.
Gamma radiation delivered to blood components inactivates lymphocytes within product.		Component should be labeled as being irradiated. RBCs and platelets are not affected.

Both GM-CSF and G-CSF are myeloid-stimulating factors. GM-CSF (sargramostin) activates mature granulocytes and macrophages and has a multilineage factor. GM-CSF is indicated for the acceleration of myeloid recovery in patients with non-Hodgkin's lymphoma, ALL, and Hodgkin's disease undergoing autologous BMT. G-CSF (filgrastim) is lineage specific and regulates the production of neutrophils within the bone marrow. It reduces the incidence of infection, as manifested by febrile neutropenia in patients with nonmyeloid malignancies who are receiving myelosuppressive anticancer drugs associated with severe neutropenia and fever.

Studies of erythropoietin in transplant patients continue. A review of the studies has shown a decrease in the need for RBC transfusions in the allogeneic population.[49] The efficacy of erythropoietin following autologous transplant remains to be seen.[49] Balance the benefit of erythropoietin compared to the cost of therapy remains a significant issue.[49, 58]

COMPLICATIONS OF MARROW AND STEM CELL TRANSPLANTATION

Transplant recipients experience toxic complications associated with the procedure. Most complications result from the effects of the conditioning regimen. The major complications characteristic of transplant are graft failure, infections, pneumonitis, veno-occlusive disease, GVHD, and recurrence of original disease (Table 25–10).

Graft Failure

Graft failure or rejection after transplant is a relatively rare occurrence, but an incidence of 5% to 15% has been reported.[1] *Graft failure* is defined as failure of marrow recovery to return or the loss of marrow function after an initial period of recovery.[2, 4] An increased risk of graft failure is seen in patients who receive T-cell–depleted marrow, a low marrow cell dose, or HLA-mismatched marrow or who have extensive marrow fibrosis before BMT. Patients with aplastic anemia who have been previously transfused or receive only cyclophosphamide for their conditioning regimen are at an increased risk for graft failure.[4]

Infection

Infection is the most common post transplant complication. Alterations in the integrity of physical barriers and severe granulocytopenia from the pretransplant regimen set up an environment for serious bacterial and fungal infections. One half of all infections occur in the first 4 to 6 weeks after transplant.[30] Usually the causative agents are from the patient's own microflora, particularly from the gastrointestinal (GI) tract and integumentary system. Common agents are gram-positive and gram-negative bacteria, such as *Staphylococcus, Streptococcus, Klebsiella,* and *Pseudomonas.*[76] Fungal infections are less common than bacterial infections, accounting for only 10% to 15% of systemic infections.[98] The use of prophylactic fluconazole has decreased the incidence of candidosis; aspergillus has become the most common posttransplant fungal infection.[89]

Viral infections occur at varying times after BMT. Herpes simplex virus (HSV) reactivation generally occurs in the early posttransplant period but the incidence can be dramatically decreased in seropositive patients who receive prophylactic acyclovir.[89] Cytomegalovirus (CMV) infection generally occurs 3 to 6 months after transplant. With the newer early detection techniques available and ganciclovir prophylaxis, the incidence of CMV disease has decreased.[89] Varicella-zoster virus (VZV) is usually not seen until later in the first year after the transplant. Viral infections, especially CMV and VZV, are also typically associated with the incidence of chronic GVHD and can occur at any time during the course of chronic GVHD.[83]

During the first 6 weeks after BMT, prevention of infections is the most important step in counteracting infections. Maintaining protective environments, providing good hygiene, frequently monitoring vital signs, and performing head-to-toe assessments are very important. The greater the speed of marrow recovery, the less is the incidence of bacterial and fungal complications.[52] For this reason, the use of growth factors to stimulate engraftment has become routine.

Pulmonary

Interstitial pneumonia accounts for 40% of transplant-related deaths.[78] During the early posttransplant neutropenic period, bacterial infections account for 20% to 50% of pulmonary infections.[62] Interstitial pneumonia typically occurs within the first 100 days after transplant. The risk factors for developing pneumonia include use of immunosuppressants, lung damage, use of TBI, and presence of opportunistic organisms.[78] Interstitial pneumonia can be caused by an infection or it can be idiopathic. The most common viral cause is CMV. It is important that all patients and donors are screened for CMV prior to transplant so patients at risk can receive the appropriate treatment. Screening consists of serologic testing for CMV antibodies. In an allogeneic transplant a seropositive donor can transmit CMV to a seronegative recipient. Patients who are CMV seropositive or have a seropositive donor generally receive ganciclovir as prophylaxis. Ganciclovir is initiated after the patient is well engrafted. Lung damage can also be caused by carmustine and TBI although this does not

TABLE 25-10

Major Complications after Transplant

Complication	Appearance	Signs/Symptoms	Management
GRAFT REJECTION	1–4 wk	Absent/prolonged neutropenia Partial marrow recovery Hypoplasia Hemolysis	Administer blood component therapy. Consider retransplantation.

INFECTION
Bacterial
Fungal
Viral
  Herpes virus
  Cytomegalovirus (CMV)
  Varicella-zoster virus
	
	1–5 wk
	1–5 wk
	
	1–3 mo
	3 mo
	1st year
		Fever
		Dry, nonproductive cough
		Change in breath sounds
		Erythema—oropharynx/catheter site
		Diarrhea
		Shortness of breath, fever
		Lesions—skin or mucous membranes
		Hypotension
			Maintain protective environment.
			
			Provide good hygiene.
			Monitor vital signs frequently.
			Perform frequent head-to-toe systems assessments.
			Administer colony-stimulating factors.
			Ensure CMV-negative blood products.
			Administer broad-spectrum antibiotics.
			Administer acyclovir and/or ganciclovir.
			Administer IV immunoglobulins.

VENO-OCCLUSIVE DISEASE (VOD)	1–3 wk	Weight gain Ascites Hepatomegaly Right upper quadrant pain Bilirubin level above 2 mg/dL	Maintain intravascular volume. Administer RBCs and IV fluids. Frequent physical assessments. Weigh twice daily. Measure abdominal girth daily. Administer low-dose dopamine, heparin, and/or recombinant tissue plasminogen activator (rTPA).
PNEUMONITIS Interstitial Toxic	 1–4 mo 1–6 mo	Fever Dry, nonproductive cough Shortness of breath Tachypnea interstitial changes on x-ray film	Ensure CMV-negative blood products. Ensure leukocyte-poor blood products. Administer colony-stimulating factors. Administer ganciclovir. Administer IV immunoglobulins.
ACUTE GVHD	3–14 wk	Maculopapular skin rash Nausea, vomiting uncontrollable diarrhea Jaundice Elevated liver function tests Hepatomegaly	Provide immunosuppression with cyclosporine, steroids, methotrexate, and/or tacrolimus (Prograf). Provide symptomatic treatment of skin, gastrointestinal tract, and/or liver.
CHRONIC GVHD Skin Mouth Eyes Sinuses Gastrointestinal tract	 Months-years	 Hyperpigmentation or hypopigmentation, patchy erythematous scaling, thickening/hardening resembling scleroderma, hair loss in involved areas White striae and erythema on mucosa, decreased salivary flow with dryness of mouth Dryness, redness, itching/burning; corneal thickening Chronic sinusitis, predisposition to gram-positive infections Difficulty swallowing, retrosternal pain, abdominal discomfort, diarrhea	Provide immunosuppression with cyclosporine, steroids, azathioprine (Imuran), and/or thalidomide (investigational). Manage symptoms of affected organ or system.

TABLE 25–10

Major Complications after Transplant *Continued*

Complication	Appearance	Signs/Symptoms	Management
Pulmonary		Productive cough, progressive dyspnea, wheezing, pneumothorax	
Vagina		Inflammation, dryness, stenosis	
Muscle		Occasional polymyositis, proximal weakness	
Genitourinary tract		Cystitis, mild nephrotic syndrome	
Hematopoietic		Eosinophilia, thrombocytopenia, hypoplastic marrow, marrow fibrosis	
Lymphoid		Hypocellularity and atrophy of lymph tissues, functional asplenia	
Endocrine		Decreased growth rates, delayed pubertal development, autoimmune hyperthyroidism	
Nervous system		Entrapment neuropathy, peripheral neuropathy, myasthenia gravis	
LATE EFFECTS			
Cataracts	1–6 y	Loss of vision	Consider surgical intervention.
		Dryness	
Gonad dysfunction	Variable	Infertility	Administer replacement sex hormones.
		Menopause	Refer for psychosexual counseling.
Growth failure	Variable	Impaired growth of facial skeleton and dentition (<6 y old)	Administer supplemental growth hormone.
		Absent growth spurts	Administer replacement sex hormones.
		No height changes	
Hypothyroidism	1–15 y	Dry skin	Administer replacement hormones.
		Hoarse speech	
		Lethargy/apathy	
		Weight gain with appetite loss	
		Increased susceptibility to cold	
Secondary malignancy	Months-years	Specific to disease	Determine by type and extent of disease and patient's physical and psychologic status.
RECURRENCE			
	Months-years	Signs/symptoms of original disease.	Determine by extent and patient's physical and psychological status.

often manifest itself until 3 to 4 months after transplant. When recognized early and treated with steroids the damage is reversible.

Veno-occlusive Disease

Veno-occlusive disease (VOD) of the liver occurs in approximately 20% of patients undergoing allogeneic BMT and 10% of patients undergoing autologous BMT. Mortality rates of up to 50% have been reported. VOD is a complication of the conditioning regimen; the risk is greater for those patients receiving TBI. VOD is the occlusion of the central veins of the liver resulting in venous congestion and stasis; this results in damage to the hepatic cells. The onset of VOD is usually early after BMT, in the first 3 weeks, but has been seen later. VOD is usually diagnosed by its classic symptoms of weight gain greater than 5% over baseline, hepatomegaly, right upper quadrant pain, total serum bilirubin level above 2 mg/dL, and ascites. Risk factors include a history of hepatitis, elevated transaminase at the time of transplant, mismatched or unrelated transplant, and the use of methotrexate as GVHD prophylaxis.

Treatment is aimed at maintaining intravascular volume to minimize further liver damage and maintain renal perfusion. Other treatment approaches remain controversial. Low-dose dopamine infusions have been used to increase renal perfusion, but this practice has been questioned. Low-dose heparin infusions also have been used for prophylaxis and treatment; some studies show favorable results in decreasing the incidence of VOD but results are inconclusive. Prostaglandin has vasodilatory, antithrombotic, and thrombolytic effects. Early studies in the use of prostaglandins for treating

VOD have shown efficacy but have also shown significant toxicity. Recombinant tissue plasminogen activator (rTPA), a thrombolytic agent, has been used to treat VOD, and early studies show it to be safe and effective in about 50% of patients.[73, 99] More recently infusions of antithrombin III concentrate have been used to treat VOD and appears promising.[64]

Graft-Versus-Host Disease

Graft-versus-host disease is a complication that can occur after allogeneic transplantation. It is an immune-mediated reaction of the newly grafted stem cells to the body of the recipient. The source of stem cells can affect the incidence of GVHD. Stem cells from UCB appear to cause less GVHD.[41] There does not appear to be a significant difference in the incidence of acute GVHD with the use of allogeneic PBSCs but the incidence of chronic GVHD may be higher.[84] Two types of GVHD have been identified: acute and chronic. They are distinguished from each other by the target organs, pathology, and timing after BMT. Chronic GVHD may occur after acute GVHD, but not always. A patient may also develop chronic GVHD without ever having had acute GVHD.

Acute GVHD. Acute GVHD is typically defined as occurring before 100 days after BMT. There is a 45% incidence in HLA-matched sibling donor transplants and greater than 75% incidence in HLA-mismatched related donor transplants.[31] The risk factors related to the incidence of acute GVHD are advanced patient age (> 45 years), HLA mismatch, and donor-recipient gender mismatch.[31, 55] The skin, GI tract, and liver are the primary target organs of acute GVHD. The occurrence of acute GVHD also prolongs immunodeficiency.

Skin involvement is characterized by a maculopapular rash that can proceed to a desquamating dermatitis. A biopsy of the skin is necessary to confirm the diagnosis and rule out other causes for the rash. In the first 20 days after BMT, this can be difficult because of changes in the skin related to the conditioning regimen. The GI involvement is typically characterized by nausea, vomiting, and diarrhea. Again, a biopsy of the GI mucosa is the only definitive way to make a diagnosis. The pathologic changes seen in the GI tract are similar to those seen in the skin. In both the skin and the GI mucosa, secondary infections can occur because the acute GVHD has altered their integrity. Liver involvement is characterized by jaundice, elevated liver function studies, and hepatomegaly.

Acute GVHD can range from mild to life-threatening and is graded to distinguish its severity (Table 25–11). In its mildest form, acute GVHD typically can be controlled and actually benefits those patients receiving transplants for malignancies. Patients with acute GVHD have a decreased incidence of disease recurrence.[25]

Because acute GVHD can be a life-threatening complication, means of preventing its occurrence are routinely administered. One of the most common means of preventing GVHD is the use of cyclosporine, steroids, and methotrexate (MTX). Tacrolimus (Prograf) is an immunosuppressant similar pharmacologically to cyclosporine but about 100 times more potent. Early studies show a lower incidence of GVHD using tacrolimus instead of cyclosporine, but randomized clinical trials are ongoing.[2] All these agents provide immunosuppression after BMT and are given according to a scheduled regimen (Table 25–12). Because GVHD is immune mediated, suppressing immune reactions after BMT should prevent its occurrence. The T cells have been identified as the primary culprit in GVHD. Depleting the marrow of T cells before infusion into the recipient has greatly reduced the incidence and severity of acute GVHD.[31] However, the incidence of graft rejection and relapse is also significantly increased.[31]

Treatment for acute GVHD centers around increasing immune suppression. Often first-line therapy for GVHD is prednisone. Antithymocyte globulin (ATG) is often used as second-line therapy. Increasing the doses of cyclosporine or tacrolimus may also be beneficial, but serum drug levels must be closely monitored. Mycophenolate mofetil an immunosuppressant used in

TABLE 25–11
Acute Graft-Versus-Host Disease (GVHD) Severity Grading

Stage	Skin	Liver	GI Tract
+	Maculopapular rash over < 25% of body surface	Bilirubin 2–3 mg/dL	Diarrhea > 500 mL/d
++	Maculopapular rash over 25–30% of body surface	Bilirubin 3–6 mg/dL	Diarrhea > 1000 mL/d
+++	Generalized erythroderma	Bilirubin 6–15 mg/dL	Diarrhea > 1500 mL/d
++++	Generalized erythroderma with bullous formation (> 2 cm vesicle) and desquamation	Bilirubin > 15 mg/dL	Severe abdominal pain with or without ileus

TABLE 25–12
Example of Immunosuppression Schedule

Day of BMT	Cyclosporine	Methylprednisolone
−2	IV 5 mg/kg/d continuous infusion	
+4	IV 3 mg/kg/d continuous infusion	
+8		IVP 0.5 mg/kg BID
+15	IV 3.75 mg/kg/d continuous infusion	IVP 0.375 mg/kg BID
+23		IVP 0.25 mg/kg BID
+29	PO 7.5 mg/kg BID	
+31		PO 0.125 mg/kg BID
+36	PO 5 mg/kg BID	
+38		PO 0.25 mg/kg × 1
+40		PO 0.25 mg/kg × 1
+42		PO 0.25 mg/kg × 1
+84	PO 4 mg/kg BID	
+98	PO 3 mg/kg BID	
+120	PO 2 mg/kg BID	
+181	Discontinue	

IV, Intravenous; IVP, IV push; PO, orally.

solid organ transplants shows promise in the treatment of GVHD.[6] About 50% of patients with grade II or III GVHD respond to treatment. The mortality rate can be as high as 50%.[2, 4]

Chronic GVHD. The onset of chronic GVHD is typically 100 days after transplant; however, it can occur at 70 days or years after transplant. It affects as many as 50% of matched sibling transplants and is life-threatening in about 5% of cases. It is characterized by scleroderma-like features and persistent immunodeficiency. It is a systemic multiorgan syndrome that resembles collagen-vascular diseases.[31] Chronic GVHD can be *Progressive,* a continuation of acute GVHD, *Quiescent,* occurring after acute GVHD has resolved, or it can be *DeNovo,* occurring without any acute GVHD preceding it.[19] The risk factors related to incidence are advanced age of recipient (> 45 years), occurrence of preceding acute GVHD, T-cell–replete marrow, and female donor to male recipient.[31]

Almost every organ in the body can be affected by chronic GVHD (see Table 25–10). The basic effect is that of dermal thickening, fibrosis, and dryness. Bacterial, fungal, and viral infections are common in patients with chronic GVHD and are the most frequent cause of death.[19] Late interstitial pneumonitis occurs frequently. Mortality is highest in patients with progressive acute to chronic GVHD and those with multiorgan involvement.[19] Currently, standard treatment for chronic GVHD is prednisone; it is effective in 50% to 70% of cases.[4] Other agents have been used such as cyclosporine, tacrolimus, azathioprine, plasmapheresis, ATG, and thalidomide.[31]

Recurrence

Disease recurrence remains the most significant problem after transplantation. It is the major factor related to patient mortality longer than 3 months after BMT. Relapse is more frequent after autologous BMT presumably because of hidden malignant cells in the transplanted stem cells.[19] In allogeneic transplantation the presence of GVHD is associated with decreased incidence of recurrence.[19] Some patients have been successfully retransplanted. Factors associated with better survival after a second transplant are a diagnosis of CML, AML in remission, good performance status, and duration of posttransplant remission of longer than 1 year. Patients with CML who relapse have been successfully treated with interferon.[2, 4]

Late Effects

Long-term effects of BMT can occur several months to several years after transplant. Late effects are a common concern as more patients survive disease-free for as long as 20 years after BMT. The more common effects are cataracts, hypothyroidism, growth failure, gonadal dysfunction, and secondary malignancies. The late effects of BMT are of particular concern in the pediatric population and for patients with the possibility of cure with less intensive treatment.[75]

Cataracts. Cataracts are of concern primarily in patients who receive TBI. Because radiation is more commonly being given in fractionated doses, the incidence of cataracts has decreased. Patients receiving TBI in a single dose have an 80% incidence of cataracts versus a 20% incidence when TBI is given in fractionated doses.[16] Patients receiving conditioning regimens of chemotherapy only do not have significant risk of developing cataracts.

Gonadal Dysfunction. Sexual development is impaired in both men and women. Older patients (> 40 years) are less likely to recover their reproductive functioning.[75] After TBI most women (75%) experience ovarian failure and require hormone replacement.[75] After TBI, most men will recover production of testosterone but have absent or abnormal spermatogenesis.[75] If TBI is not used as part of the conditioning regimen, both men and women have a better chance of recovering gonadal functioning. There are several reports of patients having children after transplant.[75]

Growth Failure. Impairment of growth is a common problem in children after transplantation. Again, the incidence is high in those children who received TBI.[16] Of children who received TBI, 50% to 60% have decreased growth hormone, causing a retardation of spinal growth and the pubertal growth spurt.[75] Administration of growth hormone has shown some effect on growth velocity, and some catch up in growth can occur.

Hypothyroidism. The incidence of hypothyroidism is also related to preparation with TBI. Thyroid function is affected in as many as 60% of patients receiving single-dose TBI and as many as 25% of those receiving fractionated TBI.[19] Patients who have received conditioning regimens of chemotherapy only usually have normal thyroid function.

Secondary Malignancy. New malignancies may develop 6 months to years after BMT. A 4% to 6% incidence of secondary malignancies has been reported in long-term survivors of allogeneic BMT.[2, 75] TBI, immunosuppression, immunodeficiency, viral infection, chronic immune stimulation, and genetic predisposition are factors that have been identified with increased risk of second malignancy after BMT.[75] Radiation appears to be the most important risk factor. Lymphoproliferative disorders such as ALL, and non-Hodgkin's lymphoma are among the most frequently reported new malignancies and develop more often in donor cells.[19] Most often the appearance of leukemia is a recurrence of the original disease.[19] Overall, BMT recipients have a sixfold to sevenfold higher tumor incidence than nontransplanted individuals.[19]

Quality of Life/Survivorship. Interest on the part of researchers in quality of life after BMT has increased in recent years. A number of studies have been done to assess quality of life at various intervals after transplant. A number of tools have been used to collect this information. Some examples are Profile of Mood States, Psychological Adjustment to Illness Scale, Functional Living Index—Cancer, and the Cancer Rehabilitation Evaluation System. There is a need for more research in this area to develop better tools and determine the best times to measure quality of life throughout the transplant process.[96, 97]

ACCREDITATION

In recent years with the increase in the number of transplant centers, there has been a call to establish standards and regulate transplant programs. In 1994, standards were developed by the Foundation for the Accreditation of Hematopoietic Cell Therapy (FAHCT). FAHCT was created by the International Society for Hematotherapy and Graft Engineering (ISHAGE) and the American Society of Blood and Marrow Transplantation

(ASBMT). The major goal of FAHCT is to promote quality transplant programs. The standards encompass all aspects of a transplant program, cell collection, processing, and transplantation. Accreditation is voluntary; however, it is likely that in the near future third-party payers will look at FAHCT accreditation as a standard for reimbursement.

FUTURE DIRECTIONS AND ADVANCES IN BONE MARROW AND STEM CELL TRANSPLANTATION

According to data from the International Bone Marrow Transplant Registry, the number of patients undergoing BMT continues to increase annually. Future advances will include the use of cord blood stem cells for gene therapy because they are more efficient at taking up genes than are stem cells from other sources; fetal therapy; transplanting stem cells in utero for patients with congenital diseases such as SCIDS; and expansion of stem cells in the laboratory so fewer stem cells will be needed. Collection of PBSC is already expanding to include allogeneic donors; we can expect this to increase. The donor pool will continue to expand with an increase in the number of donors in the NMDP.

Outpatient resources and transplantation via the outpatient mode will continue to expand. Third-party reimbursement, length of hospital stay, and financial resources for medications used in transplant recovery will have ongoing scrutiny.

Ongoing research will continue to look for better conditioning regimens and more effective treatments for infection and GVHD. Manipulation of the immune response against tumor cells following transplant using cellular therapy and cytokines is being explored. Use of peripheral blood CD34$^+$ cells for gene therapy is also under investigation, as is combining immunotherapy with transplant.

CONCLUSION

Bone marrow transplantation, regardless of the source of stem cells, offers cure and new hope for the future to many patients with life-threatening diseases. Continued expansion of the donor pool and ongoing research exploring better conditioning regimens, hematopoietic growth factors, and antibiotic/antifungal/antiviral drugs will be ongoing challenges. Financial reimbursement issues will continue to be a challenge; managed care is already having an impact. Many insurance companies are already expecting transplant centers to negotiate a fixed price; this will increase competition among transplant centers, because the lowest bidder will get the contracts and therefore the patients. Many third-party payers already require transplant centers to sign contracts as "centers of excellence" or preferred providers. Patients will no longer be able to choose a transplant center. There will be ongoing debate about which indications for transplantation are experimental. Transplantation is constantly changing but this challenging practice environment will continue to provide opportunities for skilled nurses.

The following is a list of resources and support services for patients and families undergoing bone marrow transplantation:

1. American Cancer Society, Atlanta, GA
2. Aplastic Anemia Foundation of America, Baltimore, MD
3. BMT Family Support Network, Avon, CT
4. BMT Link, Southfield, MI
5. BMT Newsletter, Highland Park, IL
6. Cancer Information Service, Bethesda, MD
7. Candlelighters Childhood Cancer Foundation, Bethesda, MD
8. Children's Transplant Association, Dallas, TX
9. Corporate Angel Network, White Plains, NY
10. Immune Deficiency Foundation, Bethesda, MD
11. Leukemia Society of America, New York, NY
12. LIFE-SAVERS Foundation of America, Covina, CA
13. National Marrow Donor Program, Minneapolis, MN
14. National Cancer Institute, Bethesda, MD
15. National Children's Cancer Society, St. Louis, MO
16. National Coalition of Cancer Survivorship, Silver Spring, MD
17. Oncology Nursing Society Bone Marrow Transplant Special Interest Group, Pittsburgh, PA
18. Ronald McDonald Houses and Children's Charities, Chicago, IL

Nursing Management

Bone marrow and stem cell transplantation is a strenuous medical treatment that in and of itself can be life-threatening. As with any major medical treatment and life-threatening situation faced by patients and families, the general stresses that affect these individuals must be addressed. These stresses are not necessarily unique to transplant; however, throughout the transplant process there are periods of transition when these general stresses increase in occurrence or intensity.

Prior experiences affect a patient/family examination of the risks and benefits of transplant. For some patients, the decision to have a transplant comes on the heels of being informed that they have a life-threatening illness and transplant must be done as soon as possible and is the only chance of cure. For other patients, the decision for transplant comes after a course or more of chemotherapy and living with their disease for a period of time pretransplant. Still other patients are informed at the time of diagnosis that a transplant is the only curative option and needs to be done within a certain time frame. Also affecting the patient's reaction to transplant is the ability to locate a donor if the patient cannot be his or her own donor and does not have a match within his or her family.

The idea of transplantation as a treatment option generally creates a wide spectrum of emotional reactions. Patients may experience anxiety, fear, depression, denial, grieving, and hopefulness all at different times. Coping styles that the patient and family have relied on in the past will be those they most likely fall back on at this time. Dysfunctional or disruptive coping behaviors, such as substance abuse, may resurface. Past or current psychiatric problems may also become intensified.

Everyday life for these patients and their families will be disrupted by transplantation. There will be changes in patients' roles within the family. When the transplant center is a distance from home, the family may be separated for several months. The relocation of the patient and a family member may be necessary. Child care as well as elder care can be affected by changes in the roles of family members. New routines also have to be incorporated into family life. Lifestyle changes after transplant may be permanent or temporary and can be a major disruption on family life.

The financial impacts of transplant can be devastating to families. Transplantation is a costly treatment. This is because of the numerous resources necessary to care for the patient. The cost of housing, food, dependent care, and transportation can seriously affect the financial status of any family. Reimbursement continues to vary based on the third-party payer and the disease being treated. Third-party payers may detail which diseases they accept as being treatable by transplantation and which are experimental. Very rarely are the costs of searching for an unrelated donor covered by third parties. They may cover the cost of the patient's care throughout the transplant, but the cost of searching for an unrelated donor is not covered.

Donors for allogeneic transplants also have special considerations that need to be addressed. The most important is the one of choice. Potential donors need to be adequately educated as to their role in a transplant if they are a match. It is the donor's choice to donate. In families with less than ideal relationships, this can be a challenge. Donors also need to be aware that agreeing to donate carries some amount of responsibility for the recipient's health. However, they must also understand that once they have donated, they have no control over what happens to the recipient. This is especially important in cases where patients develop GVHD.

Caring for patients undergoing BMT requires comprehensive and consistent nursing management. Patient/family teaching is key to providing assistance to patients and family members throughout the transplant process. The table on page 753 outlines the teaching priorities by stage of transplantation. Examples of nursing diagnoses and interventions for patients undergoing BMT follow.

Nursing Diagnosis

- *Disturbance in body image, risk for, related to treatment process*

Outcome Goals

Patient will be able to:

- Verbalize and demonstrate acceptance of appearance.
- Demonstrate a willingness and ability to resume self-care roles and responsibilities.

Interventions

- Encourage patient to verbalize feelings about appearance and perceptions of life-style changes.
- Validate perceptions and ensure that responses are appropriate.
- Promote acceptance of positive, realistic body image.
- Explore ways that the patient can cope with body image changes within his or her cultural expression.

Nursing Diagnosis

- *Alteration in comfort, pain, risk for, related to side effects of treatment regimens*

Outcome Goals

Patient will be able to:

- Identify activities that increase or decrease pain.
- Relate pain relief.

Interventions

- Assess patient's pain:
  - Location
  - Onset
  - Frequency
  - Intensity
  - Quality
- Identify effective pain control measures.
- Administer medications as ordered and needed.
- Assess for effectiveness of pain control measures.
- Intervene at onset of pain.
- Instruct patient in relaxation techniques (see Chapters 27 and 30).

Nursing Diagnosis

- *Ineffective coping, individual, related to transplant process and potential life-style changes*

Outcome Goals

Patient will be able to:

- Identify coping patterns and the consequences of the behavior that results.
- Identify personal strengths and accept support.

Interventions

- Assess patient's level of distress and anxiety related to:
  - Uncertainty of future
  - Bothersome symptoms
  - Changes in self-concept
- Assess for signs of maladaptive or risky behaviors that interfere with responsible health practices.
- Identify patient's support system, resources, and communication patterns.
- Assess patient's ability to problem solve.
- Listen attentively and provide support.
- Encourage verbalization of fears.
- Assist patient with problem solving as needed.
- Provide reassurance that anxiety or distress are common feelings among transplant patients.
- Initiate referrals to social work, psychology, or community resources as appropriate (see Chapters 28 and 33).

Nursing Diagnosis

- *Ineffective coping, family, compromised, related to transplant process and role changes*

Outcome Goals

Patient/family will be able to:

- Identify responses that are neglectful or harmful.

Patient/Family Teaching Priorities by Stage of Transplantation

Topic	Before Transplant	During Transplant	After Transplant
TRANSPLANT PROCESS			
Donor identification	X		
Tissue typing	X		
Recipient workup	X		
Donor workup	X		
Goal of transplant	X	X	
Duration of process	X	X	
Conditioning regimen	X	X	
Stem cell collection	X	X	
Immunosuppression	X	X	X
Unit environment	X	X	
CENTRAL VENOUS CATHETER			
Insertion	X	X	
Catheter care	X	X	
ROUTINE CARE			
Hygiene/skin care	X	X	
Oral care	X	X	
Nutrition	X	X	
Infection precautions	X	X	
Bleeding precautions	X	X	
SIDE EFFECTS			
Nausea/vomiting	X	X	
Diarrhea	X	X	
Alopecia	X	X	
Stomatitis	X	X	
Seizures	X	X	
Hypotension	X	X	
Cystitis	X	X	
Acral erythema	X	X	
Conjunctivitis	X	X	
Fever	X	X	
Parotitis	X	X	
COMPLICATIONS			
Graft rejection	X	X	X
Infections	X	X	X
Pneumonitis	X	X	X
GVHD	X	X	X
Late effects	X	X	X
Recurrence	X	X	X
SUPPORTIVE CARE			
Blood components	X	X	X
Antibiotics	X	X	X
Antifungals	X	X	X
Antivirals	X	X	X
Parenteral nutrition	X	X	X
PSYCHOSOCIAL			
Coping strategies	X	X	X
Sexuality	X	X	X
Socialization	X	X	X
Resources	X	X	X
DISCHARGE			
Follow-up schedule		X	X
Medications		X	X
Diet		X	X
Activity	X	X	X
Precautions	X	X	X
Work/school	X	X	X
Emergency contact	X	X	X

- Verbalize the need for assistance.
- Access available community resources.

Interventions

- Assess past family relationships and coping patterns.
- Provide opportunities for family to express feelings.
- Assist family members in adapting to changes in roles and activities as appropriate.
- Listen attentively and provide support.
- Encourage communication and positive interaction between patient and family.
- Assess cultural issues that are unfamiliar.
- Initiate referrals to social work, psychology, or community resources as appropriate.

Nursing Diagnosis

- *Fluid volume deficit or excess, risk for, related to compromised regulatory mechanisms, as evidenced by altered electrolytes*

Outcome Goals

Patient will be able to:

- Maintain normal fluid volume and electrolyte balance as evidenced by:
    Normal blood and urinary laboratory values
    Maintaining baseline weight
    Normal skin turgor
    Moist mucous membranes
    Normal mentation

Interventions

- Monitor patients:
    Intake and output
    Weight
    Abdominal girth
    Edema
    Serum electrolytes
    Blood urea nitrogen
    Hemoglobin and hematocrit
- Assess patient for signs of fluid overload or dehydration.
- Administer diuretics as ordered.
- Maintain fluid restrictions as needed.

Nursing Diagnosis

- *Altered growth and development, related to late effects of treatment*

Outcome Goals

Patient will be able to:

- Demonstrate an increase in behaviors in personal, social, language, and cognition or motor activities appropriate for age-group.

Interventions

- Monitor patient's growth according to standard growth charts.
- Assess for accomplishments of normal growth and developmental tasks.
- Monitor for learning disabilities.
- Provide referrals for educational and emotional support as needed.
- Administer growth hormone as ordered and assess for response.

Nursing Diagnosis

- *Risk for infection, related to myelosuppression and immunosuppression*

Outcome Goal

Patient will be able to:

- Be free of infection as evidenced by absence of fever (< 38.5°C) and chills, pulse within normal limits, absence of adventitious breath sounds, absence of burning on urination, absence of redness or swelling at central line site, negative cultures.

Interventions

- Assess for signs and symptoms of infection:
    Fever
    Cough
    Erythema
- Institute measures to prevent exposure to potential sources of infection:
    Meticulous handwashing
    Meticulous hygiene
    Good oral hygiene after meals
- Monitor white blood count and differential.
- Monitor vital signs and head-to-toe systems assessments frequently.
- Obtain cultures of blood, urine, stool, sputum as ordered and appropriate.
- Administer antibiotics, antifungals, antivirals, and antipyretics as ordered.
- Instruct patient and family in prevention of infections.
- Monitor culture results and serum antibiotic levels as needed.
- Implement protective isolation precautions per hospital policy.
- Minimize invasive procedures.

Nursing Diagnosis

- *Risk for injury, related to thrombocytopenia*

Outcome Goals

Patient will be able to:

- Be aware of and report signs and symptoms of bleeding.
- Demonstrate measures to prevent bleeding.
- Demonstrate absence of bleeding.

Interventions

- Monitor platelet count and anticipate nadir.
- Assess for signs and symptoms of bleeding:
  Petechiae
  Ecchymosis
  Epistaxis
  Vaginal or rectal bleeding
- Administer platelet transfusions as ordered.
- Observe patient for signs of transfusion reaction and response to transfusions.
- Teach patient to avoid:
  Shaving with razor
  Flossing teeth
  Picking nose or scabs
  Forceful nose-blowing

Nursing Diagnosis

- *Knowledge deficit related to transplant process*

Outcome Goals

Patient/family will be able to:

- Discuss knowledge or experience related to BMT.
- Discuss rationale for BMT.
- Acknowledge potential therapeutic and adverse effects of BMT.
- Describe medical and nursing interventions available and required during treatment.

Interventions

- Evaluate patient and family readiness to learn.
- Identify barriers to learning such as language, physical deficiencies, psychological deficiencies, intellectual development.
- Determine patient and family knowledge of the transplant process.
- Review information patient and family have already been given.
- Provide written or audiovisual education materials and review with patient and family; consider culture-sensitive materials.

- Allow adequate time for verbalization of questions, concerns, and fears.
- Reinforce and clarify information as needed.

Nursing Diagnosis

- *Altered nutrition, less than body requirements, related to effects of treatment process*

Outcome Goals

Patient will be able to:

- Report/maintain adequate nutritional status during periods of decreased oral intake.
- Report strategies to manage altered taste.
- Experience minimal or no nausea and vomiting.

Interventions

- Assess nutritional intake and monitor calorie counts.
- Assess for causes of decreased nutritional intake:
  Nausea and vomiting
  Xerostomia
  Taste changes
- Provide small, frequent meals.
- Determine cultural preferences and meanings of foods.
- Initiate referral to dietician for assessment of food preferences and appropriateness of diet (see Chapter 29).

Nursing Diagnosis

- *Altered sexuality patterns, related to treatment process and to late effects*

Outcome Goals

Patient/significant other will be able to:

- Share concerns regarding sexual function.
- Express satisfaction with sexual patterns.

Interventions

- Assess for physical symptoms that may affect libido.
- Assess for fear, anxiety, depression, and diminished self-concept.
- Consider culture/sensitive interventions.
- Promote open communication about sexual issues by bringing up the subject.
- Instruct patient on appropriate hygiene and contraceptive measures (see Chapter 33).

Nursing Diagnosis

• *Impaired skin integrity, risk for, related to treatment process and to GVHD*

Outcome Goal

Patient will be able to:

• Have intact skin and be free of infection.

Interventions

• Assess impaired area every shift for:
    Color
    Scaling
    Bleeding
    Drainage
    Tenderness
• Avoid use of harsh soaps, hot water, perfume, deodorant, and oil-based creams.
• Maintain meticulous hygiene with antibacterial soap.
• Instruct patient to avoid activities and clothing that irritate affected areas.
• Instruct patient to avoid exposure to the sun and to use sun screen when outdoors.
• Use therapeutic beds and pain medications as needed for severe skin GVHD (see Chapters 30 and 31).

Nursing Diagnosis

• *Ineffective management of therapeutic regimen, risk for, related to posthospitalization follow-up*

Outcome Goals

Patient/family will be able to:

• Explain and discuss treatment regimen, rationale of regimen, expectations of regimen, side effects of regimen, life-style changes needed, follow-up care needed, resources support available.
• Relate an intent to practice health behaviors needed for recovery and prevention of complications.

Interventions

• Identify factors that influence learning.
• Explain the need for close follow-up after BMT.
• Explain the need to remain close to the BMT center for 100 days or as appropriate.
• Explain the expectations of family and caregiver.
• Explain home alterations needed.
• Provide written material.
• Consider culture-sensitive materials and interventions.

Chapter Questions

1. Nonmyeloablative conditioning regimens are generally used for which patients?
   a. All patients under consideration for transplantation
   b. Only young, healthy patients
   c. All patients with significant organ damage
   d. Patients over 55 with or without organ damage
2. The side effects G-CSF when used for mobilization in peripheral stem cell transplantation are:
   a. Headache, vomiting, fatigue
   b. Headache, delirium, fatigue
   c. Bone pain, headache, fatigue, nausea
   d. Bone pain, jaundice, weight gain
3. Advantages for the use of umbilical cord blood for transplantation include all of the following *except:*
   a. Readily available stem cell source
   b. Collection poses no risk to the donor
   c. Increased risk of graft failure
   d. Decreased risk of GVHD

4. The most common side effect after transplant is:
   a. GVHD
   b. Infection
   c. VOD
   d. Secondary malignancy
5. An autologous transplant is one in which the donor is:
   a. A sibling
   b. A cord blood donor
   c. A parent
   d. The patient
6. The most appropriate method of mobilization for allogeneic stem cell collection is:
   a. Chemotherapy alone
   b. Chemotherapy plus growth factor
   c. Growth factor alone
   d. No mobilization is needed
7. Currently the only "cure" for CML is:
   a. Allogeneic transplantation
   b. Autologous transplantation
   c. Interferon
   d. There is no cure

8. All of the following are important components of the pretransplant work-up *except:*
   a. Pulmonary function tests
   b. Echocardiogram
   c. Social work consult
   d. Consultation with podiatrist

9. The most common posttransplantation complication is:
   a. Graft rejection
   b. Infection
   c. Pneumonitis
   d. Veno-occlusive disease

10. Medications used in prevention of GVHD include:
   a. Cyclosporine, methotrexate, tacrolimus, steroids
   b. Cyclosporine, tacrolimus, cytoxan, steroids
   c. Cyclosporine, tacrolimus, cytarabine, steroids,
   d. Cyclosporine, tacrolimus, foscarnet, steroids

BIBLIOGRAPHY

1. Anderlini P: The role of allogeneic peripheral blood stem cell transplantation. http://www.bmtinfo.org/bmt/topics, 1999.
2. Anderlini P, Przepiorka D: Allogeneic marrow transplantation. In Pazdur R, editor: *Medical oncology: a comprehensive review,* Huntington, NY, PRR, 1995.
3. Anderlini P and others: Blood stem cell procurement: donor safety issues, *Bone Marrow Transplant* 21(suppl 3):S35, 1998.
4. Applebaum F: Allogeneic bone marrow transplantation for treatment of malignancy. In Macdonald JS, Haller DG, Mayer RJ, editors: *Manual of oncologic therapeutics,* Philadelphia, Lippincott, 1995.
5. Attal M, Harousseau J: Standard therapy versus autologous transplantation in multiple myeloma, *Hematol Oncol Clin North Am* 11:133, 1997.
6. Basara N, Blau W, Romer E: Mycophenolate mofetil for the treatment of acute and chronic graft versus host disease in bone marrow transplant patients, *Blood* 90(suppl):105a, 1997.
7. Bearman S: The syndrome of hepatic veno-occlusive disease after marrow transplantation, *Blood* 85:3005, 1995.
8. Bell A and others: Peripheral blood stem cell autografting, *Lancet* 1:1027, 1986.
9. Bensinger W, Buckner C, Gahrton G: Allogeneic stem cell transplant for multiple myeloma, *Hematol Oncol Clin North Am* 11:147, 1997.
10. Bhatia R, Forman S: Autologous transplantation for the treatment of chronic myelogenous leukemia, *Hematol Oncol Clin North Am* 12:151, 1998.
11. Bierman P, Armitage J: Autologous bone marrow transplantation. In Macdonald JS, Haller DG, Mayer RS, editors: *Manual of oncologic therapeutics,* Philadelphia, Lippincott, 1995.
12. Bilodeau B, Fessele K: Non-Hodgkin's lymphoma, *Semin Oncol Nurs* 14:273, 1998.
13. *BMT Newsletter:* Peripheral stem cell transplants, 11:1, 1992.
14. *BMT Newsletter:* Cord blood transplants, 7:1, 1996.
15. Boiron J and others: Autologous stem cell transplantation for patients with chronic myelogenous leukemia in first chronic phase not responding to alpha-interferon, *Blood* 88(10 suppl 1):126A, 1996.
16. Boulad F, Sands S, Sklar C: Late complications after bone marrow transplantation in children and adolescents. *Curr Prob Pediat* 28:277, 1998.
17. Buchsel P, Kapustay P: Peripheral stem cell transplantation, *Oncol Nurs* 2:2, 1995.
18. Buchsel P, Leum E, Rudder-Randolph S: Nursing care of blood stem cell transplant recipients, *Semin Oncol Nurs* 13:172, 1997.
19. Buchsel P, Wroblewski E, Rudder-Randolph S: Delayed complications of bone marrow transplantation: an update, *Oncol Nurs Forum* 23:1267, 1996.
20. Buckley R and others: Hematopoietic stem-cell transplantation for the treatment of severe combined immunodeficiency, *N Engl J Med* 340:508, 1999.
21. Byrne J, Russell N: Peripheral blood stem cell transplants, *J Clin Pathol* 51:351, 1998.
22. Callaghan M: Hodgkin's disease, *Semin Oncol Nurs* 14:262, 1998.
23. Castaigne S and others: Successful haematopoietic reconstitution using autologous peripheral blood mononucleated cells in a patient with acute promyelocytic leukemia, *Br J Haematol* 62:209, 1986.
24. Caudell K: Graft-versus-host disease. In Whedon M, Wujcik D editors: *Blood and marrow stem cell transplantation,* Boston, Jones & Bartlett, 1997.
25. Crouch M, Risse C: Post-induction autologous bone marrow transplantation. In Wujcik D, editor: *Nursing care issues in adult leukemia,* Huntington, NY, PRR, 1995.
26. Crouch M, Ross J: Current concepts in autologous bone marrow transplantation, *Semin Oncol Nurs* 10:1, 1994.
27. Cuaron L, Gallucci B: Gene therapy and blood cell transplantation, *Semin Oncol Nurs* 13:200, 1997.
28. Engels E and others: Early infection in bone marrow transplantation: quantitative study of clinical factors that affect risk, *Clin Infect Dis* 28:256, 1999.
29. Flowers M, Kansu E, Sullivan K: Pathophysiology and treatment of graft versus host disease, *Hematol Oncol Clin North Am* 13:5, 1999.
30. Forman S: Stem cell transplantation in acute leukemia, *Curr Opin Oncol* 10:10, 1998.
31. Forte K: Alternative donor sources in pediatric bone marrow transplantation, *J Pediatr Oncol Nurs* 14:213, 1997.
32. Frisk P, Lonnerholm G, Oberg G: Disease of the liver following bone marrow transplantation in children: incidence, clinical course and outcome in a long term prospective, *Acta Paediatr* 87:579, 1998.
33. Gale R: Cord-blood-cell transplantation: a real sleeper, *N Engl J Med* 332:6, 1995.
34. Giralt S and others: Engraftment of allogeneic hematopoietic progenitor cells with purine analog-containing chemotherapy: harnessing graft versus leukemia without myeloablative therapy, *Blood* 89:4531, 1997.
35. Goldman J: Peripheral blood stem cells for allografting, *Blood* 85:1413, 1995.

36. Gould D, Franco T: Allogeneic bone marrow transplantation. In Wujcik D, editor: *Nursing care issues in adult acute leukemia,* Huntington, NY, PRR, 1995.

37. Gluckman E: Umbilical cord blood biology and transplantation, *Curr Opin Hematol* 2:413, 1995.

38. Gluckman E, Rocha V, Chastang C: Cord blood banking and transplant in Europe, *Bone Marrow Transplant* 22(suppl 1):S68, 1998.

39. Grigg A and others: Fludarabine based non-myeloablative chemotherapy followed by infusion of HLA identical stem cells for relapsed leukemia and lymphoma, *Bone Marrow Transplant* 23:107, 1999.

40. Hegland J: Transplant immunology: HLA and issues of stem cell donation. In Whedon M, Wujcik D, editors: *Blood and marrow stem cell transplantation,* Boston, Jones & Bartlett, 1997.

41. Janssen W: Peripheral blood and bone marrow hematopoietic stem cells: are they the same? *Semin Oncol* 20(suppl 6):5, 1993.

42. Kapustay P: Blood cell transplantation: concepts and concerns, *Semin Oncol Nurs* 13:151, 1997.

43. Kessinger A and others: Reconstitution of human hematopoietic function with autologous cryopreserved circulating stem cells, *Exp Hematol* 14:192, 1986.

44. Kessinger A and others: Cryopreservation and infusion of autologous peripheral stem cells, *Bone Marrow Transplant* 5:25, 1990.

45. King C: Peripheral stem cell transplantation: past, present, and future. In Buchsel PC, Whedon MB, editors: *Bone marrow transplantation: administrative and clinical strategies,* Boston, Jones & Bartlett, 1995.

46. Klaesson S: Clinical use of rHuEPO in bone marrow transplantation, *Med Oncol* 16:2, 1999.

47. Kletzel M, Abella E, Sanders E: Thiotepa and cyclophosphamide with stem cell rescue for consolidation therapy for children with high-risk neuroblastoma: a phaseI/II study of the pediatric blood and marrow transplant consortium, *J Pediatr Hematol Oncol* 20:49, 1998.

48. Klumpp T: Complications of peripheral transplantation for solid tumors in children, *Curr Opin Pediatr* 9:55, 1997.

49. Klumpp T and others: Granulocyte colony-stimulating factor accelerates neutrophil engraftment following peripheral-blood stem-cell transplantation: a prospective randomized trial, *J Clin Oncol* 13:1323, 1995.

50. Kurtzberg J and others: Placental cord blood as a source of hematopoietic stem cells in transplantation into unrelated recipients, *N Engl J Med* 335:157, 1996.

51. Ladenstein R, Philip T, Gardner H: Autologous stem cell transplantation for solid tumors in children, *Curr Opin Pediatr* 9:55, 1997.

52. Marks D, Goldman J: Bone marrow transplantation in chronic myelogenous leukemia, *Marrow Transplant Rev* 2:17, 1992.

53. McGlave P: Bone marrow transplants in chronic myelogenous leukemia: an overview of determinants of survival, *Semin Hematol* 27:23, 1990.

54. McGlave P: Unrelated donor transplants for chronic myelogenous leukemia, *Hematol Oncol Clin North Am* 12:93, 1998.

55. Miller A: Hematopoietic growth factors in autologous bone marrow transplantation, *Semin Oncol* 20(suppl 6):5, 1993.

56. Miller J: Innovative therapy for chronic myelogenous leukemia, *Hematol Oncol Clin North Am* 12:173, 1998.

57. Nelson J: The blood cell transplant program, *Semin Oncol Nurs* 13:208, 1997.

58. Nemunaitis J: Growth factors in allogeneic transplantation, *Semin Oncol* 20(suppl 6):5, 1993.

59. O'Connell S, Schmit-Pokorny K: Blood and marrow stem cell transplantation indication, procedure, process. In Whedon M, Wujcik D, editors: *Blood and marrow stem cell transplantation,* Boston, Jones & Bartlett, 1997.

60. *Oncology News International:* Cord blood is used as a source of stem cells for pediatric transplantation, 4:7, 1995.

61. Patton D and others: Treatment of veno-occlusive disease of the liver with bolus tissue plasminogen activator and continuous infusion of anti-thrombin III concentrate, *Bone Marrow Transplant* 17:443, 1996.

62. Perentesis J and others: Autologous stem cell transplantation for high-risk pediatric solid tumors, *Bone Marrow Transplant* 24:609, 1999.

63. Ramsey N: Bone marrow transplantation in pediatric oncology. In Pizzo PA, Poplack DG, editors: *Principles and practice of pediatric oncology,* Philadelphia, Lippincott, 1993.

64. Rivera L: Blood cell transplantation: its impact on one family, *Semin Oncol Nurs* 13:194, 1997.

65. Rowe J and others: Recommended guidelines for the management of autologous and allogeneic bone marrow transplantation, *Ann Intern Med* 120:2, 1994.

66. Rubenstein P and others: Stored placental blood for unrelated bone marrow reconstitution, *Blood* 81:7, 1993.

67. Rubenstein P, Adamson J, Stevens C: The placental/umbilical cord blood program of the New York blood center: a progress report, *Ann NY Acad Sci* 872:328, 1999.

68. Sable C, Donowitz G: Infections in bone marrow transplant recipients, *Clin Infect Dis* 18:273, 1994.

69. Safah HF, Weiner R: Veno-occlusive diseases following bone marrow transplantation, *Mediguide Oncol* 14:4, 1994.

70. Sanders J: Bone marrow transplantation for pediatric leukemia, *Pediatr Ann* 20:12, 1991.

71. Sanders J: Bone marrow transplantation for pediatric malignancies, *Pediatr Clin North Am* 44(4):1005, 1997.

72. Schiodt I and others: Early infections after autologous transplantation for haematologic malignancies, *Med Oncol* 15:103, 1998.

73. Secola R: Pediatric blood cell transplantation, *Semin Oncol Nurs* 13:184, 1997.

74. Shapiro T: Pulmonary and cardiac effects. In Whedon M, Wujcik D, editors: *Blood and marrow stem cell transplantation,* Boston, Jones & Bartlett, 1997.

75. Simone J: Autologous bone marrow transplantation in childhood cancer, *J Clin Oncol* 11:8, 1993.

76. Stadtmauer E, Schneider C, Silberstein L: Peripheral blood progenitor cell generation and harvesting, *Semin Oncol* 22:3, 1995.

77. Steven K: Umbilical cord transplants: treatment for selected hematologic and oncologic diseases, *J Perinat Neonat Nurs* 11:19, 1997.

78. Stiff P: Blood and marrow transplantation in relapsed and refractory non-Hodgkin's lymphoma, *Oncology* 12(10 suppl 8):56, 1998.

79. Stocchi R and others: Management of human CMV infection and disease after allogeneic bone marrow transplantation, *Haematologica* 84:71, 1998.

80. Storek J and others: Allogeneic peripheral blood stem cell transplantation may be associated with a high risk of chronic graft versus host disease, *Blood* 90:4707, 1997.

81. Stroncek D and others: Treatment of normal individuals with granulocyte-colony-stimulating-factor; donor experience and the effects on peripheral blood CD34+ cell counts and on the collection of peripheral blood stem cells, *Transfusion* 36:601, 1996.

82. Stuart R: Autologous bone marrow transplantation for leukemia, *Semin Oncol* 20(suppl 6):5, 1994.

83. Tilly H and others: Haemopoietic reconstitution after autologous peripheral blood stem cell transplantation in acute leukemia, *Lancet* 11:154, 1986.

84. Ueno N, Champlin R: Autologous transplantation: basic concepts and controversies. In Pazdur R, editor: *Medical oncology: a comprehensive review,* Huntington, NY, PRR, 1995.

85. Van Burik J, Weisdorf D: Infections in recipients of blood and marrow transplantation, *Hematol Oncol Clin North Am* 13:5, 1999.

86. Varterasian M: Biologic and clinical advances in multiple myeloma, *Oncology* 9:5, 1995.

87. Vose J, Armitage J, Kessinger A: High-dose chemotherapy and autologous transplant with peripheral-blood stem cells, *Oncology* 7:8, 1993.

88. Wagner N, Quinones V: Allogeneic peripheral blood stem cell transplantation: clinical overview and nursing implications, *Oncol Nurs Forum* 25:1049, 1998.

89. Wagner J: Umbilical cord transplantation, *Leukemia* 12(suppl 1):530, 1998.

90. Walker F, Roethke S, Martin G: An overview of the rationale, process, and nursing implications of peripheral blood stem cell transplantation, *Cancer Nurs* 17:2, 1994.

91. Welte K: Matched unrelated transplants, *Semin Oncol Nurs* 10:1, 1994.

92. Whedon M, Ferrell B: Quality of life in adult bone marrow transplant patients: beyond the first year, *Semin Oncol Nurs* 10:1, 1994.

93. Winer E, Sutton L: Quality of life after bone marrow transplant, *Oncology* 8:1, 1994.

94. Wingard J: Infections in allogeneic bone marrow transplant recipients, *Semin Oncol* 20(suppl 6):5, 1993.

95. Wujcik D, Ballard B, Camp-Sorrell D: Selected complications of allogeneic bone marrow transplantation, *Semin Oncol Nurs* 10:1, 1994.

96. Wujcik D: Future consideration in transplantation, *Semin Oncol Nurs* 13:216, 1997.

97. Wujcik D: Hematopoiesis. In Whedon M, Wujcik D, editors: *Blood and marrow stem cell transplantation,* Boston, Jones & Bartlett, 1997.

98. Yoder L: Diseases treated with blood cell transplants, *Semin Oncol Nurs* 13:164, 1997.

26 Cancer Clinical Trials

Mary Magee Gullatte and Shirley E. Otto

CHAPTER

Clinical trials have heralded the transformation of cancer treatment and symptom management over the last three decades. The efforts of a worldwide network of health care professionals committed to improving survival and outcomes of cancer care have resulted in paramount improvements in all aspects of cancer treatment modalities and innovations in symptom management. Oncology nurses continue to be at the piercing point of the cutting edge in efforts to offer quality cancer care for patients. The newest technology battlefield is understanding the possibilities and exploring the limits of gene therapy. Oncology nurses have established a firm presence in clinical trials and are valued as professional colleagues in partnership with other health care professionals to help fashion the future in gene therapy related to cancer prevention early detection and treatment. Oncology nurses are invaluable as independent researchers, in providing patient education and support, and in obtaining informed consent for clinical trials. This chapter focuses on a review of the history, purpose, and implementation of clinical trials. Complementary and alternative therapies are also addressed. Several controversial issues related to ethics of some gene therapy trials will be discussed related to protecting human subjects in clinical trials and advancing medical technology and treatment.*

HISTORICAL PERSPECTIVE

The U.S. government founded the National Institutes of Health (NIH) in 1887. The purpose of the NIH is to support research into the causes, diagnosis, prevention, and cure of human disease. One of the largest biomedical research facilities in the world, the NIH is part of the U.S. Department of Health and Human Services (DHHS).[36, 58]

Many of the early clinical trials in the United States focused on the prophylaxis and treatment of infectious diseases. By the 1930s, cancer was identified as a major health problem requiring a large-scale national plan of action. In 1937, Congress unanimously passed the *National Cancer Institute Act,* which appropriated $700,000 to establish the National Cancer Institute (NCI), now the largest of the 12 NIH institutes. The NCI expected to break new theoretical ground by conducting its own research, promoting research in other institutions, and coordinating cancer-related activities throughout the United States.[8, 26, 34–36, 51]

The Warren Grant Magnuson Clinical Center was established in 1953 on the NIH campus. The NIH institutes that are conducting combined laboratory and clinical studies share the center. Both inpatients and ambulatory care patients from all over the world participate in cancer clinical trials at this facility. Travel, nursing care, and medical care are provided to these patients at no cost. The trials performed within the NIH clinical center are called *intramural research studies. Extramural research studies* trials are those NCI-sponsored studies conducted at universities, medical schools, and hospitals across the United States. Extramural trials are supported by grants, contracts, or cooperative agreements and use about 80% of the funds appropriated to the NIH by the U.S. Congress.[8, 18, 35, 36, 58, 62, 63]

The years after World War II brought successes in cancer treatment with the development of new chemotherapeutic agents. The *National Chemotherapy Program,* funded through congressional appropriations in 1955, was devoted to testing new chemicals that might prove to be effective antineoplastic agents. The Cancer Chemotherapy National Service Center at the NCI functioned as a pharmaceutical house to move new drugs into both the intramural and the extramural trials. In 1965, the program expanded to include international drugs.[8, 18, 35, 36, 63]

The motivated efforts of a public and private campaign ultimately resulted in the signing of the *National Cancer Act* in 1971. This created a national cancer program administered by the NCI, with its director

---

* References 7, 21, 34–36, 43, 49, 51–54, 58.

appointed by and reporting to the president of the United States. This legislation was a landmark in the history of cancer treatment and research. Increased power and funding created new opportunities for physicians, improving the quality and increasing the accessibility of cancer care for patients across the United States.[54, 58, 63, 64]

In 1991, on the 20th anniversary of the National Cancer Act, Harold Freeman, MD, chairman of the President's Cancer Panel, testified before a house panel and listed the following accomplishments in cancer treatment[16, 34, 35, 36]:

Fewer amputations for osteosarcoma patients

A 50% survival rate for patients with acute lymphocytic leukemia, improved from 28%

Improvement in 5-year survival rate of women with breast cancer from 85% to 91%

Prostate cancer 5-year survival rate of 71%, up from 50%

The following programs, initiated by the NCI since 1971, increased the number of cancer specialists and organized a structure to coordinate national research and to translate research advances into clinical practice.

Oncology Training Programs

The NCI funded fellowship programs in medical oncology and radiotherapy. There were 100 medical oncologists in the 1960s; and by 1987, there were more than 4000. The first certifying examinations for medical oncologists were in 1974. The increased numbers of radiation therapists and medical oncologists allowed movement of this specialty from predominantly university settings into community hospitals and into many less urban settings.[34-36]

Comprehensive Cancer Centers

The National Cancer Act of 1971 formally authorized the *Cancer Centers Program.* The NCI was challenged to develop a network of specialized and comprehensive cancer centers to serve as a national resource for research and a multidisciplinary treatment approach, as well as a community resource through outreach programs and cancer control. Designation as a comprehensive cancer center requires meeting eight criteria established by the NCI: (1) basic research, (2) mechanisms for technology transfer, (3) clinical research, (4) program of high-priority clinical trials, (5) cancer prevention and control research, (6) research training and continuing education programs, (7) cancer information services, and (8) community service and outreach activities.[53, 54, 63, 64] In 2000, there were 37 NCI-designated comprehensive cancer centers, a tremendous increase

since the year of the National Cancer Act, when there were only three.[53, 54, 63, 64]

Cooperative Research Groups

Cooperative research groups are NCI-supported national networks of researchers, cancer centers, and community physicians who conduct high-quality clinical trials around the country. All cooperative group clinical trials are listed in the NCI clinical trials database at http://www.cancer.gov. These groups are funded by the NCI through cooperative agreements. The cooperative group program started with the National Chemotherapy Service Center funding in 1955. The original purpose of the groups was to test the new chemotherapeutic agents developed at the NCI. The scope of the program has broadened through the years, and current areas of research include evaluation of multimodality therapies, basic science, supportive care, quality of life, and chemoprevention trials. The results of cooperative group research are reported through group-wide meetings and published in scientific journals.*

There are five primary goals of cooperative group research:

To improve survival and quality of life for cancer patients

To conduct basic scientific research into cancer biology, pathology, epidemiology, and supportive care

To serve as a research base for the implementation of cancer control research

To conduct oncology nursing research

Cooperative groups share common goals but may differ in their clinical focus. The focus may be the multimodality treatment of all adult cancers or all pediatric cancers. Other groups focus on a specific type of cancer or specific type of treatment. The names of certain groups may imply a geographic focus such as the Southwest Oncology Group (SWOG), but they include members from across the United States as well as some international locations.[1, 18]

Cooperative groups are generally similar in structure. They are composed of an operations office, statistical center, and various standing committees. The *operations office* manages the administrative affairs of the group and houses the group chairman. The *statistical center,* which may be in a different location, houses the group biostatistician and protocol data coordinators. This office handles protocol registration, quality control of data, and ongoing statistical analysis of protocols. Each cooperative group has *standing disease and discipline committees* that represent the group's focus.[1, 18, 19, 51]

---

* References 1, 18, 19, 26, 35, 36, 53, 54, 57–59, 63, 64.

The role of oncology nurses in cooperative research groups has become more valued over the past decade. Nurses review protocols before activation to assess the impact of the proposed treatment on staffing requirements and workload. Nurses are principal investigators or co-investigators on companion studies and cancer control studies. Nurses may be involved in the research process as independent researchers, co-investigators, protocol coordinators, or clinical research associates. The NIH has now written into a number of their grant incentives for nurse principle investigators particularly in the NIH funded General Clinical Research Centers.[63–65]

Community-Based Research Programs

Cooperative Group Outreach Program. The NCI Cooperative Group Outreach Program (CGOP), implemented in 1976, was the first comprehensive effort to extend participation in clinical trials to community physicians. The objectives of the program are to make state-of-the-art cancer treatment available to patients in the community setting, enhancing the pool of patients available for clinical trials. The program consists of individual community oncologists, surgeons, or radiologists contracting with a member institution of a cooperative group to register patients for research protocols. The amount of funding the CGOPs receive is based on the number of eligible patients they enter into studies.[1, 8, 15, 18, 19, 52]

Community Clinical Oncology Program. The Community Clinical Oncology Program (CCOP) was initiated by the NCI in 1983 to disseminate state-of-the-art cancer research to patients in community settings. CCOP institutions are groups of community-based physicians who are linked to cooperative groups and cancer centers that serve as their research bases.[8, 15, 18, 19]

This mechanism is beneficial to the patients, the community, and the NCI. Patients now have access to investigational therapies without traveling to a geographically distant treatment center. The local medical community benefits through opportunities for education and exchange of information. The NCI benefits by having available more patients potentially eligible for registration on clinical trials. All studies available for CCOP participation through the 17 research bases are assigned a "credit" value by the NCI. Generally, treatment studies are assigned one to two credits per patient depending on the complexity of the study. CCOPs are required to accrue at least 50 treatment credits each year.[18, 19, 26, 63–65]

Minority-Based CCOPs. The CCOP model was expanded in 1993 when the NCI funded 13 minority-based CCOPs. These are located in areas that serve ethnic minorities and underserved populations. Minority-based CCOPs accrue patients for both treatment studies and cancer control studies. One such group initiative was the National Black Leadership Initiatives on Cancer (NBLIC). This program recently concluded. The effort of the NBLIC within Appalachian, African American, and Hispanic populations was to focus on cancer awareness, reduce cancer incidence and mortality, increase cancer survival, and improve access to health care within minority and medically underserved populations.*

Cancer Control. Cancer control is the reduction of cancer incidence, morbidity, and mortality through an orderly sequence from research or interventions (including their impact on populations) to the broad, systematic appreciation of the research results. With the National Cancer Act in 1971, cancer control activities were formalized as part of the National Cancer Program and recognized as a distinct program entity. With the creation of the Division of Cancer Control and Rehabilitation (DCPC) at the NCI in 1974, a national effort for effective intervention was made possible for the first time. DCPC research priorities include tobacco-use control; diet, nutrition, and cancer prevention; chemoprevention; early detection; and access to state-of-the-art diagnosis and treatment.[18, 19, 43, 51]

Because of the relatively large number of participants required to complete cancer control research, it is frequently implemented through the cooperative group mechanism. Each cooperative group has a standing cancer control committee composed of interested oncology nurses, physicians, epidemiologists, and statisticians. Cancer control concepts are developed and submitted to the DCPC for review. Once the concept is approved, a protocol is developed and resubmitted to the NCI for final review, approval, and eventual activation by the research group. In 1986, the NCI mandated CCOP participation in cancer control research. CCOPs are required to accrue 50 cancer control credits per year. Cancer control studies are usually assigned a portion of credit (0.1, 0.3, and 0.5) per patient registered.[43, 44, 51]

Oncology nurses, well versed in the mechanisms of clinical trials, are primarily responsible for the implementation, data collection, and conduct of the study. Oncology nurses may evolve into independent prevention investigators in trials that treat well populations with essentially toxic agents.[29, 34, 45]

Non–NCI-Sponsored Research

Although the NCI supports a large network of cancer centers, cooperative research groups, and community programs, most cancer clinical trials are not sponsored by the NCI. Comprehensive cancer centers and univer-

---

* References 14, 15, 20, 23, 24, 25, 27, 42.

sity hospitals contribute patients to NCI studies, but they also conduct their own cancer research activities. Physician investigators in their own institution develop these research studies. Studies include early trials with new chemotherapeutic or biologic agents and comparative randomized trials to identify new or more effective drug combinations. Radiation therapists in these institutions also conduct cancer clinical trials. The pharmaceutical industry sponsors many clinical trials to evaluate new agents. The pharmaceutical company contracts with institutions or individual investigators to register patients in their studies. In recent years there has been a striking increase in clinical trials conducted by private pharmaceutical firms, largely related to a marked expansion in the field of biotherapeutics.[18, 19, 43, 51]

DRUG DEVELOPMENT

The NCI is the largest single sponsor of studies using antineoplastic agents. More than 250 such agents are currently in clinical testing, and even more are in preclinical testing. New drugs are also developed by pharmaceutical companies. Agents at the NCI are developed through the Investigational Drug Branch (IDB), a division of the Cancer Therapy and Evaluation Program (CTEP). The development of new agents, whether through IDB or industry, is extremely costly in terms of labor, time, and financial resources. The research and development division in industry represents the largest capital investment, referred to as the R&D, thus, directly affecting drug cost for the consumer once the drug receives FDA approval.[53, 54, 63–65] Table 26–1 lists various CTEP-sponsored cooperative groups.

Identification

The first and most obvious step is the discovery of the new agent. Two basic approaches exist for the selection of chemicals to be tested: the empiric and the rational. The *empiric approach* is a systematic screening of chemicals from a wide variety of plant, animal, and mineral sources. For example, vincristine, an effective commercially available drug, was extracted from the *Vinca* alkaloid plant. Natural products are emphasized because of the observation that these substances successfully treat many human diseases.[2, 18, 21, 35]

Drawbacks to the traditional discovery process are that thousands of substances must be screened to find one that has activity in human cancer. After investing large amounts of time and money, it is still unknown why the response is produced or how it may be improved. *Rational drug design* addresses these shortcomings by attempting to identify the cell receptor site responsible for a given effect and, through a systematic process, specifically design compounds to stimulate or inhibit the

TABLE 26–1

National Cancer Institute: Cancer Therapy Evaluation Program Cooperative Groups

American College of Surgeons Oncology Group (ASCO-OG), www.acosog.org/
Cancer and Leukemia Group (CALGP), www-calgb.uchicago.edu/
Children's Cancer Group (CCG),* www.nccf.org/index/htm
Eastern Cooperative Group (ECOG), www.ecog.dfci.harvard.edu
Gynecologic Oncology Group (GOG), www.gog.org/
Intergroup Rhabdomyosarcoma Study Group (IRSG),* www.rhabdo.org/
National Surgical Adjuvant Breast and Bowel Project (NSABP), www.nsabp.pitt.edu/
North Central Cancer Treatment Group (NCCTG), www.ncctg.mayo.edu/
Pediatric Oncology Group (POG),* www.pog.ufl.edu/
Radiation Therapy Oncology Group (RTOG), www.rtog.org/
Southwest Oncology Group (SWOG), www.swogstat.org/
National Wilms Tumor Study Group (NWTSG),* www.nwstg.org/

These specific groups are going to be combined by the year 2003 into one cooperative group Children's Oncology Group (COG) web site. Name and web site to be announced.

receptor. Techniques of molecular biology refined in the biotechnology industry and computer technology aid in this process. The Division of Cancer Treatment at the NCI has established a grant program, the National Cooperative Drug Discovery Groups. These groups promote collaboration among scientists from academia, government, and industry in developing new antineoplastic agents.[54, 58, 63–65]

Drug Screening

Identified compounds are entered into the NCI's Division of Cancer Treatment drug testing program. Computer analysis and application of specific criteria for selection reduce the chance of duplicating drugs already under evaluation. The NCI selects approximately 10,000 of the 40,000 available substances for further testing. These 10,000 compounds then undergo a screening process that uses both animal and human tumor systems. The tumor system most frequently used from 1955 to 1975 was the murine L1210 leukemia system. Tumors of uniform and predictable behavior were transplanted into mice, and the new drugs were given to the mice to evaluate tumor shrinkage and prolonged survival. This screening system was eventually found to be effective in selecting drugs active against leukemias and lymphomas but ineffective against solid tumors. Now the initial screening is performed in a system called the *P388 mouse leukemia*. Approximately 250 agents will demonstrate antitumor effect in this system and advance to a tumor panel consisting of human tumors transplanted into immunodeprived ("nude") mice. The new agent must show efficacy against at least one of the tumors to advance to further testing. The human tumor cloning system developed in 1980 can grow human cancer cells in culture for the purpose of anticancer drug screening.*

Formulation and Production

Ten of the compounds that successfully pass through the screening system will be selected for identification, purification, and definition of chemical structure. Large amounts of the drug must be produced so that there is sufficient quantity for further testing. The agent Taxol (paclitaxel) is an example of a drug production problem. This agent, known to be effective against ovarian, lung, and breast cancers, is found in the bark of the Pacific yew tree. A large volume of yew bark must be harvested to produce even small quantities of Taxol. Because a particular type of owl, an endangered species, inhabits these trees, debate erupted among the scientific community, conservationists, and the government. The scientific community successfully responded with clinical trials aimed at the development of a synthetic paclitaxel.†

Toxicity Testing

Preclinical testing for drug toxicity is required once formulation and production problems are solved. The goals of toxicology studies are to predict the safest starting dose for clinical trials and to determine if and when organ system toxicity occurs. Toxicity testing is done in mice. Testing formerly was done in a number of larger animals, but this was expensive and did not increase the safety of the drugs. The mice are used to develop a dose-response curve. The lethal dose in 10%, 50%, and 90% of the animals is determined. The dose that is lethal in 10% of the mice, called the *LD10,* is used to establish an initial dose for human trials. To maximize safety, if an unknown compound is being given in humans, only 10% of the LD10 is used at first.‡

Investigational New Drug Application

More than 800 clinical trials are being conducted by the NIH. Before a new drug, or a drug with a new application can be tested in humans, its sponsor, either the NCI or a pharmaceutical company, submits an Investigational New Drug (IND) application to the Food and Drug Administration (FDA) to request permission to evaluate the agent in human cancer. The sponsor may begin to investigate the drug 30 days after the FDA has received the application. The development process for a new drug is lengthy and costly, taking approximately 12 years and 50 to 70 million dollars from screening to commercial availability.[53, 54, 58, 63–65]

Faster Drug Approvals for Cancer Patients

The FDA must ensure that the benefits of prescription drugs outweigh their risks while making these drugs available to patients. To shorten the usual 30-month review of a new drug application, the Prescription Drug User Free Act of 1992 and the FDA Modernization Act of 1997 were passed.* Multiple anticancer drugs have pursued this process and to date two drugs received full approval: (1) docetaxel in 1996 for locally advanced metastatic breast cancer that had previously treated with anthracycline-based chemotherapy and (2) irinotecan in 1996 for advanced or recurrent colorectal cancer following treatment with fluorouracil.†

This new clinical trials research process promises much hope to many patients and families with cancer who have long awaited improved strategies for cancer treatment implementation.[28, 45]

Physician Approval

The FDA must approve physicians who wish to participate in the human clinical trials of investigational drugs. The FDA requires that these physicians, through medical training and experience, assume responsibility for compliance with the protocol requirements for drug administration, data monitoring, and toxicity reporting. The physicians sign an agreement that outlines their responsibilities in clinical research—Form FDA 1573.

Clinical trials are carefully controlled experiments aimed at using the smallest number of subjects to determine with statistical confidence the effectiveness of treatments while maintaining patient safety. The primary goal of clinical cancer research is to identify treatments that ultimately translate into improved quality of life and improved survival. Two major steps must occur before a clinical trial is implemented: (1) the design and writing of the cancer treatment protocol and (2) the approval of regulatory boards.‡

CANCER PROTOCOLS

A protocol is a formal document written to clearly describe the proposed experiment. Both cancer treatment and cancer control experiments are written as protocol documents. *Protocols* provide the rationale for the pro-

---

* References 8, 21, 35, 43, 53, 54, 63–65.

† References 8, 18, 19, 21, 35, 43, 53, 54, 63–65.

‡ References 8, 18, 19, 21, 35, 43, 53, 54, 63–65.

* References 15, 17–19, 43, 53, 63–65.

† References 15, 18, 19, 43, 53, 54, 63.

‡ References 18, 19, 35, 36, 54, 63, 64.

posed study, the study objectives or questions to be answered, and a concise description of the treatment involved. Protocols are written in a similar format and contain the same basic elements regardless of whether the study originates in a cancer center, cooperative group, or pharmaceutical company. The protocol is written by the principal investigator and must be approved by the study sponsor before distribution to participating investigators. The protocol is then followed by everyone involved in the study, including physicians, nurses, data managers, pharmacists, sponsor, and statisticians. The protocol document may be revised or amended as needed by the study sponsor throughout the course of the clinical trial. It is sound clinical practice to have a protocol manual with all the active studies easily accessible in the area where protocol patients are evaluated and treated.[1, 3, 8, 9, 11, 21, 35]

Table 26–2 lists the basic elements of a protocol, describes the purpose of each element, and presents nursing actions to be taken in evaluating and treating protocol patients.

ETHICAL ISSUES AND REGULATIONS

Basic ethical and regulatory conditions must be met before a clinical trial can be initiated. First, the study must be approved for human use by the institutional review board (IRB), and the patient must voluntarily give consent to participate. As part of the consent, the patient must be informed that he may withdraw from the study at any time without fear of adverse treatment by the health care team. The prime objective of such review boards is to ensure the protection of human subjects.[1, 3, 4, 9, 23]

Historical Perspective

These conditions, aimed at the protection of human subjects, developed over the past 50 years. The Nuremberg Trials of 1947 exposed the horrors of human experimentation performed on Nazi prisoners in concentration camps during World War II. In 1949, the *Nuremberg Code* set forth standards for physicians and scientists conducting biomedical experiments on humans. The codes further set forth the absolute requirement of "voluntary consent of the human subject." Unfortunately, several examples of subject abuse in medical research occurred in the United States after the *Nuremberg Code* was enacted. There was no regulatory oversight of clinical research in the United States before 1960. The Tuskegee Syphilis Study, begun in Macon County, Alabama, in 1932 under the auspices of the U.S. Public Health Service, knowingly allowed hundreds of African American men with syphilis to go untreated in efforts to study the long-term effects of syphilis. This study, intended to last 6 months, continued until 1973, when

the Department of Health, Education, and Welfare halted it only after the national media exposed the story in 1972.[4, 33, 37, 39, 40]

Incentives were given to the men in Macon County, such as free medical care (other than for syphilis) and follow-up, hot meals, and hospitalization as needed. At the time the illegal study was terminated, only 72 of the study subjects remained. In 1997, the U.S. President, William Clinton, apologized on behalf of the nation for the Tuskegee Syphilis Study. In 1997, only 8 of the original unwilling study subjects were still alive. In his address at the White House, President Clinton also addressed the steps that his administration would take to increase understanding about ethical issues in research.[4]

Another example of failure to disclose research information was the Willowbrook experiment conducted between 1956 and 1970 on 700 to 800 retarded children. Consent was given by parents to enroll their children in this study to better understand hepatitis and to possibly develop more effective vaccines. Incentives were used to gain parental consent, including earlier admission of their child to the hospital and better hospitalization conditions for children in the study.[1, 3, 37, 43]

The *Helsinki Declaration,* passed by the World Health Organization in 1964 and revised in 1975, provided recommendations to guide physicians in biomedical research. In the United States in 1966 the first research regulations were issued by the Surgeon General's office requiring internal review for all research protocols. The Congress strengthened this regulation in 1974 by passing the *National Research Act* (Public Law 98-348), which required review of all research with human subjects by an IRB before any grants or contracts could be funded. The National Commission for the Protection of Human Subjects of Biomedical and Behavioral Research ("the commission") was created by the 1974 National Research Act. The commission published a series of reports and recommendations on human research. This information, known as the *Belmont Report,* was published in 1979. The three ethical principles listed below are the foundation of the IRB informed consent*:

1. Respect for persons (*autonomy*)
2. Minimization of risk and maximization of benefits to the subjects (*beneficence*)
3. Fairness in the distribution of research burdens and benefits (*justice*)

Institutional Review Boards

The IRBs were created to take a proactive initiative to ensure the protection of human subjects in research trials. To protect humans from research abuses, the DHHS requires all federally funded institutions to have

---

* References 1, 3, 8, 12, 20, 22, 54, 58, 59, 63.

TABLE 26–2
Protocol Elements, Purpose, and Nursing Interventions

Protocol Element	Purpose	Nursing Interventions
Objectives Background	Defines intent of study Describes previous studies and justification for current study	Understand objectives and background of study and incorporate them in patient/family teaching plan to ensure adequacy of informed consent process and to enhance patient's understanding and compliance.
Drug information	Describes animal toxicology studies, human toxicity previously observed, mechanisms of drug action, drug storage, preparation, administration, supplier	Have adequate knowledge of drugs, especially investigational drugs, before drug administration. Demonstrate knowledge of safe dose range, expected side effects, correct preparation, administration, and organs of drug excretion and metabolism.
Patient eligibility	Defines parameters of patient participation: Disease confirmation Major organ function Performance status Medical history	Accurately assess patient's cancer history and previous treatments applicable to eligibility. Evaluate patient's performance status. Evaluate required hematologic and chemistry results. Assess radiologic tests for bidimensionally measurable disease. Ensure all prestudy tests are performed within required time frame.
Treatment plan	Details initial and subsequent doses, administration guidelines and schedule, duration of treatment	Verify body surface area (BSA) for all doses and initial and subsequent dose calculations. Validate method of drug administration. Ensure correct dose modifications for subsequent courses based on criteria defined by protocol. Provide patient/family teaching regarding side effects, self-care, and administration schedule for drugs. Administer additional medications as needed, including antiemetics, laxatives, and antidiarrheal agents.
Study parameters	Schedule of required evaluations and treatment	Provide patient/family teaching about follow-up blood counts, office visits, hospitalizations, and appointments for scans and x-ray films. Ensure required tests are performed, with results available before ordering the next treatment. Provide patient/family with phone numbers of appropriate contacts for questions.
Criteria for response	Defines response: Complete remission Partial remission Stable disease Increasing disease	Demonstrate knowledge of current disease status. Assess patient's response at required intervals per protocol, incorporating physical examination findings and radiologic and biochemical results. Give emotional support to patient during response evaluation. Note any change in response requiring change in treatment plan.
Discipline review	Verification of correct pathologic diagnosis and radiation therapy by a designated review panel	Ensure required slides, blood samples, films, etc. are submitted to correct address within required time. Coordinate these activities with other departments (laboratory, pathology, radiation therapy).
Data submission	Defines required data forms and submission intervals	Complete data forms, ensuring all submitted information is found in patient's medical record. Verify accurate documentation of treatment, required laboratory and radiology parameters, toxicity and response evaluations. Submit within time constraints of research group.
Statistical considerations	Defines accrual goals, study design, statistical analysis	Know expected number of patients to be accrued and expected length of study. Ensure use of correct scale.
Toxicity criteria	Grading of treatment-related toxicities according to standardized scale	Accurately assess and document toxicities in patient chart. Record toxicity grade on flow sheets at required intervals. Distinguish between side effects of disease and treatment. Provide patient/family teaching regarding symptom management. Implement appropriate medical and nursing interventions to lessen morbidity of disease process or treatment or both.

TABLE 26-2
Protocol Elements, Purpose, and Nursing Interventions *Continued*

Protocol Element	Purpose	Nursing Interventions
Informed consent	Sample form that must be modified to meet institutional guidelines	Verify institutional review board (IRB) approval date before patient registration; all protocols must be initially approved, followed by annual full board review. Verify patient has given informed consent before telephone registration. Provide patient with copy of consent.
Adverse drug reaction (ADR) reporting	Defines ADR and reporting responsibilities	Demonstrate knowledge of previously reported drug toxicities. Inform physician of possible observed ADR. Do thorough clinical investigation to determine whether adverse effect is caused by study drug. Notify appropriate authorities, and submit required reporting forms according to time frame.

IRBs. The Office for Protection from Research Risks (OPRR) is the administrative subdivision of DHHS that negotiates assurances of compliance with research institutions. The *assurance program* requires that all investigational clinical protocols are subjected to full board review before human research subjects can be recruited and at least annually thereafter. Each institution must send IRB certification information to the cooperative group's operations office.*

The IRB is composed of at least five members with professional competence, experience, and qualifications. The board should include both men and women and should represent a variety of backgrounds, races, and cultural considerations. At least one member should be a nonmedical professional, and one person must have no direct affiliation with the institution performing the research. The protocol review process provides the investigator, the institution, and the patient with the assurance that the research is medically and ethically sound.[34-36]

Informed Consent

Before a research subject can be registered on an IRB-approved research study, the DHHS requires informed consent to be given by the subject. *Informed consent* is defined as "the knowing consent of an individual or his legally authorized representative so situated as to be able to exercise free power of choice without inducement or any element of force, fraud, deceit, distress, or any other form of constraint or coercion." Information must be provided in a language understandable to the subject and at an appropriate literacy level. It is not complete unless the patient understands what he has been told and is able to use the information to decide whether to participate in the study. The physician or research nurse obtaining the consent must verify that the patient understood what was read and heard. Patients must be allowed to ask questions, and the physician or research nurse should question the patient to determine the level of understanding.*

The required elements of informed consent include:

Statement of research, purpose of the research, expected duration of participation, and description of procedures, including identification of any experimental procedures

Description of risks and benefits of the study treatment

Disclosure of alternative procedures or treatments that may be advantageous to the subject

Description of confidentiality; disclosure of possibility of FDA inspection

Explanation as to whether compensation and medical treatments are available if injury occurs

Whom to contact about research, patient's rights, and research-related injury

Instruction that participation is voluntary and results in no penalty or loss of benefits to which the subject is otherwise entitled

Underrepresented Groups in Clinical Trials

To date, the cancer clinical trials that have been conducted nationally have included relatively few women, poor elderly, children, or minority participants. Lack of access to health care as well as the failure of researchers

---

* References 1, 3, 8, 17, 18, 21, 34, 35, 36.

* References 9, 18, 21, 22, 27, 29, 34, 35.

to accommodate cultural and economic variables when planning and conducting clinical trials are but a few of the cited reasons for continued underrepresentation of special populations.[20, 23, 25]

When such populations were represented in adequate numbers in clinical trials, it has been noted that by controlling for socioeconomic status, one can greatly reduce and in some instances nearly eliminate the apparent mortality and disparity of occurrence of cancer among and between ethnic groups and economic levels. This finding has provided the impetus for additional mandates from the NIH for the development of active recruitment procedures at designated comprehensive cancer centers to ensure adequate representation of women and minorities, or these centers may risk losing funding and comprehensive cancer center designation. In addition, the American Cancer Society (ACS), the American Society of Cancer Institutes, and the Association of Community Cancer Centers have come forth in recent years to endorse appropriate representation of women and minorities in clinical trials and to encourage the public and health care professionals alike to consider protocol therapy when and where it exists. The challenge to health care providers in dealing with those patients who may not have adequate insurance or access to care is to avoid segregating them from cancer clinical trial participation based on barriers that could be broken down with a committed effort by providers and administrators within health care centers.[4, 9, 12, 63, 64]

In efforts to correct this deficit in clinical and biological research, the NIH Revitalization Act of 1993 mandates the inclusion of women and minorities in clinical trials funded through that agency. In response to this Act the NIH published the NIH Guidelines on the Inclusion of Women and Minorities as Subjects in Clinical Research. These guidelines may be obtained by visiting the web site for NCI.[4, 35, 36, 54, 63]

Minority Participation in Clinical Trials

Researchers are struggling with defining strategies to increase accrual of minorities and women into clinical trials. Grants funded by NIH and NCI require inclusion of minorities, women, and children. The disparity in incidence and mortality for cancer among minority population is disproportionately high. Because minorities are underrepresented in clinical trials, results form said trials are not culturally and ethnically complete.[4, 16, 23, 25]

Some barriers to participation in clinical trials for minorities include language and culture, lack of trust in the researcher or institution, fear of harm, and lack of understanding of the process. For many African Americans the mistrust created by the historical Tuskegee Syphilis Study from 1932–1972, is more than just a tragic event in the history of medical research. In the Tuskegee Trials the U.S. Public Health Service conducted a study by withholding treatment of known syphilis patients without their consent. The study plan was to observe the long-term effects of syphilis in an untreated human host. This unconsented study continued for 40 years prior to being exposed and terminated in 1972. One beneficial outcome from this medical horror was mandatory informed consent safeguards in the United States. Unfortunately, the damage done by this and other unethical treatment of human subjects in clinical trials will live in infamy.*

To lend more scientific cross-cultural validity of clinical trials minorities should be included in clinical trials across a wide variety of cancers. Researchers can start by engaging patients early in the process through building trust and educating the patient and family in the entire treatment plan. If these efforts are genuine and consistent the reward will be increased recruitment of minorities in clinical trials. A study cited the following barriers to African American women participating in clinical trials: (1) feeling of the women that the research was unethical, (2) belief that the researchers did not care about them, (3) feeling that they would have access to better care if not participating in a trial and, finally, (4) they would be more likely to participate in a clinical trial if the researcher were African American. A prior study, published by Harris and colleagues,[23] revealed the following barriers: a general lack of awareness of trials, mistrust of the medical system, economic factors including travel expenses involving office visits, and communication gaps. A recent study by Zhu,[52] conducted in 10 public housing complexes in Nashville, Tennessee, investigating the recruitment of elderly African American women in cancer prevention and control studies, found that lack of participation may be accentuated among older single African American women partly because of financial, social, physical, and cognitive factors.[22–24, 39, 44, 45, 48, 52]

PHASES OF CLINICAL RESEARCH

There are four phases of clinical trials in humans' investigative research: I, II, III, and IV.[2, 8, 11, 18, 19, 21, 35]

Phase I

The purpose of a phase I trial is to determine the maximum tolerated dose (MTD) in humans, to determine the most effective schedule of administration, and to identify and quantify toxic effects in normal organ systems. Studying the pharmacokinetics of the agent, including drug absorption, distribution, metabolism, and

---

* References 4, 9, 14, 16, 18, 19, 22, 23.

excretion, is a primary aim of these trials. The previous animal testing helps predict human toxicities, but careful and frequent monitoring of all human organ systems is required to define the dose-limiting toxicities.

Patients eligible for phase I trials have often been heavily pretreated with available standard therapies before having entered the study. Major organ function must meet the study eligibility criteria; life expectancy is required to be at least 1 to 2 months; and toxicity from previous treatments must be resolved. Objectively measurable disease is usually not a requirement in these trials, because therapeutic response is not an endpoint of the study.

The initial drug dose in a phase I trial is one tenth of the dose that was lethal to 10% of the mice in toxicity testing. Three patients are entered at this dose, each about a week apart. Patients are then observed for toxicity for a specified period. When no irreversible, life-threatening, or fatal toxicities have occurred, three more patients are entered at the next higher dose level. The MTD is usually defined within five dose escalations; thus a phase I trial requires 15 to 20 subjects. The escalation of doses in tiers of patients is called the *Fibonacci search method*. Efforts are underway to attempt to expedite dose escalation by using pharmacologic data to determine the starting dose, to guide dose escalation, and to define the MTD using fewer subjects.

Antitumor response or lack of response does not contribute directly to moving the agent into phase II trials. Drugs are selected based on suggestion of therapeutic benefit. An effective agent may not produce responses in phase I trials because the optimal dose and schedule is unknown at the initiation of phase I studies.

Phase I trials are usually performed in single institutions so that the data can be monitored very closely by the study sponsor. Data are submitted biweekly, and study summaries are required every 6 months to comply with FDA regulations. The first occurrence of any toxic reaction is reported by telephone to the Cancer Therapy and Evaluation Program for NCI-sponsored drugs to allow rapid information dissemination to other investigators using the agent.

Not all cancer trials involve the use of chemotherapeutic agents. Trials may also investigate biologics, radiation therapies, surgical interventions, mechanical devices, or psychometric tools. Cancer control studies all progress through the three phases of clinical trials.

Phase II

Phase II evaluation of a new anticancer drug is designed to determine whether the compound has objective antitumor activity in a variety of cancers. Attention is focused on the types of tumors that respond and the dose-response relationship. Unlike phase I studies, these trials are disease oriented. It is impossible to test the new drug for all types of cancer to determine which ones respond, so the Drug Development Program of the NCI's Division of Cancer Treatment evolved the concept of signal tumors. These *signal tumors* include breast cancer, colorectal cancer, lung cancer, melanoma, acute leukemia, and lymphoma. These represent the minimum number of cancers against which the new drug must be evaluated. This panel includes tumors that are at opposite extremes in sensitivity to chemotherapy and those that are leading causes of cancer deaths. If a drug is inactive in these patients, it is likely to be inactive in other tumors.

Eligibility for a phase II study does require measurable or evaluable lesions because these areas are followed for tumor response. Depending on the drug and disease under study, previous treatment with chemotherapy and other treatment modalities may or may not be allowed. Adequate hematologic, hepatic, renal, and cardiac parameters are specified by the protocol. Life expectancy of at least 8 weeks is required, and patients must be capable of partial self-care to be eligible for most phase II trials.

The phase II study is a plan to ensure that adequate numbers of patients with the greatest probability of benefit are treated with the optimal dose and schedule of the drug. The recommended dose and schedule from phase I are tested in a variety of tumor types. The main problem in phase II trials is maintaining uniformity in treatment and study population. A phase II study will require 15 to 30 patients; each phase II drug is assigned by the NCI to two different cooperative groups. The endpoints of a phase II trial may vary with the type of disease under study. For example, an endpoint of complete remission would not be realistic for a typically treatment-resistant disease such as metastatic melanoma. Because minimal effective treatment exists for this disease, the sole endpoints may be identifying the response rate and toxicity of the new agent.

Phase III

A phase III trial establishes the value of the new treatment relative to standard treatments by a randomized or comparative study. The best role for the new drug must be defined. Different study methods that may be used to define this role are comparing the new drug with the best standard drug; using the new agent in a current, effective drug combination; and comparing combined-modality treatment with the previous best single modality. There must be reasonable evidence to suggest that the new drug or combination of drugs is equivalent to or more effective than the currently accepted standard therapy. Eligibility for a phase III trial is similar to that for phase II in that patients must have histologically confirmed disease that is bidimensionally measurable, have adequate major organ function, and be capable of performing at least partial self-care. Patients in phase III trials have received little or no previous therapy.

Phase III trials are large studies that involve hundreds of patients and generally multiple institutions. More phase III trials are being performed through the intergroup mechanism of the NCI, whereby several cooperative groups cosponsor the study. This allows patients to be accrued from a wider geographic segment, thus allowing a more rapid completion and analysis of the study. Community-based programs contribute significant numbers of patients to phase III trials. Recruitment of the underserved, minorities, and women in these trials is key to the future applicability of the agent and treatment response across race, ethnic, gender and socioeconomic differences.

These trials are often randomized, meaning that the patient is arbitrarily assigned to one of two or more possible treatments. Neither the physician nor the patient knows which treatment will be assigned until after informed consent is given and registration completed. The purpose of *randomization* is to remove potential biases in allocating patients to each treatment so that similar numbers of "like" patients receive each treatment. Another advantage of randomized trials is that treatment groups can be "balanced" according to prognostic factors by means of stratification. The *stratification process* may involve such variables as age, performance status, extent of disease, or prior therapy. This method ensures that patients with a good prognosis and those with a poor prognosis are distributed equally among all treatment arms so that valid conclusions may be drawn when the study is completed.

The primary endpoint of a phase III trial is to improve on existing treatment. Investigators measure for higher complete response rates, increased disease-free survival, and longer overall survival. As treatment results improve, long-term toxicities become an important endpoint. Recently, more attention has focused on quality of life as a study endpoint.

Phase IV

Briefly, a phase IV clinical trial is designed to determine the optimal use of a treatment as a standard therapy. In this design study large numbers of subjects are recruited. Phase IV studies build on the endpoints of successful phase III trials to enhance scientific findings. As mentioned, the primary endpoint of these "refining" protocols is the determination of optimal treatment use.

ACCRUAL ON CLINICAL TRIALS

Although the ACS and NCI, now report reductions in overall cancer incidence and mortality, more than 1 million Americans are diagnosed with cancer annually; one half of these individuals will eventually succumb to the disease. Historical data verify that fewer than 3% of patients receiving cancer therapy are treated through clinical trials. Fewer than 10% of patients eligible for NCI-sponsored studies will be registered. Elderly cancer patients account for 63% of people with cancer; yet, this group comprises only about 25% of the patients enrolled in cancer trials. In 1987, Friedman[9] reported that in NCI-sponsored cooperative group trials, only 1% to 1.5% of potentially eligible breast cancer patients, 0.5% of rectal cancer patients, and 1% of colon cancer patients were actually registered as participating in a study by their physicians. This slow accession of patients is a contributing factor to three major cooperative group studies taking 32%, 113%, and 119% longer to complete than projected. For studies in which the endpoint is reduction in mortality, 18 to 24 months should be sufficient to accrue the needed number of patients. Given the present accrual rates, however, 3 to 8 years or longer may be necessary to provide sample sizes of acceptable magnitude. In addition to the expense of keeping a trial open for an extended period, slow accrual also delays analysis of the study and therefore dissemination of new information into standard practice.[14–16, 25, 27, 42]

Strategies to Increase Accrual

Community Clinical Oncology Program. The CCOP, as discussed previously, was implemented by the NCI in 1983. A primary goal was to increase the available numbers of potentially eligible patients for clinical trials, thus improving accrual rates. Figures from the SWOG attest to the community contribution: in 1983, the year CCOP accrual began, 209 CCOP patients were registered on SWOG studies. The following year the CCOP contribution increased to 1230 patients.

Recent data indicate that 60% of patients entered in cancer clinical trials are from the community setting. Even in the community setting, however, only approximately 30% of patients are eligible for participation, and only 10% of these are registered. This number may continue to decrease in the face of managed care. In a study published by the Association for Community Cancer Centers, 484 medical oncologists were surveyed regarding patient participation in clinical trials. Results indicated that 670 patients in a 1-year period were not entered in clinical trials because of third-party payer denial.[18, 19, 35, 43]

High-Priority Trials. In 1988, the NCI implemented the High-Priority Clinical Trials Program to enhance accrual to important cooperative group phase III trials. These studies are selected from existing cooperative group protocols because they require large numbers of patients, involve common malignancies, and answer important questions, the results of which will likely lead to improved patient survival. Physicians who are not participating in clinical trials through the other available mechanisms may affiliate with a group as high-priority investigators. These physicians are reimbursed for the number of eligible patients they register into study. The High-Priority Trials program has been successful in increasing patient accrual. Historically, these trials account for only 6% of currently active phase II studies but accrue 27% of current phase III patients.[51]

Special Populations Networks

In April 2000, Richard Klausner, MD, director of the NCI, announced a $60 million dollar program to address the unequal burden of cancer within certain populations in the United States over the next 5 years. The Special Populations Networks for Cancer Awareness Research and Training is intended to build relationships between large research institutions and community-based programs. NCI further announced the award of 18 grants at 17 institutions to address the unequal burden of cancer within special populations in the United States.[53, 54, 63, 64]

As previously stated in Chapter 4, cancer is one of the six focus areas in the DHHS initiative, *Healthy People 2010,* to eliminate racial and ethnic disparities in health. More information may be obtained by viewing the web site http://raceandhealth.hhs.gov. Dr. Klausner reported that the Networks project will be carried out in three overlapping phases. Phase I: a variety of cancer awareness activities will be implemented within targeted communities, and community groups will work with private and public sector organizations to develop project plans. Phase II: researchers will focus on establishing partnerships with NCI-designated cancer centers, academic institutions, and NCI clinical trials cooperative groups to enhance minority participation in clinical trials and to improve training opportunities for minority scientists. Phase III: will be devoted to using information gleaned from the pilot projects developed in the second phase to develop full-fledged investigator-initiated research grant applications, as well as to enhance the infrastructure developed in the first and second phases.[58, 59, 62, 63]

The Agency for Health Care Quality and Research (AHCQR) has signed cooperative agreements with 11 universities and medical institutions to support centers that will study the effectiveness of medical treatment for racial and ethnic minority populations. The Medical Treatment Effectiveness Program (MEDTEP) research centers on minority populations will seek ways to improve the effectiveness of medical diagnosis and treatment and disseminate information to help both minority patients and their health care providers. A list of the centers and their population focus is listed in Table 26–3.

Obstacles to Accrual

Various reasons and explanations are cited for poor patient accrual on clinical trials. Johansen[24] and coworkers group these obstacles into patient-related, nurse-related, and physician-related obstacles.

Patient-Related Obstacles. These authors identify potential patient-related barriers as financial costs (transportation, lodging, meals, loss of income); concerns of privacy and confidentiality; lack of interest in, disapproval of, or low opinions of clinical research; fear; anxiety; denial; and family influences.

Nurse-Related Obstacles. Numerous nursing barriers to accruing patients on clinical trials also exist. Treating research patients increases the job responsibilities of nurses, and conflicts in responsibility may arise. Many nurses do not have the opportunity for education regarding clinical research and feel poorly prepared to assume these responsibilities. Lack of rewards and recognition for members of the research team and a lack of investigator/nurse and nurse/nurse collaboration may produce frustration.[22, 29]

TABLE 26–3

Universities and Medical Centers Participating in the Agency for Health Care Policies and Research Medical Treatment Effectiveness Program

Site	Target Population	City
Columbia University/ Harlem Hospital	African American	New York City
University of California	African American, Hispanic/Latino	San Francisco
University of Maryland	African American	Baltimore
University of Texas Health Sciences Center	Hispanic/Latino	San Antonio
Henry Ford Hospital	African American	Detroit
Meharry Medical College	African American	Nashville
Morehouse School of Medicine	African American	Atlanta
Pacific Health Research Institute	Asian American and Pacific Islander	Honolulu
University of California	Asian American and Pacific Islander	Los Angeles
University of Illinois	Mexican American, Puerto Rican	Chicago
University of New Mexico	American Indian, Hispanic Latino	Albuquerque

Physician-Related Obstacles. Numerous authors discuss physician obstacles to registering patients on research studies. An early trial conducted by the National Surgical Adjuvant Breast and Bowel Project studied reasons surgical principal investigators chose not to enter patients in a large, multicenter, cooperative group trial. The clinical trial compared segmental mastectomy with postoperative radiation therapy, segmental mastectomy alone, and total mastectomy. Patient accrual was so far below expected accrual that it threatened the successful completion of the trial. Of the 94 surveyed principal investigators, 91 responded to the survey. These physicians identified the following reasons for not entering eligible patients:

Concern that the physician-patient relationship would be affected by a randomized clinical trial
Difficulty with informed consent
Dislike of open discussion involving uncertainty
Perceived conflict between the roles of scientist and clinician
Practical difficulties in following procedures
Feelings of personal responsibilities
Feelings of personal responsibility if the treatments were found to be unequal

Additional factors that inhibit participation in clinical trials were identified in a 1989 American Medical Association (AMA) survey. These factors include lack of time, bureaucratic administration of research, professional liability concerns, ethics of patient care, lack of interest, and reimbursement. However, three fourths of these physicians had a positive view of clinical trials.[1, 8, 14, 18]

Financial Barriers. Financial barriers have become increasingly problematic over the past decade. There are three major areas of expense in cancer clinical trials. The first is for the actual implementation and conduct of the trial and includes research personnel, data collection and analysis, and study monitoring. The second major area of expense is direct patient care, including the cost of drugs, tests, and hospitalization. Historically, these costs were shared by treating facility, NCI- supported grants, pharmaceutical grants, insurance carriers, and the patient. With a recessionary economy, spiraling health care costs, and increased competition for fewer government dollars, the burden of covering costs is shifting. The result of these changing economic conditions is that institutions and health professionals may be less able to participate in clinical trials without adequate reimbursement. According to 1996 data, about 19% of Americans under the age of 65 have no health insurance, and about 20% of older persons have only Medicare coverage. The DHHS reports that more than 48 million persons in the United States do not have health insur-

ance, including 11 million uninsured children. For persons of Hispanic origin, approximately one in three was without health insurance coverage in 1997. Mexican Americans had one of the highest uninsured rates at 38%.[62]

The third area of financial barriers relates to expenses incurred by the patient and family. These expenses can be defined as reimbursable and nonreimbursable or "out-of-pocket" expenses associated with treatment. For patients, decisions about participation in a clinical trial may be affected by the insurer's willingness to reimburse expenses. One specific problem in reimbursement is the third-party coverage for *off-label use* of chemotherapeutic agents. When the FDA approves the commercial use of an agent, it is for the specific condition listed on the package insert. Clinical trials and years of experience, however, often indicate that these agents are effective in conditions other than those listed on the label. These drugs become "standard care" and are prescribed for many patients. In 1991, the General Accounting Office conducted a survey to determine the extent of off-label drug use in the practice of medical oncology; 680 respondents reported the recommendations they made to their last three patients and also designated agents they often use to treat specific malignancies. The survey found that one third of all prescribed drugs were for off-label indications, and 44% of all combination drug treatments were off-label. Half the respondents reported insurance reimbursement problems. The problem is that some insurers have considered off-label use of the drug to be "investigational" and therefore a nonreimbursable expense. This interpretation of off-label use has not been supported by the FDA, Health Care Financing Administration (HCFA), or current state legislation and is actively being addressed in the cancer care arena.*

Out-of-pocket expenses are the other, often overlooked, financial barrier faced by patients. A number of categories of out-of-pocket expenses have been identified in the general health care literature and in the cancer literature. These expense categories have also been referred to in literature specific to cancer clinical trials. Specifically, such expenses as loss of work, income, and leisure time by patients and caregivers associated with frequent attendance at treatment facilities have been noted. Transportation costs, food and nutritional supplements, over-the-counter medications, cosmetics, clothing, additional household expenses, child care, and home health care are all examples of nonreimbursed expenses associated with cancer treatment.[45, 49, 51, 54, 63]

---

* References 15, 17, 19, 26, 34, 42, 43, 49.

Other published works have linked these economic distresses with cancer patients' refusal to enter into a clinical trial and with treatment noncompliance. Along with unmet emotional needs, patients cite unmet financial and transportation needs as creating a significant burden for themselves and their families. Personal reports of unmet needs by cancer patients and their selected family members are positively associated with increased financial obligations. A noteworthy point discovered in this review of literature regarding out-of-pocket expenses is the apparent significant financial impact of health care on women. In almost all instances, women encounter greater out-of-pocket costs than men. This factor also is addressed in recent NCI mandates for strategic imperatives designed to enhance the accrual of women and minorities in cancer clinical trials.[39, 42, 44, 45, 48, 49]

Obstacles Related to Race, Culture, and Poverty. Obstacles and barriers related to recruitment and participation in clinical trials by individuals from diverse cultures require some investment of time on behalf of the researcher to actively recruit from these groups. Years of mistrust and real or perceived unethical treatment in the health care environment has led to the underrepresentation of these special populations who often suffer disproportionately from disease and death. In the study by Zhu,[52] the results suggest that a strategy, which targets the cultural, perceptive, and cognitive characteristics of the population, was effective in increasing the enrollment of study subjects in the African American population. Initiatives targeted at education, communication, cultural competence, and establishing a trust relationship with potential study participants will reduce some of the identified barriers to recruitment of individuals from diverse cultures.

Strategies to Overcome Clinical Trial Participation

Presently, clinical research in cancer is being threatened by inadequacies in the accrual of patients for clinical trials. A concerted effort by physicians, research nurses, professional health care organizations, and the NCI can identify solutions to these accrual crises. Education is an effective tool in overcoming many barriers. The NCI, through its *Patient to Patient* campaign, is attempting to increase public knowledge about and acceptance of clinical trials. Products of this campaign include press releases, the brochures *What are Clinical Trials All About?* and *Cancer Treatments: Consider the Possibilities,* and a videotape, *Patient to Patient: Cancer Clinical Trials and You.* Patients can also be encouraged to call the NCI Hotline (1-800-4-CANCER) to obtain information about the disease, treatment centers, and available

clinical trials. The Physicians Data Query (PDQ) database now has treatment-related information available by fax. This program is called CancerFax and is accessed by dialing 301-402-5874 from the telephone on the fax machine. Anecdotal experience, even at this early stage, suggests that enhancing public awareness of and demand for access to clinical trials may be one of the most effective means of increasing accrual rates.[54, 58, 63, 64]

In May 2000, the NCI announced the launch of the Clinical Trials Gateway Web feature. This initiative brings about a fundamental change in how the NCI develops, reviews, conducts, and supports clinical trials. The new initiatives are divided into five categories[53, 54, 58, 62–65]:

1. Broadening access—opening clinical trials to more physicians and patients will mean quicker responses to cancer research questions.
2. Generating new ideas—canvassing a broad range of basic and applied scientists from both academia and industry
3. Educating and communicating—reaching out to physicians and patients will bring more people into the clinical trials system, and reinforce that clinical trials are critical.
4. Streamlining procedures—reducing paperwork and consolidating procedures will ease clinical trials participation for physicians while maintaining safety and quality.
5. Automating data systems—virtually every component of the new system will be online. For more regarding the above information visit the NCI clinical trials web site http://www.cancertrials.nci.nih.gov.

Oncology research nurses are at the core of this patient education task. Patient education about clinical trials focuses on defining the purpose and relevance of cancer research, including the significance of control groups and randomization. Teaching is accomplished either in an individual setting with the patient and significant others or in a group setting. Participating in community-based prevention and screening programs will provide opportunities to educate the public about the benefits of clinical trials. To overcome the obstacle of increased job responsibilities for nurses in clinical trials, Johansen[24] and coworkers propose two strategies: adjusting the nurse/patient ratio when additional duties are required for clinical trial patients and demonstration of support of clinical research nurses by primary nurses and administrators. The authors also suggest the following as forms of recognition for the nurses' research involvement: coauthorships, attending educational conferences, presenting at research symposia, and developing educational material for patients and professionals related to aspects of clinical trials. Physicians may reciprocate support by supporting nursing research and other professional endeavors. It is also suggested that the type and amount of research involvement influence recognition and should be negotiated by the nurse researcher before the study is implemented.[22, 25, 27]

Oncology research nurses can help increase patient accrual by building trusting relationships with patients and providing education specific to treatment options and expectations. Physicians can be better informed of available studies and eligibility requirements through improved communication and Internet access to health care sites. Tumor registries and medical records departments can provide information on newly diagnosed patients, whose charts are then evaluated by the research nurse for protocol eligibility. Research nurses coordinate prestudy testing, evaluation of results, planning, and troubleshooting of potential barriers. These mechanisms decrease the amount of physician time required to prepare patients for registration. One of the main obstacles reported by physicians to registration of patients is lack of time. These measures may increase physician enthusiasm regarding participation and registration of patients in clinical research studies.[27]

To reduce both time involvement and costs of clinical trials, most trial sponsors have review mechanisms to ensure that studies are cost conscious but maintain the scientific integrity necessary to fulfill the clinical objectives. This action results in decreasing the frequency of expensive radiographic and nuclear scans and eliminating interesting but nonessential testing. Chemotherapy for solid tumor patients and some blood and marrow stem cell transplant patients has moved to the ambulatory care setting. Study sponsors are simplifying and standardizing data collection forms to decrease the amount of time required for manual data entry.[18, 19, 27, 43, 45, 51]

COMPLEMENTARY AND ALTERNATIVE THERAPIES

Complementary or alternative therapy may be described as treatments or supportive methods that are used by patients with cancer (only therapy) or to complement or "add to" their standard or mainstream conventional type medical treatments. Standard, mainstream, and investigational therapies (e.g., chemotherapy, radiation therapy, and biotherapy etc.) follow the scientific method of study using approved research designs, methods, implementation strategies, and evaluations. Not all of the complementary or alternative therapies have completed such a rigorous research process. Table 26–4 provides a list of types and descriptions. These therapies are often promoted as potential cures for cancer as independent treatments to be received in settings outside of the medical mainstream. Sufficient

data to document their efficacy is not widely known or available. Some of these therapies are potentially harmful and typically expensive.[6, 7, 10, 32, 41]

Most of the complementary or alternative therapies are self-prescribed and self-administered, and the information about the therapy is sought by the patient in a nonscientific approach. Despite all of these facts, complementary and alternative therapies have gained wide acceptance by patients, families, nurses, physicians, and other health professionals. Many hospitals and medical centers now have research and clinical programs in complementary therapy. Some health insurance programs cover the services and providers. In 1992, Office of Alternative Medicine (OAM) was created at the NIH by a congressional mandate. Its purpose is to investigate unconventional methods. Initially 30 pilot studies were supported and 11 Complementary Alternative Medical Research Centers were established. In late 1998, Congress approved an annual budget for OAM for $50 million dollars.[6, 7, 10, 32, 41]

In addition to the above-mentioned therapies are therapies further described as ineffective, quackery, questionable, unorthodox, unconventional, new age, or holistic. Most of these types of therapy fit the description of *unproven*. Limited information is known about each type and, like the complementary and alternative therapies, does not follow the model of rigorous research methodology. The types of therapies that are frequently sought by the patient and family with cancer include laetrile, varied dietary metabolic therapies, vaccines, and drugs that do not have scientific approval for that specific use.[31, 32]

The ACS defines unproven cancer therapies as "those diagnostic tests or therapeutic modalities which are promoted for cancer prevention, diagnosis, or treatment and which are, on the basis of careful review by scientists and/or clinicians, not deemed proven or recommended for current use." Furthermore, the American Society of Clinical Oncology's Subcommittee on Unorthodox Therapies states that the term *quackery* implies a knowing intent to misrepresent, whereas belief based on inadequate knowledge may be the underlying promotional incentive rather than the deliberate intent to defraud. The important common feature to all these treatments is *ineffectiveness*.[5–7, 31, 32]

The impact of all the previously mentioned therapies in today's society is tremendous. The number of patients subjected to these therapies may never be known, but it is known that more than $4 billion is spent annually by people with cancer and those desiring an easy method to prevent cancer. Promoters of such therapies accumulate millions every year, and the cancer patient, who may be curable through conventional or standard treatment, bears the financial burden of the promoter's financial gain. The medical professional may perceive the cancer

TABLE 26–4
Complementary and Alternative Therapies

TYPES	DESCRIPTION
Diet and nutrition	*Macrobiotic diet*—derives 50–60% of calories from whole grains, 25–30% from vegetables, and the remainder from beans, seaweed, and soups. *Meats, certain vegetables, and processed foods are prohibited.* *Metabolic therapies and detoxification*—treatments are composed of a low-salt diet, high-potassium diet with coffee enemas, and a gallon of fruit and vegetable juice daily; the specific therapy in each clinic setting. *Megavitamin therapy*—megadoses of vitamins and minerals are self-administered or self-managed. *Nutritional supplements*—variety of products self-administered to enhance dietary intake.
Mind-body techniques	*Biofeedback*—prescribed and/or self-administered mind-body techniques, e.g., via audiotapes, books, and visual imaging to facilitate positive attitude concepts. *Imagery*—use of vivid descriptions or figures of speech in speaking or writing to produce mental images. *Meditation*—prescribed and/or self-administered methods via audiotapes, books, videotapes, music and spiritual study/reflection; to promote a sense of tranquillity and peace for the body, mind, and spirit. *Relaxation/distraction techniques*—prescribed or self-administered techniques via music, audiotapes, imagery to enhance mind-body relaxation. *Yoga*—prescribed technique—a system of exercises practiced to promote control of the body and mind; a discipline aimed at training the consciousness for a state of spiritual insight and tranquillity.
Bioelectromagnets	*Therapies* that use low-frequency portion of the electromagnetic spectrum to produce magnetic fields, e.g., magnets can be purchased as arm, leg, wrist, or body bands, shoe inserts, or bed mattress.
Traditional and folk remedies	*Systems of healings* that include remedies or strategies that have a strong mind-body component and concept that human physiology and disease are interwoven; techniques that may be used include yoga, body cleansings, acupuncture, acupressure, herbal teas, relaxation, and/or other medicinal remedies.
Pharmacologic and biologic treatments	*Pharmacologic preparations* that may include antineoplastics; phenylacetate; combination of multiple protein agents; shark cartilage; and/or Cancell (FDA reports is composed of nitric acid, sodium sulfate, potassium hydrochloride, sulfuric acid, and catechol).
Manual healing methods	*Methods* that may include a variety of touch and manipulation techniques, e.g., therapeutic touch, reflexology, hands-on-massage
Herbal medicine	*Herbal remedies* that may include such products as: Essiac (4 elements of herbs: burdock, turkey rhubarb, sorrel and slippery elm); Iscador (derivative of mistletoe); Cat's Claw, chaparral tea, Comfrey, hot red peppers, willow tea, garlic preparations, multiple type of spice products commonly used in baking or cooking, etc., varieties of dried root single or combinations, and/or Wart's preparation.

Data from references 7 and 10.

patient who seeks unproven therapy as naive. However, although patients discuss the latest "cure" through the extensive and accessible "underground" of patients sitting in clinic waiting rooms, it may be the health care professionals who are naive. Fear of discontinuation of medical treatment often precludes the verbalization of these ideas to physicians and nurses.[5–7, 31, 32, 41, 46]

Historical Perspective

Unproven cancer treatments have been documented as early as 1748, when George Washington and James Madison of the Virginia General Assembly appointed a committee to evaluate Mary Johnson's recipe for curing cancer. The cure, containing sorrel, black celandine, and spring water, was so well defended by testimonials from the "cured" that Mary Johnson was indeed awarded 100 pounds by the assembly. Numerous unproven treatments flourished, and advertisements by promoters abounded.[30, 31]

In 1906, the U.S. Congress passed the *Food and Drug Act*. In 1910, the first time it was challenged, the U.S. Supreme Court ruled that it applied only to truthful labeling of ingredients in a product. The court concluded that individuals could not be prosecuted for what was termed "mistaken praise" for their treatments. In 1912, President Taft urged Congress to pass tougher legislation. This produced the *Sherley Amendment*, which made it a crime to make false or fraudulent claims of therapeutic efficacy. However, it was the prosecution's responsibility to prove intent to defraud. An important piece of legislation, passed by Congress in 1938, finally required scientific proof of drug safety before marketing. A Supreme Court ruling in 1943 determined that the responsibility for establishing safety lies with the drug manufacturer. In 1962, Congress further clarified the Food and Drug Act and added the essential element of *proof of drug efficacy*. This represents research in its current form: data are collected from animal studies evaluating safety and efficacy, an investigational new drug application is filed with the FDA, and on approval of that application the drug enters human clinical trials. When all phases of clinical trials are complete, the company can market the drug if it is indeed safe and effective. The problem is that patients can still choose to use an ineffective and unproven therapy. The FDA is responsible for enforcement of the Food and Drug Act, which is difficult at best. The FDA's legal base is interstate commerce, so promoters operating entirely within a state can totally avoid FDA laws. The U.S. government has no control over ineffective therapies outside the United States.[6, 7, 10, 31, 32, 35, 41]

It is apparent that the health care profession cannot rely solely on governmental legislation and enforcement to protect patients from unproven and possibly dangerous treatments. The health care provider must help patients recognize these methods for what they are and make informed decisions regarding their cancer treatment.[46]

Recognizing Ineffective or Unproven Cancer Therapies

The American Society of Clinical Oncologists Subcommittee on Unorthodox Therapies published its paper *Ineffective Cancer Therapy: A Guide for the Layperson* in 1983. The committee identified the following 10 ways to recognize ineffective therapy[30–32]:

1. *Is the treatment based on an unproven theory?* Promoters of ineffective cancer therapy are experts at using confusing scientific language in brochures. However, these claims are not backed with peer-reviewed publication in scientific journals. Encourage patients to use the National Library of Medicine Medlars Computer through their local reference library to determine whether the claims are published in scientific literature.

2. *Is there a need for special nutritional support when the remedy is used?* People have believed in the medicinal power of certain foods for centuries, and proper nutrition is essential for good health. However, promoters may capitalize on the notion that certain natural foods can cure or prevent cancer. Many ineffective therapies claim that spe-

cial food preparation or nutritional supplements are required to achieve the treatment's full effect.

3. *Is there a claim made for harmless, painless, nontoxic treatment?* These claims may be especially difficult to resist, particularly when the promoter reinforces this with such phrases as "burning radiation," "poisonous chemotherapy," and "mutilating surgery."

4. *Are claims published frequently in the mass media?* Although promoters' claims are not published in scientific literature, they have an attentive audience in the media, often quick to publicize a "new cure" without full investigation. Because the FDA can enforce misleading drug labels but not media claims, the belief that "they couldn't say it if it weren't true" is simply not the case.

5. *Are claims of benefit the result of the power of suggestion?* Promoters rely heavily on testimonials of their "cured" clients. This can overwhelm the cancer patient, who does not know that some of these people never had cancer and that others who gave testimonials succumbed to cancer a short time later. Predictably, the placebo effect of any treatment, when backed with faith and expectation, can result in subjective improvements for short periods. The only scientifically valid evidence, however, is objective tumor response.

6. *Are the major promoters recognized experts in cancer treatment?* Many ineffective therapy promoters look like experts; they wear white coats and have framed degrees hanging in the office. Some are physicians but lack expertise in cancer research and care. The patient should check the Directory of Medical Specialists, which lists individuals who have recognition, special training, and experience in cancer research and treatment.

7. *Do promoters back up their claims with controlled studies?* Promoters claim excellent results from their treatment. However, the demonstration may be from patients' testimonials rather than from controlled trials. Promoters may claim they do not have the staff or money to conduct such investigations. This claim is difficult to believe when they collect millions of dollars in profits every year.

8. *Is there a claim that only specially trained physicians can produce results with their drug, or is the formula a secret?* Formulations of reputable cancer drugs are published in scientific journals, and the information is available to all physicians.

9. *Do the promoters attack the medical and scientific establishment?* Promoters often voice claims of a conspiracy in the medical community to prevent

a cancer cure, thus securing the incomes of its members. However, members of the establishment also die of cancer, as do their loved ones. Ineffective promoters segregate themselves from the medical community, often performing their cures in hotel rooms and discouraging consultation with medical experts.

10. *Is there a demand for "freedom of choice" regarding drugs?* Americans revere the word "freedom," and so promoters claim the patient's freedom of choice would be limited if promoters were not allowed to sell their products. The freedom to misrepresent facts in drug labeling and selling is no freedom at all, but simply a license to steal from the public.

PATIENT MOTIVATIONS FOR THE USE OF UNPROVEN THERAPIES

Fear

The psychological factors that influence a patient to seek unproven therapies are multiple and complex, but the strongest motivator may be fear. A Gallup poll in 1976 surveyed 1548 men and women about their fear of disease; 58% of those interviewed stated cancer was the disease they feared most. Many people see cancer as a frightening, painful process ending in death. In addition to fear of death, fears of an uncertain future, pain, mutilation, loss of family, dependence, costly medical care, and alienation dominate.[30, 31, 32, 46]

Family Pressure

Pressures from family and friends may add to these psychological fears. In a sincere and well-meaning attempt to help, they look for a cure, determined to leave no stone unturned in their search. When cancer is diagnosed, people immediately relate success stories of others they know who may have been cured by conventional means, but they also tell stories of those cured by mystical and "innovative" means. Fear and pressure may lessen objectivity and increase vulnerability to the claims of ineffective therapy promoters. The family, as the patient's strongest support system, feels a responsibility to help decide on treatment, and the patient, fearing alienation from family, may succumb to their wishes.[6, 7, 10, 46]

Recurrence and Progression

Many people resort to unproven therapies when the initial diagnosis is made; others who start with conventional therapy make that same decision when they find their disease has recurred or metastasized. A period of

searching for a second opinion or reason for error in diagnosis is followed by anxiety, sometimes bordering on panic, and depression. Depression changes sleeping and eating patterns and impairs the ability to work and concentrate. The patient may reach a point of hopelessness and helplessness, knowing a cure may now be out of reach. At this time of emotional turmoil, thoughts may turn to pursuing unproven methods as a last resort.[6, 10, 46]

Mistrust of Medical System

Medical professionals would like to believe lay people hold them in high regard, but this is not always true. Today's society has a medical sophistication unknown to previous generations. Health maintenance and prevention and treatment of disease are common topics in the national and local news. News from the latest *New England Journal of Medicine* may be heard on the nightly news before the issue arrives in the mail. While people are assuming more responsibility for their own health, they are actively assimilating new information. Some of this information includes knowledge of the side effects of conventional cancer treatments. They associate alopecia, nausea, vomiting, lack of energy, and loss of appetite with chemotherapy. They see surgery that may cure but may result in disfigurement. The concept of radiation therapy is particularly frightening, because it cannot be seen or felt. The disillusionment some people feel with science and technology may carry over into the physician's office, where this authority figure speaks in a medical language not easily understood and can easily rebuff patients who are already understandably apprehensive.[6, 10, 22, 28, 45]

Promoters of unproven therapies understand well the anxieties of patients in the conventional medical system. They deal with the apprehension, loss of control, and feelings of isolation very effectively by making the patient an active part of the treatment program. Coupled with a promise for cure without discomfort, a close camaraderie soon develops between the provider and patient, both of whom are outside the medical system.[6, 10, 30–32, 46]

Nursing Role

Patients may perceive their physicians as too busy to answer questions about complementary and alternative therapies, and so they frequently direct these queries to the nurse. Angry memories of curable patients who opted for laetrile may make the nurse's first emotional reaction to lecture the patient and tell her that these people have nothing to offer and only want money. This approach may quickly confirm the distrust for the medical community and encourage the patient to seek other treatment options. Patients need factual information delivered in a calm, objective, and nonjudgmental manner. This is the appropriate time to evaluate what the patient has read or heard about the alternative therapy and what the perceived benefits are. What is the level of interest in the unproven method? What is the level of understanding about current therapy and treatment goals?

This is an important opportunity to provide accurate information about unproven methods. All currently accepted treatments were unproved at one time. The FDA and NCI protect patients by requiring proof of safety and efficacy before generalized use of a drug. The following interventions may help the patient evaluate unproved methods and improve nurse–patient relationships[6, 7, 10, 27, 41]:

1. Explain how to access the Medlars system to determine scientific testing of treatment.
2. Check resources to verify promoter's cancer expertise:
   Directory of Medical Specialists
   American Federation of Clinical Oncologic Societies
   American Association for Cancer Research
   American Society of Clinical Oncology
   National Cancer Institute Hotline (1-800-4-CANCER)
   National Center for Complementary and Alternative medicine (NCCAM) http::/chprd.sph.uth.tmc.edu/utcam
   University of Texas M D Anderson Cancer Center http://chprd.sph.uth.tmc.edu/utcam
3. Offer reliable information:
   What Are Clinical Trials All About? (NCI)
4. Examine the patient's expectation of current treatment plan.
5. Offer quality-of-life versus quantity-of-life information.
6. Help reestablish hope.
7. Identify ways to make the patient and family more involved in treatment.
8. Consider referrals for a second opinion, which may increase confidence in current treatment or identify additional therapeutic alternatives.

If unproven methods or promotional techniques seem to the nurse or physician to warrant further legal investigation, the following organizations should be notified: local health department, consumer protection office, and appropriate medical society. The federal agencies and national organizations involved in the investigation, regulation, or reporting of such practices include the FDA, Federal Trade Commission, U.S. Postal Service, Consumer Product Safety Commission, and AMA (see listings in the bibliography).

FUTURE DIRECTIONS AND ADVANCES

Through the advent of numerous medical advances through clinical research a diagnosis of cancer will not be synonymous with death in the 21st century. Combinations of surgery, radiation, biotherapy, chemotherapy, and bone/stem cell transplantation and advances in pharmacotherapeutics for symptom management have made a number of cancers curable. Even more cancers may become preventable and curable in the next decade with the addition of genetic testing, cloning, and other therapeutic and technological medical advances. Clinical trials also supply blood and tissue specimens for clinical research. This has greatly increased the knowledge of disease biology. Childhood acute lymphocytic leukemia can now be subclassified into a variety of prognostic groups and the treatment tailor-made to yield the best outcome. Human tumor tissue can be cloned for testing with a variety of drugs to determine the most effective treatment. Polyglycoprotein, identified on the cell surfaces of some patients with multiple myeloma, ovarian cancer, and acute multiple myeloma, indicates a high risk for drug resistance. New tumor markers are being studied for prognostic significance. The study of oncogenes sheds further light on the biology of cancer. Advances in cytogenetic studies may identify high-risk subsets of patients requiring more aggressive therapy. Finally, the identification and mapping of the human genome will direct cancer research in this century and the next.[18, 19, 26, 27]

One of the main emphases of the cancer control objectives is the prevention of cancer. Therefore, health professionals are faced with the potential to affect more than one half of all cancers with prevention techniques. One of the top six new DHHS *Healthy People 2010* initiatives is related to cancer control, as well as eliminating disparities among high-risk populations. The launch of the NCI Special Populations Network offers opportunities for researchers to make a difference in this new focused cancer control initiative. These studies present new challenges and opportunities for oncology nurses and researchers. The health care focus of the nation is stressing wellness rather than illness. Cancer control studies will direct oncology nurses and researchers into the community for many of the studies. New physician networks will be identified. From the NCI perspective of funding, cancer control trials will be as important as clinical trials.[49]

In recent years, gene transfer therapy has emerged as a promising cancer treatment. Currently in various stages of phase I and II trials, this treatment technique involves the manipulation of the genetic production of enzymes, which control every chemical process in the body. Studies are underway involving oncogenes and tumor suppressor genes. Innovative therapeutic treatment trials are rapidly becoming an integral part of this era of health care reform evaluations of the economic impact of novel and conventional treatment regimes. As issues of reimbursement become greater obstacles to the development of innovative treatment options, health care providers will be forced to investigate the financial as well as the physical outcomes of cancer treatment.[18, 19, 26, 49, 51]

CONCLUSION

Throughout this chapter there have been numerous references to the World Wide Web to access information for health care and oncology care professionals and the public. This information super highway increases access to a plethora of clinical trials information, including complementary and alternative therapies. Consumers, patients, family members, and health care providers will continue to be engaged in all aspects of their care including clinical trials information related to the availability and access to disease specific prevention and treatment options. Oncology nurses should continue to advocate for patient education, informed consent, and ethical research practices. The Oncology Nursing Society has published a position paper on clinical trials and have an active Clinical Trials Nursing Special Interest Group (SIG). For more information about the Oncology Nursing Society, visit their web site at www.ons.org.

There continue to be opportunities and discoveries in the area of cancer research. New antineoplastic agents as well as new indications for some tried agents are continually being sought and tested to increase cancer treatment options and better survival statistics. The cost, challenges, and complexities associated with clinical trials and human subject investigation are many-fold. However, as with the basis of many trials, the potential benefits often outweigh the risks for the patient. The prime objective to keep in mind as researchers and oncology nurses is that the decision to participate in clinical trials must be an informed decision and that decision begins and ends with the patient or legal guardian.[18, 19, 26, 49, 51]

Nursing Management

Chemotherapy research was one of the first areas that emphasized active collaboration of nurses in research. The need for skilled chemotherapy nurses stimulated the development of role expansion. Nurses provided patient education regarding the various aspects of clinical trials. More recently, the role of nurses in clinical trials has expanded from the nurse as a participant in medical research to the nurse as principal investigator for independent research. The roles of nursing in clinical trials include the areas of direct patient care, education, advocate coordination, administration, and independent research. These roles are accomplished by a variety of individuals, who may include hospital staff nurse, ambulatory care nurse, research nurse, clinical research associate, clinical nurse specialist, nurse practitioner, and unit manager. Maintaining coordinated efforts among these individuals requires skill in both organization and communication. Successful implementation and conduct of clinical trials results in safe patient care and generalizable research results.[7, 12, 27]

Greater numbers of nurses than ever are actively involved in clinical trials because of the extension of these trials into the community. Nurses practicing in institutions that do not perform clinical trials still need a working knowledge of these studies because they may refer patients to centers for possible entry into a trial. In addition, in this era of managed care, clinical trial participants who are not receiving investigational medications are frequently referred back to the community setting for treatment and follow-up. The education and support an informed oncology nurse can bring to this stressful situation are invaluable.[27]

Nursing diagnoses and interventions for patients participating in phase I, II, III, and IV clinical trials:

Nursing Diagnoses

- *Knowledge deficit related to disease pathology, new diagnosis*
- *Knowledge deficit related to clinical trials process, randomization process, informed consent process*
- *Knowledge deficit related to experimental chemotherapy, side effects*
- *Decisional conflict related to involvement in clinical trial versus standard therapy*
- *Anxiety related to new diagnosis or disease progression*
- *Anxiety related to treatment with experimental agent or procedure*
- *Anxiety related to completion of quality of life tools*
- *Ineffective individual coping related to new diagnosis or change in prognosis and new treatment*
- *Powerlessness related to involvement in a large clinical trial*

Interventions: Phase I Clinical Trials

- Assess adequacy of informed consent, and notify physician if patient does not fully understand risk-benefit relationship.
- Know mechanism of drug action, route of administration, absorption, metabolism, and excretion.
- Know results of animal toxicology studies to anticipate human toxicities.
- Assess for, evaluate, and document unexpected adverse drug events (ADEs).
- Provide nursing care to minimize disease-related and treatment-related morbidity.
- Understand disease process to distinguish between disease-related and treatment-related effects.
- Carefully document objective and subjective responses to treatment.
- Document acute, chronic, delayed, and cumulative side effects and toxicities.
- Perform and document results of pharmacokinetic studies.
- Participate in decisions concerning dose escalation, schedule manipulation, and determination of optimal dose.
- Assess patient tolerance of regimen as related to psychosocial concerns in all phases of the study.

Interventions: Phase II Clinical Trials

- Know results of phase I drug studies:
    Side effects
    Dose-limiting toxicities
    Method of administration
    Drug metabolism and excretion
- Provide patient education and support:
    Treatment plan
    Expected side effects
    Symptom management
    Disease process

Interventions: Phase III and Phase IV Clinical Trials

- Ensure correct calculation of drug doses.
- Document patient's response (i.e., toxicities and grade).
- Modify doses accurately and consistently.
- Evaluate tumor measurements appropriately for response determination.
- Ensure patient's understanding of randomization process.
- Assess for new and unexpected side effects of drug.
- Assess and document performance status.
- Administer quality of life assessment tools.

Follow-up after treatment completion:

- Teach patient importance of follow-up visits even years after treatment is completed.

- Report data on survival and long-term effects until patient is deceased.
- Develop systems to maintain contact with patients who have moved or changed physicians.
- Encourage patients to return to a healthful lifestyle in light of knowing cancer may recur.
- Teach age-appropriate recommendations for prevention, screening, and early detection (see Chapter 4)
- Counsel other family members of patients at high risk for developing cancer.

PATIENT CARE

The area of patient care includes the informed consent process, treatment administration, toxicity assessment, and documentation.

Informed Consent

In the past the nursing responsibility in the informed consent process consisted mainly of verifying that the signature on the consent document was that of the patient. Responsibility for disclosure rested entirely with the physician. Nurses answered questions to reinforce the physician's explanation.[12, 38, 46]

The changing role of the nurse and the autonomy of expanded roles, especially in ambulatory care and clinical trials bring new professional and legal responsibilities for informed consent to the oncology research nurse. Establishing the diagnosis and choosing a treatment plan are independent functions of the physician or in collaboration with the physician and oncology nurse practitioner, but administering medical and nursing treatments and diagnosing and managing human responses to health problems are independent functions of the nurse. Clinical trials are an area of collaboration. The physician or oncology nurse practitioner may introduce the idea of participation in a clinical trial and give an overview of the treatment, but often the protocol or research nurse explains the details of the consent form and obtains the patient's written signature of consent. In doing so, the protocol nurse accepts the delegated responsibility of providing information to aid the patient in decision-making. In this role the nurse assumes greater responsibility than that of witness. The individual who obtains the consent of the patient or guardian should not be the same person who witnesses the signature on the consent form. The following factors assist in the process of obtaining informed consent of the patient*:

---

* References 1, 9, 10, 12, 29, 35, 38, 44.

PATIENT TEACHING PRIORITIES

Cancer Clinical Trials and Complementary/Alternative Therapies

Review Cancer Control Study Guidelines (purpose, treatment/drug schedule, side effects of drugs), preparation and schedule for diagnostic examinations, and follow-up plan.

Assess readiness to learn, education, and literacy level.

Assess preferred learning method.

Assess cultural and spiritual needs.

Assess reading level of educational materials (recommended 5th grade).

Assess and clarify issues related to the informed consent, clinical trial, and randomization process.

Review the purpose and treatment schedule; drugs and their related side effects; symptom management (e.g., fever, pain, nausea, nutrition); appointments for diagnostic tests/procedures; monitoring of blood counts; return office/clinic visits or hospitalization; resources to contact for emergent care; and questions about clinical trials. Review information related to complementary and alternative therapies and precautions especially related to botanicals.[35, 38]

Use a nonjudgmental approach in providing or clarifying information regarding complementary, alternative, or ineffective therapies.[46]

Refer the patient and family to reliable sources such as American Cancer Society, National Cancer Institute, National Institute, and Food Drug Association for clarifying current and accurate information.

Allow patient to take the consent form home to read before making a decision.

Write down treatment information.

Draw a diagram of randomization and treatment schedule.

Provide *What Are Clinical Trials All About* pamphlet from the NCI.

Provide the patient or guardian with the NCI Clinical Trials web site.

Encourage patient to call the NCI hotline (1-800-4-CANCER) or visit the NCI web site (http://www.cancer.gov), for information regarding disease and treatment.

Show audiovisual information about treatment option (surgery, chemotherapy, radiation, etc.) and management of side effects.

Provide telephone numbers for patient to call if questions arise.

Encourage patient or guardian to write down questions for the health care provider.

Assess patient's anxiety level and integration of new information.

Question patient to determine whether he understands the treatment plan and management of side effects.

Continue to review and reinforce information throughout treatment.

See Patient Teaching Priorities and Geriatric Considerations boxes.

Treatment Administration

Protocol guidelines must be strictly followed so that results from a group of patients treated in precisely the same manner can be analyzed and the study repeated and validated. The nurse administering the treatment should always verify the body surface area (BSA) calculation, protocol dose calculations and modifications, pretreatment laboratory values, and method of administration. Nurses should be provided with protocol abstracts in the patient chart or a set of protocols in the treatment area to facilitate these activities. A staff nurse, clinic nurse, research nurse, or chemotherapy nurse may administer experimental drug therapy; an oncology certified nurse would be ideal.[38]

Toxicity Assessment

The observation skills of oncology nurses are crucial to assess treatment-related toxicities and patient response on clinical trials. The nurse's observation of the patient after treatment identifies the side effect profile and ultimately is the basis for the plan of care of patients receiving experimental treatment in the

GERIATRIC CONSIDERATIONS

Cancer Clinical Trials

The oncology nurse should be aware of age-related competencies in care of older adults and their eligibility and participation in cancer clinical trials.

Cancer clinical trials and cancer control research have established eligibility criteria for patient accrual; refer to age-related guidelines.

Consider sensory and neuromuscular deficits (e.g., visual, hearing, mobility) in selection of educational materials.

Review current prescriptions, over-the-counter medications, and botanicals that may pose drug interactions with scheduled drugs or treatments.

Initiate assessment and intervention strategies for additional limitations, such as fixed income, transportation, caregiver resources, and age-related functional status.

future. The nurse may be the first person to recognize a side effect, perhaps even before the patient is aware of the experience. Prompt assessment and intervention as well as patient and family education throughout the clinical trial process as needed will make the experience for the patient better tolerated.[35, 38]

Documentation

Accurate nursing documentation is the foundation of good clinical research. All data that are reported on flow sheets or case report forms must be verifiable in the patient's medical record. Nurses must document treatments and patient response accurately. Study investigators can extrapolate hematologic toxicity from laboratory work but cannot document other, more subjective toxicities unless nursing documentation is objective. Areas requiring precise nursing assessment and documentation include patient's level of activity, oral assessment, nausea, vomiting, anorexia, pain, diarrhea, constipation, skin condition, weight loss, changes in sexual capability, and psychological changes. Inaccurate or inconsistent assessment or documentation of toxicities may result in patients receiving ineffective low doses or toxicity-producing high doses during the subsequent course of therapy. The previous Interventions section lists specific nursing responsibilities for phase I, II, III, and IV clinical trials.[38]

Nursing Education

Generalist or advanced oncology nurses are an integral component of the research team and must be knowledgeable about research protocols in which they are participating. Areas of education include the purpose and history of the protocol treatment, design of the study, previously observed toxicity, treatment administration, and management of side effects. One must not overlook the need to support the patient and family during this process.

Chapter Questions

1. The Cancer Center's program was enacted in 1971 by which of the following?
   a. National Cancer Institute
   b. National Cancer Act
   c. Cooperative Research Groups
   d. Community Clinical Oncology Program

2. This program was initiated by the National Cancer Institute in 1983 to disseminate state-of- the-art cancer research to patients in community settings:
   a. Cooperative Group Outreach Program
   b. National Black Leadership Initiative on Cancer
   c. Community Clinical Oncology Program
   d. Comprehensive Cancer Center Research

3. The largest single sponsor of studies using antineoplastic agents is the:
   a. American Cancer Society
   b. Office of Minority Health
   c. Pharmaceutical industry
   d. National Cancer Institute

4. Before a drug can be studied in humans, its sponsor must submit a investigational New Drug Application (IND) to which of the following agencies:
   a. Food and Drug Administration (FDA)
   b. National Cancer Institute (NCI)
   c. Health Care Financing Administration (HCFA)
   d. Cancer Therapy and Evaluation Program (CTEP)

5. Which phase of the human investigation trial determines whether a compound has objective antitumor activity against a variety of cancers:
   a. Phase I
   b. Phase II
   c. Phase III
   d. Phase IV

6. In phase IV of a clinical trial the objective is to determine which of the following?
   a. Value of a new treatment relative to the standard therapy
   b. Optimal use of a treatment as standard therapy
   c. Maximum tolerated dose and schedule of the new therapy
   d. Antitumor activity against a variety of cancers

7. Complementary and alternative therapies may include the following treatments:
   a. Diet, bioelectromagnets, biotherapy, herbal medicine
   b. Diet, herbal medicine, chemotherapy, manual healing methods
   c. Diet, mind-body techniques, antimicrobials, herbal medicine
   d. Diet, herbal medicine, folk remedies, mind-body techniques

8. Patient and family motivators regarding use of unproven therapies may include:
   a. Mistrust of medical system, fear, family pressure, and disease recurrence
   b. Medical costs, fear, family pressure, convenient schedule

c. Nurse advocacy, costs, fear, and family pressure

d. Physician advocacy, convenient schedule, fear costs

9. When questioned by patient and family regarding unproven methods of cancer treatment, appropriate resource referrals include:

a. ACS, NCI, NCCAM, FBI

b. ACS, NIH, NCCAM, OSHA

c. ACS, NCI, NCCAM, FDA

d. ACS, FDA, FBI, OSHA

10. Patient teaching priorities for cancer clinical trials and complementary/alternative therapies include:

a. Assess: readiness to learn, cultural/spiritual needs, reading level, employment status

b. Assess: preferred learning method, readiness to learn, reading level, income status

c. Assess: reading level, religious faith, environmental issues, readiness to learn

d. Assess: readiness to learn, preferred learning method, reading level, cultural/spiritual needs

BIBLIOGRAPHY

1. Ad Hoc Committee on Health Literacy for the Council on Scientific Affairs, American Medical Association: Health literacy: report on the Council on Scientific Affairs. *JAMA* 281:552, 1999.

2. Augustine SC: Radiopharmaceuticals in the detection and treatment of cancer and cancer-related therapies, *Highlights Oncol Pract* 17:64, 1999.

3. *Belmont Report: Ethical principles and guidelines for the protection of human subjects of research,* DHHS Publication No. (05)-78-0012, Washington DC, US Government Printing Office, 1978.

4. Brooks J: Minority participation in clinical trials: the impact of the Tuskegee Syphilis Study. *Closing the Gap,* Washington, DC, Office of Minority Health, US Department of Health and Human Services, December 1997/January 1998.

5. *Cancer Facts and Figures 2000:* Atlanta, GA, American Cancer Society, 2000.

6. Cassileth BR: *The alternative medicine handbook: the complete reference guide to alternative and complementary therapies,* New York, Norton, 1998.

7. Cassileth BR: Complementary and alternative therapies, *Oncol Nurs Updates* 5:1, 1998.

8. Christian M, Shoemaker D, and the Cancer Therapy Evaluation Program. *Investigator's handbook,* Bethesda, MD, National Cancer Institute, Department of Health and Human Services, October 1993.

9. Closing in on a cure: solving a 5000 year old mystery, Washington, DC, 1987, US Department of Health and Human Services. Department of Health and Human Services: Protection of human subjects: informed consent, Washington DC, *Federal Register,* January 27, 1981, Part IX.

10. Decker GM, editor: *An introduction to complementary & alternative therapies,* Pittsburgh, Oncology Nursing Press, 1999.

11. DeVita VT: Principles of chemotherapy. In DeVita VT Jr, Hellman S, Rosenberg SA, editors: *Cancer: principles and practice of oncology,* ed 5, Philadelphia, Lippincott, 1997.

12. Donovan CT: Ethics in cancer nursing practice. In Groenwald S and others, editors: *Cancer nursing: practice and principles,* ed 5, Boston, Jones & Bartlett, 2000.

13. Facts and Comparisons. *The Lawrence review of natural products monograph system,* St. Louis, Walter Kluwer Company, 1998.

14. Fleming ID: Barriers to clinical trials, *Cancer* 74:2662, 1994.

15. Food and Drug Administration Act Modernization Act of 1997. *Federal Register* 64(79):20312, 1999.

16. Freeman HP: Poverty, race, racism and survival, *Ann Epidemiol* 3:145, 1993.

17. General Accounting Office: *Off label drugs: initial results of a national survey,* GAO/PEDM-91-12BR, Washington, DC, US General Accounting Office, 1991.

18. Goldspiel BL: Clinical cancer trials, *Highlights Oncol Pract* 18:1, 2000.

19. Goldspiel BL: Faster drug approvals for cancer patients, *Highlights Oncol Pract* 18:15, 2000.

20. Gorelik PB and others: The recruitment triangle: reasons why African Americans enroll, refuse to enroll, or voluntarily withdraw from a clinical trial, *J Natl Med Assoc* 90:141, 1998.

21. Grevner MR, Chapner BA: Cancer drug discovery and development. In DeVita VT Jr, Hellman S, Rosenberg SA, editors: *Cancer: principles and practice of oncology,* ed 5, Philadelphia, Lippincott, 1997.

22. Harris KA: The informational needs of patients with cancer and their families, *Cancer Pract* 6: 39, 1998.

23. Harris Y and others: Why African Americans may not be participating in clinical trials. *J Natl Med Assoc* 88:630, 1996.

24. Johansen HK, Gotzsche PC: Improving the conduct and reporting of clinical trials, *JAMA* 283(21):2787, 2000.

25. Johnson MA, Mayer DK, Hoover HC: Obstacles to implementing cancer clinical trials, *Semin Oncol Nurs* 7:260, 1991.

26. Lindley C: Treatment highlights, *Highlights Oncol Pract* 18:20, 2000.

27. Linstrom W: Scientist, educators, patients, advocates . . . clinical trial nurses play many roles. *ONS News* 15:1, 2000.

28. Looney M: Death, dying, and grief in the face of cancer. In Burke CC, editor: *Psychosocial dimensions of oncology nursing care,* Pittsburgh, Oncology Nursing Press, 1998.

29. Mayer DK: Cancer patient empowerment, *Oncol Nurs Updates* 6:1, 1999.

30. Miller NJ, Ruben JH: Unproven methods of cancer management. Part I. Background and historical perspectives, *Oncol Nurs Forum* 10:46, 1983.

31. Milstead JC, Davis JB, Dobelle M: Quackery in the medical device field. In *Proceedings from the Second National Congress on Medical Quackery,* 1963.

32. Montbriand MJ: Past and present herbs used to treat cancer: medicine, magic, or poison? *Oncol Nurs Forum* 26:49, 1999.

33. Mouton CP and others: Barriers to black women's participation in cancer clinical trials. *J Natl Med Assoc* 89:721, 1997.

34. National Cancer Policy Board, Hewitt M, Somone J, editors: *Ensuring quality cancer care.* Washington, DC, National Academy Press, 1999.

35. National Cancer Institute: *From lab to patient care: the drug approval process,* 2000.

36. National Institute of Health. National Cancer Institute, Perscription Drug Marketing Act of 1987, Perscription Drug Amendment of 1992, Food and Drug Administration HHS Final Rule, *Federal Register* 65(86):25639, 2000.

37. The Nuremburg Code, 1949. In Beauchamp T, Childress J, editors: *Principles of biomedical ethics,* ed 2, St. Louis, Mosby, 1981.

38. Oncology Nursing Society: *Cancer chemotherapy guidelines and recommendations for practice,* Pittsburgh, Oncology Nursing Press, 1999.

39. Post, DM, Weddington, WH: Racial disparities in participation in biomedical research. *J Natl Med Assoc* 92:62, 2000.

40. Reiser J, Dyck AJ, Curran WJ, editors: *Ethics in medicine: historical perspectives and contemporary concerns,* Cambridge, MA, Massachusetts Institute of Technology, 1977.

41. Richardson MA: Research of complementary/alternative medicine therapies in oncology: promising but challenging, *J Clin Oncol* 17(suppl):38, 1999.

42. Robertson N: Clinical trials participation: viewpoints from racial/ethnic groups, *Cancer* 74:2687, 1994.

43. Shalabi AM and others: Obtaining investigational agents from the National Cancer Institute: when clinical trials are not an option, *Highlights Oncol Pract* 18:8, 2000.

44. Simon R, Friedman MA The design and interpretation of clinical trials. In Perry MC, editor. *The chemotherapy source book,.* Baltimore, Williams & Wilkins, 1992.

45. Sivesind DM, Rohaly-Davis JA: Coping with cancer: patient issues. In Burke CC, editor: *Psychosocial dimensions of oncology nursing care,* Pittsburgh, Oncology Nursing Press, 1998.

46. Sparber A and others: Use of complementary medicine by adult patients participating in cancer clinical trials, *Oncol Nurs Forum* 27:623, 2000.

47. Strickland PT, Kensler TW: Chemical and physical agents in our environment. In Abeloff MD and others, editors: *Clinical oncology,* ed 2, New York, Churchill-Livingstone, 2000.

48. Sung JFC and others: Knowledge, belief, attitude, and cancer screening among inner city African American Women, *J Natl Med Assoc* 89:405, 1997.

49. US Department of Health and Human Services: *Healthy People 2010.* January 2000. 1-800-367-4725. US Government Printing Office, Stock number 017-001-00543-6.

50. Veatch RM: *Case studies in medical ethics,* Cambridge, MA, Harvard University Press, 1977.

51. Zamboni WV, Tonda ME: New clinical trial designs, *Highlights Oncol Pract* 18:2, 2000.

52. Zhu K and others: Recruiting elderly African Americans in cancer prevention and control studies: a multifaceted approach and its effectiveness. *J Natl Med Assoc* 92(4): 169, 2000.

Clinical Trial Web Sites:

53. http://www.fda.gov/fdac/special/newdrug/testtabl.html
54. http://cancertrials.nci.govunderstanding/indepth/fda/index.html
55. http://fda.gov/cder/guidance/105–115.htm
56. http://www.ons.org
57. http://www.worldoncology.net
58. http://nhgri.nih.gov/Data/ *Genomic and Genetic Data*
59. http://www.nfcr.org/html/homepage/index.html
60. http://oncolink.upenn.edu
61. http://www.omhrc.gov
62. http://www.health.gov/healthypeople/
63. http://www.nci.nih.gov/
64. http://cancernet.nci.nih.gov/trialsrch.shtml (PDQ)
65. http://ctep.info.nih.gov/

Additional Government and Regulatory Web Sites:

Agency for Health Care Policy and Research (AHCPR), www.ahcpr.gov

Centers for Disease Control and Prevention (CDC), www.cdc.gov

CDC Hospital Infections Program (HIP), www.cdc.gov/ncidod/hip/hip.html

CDC MedWatch Program, www.cdc.gov/medwatch

Food and Drug Administration, www.fda.gov

International Standards Organization, www.iso.com

Occupational Safety and Health Administration, (OSHA), www.osha.gov

United States Post Office, www.uspo.gov

World Health Organization (WHO), www.who.com

Cancer Care
Supportive Therapies

Fatigue

Margaret L. Barnett

"Whether the disease is cured, in remission, under control, or progressing, we have the privilege of watching our patients do everyday things heroically; we gain an appreciation of them and how they get the most out of living."

Mary L. Winningham, 1995

Fatigue is the most frequently experienced symptom of cancer and cancer treatment.[2, 6, 21] It is also the most undertreated symptom. It can alter functional and cognitive status, sense of well-being, and relationships. Cancer-related fatigue often influences patient decisions about treatment and physician decisions about chemotherapy or doses of biologic response modifiers.[14, 29, 48] Patients find the symptom of fatigue distressing. Lack of energy, as many patients refer to fatigue, also negatively affects quality of life. Morbidity of cancer and cancer treatment may be increased with fatigue as a result of adverse effects on appetite, impairment of role, diminished quality of life, and loss of hope.[48] Fatigue is difficult to measure, and little is understood about its mechanisms.[6, 57] The purpose of this chapter is to highlight what are presently identified as factors that relate to fatigue. By understanding these factors that relate to cancer and cancer treatment fatigue, the nurse can plan interventions to assist patients in managing fatigue more effectively, resulting in an improved quality of life.

The Oncology Nursing Society, and the Oncology Nursing Foundation jointly sponsored The Fatigue Initiative Through Research and Education project, known as FIRE. The 5-year FIRE project has been underwritten by Ortho Biotech Inc. of Raritan, NJ. This project has focused on three components: (1) a 4-day professional education course that included more than 200 nurses from the United States, Canada, and Europe; (2) a Public Education Program that included a National Cancer Awareness Day, resource kits, and a touring virtual reality road show that provided an experiential encounter with cancer-related fatigue; and (3) multifaceted research activities including three phase I multi-institutional planning grants, a phase II multi-institutional research project, a fatigue clinical research

scholar, three multi-institutional instrument development grants, and a state-of-the-knowledge conference.[17, 42, 43] Since the FIRE project there has been a rapid increase of research and education that has resulted in new tools and techniques for assessment and measurement of fatigue in a variety of clinical settings.

DEFINITION AND MEASURES OF FATIGUE

No universal definition of fatigue exists. Fatigue has been viewed in terms of both objective performance and subjective experience.[18, 35] An objective indicator would identify a point at which performance declined either physically or mentally. Exercise endurance and accuracy of completion of a mental task are examples of the use of objective indicators. In the subjective state, the patient's self-report—perception of fatigue and how it relates to that individual's functioning—is the most important indicator of fatigue.[35, 44, 49] As nurses care for the patient with cancer fatigue, the subjective view is most relevant to the assessment and development of a plan of care that will help the patient deal with the experience.[44] *Fatigue* is described as a human response to cancer and its treatment that may be characterized by subjective feelings of weakness, exhaustion, and lack of energy resulting from prolonged exertion or stress.[2, 22] The outcome is an impaired functional status. Ferrell describes four domains of life that help explore the impact of fatigue on quality of life.[14, 15] Disruption of any of the following domains—physical well-being, psychological well-being, social concerns, or spiritual well-being—ultimately has an affect on quality of life. Fatigue is not just a physical phenomenon.[15]

Fatigue can be classified as acute or chronic. Acute fatigue is an expected occurrence after energy has been expended; it has a short duration of hours, days, or weeks.[1, 2] Acute fatigue serves as a protective mechanism, which is usually alleviated by rest. In contrast, chronic fatigue is regarded as abnormal or excessive and may be described as involving the whole body. Chronic fatigue is not relieved by rest and is overwhelming.[1, 2, 52] It may also involve multiple and additive causes such as cancer treatments and their related side effects. Patients also experience fluctuating intensity of fatigue that can create frustration when the patient and family are trying to plan activities. These fluctuations in energy levels make it hard for patients to get enough rest without slowing down unnecessarily.[21] Chronic overwhelming fatigue results in decreased activity and may eventually lead to disability.[73, 74]

The North American Nursing Diagnosis Association's definition of fatigue is: "The self-recognized state in which an individual experiences an overwhelming sustained sense of exhaustion and decreasing capacity for physical and mental work that is not relieved by rest." In addition to this definition, it is important to note that fatigue is also influenced by cultural and maturational factors.[1, 6, 8, 30]

Aaronson and colleagues[1] developed a biobehavioral definition of fatigue that addresses the contribution of physiologic and psychological functioning as well as social and cultural factors related to the experience of fatigue. Fatigue is viewed as: "The awareness of a decreased capacity for physical and/or mental activity due to an imbalance in the availability, utilization, and/or restoration of resources needed to perform activity."[1] This definition is important because it may capture the complexity of this symptom, which will assist in the development of standardized measures of fatigue.

Presently measures of fatigue are tailored to the etiology of the fatigue, therefore limiting generalization of findings. Aaronson and other researchers developed the following five characteristics to better identify possible causes and consequences of fatigue. These are: (1) subjective quantification of fatigue, (2) subjective distress because of fatigue, (3) subjective assessment of the impact of fatigue on activities of daily living, (4) certain widely recognized correlates of fatigue, and (5) key biologic parameters. Measurements were then identified for each of these important characteristics to enable measures of fatigue across multiple studies that may result in more generalizable findings. Other factors that

TABLE 27–1
Nursing Theories, Models, and Frameworks

Theory/Model/Framework	Description
Accumulation hypothesis	Suggests that accumulation of waste products in the body results in fatigue.
Depletion hypothesis	Suggests that muscular activity is impaired when the supply of substances such as carbohydrate, fat, protein, adenosine triphosphate (ATP), and protein is not available to the muscle. Anemia can also be considered a depletion mechanism.
Biochemical and physiochemical phenomena	Proposes that production, distribution, use, equalization, and movement of substances such as muscle proteins, glucose, electrolytes, and hormones may influence the experience of fatigue.
Central nervous system control	Grandjean proposes that the central control of fatigue is placed in the balance between two opposing systems: the reticular activating system (RAS) and the inhibitory system, which is believed to involve the reticular formation, the cerebral cortex, and the brain stem.
Adaptation and energy reserves	Selye suggests that each person has a certain amount of energy reserve for adaptation, and that fatigue occurs when energy is depleted. Selye's hypothesis incorporates ideas from the other hypotheses but focuses on the person's response to stressors.
Psychobiologic entropy	Proposes to associate activity, fatigue, symptoms, and functional status based on clinical observations that persons who become less active as a result of disease or treatment-related symptoms lose energizing metabolic resources.
Aistars' organizing framework	This framework is based on energy and stress theory and implicates physiologic, psychological, and situational stressors as contributing to fatigue. Aistars attempts to explain the difference between tiredness and fatigue within Selye's general adaptation syndrome.
Piper's integrated fatigue model	Piper suggests that fatigue mechanisms influence signs and symptoms of fatigue. Changes in biologic patterns such as host factors, metabolites, energy substrates, disease, and treatment, along with psychosocial patterns, impact a person's perception and leads to fatigue manifestations. The fatigue manifestations are expressed through the person's behavior.
Attentional fatigue model	Use of attentional theory linked to attentional fatigue. When increased requirements or demands for directed attention exceed available capacity, the person is at risk for attentional fatigue.

Data from references 2, 14, 15, 29, 48, 70–72.

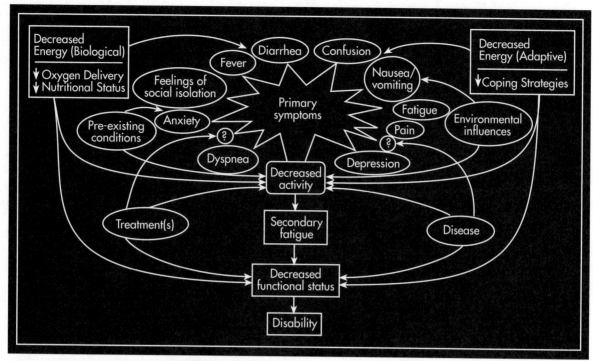

FIGURE 27-1 The psychobiological-entropy model of functioning. (Redrawn from Maryl L. Winningham. Copyright 1995. All rights reserved.)

influence the characteristic are response biases and expectations about how one does feel versus how one should feel.[1] Therefore, future studies should carefully consider how they define and measure fatigue.

Other current measures of fatigue include the Brief Fatigue Inventory, Profile of Mood States (POMS) Fatigue subscale, the Functional Assessment of Cancer Therapy-Fatigue (FACT-F), the revised Piper Fatigue Self-Report Scale, the Pearson-Byars Fatigue Feeling Checklist, Multidimensional Fatigue Inventory (MFI-20), Rhoten Fatigue Scale, and the Schwartz Cancer Fatigue Scale.* When selecting a scale to measure fatigue it's important to consider the following: (1) what aspects of fatigue are to be measured, e.g., outcomes, severity, associated factors; (2) the length of the instrument; (3) ease of scale translation from English to another language; (4) does the scale provide enough variability for the assessment of different levels of fatigue; and (5) comprehension of items on the scale. To find interventions and new treatment for fatigue it is essential to continue to research for improved methods of assessing and evaluating fatigue.

---

* References 3, 10, 15, 39, 51, 59, 61.

Pathophysiology

Because fatigue is multidimensional and multicausal, no clear support for any of the major hypotheses or models has emerged.[2, 35, 37, 73] Each of the theories, frameworks, or models in Table 27-1 represents aspects of fatigue experienced by individuals with cancer. These potential causes of fatigue assist nurses in planning interventions. Most hypotheses relating to fatigue in cancer patients remain untested. Winningham suggests that fatigue has a unique relationship to other symptoms based on how the symptoms affect the individual's level of activity (Fig. 27-1). Cancer patients who become less active as a result of disease or treatment-related symptoms lose energizing metabolic resources such as oxygen and nutrients.[74] Winningham has listed 10 propositions describing the theoretic relationships among activity level, perception of fatigue, symptom management, and functional status (Box 27-1). These propositions emphasize a need for balance between restorative activity and restorative rest.

An individual's spiritual orientation (values and meaning) determines the direction and amount of energy needed for day-to-day functioning. Quality of life in the physical, psychological, and social domains is affected by the distribution of energy among those do-

---

BOX 27-1

Ten Propositions Explaining Fatigue in Cancer

The relationship between activity, fatigue, symptom management, and functional status in people with cancer can be summarized in the following propositions:

- Too much rest as well as too little rest contributes to increased feelings of fatigue.
- Too little activity as well as too much activity contributes to increased feelings of fatigue.
- A relative balance between activity and rest promotes restoration; an imbalance promotes fatigue and deconditioning.
- Deconditioning is the adaptive energetic response whereby an organism's biologic work potential is decreased over time.
- Everyday energy expenditure in activity is the most potent known regulator of the body's energy systems. ("Use it or lose it.")
- Any symptom/condition that contributes to decreased activity will lead to deconditioning, increased fatigue, and decreased functional status.
- Any intervention that provides relief of a symptom/condition that contributes to decreased activity may simultaneously serve to mitigate fatigue and promote functioning providing that intervention does not have a sedating or catabolic effect.
- The experience of fatigue potentiates distress associated with other symptoms/conditions.
- The experience of other symptoms/conditions potentiates feelings of fatigue.
- Deconditioning and perceived fatigue interact to make every aspect of life more stressful and negatively impact quality of life, thus contributing to increased suffering.

From Winningham M: Fatigue: the missing link to quality of life, *Qual Life Res* 4:2, 1995.

---

mains.[74] Others, however, suggest that spirituality is one of the four domains that affects fatigue.[11, 14, 15]

Persons with cancer require energy to successfully manage symptoms and side effects. They may also have to deal with disruption in their usual restorative activities when nausea, pain, dyspnea, or other symptoms interfere with sleep, rest, and exercise.[15] Factors that contribute to fatigue and strategies that allay fatigue are listed in Box 27-2.[3, 4, 7, 35, 37, 72-74]

CANCER AND FATIGUE

Most patients with cancer experience some level of fatigue. Patients with lung cancer rate fatigue as severe and as the most problematic symptom.[12, 58] When Ferrell and colleagues[15] investigated how fatigue affects quality of life, they did a secondary analysis of several of their studies. The analysis revealed that fatigue is a symptom that does affect all dimensions of quality of life.[15, 61] In the physical domain individuals described the intensity of their fatigue as "bone tired." Psychological well-being was affected by feelings of uselessness, depression, or anxiety in response to fatigue. These individuals also felt that their complaints of fatigue were not taken seriously by health care providers and family members. In addition, fatigue was minimized because it was not life-threatening. When individuals spoke of social isolation they described limited leisure activity, less energy for and diminished interest in sexual activity, and less energy to continue work although many individuals had to continue to work for financial and medical insurance reasons.[15, 47, 51] Spiritual well-being was affected for individuals with fatigue. Subjects felt hopeless and abandoned by their bodies. Other subjects described fatigue

---

BOX 27-2

Propositions Relating Fatigue, Energy, Quality of Life, and Spirituality

- The cancer experience is often characterized by decreases in energy capacity and by increases in perceived fatigue.
- The cancer experience usually requires an increase in adaptive energy expenditure in responding to disease- and treatment-related exigencies, as well as an alteration of activities related to quality-of-life domains.
- Fatigue becomes a critical factor in the cancer experience when less energy is available to address everyday life challenges.
- Conflicts reflect the stress caused by energy demands of life in contrast to the individual's inability to meet those demands and contribute to increased perception of fatigue.
- An individual's spiritual orientation (values and meaning) determines direction and amount of energy focused on everyday functioning in the separate domains of quality of life.
- Coping techniques reflect appraisal of energy resources versus demands to resolve conflicts and thus reduce energy waste.
- Quality of life at any stage in the cancer experience depends on the satisfactory resolution of energy conflicts consistent with an individual's spiritual system.

From Winningham M and others: Fatigue and the cancer experience: the state of knowledge. *Oncol Nurs Forum* 2(1):23, 1994.

---

as a wasting of precious time. With respect to the concept of time, individuals generally prioritized use of their energy for family and relationships.[15, 70]

Many factors contribute to an individual's feeling of fatigue. It is not clear how all these factors interact physically and mentally to produce the symptom of fatigue (see Box 27–2). Patients with cancer are commonly advised to slow their pace and get plenty of rest.[2, 35, 45, 74] However, decreased activity may be a contributing factor to their fatigue instead of a benefit. This decrease in activity may cause an increase in energy loss resulting in decreased function of organ systems.[74] Patients with fatigue who received chemotherapy or radiotherapy showed improvement in levels of fatigue and decreased psychological distress if they followed an exercise program.[13, 41] However, it appears to be important to advise patients to monitor the intensity of fatigue and balance the activity with efficient periods of rest.[5] A recent cross-sectional descriptive survey of patterns of exercise and fatigue in physically active cancer survivors revealed that patients with non-Hodgkin's lymphoma experienced significantly decreased benefit from exercise than those patients with breast or prostate cancer.[62] More research is needed to examine the relationship between fatigue and exercise and the clinical variables that influence the response to exercise.

Pediatric studies of fatigue are scant. Fatigue in this population is not defined conceptually or empirically. Pediatric patients, their parents, and health care providers do agree that fatigue is a state of being weak or tired that is influenced by environmental and treatment-related factors that can result in difficulties with play/social activities and negative emotions or mental withdrawal. A descriptive study by Hinds and colleagues[25, 26] identified factors that contribute to or alleviate fatigue. These factors were then grouped into categories: (1) environmental, (2) personal/behavioral, (3) cultural/family/other, and (4) treatment-related from the perspective of each group of participants. Findings of the study indicated that children, adolescents, parents, and staff share similarities and differences in defining patient fatigue. The definition of fatigue reflects changes in the patient's behavior or emotional state and the recognition of the patient's desire to rest. All four perspectives identify cancer treatment as a causative or contributory factor to fatigue. Refer to Table 27–2 for details of contributing and alleviating factors in the pediatric patient.[25, 26]

Organ systems affected by fatigue often include the cardiorespiratory, musculoskeletal, and central nervous system.[20, 45, 74] Clinical signs and symptoms of these physiologic changes are listed in Box 27–3. It is a nursing responsibility to recognize those patients who are at risk for fatigue and implement appropriate nursing interventions before quality of life deteriorates.[9, 45, 56]

CANCER TREATMENTS

Surgery

Most patients with cancer usually have at least one surgery to obtain a diagnosis of cancer. Patients with cancer recovering from surgery consistently report fatigue, which may persist as long as 6 months.[44, 45, 49] Some patients have multiple surgeries related to their cancer and may experience cumulative fatigue.[45] Several physiologic mechanisms are proposed for surgery-related fatigue (Box 27–4). It is known that surgery-related fatigue does improve with time unless other cancer treatment interventions are implemented or the cancer itself progresses.[74] The relationship between fatigue and anxiety in surgical patients was examined.[8] The researchers concluded that preoperative anxiety was not a significant factor in the development of postoperative fatigue and that postoperative fatigue may be caused by physiologic rather than psychologic factors.[8] Attentional fatigue, or the decreased capacity to direct attention, was present postoperatively in women who had either mastectomy or breast conservation surgery. The attentional deficits in the postsurgical period were present regardless of the extent of the surgery.[20]

Chemotherapy

The most commonly reported side effect of chemotherapy is fatigue.* Investigators have reported that 80% to 99% of patients receiving cytotoxic agents experience fatigue.[29, 30, 35, 74] After pain, fatigue is the second most distressing symptom reported by patients receiving investigative chemotherapy.[35] In patients with lymphoma who received chemotherapy, fatigue was the most common problem second only to nausea.[62] Patients with cancer have skipped doses or withdrawn from potentially curative chemotherapy treatment because of fatigue.[74] Fatigue levels peak about 7 to 10 days after chemotherapy and then return to baseline levels before the next cycle.[48, 74] However, in women with breast cancer being treated with chemotherapy, Richardson[55] found that fatigue levels increased before subsequent cycles of chemotherapy. Fatigue was also found to be more prevalent in the late afternoon and evening. In contrast, a recent study in women with breast cancer who had completed three treatment cycles of chemotherapy found that the subjects experienced the same levels of fatigue in the first 48 hours after treatment for each cycle.[32] However, others report that chemotherapy-related fatigue is cumulative.[6, 74]

The patterns of fatigue in individual chemotherapy regimens are presently being studied. Richardson and

---

* References 6, 24, 29, 35, 45, 48, 74.

TABLE 27-2

Categories and Definitions of Contributory and Alleviating Factors in 7–12-Year-Old Patients with Cancer

Contributory	Alleviating
ENVIRONMENT	
Hospital admission or long length of stay	Protect rest or sleep patterns
Long waits involving prone positions without physical movements	Implement schedule of defined waking time and bedtime
Altered schedules or routines without designated beginning or end of day	Abbreviated clinic visit
Multiple situations of high cognitive demand	Minimize noise levels or other forms of stimulation
PERSONAL/BEHAVIORAL	
Belief that normal functioning not possible	Emphasize what the child can do instead of what he cannot
Experience of altered time or interrupted sleep pattern	Provide child with additional support and encouragement to voice any concerns
Patient's age	Encourage child to participate in activities and methods of distraction
Lack of sufficient cognitive stimulation	Allow choices
	Individualize care to specific needs of each child
CULTURAL/FAMILY/OTHER	
Being affected adversely by the emotions, moods, concerns, and expectations of family/friends	Rearranging family schedules around the time when the child has the most energy
Being urged by others to participate too vigorously in activities or to unnecessarily avoid participation	Provide more quiet activities and rest
	Encourage family members to examine expectations of child whether too demanding or too minimal
	Avoid creating dependency by allowing the child appropriate activities
	Teach parents relaxation strategies and the importance of maintaining their own health
TREATMENT-RELATED	
Experiencing invasive examinations or procedures	Careful monitoring of child's nutritional status
Repeated courses of treatment without sufficient days to recover	Monitoring of hematologic status and other treatment-related or chemotherapy-related side effects
Inadequate nutrition or metabolic changes	Evaluation of effectiveness of blood product administrations and pharmacologic interventions
Adverse effects of therapy	
Diagnosis-related factors	

Modified from Hinds P and others: Fatigue in 7- to 12-year-old patients with cancer from the staff perspective: an exploratory study. Oncol Nurs Forum 26:37, 1999, and Hinds P and others: Comparing patient, parent, and staff descriptions of fatigue in pediatric oncology patients. Cancer Nurs 22:277, 1999.

BOX 27-3

Clinical Signs and Symptoms of Physiologic Changes Related to Fatigue in Cancer

Decreased strength
Increased dyspnea
Tachycardia with exertion accompanied by frequent need to slow down or stop and rest
Difficulty concentrating
Decreased ability to perform activities
Decreased nutritional intake
Change in sleep/rest pattern

Data from references 15, 20, 45, 74.

---

colleagues[55] concluded in their study that specific chemotherapy regimens and certain methods of drug administration were associated with fatigue that was more intense and unrelenting. For example, patients receiving weekly injections experienced moderate levels of fatigue, whereas those receiving cycles every 3 to 4 weeks experienced higher levels of fatigue. The most severe fatigue was experienced with the combination of bolus plus continuous infusion chemotherapy.[55] It remains unknown how drowsiness from antiemetics, analgesics, antianxiety agents, and antidepressants affect fatigue in the person receiving chemotherapy.

Multiple factors associated with chemotherapy-related fatigue (Box 27–5) have been investigated, but no single responsible cause has been cited. Some researchers have found that a correlation exists between

---

BOX 27-4

Potential Causes of Postoperative Fatigue

Increased cardiac effort
Use of anesthetics
Route of administration of analgesics
Alteration in nutrition
Decreased physical activity
Use of variety of treatment methods

---

the presence of fatigue and the number of other symptoms experienced, such as pain, dyspnea, nausea/vomiting, or cachexia.[7, 32, 35, 53, 55, 74] Subjects who were already experiencing symptoms prior to the start of chemotherapy experienced more severe fatigue after chemotherapy.[7, 32] Most women with menopausal symptoms experienced an increase in the intensity of fatigue.[7] The duration of illness and the length of hospitalization also affect the fatigue experience.[19] However, performance status was found to be a better predictor of fatigue severity than age, gender, or extent of disease in patients receiving chemotherapy.[32]

Breast cancer patients receiving chemotherapy who described increased anxiety and depression were found to have increased levels of fatigue.[55] Women who used catastrophizing as a coping mechanism also exhibited increased levels of fatigue. Castastrophizing is characterized by negative self statements and overly negative thought and ideas about the future.[7, 32] Nursing knowledge of potential fatigue patterns is essential to develop

---

BOX 27-5

Factors Associated with Chemotherapy Fatigue

Pathologic
Environmental
Psychological
Nutritional
Duration of illness
Concurrent medical condition
Drug interactions
Age of subject
Menopausal symptoms
Performance status
Chemotherapy side effects

---

a plan of care and interventions for the patient with chemotherapy-related fatigue.

Radiation Therapy

Skin problems and fatigue are the most frequently reported side effects of radiation therapy.[64, 74] Most radiation side effects are local and predictable based on the site of the treatment field. Patients who have radiation and chemotherapy are at increased risk for fatigue whether the chemotherapy and radiation are concurrent or sequential.[36] Causes of fatigue in radiation therapy patients are not clear, but some research suggests that the risk for fatigue increases with the factors listed in Box 27-6.[23, 30] The incidence of fatigue is 65% to 100% in patients receiving radiation treatment.[45] Patients receiving radiation therapy have multiple disease sites and receive different doses for different cancers. Fatigue does not appear to be affected by the dose of radiation or fractionation; therefore, it has been suggested that a central mechanism may be responsible for the symptom of fatigue (see Box 27-2).[31, 45] Smets and colleagues[65] found that the number one predictor of posttreatment fatigue is the degree of fatigue that is present before starting radiation therapy.

Fatigue associated with radiation therapy is an important clinical problem for patients receiving treatment because of the negative impact on quality of life.[15, 29, 45] It is the only common systemic side effect of local radiation therapy with an acute onset and gradually increases in its severity during the course of radiations therapy. Fatigue is the most severe during the last week of radiation treatment.[31, 64]

Over the course of radiation therapy, the prevalence of fatigue can vary. Fatigue is usually intermittent at the beginning of treatment and then gradually increases as the treatment progresses.[29, 40, 64] The exception to this is the patient with lung cancer, whose fatigue is more severe at the beginning of radiation treatment and gradually decreases as the tumor responds to therapy. The improved energy level may be related to newly opened

---

BOX 27-6

Factors That Increase the Risk for Fatigue with Radiation Therapy

Age > 34 years	Length of treatment
Gender	Level of fatigue before
Weight loss	treatment
Psychological distress	Sleep disturbance
Pain	Advanced disease
Symptom distress	

---

airways resulting in less effort to breathe.[45] Fatigue may decline over the weekend when patients are not receiving radiation therapy treatment.[64] Early afternoon and evening are the most common times for patients to feel fatigued.[45] At 2 weeks after radiation patients report that fatigue has almost returned to preradiation level.[64] Usually within 3 months after radiation therapy is completed, fatigue decreases to pretreatment levels.[29, 30, 45] Another study showed that fatigue in disease-free patients at 9 months after radiation did not differ significantly from the general population. In this group of patients the degree of fatigue experienced after radiation was related to functional disability, pain, and intensity of fatigue prior to radiation therapy.[65]

Biotherapy

Biologic response modifiers (BRMs) are a category of biologic agents that alter the immune system by stimulating or suppressing it. Types of BRMs include interferon, interleukin-2, tumor necrosis factor, colony-stimulating factors, monoclonal antibodies, and retinoids. Each of these agents may affect the type and pattern of fatigue experienced by the individual (Table 27–3).[50, 56, 67, 74] The pattern or duration of fatigue is affected by the BRM agent, dose, and route of administration. Fatigue associated with interferon is most severe in the afternoon and evening. It is also dose related and worsens with continued therapy, and it is associated with significant depression.[11] The cause of fatigue induced by α-interferon is unknown, but it may have a neuromuscular component.[10] Another possible mechanism of fatigue during treatment with α-interferon is hormonal syndromes (e.g., hypothyroidism).[33]

Toxicity from the biotherapy agents are dose limiting, requiring reduction in dosages, postponement of treatment, or termination of treatment.[45] Biotherapy is responsible for fatigue that is more severe than the fatigue related to surgery, radiation therapy, or chemotherapy.[56] Fatigue related to biotherapy is only a part of a group of symptoms, including fever, chills, myalgia, headache, and malaise. Additional side effects include mental fatigue and cognitive deficits.[35] Because fatigue is so pervasive and severe in patients receiving BRMs, preventing and relieving the fatigue becomes a high priority in the plan of care.

Bone Marrow and Stem Cell Transplant

Fatigue is commonly reported following bone marrow/stem cell transplant and has a negative effect on overall quality of life.[4, 14, 19] Even though studies show that overall quality of life improves during the months and years after transplant, patients report fatigue as a major concern. In one study of stem cell transplant patients 1 year after transplant, evaluation showed that the mean energy rating of patients had returned to only 70% of normal.[38] Patients generally report that the intensity of fatigue lessens as time increases. However, fatigue remains a constant concern throughout the course of recovery after stem cell transplant.

Some of the factors that are thought to be associated with increased fatigue include depression, anxiety, sleep problems, older age, decreased performance status, and autologous stem cell transplant.[4, 19, 27, 28] Other variables that do not seem to correlate significantly with fatigue include diagnosis, cancer stage, or chemotherapy regimens.[19] Autologous stem cell transplant patients with breast cancer who experienced a longer time to engraftment reported more severe fatigue toward the end of treatment. In addition, prolonged hospitalization resulted in increased fatigue. Also, the patients who received total-body irradiation experienced sleep problems after transplant and also experienced increased fatigue.[4, 19, 27, 28] The issue of the intensity of fatigue related to gender after bone marrow transplant remains controversial. Future research should focus on prospective studies that identify biologic parameters associated with fatigue including psychological and physiologic mechanism that produce fatigue and interventions

TABLE 27–3
Biologic Response Modifier Agents and Common Side Effects

BRM Agent	Comments
Interferons	Physical and mental fatigue are common dose-limiting side effects. Fatigue may be worse in older patients and those receiving other BRMs concurrently. Flulike syndrome occurs.
Interleukin-2	Greater fatigue occurs than from other BRMs and is dose-limiting toxicity. Fatigue increases with length of treatment and flulike syndrome. Cognition and orientation decline.
Tumor necrosis factor (TNF)	Muscle wasting may be mediated by TNF. Flulike syndrome occurs.
Colony-stimulating factors (CSF)	Difficult to assess—fatigue is already present when most CSFs are started. Erythropoietin could reverse fatigue related to anemia. Cumulative fatigue occurs with GM-CSF, especially in the AIDS population.

GM, granulocyte-macrophage; AIDS, acquired immunodeficiency syndrome. Data from references 10, 11, 50, 56.

to alleviate fatigue in patients who receive allogeneic or autologous bone marrow transplant, stem cell transplant, or high-dose chemotherapy with stem cell transplant.

FACTORS INFLUENCING FATIGUE

Initially, patients may not notice how fatigue has changed some of their activities. But over time, they eventually reach a values-determined balance between their energy at hand and their desire to do what they want.[75] Quality of life as it relates to fatigue is a nebulous concept. What one patient deems to be quality is not the same for another. Nurses must help patients discover their own balance between fatigue, energy, quality of life, and spirituality.[14, 15]

In addition to cancer and cancer treatment, patients experience a variety of problems that may elicit mental, physical, and emotional fatigue. Physical, psychosocial, functional, and spiritual factors influence fatigue. Physical factors such as symptom distress and overall performance status, along with psychological factors such as depression and anxiety, contribute to fatigue and its impact on the life of the patient with cancer (Box 27–7).[2, 11, 12, 14, 35, 54, 74] Another factor that influences fatigue is the perception of fatigue by the oncologist. Even though the oncologist's perception and patient's report of the incidence of fatigue are very similar, only 27% of patients reported that their oncologist recommended any treatment for fatigue. This is significant because when patients used the oncologist-recommended treatment for fatigue the patients reported improvement in their level of fatigue.[47, 70]

The value and meaning that individuals give to the changes in their life that have been caused by fatigue will influence their level of functioning and their contentment with the overall situation.[7, 30, 45] Some patients find a few weeks of fatigue acceptable in light of their personal goals for a cure, remission, or relief of a symptom such as pain. Other patients may find that fatigue for any length of time is an unacceptable experience.[45] Being able to carry out the functions of everyday living are important considerations for patients, whether it be their activities at home, at work, or socializing. Attentional fatigue (decreased capacity to concentrate) affects functioning as well.[8] Patients often keep books at their hospital bedside but never seem to find the energy to read them. Mental demands are routinely placed on patients to digest complex information regarding diagnosis, tests, treatments, prognosis, and other information. Attentional fatigue may be common during and after cancer treatment.[20, 74] Patients with breast cancer who received chemotherapy experienced increased cognitive dysfunction when compared to those who did not receive chemotherapy. In addition, the higher the doses of chemo the higher the occurrence of cognitive impairment. It is not yet known if this is associated with clinical disability or inability to work.[16, 68] More research is needed in this area.

Spirituality is another aspect of personhood that affects how fatigue is managed. Winningham[75] describes spirituality as "expanding boundaries inward, outward, and upward." In trying to make sense of what has happened in their lives, patients attempt to attach some value or meaning to their diagnosis, treatment, suffering, recovery period, and possible impending death. By searching for value or meaning in their experiences, patients consider the meaning and consequences of their diagnosis. Patients also review their life and look for ways to cope by being hopeful, changing their priorities, and learning to live with their diagnosis.[14]

All these spiritual and emotional activities take energy in an already fatigued individual. In some instances patients are thought to be "depressed" but in reality they may be demonstrating an energy-saving behavior—withdrawal.[75] Patients are attempting to balance an interrelationship of fatigue, spirituality, and quality of life by their own value system. Nurses must assess where patients are in that process and not where nurses expect them (or their families) to be. Winningham's model (see Fig. 27–1) illustrates the interrelationships between energy available, energy expenditure, and quality-of-life domains. The amount of energy that healthy individuals commit to role expectations and daily activities in each domain is fairly consistent over time.[75] However, a diagnosis of cancer and the demands of cancer treatment require reallocation of the amount of energy spent on each activity. Conflict or coping will influence the energy available to the person. A patient's spiritual focus determines the direction and amount of

---

BOX 27–7

Factors That Influence Fatigue

Physical

Pain
Sleep/rest patterns
Nutrition
Gastrointestinal problems
Bone marrow suppression
Multiple medications
Overall physical condition (Performance status)

Psychosocial

Depression/isolation
Anxiety
Appearance
Control
Roles/isolation
Relationships/affection/ sexual function
Finances

Data from references 2, 6, 7, 31, 32, 34, 35, 40, 45, 74.

energy used on daily activities in the separate domains of quality of life.[75] Box 27–2, identifies relationships among fatigue, energy, quality of life, and spirituality.[75]

Fatigue in Advanced Cancer

Fatigue in patients with advanced cancer is chronic and continues without relief. This unrelenting fatigue promotes an aversion to activity with a desire to escape.[54] Significant factors that relate to fatigue in patients with advanced cancer are length of illness, intensity of pain experience, dyspnea, and mood disturbance.[6, 66] Patients with lung cancer have more severely limited physical functions than other cancer patients regardless of age.[6] Women with lung cancer seem to experience greater fatigue than men.[12] Research has demonstrated that age and morbidity are significantly correlated; however, age plays less of a role in physical function than does symptom distress associated with the cancer. Symptom distress is the amount or intensity of physical or mental distress or suffering experienced from a specific symptom. It is reflective of the individual's response to her physical, psychosocial, spiritual, familial, and cultural background experience along the cancer continuum. For example, a patient with a sedentary life-style before her illness may not be as upset at the changes fatigue might bring to an already quiet life-style. However, a young man who is married with children and active in seasonal sports would tend to be more upset in his life-style changes related to fatigue.

A recent study compared the prevalence of fatigue in patients with advanced cancer and a control group. The prevalence of severe fatigue was 75% in the advanced cancer group. The severity of fatigue was unrelated to age, sex, diagnosis, presence or site of metastasis, anemia, dose of opioid or steroid, any of the hematologic or biochemical findings (except urea), nutritional status, voluntary muscle function, or mood. Patients with advanced cancer were found to have a significant relationship between fatigue severity and the symptoms of pain and dyspnea. In the control group there was a correlation between the prevalence of fatigue with the symptoms of anxiety and depression. It is possible that fatigue may be the single most important indicator of quality of life in patients with advanced cancer.[66]

Hope or the "fighting spirit" plays a therapeutic role in the coping process of patients with cancer.[54] Hope instills an expectation of a future good that is realistically possible and significant to the patient. It may be possible to decrease fatigue and increase quality of life in the patient with advanced cancer by using nursing strategies that control physical symptoms such as pain and shortness of breath. It is also necessary to use strategies that decrease stress, anxiety, depression, and fear as a means to enhance hope.[22]

CONCLUSION

Present research documents a high incidence of fatigue in patients with cancer and those receiving cancer treatment. Presently the patient's self-report is the most satisfactory measure of fatigue. Care of the person with fatigue is based on clinical judgment rather than on research. Further research is needed to improve the care of patients with fatigue, including the measurement, interventions, economic cost, and development of education strategies.

With the present knowledge and future research data, it is hoped that outcomes in patients with fatigue will continue to improve. This will have a positive impact on quality of life for many individuals.

Nursing Management

Fatigue is the most common symptom of cancer and cancer treatment and is the least understood or researched. Because fatigue is not life-threatening, health care providers often minimize the impact that it has on patients' level of functioning and quality of life.[14, 15] At present, practice guidelines are based on clinical judgment rather than research.[45] Despite limitations in the knowledge about prevention and treatment of fatigue, nursing has much to offer in helping patients manage fatigue. Careful nursing assessment, collaboration, planning the interventions, evaluation, and modification of the nursing plan are key elements in the management of fatigue. The nursing diagnosis of *Fatigue* should focus on the patient's response to the occurrence of symptoms in the physical, psychosocial, functional, and spiritual areas. The nurse should also explore the meaning that the patient assigns to these symptoms.[15] The goal for nursing care for the patient with cancer or treatment-related fatigue is to maintain the highest possible level of functioning and quality of life by helping the patient balance energy requirements with the energy on hand.

Patients underestimate the occurrence and severity of fatigue related to cancer and cancer treatment. Patients' perceived ability to deal with symptom distress correlates with fatigue distress.[45, 48, 74] Less symptom distress will be experienced by education of patients and families about the effects of fatigue as it relates to their cancer or cancer treatment.

Nursing Diagnoses: *Cancer and Cancer Treatment-Related Fatigue*

- *Fatigue*[45, 50, 53, 56]
- *Pain*
- *Ineffective breathing pattern*
- *Mobility, impaired physical*
- *Nutrition, altered: less than body requirements*
- *Coping, ineffective individual*
- *Knowledge deficit (affects of fatigue after chemotherapy, radiation therapy, BRM or bone marrow/stem cell transplant)*
- *Social isolation (changes in roles/relationships, activity level)*
- *Anxiety*
- *Spiritual distress (distress of the human spirit)*
- *Hopelessness*

Outcome Goals

The patient, caregiver, or significant other will be able to:

- Identify factors that cause or increase fatigue.
- Describe factors that restore or conserve energy.
- Share feelings regarding the effects of fatigue on life-style.
- Establish priorities for daily and weekly activities.
- Participate in activities that stimulate and balance physical, cognitive, affective, social and spiritual domains.

Assessment

Factors to consider in assessment of the patient with fatigue:

- Assessment should not be a burden to an already fatigued patient.[20, 22, 35, 74]
- Timing of the assessment is important to gain pertinent information.
- If fatigue does not gradually decrease once the treatment had been completed, an evaluation should be done to rule out other potential medical problems.

Qualitative assessment of the cancer patient's level of fatigue:

- Assess changes in functional ability by using theoretic models such as Piper or Winningham (see Table 27–1).
- Ask the patient to describe a typical day now and before the illness.[22, 35, 41, 74]

- What has the patient stopped doing because of fatigue?
- Which of these things are most important for the patient to continue and which of these could be done by someone else?
- What time of day is the fatigue lowest and most severe?
- How does the feeling of fatigue relate to the patient's cancer treatment?
- What does the patient do to lessen the fatigue and is it beneficial?
- Ask the patient how he views the fatigue and what it means to him?
- What does the patient identify as a strength, ability, or interest?
- How is the patient/family coping with fatigue, and how has the patient coped in the past?
- Review present medical history and data for present or suspected presence of other medical conditions that might cause fatigue, e.g., pulmonary disease, sleep disruption, dehydration, anemia.

Factors to consider in measurement:

- Method of measurement should not be a burden to an already fatigued patient.
- Measurement methods should match the developmental stage of the patient.[1, 17]
- Culture and primary language will influence measurement options.
- Various self-report tools that range from a simple yes-no question to a multiple adjective checklist are used for fatigue measurement. The Rhoten Fatigue Scale is a linear 0 to 10 scale, with 0 being not tired, full of energy, or peppy and 10 representing total exhaustion.
- Measurement should be done at multiple points in time (e.g., baseline, pretreatment, nadir).
- Fatigue measurement is not well developed; however, consider the criteria just listed and find a consistent, helpful measure.

Interventions

- Facilitate rest or sleep by the following[18, 23, 63, 66]:
    Provide environmental comforts (e.g., room temperature, light/dark, noise/interruptions).
    Minimize symptoms that interfere with sleep such as pain, nausea/vomiting, dyspnea, or anxiety.
    Administer prescribed medication PRN or on schedule as indicated.
    Encourage patients to use strategies that relieve fatigue (e.g., conversation, hobbies, regular light exercise, relaxation techniques).

Sleep just long enough. Curtailing time in bed helps patient feel refreshed and avoids fragmented and shallow sleep.

Strengthen circadian cycling by regular arousal time and bedtime.

Offer bedtime snack to prevent hunger from disturbing sleep.

Explore how naps affect the patient (e.g., feel refreshed, feel more tired and listless, sleep better at night, sleep poorly).

Avoid stimulants such as cola, caffeine, and chocolate, especially after lunch.

Avoid alcohol ingestion near bedtime because it may fragment sleep.

- Prioritize activities by encouraging the patient to[35, 45, 54, 74]:

    Save energy for most important or enjoyed activities.

    Set limits (it is alright to say "no").

    Pace activities to save energy.

    Keep a log of activities (e.g., daily routines and accompanying energy levels to assist in setting priorities and planning ahead).

    Plan daily activities in advance to manage physical and emotional stressors.

- Exercise[5, 35, 41, 45, 60, 72, 73, 75]:

    Teach self-care techniques for exercising such as walking daily, pulse monitoring, and avoiding temperature extremes.

    Contraindications to exercise include unusual fatigability, unusual muscle weakness, irregular pulse, leg pain or cramps, chest pain, nausea, vomiting within previous 24 to 36 hours, dyspnea, or IV chemotherapy within the past 24 hours.

    Facilitate hospitalized patients by scheduling light activity periods and referring to occupational or physical therapy department for assistance in activity planning.

    Exercise is helpful in providing stimulation opportunities to prevent boredom-related fatigue.

- Other interventions[9, 53, 54, 66, 74]:

    Assist patient with personal hygiene to save energy for priority activities.

    Encourage small meals—less energy is needed for digestion.

    Provide nutritious, high-protein meals and snacks throughout the day.

    Collaborate with physician to treat the underlying physical causes of fatigue (e.g., pain, dyspnea).

    Collaborate with physician to treat anemia (e.g., oxygen therapy, erythropoeitin, transfusions).

PATIENT/FAMILY TEACHING PRIORITIES

Fatigue

Give all patients preparatory information about fatigue.

Teach the patient how to assess the intensity of their fatigue.

Think of energy as a bank account; deposits and withdrawals must be planned on a daily to weekly basis.

Rest when tired; sit or lie down frequently.

Avoid physical and emotional stress.

Limit environmental stressors (temperature extremes, long hot showers/baths, smoke or noxious fumes).

Pace daily activities according to energy level.

Plan workload around your best times of the day.

If fatigue increases, set priorities and reduce activities.

Solicit help for household chores, child care, errands.

Food will help energy levels; eat nutritious snacks.

Mild to moderate exercise (walking, golfing or swimming) increase energy levels; avoid heavy exercise.

Do whatever you can while sitting (use shower bench or lawn chair while in shower and to dry off).

Loose fitting clothes allow easier breathing.

Organize work space to save energy.

Use cookwear you can serve from.

To relieve mental fatigue, reading, sitting outdoors, gardening, and talking with friends are helpful.

Try to keep a balance between the activities you must do and those that make you happy.

Data from references 45, 46, 52, 56, 63, 74.

Evaluate current medications that may contribute to fatigue (e.g., antiemetics, anticonvulsants, anxiolytics).

Collaborate with physician to administer prescribed agents that alter metabolism (e.g., Megace [methylphenidate]).

Discuss psychosocial spiritual stressors (e.g., meaning of fatigue, depression, financial concerns).

As fatigue decreases, gradually reintroduce normal activities into the daily routine and monitor fatigue status.

Use assistive devices (e.g., walkers, wheelchairs) to conserve energy.

Suggest attention-restoring activities for those patients with mental fatigue, such as walking or sitting in a natural environment, tending plants or gardening, or bird watching.

If a patient's fatigue does not gradually decrease within a few months of completing the treatment, a medical evaluation should be done.

Evaluation

- Evaluate response to interventions by using the patient's subjective response and activity log. Determine if patient/family are satisfied; if so, continue nursing care plan.
- If patient/family are not satisfied; look first at the goals and goal attainment.

Are the goals reasonable?

Ask the patient/family if the importance of the intervention is understood and if the interventions are practical for them.

If goals and the patient/family understanding are adequate, repeat the nursing process starting with assessment (a different measurement tool may be helpful).

If interventions are not practical or applicable for the patient/family, modify the nursing plan and then reevaluate.

Chapter Questions

1. Fatigue has been viewed in terms of both:
   a. Objective experience, subjective performance
   b. Objective performance, subjective experience
   c. Objective performance, subjective performance
   d. Objective experience, subjective experience

2. Physiologic changes related to fatigue include:
   a. Increased dyspnea, heart rate, and strength
   b. Decreased dyspnea, heart rate, and strength
   c. Increased dyspnea, heart rate, and decreased strength
   d. Decreased dyspnea, heart rate, and increased strength

3. Patients with lung cancer generally have more fatigue at the beginning of radiation than after the treatment is completed. Which response best explains this improvement in the patient?
   a. The patient has stopped smoking recently.
   b. The tumor is decreasing in size, allowing improved breathing, which consequently decreases fatigue.
   c. Radiation therapy always decreases fatigue in patients with any type of cancer.
   d. Patients eat better while receiving radiation and consequently have more energy.

4. What cancer therapy seems to produce the most severe fatigue that may result in the patient discontinuing therapy?
   a. Biologic response modifiers
   b. Chemotherapy
   c. Radiation therapy
   d. Surgery

5. The most helpful interventions to alleviate fatigue include:
   a. Avoid going out of the house, and limit contact with friends.
   b. Rest in bed more, and limit activity.
   c. Continue normal level of activity except limit social activities.
   d. Rest periods, napping, mild exercise, and a good night's sleep

6. Compared with the fatigue experienced by healthy people, cancer treatment-related fatigue is:
   a. Not fully relieved by sleep or rest
   b. Only occurs after chemotherapy
   c. Only observed in people who are depressed
   d. Not fully relieved by activity or distraction

7. The most reliable information to assess fatigue is determined by:
   a. Assessment of the behavior of the person
   b. Muscle-function testing
   c. The self-report of the person
   d. Report from the nurse or the family regarding the person with fatigue

8. An activity log, maintained by the person, will assist in providing information from what area(s)?
   a. Prioritizing activities
   b. Setting realistic goals with the patient
   c. Identifying rest/sleep patterns
   d. All the above

9. Factors that increase the risk for fatigue for patients receiving radiation therapy include:
   a. Age > 34 years, pain, gender, duration of illness
   b. Age < 34 years, pain, gender, duration of illness
   c. Age < 34 years, pain, gender, duration of treatment
   d. Age > 34 years, pain, gender, duration of treatment

10. The primary outcome of effective management of cancer treatment-related fatigue is expected to be:
    a. Fewer phone calls and office visits
    b. Improved individual quality of life
    c. Acceptance of fatigue as an inevitable result of cancer treatment
    d. Improved exercise program for patients with fatigue

BIBLIOGRAPHY

1. Aaronson L and others: Defining and measuring fatigue, *Image J Nurs Scholar* 31:45, 1999.
2. Aistars J: Fatigue in the cancer patient: a conceptual approach to a clinical problem, *Oncol Nurs Forum* 14:25, 1987.
3. Akechi T and others: Fatigue and its associated factors in ambulatory cancer patients: a preliminary study, *J Pain Symptom Manage* 17:42, 1999.
4. Andrydowski M and others: Patients' psychosocial concerns following stem cell transplantation, *Bone Marrow Transplant* 24:1121, 1999.
5. Berger A: Patterns of fatigue and activity and rest during adjuvant breast cancer chemotherapy, *Oncol Nurs Forum* 25:51, 1998.
6. Blesch K: Correlates of fatigue in people with breast or lung cancer, *Oncol Nurs Forum* 18:81, 1991.
7. Broeckel J and others: Characteristics and correlates of fatigue after adjuvant chemotherapy for breast cancer, *J Clin Oncol* 16:1689, 1998.
8. Cimprich BE: Attentional fatigue following breast cancer surgery, *Res Nurs Health* 1:199, 1992.
9. Clark M, Lacasse C: Cancer-related fatigue: clinical practice issues, *Clin J Oncol Nurs* 2:45, 1998.
10. Dalakas M, Mock V, Hawkins M: Fatigue: definitions, mechanisms, and paradigms for study, *Semin Oncol* 25(1 suppl 1):48, 1998.
11. Dean GE, Spears L, Ferrell BR: Fatigue in patients with cancer receiving interferon alpha, *Cancer Pract* 3:164, 1995.
12. Degner LF, Sloan JA: Symptom distress in newly diagnosed ambulatory cancer patients and as a predictor of survival in lung cancer, *J Pain Symptom Manage* 10:423, 1995.
13. Dimeo F and others: Effects of physical activity on the fatigue and psychologic status of cancer patients during chemotherapy, *Cancer* 85:2273, 1999.
14. Ferrell BR and others: Quality of life in long-term cancer survivors, *Oncol Nurs Forum* 22:915, 1995.
15. Ferrell BR and others: "Bone tired": the experience of fatigue and its impact on quality of life, *Oncol Nurs Forum* 23:1539, 1996.
16. Ganz P: Cognitive dysfunction following adjuvant treatment of breast cancer: a new dose-limiting toxic effect? *J Natl Cancer Inst* 90:182, 1998.
17. Grant M and others: Developing a team for multicultural, multi-institutional research on fatigue and quality of life, *Oncol Nurs Forum* 25:1404, 1998.
18. Graydon JE and others: Fatigue-reducing strategies used by patients receiving treatment for cancer, *Cancer Nurs* 18:23, 1995.
19. Hann D and others: Fatigue and quality of life in breast cancer patients undergoing autologous stem cell transplantation: a longitudinal comparative study, *J Pain Symptom Manage* 17:311, 1999.
20. Hansen M, Kehlet H: Fatigue and anxiety in surgical patients, *Br J Surg* 79:165, 1992.
21. Harpham W: Resolving the frustration of fatigue, *CA Cancer J Clin* 49:178, 1999.
22. Held JL: Cancer care: managing fatigue—help your patients cope with persistent fatigue during their cancer treatments, *Nursing* 24:26, 1994.
23. Hickok J and others: Frequency and correlates of fatigue in lung cancer patients receiving radiation therapy: implications for management, *J Pain Symptom Manage* 11:370, 1996.
24. Hilfinger D and others: Patients' perspectives of fatigue while undergoing chemotherapy, *Oncol Nurs Forum* 24:43, 1997.
25. Hinds P and others: Fatigue in 7- to 12-year-old patients with cancer from the staff perspective: an exploratory study, *Oncol Nurs Forum* 26:37, 1999.
26. Hinds P and others: Comparing patient, parent, and staff descriptions of fatigue in pediatric oncology patients, *Cancer Nurs* 22:277, 1999.
27. Hjermstad M and others: Health-related quality of life 1 year after allogeneic or autologous stem-cell transplantation: a prospective study, *J Clin Oncol* 17:706, 1999.
28. Hjermstad M and others: Do patients who are treated with stem cell transplantation have a health-related quality of life comparable to the general population after 1 year? *Bone Marrow Transplant* 24:911, 1999.
29. Irvine D and others: A critical appraisal of the research literature investigating fatigue in the individual with cancer, *Cancer Nurs* 14:188, 1991.
30. Irvine D and others: The prevalence and correlates of fatigue in patients receiving treatment with chemotherapy and radiotherapy, *Cancer Nurs* 17:367, 1994.
31. Irvine D and others: Fatigue in women with breast cancer receiving radiation therapy, *Cancer Nurs* 21:127, 1998.
32. Jacobsen P and others: Fatigue in women receiving adjuvant chemotherapy for breast cancer: characteristics, course, and correlates, *J Pain Symptom Manage* 18:233, 1999.
33. Jones T, Wadler S, Hupart K: Endocrine-mediated mechanisms of fatigue during treatment with interferon-α, *Semin Oncol* 25(1 suppl 1):54, 1998.
34. Kalman D, Villani L: Nutritional aspects of cancer-related fatigue, *J Am Diet Assoc* 97:650, 1997.
35. Love RR and others: Side effects and emotional distress during cancer chemotherapy, *Cancer* 63:604, 1989.
36. Macquart-Moulin G and others: Concomitant chemoradiotherapy for patients with nonmetastatic breast carcinoma, *Cancer* 85:2190, 1999.
37. Mast M: Correlates of fatigue in survivors of breast cancer, *Cancer Nurs* 21:136, 1998.
38. McQuellon R and others: Quality of life and psychological distress of bone marrow transplant recipients: the "time trajectory" to recovery over the first year, *Bone Marrow Transplant* 21:477, 1998.
39. Mendoza T and others: The rapid assessment of fatigue severity in cancer patients, *Cancer* 85:1186, 1999.
40. Miaskowski C, Lee K: Pain, fatigue, and sleep disturbances in oncology outpatients receiving radiation therapy for bone metastasis: a pilot study, *J Pain Symptom Manage* 17:320, 1999.
41. Mock V and others: Effects of exercise on fatigue, physical functioning, and emotional distress during radiation therapy for breast cancer, *Oncol Nurs Forum* 24:991, 1997.

42. Mock V, Nail L, Grant M: Implementing the FIRE planning grant, *Oncol Nurs Forum* 25:1389, 1998.
43. Mock V and others: Establishing mechanisms to conduct multi-institutional research—fatigue in patients with cancer: an exercise intervention, *Oncol Nurs Forum* 25:1391, 1998.
44. Nail L, King K: Fatigue, *Semin Oncol Nurs* 3:257, 1987.
45. Nail L, Jones L: Fatigue side effects and treatment and quality of life, *Qual Life Res* 4:8, 1995.
46. Nail L: The fatigue of treatment, *Reflections Fourth Quarter:* 17, 1999.
47. Newell S and others: How well do medical oncologists' perceptions reflect their patients' reported physical and psychosocial problems? *Cancer* 83:1640, 1998.
48. Pickard-Holley S: Fatigue in cancer patients: a descriptive study, *Cancer Nurs* 14:13, 1991.
49. Piper BF, Lindsey A, Dodd M: Fatigue mechanisms in cancer patients: developing nursing theory, *Oncol Nurs Forum* 14:17, 1987.
50. Piper BF and others: Recent advances in the management of biotherapy-related side effects: fatigue, *Oncol Nurs Forum* 16:27, 1989.
51. Piper BF and others: The revised piper fatigue scale: psychometric evaluation in women with breast cancer, *Oncol Nurs Forum* 25:677, 1998.
52. Potempa KM: Chronic fatigue, *Annu Rev Nurs Res* 11:57, 1993.
53. Rhodes V, Watson P, Hanson B: Patients' descriptions of the influence of tiredness and weakness on self-care abilities, *Cancer Nurs* 11:186, 1988.
54. Rhodes VA, McDaniel RW: Fatigue and advanced illness, *Qual Life Res* 4:14, 1995.
55. Richardson A, Ream E, Wilson-Barnett: Fatigue in patients receiving chemotherapy: patterns of change, *Cancer Nurs* 21:17, 1998.
56. Robinson KD, Posner JD: Patterns of self-care needs and interventions related to biologic response modifier therapy: fatigue as a model, *Semin Oncol Nurs* 8:17, 1992.
57. Ryden M: Energy: a crucial consideration in the nursing process, *Oncol Nurs Forum* 16:71, 1977.
58. Sarna L, Brecht M: Dimensions of symptom distress in women with advanced lung cancer: a factor analysis, *Heart Lung* 26:23, 1997.
59. Schneider R: Reliability and validity of the Multidimensional Fatigue Inventory (MFI-20) and the Rhoten Fatigue Scale among rural cancer outpatients, *Cancer Nurs* 21:370, 1998.
60. Schwartz A: Patterns of exercise and fatigue in physically active cancer survivors, *Oncol Nurs Forum* 25:485, 1998.
61. Schwartz A: The Schwartz Cancer Fatigue Scale: testing reliability and validity, *Oncol Nurs Forum* 25:711, 1998.
62. Sitzia J and others: Side effects of CHOP in the treatment of non-Hodgkin's lymphoma, *Cancer Nurs* 20:430, 1997.
63. Skalla KA, Lacasse C: Patient education for fatigue, *Oncol Nurs Forum* 19:1537, 1992.
64. Smets E and others: Fatigue and radiotherapy: (A) experience in patients undergoing treatment, *Br J Cancer* 78:899, 1998.
65. Smets E and others: Fatigue and radiotherapy: (B) experience in patients 9 months following treatment, *Br J Cancer* 78:907, 1998.
66. Stone P and others: Fatigue in advanced cancer: a prospective controlled cross-sectional study, *Br J Cancer* 79:1479, 1999.
67. St. Pierre B, Kasper C, Lindsey A: Fatigue mechanisms in patients with cancer: effects of tumor necrosis factor and exercise on skeletal muscle, *Oncol Nurs Forum* 19:419, 1992.
68. van Dam F and others: Impairment of cognitive function in women receiving adjuvant treatment for high risk breast cancer: high dose versus standard dose chemotherapy, *J Natl Cancer Inst* 90:210, 1998.
69. Varricchio C: Selecting a tool for measuring fatigue, *Oncol Nurs Forum* 12:122, 1985.
70. Vogelzang N and others: Patient, caregiver, and oncologist perceptions of cancer-related fatigue: results of a tripart assessment survey, *Semin Hematol* 34(3 suppl 2):4, 1997.
71. Winningham M: Walking program for people with cancer, *Cancer Nurs* 14:270, 1991.
72. Winningham M: How exercise mitigates fatigue: implications for people receiving cancer therapy, *Biother Cancer* 16, 1991.
73. Winningham M, MacVicar M, Burke C: Exercise for cancer patients: guidelines and precautions, *Physician Sportsmed* 14:125, 1986.
74. Winningham M and others: Fatigue and the cancer experience: the state of the knowledge, *Oncol Nurs Forum* 21:23, 1994.
75. Winningham M: Fatigue: the missing link to quality of life, *Qual Life Res* 4:2, 1995.
76. Yellen and others: Measuring fatigue and other anemia-related symptoms with the Functional Assessment of Cancer Therapy (FACT) measurement system, *J Pain Symptom Manage* 13:63, 1997.

Home Care, Alternative Care Settings, and Cancer Resources

Shirley E. Otto and Leslie A. Metivier Johnston

28 CHAPTER

During the last decade, rising health care costs and the efforts to contain these costs, such as diagnosis-related groups (DRGs), resulted in increased emphasis on home care and alternative care settings. A contributing factor to the exponential growth experienced in home health care in the late 1980s and 1990s was an expectation that it could save health care dollars through prevention of repeated hospitalizations and placement in long-term care facilities. Other factors included demographic changes in America, technologic advances, and consumerism. However, recent trends have prompted the federal government to propose changes in policy and regulatory practices affecting the home health care industry related to administration of Medicare benefits and the Balanced Budget Act of 1997. The trends include increasing use of home health care to provide postacute care services, decreases in length of hospitalization for certain diagnoses, and increased percentages of the United States population enrolled in managed care programs both commercial and through Medicaid programs.[17, 43, 55, 96, 99] As a result, the home care industry started receiving Medicare reimbursement through a prospective payment system (PPS) beginning in the year 2000. The PPS system will introduce the use of home health-related groups (HHRGs) based on specific assessment information. Home care will shift its focus increasingly to cost-effective measures for the delivery of quality care with optimal outcomes for patients. In addition to measuring outcomes through the use of the Outcomes and Assessment Information Set (OASIS) currently mandated for home care, home health agencies are instituting and considering the use of specific disease management protocols, the use of patient care coordinators (PCCs) to determine care needs for specific populations, and cooperative community-based practice models for care delivery across a continuum.[7, 8, 10, 105] Past surveys have indicated that a majority of Americans prefer receiving health care in the home instead of some form of institutional care.[10, 12, 17, 36, 43] The identified advantages of home care include familiarity with surroundings and caregivers, increased sense of control, convenience for patients and families, less disruption in family life and related activities, less expensive cost of care, and overall improved quality of life.[56, 69, 72, 99]

The disadvantages of home care that need to be considered include potential for increased out-of-pocket costs, increased stress and emotional strain related to caregiver burden, loss of privacy, changes in daily routine, and competence of patients and caregivers in managing complications and emergencies. Home care has become increasingly "high tech," providing intravenous (IV) infusions, parenteral nutrition, supplemental oxygen, and respirators in the home setting. Consequently, patients are discharged after only a short hospital stay, whereas in the past, they would have remained hospitalized for ongoing assessment and evaluation of their status and response to treatment. Many cancer therapies that were previously administered only in acute care settings are now given routinely in an outpatient or home care setting. During the 1990s, 10% to 20% of cancer care was given in the traditional acute care hospital setting, and the remainder was given in alternative outpatient or postacute settings, such as home care and ambulatory clinics. Advances in cancer treatments and the availability of improved technology have made outpatient and home cancer treatment both safe and effective.*

It is important to note that accompanying the decreased hospital stay, emergency department use and subsequent rehospitalization have increased. Patients

---

*References 7, 8, 19, 36, 44, 56, 57, 59, 79, 91.

who are frequent visitors to the emergency department or who have frequent readmissions to the hospital due to exacerbations of chronic illnesses are often patients who could or should have received home health care at an earlier time. As the trend for earlier discharge continues, nurses are expected to facilitate the transition between the acute care and community or convalescent setting. This transition is a complex and challenging task that requires comprehensive data-gathering and decision-making skills. The health care professional must be able to collect and analyze pertinent information to develop an appropriate discharge plan. Elderly patients are more at risk for hospitalization and recurrent hospitalizations and home health care does reduce the number of hospital readmissions. The early discharge process limits the time during hospitalization for health professionals to instruct the patient in the self-care practices necessary to enhance their recovery in the home. This health teaching, therefore, needs to be continued after hospital discharge to lessen the chance of illness exacerbation and rehospitalization. Thus, nursing care is needed for the facilitation of the patient's self-care practices, health teaching, continuation of skilled assessments, and communication of changes in condition to the physician.[50, 94, 96, 99]

The trend for more economical, home-based, family-supported cancer care and treatment is on the increase. However, it is important to note that demographic changes in U.S. society and the decline of traditional extended family support systems necessitate use of additional community-based support services to maintain the patient in the home setting or consideration of alternative settings for care that are now more frequently available through managed care systems. It is essential that the health care professional accurately assess and identify the specific needs of the patient and, if the family is available, their ability to take on the caregiving role. Identification of the presence or absence of adequate caregiving supports is central to determining if home care or an alternative care setting is appropriate. This is particularly important because home care is a necessarily intermittent and limited service that is not meant to substitute for long-term care services. Patients and families need accurate information about home care to address their expectations of the services and ensure better satisfaction with care provided. The focus of home care is to promote independence in the management of health care needs. It is also imperative that health care providers, especially the oncology nurse, be cognizant of all the variables that will affect the patient's response to treatment when he is at home or in an alternative care setting. The goal is to ensure the patient's safety and facilitate the transition throughout a coordinated system of health care delivery. This system includes various settings within a continuum of care

in which comprehensive assessments of patient/family needs are communicated consistently to health care providers involved in the patient's care. To accomplish this, the oncology nurse must thoroughly assess and accurately identify the patient's and family's abilities and learning needs, as well as the environmental factors in the home that may interfere with the patient's safety and well-being.*

Clinical research has determined that supporting the caregiver in the caregiving role, particularly with the day-to-day management of care, is of paramount importance. The intervention most needed is the provision of assistance to family members caring for cancer patients. This intervention should be tailored to meet individual needs but must include information and skills relative to physical care, emotional support, and respite when possible.[56, 58] The discharge planning process is an organized, systematic approach used primarily in the acute care setting to facilitate the transition from the hospital to home. As health care delivery systems attempt to control costs and avoid duplication of services while maintaining high-quality care, oncology nurses have become aware that the assessment and planning process characteristic of discharge planning should not be limited to the acute care setting. Patients in outpatient oncology settings also have discharge planning needs. This process is ongoing and should continue as the patient moves through a variety of health care settings during the course of the illness. A patient-centered approach to provide continuity of care facilitates the delivery of holistic health services that serve the patient's best interests while assisting providers to plan services that are based on needs.[64, 69, 72, 80, 91, 94]

Discharge planning, an essential component of quality patient-centered care, is supported by a federal law passed in December 1994. The law requires that standards and guidelines for discharge planning contain the following seven components†:

1. The hospital must identify, at an early stage of hospitalization, patients who are likely to experience adverse health consequences if discharged without adequate discharge planning.
2. Hospitals must provide a discharge planning evaluation for patients identified under the requirement listed above and for other patients at the request of the patient or his representative or physician.
3. Any discharge planning evaluation must be made on a timely basis to ensure that appropriate arrangements for posthospital care will be made be-

---

* References 3, 7, 8, 10, 17, 23, 37, 43, 57, 59.

† References 12, 18, 28, 31, 40, 56, 58, 96, 99.

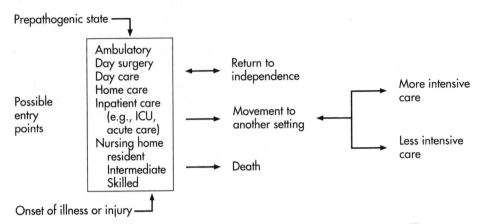

FIGURE 28–1 Illness–wellness continuum through discharge planning. (From Kelly K, McClelland E: Discharge planning: home care considerations. In Martinson IM, Widmer A, editors: *Home health nursing,* Philadelphia, Saunders, 1989.)

fore discharge and to avoid unnecessary delays in discharge.

4. This evaluation must include the patient's likely need for and availability of appropriate posthospital services.
5. The discharge planning evaluation must be included in the patient's medical record for use in establishing an appropriate discharge plan, and the results of the evaluation must be discussed with the patient or his representative.
6. At the request of the patient's physician, the hospital must arrange for the development and initial implementation of a discharge plan for the patient.
7. A registered professional nurse, social worker, or other appropriately qualified staff member must develop or supervise any discharge planning or discharge plan required under this act.

The discharge planning usually focuses primarily on the transition from the acute care setting. In practice, the process used in the hospital setting can be directly applied to the outpatient setting or any other health care setting in which a health care professional identifies unmet needs.

1. Discharge planning can begin at any entry point in the health care system.
2. Any point on the health continuum can serve as a basis for entry into the health care system.
3. Movement through the care continuum may be multidirectional.
4. The complexity and intensity of care should be flexible and adaptable to the care needs of the patient.

Figure 28–1 demonstrates the illness–wellness continuum through discharge planning.

Discharge Planning Process

Discharge planning is a process that involves assessment, identification of continuing care needs, planning, and implementation of a plan to meet those needs. Expediting patient transfers to more cost-effective levels of care at the earliest possible time necessitates not only effective tools to facilitate the process, but also adherence to professional standards of practice for discharge planning. Discharge planning is performed by a variety of health care professionals, including nurses and social workers. These professionals must have the basic skills necessary to assess, develop, and implement individualized continuing care plans. In recent years, the role of the hospital-based discharge planner has often expanded to a case coordination or case management role within a larger health care system. Therefore, the need for standards of discharge planning applicable to all settings is important. The following seven essential components outline the standards of practice for discharge planning and should be used in the discharge process (Box 28–1)[12, 13, 66, 80, 94, 103]:

- Assessment
- Needs identification
- Planning
- Documentation and communication
- Implementation
- Patient education
- Program evaluation

Adherence to standards of discharge planning and use of a systematic approach such as this example is beneficial because it not only helps to develop a comprehensive plan of care, but also provides a built-in mechanism for ongoing reevaluation and modification of the plan. Figure 28–2 is a sample of a discharge planning flow sheet.

ASSESSMENT

The oncology nurse in the acute care setting has a unique opportunity to perform a comprehensive assessment of the patient's strengths and limitations over days and sometimes weeks. This allows for the establishment of rapport between the nurse and patient. Frequently, when care is given over several days, the nurse has the ability to identify a patient care need that may not have been previously assessed. However, nursing in the inpatient setting is frequently extremely hectic, and nurses do not have the luxury of spending extended periods with patients exploring their discharge needs when other needs must be addressed immediately. Often it becomes a matter of prioritization: What needs to be done now and what can wait? It is important to understand that discharge planning *cannot* wait until the day the patient is leaving the hospital for home or for placement in an alternative care setting.[6-8, 10, 17]

Similarly, the oncology nurse in the outpatient clinic or alternative setting also has the opportunity to assess for and identify the patient's specific health care needs. The oncology nurse can quickly and effectively assess, identify, and respond to patient and family needs as they surface, if the nurse is continuously cognizant of the importance of planning for continued care and has an appropriate method to facilitate the process.

Many factors must be considered before discharge, and advance planning is imperative. Consultation with the designated home care agency and/or hospice nursing staff will facilitate an effective discharge planning transition from the acute care setting to the home setting. This process necessitates not only thorough assessment and evaluation, but also extensive planning, communication, and coordination. The chart contains the patient admission data as an initial source of data for the discharge planner to screen and identify patients that may have continuing care planning needs. The oncology nurse, using secondary sources of data such as the patient's record, also relies on first-hand observations and assessment of the patient. Specific patient components that identify patients who are in particular need for continuing care planning include the following*:

- Age (over age 65 or pediatric cases)
- Medical diagnosis, history, and prognosis
- Goal of treatment and the response to treatment
- Functional capacity and ability to perform activities of daily living (ADLs) safely; activity and exercise ability

---

* References 7, 10, 18, 23, 30, 31, 35, 48, 52, 55, 59

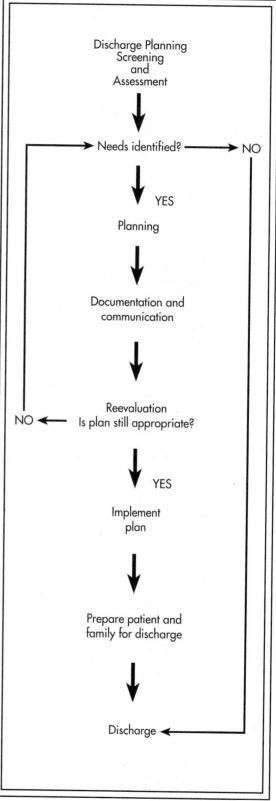

FIGURE 28–2 Discharge planning flow sheet. (Redrawn from Hamilton M: Standards of practice for discharge planning, *Contin Care,* September 1995, p. 34.)

BOX 28-1

Standards of Practice for Discharge Planning

STANDARD ONE: ASSESSMENT

Expected outcome: all patients will be screened as soon as possible after admission to identify continuing care needs. Accurate assessments are essential to development of appropriate discharge plans.

A. Assessment/screening triggers
1. Admission review
2. Case-finding criteria
3. Continued-stay review
4. Receipt of order/referral
B. Data collection sources
1. Patient/family interviews
2. Clinical/medical record
3. Physicians, nurses
4. Other health care professionals
C. Patient components
1. Physical
   a. Age (high risk: over age 65, pediatric cases)
   b. Admitting diagnoses (high risk: HIV/AIDS, cancer, cerebrovascular accident (stroke), substance abuse, psychiatric diagnoses, chronic illnesses)
   c. Medical history, prognosis
   d. Response to treatments
   e. Functional capacity and ability to perform activities of daily living (ADLs) safely (e.g., feeding, bathing, mobilizing, ambulating, vision, hearing, communicating, toileting, shopping, housekeeping, using the telephone, sleeping)
   f. Medications
   g. Nursing care/therapy needs
   h. Nutritional status
   i. Skin integrity
   j. Pain
   k. Exercise, activity tolerance
2. Emotional/cognitive/behavioral
   a. Level of consciousness, orientation, memory, competence, judgment
   b. Motivation and readiness for self-care
   c. Learning ability
   d. Personal goals, preferences
   e. Self-perception, health perception
   f. Presence of confusion, dementia, depression, anxiety
   g. Communication
   h. Coping mechanisms
3. Psychosocial
   a. Adequacy of living arrangements/caregivers
   b. Familial/social support systems
   c. Availability of community resources
   d. Roles, relationships, ability to socialize
   e. Values, beliefs, cultural/spiritual preferences
   f. Designated party for health care decisions
   g. Advance directives
4. Financial
   a. Insurance/benefits, contractual considerations
   b. Income, occupation, employment
   c. High-risk: homeless, indigent, Medicare, Medicaid, and nonfunded patients

STANDARD TWO: NEEDS IDENTIFICATION

Expected outcome: assessment data will provide a basis for indentification of actual or potential continuing care needs or problems that may affect discharge planning decisions.

A. Home with no aftercare needs identified
B. Home health care
1. Nursing services/attendant care
2. Home medical equipment
3. Therapy services (e.g., occupational/physical/speech therapies)
4. Social services
5. Nutritional support
6. Clinical laboratory, radiology
C. Transportation needs
1. Frequency
2. Distance
3. Public assistance
D. Financial assistance
1. Availability of third-party coverage
2. Family resources
3. Public assistance
E. Board and care/assisted living
F. Rehabilitation services
1. Inpatient
2. Outpatient
G. Nursing facility
1. Extended care facility (ECF)
2. Transitional care unit (TCU)
3. Subacute care facility
4. Convalescent/long-term care facility
H. Transfer to another acute care facility
1. Acute care hospital
2. Long-term acute care hospital (LTAC)
I. Hospice care/palliative care program

STANDARD THREE: PLANNING

Expected outcome: individualized plan of care will be developed from the information obtained in the assessment and needs identification processes. This plan will include input from the multidisciplinary health care team, patient, and family.

A. Prioritize identified discharge planning needs
B. Identify available resources
1. Equipment
2. Personnel
3. Facilities
4. Supportive services/agencies
C. Select actions/interventions to achieve desired goals

BOX 28-1

Standards of Practice for Discharge Planning Continued

STANDARD FOUR: DOCUMENTATION AND COMMUNICATION

Expected outcome: all aspects of discharge planning process will be documented and communicated in a timely manner.

A. Multidisciplinary care plan/discharge record (if available)
   1. Name of discharge planner
   2. Date of patient contacts
   3. Identified needs
   4. Expected outcomes
   5. Interventions
B. Progress notes
   1. Date of consultation/referral
   2. Referral source
   3. Assessment (physical, emotional, psychosocial, financial, and personal data)
   4. Updates, reassessments
   5. Needs identified
   6. Requirements to meet continuing care needs
   7. Referrals to outside agencies/services
   8. Anticipated disposition/date
C. Communicate/collaborate on plans
   1. Patient and family
   2. Attending physicians
   3. Nursing/ancillary services
   4. Community resources
   5. Insurance/utilization review (UR)/case management

STANDARD FIVE: IMPLEMENTATION

Expected outcome: individualized patient's plan of care will be implemented in a timely, effective manner to ensure postdischarge needs are met.

A. Contact appropriate and available resources
B. Coordinate placement
   1. Initiate patient transfer and referral record
   2. Initiate chart/copies process
C. Order needed equipment, supplies, transportation, services
D. Assist with referrals
   1. Social services
   2. Agencies

   3. Legal counsel
   4. Support groups
   5. Medicaid, Medicare, etc.
E. Obtain consent for authorization to release medical records (as appropriate)

STANDARD SIX: PATIENT EDUCATION

Expected outcome: health care team, patient, and family will be knowledgeable about the discharge plan and the responsibilities to meet patient's ongoing health care needs.

A. Multidisciplinary team
   1. Nursing
   2. Physical/occupational/speech therapies
   3. Pharmacy
   4. Nutritional services
   5. Social services
   6. Respiratory therapy
   7. Physicians
B. Patient/family teaching
   1. Identify learning needs/barriers
   2. Assess readiness to learn
   3. Identify resources available
   4. Verbal/written discharge instructions

STANDARD SEVEN: PROGRAM EVALUATION

Expected outcome: to meet and exceed customer expectations through an ongoing performance improvement program.

A. Periodic program evaluation
   1. Assess timeliness of screening
   2. Ensure appropriateness/accuracy of assessments
   3. Determine effectiveness of interventions
   4. Assess for preventable readmissions
B. Monitor outcome through feedback
   1. Community resources/facilities
   2. Patients/families
   3. Physicians, nursing
   4. Multidisciplinary health care team
C. Communicate outcomes through appropriate channels
   1. Financial
   2. Clinical
   3. Satisfaction indicators

Modified from Hamilton M: Standards of practice for discharge planning, *Contin Care,* September 1995, pp. 33, 34, 36.

- Medications; infusion therapy
- Nursing care and therapy needs
- Comfort; nutrition; and wound and skin status

Regardless of the mechanism used in identification of the patient for continuing care needs, a screening process should be followed by the patient interview, identification of the specific problems or needs, and development of a plan for solving patient problems or needs. These three major components of the discharge planning process have specific subcomponents that, when addressed, both clarify and simplify the continuing planning process.

Patient Interview

1. Make introduction (if necessary).[53, 57, 59, 64, 80]
2. Establish the relationship of the patient to spouse; family, including children; neighbors; church, and senior citizen support activities (if applicable).
3. Establish how the patient's illness has affected her role and function in the family, with special attention to financial support, shopping, meal preparation, transportation, and living arrangements.
4. Determine the patient's prehospital daily routine.
5. Assess the patient's learning and comprehension ability.
6. Assess the patient's interest in discharge planning services.
7. Assess the patient's goals and expectations for the treatment and rehabilitation process.

Identification of Continuing Care Problems and Needs

On completion of the patient interview, determine the needs or potential problem areas that may exist and verify the patient's interest in having continuing care planning services. Potential areas of concern that increase the risk of home care needs include*:

1. Inadequate or no support system
2. Inadequate financial resources
3. Poor environmental conditions
4. Inability to carry out treatment and medication regimen
5. Inability to carry out ADLs
6. Poor socialization
7. Potential problems related to disease progression or treatment

---

* References 33, 36, 39, 84, 86, 94, 96, 106.

PLANNING

Development of Plan for Solving Patient's Problems and Addressing Needs

After the patient's problems or needs are identified, a collaborative process involving the patient, family or significant others, and health care professionals should occur. At this time the oncology nurse should assist the patient, family, and significant others to look realistically at their goals and expectations and subsequently develop a plan for care. This may entail placement in an extended care facility or linkage with community-based agencies providing service in the home setting. With the diverse services available, it is necessary to address the following factors when assisting the patient and family in this decision-making process.[6, 8, 10, 14, 38, 40]

1. Assist patient or family to identify the specific problem(s).
2. Assist patient or family to set priorities among the problems.
3. Assist patient or family to identify the services or resources needed.
4. Interpret services of the available resources to patient or family.
5. Establish patient's financial status.
6. Work out details of selected plan with patient or family.
7. Obtain patient or family consent to contact the resources in their behalf.
8. Establish criteria for evaluation of the effectiveness of the plan.

The nurse can use the resources available in their practice setting and establish a collaborative relationship with the continuing care team to facilitate the process for the benefit of the patient. Often, because of early discharge, there is not sufficient time to initiate all the appropriate referrals to community support services. In such cases the referrals may be made after the patient is home. The professional implementing the discharge plan should make the initial contacts with the support services. A responsible family member may be willing to follow up on a referral made by the professional. Provide the family member the name of the referred agency, the telephone number, and the agency contact person.[12, 18, 19, 23, 49, 55, 57]

If the patient needs skilled nursing care in the home setting, a referral to a skilled home care agency should be made. Most hospitals have continuing patient care forms that must be completed when a referral is initiated. The nurse should include information about other identified needs and request that the home care agency's personnel assist the patient with the referral process. It is essential that all relevant patient information is communicated and documented clearly, concisely, and in a timely manner. In addition to information about identified support needs, the referral for continuing patient care in the home care setting should also include information about significant factors related to this hospitalization, relevant past medical history, current medications and treatment orders, identified nursing problems, and results of recent diagnostic tests or blood work. Concise and comprehensive referrals are essential to facilitate the transition from one setting of care to another and to promote continuity of care. The comprehensive information on the referral form is essential to make the home care nurse's job more efficient. A list of national community resources is given in the Appendix at the end of this chapter.[12, 23, 99]

Assessment of Caregiver and Informal Supports

In most institutions, assessment of supports of family, friends, and available organized institutions is routinely done if it is determined that the patient needs assistance in the home setting. Frequently, a primary caregiver, usually the spouse, has been identified, and some in-hospital teaching has been initiated by the nurses before discharge. As the trend for early discharge continues, the family support system must assume greater responsibility for maintaining what is often a very aggressive post-hospitalization treatment plan. The stress and anxieties associated with the caregiving responsibilities can be overwhelming. Often, unasked questions and feelings of inadequacy in their ability to care for their loved one properly and safely add to the caregiving burden. Teaching them not only the "what to do's" but also the "what to expect" is one of the best stress reducers.*

Family members or friends provide approximately 80% of in-home care in the United States. Often these individuals do not have the option of quitting this role because of a sense of responsibility and duty and as an expression of love and devotion to the patient. Most frequently, women over 55 years of age are the caregivers of the patient. Often these women receive assistance from other family members. Older men with cancer are usually cared for by their spouse. Elderly women with cancer, because of their longevity, are cared for by their adult children. Middle-aged cancer patients are cared for primarily by their spouse. The level of depression among caregivers is highest for wives, followed by daughters and then other female caregivers. Spousal caregivers are at particular risk for caregiver burden and illnesses associated with caregiver stress, because they maintain the caregiving role for longer periods and provide more extensive and comprehensive care.

In addition, they believe that they are obligated to do so, with or without formal or informal assistance.*

An extensive assessment of the caregiver can be conducted as part of the discharge planning process that includes the following assessment/question format:

1. Has the caregiver's age been considered as well as the patient's?
2. Does the caregiver's mental and physical condition allow that person to assume this responsibility?
3. Will the caregiver live in the patient's home?
4. If the caregiver is not in the home, how accessible will that person be?
5. Who can provide some relief or free time for the caregiver?
6. Is the caregiver aware of the patient's medical condition?
7. Has the caregiver received instructions on administering medications, observing for possible side effects, and managing them?
8. Is the caregiver aware of the expected course of treatment?
9. If there is to be a change in the patient's condition, does the caregiver know what problems to watch for?
10. If the patient's condition changes, does the caregiver know whom to call?
11. Does the caregiver know the name of the physician directing the home care plan?
12. If a home care agency will provide care at home, has the caregiver received the name and phone number of the company?
13. If the patient will be using medical equipment in the home, has the caregiver been given the name of the company that supplies it?
14. Has the caregiver been helped to develop a list of emergency telephone numbers: community emergency numbers, rescue emergency numbers, physician, home care agency, equipment supplier, and other family members?
15. Does the caregiver know about any follow-up medical appointments scheduled for the patient?
16. Has the caregiver been instructed in what *not* to do for the patient as well as what to allow the patient to do for herself?
17. If prescriptions must be filled, are there immediate funds available to do this? Also, if a prescription is difficult to obtain at local pharmacies, advise the caregiver where it is available.
18. Have questions regarding financial matters related to the patient's home care needs been ar-

---

* References 14, 27, 31, 49, 58, 69, 80, 83.

* References 14, 31, 37, 40, 41, 45, 83, 92, 93, 96, 105.

ranged before discharge? Is the caregiver attending to financial matters?

19. If the caregiver can no longer assume responsibility, whom should she notify?

20. Does the caregiver have medications for the patient's first 24 hours home? If not, is there a plan developed to obtain these medications?

21. Has the caregiver been made aware of any appropriate support groups available in the community?

22. Have you supplied the caregiver with suitable educational materials regarding the patient's diagnosis?

23. Does the caregiver have the name and telephone number of the person who arranged for home care services and who can be called to clarify issues or further explain services to be expected?

24. Has the discharge planner asked the caregiver if she has any questions or problems concerning the discharge, date, time, transportation home, or the services the caregiver and patient will be receiving?

Value of Humor

Humor as a preventive therapy for family caregivers is one type of respite that has been underused in primary prevention of caregiver burnout. Humor is not just the telling of jokes. It is a concept that includes wit, laughter, joking, comedy, kidding, teasing, mimicking, and satire. What is seen as humorous varies with different personalities, cultures, and backgrounds as well as with levels of stress and pain. Humor can help "recharge" family caregivers physically and psychologically and can improve the quality of their lives. Humor can also facilitate communication and promote positive interpersonal relationships among health care providers, patients, and their families. To use humor therapeutically, oncology nurses must first understand the family's and caregivers' coping patterns, level of anxiety, and sense of humor.[*] Table 28–1 lists the holistic effects of humor.

SETTINGS FOR CARE

In the past, the hospital was the primary setting for care. In recent years, hospitals, as well as other health care providers and payers, have created innovative alternative care sites that reduce the cost but not the income while maintaining quality care.[†]

Extended Care

Usually in the outpatient setting, extended care placement is not an identified need; however, it is wise to have a working knowledge about these resources. At times, family members may find the caregiving burden too overwhelming and request information on and assistance with extended care placement. If it is determined that the patient's care needs necessitate placement in an extended care facility, the facility that will most effectively meet the patient's needs must then be identified. The following six basic types of extended care facilities vary according to the amount and type of care needed by the patient:

1. Subacute care facilities
2. Skilled care facilities

TABLE 28–1
Holistic Effects of Humor

Human Dimension	Effects of Humor
Musculoskeletal system	Upward movement of cheeks and upper lip; vocal cords function to produce laughter sounds; movement of arms, hands, torso, head
Respiratory system	Rapid, shallow breathing; ratio of expirations to inspirations increased; ventilation increased
Cardiovascular system	Circulation stimulated; cardiac muscle stimulated; production of thrombosis-preventing plasminogen activator stimulated
Immune system	T-lymphocyte production stimulated
Endocrine system	Catecholamine production stimulated, especially epinephrine (Adrenalin); endorphin release stimulated
Behavioral system	Stress-worry cycle interrupted; effects of stress, tension, anxiety decreased; expression of emotion facilitated; learning and memory enhanced; self-concept and/or self-acceptance reflected and reinforced; consensual validation, bonding, social cohesiveness facilitated; negative feelings, attitudes, and ideas expressed in socially acceptable manner
Spiritual system	Existential paradox of God-mortal and death paradox of sad-glad played with; absurdities of life and human condition held up to jest; human spirit rescued from despair

Modified from Pasquali EA: Humor: preventive therapy for family care givers, Home Healthcare Nurse 9(3):34, 1991.

* References 16, 23, 25, 43, 45, 51, 78.

† References 1, 10, 35, 36, 41, 56, 57, 70, 72, 93, 96, 103.

3. Intermediate care facilities
4. Adult foster or sheltered care facilities
5. Residential care facilities
6. Adult day-care facilities

Subacute care facilities, also known as long-term care hospitals, are a recent development in the health care system. These are cost-efficient settings that provide a variety of medical-surgical, oncologic, rehabilitation, and additional specialty care services in an alternative setting for those patients who no longer need acute care services but are too ill to send home. This alternative care setting is preferred by case managers and managed care organizations because it offers outcome-focused care as well as cost efficiency. Many hospitals have begun to add subacute facilities to enhance revenues while still providing appropriate care to patients with specialized needs such as highly skilled nursing and therapy services. An added benefit to providing such a facility for care is that it separates the chronically ill patients from others. This enables health care providers to consider the underlying assumptions of care and the appropriateness of aggressive care measures while still providing care for chronically critically ill patients in specialized "low-tech" units without compromising prospects for recovery.

Skilled care facilities provide around-the-clock skilled nursing care and observation. In addition, there is frequent medical supervision. *Intermediate care facilities* provide around-the-clock basic nursing care for patients who are medically stable but unable to care for themselves. *Adult foster care* or *sheltered care facilities* are for individuals who require a protective living arrangement that provides general supervision and assistance with bathing, dressing, meals, and other personal needs. *Residential care facilities* are for individuals who no longer want to live alone or have no place to live. In general, these facilities also provide similar services as a sheltered care facility and occasionally, in times of illness, may provide intermediate care for their residents. These facilities often have various levels of living arrangements, ranging from independent to assisted living.

Adult day-care facilities provide various levels of care for cancer patients and much needed respite for family caregivers. Adult day-care programs serve as a bridge between traditional care services and the home where there otherwise might be a gap in service delivery. Some adult day-care programs also provide services for the caregiver, ranging from counseling to caregiver support groups.

Because many extended care facilities are available, it becomes an overwhelming task to select the best one. The long-term care ombudsman office in each state will provide lists of certified extended care facilities that offer the various levels of care. This state office will also provide information regarding reimbursement of these facilities by Medicare or Medicaid. This is a helpful starting point for patients and their family members. It is recommended that the patient or significant other tour the facilities before making a selection.[17, 66, 92]

Home Care

Home care has seen an increase in utilization for nearly two decades because of the implementation of DRGs and subsequent earlier discharges. Increased momentum of consumerism and the desire to exercise more control over personal health care have also been influencing factors. Home care is on the cutting edge of change in nursing and health care. In a time of increasing concern over federal health care expenditures, home care represents a humane, sensible alternative to institutionalized care for an increasing number of Americans. It also offers other benefits, including eliminating the risk of nosocomial infection, maintaining patients' and families' social and cultural patterns, and promoting patients' self-esteem, independence, and personal involvement in care.[15, 66, 89, 90, 98, 100]

The option of home care services is understandably attractive to cancer patients and their families, who face an illness that often strips away much of their sense of personal control. A cancer diagnosis, however, is often not easily placed within the type of disease management pathway that many case managers are adopting to control home care costs. The reasons for this are the frequency and costs of treatments required for cancer patients and the necessity for many treatments to be given during intermittent short inpatient stays over an extended period of time. Home care agencies will need to develop strategies and relevant pathways to address the needs of cancer patients. This will require using nurses with expertise in oncology as primary care nurses or case managers to coordinate the care of cancer patients in the home setting. Presumably oncology patients have an expectation that care in the home will be provided as the need arises because of the intensive nature of their treatment. The fact remains that being in the comfort of their own home and receiving care is preferred over institutionalization by 71% of Americans.*

Home care services available to health care consumers include both traditional and high-technology care. Traditional home care services generally provide skilled nursing care, including patient assessment and intervention, patient and family education; rehabilitative services such as physical, occupational, and speech and language therapies; social work intervention; and home health aide support. Rehabilitative services are espe-

---

* References 10, 12, 17, 23, 31, 35, 36, 53, 57.

cially important in ensuring quality care within the limits of home care services for patients with cancer. These patients often have significant fatigue associated with disease processes and treatments. Many treatments may also increase the risks for short or long-term disabilities. Physical and occupational therapists can provide home exercise programs, and implement use of assistive devices and home modification to maintain optimal independence. Speech and language therapists can initiate or continue programs to assist patients both with speech and dysphagia problems in the home setting. In addition, home health agencies often employ other specialists such as registered dietitians for nutrition consults, and certified enterostomal therapy nurses for wound and skin care and lymphedema management.[7, 8, 10, 57]

Recent improvements in and the increasing availability of high technology in the home setting have made home care a viable option for cancer patients at all stages of treatment and illness. High-technology home care for patients with cancer generally refers to the home management of infusion therapies such as the following: analgesia, antiemetics, antifungals, antimicrobials, hydration, electrolyte replacement, chemotherapy, blood sampling for diagnostics tests, enteral or parenteral nutrition.*

Home IV therapy is one of the most rapidly growing trends in the home care industry. Cost containment and the growing threat of communicable disease transmission in hospitals are the two major factors contributing to this trend. Not all patients with cancer are good candidates for home infusion therapy. These patients and their families must be properly screened before initiating such therapies in the home setting to ensure that the treatment is both safe and efficacious. In addition, physician support and accessibility for clear, open communications must be present to ensure continuity of care and safe infusion therapy in the home setting.†

Criteria used by home health agencies to determine eligibility for services may include the guidelines established by Medicare regulations and include: (1) be homebound; (2) require a skilled intervention; (3) have a plan of care signed by a physician; (4) receive care that is part-time and intermittent; (5) receive care that is reasonable and necessary. The "homebound status" definition is the individual is confined to his home, if that individual has a condition, due to illness or injury that restricts the ability of the individual to leave his home except with the assistance of another individual or the aid of a supportive device; or if the individual has a condition such that leaving his home is contraindicated. Additional language states that leaving

home should require a considerable taxing effort for the patient. Absences from the home should be short, infrequent, or solely to receive treatment (Fig. 28–3).*

Patients who receive infusion therapy in the home must have a venous access device to ensure a reliable, safe, and patent access site. A variety of infusion pumps that are compact, reliable, and easy to manage are available for the home setting and ensure that the prescribed medication is administered as ordered. A variety of types of central venous catheters are available. Tables 28–2, 28–3, and 28–4 present a general overview of tunneled central venous catheters and peripherally inserted central venous catheters (PICC lines), as well as guidelines for care and management. Table 28–5 provides a general overview of infusion pumps.[62, 63, 65, 76, 86]

Total parenteral nutrition (TPN) and enteral therapy for cancer patients have been controversial issues from medical, ethical, and financial perspectives. Nevertheless, this form of treatment is frequently provided in the home setting. It is generally believed that improved nutritional status improves the quality of life but does not necessarily prolong life. During the end stage of illness, however, when vital organs begin to shut down, infusion therapies are not advised. This is particularly difficult for families to accept and understand because they frequently believe that because the patient is not eating or drinking, IV lines are necessary. If the rationale for withholding, discontinuing, or decreasing fluids to keep vein open (KVO) is not clearly explained to families at this time, they may be concerned that the patient is being denied vital treatment.[7–10, 13, 31, 38]

As many as 70% of patients with cancer experience pain during their illness, and at least 90% of this cancer-related pain can be effectively relieved with existing pain management techniques. Although the oral route of pain medication is the preferred method by pain experts, high-technology pain management is a reasonable option to patients whose pain cannot be effectively controlled otherwise. The American Pain Society, a national chapter of the International Association for the Study of Pain, publishes a helpful booklet, *Principles of Analgesic Use in the Treatment of Acute Pain and Chronic Cancer Pain.* In addition, the American Pain Society may be contacted to obtain additional information regarding pain management and consult with another health care professional experienced in pain management techniques[2, 3, 16, 30, 35, 44] (see the Appendix and Chapter 30).

With the advances in anticancer therapies and the availability of portable infusion pumps, chemotherapy administration in the home setting has become both safe and effective. As a result, this has become an

---

* References 6–8, 19, 32–34, 36, 39, 54, 57, 62, 64.
† References 19, 39, 54, 57, 76, 79, 84, 99.

---

* References 17, 28, 31, 81, 96, 103, 104.

Text continued on page 822

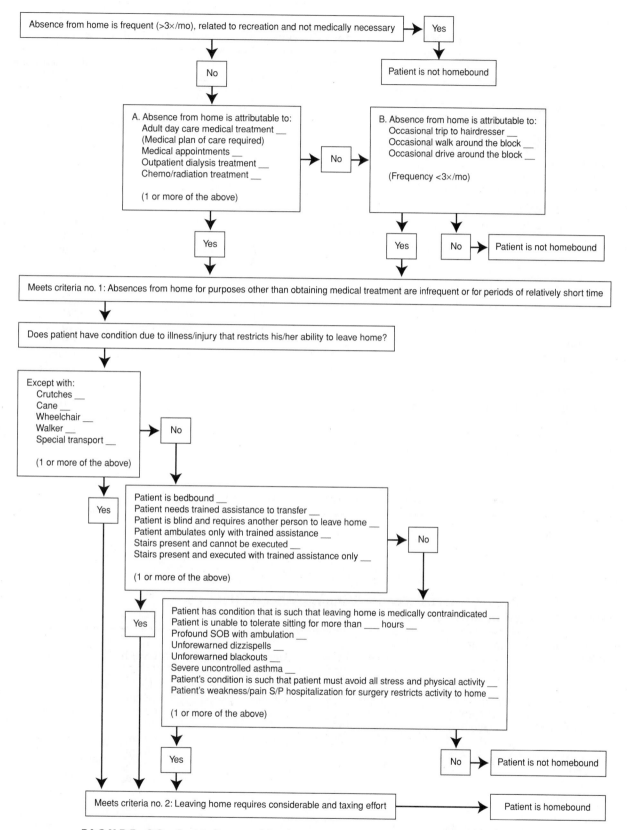

FIGURE 28–3 Medicare tool for determining homebound status. (From Weiss R, Milone-Nuzzo P: Medicare and the nurse: a tool to assess homebound status, *Home Healthcare Nurse* 17(8):489, 1999.)

TABLE 28–2

Examples of Tunneled Central Venous Catheters Currently Marketed in the United States

Model/Material (Manufacturer)	French Size	Inner Diameter	Total Lumen Volume (Priming Volume)
SINGLE-LUMEN DEVICES			
Hickman Single-Lumen Catheter/silicone (Bard)	9	1.6 mm	1.8 mL
Groshong Single-Lumen Catheter/silicone (Bard)	7 and 8	1.3–1.5 mm	0.7–1.2 mL
Quinton Single-Lumen Central Venous Access Catheter/ silicone (Quinton)	3.9–9.7*	0.75–1.5 mm	0.9–2.0 mL
Harborin Single-Lumen Central Venous Catheter/ polyurethane (Harbor Medical Devices)	7	1.5 mm	0.9 mL
DOUBLE-LUMEN DEVICES			
Hickman Dual-Lumen Catheters/silicone (Bard)	7	0.8 mm/1.0 mm	0.6 mL/0.8 mL
	9	0.7 mm/1.3 mm	0.6 mL/1.3 mL
	12	1.6 mm/lumen	1.8 mL (each lumen)
Leonard Dual-Lumen Catheter/silicone (Bard)	10	1.3 mm/lumen	1.3 mL/lumen
Groshong Dual-Lumen Catheter/silicone (Bard)	9.5	1.1 mm/1.33 mm	0.5 mL/0.8 mL
Cook TPN Double-Lumen Central Venous	5	0.5 mm/lumen	0.2 mL/lumen
Catheters/silicone (Cook Critical Care)	7	0.7 mm/1.0 mm	0.4 mL/0.6 mL
	9	1.0 mm/1.3 mm	0.6 mL/1.0 mL
	12	1.0 mm/1.6 mm	1.6 mL/2.3 mL
Quinton RAAF Dual-Lumen Central	9	1.1 mm/lumen	1.2 mL/lumen
Venous Catheters/silicone	12	1.5 mm/lumen	2.2 mL/lumen
	13.5	2.0 mm/lumen	2.5 mL/lumen
TRIPLE-LUMEN DEVICES			
Nutritional Support Catheter/polyurethane (Arrow International)	7		0.7 mL/0.5 mL/0.5 mL
Hickman Triple-Lumen Catheter/silicone (Bard)	12.5	1.0 mm/1.0/mm/1.5 mm	0.7 mL/0.7 mL/1.6 mL
Quinton Triple-Lumen Central Venous Access Catheter/ silicone	11.7	1.0 mm/1.0 mm/1.25 mm	1.0 mL/1.1 mL/1.2 mL

* Size depends on model.

Modified from Finley RS: Drug-delivery systems: infusion and access devices, Highlights Antineoplast Drugs *13(2):15, 1995.*

TABLE 28–3

Examples of Peripherally Inserted Central Venous Catheters (PICCs) Currently Marketed in the United States

Model or Trade Name/Material (Manufacturer)	French Size	Lumen Diameter	Length	Priming Volume
SINGLE-LUMEN DEVICES				
Groshong PICC/silicone (Bard)	4	0.8 mm	56 cm	0.3 mL
C-PICS/silicone (Cook Critical Care)	5	0.91 mm	60 cm	0.6 mL
V-Cath/silicone (HDC Corporation)	2	0.3 mm	40 cm	0.1 mL
	4	0.9 mm	60 cm	0.4 mL
L-Cath PICCs/polyurethane	5	1.2 mm	56 cm	0.9 mL
(Luther Medical Products)	3.5	0.7 mm	56 cm	0.4 mL
	2.6	0.5 mm	56 cm	0.2 mL
DOUBLE-LUMEN DEVICES				
D/L PICC/silicone (Bard)	5	0.8 mm/0.6 mm	55.9 cm	0.4 mL/0.3 mL
Double-Lumen Per-q-cath/silicone (Bard)	4	0.5 mm/0.3 mm	60 cm	0.1 mL/0.6 mL
	5	0.8 mm/0.4 mm	60 cm	0.3 mL/0.1 mL

Modified from Finley RS: Drug-delivery systems: infusion and access devices, Highlights Antineoplast Drugs *13(2):15, 1995.*

T A B L E   2 8 – 4

Central Venous Catheters: Recommended Nursing Management

Type	Heparinization*	Dressing	Blood Sampling
ADULT			
Central Venous Catheters, Short-Term Use, Subclavian Single/dual/triple-lumen	After each use, flush each lumen with 5 mL normal saline (N/S), then heparinized saline 2 mL (100 U/mL). For catheter *not* in use, flush each lumen with heparinized saline 2 mL (100 U/mL) *every 12 hours.*	Daily sterile dressing change at the site for duration of catheter placement. Gauze dressing change every 24 hours. Change Luer-Lok injection caps *every 72 hours.*	Shut off all IV lines for *1 to 3 minutes.* Withdraw 5 mL blood. Discard. Withdraw blood sample. Flush lumen with 5 mL N/S, then heparinize or resume IV line. *Total parenteral nutrition (TPN): shut off IV line 10 minutes.*
Peripherally Inserted Central Venous Catheters Long-line PICC† Single/dual-lumen (Use gentle pressure on syringe plunger for PICCs.)	After each use, flush lumen with 2 mL N/S, then heparinized saline 1 mL (100 U/mL). For catheter *not* in use, flush lumen with heparinized saline 1 mL (100 U/mL) every 12 hours.	Sterile dressing change after first 24 hours, then every 72 hours. Change Luer-Lok injection caps every 72 hours.	Shut off all IV lines for *1 to 3 minutes.* Withdraw 1.5 mL blood. Discard. Withdraw blood sample. Flush lumen with 2.5 mL N/S, then heparinize or resume IV line. *TPN: shut off IV line 10 minutes.*
Tunneled Catheters, Long-Term Use Hickman Quinton/Raaf Single/dual/triple-lumen	After each use, flush *each* lumen with 5 mL N/S, then heparinized saline 2 mL (100 U/mL). For catheter *not* in use, flush *each* lumen with heparinized saline 2 to 5 mL (100 U/mL) daily/biweekly.	Daily sterile dressing change at exit site for initial 14 days. Gauze dressing change every 24 hours. Thereafter, cleanse exit site daily (Betadine/alcohol). Optional daily clean dressing. Change Luer-Lok injection caps *weekly.*	Shut off all IV lines for *1 to 3 minutes.* Withdraw 5 mL blood. Discard. Withdraw blood sample. Flush lumen with 5 mL N/S, then heparinize or resume IV line. *TPN: shut off IV lines 10 minutes.*
Groshong Single/dual-lumen	Does not require heparin to maintain catheter patency. *Use force when flushing.* Flush *each* lumen with 5 mL N/S after each use, except for TPN, then flush with 30 mL N/S. For catheter *not* in use, flush with 5 mL N/S weekly.‡	Daily sterile dressing change at exit site for initial 14 days. Gauze dressing change every 24 hours. Thereafter, cleanse exit site daily (Betadine/alcohol). Optional daily clean dressing. Change Luer-Lok injection caps weekly.	Shut off all IV lines for *1 to 3 minutes.* Withdraw 5 mL blood. Discard. Withdraw blood sample. Flush lumen with 30 mL N/S vigorously, then resume IV line or apply injection cap.‡ *TPN: shut off IV line 10 minutes.*
Implantable Vascular Access Devices Davol Port Infuse-A-Port Port-A-Cath	After each use, flush *each* port with Huber needle: 10 mL N/S, followed by heparinized saline (100 U/mL).§ For port *not* in use, flush each port with 3 to 10 mL heparinized saline (100 U/mL) *every 30 days* (venous placement). Intermittent flush > 1/day use N/S and/or low-dose/low-volume heparin.‖	Sterile bio-occlusive dressing when port accessed. Steri-strips at new incision site for 3 days. When incision site healed and port not accessed, no dressing required. When port is accessed for continuous infusion, change needle and extension tubing every 5 to 7 days.	Shut off all IV lines for *1 to 3 minutes.* Withdraw 5 mL blood. Discard. Withdraw blood sample. Flush with 20 mL N/S, followed by 3 to 10 mL heparinized saline (100 U/mL)‡ or resume IV line. *TPN: shut off IV line 10 minutes.*

Table continued on following page

TABLE 28-4

Central Venous Catheters: Recommended Nursing Management *Continued*

Type	Heparinization*	Dressing	Blood Sampling
PEDIATRIC			
Short-Term Use, Subclavian Single-lumen/or multilumen	After each use, flush *each* lumen with 2 mL N/S, followed by 1 mL heparinized saline solution, 10 U/mL, after each use or at least twice a day.	Daily sterile dressing change at site for duration of catheter placement. Gauze dressing change every 24 hours. Change Luer-Lok injection caps every 24 hours.	Shut off all IV lines for *1 to 3 minutes.* Withdraw 3 mL blood. Discard. Withdraw blood sample. Flush lumen with 2 mL N/S, then heparinize or resume IV line. *TPN: shut off IV line 10 minutes.*
Peripherally Inserted Catheters Long-line PICC† Single/dual lumen (Use gentle pressure on syringe plunger for PICCs.)	After each use, flush lumen: *Pediatrics:* 2 mL N/S in 5-mL syringe or larger, followed by 1 mL heparinized saline (10 U/mL) after each use or at least twice a day. *Special care nursery (neonates):* 0.5 mL N/S, preservative free, in 5 mL syringe or larger, followed by 0.5 mL heparinized saline (4 U/mL). Intermittent flush schedule every 4 to 8 hours: consult with physician's orders.	Sterile dressing change after first 24 hours, then every 72 hours. Change Luer-Lok injection caps every 72 hours.	Shut off all IV lines for *1 to 3 minutes.* Withdraw 1.5 mL blood. Discard. Withdraw blood sample. Flush lumen with 2.5 mL N/S, then heparinize or resume IV line. *TPN: shut off IV line 10 minutes.*
Tunneled Catheters, Long-Term Use Broviac	After each use, flush lumen with 2 mL N/S, then heparinized saline 1 mL (10 U/mL). For catheter *not* in use, flush lumen with heparinized saline 1 mL (10 U/mL) daily.	Daily sterile dressing change at exit site for initial 14 days. Gauze dressing change every 24 hours. Thereafter, cleanse exit site daily with Betadine. Apply sterile 2 × 2. Change Luer-Lok injection caps weekly.	Shut off all IV lines for *1 to 3 minutes.* Withdraw 3 mL blood. Discard. Withdraw blood sample. Flush lumen with 2 mL N/S, then heparinize or resume IV line. *TPN: shut off IV line 10 minutes.*
Implantable Vascular Access Devices Port-A-Cath	After each use, flush the port with Huber needle, 5 mL N/S, followed by 2 mL heparinized saline (100 U/mL). For port *not* in use, flush port with 2 mL heparinized saline (100 U/mL) *every 30 days* (venous placement).	Sterile bio-occlusive dressing when port accessed. Steri-strips at new incision site for 3 days. When incision site healed and port not accessed, no dressing required. When port is accessed for continuous infusion, change needle and extension tubing every 5 to 7 days.	Shut off all IV lines for *1 full minute.* Withdraw 3 to 5 mL blood (depending on size of child). Discard. Withdraw blood sample. Flush with 5 mL N/S, then heparinize or resume IV line. *TPN: shut off IV line 10 minutes.*

* Heparinization of central venous catheters varies in frequency, volume of solution, concentration of the heparin dilution, type of device, and patient's age and weight. Confirm with physician managing patient's care and agency/institution for nursing management protocol regarding heparinization of central venous catheters/implantable ports.

  Consider patient with an alteration in coagulation factors and/or heparin allergy/intolerance with frequency of use of intermittent device. Potentially these patients may require low-concentration (e.g., 10 U/heparin/mL) and/or alternative flushing solution (e.g., sodium citrate, 1.4% solution).

† Use 5 mL or larger syringes when flushing and/or blood sampling from PICC.

‡ Selected oncologists use 2 to 5 mL heparinized saline (100 U/mL).

§ Check manufacturer's specific recommendations regarding volume. Oncologists use heparin, 10 mL (100 U/mL).

‖ Assess patient, disease, platelet count with frequency/volume/concentration of heparinization schedule.

From Otto SE, editor: Pocket guide to intravenous therapy, ed 4, St. Louis, Mosby, 2001.

TABLE 28-5
Features of Ambulatory Infusion Devices

AMBULATORY, SINGLE CHANNEL

Name/Model (Manufacturer)	Pumping Mechanism	Drug Reservoir/ Accessories	Battery/ Power Source	Range of Infusion Rates	Alarms/Safety Features	Keep Open Rate	Program Modes	Weight	Size
WalkMed 440 PIC (Medex, Division of Ivion)	Linear peristaltic	Disposable 65, 150, 250 mL bags; dedicated pump sets	9 V disposable battery (450–650 mL/battery)	1–30 mL/h (can also be programmed as mg/h)	Near end of program; volume limit; occlusion; system malfunction; low battery; depleted battery; end of infusion; door open; programming error; lockout levels	0–9.9 mL/h	PCA; intermittent; continuous	360 g	1.6 × 11.2 × 10.2 cm
WalkMed 350 (Medex Ambulatory Infusion Systems, Division of Ivion)	Linear peristaltic	Disposable 65, 150, 250 mL bags; dedicated pump sets	9 V alkaline battery (3–21d)	0.1–19.99 mL/h (increments of 0.01 mL)	Occlusion; system malfunction; low battery; depleted battery; prime; door open		Continuous	360 g	4.6 × 11.2 × 10.2 cm
WalkMed PCA (Medex Ambulatory Infusion Systems, Division of Ivion)	Linear peristaltic	Disposable 65, 150, 250 mL bags; dedicated pump sets	9 V alkaline battery (1–21 days depending on infusion rate)	0.1–19.99 mL/h (increments of 0.01) or 0.1–30 mL/h (increments of 0.1 mL)	Near end; volume limit; occlusion; system malfunction; low battery; depleted battery; end of infusion; total volume delivered; programming error		Continuous; continuous with patient-activated bolus; bolus only	360 g	4.6 × 11.2 × 10.2 cm

Table continued on following page

TABLE 28-5

Features of Ambulatory Infusion Devices *Continued*

Name/Model (Manufacturer)	Pumping Mechanism	Drug Reservoir/ Accessories	Battery/ Power Source	Range of Infusion Rates	Alarms/Safety Features	Keep Open Rate	Program Modes	Weight	Size
Provider One (Abbott)	Rotary peristaltic	Any collapsible IV bag; dedicated tubing	Two disposable 9 V lithium batteries (4800 mL); or 12 V rechargeable batteries (4000 mL)	1–400 mL/h	Occlusion; cartridge improperly inserted; programming error; computer error; air in line; low battery; low reservoir; end of infusion	1 mL/h	Continuous; tapering	400 g	132 × 86 × 33 cm
Provider 5500 (Pancretec/ Abbott)	Rotary peristaltic	Any collapsible IV bag	9 V alkaline battery	0.1–250 mL/h	Occlusion; air in line; low reservoir; low battery; ending infusion; system problem; latch open	0.1 mL/h	Continuous; PCA	400 g	
Pain Management Provider (Abbott)	Rotary peristaltic	Any collapsible IV bag		0.1–25 mL/h in 0.1-mL increments	Security lock box available		Continuous; loading dose; PCA (suitable for epidural injection)		
CADD-Plus (Pharmacia Deltec)	Linear peristaltic	50, 100, 250 mL custom cassettes or any collapsible IV bag with custom adapter	9 V disposable alkaline or lithium battery	0.1–75 mL/h	High pressure; low reservoir; low battery; power-up failure; pump in stop mode; programmed volume depleted; high pressure; system error	0–10 mL/h	Continuous; intermittent; delay start	425 g	2.8 × 8.9 × 16 cm

Device	Mechanism	Reservoir	Power source	Flow rate range	Alarms	KVO rate	Modes	Weight	Dimensions
CADD-I (Pharmacia Deltec)	Linear peristaltic	50, 100, 250 mL custom cassettes or any collapsible IV bag with custom adapter	9 V disposable alkaline or lithium battery	0–299 mL every 24 h or 90 mL/h in fixed high-flow mode	Power-up fault; pump in stop mode; low battery; low reservoir volume; programmed volume depleted; high pressure; system error		Continuous	425 g	2.8 × 8.9 × 16 cm
CADD-PCA Ambulatory Infusion Pump Model 5800	Linear peristaltic	50, 100, 250 mL custom reservoir or any IV bag with remote adapter	9 V alkaline or lithium battery	0–20 mL/h (may also be programmed in mg/h)	Power-up failure; low battery; depleted battery; low reservoir; programmed volume depleted; high pressure; system error		Continuous; patient-activated bolus; continuous plus patient-activated bolus	425 g	2.8 × 3.5 × 6.4 cm
CADD-TPN Ambulatory Infusion System Model 5700 (Pharmacia Deltec)	Linear peristaltic	Collapsible IV bag with dedicated adapter tubing	9 V alkaline (6 h) or lithium (18 h) battery, rechargeable battery pack (11 h), or AC adapter	10–250 mL/h with 9 V battery or 10–400 mL/h with AC adapter	Low reservoir; programmed volume depleted; infusion period completed; low battery; depleted battery; invalid rate; high pressure; power-up fault; system error	5 mL/h	Continuous; continuous with tapering up or down	369 g	2.8 × 8.9 × 13.3 cm
EZ Flow Model 80–2 (Creative Medical Development)	Displacement chamber	Disposable 100 and 250 mL cassettes or large-volume adapter	Rechargeable NiCad battery or AC power adapter	0.6–250 mL/h (16 incremental rates)	Infusion complete; occlusion; low battery	0.2 or 1 mL/h	Continuous; intermittent	14 oz	6.75 × 3.5 × 1.27 inches
MedMate 1100 (Patient Solutions)	Peristaltic	Custom cassettes or any IV bag	Two disposable 9 V alkaline or lithium batteries or external recharger	0.1–500 mL/h	Programming error; system fault; low battery; dose due; air in line; door open; dose complete; low bag; bag end	0.1–9.9 mL/h	Continuous; tapering; patient-controlled anesthesia (PSA); intermittent; delay start	17 oz	4.4 × 3.3 × 1.4 inches

Table continued on following page

TABLE 28-5
Features of Ambulatory Infusion Devices *Continued*

Name/Model (Manufacturer)	Pumping Mechanism	Drug Reservoir/ Accessories	Battery/ Power Source	Range of Infusion Rates	Alarms/Safety Features	Keep Open Rate	Program Modes	Weight	Size
Vector MTI (Infusion Technology)		Any collapsible IV bag	Two 9 V alkaline batteries or AC power	0.1–400 mL/h	Reservoir empty; infusion complete; over pressure; check cassette; dead battery; system malfunction; air in line; low battery; low reservoir	0–5 mL/h	Continuous; intermittent; PCA; taper	14.5 oz	5.6 × 3.5 × 1.4 inches
MAXX 100 (Medication Delivery Devices)	Controlled-pressure technology	100-mL custom bag	9 V alkaline battery	50, 100, or 200 mL/h	Pump malfunction; low battery; occlusion; end of infusion; overflow		Continuous	10.5 oz	6.7 × 4.7 × 1.4 inches
SideKick (I-Flow)	Spring-driven infusion	50 and 100 mL minibags; custom IV sets that determine flow rate	Self-contained spring	50, 100, or 200 mL/h	None		Continuous		
MEDFLO II (Secure Medical Products)	Elastomeric	Unit is disposable balloon reservoir: 100, 200, and 300 mL	None	50, 100, 175, and 200 mL/h	None	NA	Continuous		2.75 × 4.25 to 7.0 inches
ReadyMed (McGaw)	Elastomeric	50, 100, 250 mL reservoirs	None	50, 100, 167, and 200 mL/h	None	NA	Continuous		
Intermate LV System (Baxter)	Elastomeric	Unit is disposable balloon reservoir: 105, 275 mL	None	50, 100, 200, and 250 mL/h	None	NA	Continuous		
Infusor (Baxter)	Elastomeric	Unit is disposable balloon reservoir: 65–275 mL	None	0.5–10 mL/h or 12–240 mL/d	With patient-controlled module attachment, lockout of 15 or 60 min		Continuous;		PCA

AMBULATORY, MULTICHANNEL

Device	Mechanism	Reservoir/tubing	Power source	Flow rate	Alarms	Flow modes	Weight	Dimensions
VIVUS 4000 Infuser (I-Flow Corporation), four channel	Positive displacement	Any IV bag; dedicated tubing; manifold line to connect up to four tubings to single IV line; programmer required for operation; communicator unit for remote programming	5 (5000 mL delivery) or 10 (10,000 mL delivery) AA disposable alkaline batteries; 1.5 V DC or external 110/120 V AC adapter	0.1–200 mL/h	Low battery; dead battery; occlusion; empty reservoir; internal malfunction; runaway infusion; open door	Continuous; sequential; continuous bolus; intermittent	1.05 kg	19.7 × 11.43 × 5.1 cm
Intelliject (Ivion), four channel	Rack and pinion drive (syringe driver)	Dedicated 30-mL syringes and manifold	Two 9 V disposable batteries	5.4–40 mL/h/channel	Occlusion; low battery; low reservoir; program error; electronic fault	Continuous; bolus; continuous plus bolus; sequential; alternating	1.54 kg	25.4 × 16.5 × 7.1 cm
Verifuse (Block Medical)	Linear peristaltic	Any IV container	Two 9 V alkaline batteries; rechargeable NiCad battery, or AC power adapter	0.1–300 mL/h	Door open; barcode fault; change batteries; low batteries; pump interrupted; air in line; low reservoir; occlusion; bad batteries; pumping complete; overvoltage; end of program; malfunction	Continuous; tapering up or down; loading dose; delay start; PCA; intermittent	17 oz	6.4 × 3.1 × 1.1 inches

Modified from Finley RS: Drug-delivery system: infusion and access devices, Highlights Antineoplast Drugs 13(2):15, 1995.

increasingly common practice in the home setting. It is important that patients receive their first dose of chemotherapy in an inpatient or outpatient setting to facilitate expedient and proper treatment if any untoward reactions occur. In addition, a plan for properly disposing of all biohazardous waste should be in place (see Chapter 23).*

It is also important that antibiotic and antifungal therapies be initiated in the inpatient or outpatient setting because side effects typically occur with these medications. When considering the continuation of these two types of therapy in the home, it is important to consider the use of an infusion pump especially if the medication needs to be infused more than once a day. An electronic pump that can be programmed for intermittent dosing will decrease the number of home nursing visits required and decrease the number of connections and disconnections of the IV line, reducing the potential for infection. Thus, the overall costs savings will usually justify the expense of the pump.[32, 39, 56, 89, 103]

Once the patient's tolerance to the medication has been established, this treatment modality in the home setting is preferable to extended hospitalization if the patient is medically stable. The patient is generally more comfortable at home, and the health care cost savings are considerable when such high-technology services are provided in the home setting. In addition, patient hospitalizations are reduced, there is increased quality of life for patients and their families, and patients have a sense of control and active participation in their treatment plan.†

Geriatric Considerations

Ill older adults generally want to be home among family and familiar surroundings. Family members often feel inadequate in their abilities to care properly for their parent/spouse and may be reluctant to bring them home. This in turn may result in feelings of guilt and fears that they may be judged as uncaring. In addition, family members have feelings of guilt and helplessness associated with their parent's/spouse's illness. The nurse must provide an opportunity for family members to discuss their fears, feelings, and concerns. Consideration should be given also to how this illness is affecting the family's ability to meet their continuing needs.‡

Needs

1. What difficulties is the family experiencing with the medical treatment? (This would include management and changes in course of illness.)

2. What are the sources of financial strain from direct and indirect costs related to the illness?
3. What changes are required in ADLs for the family?
4. In what manner has the illness fostered social isolation?
5. How have relationships within the family been affected?
6. What impact has the illness or its management had on the ability to meet their continuing needs?

Coping Strategies

1. What is the level of knowledge and technical skill the family has gained concerning the illness and its treatment?
2. What strategies does the family use to help maintain a sense of normalcy in family life?
3. Who are identified supportive people or groups, and what do they provide for the family?
4. What activities do the family members use to enhance positive coping strategies?
5. Does this illness have any positive aspects or results as perceived by this family?

After the establishment of rapport with the family, it is expected that each of these areas can be explored in more depth. The nurse and the family can work together to identify and implement mutually acceptable interventions that will promote optimal family functioning. It is important to provide the family with education to enable them to care adequately for their parent/ spouse and to provide the necessary resources to support their primary caregiving role and to foster optimal family functioning. Many community resources are available to aid and support families experiencing difficulties associated with caring for an elderly person who has cancer.

Hospice

Any discussion of home care for patients with cancer would not be complete without considering hospice and the vital care provided by health care professionals within this domain of practice. Hospice offers the health care community an approach to dealing with death and dying from a familial framework. The advent of consumerism and the desire for increased control over the delivery and quality of care, particularly when all other treatment options have been exhausted or judged to be ineffective, have contributed to the increased public awareness of and interest in the hospice concept. Even though the term *hospice* is familiar to most, many do not understand the type of services provided under hospice.*

---

*References 19, 20, 29, 77, 86, 98, 100.

†References 7, 8, 20, 26, 30, 33, 39, 56.

‡References 2, 10, 18, 19, 23, 26, 44, 50, 57, 84, 105.

*References 1, 10, 16, 23, 35, 38, 42, 44, 45, 49, 67, 87, 91, 104.

Hospice is a philosophy of care that provides high-quality, comprehensive care to persons with a terminal disease and their families. Hospice care is not exclusively terminal care. It is sensitive and skilled care that addresses the physical, psychological, and spiritual needs of the patient and family and is provided by an interdisciplinary team of professionals and volunteers. The setting for this care is usually in the home; however, hospitalization is available during acute medical crisis, impending death, or to give the family a short respite (2–5 days). Medical crises may include uncontrolled pain, nausea and vomiting, or other situations that may warrant a brief hospitalization until the patient's symptoms are controlled.[1, 10, 67, 73, 88, 105]

In home care, an assessment of the family and their ability to provide care and support for the patient is essential (Box 28–2). In the early 1980s, hospice treatment was formally acknowledged through reimbursement by Medicare and private insurance companies. This official recognition has made it easier for people to die at home by providing them with some financial and professional support, by setting standards to regulate the professional care they receive, and by educating physicians, nurses, and the public about the home death alternative. In slightly more than a decade, the grassroots, volunteer-based reform movement became an integral part of the mainstream health system in America.

A goal of hospice is to enhance the quality of life for the patient who is dying and for the surviving family members. Hospice care makes it possible for dying patients to live their last days in their own homes. Hospice programs enable terminally ill patients to remain comfortable in their own homes by providing the necessary support services. Some hospice programs have expanded the range of services available to hospice patients and their families by establishing hospice daycare centers. These centers increase the continuity of care, provide additional support services such as individual counseling and support groups, and increase the patient's and family's sense of connectedness with others.[1, 10, 44, 61, 67]

Recently, in many areas of the United States, several hospice programs have been particularly innovative in reaching out to the community at large by developing educational and bereavement programs that teach others not in hospice programs how to confront and ultimately cope with loss and grief. These hospices also provide training programs and manuals to health care providers and teachers to enable them to form support groups in their community. Many hospice programs provide consultation services to other health care providers and institutions.

The hospice team is truly a multidisciplinary team of professionals, consisting of physicians, nurses, social workers, spiritual care advisors, pharmacists, nutrition-

---

BOX 28–2

Pertinent Topics Involved in Family System Assessment

1. Which family members are present during the initial evaluation?
2. Which members appear to be the decision-makers?
3. Which family member is the hospice intake worker addressing the most during the intake process?
4. Does there appear to be consent (harmony) or discontent (disharmony) among various family members? If so, which ones?
5. What position does terminal member maintain within family structure: e.g., leader/follower, contributor/bystander, hero/scapegoat (hero: family member whose role is designed to save or protect the family from internal or external conflict; scapegoat: family member whose role is designed to take the blame for family's mishaps and problems)?
6. Are there any family members who are emotionally attached to terminal member but who are not present at the meeting and/or may not be seen as part of decision-making process? This may especially focus on children, grandchildren, and siblings of terminal member who are emotionally involved and will clearly be part of bereavement process but may be overlooked by immediate family members.
7. Do family members appear to accept the terminal diagnosis? Are they open in speaking with terminal member concerning diagnosis, or do they want to protect/conceal medical data?
8. Are any of the immediate family members, including the terminal member, affected by substance abuse, gambling, or other addictive disorders?
9. Is there a history of any mental illness within the family system?
10. Is there a history of any antisocial behavior (e.g., criminal behavior) with any family members?
11. Have there been other losses experienced by family members? What was the nature of these losses? When did they occur? How did family members cope and adjust to them?
12. What impressions does family give concerning their experiences with attending physicians? This may indicate families who have difficulty in dealing with the medical community or with authority figures.

Modified from Gulla JP: Family assessment and its relation to hospice care, *Am J Hospice Palliative Care* 7:32, 1990.

ists, and volunteers. Often, attorneys are available to provide legal aid to patients and their families. Most hospice programs provide ongoing bereavement services to families after the patient's death.

Private Duty

Many home care organizations provide supplemental home care services on a fee-for-service basis. These additional services, such as nursing, nursing aides, companions, and housekeepers, can supplement available caregiving resources or provide care when there is no available caregiver, thereby preventing or delaying institutionalization. Private-duty home care is often not included in most health insurance policies as a benefit; therefore, the patient or family is responsible for paying for this service. This can be a significant financial burden, but when one considers the alternative of institutionalization, it can be well worth the expense.[12, 23, 27, 52, 60, 69]

If the cost of such services through an agency is prohibitive for the patient and family, the nurse may suggest that they make arrangements with a friend or neighbor for light housekeeping, meal preparation, or sitter/companion services for nominal compensation. As the trend for managed care continues, some supplemental home care services will be included in the patient's health insurance plan. Third-party payers have noted that paying for additional support services to maintain the patient in the home or in nonhospital settings reduces the overall cost of long-term care.

Cultural Issues

In the complex American health care system, multiculturality is a pressing, mainstream issue. For the individual with cancer, one's native language and treasured traditions can become an obstacle, especially if the skills of the health care professionals are not tempered with cultural sensitivity. One result of the absence of culturally sensitive care is the breakdown of communication and trust, often leading to the reluctance of minorities to use available health resources. Issues related to access and acceptability of care and services have also contributed to cultural barriers to cancer care in America. Many organizations have made significant efforts to reduce cultural barriers to cancer care. Innovations include the following[10, 24, 45, 74, 80, 106]:

- Establishing a minority/cultural group: task force composed of members of the target group to identify specific barriers and a plan to reduce these obstacles
- Establishing a community speakers bureau that uses members of the targeted minority or cultural group
- Involving culturally specific minority media
- Involving culturally specific spiritual and religious institutions

- Forming culturally specific minority support groups
- Recruiting diverse health care workers through employment advertising in publications aimed at ethnic groups
- Forming an informal "language bank" of bilingual employees
- Using available technology, such as the AT&T Language Line, to facilitate communication through an over-the-phone interpretation service

As community-based and home-based health care continue to grow, health care providers will encounter individuals from diverse cultures and ethnic groups. Although an important first step is to improve communication with these groups, it is imperative that health care providers be knowledgeable in issues related to cultural diversity and conceptual differences between cultures. These providers must be proficient in modifying cancer care accordingly to provide culturally sensitive care.[24]

Reimbursement Issues

In the United States, most health care has been provided through third-party payers, that is, private health insurance companies or government health care assistance at state or federal levels. In the past decade, it was estimated that more than 40 million people were without health care insurance and that 30 to 60 million people were underinsured. This inequity among U.S. citizens is still a major component of discussions regarding health care reform on all levels. Economic assessments, analysis, and outcome measures are being increasingly used to provide health care providers, payers, and policy decision-makers with the meaningful data regarding oncology studies, innovative treatments, and alternative care settings to facilitate identification of optimal treatment and care strategies. As third-party payers and health care institutions are attempting to control spiraling health care costs and implement health care reform proactively, such data will guide and direct the allocation of health care service and resource funding. Currently, *managed care* is becoming the predominant health care delivery system and is likely to remain so in the future. More and more people are receiving care in a managed care system. In 1994, approximately 51.1 million members were in a managed care system. Government health programs are also shifting to managed care. At the end of 1996, the membership in managed care systems was estimated to exceed 62 million, an increase of approximately 10% per year. It has been predicted that 90% of the U.S. population will be in the managed care market in the year 2001.[56, 72, 94, 96, 99, 103]

As a result of this shift, a dramatic increase probably will occur in the number of subacute care facilities and a variety of alternative care facilities to provide the necessary services to avoid high-cost nursing home placements. Currently the cost of subacute care is 20% to 60% less than in an acute care setting. Subacute care facilities provide care that is outcome focused, which is also a factor contributing to cost efficiency. Unlike acute care facilities, subacute care facilities are not bound by the PPS because long-term facilities generally have patients whose stay exceeds 25 days and have few short-stay, low-cost cases. Subacute care facilities can either be free-standing long-term care institutions or housed within an existing acute care hospital as long as the federal guidelines and criteria for such facilities are met.*

Although managed care has been highly praised for its efficient management of health care dollars, concerns have been raised by some health care providers and the public that high-quality, individualized care and access to some treatment modalities have been sacrificed. This dimension in the discussion concerning health care reform and resource allocation cannot be ignored. Nurses, as patient advocates, can play an important role in clinical and community-based research that includes quality measures, patient outcomes, and access to care in addition to economic assessments and analysis. Nurses should also take an active part in provider negotiations and in establishing new standards of care as part of their patient advocacy role.[6, 8, 72, 94, 96, 99, 103]

Currently, most health care insurance policies cover home care and hospice services. All require that the service be ordered by a physician and that a medical plan of care be signed by the physician. The care provided must be intermittent, and the patient must also need skilled professional care provided by a nurse, physical therapist, or speech therapist and have a medical condition that warrants ongoing assessment and evaluation. Patients must also be *homebound,* that is, unable to leave home without assistance of others and assistive devices. If the patient or caregiver requires no additional instruction regarding the disease process or its management and the patient is medically stable for more than 2 weeks, he is no longer considered in need of ongoing skilled nursing service unless specific treatments are ordered, such as monthly catheter changes or vitamin B_{12} injections. With the advent of the PPS for home care patients covered under Medicare and the growth of managed care insurance, home health agencies will be asked to deliver more intensive services in a shorter number of visits.[94, 96, 99, 103]

Insurance coverage for home care services and alternative care settings varies from policy to policy. In most cases, insurance benefits are negotiated individually for group policies and benefit packages. More frequently

now, health insurance providers are becoming more flexible regarding the services and benefits available to individuals because the cost-saving benefits have been well documented. Prior approval usually is necessary. The medical plan of care must be reviewed and updated periodically (usually 60 days) and again signed by the physician. Box 28–3 lists the home care services provided by managed care organizations.

PATIENT AND FAMILY TEACHING

The oncology nurse must be proficient in patient and family education. The trend of consumerism and the complex nature of cancer and current, often aggressive treatment modalities necessitate improved, comprehensive patient and family education. Documented evidence supports that patients and families with increased knowledge of their illness and treatment plan experience significantly less anxiety and stress. The oncology nurse must consider individual differences as well as cultural differences when initiating patient or family teaching. Important areas to evaluate are readiness, motivation, past experiences, physical and intellectual abilities, and physical and psychological comfort. Determining what the patient or family member already knows is imperative to avoid boredom and "tuning out." Simply asking the individual if she is interested in obtaining additional information is a good first step. Oncology nurses in acute, community, clinic, and outpatient settings need to emphasize more the psychosocial and informational needs of family home caregivers. Because of shorter hospitalizations, nurses must begin this educational process early and continue the counseling process, through the discharge into the home setting. Linking families to volunteer and professional community agencies with appropriate services will provide additional resources to meet a variety of needs.*

Literacy is a problem in the United States today, with more than 20% of the general population functionally illiterate. Twenty million adults can read at an eighth-grade level, and another 20 million can read at or below the fourth-grade level. Results of other studies indicate that reported reading levels are significantly higher than the actual reading levels of patients. Illiteracy is more endemic among the elderly and poor persons. Keeping this in mind, the oncology nurse should determine the patient's reading capabilities. Many adults are embarrassed about the inability to read and over the years become very skillful in covering up this deficit. Excuses such as "I don't have my glasses with me now; can you read it to me?" or "I'll read it later" may serve as cues on which the nurse should follow up. Other indicators

---

* References 10, 12, 13, 57, 72, 96, 99.

* References 6, 10, 14, 22, 43, 46, 58, 64, 68, 95.

BOX 28-3

Home Care Services Provided by Managed Care Organizations

High-Technology Service

Infusion therapy
Parenteral therapy
Enteral nutrition
Home dialysis
Home monitoring
Customized equipment

Skilled Services

Medical
Nursing (RN)
Physical therapy
Speech therapy
Occupational therapy
Vocational services
Respiratory therapy

Semiskilled Services

Nursing (LPN)
Home health aides
Therapy assistants
Personal response systems

Pharmacy

Analgesia
Antimicrobials
Chemotherapy
Infusion solutions
Nutrition

Home Medical Equipment

Basic mobility aids
Daily living assistive devices
Extensive mobility aids
Advanced high-technology equipment
Oxygen therapies
Medical supplies

Rehabilitation/Assistive Technology

Mobility aids
Adaptive equipment
Custom seating and positioning
Orthotics and prosthetics
Aids for daily living

Hospice Services

Bereavement counseling
Social work services
Palliative services

Custodial Services

Companions
Personal aides
Housekeeping
Shopping
Cooking
Transportation

From Hammill CT, Parver CP: Home health care services: a vital component of managed care, *J Home Health Care Pract* 7(4):18, 1995.

---

include lack of interest in the material, expressions of frustration, lack of reading speed, and inability to answer questions about the content of the text.[22, 43, 46, 58, 68]

Meade and colleagues[70] conducted an analysis of the readability of American Cancer Society (ACS) patient education literature in 1991 and determined that ACS publications written before 1985 had a mean reading level of grade 12.7, whereas those written during and after 1985 had a mean reading level of grade 10.9. Of the 51 booklets analyzed in this study, only 6 booklets were written at a grade level of 8.9 or below, whereas 45 were written at ninth-grade level or above. In view of these results, it is important that the oncology nurse realize the importance of a multifaceted, creative approach to patient and family education. The findings of Meade and coworkers do not negate the value of the written material available currently from ACS and institutions. The oncology nurse must be aware of the limita-

tions of these materials, individualizing the teaching plan to meet the unique needs of each patient. The nurse must also assess for the appropriate instructional method for the individual, using *all* available educational resources and modalities, such as audiovisual, pictorial, and didactic as well as written material. These can only enhance and facilitate the learning process.[22, 68, 91, 95]

Researchers have found that contract learning has had good results when used with adult learners, because it includes concepts of independent, individualized, and self-directed learning. The education process, as with the nursing process, includes the steps of assessing, planning, implementing, and evaluating. The primary learner in the family must be identified and her learning needs assessed. After this assessment, a mutually acceptable plan to meet the identified educational needs is developed by the nurse/teacher and patient/learner. Ap-

---

BOX 28-4

Top 25 Unmet Needs of Home Caregivers

1. Information about the underlying reasons for symptoms
2. Information about what symptoms to expect
3. Information about what to expect in the future
4. Information about treatment of side effects
5. Information about community resources
6. Honest and updated information
7. Ways to reassure patient
8. Ways to deal with patient's decreased energy
9. Ways to deal with unpredictability of the future
10. Information about medications (side effects, scheduling)
11. Ways to encourage patient
12. Information about patient's psychological needs
13. Methods to decrease caregiver's stress
14. Ways of coping with patient's diagnosis of cancer
15. Information about type and extent of patient's illness
16. Ways to cope with role changes
17. Information about physical needs of patient
18. Activities that will make patient feel purposeful
19. Ways to be more patient and tolerant
20. Ways to deal with caregiver's depression
21. Ways to maintain a normal family life
22. Ways to discuss death with patient
23. Ways to deal with caregiver's fears
24. Ways to combat fatigue
25. Ways to provide patient with adequate nutrition

From Hileman JW, Lackey NR, Hassanein RS: Identifying the needs of home caregivers of patients with cancer, *Oncol Nurs Forum* 19(5):775, 1992.

---

propriate teaching strategies are used to implement the plan and are mutually evaluated, with the evaluation serving as a basis for further decision making. Addressing the educational wants and needs of the family caregiver is a top priority if the patient is to receive proper care and be able to remain in the home.[12, 23, 46, 49, 58] Box 28–4 lists the top 25 unmet needs of caregivers.

ADVANCE DIRECTIVES

Since 1991, when the Patient Self-Determination Act (PSDA) became law, hospitals have responded to the mandate by creating pamphlets and educational materials regarding advance directives. These are usually presented to patients on admission to the acute care facility, which is not ideal because at that time patients are usually either ill, anxious, or under great stress. This lack of timing does not facilitate a well-reasoned health care decision. It is preferable that patients and their families collaborate with their primary health care provider well before hospitalization. Many people have misconceptions regarding advance directives, believing that these are only for elderly or terminally ill patients and that if one does have an advance directive, it will result in limited or denied care in the future. The oncology nurse must address these misconceptions. Keeping in mind the barriers to education created by illiteracy and cultural differences, the information regarding advance directives must be provided in an easily readable and clear manner. Neumark[73] developed a patient teaching tool that does an excellent job of presenting the concept of advance directives* (Box 28–5).

DISCHARGE INSTRUCTIONS

To help facilitate the transition to the home or alternative care setting and ensure continuity of care and medical follow-up, it is important to clearly convey specific discharge instructions to the patient and family members at discharge. The time of discharge is particularly hectic, and often instructions given at this time may not be remembered accurately or at all. Consequently, it is advisable to have specific written instructions to review with and give the patient and family at discharge.

Accessing the Health Care System

Many institutions have discharge instruction sheets that are completed by the nurse and include instructions regarding follow-up appointments and medications. Patients and their families need to know how to access the health care system after discharge. The following questions can facilitate prompts or potential needs of the patient or family concerning the home care or office-care issues.

- Whom should I call when questions arise that cannot wait until the next appointment?
- What should I expect?
- When do I worry?
- When should I call?
- How can I reach these professionals?
- What about after hours? Who is the contact person then?

In addition, in all settings the experienced oncology nurse should anticipate potential problems that may arise as a result of treatment or disease progression. For example, side effects specific to the chemotherapy and other medications, the nurse can provide the patient or responsible caregiver with information regarding antici-

---

* References 44, 61, 67, 73, 80, 88, 99, 105.

BOX 28–5

Making Your Own Choices: A Guide to Help You Decide About Advance Directives

This guide is to help you learn how you can make your own choices about health care. You have the right to make choices about your health care. There is a law called the Patient Self-Determination Act. This law states that most hospitals have to tell you about something called "advance directives." This guide gives you some facts about advance directives. It will explain:

- What advance directives are
- How you make advance directives
- Why advance directives are important
- What to include in your advance directive

WHAT ARE ADVANCE DIRECTIVES?

If you are ever unable to make your own health care choices or to communicate what you want to do, other people will have to make choices for you. *Advance directives* are a way to let your family, friends, and health care providers know your wishes to receive—or not to receive—medical care and treatment. An advance directive protects your right to make your own choices. It gives you the power to control your own care.

MAKING YOUR ADVANCE DIRECTIVE

To make sure that your family, friends, and health care providers understand your choices, it is important to have your advance directive in writing.

There are two common types of advance directives. One type is called a *living will*. The second type is called a *durable power of attorney for health care*. Both are legal pieces of paper that allow you to state your wishes in writing.

- *Living will:* this explains your wishes about health care and treatments. It is used only if you become terminally ill, if you are in an accident and have permanent brain damage, or if you are in a permanent coma.
- *Durable power of attorney for health care:* this names another person to make choices for you if you cannot make choices for yourself. This person is called your *agent* or your *proxy*. It is a good idea to name a second person to make decisions for you in case your first choice is not available for some reason.

Your agent should be someone whom you know and trust. It is very important to talk about your feelings and choices about health care and treatment with your agent.

To make sure your choices are clearly known, it is best to write them down. It is helpful to be as clear as possible so that your agents understand what you would want. Any advance directive can be changed or cancelled by you at any time.

- Sign your name and put the date on the advance directive. It is best to do this in front of a notary public.

- Give a copy of your advance directive to your doctor to put in your medical file.
- Give a copy of your advance directive to each of the people you have asked to be your agents.
- Put a card in your wallet that says you have an advance directive (and where to find it).
- *Review your advance directive often. Make sure it expresses your wishes clearly.*

WHY ADVANCE DIRECTIVES ARE IMPORTANT

The purpose of an advance directive is to help other people make choices for you if you cannot make your own choices. *You want them to make the same choices that you would make.* Your advance directive guides other people to follow your wishes.

PREPARE ADVANCE DIRECTIVES WHILE YOU ARE ABLE TO MAKE YOUR OWN CHOICES

You are never too young or too healthy to have an advance directive. A time may come when an accident or illness will keep you from being able to make or communicate your own health care choices.

Some times when you may not be able to decide for yourself would be if you are:

Permanently unconscious: this means there is no chance to become conscious (in a permanent coma).
Irreversibly brain damaged: this can affect your ability to think or communicate.
Brain dead: this means all brain function has stopped permanently and will not return.

WHAT TO INCLUDE IN YOUR ADVANCE DIRECTIVE

What you choose to write in your advance directive depends on things that are most important to you.

These things are your beliefs and values. The beliefs and values that may influence your health care choices may include what you think or feel about:

- Being independent and having control
- Making your own decisions
- Pain or suffering
- Being with your loved ones at death
- What makes you happy and sad
- Where you live
- Your religious background and beliefs
- Your finances
- Your health care providers
- Your health care relationships
- Prolonging life
- Donating parts of your body

BOX 28–5

Making Your Own Choices: A Guide to Help You Decide About Advance Directives Continued

WHAT ARE YOUR CHOICES?

Before you make an advance directive, it is important to think about what you might feel if you were near death. It is helpful to express your feelings about having or not having certain forms of medical treatment. *Often having these treatments will keep you alive longer.*

Some of the medical treatments that you may have to make choices about:

- *Life-sustaining treatment/extraordinary care*: this is any treatment that keeps you alive longer and delays death.
- *Cardiopulmonary resuscitation (CPR)*: this is a method that will attempt to restore stopped breathing and/or heartbeat.
- *Code*: this means calling a special team of doctors and nurses to start CPR when your heart stops beating or you stop breathing.
- *Do not resuscitate (DNR)/no code*: this is a doctor's order that lets other staff know that you do not want to receive CPR.
- *Intravenous (IV) therapy*: this is when thin tubes are put in your vein to give you food, water, and/or medicine.
- *Feeding tubes*: this is when tubes are put in your mouth, nose, or stomach to give you liquid food if you cannot eat normally.
- *Respirator or ventilator*: this is a machine that breathes for you or helps you breathe. A tube is put in through your mouth or nose, or a hole in your neck. The tube goes into your lungs and is attached to the machine.
- *Dialysis*: this means using a machine to remove waste products from your blood if your kidneys do not work the right way.

An advance directive lets you make choices about future medical care and treatments under various circumstances. You can ask your doctor or nurse to help explain the pros and cons of the different types of medical treatments.

If you make choices while you are able, your wishes about the end of your life will be honored.

SHARING YOUR BELIEFS

Talk about your beliefs and values with the people who may have to make choices for you in the future. It is hard to think about many of these issues. But, if you talk about your wishes when you are able, the people who will have to make difficult choices for you will feel relieved that they know what you would have chosen.

Even if you do not know exactly how you feel about certain types of treatments, share your feelings with your family, friends, doctor, nurse, or spiritual leader.

Remember, advance directives let you *make your own choices.*

FOR MORE INFORMATION

Laws for advance directives are different in each state. Sample forms and more information may be available from a hospital, home health service, hospice, lawyer, or your state medical society. Other good sources to learn more about advance directives:

Legal Hotline for Older Americans
PO Box 23810
Pittsburgh, PA 15222
1-800-262-5297

Choice in Dying
200 Varick St.
New York, NY 10014
212-366-5540

Legal Counsel for the Elderly
(Associated with American Association for Retired Persons)
1331 H Street NW
Washington, DC 20005
202-434-2120

From Neumark DE: Providing information about advance directives to patients in ambulatory care and their families, *Oncol Nurs Forum* 21(4):771, 1994.

---

pated problems and self-care measures to manage these problems. Consider the patient's reading ability and assess the readability of the written material provided. If the reading skills of the patient or family member are limited, it may be more appropriate and more effective to write out very simple instructions or information specifically tailored for the individual. Alternative teaching modalities such as audiotapes or videotapes may also

be effective teaching tools to augment any teaching plan.[45, 46, 58, 72, 80]

Follow-up Appointments

Central to an effective treatment of any cancer is consistent medical follow-up. Ongoing assessment and evaluation and subsequent modification of the treatment plan are critical as the trend for more aggressive posthospital treatment continues. Follow-up appointments are important but are often difficult endeavors for patients and their families. The nurse can implement several actions to facilitate keeping follow-up appointments.

First and foremost is the almost universal concern about transportation. Patients may not have transportation resources available to them, and frequently this issue is not addressed when they are given the follow-up appointment. It is important to ask the patient or family member if transportation is a problem. If so, they may be referred to local agencies that provide such services. The ACS and the American Red Cross are national organizations that have local offices that provide transportation to and from medical facilities at no charge or minimal cost. Many private companies provide transportation services for disabled persons for a fee.[12, 23]

In addition to information about transportation resources, patients need to know what assistance is available when they arrive for their follow-up appointment. If a wheelchair is needed, how do they arrange to have one available? Most hospitals and clinics have wheelchairs available for such purposes. This should be determined before the appointment. If a wheelchair is not available, the patient should be advised to arrange for one's use.

At busy oncology clinics, follow-up appointments can become an all-day endeavor. Patients frequently are scheduled for blood work before their appointment with the physician and later may receive chemotherapy or be scheduled for other tests. Patients and their families should be advised to bring the medications that they may need to take while still at the clinic, especially PRN pain medications. Patients and their families should be told what to expect at the follow-up appointment, especially if the patient is going to receive a treatment or particular diagnostic test for the first time. Knowing what to expect greatly reduces fears and anxieties associated with the unknown.

Follow-up Telephone Call

A follow-up telephone call to patients and their families should be made within 24 to 48 hours after discharge. It is helpful for the nurse to have a copy of the continuing patient care form and discharge instruction sheets to enable them to ask appropriate questions to facilitate obtaining accurate information about the patient's status.

1. How are things going since you came home?
2. Have any problems occurred?
3. Do you have any questions that I can answer for you?

TABLE 28-6
Payer Source Guidelines

Medical Insurance	Prior Authorization	Services Covered	Certification Period	Durable Medical Equipment
Medicare	No	SN, PT, ST, OT, MSS, HHA	2 mo, 60–62 d	Yes, need medical order
Medicaid	Yes	SN, PT, ST, HHA, no MSS*	2 mo	Yes, need medical order
Blue Cross Basic	Yes	SN, PT, OT, ST, MSS, HHA	30 d	No, coverage only with major medical
Blue Cross: Blue Care Network or Personal Choice	Yes	SN, PT, OT, ST, MSS, HHA, nutrition (if agency certified for this)	30 d	Yes, with approval
Federal Blue Cross: Hi-option	Yes	SN, PT, OT, ST, MSS, HHA	30 d	Yes
Federal Blue Cross: Lo-option	No, all visits reimbursed 75%	25 SN/yr; 50 PT/yr; no HHA, OT, or ST	30 d	Yes, coverage at 75%
Commerical: Aetna, Prudential, etc.	Yes	Varies with benefit plan	60 d	Yes, varies with benefit plan
Managed care: health maintenance organizations, (HMOs), Group Health Plans, Health Alliance Plans, etc.	Yes	SN, PT, OT (MSS, HHA with authorization*)	60–62 d	Yes, varies with benefit plan

SN, Staff nurse: PT, physical therapy; ST, speech therapy; OT, occupational therapy; MSS, medical social service; HHA, home health aide.

* Refer to Box 28–3 for a list of services that are often provided through managed care.

These questions can open communication, but the nurse must ask specific questions related to the patient's illness and treatment plan to ensure an accurate assessment of the home situation. If it becomes apparent that activities are not going well in the home, the nurse may recommend that the patient be brought in to see the physician. Often, home care needs are not easily identified before discharge, but once the patient is at home, this need becomes apparent. If a home care referral has not been made, the nurse may determine at this time that a referral is warranted and initiate this process.

Durable Medical and Adaptive Equipment

Durable medical equipment (DME) includes hospital beds, wheelchairs, and much more. Many assistive devices are available to patients and their families that can simplify home care management and also promote home safety. Essential equipment such as hospital beds, wheelchairs, and bedside commodes should be in the home at discharge, but some equipment and adaptive devices should not be ordered until a home evaluation can be done. Although an experienced nurse can assess and evaluate home equipment needs, a physical or occupational therapist should be consulted. These therapists have an extensive knowledge of available equipment and may be able to meet the patient's equipment needs more effectively. Most insurance policies provide coverage for some DME; however, a physician's order and an accompanying related neuromusculoskeletal diagnosis is usually required. Some insurance companies require prior approval before the equipment can be delivered to the patient. DME companies can help with this process. Table 28–6 provides a general overview of insurance coverage and the Appendix lists national resources for durable medical and adaptive equipment.*

COMMUNITY RESOURCES

Use of available community resources is low even when these services are needed. The reasons are not clear, but contributing factors may include the following:

- Service cost
- Access/availability
- Lack of awareness of available resources
- Lack of flexibility in services
- Inappropriate use of limited resources
- Consumer dissatisfaction
- Labeling of services

Further exploration into these factors is warranted to provide appropriate, well-coordinated community re-

sources in a cost-efficient manner. Many national and local community resources are available to cancer patients and their families, ranging from personal services, informational services, social services, and support services. A telephone call to the Cancer Information Service (1-800-4-CANCER) and the local ACS chapter is a good starting point when first attempting to identify resources available in the community. Local community services often include agencies that provide or assist with the following[12, 23, 29, 37]:

1. Chore or housekeeping services
2. Adult day care
3. Socialization services (e.g., Friendly Visitor, In-Home Companion)
4. Nutritional services (e.g., Meals on Wheels, nutrition sites, food supplements, food banks/cupboards)
5. Financial savings and grant program
6. Transportation services
7. Support groups and counseling services

A list of national organizations that provide assistance to cancer patients and their families is included in the Appendix. These organizations will help nurses identify local community support services, obtain educational materials, and facilitate networking within the community.

CONCLUSION

Patients with cancer move through a number of health care settings during the course of their illnesses. Inherent within this movement are encounters with many health care professionals. A successful transition through these settings depends on the collaborative efforts of the health care providers. Ongoing communication is the key to the effectiveness of these efforts.

In addition to collaboration, a thorough assessment and evaluation of the unique and specific care requirements of the patient must be performed to identify the appropriate community support services to facilitate this transition along the continuum. Subsequent reevaluation and modification of the continuing care plan must be done periodically to ensure attainment of expected outcomes and to avoid inappropriate use of limited services. It is a challenge to meet the increasingly complex, multidimensional needs of patients with cancer and their families. Nurses must be prepared and knowledgeable to meet these needs successfully. They must also remember that what most people want is *not* the power of hospital technology in their homes or alternative settings for care, but the *security* of care that a multidisciplinary team can provide.[7, 8, 94, 96, 99, 103, 106]

---

* References 6–8, 18–20, 32, 41, 82, 97, 101.

Nursing Management

Many essential steps are necessary to facilitate transition to the home setting and ensure continuity of care. Assessment with planned interventions and an evaluation of the outcomes will enhance a smooth transition for the patient and family members. Following is an example of a nursing diagnosis with multiple assessment and intervention strategies that can be adapted to meet the varied individual patient needs.

Nursing Diagnosis

- *Home maintenance management, impaired, related to:*

  Patient

  Inability to perform household activities secondary to side effects of chemotherapy
  Inability to perform household activities secondary to disease progression
  Inability to engage in self-care activities secondary to chronic debilitating disease

  Caregiver

  Inability to maintain self and patient secondary to unavailable support system
  Inability to maintain caregiver role secondary to lack of knowledge, inadequate supports/resources

Outcome Goals

Patient/caregiver will be able to:

- Identify factors that restrict self-care and home management.
- Demonstrate the ability to perform skills necessary for care of patient or home.
- Express satisfaction with home situation.
- Experience less anxiety and stress related to caregiving role.
- Identify personal strengths and receive support through nursing relationship and community resources.

Interventions

The following interventions apply to many individuals with impaired home maintenance management, regardless of etiology:

- Assess for causative or contributing factors:
  Lack of knowledge
  Insufficient funds

  Lack of necessary equipment or aids
  Inability to perform household activities (illness, sensory deficits, motor deficits)
  Impaired cognitive functioning
  Impaired emotional functioning
  Factors affecting learning
- Reduce or eliminate causative or contributing factors if possible.
- Determine with patient and family the information needed to be taught and learned:
  Monitoring skills needed (pulse, circulation, urine)
  Medication administration (procedure, side effects, precautions)[20, 33, 34, 47]
  Treatment procedures
  Equipment use/maintenance
  Safety issues (e.g., environmental)
  Community resources
  Follow-up care
  Anticipatory guidance (e.g., emotional and social needs of family, alternatives to home care)
- Be sensitive to patient's and families' time schedules.
- Reduce or eliminate barriers for learning (e.g., delay teaching until person ready, cultural barriers, health beliefs, past experiences).
- Promote patient/family learning (e.g., reduce anxiety; provide quiet, nonstressful environment; promote positive attitude and active participation in learning process).
- Initiate teaching and give detailed written instructions. Refer to a community nursing (home care) agency for follow-up.
- Determine type of equipment or aids needed, considering availability, cost, and durability:
  Seek assistance from agencies that rent or loan supplies.
  Teach care and maintenance of supplies that increase length of use.
  Consider adapting equipment to reduce cost.
- If patient/family has insufficient funds, consult with social service department and service organizations for assistance, such as American Heart Association, The Lung Association, and American Cancer Society (see Appendix).
- Determine type of assistance needed to perform household activities (e.g., meals, housework, transportation) and assist patient to obtain them.
- Discuss with family the possibility of freezing complete meals that require only heating (e.g., small containers of soup, stew, casseroles).

- Determine availability of meal services for ill persons (e.g., Meals on Wheels, church groups).
- Teach patient/family about foods that are easily prepared and nutritious (e.g., hard-boiled eggs).
- Contract with an adolescent for light housekeeping, or refer to community agency for assistance with housework.
- Determine availability of transportation for shopping and health care:
    Request rides with neighbors to places they drive routinely.
    Consult transportation resources in community.
- If patient has impaired mental processes, assess ability to maintain household safely:
    Reduce/eliminate causative or contributing factors, if possible.
    Initiate health teaching regarding impairment, and make appropriate referrals.
- Determine if patient has impaired emotional functioning:
    Assess severity of dysfunction.
    Assess causative or contributing factors.
    Assess patient's present coping strategies.
    Teach constructive problem-solving techniques and coping skills.
    Assist patient to develop appropriate strategies based on his personal strengths and previous experience.
    Find outlets that foster feelings of personal achievement and self-esteem.
    Correct lack of support systems.
    Reduce or eliminate social isolation caused by lessened contact with others.
    Initiate health teaching.
    Assist with managing new roles/responsibilities.
    Initiate appropriate referrals.

- Provide anticipatory guidance for caregivers.
- Discuss implications of caring for a chronically ill family member:
    Amount of time involved
    Effects on other role responsibilities (spouse, children, job)
    Physical requirements (lifting)
- Share alternatives to reduce strain and fatigue of caregiving responsibilities:
    Acquire relief from responsibilities at least twice a week for at least 3 hours (sitter, neighbors, relatives).
    Enlist aid of others to meet some of patient's needs (e.g., hairdresser, transporting to physician's office).
    Plan to set aside at least 1 hour a day as leisure time (after patient asleep).
    Maintain contacts with friends and relatives even if only by telephone. Caregivers should inform friends that they do use sitters so friends can include them in some social activities.
    Give caregivers the opportunity to share problems and feelings.
    Include humor therapy strategies to help patient/caregiver relieve stress and anxiety and enhance feelings of well-being.
- Commend caregivers for their concern, diligence, and perseverance in caring for patient at home.
- Initiate health teaching and referrals as indicated:
    Refer to support groups (e.g., American Cancer Society, Encore, Y-Me).[12, 23]
    Refer to community nursing agency.
    Refer to community agencies (e.g., volunteer visitors, meal programs, homemakers, adult day care).

Chapter Questions

1. Factors influencing increased emphasis on home care and alternative care settings include all the following *except:*
   a. Balanced Budget Act 1997
   b. Implementation of diagnosis-related groups (DRGs)
   c. Increased elderly ill population
   d. Extended care facility setting availability
2. Patient characteristics that indicate high risk/need for discharge planning include:
   a. New cancer diagnosis, infusion therapy, age over 65 years
   b. Weight loss, nutrition deficits, adult 40 to 55 years old
   c. New cancer diagnosis, new diabetes diagnosis, new parent
   d. Infusion therapy, rehabilitation, new parent
3. In the United States, family members and friends provide approximately what percentage of in-home care?
   a. 50%
   b. 65%
   c. 80%
   d. 90%
4. The primary reason more people do *not* have an advance directive is:
   a. Belief that advance directives are for elderly and terminally ill patients

   b. Fear that having an advance directive will limit care in the future

   c. Poor timing of health care provider in offering information to patient

   d. Lack of information provided by health care personnel

5. Definition of Medicare guideline regarding "homebound status" includes:

   a. Confined to home only on occasion that restricts ability to leave

   b. Confined to home unless use of assistive device and ability to leave

   c. Confined to home on intermittent basis that restricts ability to leave

   d. Confined to home due to injury, illness, that restricts the ability to leave

6. All of the following statements regarding hospice goals and objectives are true *except:*

   a. Hospice strives to enhance the quality of life for the patient who is dying.

   b. Hospice provides a setting for care that is supportive of both the terminally ill individual and the family.

   c. Hospice enhances the quality of life for the surviving family through ongoing bereavement services.

   d. Hospice provides a comprehensive and multidisciplinary approach to terminal and palliative care.

7. The primary goal of patient education is to:

   a. Provide individuals and families with skills for extensive wound care management

   b. Provide individuals and their families financial management for infusion therapy

   c. Provide individuals and caregivers with infusion technology management

   d. Provide a competent alternative for care delivered by a health care worker

8. Caregiver and patient home-care education needs include:

   a. Drug administration, monitoring, and reporting drug side effects

   b. Drug and infusion information regarding problem-solving, who, when to notify

   c. Drug and infusion administration, reporting drug side effects

   d. Drug and infusion administration, physician notification, reporting side effects

9. The basic elements for the Standards of Practice for Discharge Planning include:

   a. Assessment, needs identification, planning, documentation, implementation, patient education, and program evaluation

   b. Assessment, communication, documentation, implementation, patient and program education

   c. Assessment, needs identification, communication, patient evaluation, program education

   d. Assessment, communication, documentation, patient education, program presentation

10. Advantages of home for the patient and family with cancer includes:

   a. Infusion therapy for antiemetics, analgesia, antimicrobials, and supplemental oxygen

   b. Infusion therapy for analgesia, antiemetics, antifungals, and decreased caregiver needs

   c. Infusion therapy for analgesia, antiemetics, chemotherapy, and decreased out-of-pocket expenses

   d. Infusion therapy for analgesia, chemotherapy, blood sampling, and minimal eligibility issues

BIBLIOGRAPHY

1. Amenta MO, Lippert C: Hospice is a concept, not a place, *Home Healthcare Nurse* 12:71, 1994.
2. American Geriatric Society: Clinical practice guidelines: the management of chronic pain in older patients, *J Am Soc Geriatrics* 46:635, 1998.
3. American Pain Society: *Principles of analgesic use in the treatment of acute pain and cancer pain,* ed 4, Glenview, IL, American Pain Society, 1999.
4. Angeles T: Removing a nontunneled central catheter, *Nursing98* 28:52, 1998.
5. Bagnall-Reeb H: Diagnosis of central venous access device occlusions: implications for nursing practice, *INS* 21(5S):Sll5, 1998.
6. Beach DL: Caregiver discourse: perceptions of illness-related dialogue, *Hospice J* 10:13, 1995.
7. Bean CA and others: High-tech homecare infusion therapies, *Crit Care Nurs Clin North Am* 10:287, 1998.
8. Benefield LE: Home Care in the millennium: critical competencies for nurses in the new millennium, *Home Healthcare Nurse,* 18:17, 2000.
9. Brown SL and others: Infusion pump adverse events: experience from medical device reports, *INS* 20:41, 1997.
10. Callahan R: Patient care coordination of adult oncology patients in home health, *Home Health Care Management & Practice* 10:33, 1999.
11. Camp-Sorrell D: Developing extravasation protocols and monitoring outcomes, *INS* 21:232, 1998.
12. Cancer resources in the United States, *Oncol Nurs Forum* 26:1525, 1999.
13. Capone LJ: The twelve C's of clinical documentation, *Home Healthcare Nurse* 17:382, 1999.
14. Carter R, Golant S: *Helping yourself help others: a book for caregivers,* New York, Times Books, 1996.
15. Centers for Disease Control and Prevention: Recommendations for prevention and control of hepatitis C virus(HCV) infection and HCV-related chronic disease, *MMWR* 47(RR-1 9):1, 1998.
16. Chaly PS, Loriz L: Ethics in the trenches: decision making in practice, *AJN* 98:17, 1998.

17. Chemey A: Alternative delivery sites: where does home care fit? *Home Health Management & Practice* 10:1, 1997.

18. Chung M, Akahoshi Ni: Reducing home nursing visit costs using a remote access infusion pump system, *INS* 22:309, 1999.

19. Cole D: Selection and management of central venous access devices in the home setting, *INS* 22:315, 1999.

20. Cohen MR: *IV drug safety,* Huntington, Valley, PA, Institute for Safe Medication Practice, 1999.

21. Cohen MR, editor: Medication errors, American Pharmaceutical Association, Washington, DC, American Pharmaceutical Association, 1999.

22. Cooley NE and others: Patient literacy and the readability of written cancer educational materials, *Oncol Nurs Forum* 22:1345, 1995.

23. Coping Magazine's guide to educational information and support services, *Coping* 14:30, 2000.

24. Cuthbert-Allman C, Conti PA: VNA of Boston addresses: cultural barriers in home-based care, *Caring Magazine* 14:22, 1995.

25. Davidhizer R, Giger JN: Humor-care for the caregiver, *Caring Magazine* 14:64, 1995.

26. Davis L, Drogasch NT: Triple check procedure prevents chemotherapy errors, *Oncol Nurs Forum* 24:641, 1997.

27. Deets H: Home care in the 21st century, *Caring Magazine* 14:50, 1995.

28. Discharge planning: conditions of participation, *Fed Reg* 59(238), December 1994, Rules and regulations, final rule, Health Care Financing Administration, 42 CER, Pts 405 and 482, Medicare and Medicaid Programs; Revisions to conditions of participation for hospitals, p. 64141.

29. Fall-Dickson JM, Rose L: Caring for patients who experience chemotherapy-induced side effects: the meaning for oncology nurses, *Oncol Nurs Forum* 26:901, 1999.

30. Fiesta J. Legal aspects of medication administration, *Nurs Manage* 29:22, 1998.

31. Finkelstein S: The role home health in disease management, *Home Health Care Management & Practice* 10:20, 1998.

32. Finley RS: Drug-delivery systems: infusion and access devices, *Highlights Antineoplast Drugs* 13:15, 1995.

33. Freidman MM: Risk management strategies for home infusion therapy, *INS,* 20:179, 1997.

34. Gahart BL, Nazareno AR: *Intravenous medications,* ed 16, St. Louis, Mosby, 2000.

35. Given BA: Believing and dreaming to improve cancer care, *Oncol Nurs Forum* 22:929, 1995.

36. Gorsld LA, editor: Best practices in home infusion therapy, Fredrick, MD, Aspen, 1999.

37. Greenlee RT and others: Cancer statistics, 2000, *CA Cancer J Clin* 50:7, 2000.

38. Haddad A: Ethical problems in home health, *JONA,* 22:46, 1992.

39. Hadaway LC: Vascular access devices: meeting patients' needs, *MEDSURG Nurs* 8:296, 1999.

40. Hamilton M: Standards of practice for discharge planning, *Contin Care,* September 1995, p. 33.

41. Hammill CT, Parver CP: Home health care services: a vital component of managed care, *J Home Health Care Pract* 7:16, 1995.

42. Harper BC: Report from the National Task Force on Access to Hospice Care by Minorities, *Hospice J* 10:1, 1995.

43. Harris KA: The informational needs of patients with cancer and their families, *Cancer Pract* 6:39, 1998.

44. Hasrey-Dow K and others: The meaning of quality of life in cancer survivorship, *Oncol Nurs Forum* 26:519, 1999.

45. Heineken J: Establishing a bond with clients of different cultures, *Home Healthcare Nurse* 18:45, 2000.

46. Hiromoto BNL Dungan J: Contract learning for self-care activities, *Cancer Nurs* 14:148, 1991.

47. Hodgson BB, Kizior RJ: *Saunders nursing drug handbook,* Philadelphia, Saunders, 2000.

48. Hoffman-Terry ML and others: Adverse effects of outpatient parenteral antibiotic therapy, *Am J Med* 106:44, 1999.

49. Horton JR, Gosey NL, Fay A: Cancer support services: a working prototype, *J Oncol Manage* 3:10, 1994

50. Hoskins M and others: Predictors of hospital readmission among the elderly with congestive heart failure, *Home Healthcare Nurse* 17:373, 1999.

51. Hutchison CP: Healing touch an energetic approach, *AJN* 99:43, 1999.

52. Jacobs P: *The economics of health and medical care,* ed 3, Gaithersburg, Md, Aspen, 1996.

53. Jaime AJ: Putting the pieces together: effective case management in long-term rehabilitation essential for positive outcomes, *Contin Care* 15:5, 1996.

54. Johndrow P: Phlebotomy techniques in the home, *Home Healthcare Nurse* 17:246, 1999.

55. Kaye LW: Telemedicine: extension to home care, *Telemed J* 3(3):243, 1997.

56. Kaye LW, Davitt JK: Comparison of the high-tech service delivery of hospice and non-hospice home health providers, *Hospital J* 13(3):1, 1998.

57. Kaye LW, Davitt JK: *Current practices in high-tech home care,* New York, Springer, 1999.

58. Kennis N: Maximizing your patient teaching potential, *RN* 59(2):21, 1996.

59. Kozachik SL, Given BA, Given CW: Cancer patients at home: activating nurses to assist patients and to involve families in care at home, *Oncol Nurs Updates* 6:1, 1999.

60. Lamb KV and others: Help the health care team release its hold on restraint, *Nurs Manage* 30:19, 1999.

61. Leach SA: Survivorship: what does it mean to nurses? *Innovation in Breast Cancer Care* 4:1, 1999.

62. Macklin D: Removing a PICC, *AJN* 100:52, 2000.

63. Masoorli S: Removing a PICC? Proceed with caution, *Nursing98* 28:56, 1998.

64. Mayer DK: Cancer patient empowerment, *Oncol Nurs Updates* 6:1, 1999.

65. Mazzola JR, Schott-Baer D, Addy L: Clinical factors associated with the development of phlebitis after insertion of a peripherally inserted central catheter, *INS* 22:36, 1999.

66. McClinton DR, Oncology care management, *Contin Care* 15:8, 1996.

67. Millan SC, Mahon M: The impact of hospice services on the quality of life of primary caregivers, *Oncol Nurs Forum* 21:1189, 1994.

68. Meade CD, Diekmann J, Thornhill DG: Readability of American Cancer Society patient education literature, *Oncol Nurs Forum* 19:51, 1992.

69. Moore K: Out-of-pocket expenditures of outpatients receiving chemotherapy, *Oncol Nurs Forum* 25:1615, 1998.

70. Murer CG, Brick LL: Long-term hospitals add revenues, *Contin Care* 14:25, 1995.

71. NANDA: *NANDA nursing diagnosis: definitions and classification,* Philadelphia, Author, 1999.

72. National Association for Home Care: *Basic statistics about home care,* Washington, DC, Author, 1997.

73. Neumark DE: Providing information about advance directives to patients in ambulatory care and their families, *Oncol Nurs Forum* 21:771, 1994.

74. Noggle BJ: Identifying and meeting needs of ethnic minority patients, *Hospice J* 10:85, 1995.

75. Nottingham JA: Navigating the seas of caregiving; allies and ideas for success, *Caring Magazine* 14(4), 1995.

76. Oncology Nursing Society: *Access device guidelines,* Pittsburgh, Oncology Nursing Press, 1996.

77. Oncology Nursing Society: *Cancer chemotherapy guidelines and recommendations for practice,* Pittsburgh, Oncology Nursing Press, 1999.

78. Pasquali EA: Humor: preventive therapy for family caregivers, *Home Healthcare Nurse* 9:13, 1991.

79. Perry AG, Potter PA: *Clinical nursing skills & techniques,* ed 4, St. Louis, Mosby, 1998.

80. Phillips LD: Patient education: understanding the process to maximize time and outcomes, *INS,* 22:19, 1999.

81. Pillifteri A: Child health nursing: care of the child and family, Philadelphia, Lippincott, 1999.

82. Poole SK Nowobilski-Vasilios A, Free F: Intravenous push medication in the home, *INS* 22:209, 1999.

83. Powell SK, Dalton ME: Shifting roles, *Contin Care* 15:10, 1996.

84. Powers FA: Your elderly patient needs IV therapy . . . Can you keep her safe? *Nursing* 29:54, 1999.

85. Rogers JS, Soud TE: *Manual of pediatric emergency nursing,* St. Louis, Mosby, 1998.

86. Saladow J: Infusion devices, the newest products and features, *Infusion* 2:15, 1996.

87. Sankar A: *Dying at home: a family guide for caregiving,* Baltimore, Johns Hopkins University Press, 1992.

88. Schonwefter RS, Walker RK Robinson BE: The lack of advance directives among hospice patients, *Hospice J* 10:1, 1995.

89. Schulman KA, Yabroff KR: Measuring the cost-effectiveness of cancer care, *Oncology* 9:523, 1995.

90. Sheff B: VRE and NIRSA: putting bad bugs out of business, *Nurs Manage* 30:42, 1999.

91. Springhouse: *Little black book of home care cues,* Springhouse, PA, Springhouse, 1997.

92. Stahl DA: Managed care and subacute care: a partnership of choice, *Nurs Manage* 26:16, 1995.

93. Stahl DA: Accreditation, managed care and subacute care, *Nurs Manage* 27:16, 1996.

94. Stoker J: Defining homebound status, *Home Healthcare Nurse* 17:119, 1999.

95. Straw LJ, Conrad KJ: Patient education resources related to biotherapy and the immune system, *Oncol Nurs Forum* 21:1223, 1994.

96. St. Pieffe M: Major home health regulatory changes in 2000, *Home Healthcare Nurse* 18: 27, 2000.

97. Terry J and others, editors: *Intravenous therapy, clinical principles and practice,* Philadelphia, Saunders, 1995.

98. Thomas CS: Management of infectious waste in the home care setting, *INS* 20:188, 1997.

99. US Department of Health and Human Services, Division of Nursing: *Resource and information guide,* Washington DC, Author, 1999.

100. US Department of Labor, Office of Occupational Medicine, OSHA: *Controlling occupational exposure to hazardous drugs,* CPL 2-2.20B CH-4, Washington, DC, US Government Printing Office, 1995.

101. Weinstein SM: *Plummer's principles & practice of intravenous therapy,* ed 6, Philadelphia, Lippincott-Raven, 1997.

102. Weeks JC: The Schulman/Yabroff article reviewed, *Oncology* 9:529, 1995.

103. Weiss RL, Mlone-Nuzzo P: A tool to assess homebound status, *Home Healthcare Nurse* 17:486, 1999.

104. Whaley LF, Wong DL: *Nursing care of infants and children,* ed 6, St. Louis, Mosby, 1999.

105. Woodward W, Thobaben M: Special home healthcare nursing challenges: patients with cancer, *Home Healthcare Nurse* 12:33, 1994.

106. Zanca J: The challenge of multiculturality or, how do you say cancer care in American? *Cancer News* 48:8, 1994.

APPENDIX: CANCER RESOURCES, NATIONAL RESOURCES, EQUIPMENT, PRODUCTS, INFUSION THERAPY, AND PHARMACEUTICAL COMPANIES

National, Public, Professional, and Patient Resources

American Brain Tumor Association

2720 River Road, Suite 146
Des Plaines, IL 60018
800-886-2282 (patient line)
FAX: 847-827-9918
This organization provides written information about brain tumors and treatment options, patient education materials, support group referrals, CONNECTIONS Pen-Pal program, and information about nationwide treatment facilities. Also available is a triannual newsletter, *Message Line.*

American Cancer Society

1599 Clifton Road, NE
Atlanta, GA 30329
800-ACS-2345
FAX: 512-927-5791
The ACS provides a wide range of services encompassing the following: Information to the public on all sites of cancer, community resources, rehabilitation programs

- Home care items for use by patients
- Transportation to assist cancer patients to and from medical appointments
- Patient and family education programs to provide a better understanding of the disease and its managements

- *Cancer Nursing News:* newsletter mailed to nurses, free on request
- Housing: local divisions near cancer treatment centers, providing housing for patients with cancer and a family member at a Hope Lodge or local hotel/motel.

The following programs are offered by the American Cancer Society:

- *CanSurmount:* short-term visitor program for patients with many types of cancer and for families of patients. The one-on-one visit by a person who has experienced the same type of cancer offers functional, emotional, and social support.
- *I Can Cope:* structured educational program provides information and supportive materials to persons with cancer and their families.
- *International Association of Laryngectomees:* program provides information and supportive materials to laryngectomy patients. Laryngectomy visitors provide preoperative and postoperative support to patients who have recently undergone laryngectomy surgery.
- *Look Good, Feel Better:* joint venture of ACS and The Cosmetic, Toiletry, and Fragrance Association Foundation; assists those recovering from cancer by improving their quality of life through personal appearance and body image.
- *Reach to Recovery:* program provides emotional support and practical information to women with breast cancer, especially those who have had a mastectomy. Postoperative visits are provided by women who have had a mastectomy, and literature and a temporary prosthesis are provided.
- Ostomy rehabilitation program
- Cancer prevention and early detection programs for general public
- Resources, information, and guidance for general public and health care professionals

American Foundation for Urologic Disease, Inc.

www.afud.org
1128 North Charles Street
Baltimore, MD 21201-5559
410-468-1800
FAX: 410-468-1808
This national nonprofit organization focuses on prevention and cure for urologic diseases, offering material for men, women, and children; national awareness programs; research funding; and prostate cancer support groups for patients and their families.

Cancer Hot-Line

800-525-3777
800-638-6070 (in Alaska)
800-636-5700 (in Washington, DC)
808-524-1234 (in Hawaii, neighboring islands, call collect)

Corporate Angel Network

www.corpangelnetwork.org
One Loop Road
White Plains, NY 10604
914-328-1313
This network helps cancer patients by providing air transportation to and from cancer treatment centers.

Gynecological Cancer Foundation

401 North Old Michigan Avenue
Chicago, IL 60611
800-444-4441
FAX: 312-527-6640
This organization's primary focus is an aggressive campaign to disseminate information to the medical community and the public about current trends and techniques in gynecologic cancer.

International Myeloma Foundation

2120 Stanley Hills Drive
Los Angeles, CA 90046
800-452-CURE
This organization provides information about myeloma and its treatment and management to physicians and patients.

Johanna's of Albany Ltd.

Cancer Rehabilitation Nurse Consultants
4 Executive Park Drive
Albany NY 12203
518-459-2252
This nonprofit cancer rehabilitation nursing service provides a wide range of preventive, restorative, supportive, and palliative nursing interventions for individuals with cancer. It also publishes audiovisual and written material for public and professional education.

Legal Counsel for the Elderly (in association with American Association for Retired Persons, AARP)

1331 H Street NW
Washington, DC 20005
202-434-2120

Leukemia Society of America

600 Third Ave. New York, NY 10016
800-955-4LSA
FAX: 212-573-8484
National and local organization for support of patients and families with leukemia and related disorders. Services include financial counseling, assistance with payment for outpatient drugs, laboratory costs, transportation, radiation therapy, and patient/family support groups.

Look Good, Feel Better

The Cosmetic, Toiletry, and Fragrance Association Foundation
1101 17th Street NW, Suite 300
Washington, DC 20036
800-395-LOOK
FAX: 202-331-1770
This is a free, national, public service program focusing on teaching women with cancer (through hands-on-experience) beauty techniques that will help them restore their appearance and self-image during chemotherapy and radiation treatment. This organization provides a trained and certified cosmetologist for individual or group sessions. Also available are complimentary makeup kits, pamphlets, and videotapes. This is a joint venture of the ACS, the Foundation, and the National Cosmetology Association. Contact your local ACS office or call the toll-free number.

LymphEdema Foundation
PO Box 834
San Diego, CA 92014-0834
800-LYMPH-DX
This large, nonprofit, all-volunteer, educational organization provides information and resources to patients with lymphedema and health care professionals who treat them. Membership and quarterly publication, *LymphEdema Digest,* are free.

Medical Insurance Claims, Inc.
Kinnelon Professional Complex
170 Kennelon Road, Suite 10
Kinnelon, NJ 07405
This organization was established in response to the perceived need by the public for assistance in handling insurance claims. These services can be used by senior citizens and family members too involved with the patient's illness to deal with paperwork. It has a full range of services for a fee, including filing claims and pursuing any missing information from health care providers to complete a claim.

National Brain Tumor Foundation
785 Market Street, Suite 1600
San Francisco, CA 94103
415-284-0208
FAX: 415-284-0209
800-934-CURE
This organization supports research into causes and treatments of brain tumors and offers information and support group referrals for patients and their families. An informational publication for brain tumor patients. *The Resource Guide,* and a newsletter, *Search,* are available through the foundation. A telephone consultation with a brain tumor survivor, nurse, or family member of a brain tumor patient can be arranged by calling this organization.

National Breast Cancer Coalition (NBCC)
1707 L Street, NW, Suite 1060
Washington, DC 20036
202-296-7477
FAX: 202-265-6854
A grass-roots advocacy group, whose members consist of women and concerned others, is a leader in the national movement to bring changes in public policy that benefit breast cancer patients and their survivors. This organization also has a National Alert Network that provides up-to-date information regarding breast cancer and related issues.

National Cancer Institute (NCI)
Cancer Information Service
301-496-8664
1-800-4-CANCER
The Cancer Information Service is available to answer questions by telephone from the general public, patients and their families, and health professionals. Also available are referrals to local resources and printed materials on many topics related to cancer. Callers can also be connected to the NCI's PDQ clinical trial database for health professionals, which is a comprehensive service providing state-of-the-art cancer treatment. See Professional Organizations and Resources for more about PDQ.

National Hispanic Leadership Initiative on Cancer
En Accion Coordinating Center
South Texas Health Research Center
University of Texas Health Sciences Center at San Antonio
7703 Floyd Curl Drive
San Antonio, TX 78284-7791
210-567-7826
FAX: 210-567-7855
This national network of experts in public health and medicine, in collaboration with grass-roots community-based organizations, has conducted a comprehensive assessment of cancer risk factors for all Hispanic/Latino populations. The goal is to provide these targeted populations with the knowledge and the resources to prevent and control cancer among their own people.

National Lymphedema Network
www.lymphnet.org
2211 Post Street, Suite 404
San Francisco, CA 94115-3427
This organization provides educational information, exercise programs, a quarterly newsletter, Internet service, a computer data bank, a resource guide of lymphedema support groups, and health care list and U.S. treatment centers.

National Neurofibromatosis Foundation, Inc.
141 Fifth Avenue, Suite 7-S
New York, NY 10010
800-323-7938
FAX: 212-460-8980
This organization sponsors research, publishes educational materials, and assists in the development of clinical centers and diagnostic protocols. Information packets about neurofibromatosis and support groups are available.

Oley Foundation
214 Hun Memorial, A 23
Albany Medical Center
Albany, NY 12208
800-776-OLEY
FAX: 518-445-5079
This foundation offers support to individuals receiving home parenteral and enteral nutrition therapy and to their families. It has patient/family support groups and publishes a quarterly newsletter, *Lifeline Letter.* Services are provided free of charge to patients and families.

R.A. Bloch Cancer Foundation, Inc.
4410 Main Street
Kansas City, MO 64111
800-433-0464
FAX: 816-931-7486
This community cancer resource center offers a cancer information hotline that provides information regarding national resources, peer counseling, medical second opinions, and support groups.

Skin Cancer Foundation
245 Fifth Avenue, Suite 2402
New York, NY 10016
800-SKIN-490
FAX: 215-725-5751

This foundation provides patient education materials, a newsletter, books, brochures, pamphlets, and slide and video presentations and supports research on skin cancer.

Susan G. Komen Breast Cancer Foundation

5005 LBJ Freeway, Suite 370
Dallas, TX 75244
972-855-1600
FAX: 972-855-1600
800-IM-AWARE

This national organization focuses on advocacy, research, screening, and treatment for breast cancer. It also funds research and programs for medically underserved women. The national hotline provides information and referral to treatment centers.

United Ostomy Association (UOA)

19772 MacArthur Boulevard, Suite 200
Irvine, CA 92612-2405
800-826-0826

This nonprofit organization provides speakers, literature, and monthly information meetings for people with ostomies. Volunteers, most of whom are ostomates, may visit patients with ostomies in the hospital or home with the consent of the patient's physician.

United Way of America Mid-America Region

1400 East Touhy Avenue, Des Plaines, IL 60018-3305
1-800-707-6160

The staff of local offices of this organization are very knowledgeable about the support services available to cancer patients in the surrounding communities and can provide referrals to such resources.

US TOO International, Inc.

930 North York Road, Suite 50
Hinsdale, IL 60521-7866
630-323-1002
FAX: 630-323-1003
800-80-USTOO

This organization offers information, counseling, and educational programs related to prostate cancer, surgery, radiation, medicine, nutrition, and psychology. Chapters across the United States and Canada have monthly meetings for patients and their families.

Y-Me National Organization for Breast Cancer Information and Support, Inc.

212 West Van Buren, 5th Floor
Chicago, IL 60607-3908
800-221-2141 (Hispanic-800-986-9505)
FAX: 312-294-8597

This organization provides information, telephone counseling, educational programs, and support groups for patients with breast cancer and their families and significant others. It maintains a "bank" of donated prostheses and wigs for patients with limited financial resources.

YWCA of the USA EncoreP- Program

Office of Women's Health Initiatives
624 9th Street, 3rd Floor
Washington, DC 20001

202-628-3636
FAX: 202-723-7123

Encore, the national YWCA, offers a systematic approach to women's health promotion, especially related to breast and cervical cancer education and control. Program is designed to meet the needs of all women, including minorities, those with limited incomes, and elderly women who do not use appropriate health care and preventive services. Also included are health education programs, support groups, and exercise programs for women who have had breast cancer surgery. The exercise program consists of floor and pool exercises and group discussion sessions that provides opportunities for sharing common concerns.

Wellness Community

2716 Ocean Park Boulevard, Suite 1040
Santa Monica, CA 90405
888-793-WIELL

AIDS

AIDS Action Council, 202-530-8030, FAX: 202-986-1345
AIDS Clinical Trials and Information Service (ACTS), www.actis.org

Genetics

Alliance of Genetic Support Groups, www.geneticsallaiance.org
Ethical Legal Social Implications Research Program, www.nhgri.nih.gov/About_NHGR1/Dev/Elsi
International Society of Nurses in Genetics (ISONG) nursing, creighton.edu/isong/index.html
National Society of Genetic Counselors, www.nsgc.org

Pediatrics

Association for Research of Childhood Cancer
PO Box 251
Buffalo, NY 14225-0251
716-681-4433

Association for the Care of Children's Health
acchhq@talley.com

Candlelighters Childhood Cancer Foundation
candlelighters.org

Children's Hopes and Dreams Foundations
280 Route 66
Dover, NJ 07801
973-361-7366;
FAX: 973-361-6627

Children's Hospice International
800-24-CHILD

Make-A-Wish Foundation
www.wish.org

Ronald McDonald Houses
www.rmhc.com

We Care Foundation/Camp Dream Street
PO Box 3431
Fort Smith, AR 72913
501-441-6292

Palliative Care Resources

American Academy of Hospice and Palliative Medicine,
   www.aahpm.org
Americans for Better Care of Dying,
   www.ABCD-CARING.com
Caregiver Newsletter, www.caregiver.com
GriefNet, www.rivendell.org (A collection of resources for
   those experiencing loss or grief.)
Growth House Inc., www.growthhouse.org. (Resources for
   those who have specific forms of bereavement [e.g., preg-
   nancy, grieving children etc.].)
Infoseek,
   www.insoseek.com/Hobbies_and_Interests/Family/
   Death/Grief. (An extensive list of on-line resources for
   grieving parents, grandparents, and children, and for
   grief and coping advice.)
Last Acts: Care and Caring at the End of Life,
   www.lastacts.org
National Hospice Organization, www.nho.org
On Our Own Terms: Moyers on Dying, www.pbs.org/wnet
Palliative Care Letter, www.roxane.com
Physicians End-of-Life Education EPEC,
   www.ama-assn/ethic/epec.org
Project on Death in America, www.soros.org/death.html
WidowNet, www.fortnet.org/WidowNet. (Information and
   self-help for widows/widowers.)
grief-chat@mailserv.ic.net
grief@listserv.prodigy.com
grief-parents@mailserv.ic.net
grief-men@mailserv.ic.net
grief-widowed@mailserv.ic.net
grief-pets@mailserv.ic.net
right_to_die@efn.org
HOSPIC-L@listserv.acsu.buffalo.edu

Professional Organization Web Sites

American Brain Tumor Association (ABTA), www.abta.org
American Association of Blood Banks, www.aabb.org
American Association for Cancer Education (AACE),
   gkrawiec@cancer.org
American Cancer Society www.acs.org
American Lung Association info@lungusa.org
American Medical Association, www.ama.org
American Nursing Association, www.ana.org
American Red Cross, www.arc.org
American Society Of Clinical Oncology (ASCO),
   www.asco.org
American Society of Enteral and Parenteral Nutrition,
   www.aspenpubl.com
American Society of Plastic and Reconstructive Surgeons
   (ASPRS), www.plasticsurgery.org
American Society for Therapeutic Radiology and Oncology,
   www.astro.org

Association of Critical Care Nurses, Inc, www.accn.org
Association of Nurses in AIDS Care (ANAC),
   AIDS-NURSES@aol.com
Association of Oncology Social Work (AOSW),
   aoshello@worldnet.att.net
Association of Operating Room Nurses, Inc, www.aorn.org
Association or Pediatric Oncology Nurses, www.apon.org
Hospice and Palliative Nurses Association, www.hpna.org
Hypertension Dialysis Clinical Nephrology, www.hdch.com
Intravenous Nurses Society, www.insl.org
Joint Commission on Accreditation of Healthcare Organiza-
   tions, www.jcaho.org
National Alliance of Breast Cancer Organizations
   (NABCO), www.nabco.org
National Association of Home Care, www.nahc.org
National Foundation for Cancer Research (NFCR),
   www.nfcr.org
Oncology Nursing Society, www.ons.org
   ONS Online: Information: Cancer Prevention, Diagnosis,
   Treatment, Detection Screening
Oncology Education Services, www.oesweb.com
PDQ cancer, net.nci.nih.gov
Resource Center of the American Alliance of Cancer Pain
   Initiatives, www.aacpi.org
Society of Gynecologic Oncologists, www.sgo.org
Society of Surgical Oncology, www.surgonc.org

Public General Information

Agency for Health Care Policy and Research (AHCPR),
   www.ahcpr.gov
Cancer FAX 301-402-5874
Cancer Hope Network, www.cancerhopenetwork.org
Cancer Information Service (CIS), 800-422-6237
Centers for Disease Control (CDC),
   www.cdcnac.org; www.cdc.gov
CDC Hospital Infections Program, (HIP),
   www.cdc.gov/ncidod/hip/hip/html
CDC MedWatch Program, www.cdc.gov/medwatch
Coping, Copingmag@aol.com
Combined Health Information Database (CHD),
   www.chid.nffi.gov
Food and Drug Administration, www.fda.com
International Standards Organization, www.iso.com
National Cancer Institute, 800-NCI-7890
National Cancer Survivors Day (NCSD) Foundation,
   www.NCSDF.org
National Institutes of Health (NUJ), www.nih.gov
National Marrow Donor Program (NMDP),
   www.bmtitifo.org
Office of Minority Health Resource Center (OMH-RC),
   www.omhre.gov
United States Post Office, www.uspo.gov
U.S. Department of Labor Occupational Safety and Health
   Administration (OSHA), www.osha.gov
World Health Organization (WHO), www.who.com

IV Therapy Pumps and Products Resources

Abbott Laboratories, Hospital Products Division, Abbott
   Park, IL, 847-937-6100

ALARIS Medical Systems (formerly DAM/IVAC), San Diego, CA, 800-854-7128
Arrow International Inc., Reading PA, 800-523-8446
Baxa Corporation, Englewood, CO 800-525-9567
Clinitee Nutrition Company, Deerfield, IL, 708-317-2800
Pall Corporation, www.pall.com/industrv/health/asp
Gish Biomedical, Inc., Irvine, CA, 800-938-503, www.gish.com
I-Flow Corporation, Irvine, CA, 800-448-3569
McGaw, Inc., Irvine, CA, 714-660-2000
Medex, Inc., Hilliard, OK, 800-848-1757, www.medex.com
Medtronic, Inc., Columbia Heights, MN, 800-328-0810
Metrix Company, Dubuque, IA, 800-752-3148
MicroJect, Salt Lake City, UT, 888-642-7646
Sabratek, Niles, IL, 800-556-7722
Sherwood Medical, St. Louis, MO, 800-325-7472, www.sherwoochnedical.com
SIMS Deltec, Inc., St. Paul, MN, 800-426-2448
SoloPak Pharmaceuticals, Boca Raton, FL, 800-267-5672

Infusion Products: Central Venous Catheters, PIC Catheters, and Miscellaneous Catheters

Arrow International Inc., 800-523-8446
Bard Access Systems, 800-545-0890
Becton Dickinson, 800-453-4538
B. Braun Medical Inc., 800-523-9695
CONMED, 800-527-2462
Cook Critical Care, 800-457-4500
HDC Corporation, 800-227-2918
Luther Medical Products Inc., 800-227-2918
SM Deltec, Inc., 800-426-2448
SoloPak Pharmaceuticals, 800-267-5672
Venetec International, 800-833-3895
Vygon Corporation 800-544-4907

Pharmaceutical Companies

Abbott/Ross Laboratories, 800-922-3255
Adria Laboratories, 800-795-9759
Allergan prescripton, 800-347-4500 (X6219)
Amgen, Inc, 800-272-9376
Astra FAIR Program, 800-488-3247
Baxter Biotech NA, 800-548-IGIV
Berlex, Inc., 800-473-2239
Boehringer Ingleheim, 203-798-4131
Boots, 800-323-1817
Bristol-Myers Oncology Division, 800-872-8718
Bristol-Myers Squibb Oncology Access Program, 800-272-4878
Burroughs Wellcome Co., 800-423-6869
Cerenex Pharmaceuticals, 800-745-2967
Cetus Corp., 800-755-7533
Chiron Therapeutics, 800-775-7533
Ciba-Geigy Pharmaceuticals, 800-257-3273
DuPontMerck, 302-992-4240
Fisons; 800-234-5535
Fujisawa, 800-366-6323
Genentech, 800-879-4747
Glaxo, 800-GLAX077

Hoechst-Roussel, 800-422-4779
Hoffman-LaRoche: 800-443-6676
EMRB Corp., 800-635-4673
Immunex Corporation, 800-321-4669
Janssen Pharmaceuticals, 800-253-3683
Knoll Pharmaceuticals, 800-526-0710
Lederle Laboratories, 800-533-2273
Eli Lilly & Co., 317-276-2950
Marion Merrell Dow, Inc., 800-362-7466
McNeil Pharmaceuticals, 215-628-7803
Medi-Physics, Inc., 800-204-5678
Merck, Sharp & Dohme, 800-637-2579
Miles, 800-998-9180
Norwich-Eaton Pharmaceuticals, 800-447-3437
Ortho Biotech, Inc., 800-553-3851
Parke, Davis & Co., 210-540-2000
Pfizer Labs, Roerig Division, 212-573-3954
Purdue Frederick, 203-853-0123 (X4800)
Reed and Camrick/Block Drug, 908-981-0070
Rhone-Poulenc-Rorer Pharmaceuticals, Inc., 800-996-6626
Roche Laboratories, 800-443-6676
Roxane Laboratories, Inc., 800-848-0120
Sandoz Pharmaceuticals Corp., 800-772-7556
Schering, 800-521-7517
G.D. Searle & Co., 800-542-2526
Snofi Winthrop Pharmaceuticals, 212-907-2000
Sigma-Tau Pharmaceuticals, 800-999-6673
SmithKline Beecham, 800-866-6273
Syntex Laboratories, Inc., 800-444-4200
TAP Pharmaceuticals Inc., 800-453-8438
Therabite Corp., 800-322-9500
Upjohn Co., 616-323-6004
U.S. Bioscience, 800-887-2467
Wyeth-Ayerst Laboratories, 800-568-9938
Zeneca Pharmaceuticals, 800-456-5678

Dressings, Tapes, and Skin Care Products Resources

Alba Health Products, 800-262-2404
Aloe Life International, 800-414-2563
Amerx Health Care Corp., 800-448-9599
Bard Medical Division, 800-526-4455
Beiersdorf-Jbbst Inc., 800-537-1063
B. Braun/McGaw, 800-227-2862
Brennen Medical, Inc., 800-328-9105
Brown Medical Industries, 800-843-4395
Care-Tech Laboratories Inc., 800-325-9681
Carrington Laboratories, 800-358-5205
Centurion Specialty Care, 800-248-4058
Coloplast Corporation, 800-533-0464
ConvaTec, 800-422-8811
Denna Sciences, Inc., 800-825-4325
DeRoyal, 800-337-6925
Dumex Medical, 800-463-0106
Ferris Manufacturing Corporation, 800-765-9636
FNC Medical Corporation, 800-440-2888
Genelogic, Inc., 800-976-9090
Glenwood, 800-542-0772
GOJO Industries, Inc., 800-321-9647

Hollister, Inc., 800-323-4060
Hyperion Medical Inc., 800-743-8111
Johnson & Johnson, 800-255-2500
Kendall Healthcare Products Co., 800-962-9888
Lantiseptic Division Summit Ind, 800-241-6996
3 M Health Care, 800-228-3957
Medicom Inc., 800-361-2862
Mohmlcke Health Care, 800-992-9939
Nu-Hope Laboratories, 800-899-5017
Orion Medical Products, 800-669-5079
Rynel Inc., 800-945-4992
Sage Products, Inc., 800-323-2220
Silipos Inc., 800-229-4404
Smith & Nephew, Inc., 800-876-1261
Ulmer Pharmacal Comp., 800-848-5637
Winfield Laboratories, Inc., 800-527-4616

Support Surfaces Resources

AirCare Therapy Inc., 800-942-7678
AliMed, Inc., 800-225-2610
Anatomic Concepts, Inc., 800-874-7237
B. G. Industries, 800-822-8288
Blue Chip Medical Products, Inc., 800-795-6115
Comfortex Inc., 800-445-4007
Creative Bedding Technologies, 800-526-2158
Crown Therapeutics, Inc., 800-851-3449
EROB, Inc., 800-966-3462
FloCare, 800-356-2337

Gaymar Industries, Inc., 800-828-7341
Grant Airmass Corporation, 800-243-5237
Heelbo, Inc., 800-323-5444
Hermell Products, Inc., 800-233-2342
Hill-Rom, 800-638-2546
Huntleigh Healthcare, Inc., 800-223-1218
Incacare Corporation, 800-333-6900
James Consolidated Inc., 800-884-3317
KCI (Kinetic Concepts Inc.), 800-531-5346
Lunax Corporation, 800-264-4144
Marcon Group Inc., 800-547-5021
Mason Medical Products, 800-233-4454
Mastex Industries, Inc., 800-343-7444
Mediq FST, 800-490-4744
Medline Industries, Inc., 800-633-5463
Neuropedic, 800-327-6759
Next Generation Co. Inc., 800-598-4303
Pegasus Airwave Inc., 800-443-4325
Plexus/Medical, 800-690-6113
Precision Dynamics Corporation, 800-847-0670
Regency Products International, 800-845-7931
Restorative Care of America, Inc., 800-627-1595
SenTech Medical Systems, 800-474-4225
Sleepmet Corporation, 800-742-3646
Span-America Medical Systems, 800-888-6752
Standard Textile Co Inc., 800-999-0400
Sunrise Medical Inc. Bio Clinic, 800-333-4000
Tempar-Medical, Inc., 800-878-8889
Tetra Medical Supply Corporation, 800-621-4041
Tumsaft, Inc., 800-944-8876

Nutrition

Lisa Schulmeister

Cancer and its treatment may affect the nutritional status of the patient in a variety of ways. Besides being subject to metabolic effects, patients are emotionally stressed when nutritional intake is impaired. Because eating is a basic body function and often a social activity, inability to eat or difficulty in eating may have a profound physical and psychological impact on the individual with cancer and the family.

Weight loss is present in half of patients at diagnosis and two thirds of patients with advanced cancer. It has a negative impact on the ability to tolerate cancer treatment and has been associated with decreased survival and quality of life.[83] Malnutrition is reported as the cause of death in as many as 20% of cancer patients.[65, 94] Early assessment of nutritional status and interventions as needed are basic components of oncology nursing care.

Nutrition also plays a role in cancer prevention. Cancer is largely a preventable illness and worldwide evidence indicates that diets high in fruits and vegetables reduce the risk of developing at least 10 different cancers. Likewise, decreasing total fat and saturated fat intake decreases the occurrence of hormone-related, lung, and colorectal cancers.[14]

EFFECTS OF CANCER ON NUTRITIONAL STATUS

Nutritional Components and Their Functions

Cancer may affect the metabolism of the nutritional components necessary to sustain life: carbohydrates, proteins, fatty acids, vitamins, minerals, and electrolytes. An alteration in the metabolism of these components affects the nutritional status of an individual, that is, the degree to which an individual's need for nutrition is met by intake.

Carbohydrates are the sugars that provide energy for immediate use. They are converted to glycogen or fat for long-term storage or are converted to other molecules in the body. Carbohydrates can be divided into three classes: monosaccharides, disaccharides, and polysaccharides. *Monosaccharides* are simple one-molecule sugars; examples are fructose and dextrose (glucose). *Disaccharides* are two-molecule sugars; an example is sucrose (table sugar). *Polysaccharides* are complex sugars characterized by many molecules; examples are starch and dextran.

Glucose is the fuel for most of the cells of the body. It is metabolized rapidly in the presence or absence of oxygen. Each gram of glucose provides 3.4 kilocalories (kcal). Carbohydrates are also a long-term source of energy. When glucose intake exceeds demand, it is converted into glycogen or fat. Both sources of energy are stored in the body and used when a glucose shortage occurs. When metabolized by certain processes, the glucose molecule can be used as the basis for other molecules, including amino acids and fatty acids.

Amino acids are the building blocks of the body. Proteins are many amino acids joined into one molecule. Amino acids are divided into two categories: essential and nonessential. *Essential* amino acids must be supplied from the diet because the body is unable to synthesize them from glucose or other amino acids. *Nonessential* amino acids need not be supplied from the diet because the body is able to synthesize them.

Functions of amino acids include maintenance and growth. When tissue breakdown exceeds synthesis or when glucose for energy is lacking, the result is wasting of protein from muscles and loss of mass. Amino acids assist in the regulation of body processes and make up many enzymes found throughout the body. Enzymes are the chemical regulators of many of the synthetic processes in the body. During starvation the body uses proteins as a source of energy. Each gram provides 4 kcal.

Lipids and fatty acids serve many roles in the body. *Fatty acids* are basic molecules, and *lipids* are long chains of fatty acids. Lipids may be saturated or unsaturated, depending on the number of double-bonded carbons in their structure. Lipids are an excellent source of energy, supplying 9 kcal/g. They are also the long-term storage form of glucose. Fat-soluble vitamins are transported by lipids. Many fat-soluble vitamins (A, D, E, and K) are transported throughout the body bound to fatty acids. The fat content of food is responsible for the taste of many foods and the feeling of fullness that results from eating. Lipids also provide insulation and padding. The fatty acids are precursors to many hormones, including testosterone and estrogen. They are also the basis for cholesterol.

Vitamins are compounds used in a number of enzymatic steps that regulate many processes. Normal amounts of the adult daily requirements (ADRs) of vitamins are obtained by consuming a balanced diet. Vitamins can be divided into two groups: fat-soluble and water-soluble. *Fat-soluble vitamins* are stored by the body in fat. Deficiencies take a long time to develop because these vitamins are stored. Vitamin A is important in maintaining vision and in tooth and skeletal development, and it acts as a precursor to cholesterol. Vitamin D acts to regulate protein and calcium metabolism. Vitamin E is an antioxidant; that is, it prevents or lessens damage to body tissue caused by atmospheric oxygen. Vitamin K helps maintain the clotting ability of blood.

Water-soluble vitamins are not stored in the body and are readily eliminated in the urine. Deficiencies may develop quickly if inadequate quantities are consumed. Vitamin C is used in the formation of collagen, enhances iron absorption, and serves as an antioxidant. B-complex vitamins are cofactors in many enzymatic reactions.

Macro elements, or *electrolytes,* maintain osmotic pressure and water balance, facilitate nerve conduction and muscle contraction, and perform other functions. The macro elements are sodium, potassium, chloride, calcium, magnesium, phosphorus, and sulfur.

Trace elements are so named because they are needed by the body in small quantities. Deficiencies can develop quickly, but clinical signs of deficiency may not be apparent for a long time. Trace elements include zinc, manganese, copper, chromium, selenium, iron, and cobalt, among others.

Systemic Effects of Cancer

The *anorexia-cachexia syndrome* of advanced cancer, present in up to 80% of patients with cancer,[2] is a complex response of the body to the presence of tumor caused by the body's production of inflammatory *cytokines.* Cytokines, such as interleukin-1, tumor necrosis factor-α, and in particular, interleukin-6 appear to play central roles in the initiation of the acute phase response to inflammation, utilization of exogenously administered nutrients, and loss of skeletal muscle protein.[79, 100, 105] High serum levels of these cytokines have been found in patients with cancer and appear to correlate with tumor progression.[69] However, a number of clinical and laboratory studies suggest that the action of cytokines alone is unable to explain the complex mechanism of wasting in cancer cachexia.[120] An increase in basal energy expenditures appears to play an additional contributory role in many patients.[8] The roles of leptin, a hormone secreted by adipose tissue, and neuropeptides as anorexia-cachexia syndrome mediators are currently being studied.[53, 99]

The cancer anorexia-cachexia syndrome is characterized by wasting, weight loss, weakness, fatigue, poor performance status, and impaired immune function,[100] and increasing nutrient intake is unable to reverse the wasting syndrome.[121] Alterations in the normal metabolism of carbohydrates, proteins, and fats result in increased energy expenditures. A normal body's response is to increase appetite and therefore intake, but the person with cancer experiences anorexia and has further decline in ability to meet demands. The process can be exacerbated by psychological responses: anxiety about cancer, its possible progression, depression, anticipatory phenomena, and learned food aversions.

Vitamin deficiencies observed in cancer patients include a deficiency of vitamin A in many individuals with cancer of the lung and alimentary tract. Thiamin and vitamin C deficiencies have also been reported in various malignancies. Iron deficiency may result from the unavailability of iron in the diet, malabsorption, or chronic bleeding.

Fluid and electrolyte imbalances may result from direct and indirect effects of tumors. Parathyroid, lung, kidney, and colon tumors may produce an ectopic parathyroid-like hormone that deposits calcium in the renal tubules and may result in renal failure. Hypercalcemia may also cause a concentrating effect that leads to polyuria and water depletion. Leukemia and lymphomas may induce hyperuricemia, hyperphosphatemia, and hyperkalemia as a result of electrolytes released by cellular breakdown. A common presentation of bronchiogenic carcinomas, such as small-cell cancer, is the *syndrome of inappropriate secretion of antidiuretic hormone* (SIADH). This syndrome is characterized by urinary loss of sodium and excessive retention of water by the renal tubules.[35] Renal tumors may secrete renin and in turn cause increased secretion of aldosterone, resulting in hypokalemia. Treatment with platinum-based chemotherapeutic agents may deplete magnesium and potassium.

Patients who are nutritionally depleted can have decreased immunocompetence, which becomes more severe as the disease progresses. Malnutrition decreases the size of the lymphoid tissues. Lymphatic structures such as the spleen, lymph nodes, and thymus participate directly in the immune response, and a decrease in their size contributes to immunosuppression. Decreased function of B-cell and T-cell lymphocytes will also result from malnutrition. Fewer T cells, especially helper T cells, and phagocyte dysfunction are common. The greater the malnutrition, the greater is the deficiency of T lymphocytes. This produces a delayed hypersensitivity response. The immune system works with cancer treatment to destroy tumor cells. Preservation of both nutritional status and immune system function are thus important considerations in cancer therapy.[116]

Effects of Cancer

Several local effects of cancer may alter the nutritional intake of the affected individual. Impaired ingestion may be caused by mechanical and anatomic alterations. Patients with cancer of the head and neck area, esophageal cancers, and brain tumors may have trouble with opening the mouth, chewing, and swallowing as well as with peristalsis. Patients with head and neck cancers also often have trace element deficiencies.[28] Obstruction of the esophagus can inhibit the passage of food. Gastric tumors often cause pain[91] and distention. Cancers along the alimentary tract may cause obstructions, and they often inhibit the absorption of nutrients.[77] Pancreatic cancer can cause endocrine and exocrine hormonal insufficiencies that affect nutrient consumption and absorption.[92, 93] Cancer of the small intestine affects the digestion and absorption of food. A fistula of the bowel may develop as a result of tissue necrosis from a gastrointestinal (GI) tract tumor and induce electrolyte imbalance and malabsorption.

Effects of Aging

The older adult has special nutritional needs and requirements that differ from those during other stages of life. Physiologic changes of decreased ingestion and digestion and decreased metabolic rate and excretion can adversely affect nutritional intake, and the presence of impaired mobility or visual impairment can affect the older adult's ability to obtain, prepare, and consume food. Chronic illnesses, such as cancer, medication use, and economic factors can further affect the nutritional status of the older adult.[57, 98]

Weight loss and cachexia in elderly patients may have profound consequences. Weight loss and wasting in the elderly diminish self-reliance in activities of daily living and often lead to hospitalization and the need for skilled care. Cachexia has been associated with infections, decubitus ulcer formation, and even death in the elderly.[139]

NUTRITIONAL CONSEQUENCES OF CANCER TREATMENT, ASSESSMENT, AND INTERVENTIONS

Effects of Various Modes of Treatment

Surgical alterations in any area of the alimentary tract from the mouth to the anus may cause temporary or occasionally permanent alterations in nutritional intake or absorptive capabilities. Surgical procedures that alter the patient's ability to chew or swallow may prompt the need for soft or blenderized foods, and tube feedings may be required. Assessment and correction of malnutrition have led to improvements in the preoperative and postoperative management of patients with head and neck cancers over the past 20 years.[9] Partial or total gastrectomy can cause severe nutritional problems. When the greater portion of the stomach is removed, the intrinsic factor is not produced in quantities sufficient for the absorption of vitamin B_{12}, and pernicious anemia develops. With resection of the stomach, the quantity of food that can be consumed at one time is limited, and frequent, small feedings are necessary. *Dumping syndrome* may also appear after gastrectomy; a few minutes after ingestion, food is dumped into the jejunum, and nausea, cramping, and diarrhea follow. Malabsorption of fat occurs in patients who have undergone a gastrojejunostomy. The duodenum is bypassed, and pancreatic insufficiency results. Malabsorption of fat impairs absorption of fat-soluble vitamins and calcium. Iron absorption is also decreased, and anemia occurs.[109]

Radiation therapy may affect the normal tissues surrounding the treatment areas. Patients with cancer of the head and neck have both acute and chronic symptoms. Specifically, the normal tissues of the salivary gland, oral mucosa, muscle, and occasionally bone may be affected.[52] In the acute phase, inflammation and swelling of tissues with resulting discomfort may affect nutritional intake. Stomatitis can be complicated with candidiasis (moniliasis), an oral infection with *Candida albicans* that requires antifungal medications. Taste changes, such as a diminished sense of taste or metallic taste when eating red meats, may cause aversion to food and decreased intake. Xerostomia, or diminished production of saliva, is a long-term side effect of radiation therapy. Pain and difficulty swallowing often occur. Saliva substitutes and topical anesthetics for oral use may be helpful, and eating moist foods is recommended. Dental caries may occur as a late effect of head and neck radiation. Radiation therapy to the mediastinum for lung or esophageal cancer can cause esophagitis. Dysphagia usually begins within 2 weeks of treatment and can continue for several months afterward. Interventions include topical anesthetics such as liquid antacid mixed with lidocaine viscous, nonsteroidal anti-inflammatory drugs (NSAIDs), systemic analgesics, and histamine blockers to reduce stomach acid reflux. Dietary modifications, such as soft, bland food and liquid supplements, may help maintain intake.[48] Enteral feeding is sometimes necessary during the acute phase if symptoms are severe. Long-term strictures of the esophagus may require periodic dilation.

Irradiation of the stomach and small intestine produces vomiting, anorexia, diarrhea, and gastric distention.[48] Antiemetics taken 30 minutes before treatment, a low-residue and lactose-free diet, and adequate hydration may alleviate or minimize these side effects. Antidiarrheal medications may be necessary to minimize fluid loss and permit oral intake. Generally, these acute effects resolve with the completion of therapy. Long-term side effects of radiation to the intestines that affect nutrition may be chronic obstruction, malabsorption, and fistula formation.[48]

Chemotherapy may produce side effects that impair the patient's nutritional status. Chemotherapy causes nutritional deficiencies by promoting anorexia, stomatitis, taste alterations, and alimentary tract disturbances.[133] Deficiencies of vitamins B_1, B_2, and K and of niacin, folic acid, and thiamine may also result from chemotherapy. Some chemotherapeutic regimens, such as induction therapy for acute leukemia, can cause significant weight loss and hypoalbuminemia.[32] Taste alterations, such as an aversion to red meat, are common with platinum-based products. Cool foods with little aroma and bland foods are often tolerated well. Topical application of analgesics often minimizes the discomfort of stomatitis.

Other common side effects of chemotherapy are nausea and vomiting. The severity of symptoms and their effect on nutritional status varies from patient to patient. Use of antiemetics and dietary measures may help. Prophylactic antiemetic therapy with 5-HT_3 receptor antagonists have significantly reduced the acute effects of nausea and vomiting, but some patients continue to experience nausea several days after chemotherapy.[29] Nausea and vomiting may have a psychogenic component; anticipatory nausea and vomiting before a chemotherapy treatment may occur. Odor, sight, and even thought of food may produce emesis in some patients. Relaxation and diversion therapy is sometimes indicated. Aversions to specific foods may occur as a result of the association of those foods with nausea and vomiting.

Peripheral blood stem cell transplantation and bone marrow transplantation conditioning regimens typically include high-dose chemotherapy and sometimes total-body irradiation that cause macro and micronutrient deficiencies. Specialized nutrition management, such as parenteral hydration and total parenteral nutrition, is often required.[72, 112] In one study, however, parenteral nutrition was found to prolong resumption of oral calorie intake by contributing to early satiety.[20]

Although chemotherapy is most often associated with effects that contribute to impaired nutritional intake and weight loss, weight gain has been reported to occur in women with breast cancer who receive adjuvant chemotherapy. In a study of 1100 women with breast cancer, 60% had gained weight after diagnosis and a 6-lb weight gain was common. The women also appeared to gain weight at a faster rate than women in the general population.[104]

The side effects of *biotherapy* are generally less severe than those of chemotherapy. Anorexia is a common complaint, and nausea and vomiting occur occasionally. Diarrhea may occur, depending on the agent used. Long-term low-dose treatment may result in fatigue that is intense enough to preclude fixing meals and eating. Interventions may include meal planning for quick, small meals and shopping assistance.[22] Although the effects of biotherapy are typically mild, patients treated with high doses of interleukin-2 often develop profound anorexia, malaise, loss of energy, mucositis, nausea, and vomiting.[106]

Fatigue is a side effect associated with all cancer treatment modalities. Many believe that is the most common experience of patients with cancer. Fatigue is a complex phenomenon and its effect on nutritional status is not fully understood, but use of fatigue models, such as the Piper's Fatigue Model, can assist in identifying potential causes of fatigue and promote early intervention.[60]

Nutritional Assessment

A nutritional assessment can easily be integrated in clinical practice to screen for potential or existing problems in nutritional status, provide a database for individuals at high risk, and determine response to treatment or dietary interventions.[73] Although all patients should be assessed, particular attention should be given to the elderly patient. Older adults experience physiologic effects of aging that impair their nutritional status. For instance, one in five older adults experiences xerostomia.[57] Assessment of the patient's eating patterns, nutrient intake, and supplement use and influences on eating habits should be completed before initiation of cancer treatment.

Several methods can be used to estimate or quantify the patient's nutritional status (Box 29–1). A simple method is clinical observation. A thorough nursing history will identify concurrent health problems that may affect nutrition, such as diabetes, hypertension, and malabsorption. Psychosocial factors, including the home environment, food preparation methods, and the patient's body image, should be noted. Ability to purchase food and supplements should be addressed. A physical assessment will reflect the patient's overall nutritional status. Specifically, examination of the hair, teeth, gums, and general muscle tone may provide an early indication of nutritional deficiencies. Poorly fitting dentures after weight loss may impair ability to chew. A functional assessment will determine patients' ability to prepare meals and feed themselves. Uncontrolled pain can significantly impair appetite and should be addressed.[36]

BOX 29-1

Components of Nutritional Assessment

Nursing History

Date diagnosed
Type of cancer
Type and duration of therapy
Concurrent medications
Concomitant medical conditions
Surgical procedures
Side effects of therapy
Allergies

Psychosocial Assessment

Home environment
Family support
Coping abilities
Self-image
Perceptions of role of nutrition
Cultural/religious considerations

Physical Assessment

General overall appearance
Hair texture
Skin turgor and integrity
Condition of mouth and gums
Performance status
Alterations in elimination, comfort, etc.

Dietary Evaluation

24-hour recall of intake
Food preferences
Food allergies
Use of vitamin supplements
Changes in diet or eating on life-style patterns
Observation of intake
Evaluation of nutrient composition

Biochemical Measurements

Serum albumin
Hemoglobin, hematocrit
Serum transferrin
Total lymphocyte count
Creatinine
Urine urea nitrogen
Creatinine-height index
Skin testing

Anthropometric Data

Height
Weight
Weight change over time (actual weight compared
    with ideal body weight)
Triceps skinfold thickness
Midarm muscle circumference
Subscapular skinfold thickness

Fatigue should be assessed for its impact on the ability to obtain food and eat.

Dietary evaluation is a simple and effective tool for assessing nutritional intake. A 24-hour food diary, a complete dietary history with notations of food allergies and preferences, and direct observation of intake coupled with evaluation of nutrient composition are methods for dietary evaluation. Much of this information can be collected from the patient; however, the patient may not report accurately. Direct observation of the patient's intake by a consistent nurse or dietitian is more precise but has limitations for patients who are not hospitalized.[30] Family members can be enlisted to help keep a record at home.

Biochemical measurements include laboratory values such as serum albumin, which is used to estimate visceral protein levels; serum transferrin, which reflects the body's ability to make serum proteins; and total lymphocyte count, which tests immunocompetence. Skin testing can reveal T-cell–mediated immunocompetence, and urine urea nitrogen may be measured to estimate skeletal muscle mass. Serum prealbumin level is a sensitive indicator of changes in nutritional status. Albumin levels take longer to respond to increased intake.[88, 107]

Anthropometric measurements are the patient's midarm muscle circumference (MAMC), triceps skinfold thickness (TSF), subscapular skinfold thickness (SST), and weight for height as compared with reference standards. The measurements estimate subcutaneous fat stores, energy reserves, and skeletal muscle protein mass. Moreover, measuring weight and comparing it with the patient's ideal body weight and monitoring changes in weight over time will assist in identifying any downward trend in nutritional status. The nurse must adjust for obvious changes from edema or effusions. Weighing the patient weekly can help assess changes. Daily weights are more appropriate to assess changes in fluid status.

A new nutritional assessment method consisting of three nutritional parameters has been developed for use in patients with oral and maxillofacial malignancies. A mathematical model based on body weight, mid-upper arm circumference, and hand grip strength has been shown to be a simple and accurate method for determining nutritional status in this patient population.[46]

Standardized nutritional assessments and interventional pathways for use in oncology have been developed. A standardized approach resulted in a high success rate of patients maintaining or gaining weight during cancer therapy while being managed solely by oral intervention and aggressive symptom management.[95]

Nutritional Intervention

The extent of nutritional intervention depends on the cause of weight loss and the overall goals of the patient and health care team. It may be palliative or quite aggressive.[9] The oral route is always preferred when available. Enteral feedings may be considered when a mechanical defect precludes ingestion of food. The indications for total parenteral nutrition (TPN) in patients with cancer have been liberalized over the past 20 years; however, TPN is indicated only when the gut cannot digest, absorb, and excrete nutrients.[23, 37, 55] For instance, in patients with gynecologic malignancies and irreversible bowel obstruction, TPN has been shown to prolong life, but also led to TPN-related complications.[1, 96]

Because the enteral route of nutritional support has been found to be as good as or preferable to parenteral nutrition in terms of maintenance of nutritional status and immune function, prevention of bacterial translocation, and maintenance of normal gut flora, it is always preferable in terms of physiologic response, quality of life, and cost, and should be the method of choice for the nutritional support of patients with cancer.[10, 62, 78, 103, 113] Enteral or parenteral nutrition should be considered only for patients who demonstrate most of the following conditions: (1) inability to eat for a long period, (2) weight loss from inability to eat rather than tumor-induced metabolic changes, (3) availability of professional support to reduce complications of therapy, and (4) cancer that can be expected to respond to treatment.[41] For example, enteral nutrition support for patients undergoing major abdominal surgery,[11, 41] patients with esophageal cancer being treated with concurrent chemotherapy and radiation therapy,[9] children after bone marrow transplantation,[38] and patients with acquired immunodeficiency syndrome (AIDS) experiencing dysphagia[89] has been shown to prevent further nutritional deterioration and is well tolerated. In a meta-analysis of 11 randomized controlled trials comparing enteral nutritional support supplemented by with key nutrients to standard enteral support, the supplemented enteral nutrition was found to significantly reduce the risk of infectious complications and reduced overall length of hospital stays.[47]

Health care providers are increasingly asked to consider the cost of various nutritional interventions. Nutrition counseling, liquid homemade or commercially available supplements, and appetite stimulants are relatively low-cost, effective means of nutritional support. Enteral nutrition requires invasive procedures, is more expensive, and is associated with several potential complications. TPN also requires invasive procedures, is very expensive, and is associated with numerous potential, and severe, complications.[119]

Early nutritional intervention has been found to reduce costs. When patients at risk for malnutrition receive counseling and oral nutritional support, the net savings per patient has been estimated to be $1000.

In addition, high-risk patients receiving nutritional counseling had significantly shorter hospital length of stays.[114]

NUTRITIONAL SUPPORT

Oral Nutrition

After the need for nutritional support has been established, the next step is to determine the method of delivery. The oral route is most desirable. The degree of intervention is based on the severity and etiology of the nutritional deficiency. Individuals with mild anorexia often respond to dietary counseling. Positive outcomes of dietary counseling have been demonstrated; in a study of 400 patients referred for counseling, 57% felt better emotionally, 37% felt better physically, and 64% felt more in control of their condition after talking with a dietitian.[108] In settings that do not have dietitians available for consultation and counseling, case managers or nurses providing direct care may need to provide nutrition education and counseling.[43]

Patients experiencing mild anorexia may benefit from frequent small meals and snacks. Foods high in protein, such as cheese, fish, and poultry, and foods high in calories are recommended. Family members and caregivers should offer a variety of foods; foods not appealing at one time may be favorites at another. Milkshakes, peanut butter on crackers, and prepackaged puddings are snacks that are not only nutritious, but also easy to prepare. Supplements such as Instant Breakfast (Carnation) can be taken between meals. Adding dry milk powder to cream soups or milk can increase calorie and protein content. Providing lists of recommended foods or prepared booklets can give caregivers concrete ideas to implement at home. Teaching may be necessary to overcome previous avoidance of high-calorie foods. If indicated, caregivers should provide high-calorie, high-protein supplements such as Sustacal (Mead Johnson), Ensure (Ross), or Citrotein (Sandoz). A wide range of specialized supplements also are available, such as nutritional supplements for patients with cancer with renal or pulmonary impairment.[132] The nurse should monitor for alterations in elimination when using lactose-based products; some patients experience diarrhea and do not tolerate these formulas. Fruit-flavored supplements may be well tolerated by patients who do not like milk.

Consideration needs to be given to *cultural issues* in our increasingly diverse society, because some hospitalized patients may find standard American food not suited to their taste. Family members may be encouraged to bring in favorite foods. Written materials may need to be developed in languages other than English and should include food choices familiar to the targeted population. Likewise, consideration needs to be given to *life-style preferences.* Not all patients are able to adhere to hospital-designated mealtimes. Assessing mealtime preferences can assist with planning and promote optimal intake. Offering 24-hour room service has been shown to improve food intake and satisfaction with hospital food among patients with cancer.[135]

Individuals who have a mild weight loss because of alterations in skin integrity of the oral mucosa (*stomatitis*) or taste alterations may benefit from a high-calorie bland diet. Avoidance of seasoning and experimentation with alternative flavorings such as vanilla may be beneficial. Use of a topical analgesic for stomatitis may reduce discomfort. Good mouth care cannot be overlooked; slight modifications may be needed. Substitution of baking soda or use of toothpaste specifically for sensitive mouths may be indicated. Patients should avoid commercial mouthwashes because they contain additives and flavorings that are often painful for those with altered oral mucosal integrity. Cold foods, particularly popsicles, ice cream, and frozen yogurt, often have a numbing effect and may be well tolerated. Liquids that are known to have high acidity, such as orange and lemon juice, should be avoided. Patients experiencing xerostomia may encounter difficulties maintaining adequate nutritional intake. The addition of liquids, particularly sauces and gravies, may be helpful.

Psychosocial support is indicated in addition to dietary interventions. Ineffective individual and family coping often occurs when the patient begins to lose weight. Efforts by family members to encourage a better intake are sometimes met with resistance. Frustration for both patient and family results as the patient perceives the relatives to be unsympathetic and lacking in understanding. Family members often perceive a lack of effort by the patient and become frustrated at their inability to do more. Nurses should listen to problems with nutrition and provide guidance and instruction when indicated. It may be helpful to teach families about biologic causes of anorexia to increase understanding of why the patient finds eating so difficult.

Nondietary interventions for patients with a mild weight loss include varying surroundings, eating at the table with family and friends, and arriving at the table immediately before meals to minimize the effect of food odor on appetite. Using small plates and eating more often may be helpful. Relaxation techniques may be useful for some patients.

Medications may be necessary to control the side effects of the disease or treatment that may be affecting intake. Serotonin (5-HT$_3$) blockers have demonstrated effectiveness as prophylactic antiemetic therapy.[29] Antiemetics given 30 minutes before meals and use of artificial saliva to control the symptoms of xerostomia are other examples of pharmacologic interventions. Several

randomized, controlled studies also have suggested that use of megestrol acetate with a dose range of 320 to 1600 mg/d improves appetite and prevents or decreases weight loss in patients with advanced cancer and in those undergoing various treatment modalities, such as radiotherapy and chemotherapy.* When combined with ibuprofen, megestrol acetate reversed weight loss and improved quality of life in a randomized prospective study of patients with advanced GI cancer.[75] Megestrol acetate has glucocorticoid-like activity and has been linked to the development of Cushing syndrome, new-onset diabetes, and adrenal insufficiency.[68] Clinicians need to be aware of these associations as these complications can be life-threatening if not recognized.

Dronabinol, δ-9-tetrahydrocannabinol (THC), the active ingredient in marijuana, has also been found to be an effective appetite stimulant in selected patients with advanced cancer and human immunodeficiency virus (HIV) infection. It has been used as an antiemetic for chemotherapy-associated nausea and vomiting.[44, 86]

A variety of *gut-protective nutrients,* such as the amino acid glutamine, are currently being studied to assess their role in stimulating mucosal growth, promoting gut health, and preventing dose-limiting GI symptoms during chemotherapy treatment.[136] New appetite-boosting peptides also have been identified and are being evaluated in clinical trials.[4]

Enteral Nutrition

Although oral nutrition is preferred, adequate intake may not be possible for patients who have a mechanical impairment. For these patients, it may be necessary to use a feeding tube (enteral nutrition). The enteral route is preferable because it uses the GI tract. Using the gut for feeding maintains the GI tract's digestive and absorptive capabilities and assists in maintaining GI motility. Metabolic comparisons show a more nearly normal use of some nutrients with the enteral route than with the parenteral route. A thorough assessment is essential for determining which patients are candidates for enteral nutrition. Mechanical obstruction is the only absolute contraindication to enteral nutrition.[61] Generally, patients with functioning GI tracts who are unable to ingest adequate nutrients to meet their metabolic demands are likely to benefit from tube feedings. They should have a reasonable expectation for improvement through increasing delivery of nutrients, a good support system to help with feedings at home, and reasonable life expectancy. Parenteral (intravenous) feeding is indicated only for patients who have totally nonfunctioning

---

* References 12, 13, 21, 27, 67, 69, 74, 87, 118, 125, 131.

GI tracts, who require bowel rest, or who are intolerant of enteral nutritional support.[23]

Tube feedings can be administered by the nasogastric, nasoduodenal, nasojejunal, esophagostomy, gastrostomy, and jejunostomy routes (Fig. 29–1). Passage of the feeding tube through the nose into the stomach or intestine is indicated for short-term feeding. It is best tolerated when a small, flexible feeding tube is used. Larger, stiffer tubes may damage the mucosa of the GI tract and irritate the nose. A feeding ostomy is indicated for long-term therapy, whenever obstruction makes insertion through the nose impossible, or after GI surgery. Ostomy tubes eliminate nasal irritation and are more cosmetically acceptable to the patient. Possible complications include infection or skin irritation around the feeding tube site; however, this risk is lessened with appropriate skin care.[90] Percutaneous endoscopic gastrostomy (PEG) or jejunostomy (PEJ) tubes are inserted by GI endoscopy and require a patent esophagus. It is a relatively simple procedure, with the tube being threaded through the abdominal and stomach or jejunal wall over a guidewire. The tube can be used soon after placement. Recovery time is short. It may be possible to place a button gastrostomy into a mature gastrocutaneous fistula and thereby eliminate the need for a protruding tube.[111] If GI endoscopy is not possible, place-

ment is more complicated, requiring laparotomy and a longer recovery time. A new enteral access system consisting of a subcutaneously implanted enteral nutrition port (Infuse-a-Port, SMAP Snaplock Macro-Port Venous Access System, Strato Medical Co.) connected to an enteral nutrition tube (Enteral Tube 8F, 75 cm, Zeon Co.) has demonstrated safety, efficiency, and improved cosmesis in 7 patients with advanced esophageal cancers who required long-term nutrition support.[70]

Nasogastric, esophagostomy, and gastrostomy feedings allow the digestive process to begin in the stomach. Aspiration may occur more easily with gastric feedings than with intestinal feedings because only the gastroesophageal sphincter is functioning to prevent gastric reflux. Alteration of the gastroesophageal sphincter by tumor or surgery may increase the risk of aspiration. Nasoduodenal, nasojejunal, and jejunostomy feedings, which are delivered directly into the small intestine, may be preferred in these selected patients because they then have the pyloric sphincter to prevent reflux. Tube selection is based on several factors, including the duration of therapy, history of abdominal procedures, GI function, level of debilitation, and the discharge plan. Adequate digestion and absorption occur in the small intestine; however, when feedings are improperly selected or administered, nausea, diarrhea, and cramps can result.[18]

A cervical esophagostomy is a surgically created, skin-lined canal extending from the border of the neck to the area below the cervical esophagus. The feeding tube is passed through this opening to the stomach for each feeding and removed after the feeding is finished.

Administration of Tube Feeding. The size of the tube selected for enteral feedings should be the smallest through which the food will flow. A variety of tubes are available. Most are made of soft, flexible material such as polyurethane or silicone rubber. These tubes do not stiffen when exposed to gastric juices and are more comfortable for the patient than are stiff tubes. The tubes are available in different French sizes and lengths, and most are radiopaque.

The volume and concentration of nutriment delivered by tube feeding should meet the individual's specific needs. A patient who has been without adequate food intake before tube feeding requires a period of adaptation before full volume and strength can be tolerated. Isotonic formulas are more easily tolerated than hypertonic formulas and do not require dilution. The duodenum and jejunum are more sensitive than the stomach to both volume and osmolality. Therefore, duodenal or jejunal feeding should be low in osmolality and delivered by continuous drip or pump.

Consultation with the dietary department is usually done to determine the caloric needs and most suitable

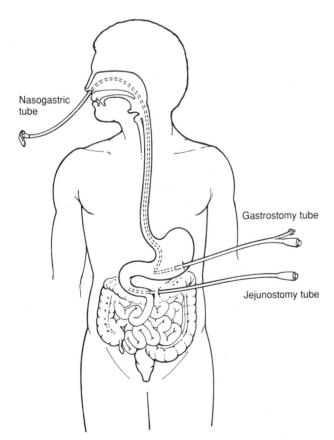

FIGURE 29–1 Three routes for tube feeding.

Nasogastric tube

Gastrostomy tube

Jejunostomy tube

formula. Water requirements are also calculated. Generally, patients need at least 1 mL fluid per calorie. Formulas range from 75% to 85% water (check exact amount on can or literature). It is usually adequate to presume about 80% for most formulas. Additional water needs to be given to meet demands. For instance, a patient with 1800 calories delivered by formula needs at least 1800 mL water, 1440 of which will be delivered in the formula (80% of 1800). The remainder must be given as flushes or extra boluses of water. Dehydration is known to occur with tube-fed patients. Additional fluid may be needed to replace fluid losses from diarrhea, sweating, or wound drainage. Patients who cannot swallow their own saliva because of obstruction may also require extra fluid replacement.

Feedings into the stomach can be done by bolus, gravity, or pump methods. Bolus feedings of enteral formulas are usually administered at 250 to 400 mL over a few minutes, five to eight times daily. Patients who are intolerant of bolus feedings may have nausea, diarrhea, aspiration, abdominal distention, and cramps. Generally, only relatively healthy individuals can tolerate bolus feedings.

Gravity feedings may be intermittent or continuous. Gravity flow rates may be inconsistent and thus must be assessed frequently. Even if checks are made as frequently as every half hour, accidental bolus delivery is possible. Ideally, the tube position should be checked two to three times daily, and gastric residual should be checked every 2 to 4 hours.

Continuous feedings may be given during the night over 10 to 12 hours or around the clock. Feedings to the distal duodenum or jejunum should be given by continuous pump infusion to prevent dumping syndrome. They should be started at 50 mL or less and advanced only if the patient shows no diarrhea, cramping, or other signs of intolerance. When the desired rate has been reached, the strength can be increased as tolerated. Generally, an isotonic or nearly isotonic formula can be started at full strength; hypertonic or concentrated formulas are usually started at half strength (half formula, half water) or at half speed. Adding water or other liquids such as dye can contaminate feedings and should be done as carefully as possible. Table 29–1 compares oral supplements and tube-feeding formulas.

Various feeding sets, containers, and pumps are available for tube feeding. Selection of equipment and supplies is based on the formula to be given, rate and frequency of feedings, tube site, and other considerations, including the caregiver's preference. Most feeding bags and administration sets are large enough to accommodate 500 to 1000 mL of formula. To prevent bacterial contamination when a large container is used, the amount of formula in the bag should approximate that which can be given over 8 hours. In warm environments a feeding bag with a pouch for an ice bag is desirable to prevent curdling of the formula and bacterial growth. New formula should not be added to formula that has already been hanging for 8 hours at room temperature. The container and tubing should be rinsed well before adding formula. With very careful cleaning, a feeding bag may be used for 2 days; however, discarding the bag after 24 hours is recommended. Ready-to-hang enteral feedings can be used for patients who are on stable regimens. They can provide approximately 1000 to 1500 mL of formula in a container that is stable for 24 hours and are as cost effective as using a bag and multiple cans of formula. They are available in screw-top or spikable prefilled bottles or bags, which decrease the chance for bacterial contamination.

Several enteral pumps can provide a controlled rate of administration. Most have internal batteries to allow limited mobility and have alarm systems that indicate problems or completion of feeding. Most pumps have occlusion and low-battery alarms and are simply designed to allow easy troubleshooting. An enteral pump is usually indicated if the patient is being fed by the small intestine, if the feedings are given continually around the clock, or if the desired rate is less than 200 mL/h.

Psychological Impact of Tube Feeding. Recognition of the psychological and social needs of the patient receiving tube feedings is an important component of nursing care. Patients facing long-term feedings must adapt to the loss of control over food selection and consumption. Because eating is a social, cultural, and sometimes religious activity, adaptation may be difficult. In addition, alterations of body image related to the presence of a nasogastric or percutaneously inserted feeding tube may cause distress.

Thirst, taste deprivation, and inability to satisfy the appetite are common complaints of tube-fed patients. Patients may feel self-conscious surrounded by the equipment and supplies needed for formula administration and may find mobility limited by the feeding pump and pole. Limiting tube feedings to night hours or using gravity administration may enhance adaptation.

An assessment of the patient's life-style, home environment, body image, and motivation for tube feeding is critical before implementing therapy. Exploration of the patient's perceptions of the importance of food and eating will assist in identifying areas of concern and is a good starting point for teaching. Involvement of the patient and family in the tube feedings is helpful. The rationale for all procedures should be described, and the patient and family should be encouraged to assist in the feeding.

Occasionally, patients are allowed some oral intake, usually fluids and soft, bland foods. Patients receiving

TABLE 29–1
Common Supplements and Tube-Feeding Formulas

	Ensure (Ross)	Ensure Plus (Ross)	Pulmocare (Ross)	Instant Breakfast (Carnation)	Jevity (Ross)	Glucerna (Ross)	Peptamen (Clintec)
Calories (kcal/mL)	1.06	1.5	1.5	0.93	1.06	1.0	1.0
Protein (g) (L/can)	37.2/8.8	55/13	62.6/14.8	58/15	44.4/10.5	41.8/9.9	40/10
Fat (g) (L/can)	37.2/8.8	53.3/12.6	92.1/21.8	35/8	36.8/8.7	55.7/13.2	39/9.2
CHO (g) (L/can)	145/34.3	200/47.3	106/25	136/35	151.7/35.9	97.3/22.2	127/32
Sodium (mEq/L)	36.8	49.6	57	11.3/8 oz	40.4	40	21.7
Potassium (mEq/L)	40	54	48.6	18.7/8 oz	40	40	32.1
Osmolality	470	690	475	720	300	375	270–380
Similar to:	Sustacal (Mead Johnson) Resource (Sandoz)	Sustacal Plus (Mead Johnson) Resource Plus (Sandoz)	NutriVent (Clintec) Respalor (Mead Johnson)	—	ProBalance (Clintec) FiberSource (Sandoz)	Glytrol (Clintec)	Vivonex (Sandoz)
Comments	Lactose free, low residue	Lactose free, low residue, high calorie	55% fat, 28% carbohydrates Good for pulmonary patients, reduced carbon dioxide production	Contains lactose Above analysis mixed with whole milk	Contains fiber, lactose and glucose free	Low carbohydrates for abnormal glucose tolerance, contains fiber, lactose free	Elemental for easy digestion
Route	Tube/oral	Tube/oral	Tube/oral	Oral	Tube	Tube/oral	Tube

all their nutrition from tube feedings may be permitted to chew gum or suck on hard candies, thus satisfying their sense of taste and their desire to chew. Some patients may satisfy a craving for a particular food by chewing and then spitting it out if they cannot swallow.

Patients requiring long-term enteral therapy may benefit from meeting with other tube-fed patients. The support and role models provided often ease the transition to tube feeding.

Monitoring the Patient. The patient's weight is a simple test for assessing whether caloric and fluid needs are met. Weighing the patient every 2 or 3 days to start will alert the caregiver to a deviance from the anticipated weight gain or maintenance. If the patient loses weight during tube feeding, adjustments in the rate, formula, or calorie content may be made quickly.

Serum proteins may also be monitored, usually every 7 to 10 days to start. In the presence of malnutrition, decreased albumin synthesis occurs. With optimal enterally provided nutritional support, serum prealbumin and protein levels may increase as the patient receives ade-

quate calories and protein; however, abnormal metabolism of nutrients in patients with advanced cancer may preclude significant gains.

Nasal tube placement should be verified by aspirating gastric contents and by listening to the area over the stomach while injecting air through the tube. Gastric contents should be checked for residual and feeding delayed if more than 100 mL is obtained (Box 29–2).

Complications of Tube Feeding. Many of the complications of tube feedings are preventable through appropriate selection of formula and tubes, proper administration, and frequent monitoring. Complications may be mechanical or metabolic and may affect the GI and respiratory systems[15, 80, 115, 138] (Table 29–2).

A common complication is tube clogging as a result of inadequate flushing or improper administration of medication. As a rule, tubes should be flushed with 30 to 60 mL water at these times: before and after intermittent feedings, every 4 hours during continuous feedings, before and after medication administration, after checking tube placement, and after checking gas-

---

BOX 29–2

Care of the Tube-Fed Patient at Home

TUBE CARE

Nasogastric

1. Change tape every other day.
2. Clean edges of both nostrils at least once a day. Lubricate with K-Y Jelly if desired.
3. Brush teeth and tongue twice daily.
4. Use lanolin-based cream to moisturize lips.

Gastrostomy

Perform gastrostomy care daily:

1. Inspect skin.
2. Observe for tube migration.
3. Clean with soap and water, starting at tube and moving outward.
4. Place transparent or hypoallergenic tape dressing.

FEEDING ADMINISTRATION

1. Elevate patient's head at least 30 degrees during feeding and for 1 hour after feeding.
2. Check tube placement. Listen with stethoscope while injecting air into tube or aspirate gastric contents.
3. Check amount of gastric residual before each intermittent feeding or approximately every 2 to 4 hours during continuous feeding. If residual is more than 100 mL, delay feeding for 1 hour and check again.
4. Flush tube with 20 to 30 mL of room-temperature water or carbonated drink before and after each intermittent feeding or every 3 to 4 hours during continuous feeding.

ASSESSMENT OF COMPLICATIONS

1. Observe for signs of complications, including nausea, cramps, diarrhea, and aspiration.
2. Inspect hands and feet for signs of fluid retention.

ASSESSMENT OF GOAL ACHIEVEMENT

1. Weigh daily or every other day.
2. Report weight loss of 2 lb or more to physician.

---

290 mOsm) begun at half rate and slowly increased may be well tolerated. The use of fiber-containing formulas can help provide more normal intestinal function. Infection may occur from contaminated feeding or *Clostridium difficile* infection if the patient has been taking antibiotics. Stool culture can help rule out infectious causes of diarrhea.

Home Enteral Therapy. The number of home enteral nutrition (HEN) patients has increased exponentially since 1988; it is estimated that at least 152,000 patients receive HEN for an average of 3 to 32 months at a cost

TABLE 29–2
Common Complications of Enteral Nutrition

Complication	Etiology
MECHANICAL	
Local skin irritation and erosion	Use of rigid, large-bore tubes
Esophagitis, pharyngitis	Use of rigid, large-bore tubes
Tube dislocation	Coughing or pulling on tube, tube migration
Tube occlusion	Kinked tube, inadequate irrigation, formula incompletely crushed, incompatible medications
GASTROINTESTINAL	
Abdominal distention	Rapid infusion rate, delayed gastric emptying, formula intolerance
Nausea, vomiting	Rapid infusion rate, delayed emptying, formula intolerance, malabsorption, electrolyte imbalance, contaminated formula
Diarrhea	Rapid infusion rate, formula intolerance, malabsorption, contaminated formula
Constipation	Long-term use of low-residue solutions, inadequate fluid intake
RESPIRATORY	
Aspiration pneumonia	Gastric reflux of aspiration (especially with large-bore tubes), improper tube placement, large gastric residuals, patient's head elevated less than 30 degrees
METABOLIC	
Hyperglycemia	Underlying diabetes, sepsis, stress, intolerance to infusion rate
Hypokalemia	Concurrent diuretic, insulin, or antibiotic therapy
Hyperkalemia	Metabolic acidosis, renal insufficiency, excessive potassium in formula
Hypernatremia, dehydration	Insufficient water (especially if hyperosmolar, high-protein formulas used)

tric residual and returning contents. Patency of clogged tubes can often be restored by irrigating the tube with carbonated beverages, such as colas and ginger ale.[39] Box 29–3 lists the factors to consider for delivering medication via enteral tubes.

Diarrhea is a common problem in tube-fed patients, especially when first begun. If the patient has not been eating, the gut may be intolerant of feeding and feeding should be started slowly. Isotonic formulas (near

---

B O X 2 9 – 3

Delivery of Medications via Feeding Tube

Use liquid preparation when possible.

Crush medications as finely as possible and mix with warm water.

Check with pharmacist if in doubt or for sustained-release products.

Flush tube with warm water before and after administering medications.

Do not mix medications; flush between administration of each drug.

Do not mix medications with formula.

Hold feeding 2 hours before and 1 hour after medications that need to be given on an empty stomach (e.g., phenytoin).

Do not crush or open enteric-coated preparations.

Blood levels may need to be checked with certain medications (e.g., theophylline, warfarin) because drug absorption may differ with various enteral formulas.

---

of $20 to $50 per day. Medicare-allowable charges for HEN represent a 90% to 95% cost savings over enteral nutrition provided in the hospital setting.[58, 63, 102]

Once it is determined that a patient needs enteral therapy and discharge is anticipated, the patient is assessed. A coordinated effort among the patient, caregivers, and health care team is essential for the successful discharge and management of patients receiving home enteral nutrition.[63] A caregiver is selected if the patient is unable to perform self-care. The capabilities of the caregiver are assessed, the home environment is discussed, and the caregiver is trained until she can independently care for the tube-fed patient. A home care referral for nursing visits to continue teaching and supervise care should be made. General care of the tube-fed patient at home includes tube care, feeding, and assessment of complications and goal achievement (see Box 29–2).

Parenteral Nutrition

Parenteral nutrition therapy supplies all of the essential nutrients by means of the intravenous (IV) route. Parenteral therapy may be called hyperalimentation and may be partial or total. Many patients receive partial parenteral nutrition in the form of dextrose solutions as part of their usual care. Total parenteral nutrition (TPN) supplies all the daily requirements for protein and calories directly into the bloodstream. Parenteral nutrition is indicated for patients who have totally nonfunctioning GI tracts, require bowel rest, or are intolerant of enteral therapy. Cancers of the GI tract and related obstructions are often indications for TPN. Because absorption of nutrients is impaired in such patients, TPN is often the only option available.[23]

The delivery routes for TPN are peripheral and central veins. Peripheral administration of TPN solutions is accomplished by using the veins of the arm. The external jugular vein in the neck may also be used. With the peripheral route the following factors should be considered[126, 127]:

- Peripheral administration provides limited calories, generally fewer than 2500 kcal/d, as well as a limited amount of protein, less than 100 g/d.
- Solutions administered peripherally can be very irritating to the vein, especially if dextrose is more than 10%.
- Solutions may be stopped quickly; tapering and weaning are not needed.
- Peripheral administration is useful for short-term nutritional support.

Administration of TPN via the central route is done using a central venous access device placed into a major vein such as the superior vena cava. Central venous access devices used for TPN include implanted ports; triple-lumen catheters; Broviac, Hickman, and Groshong catheters.[7, 40] With the central route the following factors should be considered:

- Central administration can provide a large amount of calories and protein.
- Final dextrose concentrations can be as high as 35% and final amino acid concentrations more than 5%.
- These solutions cannot be discontinued suddenly. Abrupt cessation may induce profound hypoglycemia. Tapering down the rate and concentration is the most effective method for discontinuation.

Components. The three main components of TPN are glucose, amino acids, and fats. The glucose content of TPN, usually in the form of dextrose 50%, provides both immediate and long-term energy. Amino acids or proteins are provided with or without electrolytes and are usually ordered in concentrations of 5.5% or 8.5%. The lower concentration is indicated for patients with hepatic or renal dysfunction or failure. Administration of fats with TPN is required because the TPN solution stimulates the production of insulin, which in turn prevents fat from being metabolized. A fatty acid deficiency may result. Fat is provided through lipid emulsions formulated from safflower and soybean oils emulsified with egg phospholipid. Therefore, lipids are not administered to patients with a history of allergy to eggs.[126] Lipid emulsions usually come in a concentration of 10% or 20% and may be "piggybacked" or added to the TPN solution. Exact formulations are specific to the patient;

they depend on individual requirements, tolerances, body chemistry, and disease processes (Table 29–3).

A TPN formula that combines the dextrose, amino acids, and fat emulsion in one container is often called a *three-in-one* or *total nutrient admixture.* Eliminating the need for piggybacking lipids allows for a closed system that reduces the risk of infection, minimizes manipulations, and cuts waste. Often, three-in-one solutions are ordered for patients receiving TPN at home because they are convenient and easy to administer. If lipids are piggybacked, they generally are given two or three times per week.

Many patients receiving TPN have a multilumen central venous catheter inserted. The additional lumens provide access for drug administration and blood sampling. Patients with single-lumen catheters who require medications must either have the line flushed before and after administration of medication or have the medication added to the TPN bag. Several drugs have been

tested to be compatible with TPN formulas for at least 12 hours[85, 123, 124] (Box 29–4).

Administration. TPN solutions may be given continuously or by cycling the infusion over 12 to 20 hours per day. Cycling is most often used for patients receiving TPN at home during the night because it allows them to be mobile during the day. The disadvantage of cycling TPN is that patients must be able to tolerate a high-volume load. Cyclic TPN may be increased slowly at the start and then tapered at the end of the cycle. Programmable pumps are widely used to prevent or minimize hyperglycemia and hypoglycemia as blood sugar levels rise and fall. Compact, portable TPN pumps are also available with programmable functions. The portable pump, worn in a backpack-type carrying bag, is best suited for the ambulatory patient.

Patients requiring long-term parenteral nutrition face different challenges than those needing TPN for only a

TABLE 29–3
Adult and Pediatric Parenteral Solution Formulas

Formula	Amount	Formula	Amount
ADULT		**PEDIATRIC**	
Base Solution		*Base Solution*	
40%–50% dextrose in water	500 mL	40% dextrose in water	500 mL
8.5%–10% crystalline amino acids	500 mL	8.5% crystalline amino acids	500 mL
Additives to Each Unit		*Additives to Each Unit*	
Sodium chloride, acetate, or lactate	40–50 mL	Sodium chloride	3–4 mEq/kg/daily
Potassium chloride	20–30 mEq	Potassium acid phosphate	2–3 mEq/kg/daily
Potassium acid phosphate (10–20 mM phosphorus)	15–30 mEq	Magnesium sulfate	0.25–0.5 mEq/kg/daily
Magnesium sulfate	15–18 mEq	Calcium gluconate	0.5–1 mEq/kg/daily
Multivitamin infusion	10 mL	Multivitamin infusion	
A	3300 IU	A	2300 IU
D	200 IU	D	400 IU
E	10 IU	E	7 IU
Ascorbic acid	100 mg	K	200 μg
Folic acid	400 μg	Ascorbic acid	80 mg
Niacin	40 mg	Folic acid	140 μg
Riboflavin	3.6 mg	Niacinamide	17 mg
Thiamine	3 mg	Riboflavin	1.4 mg
B$_6$ (pyridoxine)	4 mg	Thiamine	1.2 mg
B$_{12}$ (cyanocobalamin)	5 μg	B$_6$ (pyridoxine)	1 mg
Pantothenic acid	15 mg	B$_{12}$ (cyanocobalamin)	1 μg
Biotin	60 μg	Dexpanthenol	7 mg
Additive to Any One Unit Twice Weekly		Biotin	20 μg
Vitamin K	10 mg	IV fat emulsion 10%, 3–7 times weekly	50–75 mL/kg
IV fat emulsion	10% or 20%		
500 mL 2–7 times weekly	50–100 g	**INFUSION RATE**	115 mL/kg/d
Carbohydrate calories	850 kcal		115 kcal/kg/d
Protein calories	150 kcal		3 g protein/kg/d
Fat calories	1000–2000 kcal		
Nitrogen	6.5–8 g		
Amino acids	40–50 g		

BOX 29–4

Drugs Tested to Be Compatible with Total Parenteral Nutrition (TPN) Formulas for at Least 12 Hours

Aminophylline
Antibiotics
  Cephalothin
  Clindamycin
  Erythromycin
  Gentamicin
  Methicillin
  Oxacillin
  Penicillin G
  Tetracycline
  Tobramycin
Antineoplastics
  Cyclophosphamide
  Cytarabine
  Fluorouracil
  Methotrexate

Corticosteroids
H_2-receptor antagonists
  Cimetidine
  Ranitidine
Heparin
Insulin
Iron dextran
Metoclopramide
Narcotic analgesics
  Hydromorphone
  Meperidine
  Morphine

---

short time. Long-term therapy is most often accomplished in the home with the patient or designated caregiver performing many of the procedures.[5] Patients must be motivated to receive TPN at home, must be able to provide competent self-care, and have a home with essential resources, such as a telephone, running water, and electricity. Consideration must also be given to the geographic location of the patient's home; patients on home TPN ideally should be able to easily access emergency medical services. Another geographic consideration involves the transportation time between the home and TPN provider; long driving times may adversely affect the stability of TPN.[137]

Assessment of capabilities before implementing home TPN is critical, because many patients are extremely anxious about performing highly technical procedures. Anxiety usually resolves with education and time. Geriatric patients receiving home TPN generally have a good clinical outcome but do not do as well clinically as their younger counterparts, perhaps because of comorbid conditions; however, they experience fewer therapy-related complications than younger patients.[51]

Many patients note an altered self-image with long-term TPN. Their self-perceptions are undermined by being underweight or even cachexic, and this is compounded by the presence of a central venous access device connected to the TPN formula and equipment. Sleep disturbances may be induced by depressive illness, anxiety, nocturnal urination, and occasionally pump alarms.

When TPN is given to those requiring complete bowel rest, the absence of food intake may be traumatic. Eating is a major social and cultural event, and prohibiting food for several weeks disrupts the patient's life.

Monitoring the Patient and Complications of Therapy. Patients beginning TPN must be monitored frequently to assess side effects and complications of the treatment. Daily monitoring of vital signs, weight, and laboratory values may indicate metabolic changes requiring the adjustment of TPN formula or its rate of administration. The metabolic and technical problems sometimes associated with TPN are numerous. Some are related to the insertion of the central venous access device. Other problems include electrolyte imbalance, infection, and volume overload[42] (Table 29–4).

TABLE 29–4
Common Complications of Parenteral Nutrition

Complication	Etiology
NONMETABOLIC	
Allergy or sensitivity	Sensitivity to either amino acid solution or lipid emulsion
Infection	Catheter-related sepsis
Volume overload	Improper pump rate
Catheter placement	Puncture of or injury to nearby organs or vessels
Pneumothorax	
Arterial puncture	
Hematoma	
Thoracic duct puncture	
Brachial plexus injury	
Pulmonary embolism	
METABOLIC	
Hyperglycemia/ hyperosmolarity	Inability to metabolize high glucose concentration of formula
Hypoglycemia	When TPN is abruptly discontinued, high insulin levels cause rebound drop in blood sugar
Vitamin or mineral deficiencies	Administration of formulas lacking sufficient vitamins or micronutrients
Fatty acid deficiencies or overload	Insufficient or excessive administration of lipids
Hyponatremia	Formulas without sufficient sodium content
Hypokalemia, hyperkalemia	Insufficient or excessive potassium content
Hypocalcemia, hypercalcemia	Insufficient or excessive calcium content
Hypomagnesemia	Insufficient magnesium or increased metabolism of magnesium

Hypersensitivity reactions to lipid emulsion containing long-chain fatty acids have been reported. Symptoms of hypersensitivity include flushing, dyspnea, tachycardia, hypotension, and back pain. In patients with cancer, hypersensitivity to lipid emulsion can be mistaken for chemotherapy toxicity.[128] *Refeeding syndrome,* characterized by a rapid drop in levels of potassium, magnesium, and phosphorus, may be precipitated by the introduction of TPN in the severely malnourished patient. Excess amino acid intake can cause elevations in blood urea nitrogen (BUN) and creatinine levels. *Cracking* of the solution can occur in TPN/lipid formulas with a high content of calcium or phosphorus or those containing salt-poor albumin. An oily layer or oily globules within the solution indicate cracking has occurred, and the infusion should not be used.[126] With frequent monitoring by an experienced staff or well-educated patient performing self-care, the risk of complications is greatly reduced.

Home Parenteral Nutrition. The shift in care from inpatient to outpatient settings, combined with technologic advances in venous access devices, monitoring devices, and infusion pumps, and the availability of experienced home infusion therapy services has led to greater utilization of home TPN.[26] However, the annual growth rate of home TPN has dropped recently because the home infusion therapy market has become highly competitive and reimbursement from government and managed health care plans has declined.[81]

Standards for home nutrition support have been delineated by the American Society for Parenteral and Enteral Nutrition (ASPEN), a professional society of physicians, nurses, pharmacists, and nutritionists committed to promoting quality nutrition support. Their standards aim to ensure sound and efficient home nutrition support care and represent care that should be subscribed to by any home care organization providing home nutrition support therapies.[3] Clinical pathways specific to the care of the home TPN patient have been developed and can be used to facilitate cost-effective care.[54]

Screening patients for home TPN includes assessment of the home environment, availability of a caregiver, learning abilities or disabilities, physical limitations, and motivation to learn procedures. Ideally, education of the caregiver is begun before discharge. Teaching sessions over several days are best for teaching the complex procedures of TPN home administration (Box 29–5). Provision of a take-home booklet is recommended, and return demonstrations performed by the caregiver are often beneficial. One key aspect of at-home care is assessment of the central venous access device and dressing change procedure.[34]

Infectious complications of long-term central venous catheters include infections of the tunnel and exit site,

---

BOX 29–5

Care of the Patient Receiving Parenteral Nutrition at Home

Catheter Care
1. Change dressing and assess venous access device per frequency ordered by physician or institution or agency policy.
2. Flush with saline or heparin if cyclic schedule.

Preparation of Medication
1. Inject additives (e.g., vitamins) into premixed bags.
2. Assemble bag and connect tubing.

Operation of Equipment
1. Connect and disconnect pump.
2. Program pump if cyclic schedule or enter rate, volume, and other data.
3. Perform equipment troubleshooting.

Assessment of Complications
1. Assess for electrolyte imbalance and presence of hyperglycemia.
2. Observe feet and fingers for edema.
3. Monitor temperature and urine for sugar and acetone.

Assessment of Goal Achievement
1. Weigh daily or every other day.

---

catheter-related bacteremia, and septic thrombophlebitis. Despite several studies examining central line dressing change procedures and frequency, standardization for these procedures currently is lacking. However, astute assessment and meticulous dressing change technique by the caregiver minimize these complications.[64, 71, 122]

Follow-up visits in the home are essential. Although many patients may appear quite competent in the hospital, a home visit ensures that procedures are followed appropriately. During home visits, the patient's response to home TPN can be assessed. Weighing the patient combined with a subjective clinical assessment has been found to be sufficient for evaluating the nutritional status of patients on home TPN; these two simple measures were found to be as reliable as more sophisticated anthropometry and bioelectrical impedence measurements and laboratory protein and lymphocyte counts.[31] Oral care for patients receiving home TPN is important, and vital for those patients who have been instructed to take nothing by mouth.[59] Psychosocial support can be rendered to both the patient and family caregiver during home visits.[50] A home assessment also provides the opportunity to determine whether TPN formulas and supplies are stored correctly and whether infection control measures are observed.

Patients vary in the number of teaching sessions and follow-up visits required to assess compliance. Many need a visiting nurse to obtain blood samples and monitor on a schedule. The frequency of clinic visits for evaluation by the physician varies according to the patient's needs, ranging from once a week to every 6 months.

Patients may voice concerns about the cost of TPN therapy. Home TPN is usually covered by health insurance, managed care plans, and Medicare for patients experiencing bowel obstruction. Annual costs for adult home TPN have recently been estimated to range from $55,000 to $250,000 per patient, but continue to be half the cost of inpatient TPN.[101, 102, 134]

COMPLEMENTARY AND ALTERNATIVE NUTRITIONAL THERAPIES

Dietary supplements and herbs were the most commonly used complementary therapies reported by patients with cancer in 26 surveys.[33] The wide use of these therapies has been attributed to, among other things, the passage in 1994 of legislation allowing herbal medicines and other food supplements to be sold over the counter without review by the Food and Drug Administration (FDA).[17]

The FDA has officially approved six herbs: aloe, cascara, psyllium, and senna as laxatives, capsicum as a topical anesthetic, and witch hazel as an astringent.[84] More than 500 different herbs and nutritional supplements are currently on the market in the United States, and patients often obtain herbs from other countries via the Internet or other means. Patients who use herbal and related remedies do so because of belief in their efficacy, perceived safely, and reasonable cost.[6, 129] However, not all herbs, dietary supplements, and related nutritional therapies are safe and effective. Examples include Essiac, comprised of four herbs (Burdock, Turkey rhubarb, sorrel, and slippery elm), which is one of the most popular herbal cancer alternatives in North America. Researchers at the National Cancer Institute and elsewhere have not found Essiac to have any anticancer effect.[17] Herbal products with toxic effects include chapparal tea (liver failure); feverfew, ginko, and ginger (anticoagulation); Ma huang or ephedra (central nervous system stimulation); and Lobella (coma and death at high doses).[16]

The potential for herb–drug interaction is sufficiently problematic that patients on chemotherapy should be cautioned to discontinue using herbal remedies during treatment. Similar advisories are necessary for patients receiving radiation therapy because some herbs photosensitize the skin and cause severe reactions. The risk of herb–drug interactions appears to be greatest for patients with kidney or liver impairment.[17]

Other related nutritional therapies include megavitamin therapy. However, there is no scientific evidence that megavitamin therapy is effective in treating any disorder.[17] The macrobiotic diet, rooted in ancient Chinese medicine, has been used by patients with cancer and is perceived by some to be a way of life as opposed to a diet. The basic macrobiotic diet consists of 40% to 60% whole cereal grains, 24% to 30% vegetables, 10% to 15% beans and sea vegetables, 5% to 10% fish, and 5% soup. Concerns about this diet include inadequate caloric intake for patients with cancer, and the potential for protein and calcium deficiencies.[82]

ETHICAL CONSIDERATIONS

As patients with cancer enter the end-stage of disease, poor appetite becomes a distressing problem for both patients and families. Poor or absent appetite affects not only physical symptoms but also affects functional, social, and psychological aspects of patients' quality of life. A number of approaches can be used when appetite declines in the end-stage of disease, including education, dietary changes, and appetite stimulants.[110] However, these approaches often are met with minimal or no success and caregivers may voice concern that the patient will "starve to death." When dying patients are unable to take food or drink, health care providers and caregivers must help the patient decide whether to receive nutrition or hydration by artificial means. Providing this support is an area of ongoing controversy because of the difficulties associated with determining life expectancy, the current emphasis on symptom management, and emerging data that suggests that end-of-life cessation of fluid intake decreases secretions and level of consciousness and thereby improves comfort levels.[24, 45] Decisions about providing nutritional support need to be based on the needs, wishes, and expectations of both patients and their families. These decisions also must consider the legal and ethical dilemmas of care provision and the need to ensure that the care provided is based on a true examination of the risks, benefits, and burden to the patient.*

Nursing interventions for patients with end-stage disease should be directed at structural or functional deficits, such as stomatitis, nausea, and vomiting, and managing concurrent symptoms, such as pain, fatigue, and dyspnea. The use of IV hydration may be helpful in loosening pulmonary secretions, decreasing gastric secretions, and correcting fluid and electrolyte imbalances in select patients who are not imminently near death.

---

* References 25, 45, 49, 56, 66, 97, 117, 130.

However, the potential benefits of IV hydration must be carefully weighed against the potential risk of infection, the effect of the therapy on the patient's quality of life, and the cost of IV therapy. In patients with end-stage disease, dehydration decreases pulmonary secretions and level of consciousness, acting as a natural anesthetic. Maintaining moisture of oral tissues with ice chips and lubricants reduces the most distressing side effect of dehydration.

When a patient at the end-stage of disease refuses to eat or drink, the effect can be profound on the patient's caregivers as well, and their needs should not be overlooked by nurses. In one study, caregivers of patients with cancer receiving hospice care reported that their own nutritional intake declined substantially. Other issues also arose from the experience, including caregivers grappling with the meaning of food, their roles as sustainers, and feelings of loss.[76] Nurses can assist caregivers by providing information and support, and by encouraging them to optimize their own nutritional intake while caring for their loved ones.

Patients' decisions to forgo nutritional support or refuse to eat can become ethical dilemmas for families and caregivers. In situations where a patient is not at the end-stage of disease, many ethical considerations arise. For instance, in a case report, a patient with a carcinoid tumor who was not considered terminally ill became unable to tolerate jejunostomy feedings. He was determined to be a reasonable candidate for home TPN, but despite lengthy discussions about the potential benefits of home TPN, the patient declined nutritional support because he felt it was an "excessive measure," and was sent home for hospice care.[19]

Termination of nutritional support should occur when the patient, family, physician, and nurse judge that the patient no longer benefits from the nutritional support. The decision must be made in accordance with accepted community standards of care and in compliance with applicable law.

CONCLUSION

Cancer and its treatment affect nutritional status to varying degrees. Patients with local and systemic effects require ongoing assessment and prompt intervention. Nutritional support ranges in complexity depending on needs, and those needs change over time. Oral supplementation, the simplest type of support, is most effective when the patient is highly motivated, has manageable or temporary side effects, and can ingest and digest nutrients. Enteral and parenteral nutrition may be required for individuals with more severe symptoms and for those with demonstrated physical impairments of the GI tract. Despite their complexity, enteral nutrition and parenteral nutrition are often administered in the home, with family members as caregivers. Advances in home therapies and nutritional support have enabled individuals with cancer and nutritional deficiencies to remain at home and have promoted an improved quality of life.

Nursing Management

The additional nursing interventions listed below and stated as directed to the patient can be made depending on the specific alteration in intake or the patient's digestive abilities.

Nursing Diagnosis

- *Nutrition, altered: less than body requirements, related to taste/olfactory changes, dysphagia, dyspepsia, anorexia, gastrointestinal mucositis, nausea, and vomiting*

Outcome Goals

Patient will be able to:

- Maintain or improve nutritional intake, as evidenced by maintaining or gaining weight, depending on stage of disease or response to treatment.
- Safely receive enteral or parenteral support when appropriate.

Interventions: Taste/Olfactory Changes

- Use tart food to stimulate taste buds.
- Use extra seasoning.
- Try sauces and flavor additives.
- Substitute fish and chicken for red meat.

Interventions: Dysphagia

- Eat soft or liquid foods.
- Use sauces and gravies.
- Eat small meals frequently.
- If eating is painful, eat bland foods.

Interventions: Dyspepsia

- Avoid fatty and spicy foods.
- Avoid gas-producing foods.
- Use antacids.
- Avoid lying down after meals.

Interventions: *Anorexia*

- Vary surroundings.
- Eat with family and friends.
- Try new foods and recipes.
- Use smaller plates.
- Eat high-calorie snacks.
- Drink high-protein shakes.
- Try hard candy.
- Use distraction: radio, TV, etc.

Interventions: *Gastrointestinal Mucositis*

- Avoid acidic fruits and juices.
- Eat cool foods.
- Use a topical analgesic before eating.

Interventions: *Nausea and Vomiting*

- Drink clear liquids and advance diet as tolerated.
- Drink flat beverages.
- Avoid sweet, rich, and fatty foods.
- Try dry foods (e.g., toast, crackers).
- Try easily digested foods (e.g., rice).
- Avoid food odors.
- Eat cool foods.
- Eat small, frequent meals.
- Use antiemetics 30 minutes before meals.

Nursing Diagnosis

- *Constipation*

Outcome Goals

Patient will be able to:

- Identify factors that influence elimination.
- Demonstrate adequate nutritional/fluid intake.
- Maintain appropriate level of physical mobility.

Interventions

- Drink adequate fluids.
- Eat high-fiber foods.
- Exercise regularly.
- Avoid cheese and concentrated foods.

Nursing Diagnosis

- *Diarrhea*

Outcome Goals

Patient will be able to:

- Verbalize signs and symptoms of diarrhea.
- Identify potential causes of diarrhea.
- Demonstrate adequate nutritional/fluid intake.
- Eliminate foods/medications that cause/increase diarrhea.

Interventions

- Drink adequate amounts of fluid.

Chapter Questions

1. The anorexia-cachexia syndrome of advanced cancer is caused by the production of:
   a. Calcium
   b. Cytokines
   c. Lactic acid
   d. Trace elements
2. Patients undergoing total gastrectomies are at high risk for developing:
   a. Osteoporosis
   b. Fungal infections
   c. Pernicious anemia
   d. Renal failure
3. Which of the following is a late effect of head and neck irradiation?
   a. Pain
   b. Taste changes
   c. Mucositis
   d. Dental caries
4. Which of the following patients will most likely require parenteral hydration and total parenteral nutrition?
   a. An 80-year-old man on hormonal therapy for prostate cancer
   b. A 44-year-old woman on adjuvant chemotherapy for breast cancer
   c. A 60-year-old man receiving palliative care for pancreatic cancer
   d. A 36-year-old woman undergoing a peripheral blood stem cell transplant
5. Total parenteral nutrition is indicated for patients who:
   a. Have lost 10% or more of their body weight
   b. Refuse enteral feedings via gastrostomy tube
   c. Cannot digest, absorb, or excrete nutrients
   d. Dislike the taste of oral nutritional supplements
6. A risk associated with use of megestrol acetate as an appetite stimulant is the development of:
   a. Adrenal insufficiency
   b. Hyperparathyroidism

c. Addison's disease.

d. Syndrome of inappropriate ADH secretion

7. Tube feedings should be initiated slowly to minimize the risk of:

a. Aspiration

b. Malabsorption

c. Infection

d. Fluid volume overload

8. Dehydration in a terminally ill patient may result in:

a. Loss of appetite

b. Increased urination

c. Decreased level of consciousness

d. Increased pulmonary secretions

9. Biochemical nutritional assessment measures include:

a. Serum albumin, serum transferrin, total lymphocyte, BUN

b. Serum albumin, serum transferrin, total lymphocyte, CBC

c. Serum albumin, serum potassium, total lymphocyte, BUN

d. Serum albumin, serum transferrin, serum creatinine, WBC

10. Anorexia-cachexia syndrome associated with advanced cancer is characterized by:

a. Wasting, weight loss, weakness, normal immune function

b. Wasting, weight loss, weakness, impaired immune function

c. Wasting, weight gain, weakness, impaired immune function

d. Wasting, weight gain, weakness, normal immune function

BIBLIOGRAPHY

1. Abu-Rustum NR and others: Chemotherapy and total parenteral nutrition for advanced ovarian cancer with bowel obstruction, *Gynecol Oncol* 64:493, 1997.

2. Albrecht JT, Canada TW: Cachexia and anorexia in malignancy, *Hematol Oncol Clin North Am* 10:791, 1996.

3. ASPEN Board of Directors: Standards for home nutrition support, *Nutr Clin Pract* 14:151, 1999.

4. Barinaga M: New appetite-boosting peptides found, *Science* 279:1134, 1998.

5. Barnadas G: Preparing for parenteral nutritional therapy at home, *Am J Health Sys Pharm* 56:270, 1999.

6. Bartels CL, Miller SJ: Herbal and related remedies, *Nutr Clin Pract* 12:5, 1998.

7. Beau P, Matrat S: A comparative study of polyurethane and silicone cuffed-catheters in long-term home parenteral nutrition patients, *Clin Nutr* 18:175, 1999.

8. Body JJ: The syndrome of anorexia-cachexia, *Curr Opin Oncol* 11:255, 1999.

9. Bozzetti F and others: Nutritional support in patients with cancer of the esophagus: impact on nutritional status, patient compliance to therapy, and survival, *Tumori* 84:681, 1998.

10. Bozzetti F and others: Artificial nutrition in cancer patients: which route, what composition? *World J Surg* 23:577, 1999.

11. Braga M and others: Artificial nutrition after major abdominal surgery: impact of route of administration and composition of the diet, *Crit Care Med* 26:24, 1998.

12. Bruera E: Pharmacological treatment of cachexia: any progress? *Support Care Cancer* 6:109, 1998.

13. Bruera E and others: Effectiveness of megestrol acetate in patients with advanced cancer: a randomized, double-blind, crossover study, *Cancer Prev Control* 2:74, 1998.

14. Byers T: What can randomized controlled trials tell us about nutrition and cancer prevention? *CA Cancer J Clin* 49:353, 1999.

15. Cabre E, Gassull MA: Complications of enteral feeding, *Nutrition* 9:1, 1993.

16. Cassileth BR: *The alternative medicine handbook: the complete reference guide to alternative and complementary therapies,* New York, Norton, 1998.

17. Cassileth BR: Evaluating complementary and alternative therapies for cancer patients, *CA Cancer J Clin* 49:362, 1999.

18. Cattan S, Cosnes J: Enteral feeding techniques, *Curr Opin Clin Nutr Metab Care* 1:287, 1998.

19. Chapman G: An oncology patient's choice to forgo nonvolitional nutrition support: ethical considerations, *Nutr Clin Pract* 11:265, 1996.

20. Charuhas PM and others: A double-blind randomized trial comparing outpatient parenteral nutrition with intravenous hydration: effect on resumption of oral intake after marrow transplantation, *JPEN J Parenter Enteral Nutr* 21:157, 1997.

21. Chen HC and others: Effect of megestrol acetate and prepulsid on nutritional improvement in patients with head and neck cancers undergoing radiotherapy, *Radiother Oncol* 43:75, 1997.

22. Coleman C: Overview of biotherapy and nursing considerations, *J Intraven Nurs* 21:367, 1998.

23. Copeland EM: Historical perspective on nutritional support of cancer patients, *CA Cancer J Clin* 48:67, 1998.

24. Cox MJ: A compassionate response toward providing nutrition and hydration in vulnerable populations, *J Gerontol Nurs* 24:8, 1998.

25. Craig GM: Nutrition, dehydration and the terminally ill, *J Med Ethics* 21:184, 1995.

26. Crocker KS and others: Should total parenteral nutrition be initiated in the home or hospital? Point-Counterpoint, *Nutr Clin Pract* 14:124, 1999.

27. De Conno F and others: Megestrol acetate for anorexia in patients with far-advanced cancer: a double-blind controlled clinical trial, *Eur J Cancer* 34:1705, 1998.

28. Doerr TD and others: Effects of zinc and nutritional status on clinical outcomes in head and neck cancer, *Nutrition* 14:489, 1998.

29. Doherty KM: Closing the gap in prophylactic antiemetic therapy: patient factors in calculating the emetogenic potential of chemotherapy, *Clin J Oncol Nurs* 3:113, 1999.

30. Edington J: Problems of nutritional assessment in the community, *Proc Nutr Soc* 58:47, 1999.

31. Egger NG and others: Nutritional status and assessment of patients on home parenteral nutrition: anthropometry, bioelectrical impedance, or clinical judgment? *Nutrition* 15:54, 1999.

32. Eriksson KM and others: Nutrition and acute leukemia in adults: relation between nutritional status and infectious complications during remission induction, *Cancer* 82:1071, 1998.

33. Ernst E, Cassileth BR: The prevalence of complementary/alternative medicine in cancer, *Cancer* 83:777, 1998.

34. Evans-Stoner N: Guidelines for the care of the patient on home nutrition support, *Nurs Clin North Am* 32:769, 1997.

35. Ezzone SA: SIADH, *Clin J Oncol Nurs* 3:187, 1999.

36. Feuz A, Rapin CH: An observational study of the role of pain control and food adaptation of elderly patients with terminal cancer, *J Am Diet Assoc* 94:767, 1994.

37. Forchielli ML and others: Total parenteral nutrition and home parenteral nutrition: an effective combination to sustain malnourished children with cancer, *Nutr Rev* 57:15, 1999.

38. Ford C, Pietsch JB: Home enteral tube feeding in children after chemotherapy or bone marrow transplantation, *Nutr Clin Pract* 14:19, 1999.

39. Frankel EH and others: Techniques and procedures. Methods of restoring patency to occluded feeding tubes, *Nutr Clin Pract* 13:129, 1998.

40. Freytes CO: Vascular access devices in cancer patients: towards the next step, *Eur J Cancer* 33:1171, 1997.

41. Gianotti L and others: Effect of route of delivery and formulation of postoperative nutritional support in patients undergoing major operations for malignant neoplasms, *Arch Surg* 132:1222, 1997.

42. Goff K: Metabolic monitoring in nutrition support, *Nurs Clin North Am* 32:741, 1997.

43. Goff K: Enteral and parenteral nutrition transitioning from hospital to home, *Nurs Care Manage* 3:67, 1998.

44. Gralla RJ: Antiemetic therapy, *Semin Oncol* 25:577, 1998.

45. Gray R: Palliative care. To hydrate or not to hydrate? *Nurs Times* 95:36, 1999.

46. Guo C and others: A new nutritional assessment in patients with oral and maxillofacial malignancies, *Auris Nasus Larynx* 24:385, 1997.

47. Heys SD and others: Enteral nutritional supplementation with key nutrients in patients with critical illness and cancer: a meta-analysis of randomized controlled clinical trials, *Ann Surg* 229:467, 1999.

48. Holmes S: Nutrition in patients undergoing radiotherapy, *Prof Nurse* 12:789, 1997.

49. Holmes S: Professional considerations. The challenge of providing nutritional support to the dying, *Int J Palliat Nurs* 4(1):26, 1998.

50. Howard L, Hassan N: Home parenteral nutrition: 25 years later, *Gastroenterol Clin North Am* 27:481, 1998.

51. Howard L, Malone M: Clinical outcome of geriatric patients in the United States receiving home parenteral and enteral nutrition, *Am J Clin Nutr* 66:1364, 1997.

52. Hunter AM: Nutrition management of patients with neoplastic disease of the head and neck treated with radiation therapy, *Nutr Clin Pract* 11:157, 1996.

53. Inui A: Cancer anorexia-cachexia syndrome: are neuropeptides the key? *Cancer Res* 59:4493, 1999.

54. Ireton-Jones C and others: Clinical pathways in home nutrition support, *J Am Diet Assoc* 97:1003, 1997.

55. Ireton-Jones CS, Stiller DL: Evaluation of outcomes for patients with AIDS receiving home parenteral nutrition, *Nutrition* 14:731, 1998.

56. Jackonen S: Dehydration and hydration in the terminally ill: care considerations, *Nurs Forum* 32:5, 1997.

57. Jaffe M: *Geriatric nutrition & diet therapy*, ed 2, El Paso, Skidmore-Roth, 1995.

58. Jewell KE: Coverage and reimbursement for enteral feeding devices in nutrition support, *Nutr Clin Pract* 13:S28, 1998.

59. Jones CV: Nutrition. The importance of oral hygiene in nutritional support, *Br J Nurs* 7:74, 1998.

60. Kalman D, Villani LJ: Nutritional aspects of cancer-related fatigue, *J Am Diet Assoc* 97:650, 1997.

61. Kirby DF, Teran JC: Enteral feeding in critical care, gastrointestinal diseases, and cancer, *Gastrointest Endosc Clin North Am* 8:623, 1998.

62. Klein S and others: Nutrition support in clinical practice: review of published data and recommendations for future research directions. Summary of a conference sponsored by the National Institutes of Health, American Society for Parenteral and Enteral Nutrition, and American Society for Clinical Nutrition, *Am J Clin Nutr* 66:683, 1997.

63. Klein GL and others: A multidisciplinary approach to home enteral nutrition, *Nutr Clin Pract* 13:157, 1998.

64. Lau DE: Transparent and gauze dressings and their effect on infection rates of central venous catheters: a review of past and current literature, *J Intraven Nurs* 19:240, 1996.

65. Laviano A, Meguid MM: Nutritional issues in cancer management, *Nutrition* 12:358, 1996.

66. Lennard-Jones JE: Ethical and legal aspects of nutrition and hydration, *Nurs Stand* 13:33, 1998.

67. Loprinzi CL and others: Randomized comparison of megestrol acetate versus dexamethasone versus fluoxymesterone for the treatment of cancer anorexia/cachexia, *J Clin Oncol* 17:3299, 1999.

68. Mann M and others: Glucocorticoidlike activity of megestrol. A summary of Food and Drug Administration experience and a review of the literature, *Arch Intern Med* 157:1651, 1997.

69. Mantovani G and others: Cytokine activity in cancer-related anorexia/cachexia: role of megestrol acetate and medroxyprogesterone acetate, *Semin Oncol* 25(2 suppl 6):45, 1998.

70. Maruyama M and others: Subcutaneously implanted enteral nutrition port, *JPEN J Parenter Enteral Nutr* 21:238, 1997.

71. Masoorli S: Central lines: controversies in care, *Nursing* 27:72, 1997.

72. Mattox TW: Specialized nutrition management of patients receiving hematopoietic stem cell transplantation, *Nutr Clin Pract* 14:5, 1999.

73. McMahon K and others: Integrating proactive nutritional assessment in clinical practices to prevent complications and cost, *Semin Oncol* 25(2 suppl 6):20, 1998.

74. McMillan DC and others: A pilot study of megestrol acetate and ibuprofen in the treatment of cachexia in gastrointestinal cancer patients, *Br J Cancer* 76:788, 1997.

75. McMillan DC and others: A prospective randomized study of megestrol acetate and ibuprofen in gastrointestinal cancer patients with weight loss, *Br J Cancer* 79:495, 1999.

76. Meares CJ: Primary caregiver perceptions of intake cessation in patients who are terminally ill, *Oncol Nurs Forum* 24:1751, 1997.

77. Mercadante S: Nutrition in cancer patients, *Support Care Cancer* 4:10, 1996.

78. Mercadante S: Parenteral versus enteral nutrition in cancer patients: indications and practice, *Support Care Cancer* 6:85, 1998.

79. Moldawer LL, Copeland EM: Proinflammatory cytokines, nutritional support, and the cachexia syndrome interactions and therapeutic options, *Cancer* 79:1828, 1997.

80. Moller P and others: Gastrostomy by various techniques: evaluation of indications, outcome, and complications, *Scand J Gastroenterol* 34:1050, 1999.

81. Monk-Tutor MR: The US home infusion market, *Am J Health Syst Pharm* 55:2019, 1998.

82. Murray M, Decker GM: Diet, nutrition, and lifestyle changes. In Decker GM, editor: *An introduction to complementary and alternative therapies,* Pittsburgh, Oncology Nursing Press, 1999.

83. Murry DJ and others: Impact of nutrition on pharmacokinetics of anti-neoplastic agents, *Int J Cancer* 11(suppl):28, 1998.

84. Myers JS: Herbal medicine. In Decker GM, editor: *An introduction to complementary and alternative therapies,* Pittsburgh, Oncology Nursing Press, 1999.

85. Najari Z, Rusho WJ: Compatibility of commonly used bone marrow transplant drugs during Y-site delivery, *Am J Health Syst Pharm* 54:181, 1997.

86. Nelson K and others: A phase II study of delta-9-tetrahydrocannabinol for appetite stimulation in cancer associated anorexia, *J Palliat Care* 10:14, 1994.

87. Neri B and others: Effect of medroxyprogesterone acetate on the quality of life of the oncologic patient: a multicentric cooperative study, *Anti-Cancer Drugs* 8:459, 1997.

88. Niyongabo T and others: Comparison of methods for assessing nutritional status in HIV-infected adults, *Nutrition* 15:740, 1999.

89. Noble C: Nutritional support in HIV infection: the use of enteral feeding to achieve weight gain and meet nutritional requirements in a patient with AIDS, *J Hum Nutr Diet* 9:69, 1996.

90. O'Brien G and others: G-tube site care: a practical guide, *RN* 62:52, 1999.

91. O'Connor KG: Gastric cancer, *Semin Oncol Nurs* 15:26, 1999.

92. Okusaka T and others: Prognosis of advanced pancreatic cancer patients with reference to calorie intake, *Nutr Cancer* 32:55, 1998.

93. Ottery F: Supportive nutritional management of the patient with pancreatic cancer, *Oncology* 10(9 suppl):26, 1996.

94. Ottery FD: Cancer cachexia: prevention, early diagnosis and management, *Cancer Pract* 2(2):123, 1994.

95. Ottery FD: Definition of standardized nutritional assessment and interventional pathways in oncology, *Nutrition* 12(1 suppl):S15, 1996.

96. Philip J, Depczynski B: The role of total parenteral nutrition for patients with irreversible bowel obstruction secondary to gynecological malignancy, *J Pain Symptom Manage* 13:104, 1997.

97. Phipps E: Nutrition and hydration for the terminally ill, *JAMA* 273:1736, 1995.

98. Pironi L: Nutritional aspects of elderly cancer patients, *Rays* 22(1 suppl):42, 1997.

99. Plata-Salaman CR: Cytokines and anorexia: a brief overview, *Semin Oncol* 25(1 suppl 1):64, 1998.

100. Puccio M, Nathanson L: The cancer cachexia syndrome, *Semin Oncol* 24:277, 1997.

101. Puntis JW: The economics of home parenteral nutrition, *Nutrition* 14:809, 1998.

102. Reddy P, Malone M: Cost and outcome analysis of home parenteral and enteral nutrition, *JPEN J Parenter Enteral Nutr* 22:302, 1998.

103. Rivadeneira DE and others: Nutritional support of the cancer patient, *CA Cancer J Clin* 48:69, 1998.

104. Rock CL and others: Factors associated with weight gain in women after a diagnosis of breast cancer. Women's Healthy Eating and Living Study Group, *J Am Diet Assoc* 99:1212, 1999.

105. Sakurai Y, Klein S: Metabolic alteration in patients with cancer: nutritional implications, *Surg Today* 28:247, 1998.

106. Samlowski WE and others: Effects of total parental nutrition (TPN) during high-dose interleukin-2 treatment for metastatic cancer, *J Immunother* 21:65, 1998.

107. Say J: Nutritional assessment in clinical practice: a review, *Nurs Crit Care* 2:29, 1997.

108. Schiller MR and others: Patients report positive nutrition counseling outcomes, *J Am Diet Assoc* 98:977, 1998.

109. Scolapio JS and others: Gastrointestinal motility considerations in patients with short bowel syndrome, *Dig Dis* 15:253, 1997.

110. Seligman PA and others: Approach to the seriously ill or terminal cancer patient who has a poor appetite, *Semin Oncol* 25(2 suppl 6):33, 1998.

111. Shike M: Percutaneous endoscopic stomas for enteral feeding and drainage, *Oncology* 9:39, 1995.

112. Sigley T: Nutrition support of the bone marrow transplant patient, *Top Clin Nutr* 13:35, 1998.

113. Sikora SS and others: Role of nutrition support during induction chemoradiation therapy in esophageal cancer, *JPEN J Parenter Enteral Nutr* 22:18, 1998.

114. Smith PE, Smith AE: High-quality nutritional interventions reduce costs, *Healthcare Financial Manage* 51:66, 1997.

115. Snider RD, Kruse JA: Catheter breakage: an unusual complication of nasoenteric feeding tubes, *Am J Gastroenterol* 90:1171, 1995.

116. Souba WW: Nutritional support. In DeVita VT, Hellman S, Rosenberg SA, editors: *Cancer: principles and practice of oncology,* ed. 5, Philadelphia, Lippincott-Raven, 1997.

117. Steiner N, Bruera E: Methods of hydration in palliative care patients, *J Palliat Care* 14:6, 1998.

118. Strang P: The effect of megestrol acetate on anorexia, weight loss and cachexia in cancer and AIDS patients, *Anticancer Res* 17:657, 1997.

119. Tchekmedyian NS: Pharmacoeconomics of nutritional support in cancer, *Semin Oncol* 25(2 suppl 6):62, 1998.

120. Tisdale MJ: Biology of cachexia, *J Natl Cancer Inst* 89: 1763, 1997.

121. Tisdale MJ: Wasting in cancer, *J Nutr* 129(1S suppl): 243S, 1999.

122. Treston-Aurand J and others: Impact of dressing materials on central venous catheter infection rates, *J Intraven Nurs* 20:201, 1997.

123. Trissel LA and others: Compatibility of parenteral nutrient solutions with selected drugs during simulated Y-site administration, *Am J Health Syst Pharm* 54:1295, 1997.

124. Trissel LA and others: Compatibility of medications with 3-in-1 parenteral nutrition admixtures, *JPEN J Parenter Enteral Nutr* 23:67, 1999.

125. Vadell C and others: Anticachectic efficacy of megestrol acetate at different doses versus placebo in patients with neoplastic cachexia, *Am J Clin Oncol* 21:347, 1998.

126. Viall CD: Taking the mystery out of TPN, Part I, *Nursing* 25:34, 1995.

127. Viall CD: Taking the mystery out of TPN, Part II, *Nursing* 25:57, 1995.

128. Weidmann B and others: Hypersensitivity reactions to parenteral lipid solutions, *Support Care Cancer* 5:504, 1997.

129. Weitzman S: Alternative nutritional cancer therapies, *Int J Cancer* 11(suppl):69, 1998.

130. Welk TA: Clinical and ethical considerations of fluid and electrolyte management in the terminally ill client, *J Intravenous Nurs* 22:43, 1999.

131. Westman G and others: Megestrol acetate in advanced, progressive, hormone-intensive cancer. Effects on the quality of life: a placebo-controlled, randomized, multi-centre trial, *Eur J Cancer* 35:586, 1999.

132. White G: Nutrition update. Nutritional supplements and tube feeds: what is available? *Int J Palliat Nurs* 4:176, 1998.

133. Wilkes JD: Prevention and treatment of oral mucositis following cancer chemotherapy, *Semin Oncol* 25:538, 1998.

134. Williams DM: The current state of home nutrition support in the United States, *Nutrition* 14:416, 1998.

135. Williams R and others: Room service improves patient food intake and satisfaction with hospital food, *J Pediatr Oncol Nurs* 15:183, 1998.

136. Wilmore DW: Metabolic support of the gastrointestinal tract: potential gut protection during intensive cytotoxic therapy, *Cancer* 79:1794, 1997.

137. Wormleighton CV: Stability issues in home parenteral nutrition, *Clin Nutr* 17:199, 1998.

138. Yagi M and others: Complications associated with enteral nutrition using catheter jejunostomy after esophagectomy, *Surg Today* 29:214, 1999.

139. Yeh SS, Schuster MW: Geriatric cachexia: the role of cytokines, *Am J Clin Nutr* 70:183, 1999.

Pain Management

Carol J. Swenson

The time has arrived for nurses to step forward and implement quality pain management. As Dahl writes, "Despite two decades of work by health professionals from all disciplines, the undertreatment of cancer pain remains a major public health problem."[3]

Nurses play a major role in the successful management of the person who is experiencing cancer pain. One of the Oncology Nursing Society's (ONS) position statements on cancer pain is that *"nurses are responsible and accountable for implementation and coordination of the plan for management of cancer pain."*[126-128] In all health care settings this is important, because the nurse is the professional person who most often conducts the ongoing assessment and therefore can determine whether the pain has increased, whether side effects are being managed effectively, and, most importantly, whether the patient and family are satisfied with the pain relief provided. Nurses must accept the responsibility and accountability for the plan of care in the management of cancer pain.

With the pharmacologic agents and technology currently available, it is unfortunate when untreated cancer pain causes patients to suffer unnecessarily. It is estimated that 90% to 95% of pain can be relieved in the highly controlled settings of hospices or palliative care units, yet the question remains whether medications and technology are being adequately used to control cancer pain. Pain affects a person's sleeping pattern, family, work, and social relationships. Ultimately, it affects a patient's quality of life and possibly the will to live.

DEFINITIONS

Pain—"Whatever the experiencing person says it is, existing whenever the experiencing person says it does"[80] is the most global and patient-centered pain description. The American Pain Society (APS)[6] and the ONS position paper on pain[126-128] both use Merskey's definition of pain: "an unpleasant sensory and emotional experience associated with actual or potential tissue damage, or described in terms of such damage."[89] From these two descriptions of pain, it becomes apparent that pain is multidimensional and subjective. Because pain is a subjective experience, the patient is the only authority on its existence—not the health care professional.

Other definitions that assist in understanding the pain experience are suffering, tolerance, addiction, and dependence.

Suffering—a physical or mental experience, that the person dislikes (e.g., adversity, agony, anguish, torment, trouble). Suffering is more global than pain, because pain implies only the physical sphere, whereas suffering may be spiritual, emotional, or social as well as physical. Suffering is distinct from pain and can occur with or without the presence of pain.

Drug tolerance—the involuntary need for increasing doses of analgesic to achieve the same level of pain relief. The actual incidence of tolerance is not known, and many people will never develop it. According to Cherny, "true pharmacological tolerance to the analgesic effects of opioids is not a common clinical problem."[26] When an increase of medication is required, it is most often an event of disease progression, but tolerance must be considered. When drug tolerance develops, first the duration of relief decreases and then the level of pain relief decreases. Tolerance may occur with any route of analgesic administration. Sallerin-Caute and colleagues[116] studied 159 patients with refractory cancer pain and treated them with intrathecal morphine. There was a two- to threefold increase in dose over 90 days; they concluded that this may have been tolerance, but it did not interfere with satisfactory pain management. If tolerance is suspected, another opioid can be used. When another opioid is used, one third to one half of the equianalgesic dose should be given because cross-tolerance between narcotics is incomplete and the person may otherwise be overmedicated.[6]

Addiction—the use of narcotics for the psychological euphoric effect and not for the analgesic effect; there is overwhelming involvement with obtaining and using drugs for other than approved medical reasons. Addiction as a result of medically prescribed narcotics is rare (<1:1000). Porter and Jick[110] report that of 11,882 hospitalized patients who had received at least one opioid injection during hospitalization, there were only four cases of documented addiction in patients with no previous history of addiction. Most often health care professionals overestimate the incidence of addiction after prescribed opioids for medical purposes. The lay public is often also frightened of potential addiction and need education about the appropriate use of opioids and assurance that addiction is a nonissue in the management of cancer pain.

Physical dependence—the body's adaptation to the use of opioids without which abstinence syndrome (or withdrawal symptoms) will occur based on physiologic changes. The person with cancer who uses opioids for longer than 3 to 4 weeks will be physically dependent but is not addicted.[6,137] The physically dependent person will not have the craving for the euphoric effect and will not be engaging in drug-seeking behaviors. (See page 883 for directions on "weaning" the physically dependent person from opioids.)

According to McCaffery's definition, nurses must believe every patient who says that he has pain to not inadvertently miss treatment of pain. Lack of observable pain does not mean lack of pain.

PHYSIOLOGY OF PAIN TRANSMISSION

The complex neurophysiologic activity that results in pain comprises four steps (Fig. 30–1)[137]:

1. *Transduction* is the process by which noxious (i.e., painful) stimuli lead to electrical activity in the endings of the primary afferent fibers. The stimulus may be mechanical, thermal, or chemical, causing the release of biochemical substrates that lead to the generation of an action potential (influx of sodium, efflux of potassium, change in the charge along cellular membrane) and electrical changes in the neuron. The primary afferent pain fibers are:

   A—large myelinated fibers that have rapid conduction, and

   C—small unmyelinated fibers that have slower conduction.[56,95]

2. *Transmission* is the relay by which impulses are sent from the primary afferent nerves to the dorsal horn of the spinal cord. The primary afferent nerve terminates, and the spinothalamic tract neuron carries the message across to the contralateral side of the spinal cord, where it joins a group of fibers that carry pain messages.[137]

3. *Perception* is the translation of neural response into sensation in the cerebral cortex; the person recognizes the feeling as pain.

4. *Modulation* is the control of pain transmission and may include both inhibition and enhancement of nociceptive stimuli. Modulation involves opiate receptors in the cortex, midbrain, spinal cord, gastrointestinal (GI) tract, bladder, and uterus. They bind endogenous and exogenous opiates to block pain transmission.

In the past, theories of pain were developed because of the lack of the capability to determine precisely what occurs physiologically during the pain experience. Some of the past theories were as follows[84]:

- *Specificity*—the intensity of nociceptive stimulus and perception of pain are directly correlated and travel along specific pathways from the pain receptors to the spinal cord.
- *Gate control theory*—nociceptive impulses are transmitted via the spinothalamic tract but can be modulated in the spinal cord, brain stem, or cerebral cortex. Two types of afferent fibers have been identified: thinly myelinated A-delta fibers and unmyelinated C fibers. The substantia gelatinosa in the dorsal horn of the spinal cord is the proposed site of the "gating" mechanism.

Endorphins and enkephalins—in the mid-1970s these "morphine within" opioid-like substances in the brain and spinal cord were discovered.

Today studies are involved with the exact physiology of pain and people are researching the neurodynamics of pain. Paice,[95] writes of "unraveling the mystery of pain" and describes the primary afferent fibers, dorsal horn of the spinal cord, spinothalamic tract, cortex, and modulator systems and their interactions in the transmission and interpretation of pain.

Science may have progressed beyond the theory stage, but much is yet to be learned of this complex phenomenon called *pain*.

TYPES OF PAIN

Some of the ways that pain can be categorized are as follows (Table 30–1):

Acute pain—acute pain is brief in duration (<3–6 months), the cause is usually known, the intensity may range from mild to severe, and the treatment is aimed at elimination of the cause.

Chronic pain—chronic pain extends beyond 3 months, the cause may or may not be known, it has not responded to treatment, or it does not subside after the injury heals. The intensity may range from mild to severe, and treatment varies.

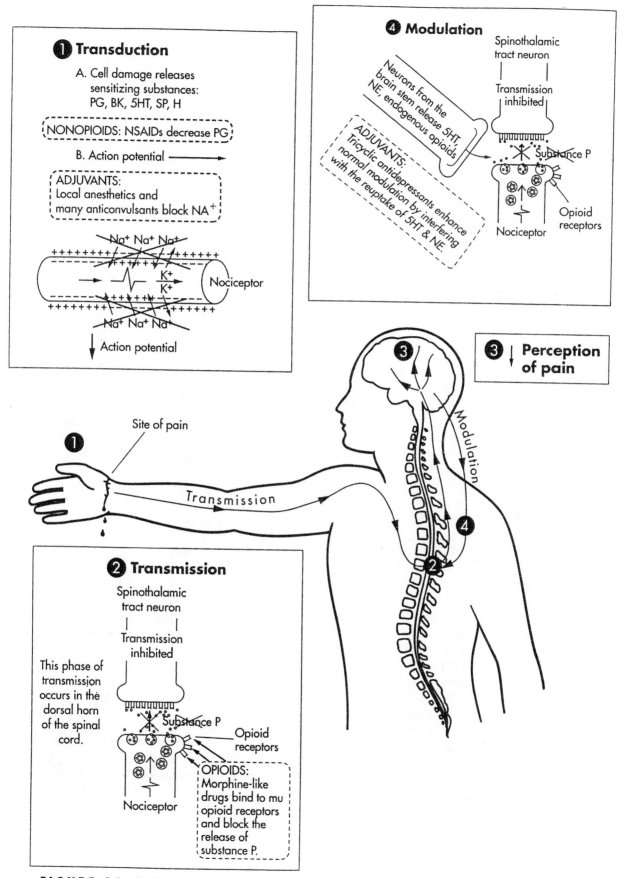

❶ Transduction

A. Cell damage releases sensitizing substances: PG, BK, 5HT, SP, H

NONOPIOIDS: NSAIDs decrease PG

B. Action potential ⟶

ADJUVANTS: Local anesthetics and many anticonvulsants block NA$^+$

Na^+ Na^+ Na^+

K^+ K^+

Nociceptor

Na^+ Na^+ Na^+

↓ Action potential

❹ Modulation

Spinothalamic tract neuron

Transmission inhibited

Neurons from the brain stem release 5HT, NE, endogenous opioids

ADJUVANTS: Tricyclic antidepressants enhance normal modulation by interfering with the reuptake of 5HT & NE.

Substance P

Nociceptor

Opioid receptors

Site of pain

❶

Transmission

❸ ↓ Perception of pain

❸

Modulation

❹

❷

❷ Transmission

Spinothalamic tract neuron

Transmission inhibited

This phase of transmission occurs in the dorsal horn of the spinal cord.

Substance P

Opioid receptors

OPIOIDS: Morphine-like drugs bind to mu opioid receptors and block the release of substance P.

Nociceptor

FIGURE 30–1 Mechanism of action. (From McCaffery M, Pasero C: *Pain: clinical manual,* ed 2, St. Louis, Mosby, 1999.)

TABLE 30-1

Characteristics of Acute and Chronic Pain and Chronic Cancer Pain

Acute Pain	Chronic Pain	Chronic Cancer Pain
Identifiable cause	Cause hard to find	Usually identifiable cause
Short duration	Lasts longer than several months	Duration varies
Sudden onset	Begins gradually and persists	Onset varies
Well defined	May or may not be well defined	May or may not be well defined
Limited	Unlimited	Unlimited
Decreases with healing	Persists beyond healing time	May persist beyond healing
Reversible	Exhausting and useless	Exhausting and useless
Objective signs and symptoms	Objective signs absent	Objective signs absent
Anxiety	Depression and fatigue	Depression, fatigue, and anxiety
Mild to severe	Mild to severe	Mild to severe
Presence of autonomic responses:	Absence of autonomic responses	Absence of autonomic responses
$\uparrow$ Heart rate		
$\uparrow$ Blood pressure		
$\uparrow$ Pupillary dilation		
$\uparrow$ Muscle tension		
$\downarrow$ GI motility		
$\downarrow$ Salivary flow		

Chronic cancer pain—cancer pain may be both acute and chronic. There is the time element of chronic pain, the intensity may be severe, the pain can be described as "intractable" (i.e., cannot be relieved), and it may be have several etiologies.

Breakthrough pain—sometimes referred to as *incident pain,* breakthrough pain is characterized as a transient increase in pain to greater than moderate intensity. Ferrell, Juarez, and Borneman define 'breakthrough pain' as "transitory episodes or flares of moderate to severe pain occurring in conjunction with chronic, persistent pain that is otherwise controlled."[52] They define 'incident pain' as "breakthrough pain that occurs in relation to specific activities (e.g., walking coughing). Petzke and coworkers[105] identified 39% of 613 cancer patients experienced transitory, incident, or breakthrough pain; Portenoy, Payne, and Jacobsen[108] found the incidence pain to be 51.2% in an oncology population. Petzke and colleagues identified these flares of pain as occurring spontaneously in 40% of the time, in relation to movement in 36% of the time, with coughing in 11% of the time, and related to other factors in 18% of 243 cancer patients.[105] Patients must be alerted that this can occur and to report it to health care providers so that appropriate medications can be ordered. Ferrell and coworkers found that 27% of a home care population with cancer did not have an order for any breakthrough analgesic.[52] Nurses can be strong advocates for patients in this instance and obtain analgesic orders to manage these events, which appear to occur in 39% to 51% of the oncology population.

INCIDENCE OF CANCER PAIN

Not all people with cancer experience pain. The incidence of cancer pain is difficult to determine, but several experts agree that the figure is 40% to 80% when considering all types and stages of cancer and Cherny states that pain is the most prevalent symptom experienced by cancer patients.[26] Levy states that 65% to 85% of patients with advanced cancer experience moderate to severe pain.[76] In 2000, the American Cancer Society (ACS) estimates cancer deaths at 552,200, which means that between 358,930 to 469,370 people in the United States may experience pain related to their diagnosis of cancer during 2000. Surveys have shown that 40% to 50% of patients fail to achieve adequate relief of cancer pain. Berry and coworkers found that 90% of 'worst pain' was not adequately controlled in a survey of 125 patients.[16] In a population of patients undgoing bone marrow transplantation, McGuire and coworkers found a pain incidence rate of 86% due to mucositis.[86]

Whether pain occurs in cancer depends on several factors. The major factors include the following:

Location of the primary or metastatic site of cancer. If there is bony involvement (as occurs with spinal metastases) or neural involvement (by direct tumor invasion or compression of any nerve tissue), the pain will be more severe than pressure caused by organ involvement.

Stage of the tumor activity. A patient in a later stage of cancer experiences pain more often and at a more severe intensity than a person who is in an early stage of disease.

ETIOLOGIES OF CANCER PAIN

There may be many causes for pain in the person with cancer. It is common that there are multiple pain sites; Caraceni and associates found that almost 25% of 1095 patients from 24 countries had two or more pains.[22]

Direct Tumor Involvement

Direct tumor involvement (e.g., proliferation of malignant cells within bone, nerves, viscera, soft tissue) is a cause for pain. The site of the pain produces different sensations and intensities. Also, the location of the site affects the type of analgesic indicated. A Memorial Sloan Kettering Cancer Center (MSKCC) survey found direct tumor involvement as the source of 78% and 62% of inpatients and outpatients, respectively.[56] The types of pain produced by direct tumor involvement may include the following:

Somatic pain (nociceptive)—results from stimulation of afferent nerves in the skin, connective tissue, muscles, joints, or bones. It is usually localized and described as throbbing, sharp, or aching and is localized. Caraceni and coworkers found the incidence to be 71.6% of cancer patients experiencing somatic pain[22]; Grond found an incidence of 64%.[61] The response to analgesics is usually good.

Visceral pain (nociceptive)—involves organs in the thoracic or abdominal area. It can be caused by infiltration, pressure, or distention. The pain is more diffuse and is often described as gnawing, crampy, constant, aching, or deep. This type of pain may be referred to cutaneous areas. Visceral pain may be seen in advanced pancreatic or liver cancer. Caraceni and coworkers found the incidence of visceral pain to be 34.7% of patients experiencing cancer pain.[22] In a study by Burrows and colleagues of patients with somatic and visceral pain, fatigue, physical well-being, nutrition, and total quality of life scores were negatively affected by the presence of pain.[21]

Neuropathic pain (deafferentation)—results from peripheral or central sensory nerve trauma injury causing abnormal firing. It is usually described as burning, shooting, lancinating, or tingling. Several neuropathic pain syndromes originate in the central or peripheral nerves. Caraceni and coworkers found the incidence of neuropathic pain to be 39.7% of patients experiencing cancer pain.[22] Grond found an incidence rate of 5% due to pure neuropathic pain, but when added to his mixed pain population (nociceptive and neuropathic, 31%), the total rate was 36%.[61] Response to analgesics is usually less predictable and coanalgesics are most often required.

Cancer pain syndrome—by definition, a syndrome is a number of different types of pain, different etiologies of pain, and different methods of treatment. Caraceni and colleagues identified types of pain syndromes.[22] Some of the known pain syndromes caused by direct tumor involvement are the following:

Bone involvement—multiple bony metastases are the most common cause of generalized bone pain. In the case of vertebral involvement, it is imperative that the nurse report this occurrence, because pain alone will precede nerve compression and prompt intervention may prevent neurologic deficit formation.

Peripheral nerves—sites where this may occur include the chest wall and retroperitoneal space, which may produce pain in the back, abdomen, or legs.

Brachial plexus—this is usually a result of a primary lung tumor (Pancoast syndrome), and aching is present in the shoulder and upper back. Patients with Pancoast syndrome may go on to develop cord compression if left untreated. Again, it is imperative that pain is assessed thoroughly, reported accurately, and treated promptly.[106]

Epidural spinal cord compression—patients with epidural spinal cord compression report pain, which may be focal or referred. The pain will precede any sensory or motor deficit, and again it is mandatory that any new back pain be communicated immediately.[106]

Cancer Treatment

Surgery, radiation therapy, or chemotherapy may exacerbate pain. An MSKCC survey found that treatment was the source of pain in 19% and 25% of inpatients and outpatients, respectively.[56] Some of the syndromes that may follow cancer treatment include the following:

Postthoracotomy pain syndrome—the intercostal nerve may be damaged at the time of surgery. This will usually be described as a burning pain (neuropathic).

Postmastectomy pain syndrome—the intercostobrachial nerve may be damaged at the time of surgery. This is usually described as a burning pain (neuropathic) and may occur soon after surgery or months later. Foley estimates that 4% to 10% of all women undergoing a breast surgical procedure are at risk to develop this syndrome.[56] Stevens and coworkers found a prevalence rate of 20% in a study of 95 women who had undergone breast cancer surgery; of this group 78.9% had a mastectomy and 21.1% had a lumpectomy.[129] Kwekkeboom[75] reviewed eight studies (1974–1993) on postmastectomy pain and found incidence rates of 8% to 100%; presence of pain was correlated with the extent of surgery (i.e., lumpectomy, modified radical mastectomy, traditional radical mastectomy), whether the intercostobrachial nerve was spared, and the number of axillary lymph nodes removed. There was a minor decrease of the incidence of pain over time, although for many it did persist for years.

Postamputation syndrome—this may be caused by the formation of a neuroma that has both lancinating (shooting) and "burning" components, or it may be a phantom sensation that exhibits both continuous dysesthesia and "shooting" pain.[106]

Multiple neural involvement—several neural areas may be affected by chemotherapy (principally the vinca alkaloids [e.g., vincristine] or cisplatin). This paresthesia or dysesthesia tends to be dose-related and will generally improve over 6 to 12 months.

Mucositis—the inflammation of the oral mucosa as a side effect of some of the chemotherapeutic agents (especially the antimetabolites) can produce intensely painful ulcerations. It is not uncommon for patients to require opioids to relieve pain during this period.

Postradiation pain—there may be unintentional damage to the spinal cord, mucosa, or bone as a result of radiation fibrosis.

The pain associated with cancer therapies may occur immediately or long after the therapy is started, making it more difficult to determine whether the pain is the result of a complication of therapy or recurrent disease.

Pain Unrelated to Cancer

Conditions unrelated to cancer (e.g., arthritis, decubitus, tension headache, diabetic neuropathy) can cause pain for the cancer patient. An MSKCC survey found 3% and 10% of inpatients and outpatients, respectively, had pain unrelated to their cancer.[56]

If someone is immunocompromised, it is not unusual for the person to develop herpes zoster (shingles). After the treatment and healing phase, a postherpetic neuralgia can remain that can be difficult to manage and needs to be addressed as a neuropathic pain in origin.

Any pain usually has special significance for the patient with cancer. Whether it is a "routine" headache or gastritis, the fear is that the pain represents an extension of the cancer. All reports of pain must be evaluated.

When there is obvious trauma to a body part, the source of one's pain is evident, but with cancer it is often difficult to determine the anatomic injury that may be occurring, and full assessment and evaluation is warranted.

FACTORS AFFECTING RESPONSE TO PAIN

An individual's response to pain is influenced by several factors, which helps explain why pain is such a complex experience.

Anxiety

In a Gallup poll conducted in the late 1990s, 70% of the people feared dying in pain or alone.[57] This fear of pain may be a cause for stress and anxiety for cancer patients. Anxiety is considered to be the most important factor affecting an individual's response to pain because it affects a person's ability to tolerate and cope with pain. One of the causes of anxiety is the belief that the pain is due to the cancer. Smith and coworkers found that patients who believed that the cause of their pain was cancer had a significantly higher intensity of pain than those who did not believe that their cancer was the cause of the pain.[123] A study of cancer pain patients and chronic noncancer pain patients was conducted by Turk and coworkers[135, 136] and they found many shared features between the two groups. One difference, however, was the higher level of support given by significant others to those who had cancer. Measures of support from loved ones can indeed have an impact on reducing anxiety, thus resulting in better pain management. Nurses can be important in eliciting those behaviors from family and friends.

Because increased anxiety increases pain, any strategy nurses can use to decrease a patient's anxiety will help control pain. Measures to decrease anxiety (e.g., distraction, relaxation) will be covered in a later section of this chapter. It is important to ask the patient and family members what has helped control the patient's anxiety in the past. Many of these measures can be incorporated into the patient's individual plan of care.

Personal Life Experience

In general, the more experience of pain one has in childhood, the greater the perceptions of pain in adulthood. It is important for the nurse to discuss past pain with the patient. Smith and coworkers studied 32 cancer patients before and after a physical therapy session.[123] They found that recall was assimilated to present pain levels and there was a positive correlation between past recall of pain intensity and present pain intensity. The nurse should also determine what measures have helped relieve pain in the past. Even though some measures may seem unlikely to help, if they are not harmful or contraindicated, they may aid the patient's pain treatment plan. The nurse should also determine what measures have not helped relieve pain in the past.

Nurses must be cognizant of what personal values and preferences may influence their professional practice. McCaffery and Ferrell found that nurses' judgment in accepting a patient's self-report of pain and in deciding what dose of analgesic they would administer was dependent on which role they assumed, as nurse or sibling, in pain scenarios.[81] As a sibling they were more ready to accept the patient's self-report of pain and to administer a higher, more appropriate analgesic dose than when they identified with the nurse role.

Over the years the question of whether gender influences response to pain has been explored. Turk and Okifuji found no significant difference between men and women on past analgesic treatment, current analgesic use, pain or disability.[136]

Culture and Religion

Acceptable responses to pain are learned at a very early age. Cultural and religious practices in one's family play an important role in the pain experience. Some cultures may view the expression of pain or suffering as a weakness, so they tend to minimize pain. Other cultures expect expression of pain, so they may have greater overt manifestations of pain. The issue of ethnicity and its relation to pain is not resolved.[118]

In a multicultural study of beliefs about reporting cancer pain and using analgesics, Ward and coworkers identified cultural barriers to pain management.[141] The three top fears among three cultures were found to be as follows:

Non-Hispanic White	Hispanic	Taiwanese
Addiction	Tolerance	Tolerance
Disease progression	Disease progression	Disease progression
Side effects	Addiction	Addiction

It is of interest that the non-Hispanic white group was the only group to identify side effects as a fear and that all groups identified addiction as a fear. It is important to realize that not all people manifest pain in the same way and that there is no right or wrong way. The nurse should accept all patients' expressions of pain, regardless of their cultural or religious backgrounds.

BARRIERS TO ADEQUATE CANCER PAIN MANAGEMENT

Lack of Knowledge

It is well documented that there is a lack of professional health care education regarding pain management that has resulted in less than optimal pain management for the person with cancer. Carron and colleagues[24] reviewed four general medical textbooks for end-of-life content, including symptom management, and found that most included some information, but none of them was rated as having helpful information on how to care for a dying patients. In a review of 50 textbooks from multiple specialties, Rabow and coworkers also found

an absence of end-of-life content; in 56.9% of the textbooks, expected content was absent.[111]

Whether in basic or continuing educational opportunities, nurses often have not been taught how to assess pain or to use different treatment modalities, especially medications, appropriately. Many nurses are not familiar with the pharmacokinetics of analgesics, the types of analgesics available, equianalgesic dosages, novel routes of delivery, or principles of scheduling administration.

Inadequate pain management education is not limited to the nursing professions. Mortimer and Bartlett[91] report a survey of internal medicine house staff, radiation oncology residents and hematology/oncology fellows who found that only 5% of them were able to convert correctly from parenteral to oral morphine. In addition 15% of the subjects "believed that addiction occurred in more than 50% of patients."[91(p 23)] Breitbart and coworkers found an inverse correlation between pain management expertise and negative attitudes and barriers.[18] Thus, provider education in the area of pain management will help to reduce the barrier of negative attitudes. According to Hill, cancer pain management has had only limited and unsatisfactory results.[64] He proposes that pain education should be included in undergraduate curriculum and not be left to the postgraduate level. He describes undergraduate nursing as "more effective," because they are more intimately involved with patients and are present on an ongoing basis.

McCaffery and Ferrell reviewed nurses' pain knowledge through surveys conducted 1988–1995.[82, 83] They found that there was an increase in nurses who accepted the patient's self-report of pain (i.e., 40.7% to 72.0%). There was also an increase in the nurses who increased an ineffective dose of morphine (i.e., 32.8% to 46.8%). Analysis of nurses' responses regarding the incidence of addiction being less than 1% also showed an increase in correct answers (i.e., 43.0% to 62.7%). Overall the correct responses to all questions also increased (i.e., 32.8% to 46.8%); thus, the total correct was still less than 50%.

There is a call for continuing education of all health care team members so that adequate pain control can be achieved. Grant and colleagues describe a 3-day pain education program for nurses.[60] The goal of the project is process improvement to provide quality patient care through adequate pain management. Positive advances have been made in recent years, and nurses have been instrumental in the development of the hospice movement, oncology nursing's focus on symptom management (i.e., pain), and individual state cancer pain initiatives.

Pederson and Parran report that a population of bone marrow transplant nurses had a knowledge score of 79% and that some nurses are more expert than others are.[103]

Nurses with more knowledge have the opportunity to mentor colleagues in need of more information to better meet patient needs.

With today's knowledge and technology, nurses can assist the patient and family to achieve better pain management outcomes.

Regulatory Issues

False perceptions exist about narcotic regulations, both nationally and in many states. Von Roenn and coworkers conducted a study among Eastern Cooperative Oncology Group (ECOG) physicians and found that 18% identified excessive state regulation of analgesics as a barrier to cancer pain management.[140] Weissman,[144] in an article on the history of narcotic control in the United States, explores the development of legal issues. He concludes with the statement that "physicians need to work with their state regulatory agencies" to identify impediments to patient care. In 1998, the Federation of State Medical Boards of the United States developed a policy document entitled "Model Guidelines for the Use of Controlled Substances for the Treatment of Pain." It promotes the principle that quality medical practice dictates that people have access to appropriate and effective pain relief. Many states allow advanced-practice nurses to prescribe analgesics, but some do not permit this and others have multiple restrictions related to pain management. Each state's practice act must be studied for nursing and physician barriers.

Myths and Misconceptions

The lay public and some health care professionals have held many myths and misconceptions about cancer pain management that are now being addressed. Some of these myths and misconceptions follow:

The person taking pain medications will easily become addicted. In a study by Paice and coworkers, 55.6% of patients reported being concerned about addiction.[97]
Cancer pain cannot really be relieved; it is part of the disease.
The "strong stuff" must be saved for later when the pain gets "really bad," or nothing will be available. Riddell and Fitch report on a study of patients' knowledge of pain management.[112] The mean score was 536.3 (of a possible 1000) and the item that showed the greatest knowledge deficit was "It is important to give the lowest amount of medicine possible to save the larger doses for later when the pain is worse." Paice and coworkers found that 39.4% of patients expressed this same concern.[97]
"Shots" are stronger than pills.
If opiates are administered routinely, death will be hastened as a result of respiratory depression.

In a study of 239 patients, Thomason and colleagues[132] identified two concerns shared by more than 50% of the subjects: (1) should be able to tolerate pain without medication and (2) side effects. The myth here is that a person should just put up with the pain and the misconception is that side effects cannot be managed; if the side effect of concern is respiratory depression, the fear may be that death would result. Patient education can alleviate both of these myths. Pain management education is important to patients and families. Effective teaching can improve patient compliance with analgesic regimens and improve quality of life.[50]

Denying the existence of pain may function as a coping mechanism because any presence of pain may be viewed as disease progression. This must be evaluated in light of other factors (e.g., personality trait of stoicism, cultural beliefs, attitudes). Myths and misconceptions must be addressed by the health care professional in the initial assessment of pain and in subsequent reassessments.

DEVELOPMENTS IN CANCER PAIN MANAGEMENT

During the 1970s the hospice movement established itself in the United States. Throughout the country in large and small communities, home care, free-standing, hospital-based, or agency-affiliated programs started serving the population who had a life expectancy of 6 months or less. With this focus of care delivery, pain became one of the central symptom management issues. Hospice nurses led the way in recognizing the uniqueness of cancer pain and became the nursing profession's experts through hands-on practice.

1974—The International Association for the Study of Pain (IASP) was formed. The APS is a national chapter of IASP.

1982—The World Health Organization (WHO) established a program in the cancer unit to study the incidence of cancer pain and to provide guidelines for cancer pain management. A 1984 meeting resulted in the publication of the booklet *Cancer Pain Relief* in 1986. The international WHO three-step analgesic ladders has been implemented in a number of countries (Fig. 30–2). This ladder provides logical steps of progression of analgesics to treat the needs of the person who has pain. The WHO published a revised edition, *Cancer Pain Relief and Palliative Care*, in 1990. Continuing with a focus on pain, in 1997 the WHO published *Looking Forward to Cancer Pain Relief for All*.

1986—The WHO established the Wisconsin Cancer Pain Initiative as the demonstration project site of the United States to "develop a comprehensive program to reduce cancer pain in the state of Wisconsin." Dahl describes the initiatives as based on a collaborative approach that depends on mutual respect and listening.[32]

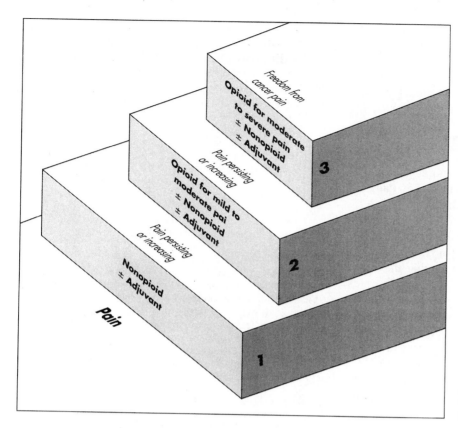

FIGURE 30-2 The World Health Organization (WHO) three-step analgesic ladder. (From World Health Organization: *Cancer pain relief,* ed 2, Geneva, Switzerland, Author, 1996.)

All of the established state cancer pain initiative programs have nurse involvement, and a nurse leads some state programs. State cancer pain initiatives address the issues of government regulations, myths and misconceptions of lay people and professionals, and professional education of pain management strategies. Education also includes assertiveness and a cancer pain role model education program has been implemented by the Wisconsin Cancer Pain Initiative. Weissman and Dahl[145] found that interdisciplinary team participants demonstrated a significant improvement in cancer pain knowledge as a result of the 1-day conference and that the teams had completed 227 educational or clinical practice projects.

1990—The APS published its "Standards on Acute and Cancer Pain." This interdisciplinary professional pain organization recognized that there was a means of setting criteria against which quality of practice could be measured. (See section on Quality Assessment and Improvement.)

1990—The ONS published its detailed document, "Oncology Nursing Society Position Paper on Cancer Pain,"[126-128] which includes the following:

- Introductory material
- Scope of nursing practice regarding cancer pain
- Ethics
- Practice (problem identification, assessment, planning, implementation and coordination, evaluation)

- Education (basic, graduate, continuing, patient, public)
- Research
- Resources
- Nursing administration
- Social policy
- Pediatric cancer pain

This document is a thorough and concise paper on quality pain management and nursing's role in providing this management.

1990—The American Society of Pain Management Nurses (ASPMN) was formed. This professional organization addresses acute, chronic, and cancer pain with a goal of the education of nurses in pain management. Position statements developed by ASPMN include "Assisted Suicide," "End of Life Care," and the "Use of Placebos for Pain Management."

1991—The American Nurses Association (ANA) published a "Statement on Promoting Comfort and Relieving Pain in Dying Patients" on September 5, 1991. This position statement underscores the difference between relieving pain and mercy killing.[30] It stresses the vital role and responsibilities of the professional nurse in the management of pain.

1991—The governmental Agency on Health Care Policy and Research (AHCPR) formed an expert panel to develop guidelines on pain management. The AHCPR was established in 1989 to enhance the quality, appropriateness, and effectiveness of health care services and access to those services. It was decided that there would indeed be the need for two separate documents: one on acute operative and trauma pain and one on cancer pain. In 1992, the acute pain guideline was published, and the cancer pain guideline followed in 1994. There has been legislation passed by the House of Representatives to rename AHCPR; the proposed new name is Agency for Health Research and Quality (AHRQ), but at the time of writing this is not yet official.

1992—The Ad Hoc Committee on Cancer Pain of the American Society of Clinical Oncology (ASCO) published "Cancer Pain Assessment and Treatment Curriculum Guidelines," which can guide systematically designed educational programs.[106] In 1998, ASCO adopted the policy of "Cancer Care During the Last Phase of Life." The document addresses the multiple issues at the end of life; regarding pain, it states "Trustworthy assurance that physical and mental suffering will be carefully attended to and comfort measures intently secured. The technology exists to relieve pain and other symptoms in nearly all of our patients, if we use it."[9]

1992—The Joint Commission on Accreditation for Healthcare Organizations (JCAHO) included pain management as a component of the Patients' Rights chapter. In 2000, JCAHO implemented comprehensive standards that are scored starting in 2001. (See section on Quality Assessment and Improvement.) In July 2000, the Board of Commissioners of JCAHO approved the implementation of new pain standards, which are within six chapters and are included in all manuals (i.e., hospitals, home care agencies, long-term care facilities, behavioral health facilities, outpatient clinics, and health plans).

1998—The ONS adopted the position statement on "Cancer Pain Management." The document states that "There is no defensible reason why people with cancer should suffer from unrelieved pain, yet undertreatment of pain persists."[94]

1998—The Federation of State Medical Boards of the United States published their policy statement "Model Guidelines for the Use of Controlled Substances for the Treatment of Pain." This meaningful document is designed to allay concerns of the medical community regarding prescribing opioids for pain management. It contains a strong statement that the principles of quality medical practice dictate that people have access to appropriate and effective pain relief.

1998—The American Geriatrics Society adopted clinical practice guidelines "The Management of Chronic Pain in Older Persons." It was recognized that pain is common in older people and that chronic pain produces many numerous consequences[4] (Table 30–2).

Much time and effort have been spent studying the problem of cancer pain; identifying barriers, and establishing practice guidelines and standards. It is time to implement what is already known and make an impact on patients who experience cancer pain. Nurses do have an active role in pain teams.

PHARMACOLOGIC INTERVENTIONS

With optimal pharmacologic management alone, 70% to 90% of cancer pain can be adequately relieved.

Nonopioid Analgesics

The nonopioids work primarily at the peripheral nervous system level and are used for mild to moderate pain, especially of bone metastases, soft-tissue infiltration, or arthritis (i.e., somatic pain). The categories of nonopioids include aspirin, acetaminophen, and the nonsteroidal anti-inflammatory drugs (NSAIDs).

Most NSAIDs block the production of prostaglandins, which are chemicals produced when cells are damaged. Until the discovery of COX-2 inhibitors, all NSAIDs had potential GI side effects, and this limited their use over time. Most NSAIDs interfere with platelet aggregation and therefore are not appropriate for someone who is thrombocytopenic; there are now platelet-sparing NSAIDs (e.g., chorine magnesium trisalicylate,

---

TABLE 30-2
American Geriatrics Society—Clinical Practice Guidelines on Chronic Pain in Older Persons

RECOMMENDATIONS

I. All older patients with diminished quality of life as a result of chronic pain are candidates for pharmacologic therapy.
II. The least invasive route of administration should be used (this is usually the oral route).
III. Fast-onset, short-acting analgesic drugs should be used for episodic (i.e., chronic recurrent or noncontinuous) pain.
IV. Acetaminophen is the drug of choice for relieving mild to moderate musculoskeletal pain. The maximum dosage of acetaminophen should not exceed 4000 mg/d.
V. NSAIDs should be used with caution.
VI. Opioid analgesic drugs may be helpful for relieving moderate to severe pain, especially nociceptive pain.
VII. Fixed-dose combinations (e.g., acetaminophen and opioid) may be used for mild to moderate pain.
VIII. Patients taking analgesic medications should be monitored closely.
IX. Nonopioid analgesic medications may be appropriate for some patients with neuropathic pain and some other chronic pain syndromes.

From American Geriatrics Society Panel on Chronic Pain in Older Persons: The management of chronic pain in older persons, J Am Geriatr Soc 46(5):635–651, 1998. Reprinted by permission of Blackwell Science, Inc.

nabumetone, celecoxib, rofecoxib) and drug side effect profiles must be read carefully before using when potential bleeding is to be avoided.

The NSAID mechanism of action is believed to be inhibition of cyclooxygenase activity and prostaglandin synthesis, but other mechanisms may exist. It is now known that there are two cyclooxygenase enzymes known as COX-1 and COX-2. Inhibition of COX-1 produces the GI side effects of the traditional NSAIDs, but inhibition of COX-2 inhibits prostaglandin synthesis, and thereby the resulting pain, with reduced gastric irritation. Celecoxib (Celebrex) is the first of the COX-2 drugs approved; it is contraindicated in patients with sulfa allergies. A second COX-2 inhibitor, rofecoxib (Vioxx) is also available. There is no effect on platelet aggregation or bleeding time and therefore a COX-2 inhibitor is the choice of NSAIDs, in the thrombocytopenic patient, although there have not been trials done specifically with an oncology population. NSAIDs appear to be effective on both somatic and visceral pain sources.[87] Food decreases the rate of absorption and may delay the time to reach peak levels; therefore, NSAIDs should be taken between meals.

Nonopioids are often given together with opioids, and therefore a lower dose of opioid may be effective. Reduced morphine requirements were noted when ketorolac was administered to patients who had metastatic bone pain and/or opioid bowel syndrome; an H2 blocker was also administered to reduce GI side effects.[70]

An analgesic that does not fit the usual categories is capsaicin (Zostrix). It is derived from the Hungarian red pepper and is an antagonist that acts by depleting substance P. It is theorized that it may reduce the central transmission of information about pain and has been used in postmastectomy and postherpetic syndromes.[30] The 0.025% topical ointment is applied three or four times per day for several weeks. It does cause a burning sensation on application, and for some people this is distressing enough for them to stop the treatment (Table 30–3).

NMDA Analgesics

The N-methyl-D-aspartate (NMDA) receptor antagonists are the first new class of analgesics in 30 years.[138] These drugs do not act as analgesics directly, but in response to tissue injury and inflammation they enhance the response to opioids and prevent the development of tolerance. Two drugs being studied as analgesics in neuropathic pain states are dextromethorphan and ketamine. NMDA agents are also being developed in combination with opioids (e.g., morphine, oxycodone). In a study of patients with cancer pain, Mercadante and co-workers[88] found that there were no significant analgesic effects with the use of dextromethorphan at a dose of

30 mg three times a day. Bell[13] and Fine[53] both describe the use of low-dose ketamine (0.1–0.2 mg/kg) in cases where high-dose opioids were ineffective or intolerable side effects had developed. Opioid doses could be dramatically reduced without withdrawal symptoms. The future role of these agents as coanalgesics has not been established and additional research is required.

Opioid Analgesics

The opiates work primarily at the central nervous system (CNS) level. Those opioids used for mild to moderate pain often have acetaminophen or aspirin together with the opiate. The nurse should be aware of the total dosage of aspirin/acetaminophen consumed per 24 hours. The maximum dose of either should not exceed 6000 mg/24 h. If two tablets containing 500 mg each are taken every 3 hours, the total is 8000 mg/24 h. Tables 30–4 and 30–5 present specifics for those weighing more than 50 kg and those weighing less than 50 kg.

It has been found that there is no ceiling effect of morphine, which means that the dose can continue to be escalated to provide analgesia with increased pain levels. Some drugs have a ceiling, and beyond that ceiling dose there is no added analgesic benefit. In exceptional instances, patients may require 1000 to 2000 mg morphine, or even more, per 24 hours, and the person will be alert, ambulatory, and participating in activities of daily living.

After many years of experience with meperidine (Demerol), caution has been expressed in two areas. First, it should never be used on a continuous basis for treatment of cancer pain because the metabolite (normeperidine) is a CNS stimulator,[71] and this hyperexcitability can lead to tremors, restlessness, negative mood alterations with irritability, myoclonus, hyperreflexia, and grand mal seizure activity with repeated dosing.[17] Second, the AHCPR Clinical Practice Guidelines include the warning against the use of meperidine for people who are taking monoamine oxidase inhibitors. "Severe adverse reactions, including death through mechanisms that mimic malignant hyperthermia, have been reported when these drugs are used together."[2]

Oxycodone is an agonist that at one time was available only in combination with acetaminophen or aspirin. It is now available as a single agent in a 5-mg tablet, solutions of 5 and 20 mg/mL, and as a time-release 12-hour preparation in 10-, 20-, 40-, and 80-mg tablets. As a single agent there is no ceiling effect, and the equianalgesic conversion is 1:1 to oral morphine. Zhukovsky and associates studied the potency of high-dose oral oxycodone and oral morphine and supported a 1:1 ratio of oral morphine to oxycodone.[151]

Methadone may be an alternative opioid if a patient is not controlled by conventional analgesics (e.g., mor-

Text continued on page 883

TABLE 30-3
Nonopioid Analgesics

Drug	Recommended Dose and Interval	Comments
PARA-AMINOPHENOL DERIVATIVE		
Acetaminophen (Tylenol, Panadol, Anacin-3, Excedrin, Midol, Sine-Aid)	500–1000 mg q 4–6 h	Similar to aspirin in analgesic and antipyretic effects, but only slight anti-inflammatory effects[28]; may not have effect on platelet aggregation; may cause liver toxicity in doses 4–6 g/d.[6]
ACETYLSALICYLIC		
Acetylsalicylic acid (aspirin)	500–1000 mg q 4–6 h	Standard anti-inflammatory; increased bleeding time caused by inhibition of platelet aggregation. Recommended maximum daily dose is 4–6 g/d.
NONACETYLATED SALICYLATE		
Choline magnesium Trisalicylates (Trilisate)	1000–1500 mg q 8–12 h	Minimal effect on platelet aggregation (platelet-sparing); available in liquid; minimal GI toxicity.
Diflunisal (Dolobid)	500–1000 mg q 8–12 h	Minimal antipyretic effect; minimal GI side effects.
Salsalate (Disalcid, Salsitab)	750–1000 mg q 8–12 h	Minimal GI side effects; may have minimal effect on platelet aggregation.
NSAID		
Propionic Acid Derivatives		
Ibuprofen (Motrin, Nuprin, Advil, Medipren)	400–800 mg q 8 h	Available as oral suspension; may require escalation.
Fenoprofen (Nalfon)	200–400 mg q 4–6 h	May require escalation.
Flurbiprofen (Ansaid, Froben)	100 mg q 12 h	Available as oral liquid. Maximum daily dose 1250 mg.
Naproxen (Naprosyn)	250–500 mg q 6–8 h	Faster onset than naproxen. Aleve is available in a 220-mg dose taken q 12 h. Maximum daily dose is 1375 mg.
Naproxen sodium (Anaprox)	275–550 mg q 6–8 h	
Ketoprofen (Orudis)	25–50 mg q 6–8 h	Available for rectal administration and as a topical gel.
Oxaprozin (Daypro)	600 mg q 12 h	Maximum daily dose is 1800 mg; used for arthritis.

Drug	Dose	Comments
Acetic Acid Derivative		
Indomethacin (Indocin)	25–50 mg q 8–12 h	Available as oral suspension and rectal suppository; high incidence of GI side effects.
Sulindac (Clinoril)	150–200 mg q 8–12 h	GI side effects common; lower incidence of renal toxicity.
Tolmetin (Tolectin)	200 mg q 6–8 h	Weak analgesic effect.
Ketorolac (Toradol)	30 mg q 6 h IM or IV 10 mg q 6 h PO	Only injectable NSAID; not recommended for use longer than 5 days; equivalent to 10 mg parenteral morphine.[70]
Phenylacetic Acid		
Diclofenac (Voltarem)	50 mg q 8 h	Used for dysmennorhea and arthritis.
Fenamate		
Mefenamic acid (Ponstel)	250 mg q 6 h	Not recommended for use longer than 7 days.
Meclofenamate (Meclomen)	50–100 mg q 6–8 h	Diarrhea may occur as well as other GI side effects.
Oxicam		
Piroxicam (Feldene)	20 mg q day in divided doses	Not recommended for patients with renal or liver dysfunction; effect may not be seen for 7–12 days.
Pyranocarboxylic		
Etodolac (Lodine)	200–400 mg q 6–8 h	May increase the serum levels of methotrexate if there is reduced renal excretion. Maximum daily dose is 1200 mg
Other		
Nabumetone (Relafen)	750–1000 mg q 24 h	Minimal effect on platelet aggregation (platelet-sparing). Used for arthritis. Maximum daily dose 2000 mg.
COX-2 Inhibitors		
Celecoxib (Celebrex)	100 mg BID or 200 mg qd	Approved for arthritis; reduced incidence of GI side effects; is platelet-sparing.[138]
Rofecoxib (Vioox)	12.5–25 mg qd	Approved for arthritis; reduced incidence of GI side effects; is platelet-sparing.

Data from Agency for Health Care Policy and Research (AHCPR): Management of cancer pain, 1994, Publication No. 94-0592; American Pain Society: Principles of analgesic use in the treatment of acute pain and chronic cancer pain, ed 4, 1999; McCaffery M, Portenoy RK: Nonopioids, acetaminophen, and nonsteroidal anti-inflammatory drugs (NSAIDs). In McCaffery M, Pasero C, editors: Pain: clinical manual, ed 2, St. Louis, Mosby, 1999.

TABLE 30-4
Dose Equivalents for Opioid Analgesics in Opioid-Naive Adults > 50 kg*

Drug	Approximate Equianalgesic Dose		Usual Starting Dose for Moderate to Severe Pain		Comments
	Oral	Parenteral	Oral	Parenteral	
OPIOID AGONIST†					
Morphine‡	30 mg q 3–4 h (repeat around-the-clock dosing)	10 mg q 3–4 h	5–10 mg q 3–4 h††	15–30 mg q 3–4 h (adults) 0.30 mg/kg (children)	Standard of comparison for narcotic analgesics; 3- to 4-h duration; the metabolite morphine-6-glucuronide may accumulate in patients with renal insufficiency[84]
Morphine controlled-release‡,§ (MS Contin, Oramorph SR)	90 mg q 12 h	N/A	30–60 mg q 12 h	N/A	12-h sustained-released preparation; available in 30-, 60-, 100-, and 200-mg tablets
Kadian	100 mg QD	N/A			Available as 24-h time-release tablets (20, 50, and 100 mg)
Hydromorphone‡ (Dilaudid)	7.5 mg q 3–4 h	1.5 mg q 3–4 h	2–4 mg q 3–4 h	1.5 mg q 3–4 h	Available R; high concentration is available for parenteral use
Methadone (Dolophine)	20 mg q 6–8 h	10 mg q 6–8 h	5–10 mg q 6–8 h	10 mg q 6–8 h	Good oral potency; long plasma half-life[88] accumulates with repetitive dosing
Levorphanol (Levo-Dromoran)	4 mg q 6–8 h	2 mg q 6–8 h	2 mg q 8 h	2 mg q 6–8 h	Long plasma half-life
Oxycodone (Roxicodone)	20 mg q 3–4 h	N/A	10–30 mg q 3–4 h	N/A	No ceiling effect; is available as 5-mg tablet and as 5 mg/mL and 20 mg/mL solution[117]
(OxyContin)	30 mg q 12 h	N/A	30 mg q 12 h	N/A	12-h sustained-released tablet; available in 10-, 20-, and 40-mg tablets; food has no significant effect on absorption; oral oxycodone is equal to morphine PO
Oxymorphone‡ (Numorphan)	N/A	1 mg q 3–4 h	N/A	1 mg q 3–4 h	5 mg R suppository = 5 mg parenteral morphine

Drug					Comments
Meperidine (Demerol)||	300 mg q 2–3 h	75 mg q 3 h	N/R	100 mg q 3 h	Shorter acting than morphine (2–3 h); toxic metabolite (normeperidine) accumulates with repeated dosing, causing central nervous system (CNS) excitation, which can lead to seizures; avoid use in patients on monoamine oxidase (MAO) inhibitors because of potential adverse reaction that mimics malignant hyperthermia and may lead to cardiovascular collapse[71]
Fentanyl (Sublimaze) (Duragesic)§	N/A *Transdermal conversion*	0.1 mg	N/A	N/A	Transdermal patch; 8- to 12-h delay[40,122] in onset and offset of patch; fever increases dose delivery rate
	Morphine parenteral (24 hs)	*Morphine PO (24 h)*		*Patch*	
	5–20 mg	15–60 mg		25 µg	
	25–35 mg	75–105 mg		50 µg	
	40–50 mg	120–150 mg		75 µg	
	55–65 mg	165–195 mg		100 µg	

COMBINATION OPIOID NSAID PREPARATION

Drug					Comments
Codeine (with aspirin or acetaminophen)**††	180–200 mg q 3–4 h	130 mg q 3–4 h	30–60 mg q 3–4 h	60 mg q 2 h IM/SC	
Hydrocodone (in Lorcet, Lortab, Vicodin, Norco, others)	30 mg q 3–4 h	N/A	5–10 mg q 3–4 h	N/A	
Oxycodone (Roxicodone, also in Percocet, Percodan, Tylox, others)	30 mg q 3–4 h	N/A	5–10 mg q 3–4 h	N/A	

MIXED AGONIST-ANTAGONIST

Drug			Comments
Pentazocine (Talwin)	180 mg q 3–4 h	60 mg q 3–4 h	May cause psychomimetic effects at high dose; may precipitate withdrawal in opioid-dependent patients; not recommended for cancer patients.

Table continued on following page

TABLE 30–4

Dose Equivalents for Opioid Analgesics in Opioid-Naive Adults > 50 kg* *Continued*

Drug	Approximate Equianalgesic Dose		Usual Starting Dose for Moderate to Severe Pain		Comments
	Oral	Parenteral	Oral	Parenteral	
Nalbuphine (Nubain)	N/A	10 mg q 3–4h			Not available orally; incidence of psychomimetic effects lower than that associated with pentazocine.
Butorphanol (Stadol)	N/A	2 mg q 3–4 h			Not available orally; incidence of psychomimetic effects lower than that associated with pentazocine; nasal spray is available.
Dezocine (Dalgan)		10 mg			Same profile of effects as that associated with nalbuphine.
PARTIAL AGONIST Buprenorphine (Buprenex)	N/A	0.3–0.4 mg q 6–8 h			May precipitate withdrawal in opioid-dependent patients; not readily reversed by naloxone.

* Caution: Recommended doses do not apply for adult patients with body weight < 50 kg. For recommended starting doses for adults < 50 kg body weight, see Table 30–5.

† Caution: Recommended doses do not apply to patients with renal or hepatic insufficiency or other conditions affecting drug metabolism and kinetics.

‡ Caution: For morphine, hydromorphone, and oxymorphone, rectal administration is an alternate route for patients unable to take oral medications. Equianalgesic doses may differ from oral and parenteral doses because of pharmacokinetic differences.

§ Transdermal fentanyl (Duragesic) is an alternative option. Doses above 25 μg/h should not be used in opioid-naive patients.

‖ Not recommended. Doses listed are for brief therapy. Switch to another opioid for long-term therapy.

** Caution: Doses of aspirin and acetaminophen in combination opioid/NSAID preparations must also be adjusted to the patient's body weight.

†† Caution: Codeine doses above 65 mg often are not appropriate because of diminishing incremental analgesia with increasing doses but continually increasing nausea, constipation, and other side effects.

Note: Published tables vary in the suggested doses that are equianalgesic to morphine. Clinical response is the criterion that must be applied for each patient; titration to clinical responses is necessary. Because there is not complete cross-tolerance among these drugs, it is usually necessary to use a lower than equianalgesic dose when changing drugs and to retitrate to response.

q, Every; N/A, not available; R, rectally; NR, not recommended.

Data from Agency for Health Care Policy and Research (AHCPR): Management of cancer pain, 1994, Publication No. 94-0592; American Pain Society: Principles of analgesic use in the treatment of acute pain and chronic cancer pain, ed. 4, 1999; Pasero C, Portenoy RK, and McCaffery M: Opioid analgesics. In McCaffery M, Pasero C, editors: Pain: clinical manual, ed 2, St. Louis, Mosby, 1999.

Dose Equivalents for Opioid Analgesics in Opioid-Naive Adults < 50 kg

Drug	Approximate Equianalgesic Dose		Usual Starting Dose for Moderate to Severe Pain		Comments
	Oral	Parenteral	Oral	Parenteral	
OPIOID AGONIST*					
Morphine[†]	30 mg q 3–4 h (repeat around-the-clock dosing) 60 mg q 3–4 h (single dose or intermittent dosing)	10 mg q 3–4 h	0.3 mg/kg q 3–4 h	0.1 mg/kg q 3–4 h	Standard of comparison for narcotic analgesics; 3- to 4-hour duration; the metabolite morphine-6-glucuronide may accumulate in patients with renal insufficiency[84]
Morphine, controlled-release[†,‡] (MS Contin, Oramorph SR)	90–120 mg q 12 h	N/A	N/A	N/A	12-h sustained-released preparation; available in 30-, 60-, 100-, and 200-mg tablets
Hydromorphone[†] (Dilaudid)	7.5 mg q 3–4 h	1.5 mg q 3–4 h	0.06 mg/kg q 3–4 h	0.015 mg/kg q 3–4 h	Available R; high concentration is available for parenteral use
Levorphanol (Levo-Dromoran)	4 mg q 6–8 h	2 mg q 6–8 h	0.04 mg/kg q 6–8 h	0.02 mg/kg q 6–8 h	Long plasma half-life
Meperidine§ (Demerol)	300 mg q 2–3 h	100 mg q 3 h	N/A	0.75 mg/kg q 2–3 h	Shorter acting than morphine (2–3 h); toxic metabolite (normeperidine) accumulates with repeated dosing, causing central nervous system (CNS) excitation, which can lead to seizures; avoid use in patients on monoamine oxidase (MAO) inhibitors because of potential adverse reaction that mimics malignant hyperthermia and may lead to cardiovascular collapse[71]

Table continued on following page

TABLE 30–5

Dose Equivalents for Opioid Analgesics in Opioid-Naive Adults < 50 kg *Continued*

Drug	Approximate Equianalgesic Dose		Usual Starting Dose for Moderate to Severe Pain		Comments
	Oral	Parenteral	Oral	Parenteral	
Methadone (Dolophine, others)	20 mg q 6–8 h	10 mg q 6–8 h	0.2 mg/kg q 6–8 h	0.1 mg/kg q 6–8 h	Good oral potency; long plasma half-life; accumulates with repetitive dosing
COMBINATION OPIOID NSAID PREPARATION‖					
Codeine (with aspirin or acetaminophen)‖	180–200 mg q 3–4 h	130 mg q 3–4 h	0.5–1 mg/kg q 3–4 h	N/A	Only available with acetaminophen
Hydrocodone (in Lorcet, Lortab, Vicodin, Norco, others)	30 mg q 3–4 h	N/A	0.2 mg/kg q 3–4 h	N/A	
Oxycodone (Roxicodone, also in Percocet, Percodan, Tylox, others)**	30 mg q 3–4 h	N/A	0.2 mg/kg q 3–4 h	N/A	Elixir available 5 mg/mL and 20 mg/mL; caution with impaired ventilation, asthma, increased intracranial pressure, and liver failure.
OxyContin					12-h time release; available in 10-, 20-, 40-, and 80- mg tablets
Dihydrocodeine 16 mg + acetaminophen 356.4 mg + caffeine 30 mg (DHC Plus)			1–2 tabs q 4 h	N/A	Is a schedule III product

Caution: Recommended doses do not apply to patients with renal or hepatic insufficiency or other condition affecting drug metabolism and kinetics.

†*Caution: For morphine, hydromorphone, and oxymorphone, rectal administration is an alternate route for patients unable to take oral medications. Equianalgesic doses may differ from oral and parenteral doses because of pharmacokinetic differences.*

‡*Transdermal fentanyl (Duragesic) is an alternative option. Doses above 25 µg/h should not be used in opioid-naive patients.*

§*Not recommended. Doses listed are for brief therapy. Switch to another opioid for long-term therapy.*

‖*Caution: Doses of aspirin and acetaminophen in combination opioid/NSAID preparations must also be adjusted to the patient's body weight.*

**Caution: Some clinicians recommend not exceeding 1.5 mg/kg of codeine because of an increased incidence of side effects with higher doses.*

Note: Published tables vary in the suggested doses that are equianalgesic to morphine. Clinical response is the criterion that must be applied for each patient; titration to clinical responses is necessary. Because there is not complete cross-tolerance among these drugs, it is usually necessary to use a lower than equianalgesic dose when changing drugs and to retitrate to response.

q, Every; N/A, not available; R, rectally; N/R, not recommended.

phine or hydromorphone). It is generally administered orally, but in the instance when someone is not able to take anything by mouth, a continuous infusion by the subcutaneous (SC) route could be tried.[55] Local inflammation may occur and the remedy may be the addition of dexamethasone (1–2 mg/24 h) added to the infusion.[78] Changing the infusion site every 3 to 4 days can also reduce the incidence of inflammation.

A newer opioid in the United States for moderate to severe pain is tramadol (Ultram). It acts centrally but is not related chemically to the opiates; it may bind to mu opioid receptors and inhibit reuptake of norepinephrine and serotonin.[76] It has been used in Germany and a study of cancer patients there. Grond[62] demonstrated that with high doses (≥300 mg/d), antiemetics, laxatives, neuroleptics, and steroids were needed less than with a patient group receiving morphine. More clinical trials are needed to establish its place in cancer pain management.

The question as to the efficacy of heroin over morphine has been studied with the conclusion that heroin does not offer any advantage over morphine when an equianalgesic conversion is done.[137] Heroin (diamorphine) is metabolized to morphine before it reaches the opiate receptors of the brain. Before the studies were done, heroin was most often the narcotic of choice in the Brompton's cocktail in hospice programs in England; now oral morphine is routinely used.

Mixed agonist-antagonists may also be used for moderate to severe pain. Using mixed agonist-antagonists to manage cancer pain should be done with caution for the following reasons:

- After using agonists (e.g., morphine), withdrawal-like symptoms can be precipitated when a mixed agonist-antagonist is given.
- If given with an agonist, the mixed form will antagonize and give poor pain relief with possible increase in psychomimetic effects.

Special Issues of Opioids

Titration/Escalating Doses. Most often an increasing need for medication is indicative of progressive disease or a developing complication, and thorough assessment is warranted. When it is determined that more medication is needed to manage an individual's pain, the safe plan of increasing the dose is to *increase 25% to 50% of the previous dose.*[106] Ferrell and McCaffery identified that almost half of a group of nurses did not correctly escalate an ineffective analgesic dose.[51] This is an area where nurses must develop their skills.

Example:

Current dose: 60 mg PO morphine q 4 h;
add: 15–30 mg PO morphine q 4 h; thus
new prescription: 75–90 mg PO morphine q 4 h.

Continue assessment to determine whether additional increases are needed.

Rescue Doses. An order should be obtained for an immediate-release analgesic to offer every 1 to 2 hours for breakthrough pain. The "rescue" medication should be the same drug (e.g., morphine) as the scheduled analgesic; a liquid immediate-release formula will act more rapidly than a tablet form. This dose should equal 33% to 50% of the regularly scheduled every-4-hour dose or 10% of the total 24-hour requirement. The rescue dose may be 5% to 15% of the 24-hour baseline dose.[36]

Example:

If 180-mg oral morphine were required per 24 hours, at 10% the rescue dose would be 20 mg.
If 30-mg oral morphine is scheduled q 4 h, at 50% the rescue dose would be 15 mg.

If three or more rescue doses are required per 24 hours, an order should be obtained that includes that rescue amount in the around-the-clock (ATC) dosing. The order for rescue dosing should be maintained. (See General Principles of Analgesic Administration, no. 4, page 888.)

Decreasing Doses. If a person's pain decreases (e.g., after palliative radiation to bone metastases, nerve block), the opioid requirements may indeed decrease dramatically. Abstinence syndrome (withdrawal) will occur if someone has required opioids multiple times per day for 1 month,[6] although the "Management of Cancer Pain" AHCPR guideline states that abstinence syndrome may occur after 2 weeks of opioid therapy.

S & S withdrawal during first 24 hours:

- Restlessness
- Lacrimation
- Rhinorrhea
- Yawning
- Perspiration
- Gooseflesh
- Restless sleep
- Mydriasis

S & S withdrawal during 24 to 72 hours:

- Twitching/muscular spasms
- Kicking movements
- Severe aches in back, abdomen, and legs
- Nausea, vomiting, diarrhea
- Coryza and severe sneezing
- Increase in all vital signs (temperature, pulse, respiration, and blood pressure)

To safely "wean" the person from the opioids and prevent abstinence syndrome from occurring, the following formula is used:

Give 50% of the previous order for 48 hours and then reduce by 25% every 48 hours until less than 10 to 15 mg (parenteral morphine equivalent) per 24 hours.[6]

Example: Patient has been receiving 180 mg morphine sulfate PO/24 h (at a 3:1 ratio, this is 60 mg parenteral morphine/24 h).

Days 1 and 2: 90 mg PO morphine sulfate/24 h
Days 3 and 4: 70 mg PO morphine sulfate/24 h
Days 5 and 6: 50 mg PO morphine sulfate/24 h
Days 7 and 8: 40 mg PO morphine sulfate/24 h
Days 9 and 10: 30 mg PO morphine sulfate/24 h (all preceding doses are 10 mg parenteral morphine equivalents)
Day 11: nothing

Duration of Opioids. Not all opioids have the same duration of effectiveness; some opioids are short acting, some are long acting, and some are in the middle. Scheduling must be according to how long the medication is actually lasting, or pain will occur.

Short-acting Opioids

Fentanyl (Sublimaze) ½ h

Intermediate-acting Opioids

Meperidine (Demerol) 2–3 h
Morphine 3–4 h
Hydromorphone (Dilaudid) 3–4 h
Codeine 3–4 h
Oxycodone 3–4 h
Propoxyphene (Darvon) 3–4 h

Long-acting Opioids

Methadone (Dolophine) 6–8 h
Levorphanol (Levo-Dromoran) 6–8 h

Controlled-release oral formulations allow an extended schedule. Current formulations now available include morphine (MS Contin, Oramorph SR) every 12 hours, oxycodone (OxyContin) every 12 hours, and fentanyl transdermal (Duragesic patch) every 3 days. Studies of controlled-release oxycodone, have shown that the dose of the long-acting agent is equivalent to intermittent dosing per 24 hours.[99, 117]

Equianalgesia is the conversion of one route to another or of one opioid to another in an equivalent amount. Converting from one route of administration to another or from one opioid to another must be done in such a manner as to not undermedicate or overmedicate the patient. For instance, the potency of oral morphine and oxycodone has been determined to be 1:1.[151] The practice has been that when switching from one opioid to another opioid, one third to one half of the analgesic drug dose of the new opioid was given as the initial starting dose. The APS currently does not support that a reduction is necessary.[6] When opioids are changed or a dose adjustment is made, it is advisable to monitor the patient closely. This concept is just beginning to be realized, and nurses can do much to educate other health care professionals in the process of equianalgesic conversion.

Opioid Side Effect Management. With the administration of opioids, side effects may occur. According to Inturrisi,[68] "Patients with renal impairment are more sensitive to morphine and liable to develop toxic effects, as a result of delayed elimination of the active metabolite morphine-6-glucuronide (M-6-G)." In addition, patients with severe hepatic dysfunction require decreased doses, and caution must be used with opioids because CNS signs and symptoms may be exacerbated. Concerns about the control of side effects were identified by 65% of physicians in an ECOG study.[140] An interesting procedure to manage opioid side effects is the rotation of medications. De Stoutz and others[37] found that a dose significantly lower than the equianalgesic amount could manage the pain with decreased side effects. The questions then become: Are expected side effects being managed effectively? Are there any unexpected side effects?

A discussion of the expected side effects follows.

Constipation. Constipation does not diminish over time. The opioid effects on the GI system produce a decrease in intestinal secretions and peristalsis. All patients receiving opioids should be given stool softeners and agents to increase bowel motility to prevent constipation because opioids inhibit peristalsis in the GI tract. Vanegas and colleagues report that more than 50% of patients admitted to palliative care units are experiencing constipation.[139] Preventing severe constipation requires treating consistently and prophylactically. Often the discomfort of constipation is more distressing to the patient than other pain. If there are not orders for a bowel regimen, the nurse should obtain them immediately (see interventions for constipation, page 885).

Nursing Management

Nursing Diagnosis

- *Constipation*

Outcome Goals

Patient will be able to:

- Verbalize understanding of constipation as a continuous side effect of opioids.
- Report bowel activity.
- Drink 2 to 3 liters of fluids per day.
- Verbalize understanding of dietary bulk and exercise needs.
- Take medication as prescribed.

Interventions

- Assessment at regular intervals:
    Are bowel sounds present?
    What is the normal elimination pattern?
    Is there an established bowel elimination pattern of every 3 days or less?
    Number of stools per day?
    Character of stool?
    Absence of stool elimination?
- Action:
    Treat prophylactically.
    General nursing measures: Promote adequate fluid intake of 2 to 3 L/d. Encourage high-fiber diet. Promote exercise/activity as tolerated.
- Obtain orders for medications and administer:
    Docusate sodium (e.g., Colace, Modane Soft) range: 1 to 2 tablets TID
    Senna (e.g., Senokot) range: 2 to 4 tablets BID
    Docusate sodium + senna (e.g., Senokot-S) range: 2 to 4 tablets BID
    Bisacodyl (e.g., Dulcolax; a bisacodyl [Fleets] enema) range: 2 to 3 tablets HS
    Colyte range: 8 oz QD or BID

Rationale

- The opiate side effect of diminished neural stimulation resulting in constipation will *not* diminish over time.
- Provide hydration to bowel contents.
- Increase bulk.
- Improve general tone and stimulation.
- Routine administration required if equivalent of 30 mg PO morphine per 24 hours.
- Stool softener that lowers surface tension, permitting water and fats to penetrate and soften stools.
- Mild natural laxative derivative from the Cassia plant; it induces peristalsis.

- Stool softener plus mild laxative (see above).
- A contact laxative that stimulates sensory nerves to produce parasympathetic reflexes resulting in increased peristaltic contractions of the colon.
- An electrolyte lavage; a glycol acts as an osmotic agent, and there is virtually no net ion absorption or loss.

Nursing Diagnosis

- *Altered nutrition: less than body requirements related to nausea and/or vomiting as a side effect of opioids*

Outcome Goals

Patient will be able to:

- Verbalize understanding of temporary nature of nausea/vomiting.
- State techniques to reduce impediments to nutritional intake.
- Take antiemetics as prescribed, based on need.

Interventions

- Monitor and record intake and output.
- Weigh every 3 to 5 days, if appropriate.
- Record number of episodes of emesis per 24 hours.
- Teach patient/family techniques to improve nutritional intake:
    Small, frequent meals.
    Reduce odors.
    Eat in pleasant surroundings.
    Do not lie flat immediately after a meal.
- Administer antiemetics as needed:
    Hydroxyzine (e.g., Vistaril, Atarax) range: 25 to 50 mg q 4 to 6 h
    Prochlorperazine (e.g., Compazine) range: 10 mg q 4 to 6 h
    Thiethylperazine (Torecan, Norzine) range: 10 mg q 8 hr
    Chlorpromazine (e.g., Thorazine) range: 10 to 25 mg q 4 h
    Metoclopramide (e.g., Reglan) range: 10 to 20 mg q 6 h
    Haloperidol (Haldol) range: 0.5 to 1.0 mg q 4-8 h

Rationale

- The side effect of nausea/vomiting is usually transitory and will subside within 3 to 7 days.
- Has antiemetic, analgesic, and mild sedative activity[8] as well as being an antihistamine.

- Antiemetic; use if sedation is desired, may reduce hiccups.
- Promotes gastric emptying.
- Antiemetic; use if patient is too sedated.

Nursing Diagnoses

- Sleep pattern disturbance related to sedation
- Altered thought processes related to confusion

Outcome Goals

Patient will be able to:

- Verbalize understanding of the temporary nature of sedation and confusion.
- Take stimulants as prescribed, based on need.

Interventions

- Assess and document:
  Patient's ability to communicate and comprehend.
  Patient's disorientation/confusion, agitation, or impaired memory.
- Interview patient/family:
  Are they comfortable with the level of alertness, or is it troublesome in any way?
  Discuss other possible causes with other members of the health care team.
- Administer stimulants as needed:
  Caffeine range: 65 mg (to 200 mg/d)
  Methylphenidate (e.g., Ritalin) range: 10 to 15 mg (divide between early AM and noon)
  Dextroamphetamine (e.g., Dexedrine) range: 5 to 10 mg AM; 2.5 to 10 mg
- Orient to person, place, and time as needed.

Rationale

- Sedation and/or confusion caused by opiates will decrease with repeated dosing.
- The individuality of each person is to be respected.
- Impaired renal function, hypercalcemia, or brain metastases can be the cause of confusion/sedation rather than the opiates.
- Stimulant; has been shown to increase analgesia when given with aspirin-like drugs
- Stimulant; has analgesic properties; low toxicity (4%) includes hallucinations and paranoia; tolerance may develop within 1 month and dose require escalation.

- Stimulant; side effects may include anxiety, anorexia, or nervousness.
- Confirm reality.

Nursing Diagnosis

- Ineffective breathing pattern related to respiratory depression secondary to use of opioids

Outcome Goals

Patient will be able to:

- Verbalize understanding of the rare occurrence of respiratory depression with ongoing use of opioids.
- Exhibit absence of true respiratory depression.

Interventions

- Assess rate, depth, and quality of respirations, especially after dose escalation:
  Respiratory rate 10 or greater
  Breathing pattern is even and unlabored
- If respiratory depression is questioned, assess for hypoxia:
  Labored respirations
  Tachypnea
  Tachycardia
  Cyanosis
  Position is semi- or high-Fowler's.
- Distinguish between respiratory depression caused by opiates and a natural change if patient is terminal.
- Administer naloxone (Narcan) *only after determination of true respiratory depression.*
- Discuss rare occurrence of true respiratory depression with patient/family.

Rationale

- True respiratory depression related to opiates is rare in the person who is not opiate-naive because the body develops a tolerance to the side effects.
- Physiologic changes that occur with hypoxia.
- A natural change in respiratory pattern (Cheyne-Stokes) occurs as death approaches.
- Opiate antagonist; use with caution to avoid profound withdrawal, seizures, and severe pain. The APS[8] recommends a dilute solution (0.4 mg in 10 mL saline) administered as 0.5 mL IV push every 2 minutes.
- Provide education and support to reduce fears of causing death rather than providing pain relief.

It has been found that opioid rotation may have an effect on reducing constipation by reducing the equivalent dose of opioid required. A review of case studies found that rotation to methadone significantly reduced the laxative requirements of patients.[31]

Nausea/Vomiting. As many as 40% to 70% of patients receiving narcotics will develop mild to moderate nausea, although it will decrease over time.[139] The intensity of nausea or vomiting in patients receiving opioids varies from patient to patient and from opioid to opioid. The etiology of the nausea/vomiting appears to be the result of the effect of opioids on the chemoreceptor trigger zone in the medulla, increased vestibular sensitivity, and delayed gastric emptying. This side effect generally decreases after 2 to 3 days of repeated dosing as tolerance to the side effect develops. The side effect should be treated aggressively; it may require ATC management for 1 to 2 weeks. Antiemetic trials are warranted if nausea/vomiting is a problem.

Sedation. Because opioids have a depressant effect on the CNS, some drowsiness can be anticipated. Once pain management is achieved, normal extended sleep patterns should not be confused with sedation; the person may have been exhausted from interrupted sleep patterns caused by previous pain and may, in fact, sleep for extended periods initially just to "catch up." The questions to ask follow:

- Is the person alert and oriented when awake?
- Has the person established a good nighttime sleep pattern?
- Is the person arousable from sleep?

This side effect generally subsides over 2 to 3 days.[139] If sedation persists for more than 3 to 5 days, possible added stimulation might be required; methylphenidate counteracts sedation related to opioids.

Confusion and Hallucinations. These are most often temporary, lasting a few days to a week or two. The nurse should be aware of impaired renal function (because it will have an impact on the clearance of the narcotics); some other possible causes of confusion to be ruled out are cerebral metastases, hypercalcemia, and sepsis. Because the source of the impaired mental status (IMS) may be multicausal, all possible causes must be evaluated. The active morphine metabolite, M-6-G, has been implicated in both IMS and myoclonus in patients receiving morphine. A study reported in 1995 by Tiseo and others[133] found that neither IMS nor myoclonus was significantly associated with M-6-G/morphine ratio when adjusted for other variables. The study did confirm the correlation between decreased renal function and increasing M-6-G/morphine ratio. Active metabolites of opioids can be a source of IMS, and Bruera and colleagues[19] demonstrated a lower incidence of IMS with hydration of 1 liter and opioid rotation in terminal cancer patients. Tolerance to these side effects usually develops within 48 to 72 hours. Haloperidol in low doses (0.5–1.0 mg) is often recommended because of its efficacy and low incidence of cardiovascular and anticholinergic effects, which may be caused by morphine-induced histamine release.[26, 139]

Pruritus. This intense itching is more often observed with the administration of intraspinal narcotics and is not frequently seen with the other routes of administration. The person will exhibit this first on the face and may be unconsciously rubbing or scratching at the nose or cheeks. This can be managed with an antihistamine or with even a dilute infusion of a mixed agonist/antagonist or naloxone. Pruritus is not life-threatening but is certainly bothersome. Rapid nursing intervention will enhance the comfort level of the patient.

Myoclonus. This spasm can be opioid-induced and is usually dose-dependent. Levy suggests the use of clonazepam 0.25 to 0.5 mg orally three times a day.[76] Cherny suggests a trial with a different opioid or the use of a benzodiazepine or anticonvulsant for symptomatic treatment.[26]

Respiratory Depression. Tolerance to this potential side effect develops rapidly.[139] Pain is a natural antagonist to the respiratory depressant effects of opiates, and therefore pain provides a natural stimulant. "Clinically important respiratory depression is a very rare event in the cancer patient whose opioid has been titrated against pain."[26] Pasero and McCaffery identify the rate of clinically significant respiratory depression in hospitalized adults receiving opioids as 0.09%.[100] A sleeping rate of six to eight respirations per minute may be normal in the totally relaxed person. The "arousable factor" is a satisfactory guide: Can the person be aroused rather quickly from sleep? This will stimulate respirations. When doses are escalated, respirations should be monitored for any drastic change even though it is unlikely. The patient/family should understand that respiratory depression is a rare occurrence with continued use of opioids and that death is not being promoted.

Naloxone (Narcan) is an opiate antagonist but must be used with caution to avoid profound withdrawal, seizures, and severe pain. The APS recommends diluting 0.4 mg in 10 mL saline and giving 0.5 mL by intravenous (IV) push every 2 minutes.[6] Slow, downward titration of the opioid may be preferred.[72]

Potentiators

By definition, to potentiate is to endow with power or make potent. A word of caution is required regarding what is referred to as the use of "potentiators" to increase the effectiveness of an analgesic. Medicine and nursing have long taught that when the phenothiazine promethazine (Phenergan) is added to a narcotic, it will intensify (or potentiate) the analgesic effect of the narcotic. Studies by McGee and Alexander[85] and Dundee and Moore[43] show that, in fact, promethazine may only increase the intensity of one's pain. McCaffery calls this an antianalgesic effect. What is observed in the patient is more a potentiation of the side effects: increased sedation, hypotension, and respiratory depression. The APS[6] states that "except for methotrimeprazine (Levoprome 10–20 mg available in parenteral formulation only), *phenothiazines neither relieve pain nor potentiate opioid analgesia.*" Benzodiazepines (diazepam [Valium], lorazepam [Ativan]) are effective for anxiety or muscle spasm.[6]

GENERAL PRINCIPLES OF ANALGESIC ADMINISTRATION

1. *Choose the analgesic appropriate to the type and level of pain.* The choice of a nonopioid or weak, moderate, or strong opioid should be based on pain intensity that is determined through careful assessment (see Fig. 30–2). The concept of an orderly progression from the occurrence of pain to its successful management can be visualized as the rungs of a ladder in the following sequence:

- Pain exists.
- Use a nonopioid with or without an adjuvant drug.
- If pain persists or increases . . . Use an opioid for weak to moderate pain, with or without a non-opioid, and with or without an adjuvant drug.
- If pain persists or increases . . . Use an opioid for moderate to strong pain, with or without a nonopioid, and with or without an adjuvant drug. The top rung of this ladder is freedom from cancer pain. This orderly progression allows for trials of various medications at all levels and ensures that everything is being attempted to control the pain across the spectrum.

2. *Choose the easiest and most cost-effective route of administration.* Based on the KISSING principle (Keep It Sanely Simple In Narcotic Giving)—use the oral route whenever possible! If nausea or vomiting prohibit this route, try the rectal route. Consider the following progression of routes:

- Oral
- Rectal
- Transdermal
- Subcutaneous
- Intramuscular
- Intravenous
- Intraspinal (epidural or intrathecal)

3. *Schedule administration.* ATC dosing is mandatory to achieve a steady state of analgesia and avoid the peaks and valleys that produce cycles of pain periods alternating with sedation. A PRN schedule should never be used because the pain level then escalates and the patient must spend time just to "catch up" to prior levels of analgesia. The important feature here is to stay ahead of the pain, and this principle requires teaching and reinforcement by nurses because it differs from usual pain management to which patients are accustomed.

4. *Be prepared for breakthrough pain.* Whatever the medication, route, or frequency of administration, an order should be available for "breakthrough" pain. This is a sudden, and sometimes brief, increase in pain that may be the result of increased activity or a particular motion. This "rescue dose" is administered over and above the regularly scheduled ATC medication. If three to four analgesic doses are required each 24 hours, the ATC regularly scheduled doses should be increased to include the amount used for previous breakthrough pain while still maintaining a PRN dose for future breakthrough pain.

5. *Plan treatment of side effects.* Management of side effects must be done aggressively and often should be prophylactic. Be aware that the following side effects may occur with the repeated administration of opioids:

- Constipation (does *not* decrease over time)
- Nausea/vomiting (usually temporary, lasting about 1 week)
- Sedation (usually temporary)
- Respiratory depression (rarely occurs)
- Other (confusion/hallucinations, dizziness, urinary retention)

6. *Never use placebos.* Placebos have no place in the oncology patient population. As McCaffery[80] states, "Pain is whatever the client says it is, whenever he says it does."[84] The ONS developed a "Position Statement on the Use of Placebos for Pain Management in Patients with Cancer." This position is: Placebos should not be used:

1. To assess or manage pain
2. To determine if the pain is "real," or
3. To diagnose psychological symptoms, such as anxiety associated with pain. The document goes on to say that "nurses should not administer placebos in these circumstances even if there is a medical order."

The ASPMN also has a position statement, "Use of Placebos for Pain Management."[10] This position is "that placebos should not be used by any route of administration in the assessment and management of pain in any patient regardless of age or diagnosis." The APS states that the use of placebos is unethical and should be avoided.[6]

Adjuvant (Coanalgesic) Drugs

Several medications have been found to be analgesic for particular types of pain. These drugs may be ordered for other than their usual indications (Table 30–6). They should be used after an adequate trial of opioids has proven ineffective. Table 30–7 lists the drugs and routes of administration not recommended for treatment of cancer and pain.

Antidepressants. These can produce analgesia in particular circumstances and are appropriate despite a lack of emotional depression; they seem to act by increasing the serotonin level. Indications are neuropathic pain (especially burning), depression, or insomnia.[6, 26] The analgesic therapeutic dose of antidepressants is only one eighth to one sixth of the dose required to treat clinical depression.

Anticonvulsants. Indications are for neuropathic pain (especially shooting or stabbing), lancinating pains (e.g., postherpetic pain), tics, or myoclonic jerks. The mechanism of action is presumably suppression of paroxysmal neural discharges.[106] Caraceni and coworkers report significant reduction in burning and shooting pain scores with the use of gabapentin.[23]

Stimulants. Indications are to increase analgesic effect of other medications or to reduce the sedative effect of opioids.

Corticosteroids. Indications are for nerve infiltration or compression, bone pain, increased intracranial pressure, anorexia, or mood disorders.

Local Anesthetics. Local anesthetics may be injected locally, applied topically, or taken orally. They block sodium channels and therefore block the action potential and impede the transduction of pain. All oral local anesthetics must be used cautiously in patients with cardiac diagnoses. The use of eutectic mixture of local anesthetics (EMLA) was demonstrated by Taddio and colleagues to significantly lower pain scores in infants on whom it was applied before immunization.[130]

Radiation Therapy. Radiation therapy is often used for palliation of bone pain. Levitt states that "radiation therapy is both efficacious and cost-effective, but that it is underused as a means to control pain and improve the quality of life for patients with cancer."[77] The therapy is usually given over 2 weeks (in contrast to 5–7 weeks for curative treatment). It may take 2 to 4 weeks to achieve pain relief with marked improvement of lytic bone lesions.[90, 113] Patients will need to continue their analgesics with titration downward over time until the radiation achieves results and nursing can educate patients and families concerning this.

Radiopharmaceuticals. Specifically used in metastatic osteoblastic bone lesions related to prostate or breast cancer, strontium-89 provides pain relief in as many as 80% of patients, with a median response of 6 months.[109] It is administered intravenously over 2 minutes by radia-

tion oncologists. One side effect to monitor is bone marrow suppression, which may temporarily result in reductions in leukocyte and thrombocyte counts. This agent does not appear to affect tumor activity, and therefore the current objective is pain palliation with an improvement in quality of life.

Other. Patients with metastatic bone pain have been treated with biphosphonates (e.g., pamidronate, zoledronate) with good results shown with repeated dosing. Analgesic requirements may be reduced by 20% to 50% with the use of biphosphonates for bone pain.[76] Calcitonin has also been shown to be effective in the management of bone pain due to metastatic disease.[74] Both have a direct effect on bone resorption by inhibiting osteoclasts.

Routes of Administration

Box 30–1 presents the routes of administration. Each of these routes is described in the discussion that follows.

Oral. Oral is the route of choice for economy, safety, and ease in pain management. Even severe pain requiring high doses of narcotics can be managed orally as long as the patient is able to swallow medication without difficulty. It has been shown that 70% to 90% of pain experienced by cancer patients can be controlled by oral administration of analgesics. It is very important to convert the parenteral to oral doses correctly because they are different and the amounts cannot be interchanged (see Tables 30–4 and 30–5). Education may be required to convince the patient/family that they do not need "shots" to control the pain and that parenteral administration does not mean stronger medication. As long as the equianalgesic amount is the same, the analgesic effect will be the same. Sustained-release morphine is now available, which makes 12-hour dosing effective.

Buccal/Transmucosal—the space between the cheek and gum of the upper molars; this does not stimulate salivation. The buccal or sublingual surface may be used for absorption of liquid analgesics in small quantities. Data from controlled clinical studies are not available, but anecdotes from practice support the idea. Oral transmucosal fentanyl citrate (OTFC) is available for breakthrough, or incident, pain. It comes on a stick and the patient swabs the buccal cavity allowing it to dissolve. Analgesic effects are noted in 9 to 15 minutes. There does not appear to be a correlation between daily opioid requirements and effective breakthrough dose,[107] and titration with the available unit doses of 200, 400, 600, 800, 1200, and 1600 will be required. It may be used for children to suck preoperatively; it is contraindicated for a child weighing 15 kg or less and the recommended dose above that weight is 5 to 10 μg/kg. This product should only be used in patients who are opioid-tolerant; it should not be used for acute or postoperative pain.

T A B L E   3 0 - 6
Adjuvant Co-analgesics

Drug	Dose	Indications	Comments
TRICYCLIC ANTIDEPRESSANT			
Amitriptyline (Elavil)	25–150 mg daily (hs); start at low dose and titrate upward to effect	Neuropathic and postherpetic neuralgia (especially burning pain)	Side effects include dry mouth, urinary retention, sedation, orthostatic hypotension, delirium; may potentiate narcotics by blocking reuptake of serotonin (a neurotransmitter)
Nortriptyline (Pamelor, Aventyl)	25–100 mg	Same	Same; less orthostatic hypotension; available in liquid form
Desipramine (Norpramin)	25–150 mg	Same	Same; less sedation and anticholinergic effects
Imipramine (Tofranil)	25–100 mg	Same	
Doxepin (Sinequan)	25–150 mg	Same	
The analgesic therapeutic dose of antidepressants is 1/8 to 1/6 of dose required to treat clinical depression. Tricyclic antidepressants are to be used with caution with coronary artery disease due to potential worsening of arrhythmias.			
ANTIHISTAMINE			
Hydroxyzine (Vistaril, Atarax)	25–50 mg PO or IM q 4–6 h	Pain together with nausea, anxiety	Has analgesic effects (50 mg IM = 5 mg morphine) as well as antianxiety, antiemetic, and antihistamine effects; irritating to tissue.
ANTICONVULSANT			
Carbamazepine (Tegretol)	100 mg q 6–8 h	Neuropathic lancinating pain (shooting/stabbing) (e.g., postherpetic neuralgia, ticlike pain caused by nerve injury)	Side effects include vertigo, sedation, confusion, and bone marrow suppression; contraindicated in leukopenia
Clonazepam (Klonopin)	0.25 mg q 12 h	Same	Reduce dose if there is renal insufficiency.[23]
Gabapentin (Neurontin)	900–3600 mg/d	Same	Side effects include ataxia, skin rash, liver dysfunction; plasma levels should be monitored
Phenytoin (Dilantin)	3–5 mg/kg/d	Same	
Valproic acid (Depakene)	15 mg/kg/d	Same	Hepatotoxic; available in liquid form
STEROID			
Dexamethasone (Decadron)	10–20 mg × 1; then 4 mg q 6 h; up to 96 mg if spinal cord compression	Neuropathic pain caused by infiltration or compression (e.g., brachial or lumbosacral plexus); increased intracranial pressure; spinal cord compression	Reduces edema in tumor and nerve tissue; chronic use may cause weight gain, Cushing's syndrome, increased risk of GI bleed with NSAIDs
Prednisone	20–80 mg/d		

Drug	Dose	Indication	Comments
BENZODIAZEPINE			
Diazepam (Valium)	5–10 mg PO or IV TID	Acute anxiety or muscle spasm associated with acute pain	Side effects: sedation, respiratory depression (also used in terminal dyspnea); not effective analgesic except for muscle spasm
Lorazepam (Ativan)	0.5–2 mg PO or IV TID	Same	
STIMULANT			
Caffeine	65 mg	Lethargy; counteract sedative effect of opioids	Side effects: insomnia, tachycardia, palpitations, anorexia; may produce additive analgesia
Dextroamphetamine (Dexedrine)	2.5–7.5 mg AM & noon	Same	Same
Methylphenidate (Ritalin)	5–20 mg/d	Same	Same; tolerance may develop over 1 month, requiring dose escalation
LOCAL ANESTHETIC			
Mexiletine (Mexitil)	150 mg/d in divided doses	Neuropathic pain	Clinical trials done in diabetic neuropathy; is a cardiac dysrhythmic agent
Tocainide (Tonocard)	20 mg/kg/d	Neuropathic pain	Is a cardiac dysrhythmic agent
Lidocaine 2.5% and prilocaine 2.5% (EMLA)	Topical cream applied thickly	Postherpetic neuralgia; before procedure	Must be applied 1 hour before procedure; use only on *intact skin*[73]
RADIOPHARMACEUTICAL			
Strontium-89 (Metastron)	4 mCi	Prostatic and breast metastasis to bone; osteoblastic sites	Administered IV; effect lasts several months; side effects include myelosuppression and pain flares
BIPHOSPHONATE			
Pamidronate (Aredia)	60 mg over 4 h; 90 mg over 24 h	Bone metastases	Inhibits osteoclastic bone resorption; effect lasts 2–4 wk[26]
Zoledronic acid (Zoledronate)	4–8 mg	Bone metastases	Promotes hydration; infuse over 15 min[26]
α-ADRENERGIC AGONIST			
Clonidine (Catapres)	0.1 mg/d PO	25 μg/h epidural	Neuropathic pain; Monitor for hypotension, bradycardia and tachycardia
GABA AGONIST			
Baclofen (Lioresal)	10 mg PO BID	Skeletal muscle relaxant	Administer with food to decrease gastric irritation

hs, Bedtime; PO, by mouth; IM, intramuscular; TID, three times a day; IV, intravenous; GI, gastrointestinal; NSAIDs, nonsteroidal anti-inflammatory drugs; GABA, γ-aminobutyric acid.

Data from Agency for Health Care Policy and Research (AHCPR): Management of cancer pain, 1994, Publication No. 94-0592; American Pain Society: Principles of analgesic use in the treatment of acute and chronic cancer pain, ed 4, 1999; Portenoy RK, McCaffery M: Adjuvant analgesics. In McCaffery M, Pasero C, editors: Pain: clinical manual, ed 2, St. Louis, Mosby, 1999.

TABLE 30-7
Drugs and Routes of Administration Not Recommended for Treatment of Cancer Pain

Class	Drug	Rationale for Not Recommending
Opioid	Meperidine	Short (2–3 h) duration; repeated administration may lead to central nervous system (CNS) toxicity (tremor, confusion, or seizures); high oral doses required to relieve severe pain, and these increase the risk of CNS toxicity.
Miscellaneous	Cannabinoids	Side effects of dysphoria, drowsiness, hypotension, and bradycardia preclude its routine use as an analgesic.
	Cocaine	Has demonstrated no efficacy as an analgesic or coanalgesic in combination with opioids.
Opioid agonist-antagonist	Pentazocine Butorphanol	Risk of precipitating withdrawal in opioid-dependent patients; analgesic ceiling.
	Nalbuphine	Possible production of unpleasant psychomimetic effects (e.g., dysphoria, hallucinations).
Partial agonist	Buprenorphine	Analgesic ceiling; can precipitate withdrawal.
Antagonist	Naloxone Naltrexone	May precipitate withdrawal; limit use to treatment of life-threatening respiratory depression.
Combination preparation	Brompton's cocktail	No evidence of analgesic benefit to using Brompton's cocktail over single opioid analgesics.
	DPT (meperidine, promethazine, and chlorpromazine)	Efficacy is poor compared with that of other analgesics; high incidence of adverse effects.
Anxiolytic alone	Benzodiazepine (e.g., alprazolam)	Analgesic properties not demonstrated except for some instances of neuropathic pain; added sedation from anxiolytics may limit opioid dosing.
Sedative/hypnotic drug alone	Barbiturates Benzodiazepine	Analgesic properties not demonstrated; added sedation from sedative/hypnotic drugs limits opioid dosing.

ROUTES OF ADMINISTRATION	RATIONALE FOR NOT RECOMMENDING
Intramuscular (IM)	Painful; absorption unreliable; should not be used for children or patients prone to develop dependent edema or for patients with thrombocytopenia.

Data from Jacox A and others: Management of cancer pain: clinical practice guideline, *No. 9, AHCPR Publication No. 94-0592, Rockville, MD, Agency for Health Care Policy and Research, U.S. Department of Health and Human Services, Public Health Service, March 1994.*

A Dutch group report on the use of morphine gel applied to *open* lesions due to infiltrating cutaneous tumors, mucositis, and tenesmoidal pain.[73] In the cases presented, 2 to 5 mL of a 0.3% to 0.8% morphine gel was used and showed a lasting effect that required application two to three times per day without apparent systemic side effects. In painful sites, which are not responding well to systemic analgesics, this may provide an option.

Sublingual—beneath the tongue; administration guidelines are 1 mL every 3 minutes. Robison and co-workers[114] reviewed the absorption, bioavailability, and tolerance of sublingual versus oral morphine. They state that there is no significant advantage of sublingual over the oral route and that nurses must continue to evaluate their actions through comprehensive pain assessment and base their decisions on the individual response of patients (i.e., efficacy and tolerance to taste).

Transmucosal—a convenient unit of fentanyl is prepared as a lollipop for children to suck preopera-tively. Although contraindicated for a child 15 kg or less, the recommended dose above that weight is 5 to 10 μg/kg.

Rectal. If oral administration is not possible because of the presence of nausea/vomiting, if the person is unable to swallow, or if dysphagia is present, the same dose of oral medication administered rectally can also achieve pain relief. Controlled studies are not available to support the practice fully, but it appears that the rectal mucous membrane absorbs equally to the oral cavity (thus a 1:1 ratio) and may prevent the necessity of changing to a parenteral route. The limitations for this route include the presence of diarrhea, anal/rectal fissures, or thrombocytopenia.

Available prepared suppositories include:

- Morphine: 5, 10, 20, or 30 mg
- Hydromorphone (Dilaudid): 3 mg
- Oxymorphone (Numorphan): 5 mg

BOX 30-1

Routes of Administration

ORAL

- Preferred route for analgesics; patients maintain control
- Allows greater mobility
- Drug levels peak in 1–2 hours
- Ease in administration
- Cost efficient

ORAL TRANSMUCOSAL

- Indicated for: (1) preanesthetic; (2) conscious sedation (3) breakthrough cancer pain of cancer
- Unit is constructed as a "lollipop" to suck (not chew)
- Available as oral transmucosal fentanyl citrate (OTFC)

RECTAL

- Good for patients who are NPO, nauseated, or unable to swallow
- May be more expensive than oral route and more difficult to obtain
- Starting dose is 1:1 ratio with oral
- Currently morphine, oxymorphone, and hydromorphone are commercially available

TRANSDERMAL

- Good for patients who are NPO, nauseated, or unable to swallow
- Takes 14–24 hours to peak initially; lasts approximately 17 hours after removal
- A fentanyl patch lasts 2–3 days
- Ease in administration
- Difficult to titrate
- Local anesthetics (2.5% lidocaine and 2.5% prilocaine [EMLA]) can be used for cutaneous and mucosal lesions (e.g., postherpetic neuralgia, ulcers)
- Capsaicin (0.025%) may cause a burning sensation after application; apply four times per day

SUBCUTANEOUS INFUSION

- Provides prolonged parenteral administration of narcotics and/or intermittent bolus
- Avoids repetitive injections
- Avoids peaks and valleys in bloodstream
- Avoids need for IV access
- Readily managed at home
- Recommended for cancer patients who cannot take anything by mouth
- Requires use of infusion pump with alarms
- Morphine and hyrdromorphone are most commonly used

PATIENT-CONTROLLED ANALGESIA (PCA)

- Allows patient to receive a predetermined IV bolus of a narcotic by a pump mechanism
- Gives patient sense of control, less anxiety
- Provides quick pain relief
- Patient may require less narcotic
- Eliminates the need for repeated injections

IV CONTINUOUS INFUSION

- Provides constant narcotic intravenous infusion to maintain constant blood levels
- No peaks and valleys in blood levels
- Recommended when unable to achieve pain control through oral or rectal routes with high dosages of narcotics or unable to use oral/rectal route
- Requires use of infusion pump with alarms

IV BOLUS

- Provides the ability to titrate rapidly
- Good for acute pain and/or procedures
- Provides most rapid onset but shortest duration
- Not recommended for constant pain because of peaks and valleys in bloodstream

IM INJECTION

- Should be used mainly for acute short-term pain
- Painful administration; rotate sites
- Not recommended for chronic long-term pain—especially cancer pain
- Not recommended for use with children, emaciated patients, or patients with a decrease in muscle mass

SPINAL ADMINISTRATION

Epidural
Dose: 5–10 mg morphine
Pain relief: 12–24 hours

Intrathecal (subarachnoid)

Dose: 0.5–1.0 mg morphine
Pain relief: up to 36 hours
- Narcotic (usually preservative-free morphine) administered through catheter into epidural or intrathecal space
- Local anesthetics are often added
- May be intermittent bolus or by continuous infusion pump
- Careful selection of the patient necessary because procedure is expensive and may be risky
- Side effects include nausea, vomiting, pruritus, sedation, urinary retention, respiratory depression
- Possible complication of infection and/or meningitis

Transdermal. Duragesic is fentanyl, a short-acting narcotic, which is available as a 72-hour continuous-release product and patients/families can manage this with ease. There will be a delay of approximately 12 to 24 hours until the peak serum level of fentanyl is reached; therefore, supplemental medications will be required. A trial period may be needed to make certain that the dose is correct and that the product does indeed provide analgesia for a 72-hour duration for the patient; a subset of patients (up to 25%) will require patch exchange in less than 72 hours.[40] After removing the patch, it takes an average of 17 hours for the fentanyl serum concentration to fall by 50%; therefore the patient should be monitored for 24 to 36 hours after discontinuation. In a study of cancer patients, Sloan and colleagues found that 82% of patients rated their pain relief as good or excellent; adverse events were experienced by 30% of the patients and 17% discontinued the use of the patch.[122]

Subcutaneous. This is an often-overlooked route because IV administration has become customary. The ratio of dosing for SC versus intramuscular (IM)/IV is 1:1. A small gauge (25 or 27 gauge) butterfly needle can be placed anywhere there is adequate SC tissue (e.g., abdomen or even thigh if the individual is not ambulatory), and the line may be used continuously or intermittently. The site should be inspected every 8 hours for redness, edema, and tenderness, but the butterfly needle can be left in place for 5 to 7 days without changing sites if there are no complications. Ideally, the medication should be concentrated so that there is 1 mL or less infused per hour, but it is possible to administer even larger amounts if absorption is adequate. Bruera and coworkers describe the successful SC infusion of narcotics and fluids at the rate of 20 to 100 mL/h with the addition of hyaluronidase and potassium chloride (KCl).[20] Any medication with a parenteral formulation can be used for SC infusion.

Moulin and colleagues compared the efficacy of SC and IV routes and found no statistically significant differences in pain intensity, pain relief, mood, or sedation between the two routes.[92] Most often morphine and hydromorphone are used for SC infusion; SC fentanyl has also been described as being efficacious in managing cancer pain as well as reducing side effects of the traditional opioids.[67, 142]

Intravenous. For home use, a permanent central venous access device would probably be required. Unless the patient requires the access for other purposes (e.g., hydration, nutrition, antibiotics), it adds considerable cost (the device, surgeon's fee, surgical suite costs, maintenance) without additional benefit over other routes for pain management. If the patient cannot swallow, has diarrhea, and has inadequate SC tissue, this may be the route of choice. It can be used intermittently (with a flushing schedule) or continuously via a patient-controlled analgesia (PCA) system.

Patient-Controlled Analgesia. This method of pain control involves a machine-delivery system that is programmed by the nurse and can deliver a basal (continuous) amount with an incremental/bolus (intermittent) amount, or a combination of both. Ideally, a PCA system will be programmed to have a continuous (basal) infusion that covers the usual analgesic requirements and a bolus option available to treat breakthrough pain incidences. This type of technology can be used either SC or IV and allows the patient to have control over this area of life, namely, pain management. PCA is also a term used to describe oral consumption; the stress is on the fact that the patient has control of the analgesic.

Intramuscular. Although this route has been used over time for pain management, it is least preferred for the person with cancer, who may require medications for an extended period. Sites may become limited; absorption may become erratic, and, more important, it requires the added pain of an injection when the intent is to relieve pain.

Direct CNS Administration. When the other methods of analgesic administration have been tried and they are not effective (e.g., intolerable side effects, high dose levels), a route that may indeed provide relief is via the opiate receptors of the spinal column. The analgesia is produced by the direct effect on the opiate receptors in the dorsal horn of the spinal column The sites may be the following:

Epidural—a catheter is placed between the vertebral column and the dura. The patient will require about one tenth the amount of opioid as required parenterally. An advantage of spinal opioids is pain relief with minimal side effects. Local anesthetics may be added to opioids if the dose requirement is such that unacceptable side effects occur. Douglas and Bush describe the successful management of a complex pain syndrome; the patient used a PCA system to administer a bolus of 25 mL of 0.123% bupivacaine as needed; there was a lockout time of 6 hours.[41]

Intrathecal—a catheter is placed in the subarachnoid region. The patient will require about one hundredth of the narcotic as required parenterally.

The placement of the catheter requires strict aseptic technique by a skilled physician. The epidural or intrathecal catheter may be tunneled to the exterior for intermittent injection, or a port/pump may be implanted for continuous infusion with a bolus option. Pain relief is extended (12–24 hours) after a single injection, but for some individuals a continuous infusion may be more efficacious. As with epidural analgesia, a local anesthetic may be added.[131, 134]

Direct CNS analgesia is a relatively new area in nursing practice, and it requires that each state determine what its nurse practice act allows in regard to an intraspinal catheter (e.g., inject [and if nurses may inject, which medications may be injected?]). Nurses working with spinal administration of narcotics must have documentation of adequate educational preparation for care. The agency/institution must have policies and procedures to govern practice.

Absolute sterile technique is required in the care and management of any epidural or intrathecal pain management. One other area of question is whether to use alcohol or povidone-iodine to cleanse the injection port. Most of the guidelines specify povidone-iodine because of the known toxic effect of alcohol to the spinal cord. Paice and coworkers studied the tool used to swab the port and concluded that pledges impregnated with povidone-iodine may introduce less, if any, of the disinfectant.[98]

Because this pain management modality is costly, it is usually not considered unless life expectancy is at least 3 months. It falls into the category of "high tech," and the other modalities warrant trials first.

NONPHARMACOLOGIC PAIN RELIEF TECHNIQUES

Nurses can teach the patient/family many activities that aid in the reduction of pain. These interventions are most effective when the pain level is low, but they can also be used as an adjunct to medications when the pain is moderate. Research to support many of these mechanical or psychosocial interventions is lacking, but in many instances they have merit and warrant a trial basis.

Most of the interventions are inexpensive and easy to perform. As Spross states, "They may appear too simple or too 'low tech' to be of use in the 'high tech' settings in which cancer patients receive care."[125] Most have low risks and few side effects, and, very importantly, they provide the ability for patients to have some control over this aspect of their pain management.

Noninvasive pain relief techniques can be useful alone or as adjuncts to the management of pain. The mechanical techniques consist of cutaneous stimulation (therapeutic touch, pressure, heat, cold, massage, and transcutaneous electrical nerve stimulation [TENS]). Behavioral pain relief techniques include distraction, imagery/visualization, music, humor, prayer, education, play therapy, biofeedback, and hypnosis.

Mechanical Interventions	Behavioral Interventions
Cutaneous stimulation	Relaxation
Therapeutic touch	Distraction
Pressure	Imagery/Visualization
Massage	Music
Heat/cold	Humor
TENS	Prayer
	Education
	Play therapy
	Biofeedback
	Hypnosis

Noninvasive Mechanical Interventions

Cutaneous Stimulation. Cutaneous stimulation is any activity that stimulates the skin for the purpose of relieving pain. Massage is one form of this intervention.

Heat and Cold. Because applications of heat and cold are so common and because they have been used for so long, nurses may underestimate their value in pain control. Heat may provide comfort and relaxation, whereas cold may produce numbness and decrease pain-causing substances (e.g., bradykinin, potassium, and lactic acid).[125] Both heat and cold decrease pain and muscle spasm. Deciding which therapy to use should be based on the physiologic effects desired.

Important factors that the nurse should remember when using heat or cold therapy are the age of the patient, medical history, condition of the skin, and any discomfort. Some patients may benefit from alternating heat and cold therapy. However, if the patient cannot tolerate heat or cold therapy, it should be discontinued.

Transcutaneous Electrical Nerve Stimulation. TENS consists of a pocket-sized, battery-operated device that provides a continuous mild electrical current to the skin via electrodes. The electrodes are generally placed on or near the painful site. The stimulation is again of the large nerve fibers, which will "close" the gate. Most often the units are used for mild to moderate pain of musculoskeletal or neuropathic origin.[26]

The TENS units have different dials so that the patient can adjust the intensity, rate, and pulse width (duration) to achieve a soothing, pleasant sensation.

The nurse plays an important role in teaching these techniques, assessing whether they are being done correctly, and evaluating whether they are effective.

Behavioral Interventions

Behavioral interventions focus the person's mind on something other than the pain sensation. They may be effective because they assist to decrease the person's anxiety. These techniques are very individual as to the person's preference and will be effective only when the person believes that they will work. They are complementary and can enhance analgesic effects.

For behavioral interventions to be effective, the nurse must explore the interest areas of the patient, determine which areas may have meaning for the patient, and determine if the patient believes the approach will make a difference in relieving pain. Each technique requires time to teach and practice to become effective. Briefly, the techniques are described below:

Relaxation. Relaxation is the state of relative freedom from both anxiety and skeletal tension. Some examples include distracting thoughts, rhythmic breathing, peaceful images, quiet environment, and repetition.

Distraction. Distraction is focusing on stimuli other than the pain sensation. This is often done without realizing that it is a form of analgesia and is reducing the sensation of pain. Distraction helps alter the patient's ability to tolerate pain. Some examples include music (auditory distraction), tapping (tactile distraction), television or flowers (visual distraction), people, and humor. Each of these activities may easily be used with little or no cost and used as an adjunct to medications, but distraction has a short duration and does not replace pharmacologic analgesics.

Imagery/Visualization. Mentally creating a picture is the use of one's imagination. This may be a focus on a close person, a place of enjoyment, a past event, or anything that is thought to bring pleasure. Examples of imagery include emptying the sandbag, breathing out pain, and a ball of healing energy. The mind is occupied, and therefore the pain is reduced in focus.

Music. Music (tapes, records, CDs, live performances) is used to take the thoughts away from the painful sensation. This is very individual as to the person's preference, and the patient's choice must be explored. A teenager's choice of music would probably not be the choice of the person over 70, and the person trained in classical music may not be a country/western fan.

Humor. Laughter is used as a distraction. Humor can provide immediate distraction, but it also can provide prolonged pain relief even up to 2 hours. Does the person have a favorite comedian? Are there audio or visual recordings available of that person performing? Is there a joke book that would match the person's sense of humor? Encourage the use of humor because many people who experience an ongoing pain find that they have little to laugh about.

Prayer. Prayer is the use of communication with a higher power. Obviously the patient's religious beliefs need to be explored. Is the person a Christian and accustomed to talking with God? Is the person a Hindu for whom there are many gods? Is the person a Moslem who prays to Allah? Is the person an atheist for whom there is no god or higher power and for whom this would not be an option?

Play Therapy. Play therapy is the use of games or toys. This can be especially useful for children, but it is also useful for adults. To play is to involve the person physically and mentally in an activity and thus provide distraction. To a child, dolls can become the object taking on the pain. To adults, a board game may provide a scene of competition and temporarily shift their focus away from their pain.

Biofeedback. Biofeedback is the ability to alter the body functions (e.g., heart rate, blood pressure, muscle relaxation) by intentional mental focusing. It requires the skill of a professional person trained in the technique. It may be more difficult in the home setting, but the person may have used this approach in the past and it is worth exploring as an adjunct during this time of pain.

Hypnosis. Hypnosis is the use of psychotherapy to alter the affective component as well as the sensory component of pain; the patient's perception of pain is modified. Hypnosis has been used to decrease stress, but studies on its efficacy in pain control are lacking. Hypnosis requires a professional who is skilled in teaching hypnosis, and again, it may not be feasible for the home setting.

Invasive Techniques

Cherny states that 10% to 30% of patients may not achieve adequate pain relief and may require anesthetic or neurosurgial techniques.[26] Jacox states the number to be much lower: "In a substantial minority of patients, estimated at 1% to 15%, the use of these invasive procedures is necessary."[69] A discussion of invasive procedures follows.

Nerve Blocks. The nerve block is an injection of an anesthetic agent into or near a nerve to numb pain pathways. The nerve block can be performed with either a local temporary anesthetic agent or a permanent neurolytic agent. Local anesthetic agents provide pain relief for several hours to days. The celiac plexus block can be used for pain arising from the pancreas, upper retroperitenum, liver, gallbladder, and proximal small bowel. Response rates in pancreatic cancer are 50% to 90% and response lasts 1 to 12 months, according to Cherny.[25] In a meta-analysis of celiac plexus blocks by Eisenberg and coworkers,[45] good to excellent response rates were identified in 89% of patients during the first 2 weeks and in 90% of patients alive at 3 months. The pain source determines the appropriate nerve block.

Anesthetic Techniques*

- Epidural and intrathecal opioids
- Celiac plexus block
- Sympathetic block for visceral pain
- Sympathetic block of somatic structures

Neurosurgical Procedures. Neurosurgical procedures for pain relief are surgical or chemical (alcohol) interruption of pain pathways. It is essential that patients be carefully selected for these procedures and that they completely understand the potential risks and benefits.

Neurosurgical Procedures*

- Intraventricular opioids
- Rhizotomy
- Neurolysis of primary afferent nerves
- Cordotomy
- Pituitary ablation

Acupuncture. Acupuncture, the insertion of needles at various points into the body to relieve pain, comes from the Latin words *acus, needle,* and *pungere,* puncture. This invasive technique is based on an ancient Chinese theory of two opposing forces, *yin* and *yang;* the Chinese theory says that pain and illness are caused by an imbalance of yin and yang. It is theorized that acupuncture works because it stimulates large nerve fibers to close the gate in the spinal cord to pain impulses. It is also postulated that acupuncture causes the release of endorphins.

QUALITY ASSESSMENT AND IMPROVEMENT

Pain, as well as other aspects of health care, must be assessed for quality management. Singer and colleagues interviewed 126 patients regarding quality end-of-life care and one of the five domains identified was "receiving adequate pain management."[121] Patients rate quality pain management as important in their care. A basic first step is the development of policies and procedures related to pain. Accurate evaluation of improvement of pain management must incorporate measurement of outcomes, which for pain includes patient satisfaction. Several groups have addressed this issue and have set standards that can be applied to an individual health care agency.

1. 1987—The ONS together with the ANA published the "Standards of Oncology Nursing Practice." The "standards are primarily intended to help nurse generalists provide effective care and pursue professional development."

2. 1992—JCAHO included in their manual for hospitals the following section under Patient Rights:
   - The organization supports the rights of each patient.

     Organizational policies and procedures describe the mechanism by which the following rights are protected and exercised: The care of the dying patient optimizes the comfort and dignity of the patient through effectively managing pain.

   In 1994, JCAHO expanded the statement to cover all patients, not just the dying.

   The new standards for pain management are in all six manuals. They are the first standards developed from research-based evidence of insufficient pain management.[102, 146] The comprehensive standards implemented in 2000 call for organizations to (Table 30–8):
   - Recognize the right of patients to appropriate assessment and management of their pain.
   - Assess pain in all patients; this is to include pain intensity and quality (i.e., character, frequency, location, duration). The assessment is to be appropriate to the patient's age and recorded in a way which facilitates regular reassessment and follow-up.
   - Educate relevant providers in pain assessment and management.
   - Determine competency in pain assessment and management during the orientation of all new clinical staff.
   - Establish policies and procedures that support appropriate pain medications and their administration (i.e., PCA, IV, epidural).
   - Ensure that pain does not interfere with participation in rehabilitation through postprocedure monitoring of pain and response to treatment.
   - Educate patients and their families about the importance of effective pain management as a part of their treatment.
   - Include patients' needs for symptom management in the discharge planning process.
   - Collect data to monitor the appropriateness and effectiveness of pain management (i.e., use of clinical practice guideline, pain pathway).

3. 1995—The APS developed "Standards for Monitoring Quality of Analgesic Treatment of Acute Pain and Cancer Pain." (See Appendix A.) Each of the standards is identified as structure, process, or outcome and can be used in an agency's Quality Assessment and Improvement program. The document includes a patient interview tool to measure patient satisfaction. The APS Quality of Care

---

* Data from Cherny N: The management of cancer pain. *CA Cancer J Clin* 50:70, 2000.

TABLE 30–8
JCAHO (Joint Commission on Accreditation of Healthcare Organizations) Pain Standards 2000

Standard Number	Content
PATIENT RIGHTS RI.1.2 RI.1.2.8	All patients have a right to pain assessment and management. All patients have a right to have their pain managed effectively.
ASSESSMENT OF PATIENTS PE.1.4	Pain is assessed. This assessment and a measure of pain intensity and quality (i.e., pain character, frequency, location, duration), appropriate to the patient's age, are recorded in a way that facilitates regular reassessment and follow-up according to criteria developed by the organization.
CARE AND TREATMENT OF PATIENTS TX.3.3 TX.5.4	There is a policy and procedure on the use of patient-controlled analgesia (PCA). Pain intensity and quality (i.e., character, frequency, location, and duration of pain) are recorded in post-procedural care patients.
PATIENT EDUCATION PF.1.7	Patients are taught that pain management is a part of treatment; patients are made aware of community resources related to pain management.
CONTINUUM OF CARE CC.6.1	Discharge planning focuses on patients' health care needs including adequate symptom management.
IMPROVING ORGANIZATION PERFORMANCE	The organization collects data to monitor its performance in relation to: appropriateness and effectiveness of pain management and the outcomes of pain clinical practice guidelines.

Committee[8] conducted studies of the implementations of the guidelines at three medical centers and identified five key elements of quality improvement pain programs.
- Ensuring that a report of unrelieved pain raises a "red flag" that attracts clinicians' attention
- Making information about analgesics convenient where orders are written
- Promising patients responsive analgesic care and urging them to communicate pain
- Implementing policies and safeguards for the use of modern analgesic technologies
- Coordinating and assessing implementation of these measures
4. 1994—The AHCPR published "Cancer Pain Management."

The implementation of any of the guidelines/standards requires an interdisciplinary collaborative effort. Duncan and Otto describe the process, starting with a task force consisting of four physicians, four nurses, and one pharmacist with a nurse facilitator.[42]

Thus there are now a national accrediting body, national professional organizations, and the federal government that have developed and published information that asks the basic questions:

- Is pain being addressed as a symptom?
- How well is pain being managed?
  - . . . from the patient's point of view?
  - . . . from the health care professional's point of view?
- Quality Assessment and Improvement (QAI) audits are important to be able to document current status and future improvements in pain management.

One outcome, which can be monitored, is readmission for pain. Grant and coworkers[59] report a study in which 12.8% of 804 unscheduled readmissions were for pain. Of the 103 unscheduled readmissions related to pain, 54% of those were within 12 days of discharge. After implementing a pain education program, identifying pain as a quality improvement focus, and providing additional personnel, the total percent of admissions for uncontrolled pain was reduced from 4.4% to 3%.

Another outcome, which can be measured as a quality indicator, is the utilization of meperidine in the oncology population. Because the recommendation is to not use this analgesic in this group of patients, it becomes a measure of whether guidelines are being followed. Figure 30–3 presents a sample outcome.

By establishing a pain quality improvement project, nursing can assist in the improvement of patient care

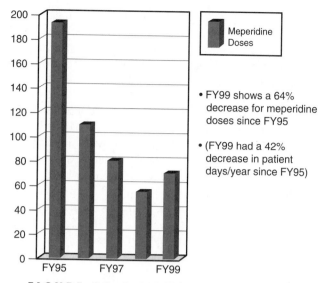

FIGURE 30–3 Meperidine doses in oncology.

- FY99 shows a 64% decrease for meperidine doses since FY95

- (FY99 had a 42% decrease in patient days/year since FY95)

and enhance quality of life. Holzhimer and coworkers described a hospice program that included education for the nurses, development and implementation of pain policies and procedures, changes in assessment and documentation, and establishment of pain quality monitors.[65] They found significant improvement in pain relief. Quality improvement is vital to good nursing practice. Pasero and colleagues have identified a comprehensive interdisciplinary approach to quality pain management.[101] They call for a total institutional commitment involving all health care providers.

Is there adequate documentation? Lack of documentation is a universal problem. In a study of German physicians, Weber and Huber found that pain severity was only documented in 37.1% of cases and opioid dose was only documented in 51.8% of patient charts.[143] In a review of 200 patient charts, Fins and associates found that only 52.4% of the 63 cancer patients had a documented comfort care plan, although 88.9% were identified as dying.[54] Not only must nurses plan for comfort care, there must be a record of it.

What education is needed (professional and lay)? Max proposes that education alone may not be sufficient to change behaviors and that guidelines and tools need to be developed to ease assessment and communication between and among patients and health care professionals.[79] Dalton and coworkers describe an educational program for rural nurses in North Carolina.[34] The interactive program was conducted 1 day a week for 6 weeks. There were demonstrated improvements in documentation, descriptions of pain, use of pharmacologic and nonpharmacologic treatment, follow-up evaluation, and use of pain-related consultants. This program incorporated didactic and practice experiences and used guidelines for documentation that were updated during the course.

The issue of the quality (or the lack of quality) of pain management has also become a legal issue. According to Frank-Stromborg and Christiansen, "the legal theory of negligence in medication error lawsuits can be applied to cases claiming inappropriate management of pain."[58] Angarola and Donato report that a jury awarded $15 million in damages to a family as a result of nursing actions that caused increased pain and suffering through withholding narcotics during the terminal illness of a man with prostate cancer metastasized to the spine and femur.[11] Shapiro states that the jury award was later resolved, and an undisclosed amount was settled among the parties.[120] With the availability of the AHCPR guidelines, the WHO guidelines, the APS standards, and many professional organizations educating about pain management, the standard of care has been set and failure to fulfill those practices may influence a jury to find that a nurse breached the standard of care. "Nurses are legally liable for the undertreatment of pain."[58] Yes, pain management has become a quality-of-care issue as well as a legal issue.

A second legal issue, which has been potentially associated with inadequate pain management, is physician-assisted suicide. Oregon legalized physician-assisted suicide in 1997. In a review of 15 patients who died after receiving prescriptions for lethal medications, Chin and colleagues found that only one patient had expressed concern about inadequate pain control.[27] The statistically significant concerns were loss of autonomy and loss of control of bodily functions. Hopefully this is a positive statement of the effectiveness of health care providers educating the public about the current ability to manage pain effectively.

THE NURSING ROLE IN PAIN MANAGEMENT

Although the care of patients with pain is multidisciplinary, in most cases nursing care is the cornerstone.[84] Pain management is a challenge that every nurse must face when caring for a patient with cancer. Regardless of the setting, the nurse has a vital role in pain management because the nurse has the ongoing contact with the patients in pain. Nurses must be vocal in the area of cancer pain. A nurse who is an advocate for cancer pain management need not be a pain expert, but rather one who is dedicated to the problem of cancer pain relief. An algorithm (decision-making tree) for the progression of pain management through the WHO ladder has been developed by Hudzinski.[66] Supporting the use of a pain algorithm DuPen and coworkers conducted a prospective study of 81 cancer patients.[44] Patients who were randomized to the algorithm group achieved a statistically significant reduction in usual pain intensity.

Patient Education. Nurses have a major role in pain management education. Some of the content includes:

- Types of pain
- Tolerance versus addiction
- Appropriate use of analgesics according to the WHO ladder
- ATC dosing
- Expected side effects and how to manage them
- When to call a healthcare provider and whom to call

A structured pain education program provided by nurses for patients and families can increase knowledge and result in decreased pain intensity.[38] It has been shown that patients can successfully use a pain diary to record their experience and the relief obtained.[39] This affords a measure of control over their situation when there may not be many areas over which they can exercise control. Benor and colleagues measured the impact of structured nursing intervention on 48 ambulatory cancer patients.[14] They found that there was a great reduction in the intensity of pain among the experimental patients with whom the nurses met 10 times to enhance self-care through education and support.

Assessment Issues in Pain Management

Nursing is involved in obtaining a detailed quantitative and qualitative assessment of the patient's pain experience. Pain is a subjective experience, and it is only the person who has the pain who is able to legitimately describe the event in detail. In a study reported by Yeager and coworkers several differences were found between patients and their caregivers, with caregivers viewing the experience more negatively than the patients.[150] Family caregivers reported the following:

1. Patients had significantly higher levels of pain than patient reports.
2. Patients experienced significantly greater distress than the patients reported.
3. The caregivers experienced greater distress from the patients' pain than the patients reported.

Again, the most meaningful and accurate assessment of pain is directly from the patient.

As early as 1987, the NIH Consensus Development Conference stated that "nurses have well-established pivotal roles in the assessment and management of pain." The importance of a thorough pain assessment was emphasized in the ECOG cancer pain study, in which 76% of the physicians identified inadequate pain assessment as a barrier to cancer pains management.[140]

Nursing qualitative assessment includes observations of behavior and appearance and the patient's description of sensations and personal impact of the pain. The quantitative assessment includes the patient's descrip-

tion of the intensity of the pain and the analgesic requirements over time. Many assessment tools are available, but care must be taken to select one that the patient can use. Shannon and coworkers recommend (1) beginning pain assessment while the patient is able to respond and (2) monitoring behaviors specific to that person that indicate pain.[119] This study found that 44.8% of patients were unable to use the McGill-Melzack Pain Questionnaire, the Memorial Pain Assessment Card, or the Faces Pain Rating Scale because of cognitive impairment, a communication barrier, or other reasons. Dalton and McNaull recommend that a universal scale (i.e., 0-10) be adopted so that patients are not confused by different providers changing from 0 to 5, 0 to 10, or 0 to 100 when asking about pain intensity.[35]

Qualitative assessment includes the following:

- Reported symptoms associated with moderate to severe pain
    Mood disturbances: anxiety, depression, anger, and irritability
    Decreased ability to concentrate/communicate
    Loss of appetite, nausea, and vomiting
    Sleep disturbances/sleep deprivation
    Sexual dysfunction/lack of interest
    Splinting, limited mobility, disuse syndromes
    Fatigue
    Behavioral changes
- Classification of pain
    Acute: less than 3 to 6 months
    Chronic: longer than 3 to 6 months
- Location
    Is it confined to one area, or does it radiate?
    Has it changed from a previous location or extended beyond a previous site?
- Quality: Because the source of pain can vary, it is imperative that the nurse elicit a description that describes the pain most accurately. Use the patient's own words for what the pain feels like. Keep in mind that the following descriptors may indicate a particular type of pain:
    Burning: possibly neuropathic pain
    Stabbing: possibly neuropathic pain
    Dull or sharp: possibly somatic pain
    Constant or deep: possibly visceral pain
- Duration
    Onset: when did it start?
    Intermittent: does it last briefly after movement?
    Constant: does it never go away?
- Aggravating and relieving factors
    What makes the pain worse? . . . better?
    Does it help to lie down, stand, and sit up?
    What has person tried? Analgesics?
        Type?
        Dose?

Frequency?

Positioning?

Heat/cold?

Massage?

Does the pain interfere with activities of daily living (ADLs)? Is sleep affected (awakens because of pain)? Is sociability limited?

What is the expectation for pain relief?

An acceptable level that is tolerable

No pain

Quantitative assessment includes the following:

• Intensity—0 to 10 with 0 being no pain and 10 the worst pain imaginable. The intensity may be a verbal or visual identification. Figure 30–4 presents an assessment scale. A conversion of numbers into word descriptors for the levels may include the following:

0 = None

2 = Mild; pain unnoticed with activity

4 = Discomforting; sometimes interferes with activities or sleep

6 = Distressing; usually interferes with activities or sleep

8 = Severe; severely "restricts" person

10 = Excruciating; the worst pain imaginable.

The use of a verbal numeric rating scale (0–10) was found by Paice and Cohen to have validity, and to be a simple tool to use with their population.[96]

• Equianalgesic amounts per 24 hours—it is important for the nurse to calculate what the total amount of analgesics required per 24 hours has been and convert this into the common language of morphine equivalents (see Tables 30–4 and 30–5 for details). Figures 30–5 and 30–6 are examples of pain assessment tools that contain both qualitative and/or quantitative elements. Assessment tools are valuable for the initial pain assessment as well as for ongoing reassessments.

GERIATRIC PAIN ISSUES

A segment of our population that has been often overlooked in the management of pain is the elderly. With the increase in longevity and the resultant aging population, health care professionals must develop a more acceptable attitude toward administering pain medications and controlling pain in the elderly. Ferrell reports two reviews of geriatric textbooks and their sparse content on pain management.[49] Of 11 medical textbooks, only 2 had chapters addressing pain, and of 5000 pages of nursing geriatric texts, fewer than 18 pages dealt solely with pain. In addition, little pain research has been designed specifically for the elderly.

Bernabei and coworkers report on a study of 13,625 cancer patients aged 65 years and older from 1492 nursing homes in five states.[15] A total of 4003 patients (29.3%) reported daily pain. Twenty-six percent of those

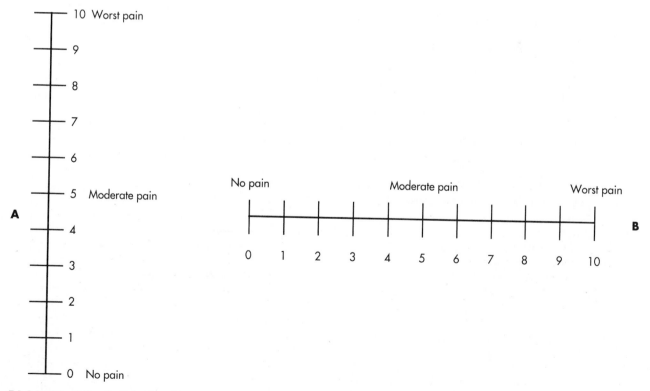

FIGURE 30–4 Pain: intensity scales. (From McCaffery M, Pasero C: *Pain: clinical manual,* ed 2, St. Louis, Mosby, 1999.)

FORM 3.1 **Initial Pain Assessment Tool**

Date _____

Patient's Name _____ Age _____ Room _____

Diagnosis _____ Physician _____

Nurse _____

1. LOCATION: Patient or nurse mark drawing.

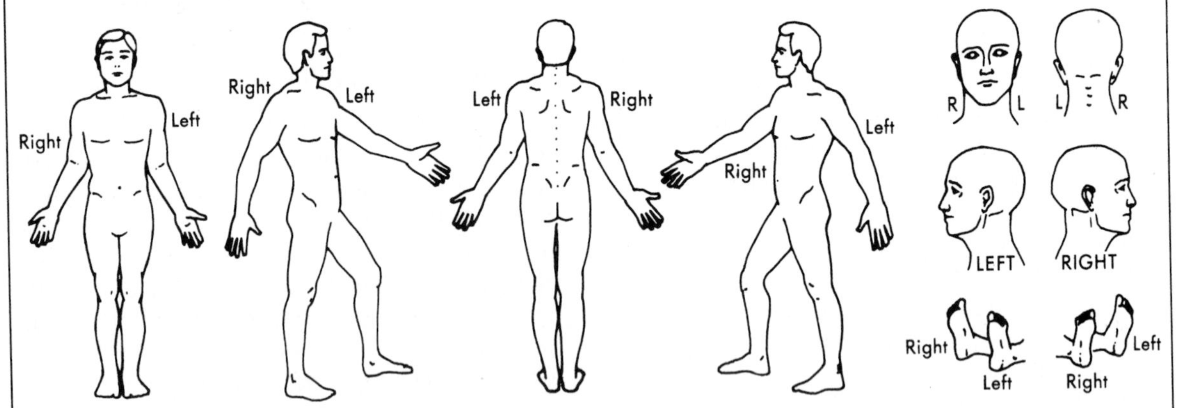

2. INTENSITY: Patient rates the pain. Scale used _____

   Present: _____
   Worst pain gets: _____
   Best pain gets: _____
   Acceptable level of pain: _____
3. QUALITY: (Use patient's own words, e.g., prick, ache, burn, throb, pull, sharp) _____
   _____
4. ONSET, DURATION, VARIATIONS, RHYTHMS: _____
   _____
5. MANNER OF EXPRESSING PAIN: _____
   _____
   _____
6. WHAT RELIEVES THE PAIN? _____
   _____
   _____
7. WHAT CAUSES OR INCREASES THE PAIN? _____
   _____
   _____
8. EFFECTS OF PAIN: (Note decreased function, decreased quality of life.)
   Accompanying symptoms (e.g., nausea) _____
   Sleep _____
   Appetite _____
   Physical activity _____
   Relationship with others (e.g., irritability) _____
   Emotions (e.g., anger, suicidal, crying) _____
   Concentration _____
   Other _____
9. OTHER COMMENTS: _____
   _____
10. PLAN: _____
    _____

FIGURE 30-5   Initial pain assessment tool. (From McCaffery M, Pasero C: Assessment—underlying complexities, misconceptions, and practical tools. In McCaffery M, Pasero C, editors: *Pain: clinical manual,* ed 2, St. Louis, Mosby, 1999.)

FORM 3.2 Brief Pain Inventory

Date ____ / ____ / ____   Time: _____

Name: _____ _____ _____
　　　　　　Last　　　　First　　Middle Initial

1) Throughout our lives, most of us have had pain from time to time (such as minor headaches, sprains, and toothaches). Have you had pain other than these everyday kinds of pain today?
1. Yes   2. No

2) On the diagram, shade in the areas where you feel pain. Put an X on the area that hurts the most.

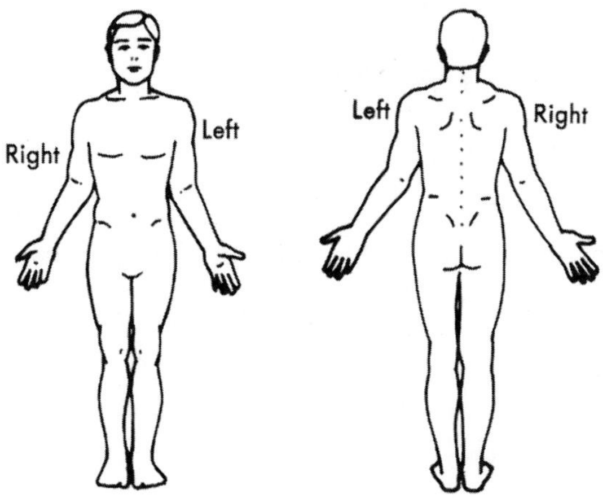

Right   Left   Left   Right

3) Please rate your pain by circling the one number that best describes your pain at its **worst** in the past 24 hours.

0 1 2 3 4 5 6 7 8 9 10
No pain   Pain as bad as you can imagine

4) Please rate your pain by circling the one number that best describes your pain at its **least** in the past 24 hours.

0 1 2 3 4 5 6 7 8 9 10
No pain   Pain as bad as you can imagine

5) Please rate your pain by circling the one number that best describes your pain on the **average.**

0 1 2 3 4 5 6 7 8 9 10
No pain   Pain as bad as you can imagine

6) Please rate your pain by circling the one number that tells how much pain you have **right now.**

0 1 2 3 4 5 6 7 8 9 10
No pain   Pain as bad as you can imagine

7) What treatments or medications are you receiving for your pain?

_____

_____

8) In the past 24 hours, how much **relief** have pain treatments or medications provided? Please circle the one percentage that most shows how much relief you have received.

0% 10 20 30 40 50 60 70 80 90 100%
No relief   Complete relief

9) Circle the one number that describes how, during the past 24 hours, pain has **interfered** with your:
A. General activity

0 1 2 3 4 5 6 7 8 9 10
Does not interfere   Completely interferes

B. Mood

0 1 2 3 4 5 6 7 8 9 10
Does not interfere   Completely interferes

C. Walking ability

0 1 2 3 4 5 6 7 8 9 10
Does not interfere   Completely interferes

D. Normal work (includes both work outside the home and housework)

0 1 2 3 4 5 6 7 8 9 10
Does not interfere   Completely interferes

E. Relations with other people

0 1 2 3 4 5 6 7 8 9 10
Does not interfere   Completely interferes

F. Sleep

0 1 2 3 4 5 6 7 8 9 10
Does not interfere   Completely interferes

G. Enjoyment of life

0 1 2 3 4 5 6 7 8 9 10
Does not interfere   Completely interferes

FIGURE 30-6 Brief pain inventory. (Copyright 1991 Charles S. Cleeland, PhD. Pain Research Group. All rights reserved. Used by permission.)

with daily pain did not receive any analgesic agent. Cleeland states that not providing pain management for the elderly is costly in terms of impaired function and decreased quality of life.[28] Analysis showed that those over 85 years old, women, and those in minority groups were the most likely not to receive anything for pain. Rochon and Gurwitz describe that older patients are more likely to report inadequate pain management, which may contribute to the undertreatment of pain in this population.[115] Clotfelter describes an educational intervention with people with cancer, over the age of 65.[29] One-half received a booklet and a video presentation on pain management. The experimental subjects had a statistically significant difference in lower pain intensity. This serves as a reminder not to exclude the elderly in our patient education on pain management. With the better informed consumer, and the implementation of the JCAHO standards addressing the issue of pain management in nursing home settings, the situation will undoubtedly improve, but there is a strong indication that nurses must act quickly and forcefully with the geriatric population.

Some of the myths that impede health care professionals in adequately managing pain in the elderly are the following:

- Pain is a natural outcome of growing old.
- Pain perception, or sensitivity, decreases with age.
- The potential side effects of narcotics make them too dangerous to use to relieve pain in the elderly.
- If the elderly patient appears to be occupied, sleeps, or can be otherwise distracted from pain, she does not have much pain.
- If the older person is depressed, especially if there is no known cause for the pain, depression is causing the pain. Pain is a symptom of depression and would subside if the depression were effectively treated.
- Narcotics are totally inappropriate for all patients with chronic nonmalignant pain.

With so many myths regarding pain in the elderly, what physiologic realities does the nurse need to keep in mind when addressing pain in the elderly?

Nursing Issues Related to the Care of Geriatric Patients

Geriatric patients are at risk for experiencing pain and not having it managed appropriately. In 1998, the American Geriatric Society published their guidelines on the management of pain in older persons (see Table 30–2). As a basis for their recommendations, the panel states that chronic pain is a common problem in this population. Of older people living in the community, 25% to 50% have pain problems, while 45% to 80% of nursing home patients have pain, which are undertreated.[4]

There are differences in managing the pain of the geriatric population and nurses need to be aware of those differences and make accommodations to safely intervene in managing that pain. Some points to keep in mind are:

Distribution of drugs—there are changes in the body composition (an increase of fat and decrease in heart, kidney, and muscle mass) as aging occurs; therefore usual adult doses may need to be decreased to avoid toxic drug levels in the blood and tissue. Decreased circulating proteins as a result of serum proteins, malnutrition, or chronic disease potentially result in greater drug effect from higher concentrations of unbound drug, with a greater risk of toxic effect.

Metabolism of drugs—there is limited research in the area of hepatic metabolic rates in relation to aging, but it may be safer to allow for longer intervals between doses in the elderly.

Excretion of drugs—a decrease in renal mass, renal blood flow, glomerular filtration rate, and tubular secretion can all occur in the kidney because of aging. With reduced function, the drugs or their active metabolites may remain in the body longer.

For an elderly population, analgesics are appropriate for pain management with the following considerations:

- The dose may need to be decreased.
- The interval between doses may need to be lengthened.
- The frequency of assessment and evaluation is increased.
- The responses cannot be predicted or generalized.

PEDIATRIC PAIN ISSUES

Hester states that pain in children is underdressed.[63] She also reports on several studies that have shown that pain is often a presenting symptom when children are diagnosed with cancer; more than half of the cases of leukemia, lymphoma, and soft-tissue sarcomas and *all* of the cases of Ewing's sarcoma, osteosarcoma, and neuroblastoma presented with pain. Pederson and Parran examined the pattern of opioids administered to patients undergoing a peripheral blood stem cell or bone marrow transplant.[104] They compared adult and children and found that the "total daily morphine equivalents/kg given to children ranged from 3–5.[6] times greater than the morphine equivalents/kg given to adults" although the self-reported pain scores were almost identical. They conclude that children may require proportionately higher amounts of opioids to maintain comparable comfort levels. Wolfe and colleagues interviewed 103 parents of pediatric oncology patients who died between 1990 and 1997.[147] From the parents' perspective, only 27% of the children with pain were treated successfully and a strong factor was whether the child's physician was actively involved in end-of-life care. There continues to be room for improvement in pain management of the pediatric population, especially in palliative care.

Banos and Barajas noted in a letter to the editor that there are now a number of pain assessment tools with established validity and reliability.[12] The question then becomes: Are the current assessment tools being used?

See Table 30–5 for medications and doses for people less than 50 kg.

Guideline:

Older than 12 years: full adult dose
7 to 12 years: 50% of adult dose
2 to 6 years: 20% to 25% of adult dose

For more information on the care of children, see Chapter 19.

Nursing Issues Related to the Care of Pediatric Patients

- Assess accurately
- Approach preventively
- Titrate to effect

In other words, intervene exactly as you would for other age groups; the analgesics are the same, but the doses, based on body weight, are different. When a child in the family has cancer, it is difficult for everyone. Ferrell and colleagues reported a study of families with a child who had cancer.[48] They found that the experience of pain was distressing to family members (x = 79.03 on a 0–100 scale) and that there was a need for basic knowledge of pain principles.

CONCLUSION

Nurses are central to the successful management of cancer pain. As Spross stated in her 1985 ONS/Schering Clinical Lecture, "Pain is an emergency for the person with cancer and, because of the distress it causes, nurses should respond with the same sense of urgency that exists when nurses respond to spinal cord compression or hypercalcemia."[124] *Not only can you make a difference in successful cancer pain management for the patient who is experiencing pain, you do make the difference.*

Nursing Management

Nursing Diagnoses: *Related to Pain*

Once the assessment of pain is completed, appropriate nursing diagnoses may include the following:

- *Altered thought processes*
- *Impaired physical mobility*
- *Constipation*
- *Diarrhea*
- *Knowledge deficit related to etiology of pain, action of analgesics, schedule of administration, potential side effects*
- *Anxiety and/or death anxiety*
- *Fear*
- *Fatigue*
- *Spiritual distress*
- *Hopelessness*

Outcome Goals: *Qualitative Components*

Patient will be able to:

- Participate in ongoing pain assessment.
- Identify qualitative components of pain.
- State the quality of the pain in descriptive terms.
- Identify previous aggravating and alleviating factors.
- State expectation of pain relief.

Interventions: *Qualitative Components*

- Assessment:
    Conduct on a systematic, ongoing basis.
    Use a tool that addresses *qualitative* components:
    Reported symptoms
    Mood disturbances (anxiety, depression, anger, irritability)
    Decreased ability to concentrate/communicate
    Loss of appetite, nausea, and vomiting
    Sleep disturbances/sleep deprivation
    Sexual dysfunction/lack of interest
    Splinting, limited mobility, disuse syndromes
    Fatigue
    Behavioral changes
    Interference with activities of daily living (ADLs)
    Location (one or more sites)
    Quality:
    Burning (neuropathic)
    Stabbing (neuropathic)
    Dull or sharp (somatic)
    Constant or deep (visceral)
    Duration:
    Onset
    Intermittent or constant

Aggravating and relieving factors:
　Standing, sitting, lying down
　What has the person tried (analgesics, heat/cold, massage, positioning)?
　Expectation for pain relief (an acceptable level or no pain)?

Rationale

- For accurate knowledge of patient's pain status and outcome of previous analgesic interventions.
- A change in location may be a new pain or a referred pain.
- Particular descriptor may indicate a specific type of pain. Use the patient's own words for what the pain feels like.
- Incorporating previously effective methodologies into the plan of care recognizes the past involvement of patient and family, strengthening a sense of personal control.
- If the patient's expectations are not realistic (i.e., total pain relief and no side effects), disappointment in the health care system could arise.

Outcome Goals: *Quantitative Components*

Patient will be able to:
- Use a consistent method of quantifying pain intensity.
- Identify effective pain relief strategies.
- Accept pain medication as prescribed.
- Participate with members of the interdisciplinary pain management team.
- Discuss documentation tools and be aware of their content.
- Report accurately whether pain relief has occurred.

Interventions: *Quantitative Components*

- Assessment:
　Conduct on a systematic, ongoing basis.
　Use a tool that addresses quantitative components:
　Intensity (0–10 scale)
　Equianalgesic amount required per 24 hours
- Planning (qualitative and quantitative):
　Determine whether current treatment is adequate and whether patient is satisfied with the pain relief.
- Interventions (qualitative and quantitative):
　Administer analgesics according to pain requirements and based on the principles of cancer pain management.
　Investigate the possible use of behavioral interventions in addition to analgesics.

Instruct patient on behavioral pain management interventions.
Collaborate with other health care professionals (e.g., physician, pharmacist, social worker) to use team approach to care.
- Evaluation and documentation (qualitative and quantitative):
　Use tools to measure:
　Intensity
　Satisfaction
　Quality of life
Conduct evaluation at intervals appropriate for severity of pain as a problem.

 PATIENT TEACHING PRIORITIES

Pain Management

Nurses play a major role in the teaching process. It may be spontaneous and informal or a lengthy session with resources (see Appendix 30-B for available printed materials.) Some of the areas of patient education are the following:

Cause of pain
Anticipated outcome (pain relief)
　Is the patient expecting no pain or manageable pain?
What to report to MD/RN
　Unmanaged side effects
　Uncontrolled pain
Medication information (schedule, dose, refills, drug interactions)
Side effects of medications and what to do to prevent or treat them (e.g., patient may be drowsy the first few days of narcotic use, but this effect will pass)
Information to restructure attitudes and beliefs regarding addiction, medications, etc.
Plan for follow-up and who to call for emergency assistance

PATIENT'S AND PROVIDERS' RESPONSIBILITIES FOR PAIN MANAGEMENT PLAN

According to Jacox and coworkers,[69] patients should receive a written pain management plan of care whenever possible and this does reinforce verbal instructions. The public is receiving more information about pain management. Lay literature has articles addressing the myths and misconceptions and where to call for information (e.g., NCI, APS, ACS). Successful pain management may depend on empowering patients to demand adequate pain treatment and that empowerment requires teaching the public about pain. Nurses are knowledgeable and are in a position to provide that education.

Rationale

- Consistency in measurement gives a measurable means to determine an increase or decrease in severity.
- A common base of amounts (i.e., morphine) provides a consistent measurement of analgesic requirements.

  See Tables 30–3 to 30–6 for specific medication information.

  Active participation in pain relief measures will increase the sense of personal control.

  An interdisciplinary team approach will address the total spectrum of pain.

  Written information is available to the interdisciplinary team.

  The evaluation frequency depends on whether pain is an active patient problem.

Planning: *Qualitative and Quantitative*

- Where is the patient on the World Health Organization (WHO) stepladder of pain management? (See Fig. 30–2.)
- Is current treatment adequate?

- Does physician need to be contacted for additional orders?
- Do the patient and family understand (and agree with) the current treatment plan?
- Is the patient satisfied with pain relief, or is more pain relief desired?

Evaluation: *Qualitative and Quantitative*

Once assessment, planning, and interventions have been implemented, evaluation then proceeds to determine effectiveness of pain management. Evaluation includes keeping a daily pain diary in which the patient/family record the following data on an ongoing basis:

- Intensity—is the pain rating score lower than it was before?
- Analgesic intake (per 24 hours)
- Satisfaction—is the patient/family pleased with the effect of the analgesic therapy? What more can be done?
- Quality of life—is the patient doing what she or he wants to do? Is pain interfering in any way with activities or personal interactions?

See Patient Teaching Priorities box (page 906).

Chapter Questions

1. Factors considered to be important affecting the response to pain include:
   a. Anxiety, personality, personal life experience
   b. Anxiety, culture and religion, personality
   c. Anxiety, personal life experience, culture and religion
   d. Anxiety, culture and religion, age
2. General principles of analgesic administration include all of the following *except:*
   a. Analgesic appropriate to type and level of pain
   b. Select the easiest and most cost-effective administration route
   c. Schedule administration frequency
   d. Schedule intermittent placebo use
3. All of the following may be used as adjuvant or coanalgesics for neuropathic pain *except:*
   a. Dexamethasone
   b. Dextroamphetamine
   c. Carbamazepine
   d. Amitriptyline
4. Nerve blocks that use a variety of anesthetic techniques to provide pain relief include:
   a. Epidural and intrathecal opioids, rhizotomy, sympathetic blocks

   b. Epidural and intrathecal opioids celiac plexus block, cordotomy
   c. Epidural and intrathecal opioids, celiac plexus block, sympathetic blocks
   d. Epidural and intrathecal opioids, cordotomy, sympathetic blocks
5. Incidence of pain in patients with cancer ranges between __% and __%:
   a. 25% to 65%
   b. 40% to 80%
   c. 50% to 75%
   d. 65% to 90%
6. The 2000 JCAHO new standards for pain management require all the following components:
   a. Assess pain in all patients, establish policies and procedures, educate relevant providers and vendors
   b. Assess pain in all patients, establish policies and procedures, educate patients and families only
   c. Assess pain in all patients, establish policies and procedures, educate patients, families and media
   d. Assess pain in all patients, establish policies and procedures, educate relevant providers, patients, and families
7. The side effect of opioid administration that does *not* diminish with repeated dosing is:
   a. Constipation
   b. Nausea

c. Pruritus

d. Sedation

8. The equianalgesic conversion from the oral to rectal route of morphine administration is:

a. 1:1

b. 1:2

c. 1:5

d. 1:10

9. Factors to consider in geriatric pain management include:

a. Drug administration, distribution, metabolism, and excretion

b. Drug distribution, metabolism, excretion and assessment frequency

c. Drug distribution, metabolism, assessment frequency, and increased dosage

d. Drug distribution, metabolism, excretion, and increased dose intervals

10. The complex neurophysiologic activity that results in pain comprises four steps:

a. Transduction, transmission, sensation, mobility

b. Transduction, transmission, perception, communication

c. Transduction, transmission, perception, sensation

d. Transduction, transmission, perception, modulation

BIBLIOGRAPHY

1. Ad Hoc Committee on Cancer Pain of the American Society of Clinical Oncology: Cancer pain assessment and treatment guidelines, *J Clin Oncology* 10:1976, 1992.

2. Agency for Health Care Policy and Research (AHCPR): *Management of cancer pain,* Publication No. 94-0592, Rockville, MD, US Department of Health and Human Services, 1994.

3. American Cancer Society: *Cancer statistics 2000, CA Cancer J Clin* 50:12, 2000.

4. American Geriatrics Society: The management of chronic pain in older persons, *J Am Geriatr Soc* 46: 635, 1998.

5. American Nurses Association Position Statement on the Role of the Registered Nurse in the Management of Analgesia by Catheter Techniques, *Am Nurse,* 67:7, 1992.

6. American Pain Society: *Principles of analgesic use in the treatment of acute pain and chronic cancer pain,* ed 4, 1999. (Copies available through the American Pain Society, 4700 West Lake Avenue, Glenview, IL 60025.)

7. American Pain Society Subcommittee on Quality Assurance Standards: Standards for monitoring quality of analgesic treatment of acute pain and cancer pain, *Oncol Nurs Forum* 17:952, 1990.

8. American Pain Society Subcommittee on Quality of Care Committee, *JAMA* 274:1874, 1995.

9. American Society of Clinical Oncology Task Force: Cancer care during the last phase of life, *J Clin Oncol* 16:1986, 1998.

10. American Society of Pain Management Nurses (ASPMN) Position statement: Use of placebos for pain management. Pensacola, FL, Author, 1997.

11. Angarola RT, Donato BJ: Inappropriate pain management results in high jury award (letter), *J Pain Symptom Manage* 6:407, 1991.

12. Banos J, Barajas C: Assessment of pediatric pain: time for an agreement, *J Pain Symptom Manage* 10:181, 1995.

13. Bell RF: Low-dose subcutaneous ketamine infusion and morphine tolerance, *Pain* 83:101, 1999.

14. Benor DE, Delbar V, Krulik T: Measuring impact of nursing intervention on cancer patients' ability to control symptoms, *Cancer Nurs* 21:320, 1998.

15. Bernabei R and others: Management of pain in elderly patients with cancer, *JAMA* 279:1877, 1998.

16. Berry DL and others: Cancer pain and common pain: a comparison of patient-reported intensities, *Oncol Nurs Forum* 26:721, 1999.

17. Brant J: What every clinician needs to know about meperidine, *Pain Management Special Interest Group Newsletter,* p. 3, Oncology Nursing Society, August, 1999.

18. Breitbart W, Kaim M, Rosenfeld B: Clinicians' perceptions of barriers to pain management in AIDS, *J Pain Symptom Manage* 18:203, 1999.

19. Bruera E and others: Changing pattern of agitated impaired mental status in patients with advanced cancer: association with cognitive monitoring, hydration, and opioid rotation, *J Pain Symptom Manage* 10:287, 1995.

20. Bruera E and others: Hypodermoclysis for the administration of fluids and narcotic analgesics in patients with advanced cancer, *J Pain Symptom Manage* 5:218, 1990.

21. Burrows M, Dibble SL, Miaskowski C: Differences in outcomes among patients experiencing different types of cancer-related pain, *Oncol Nurs Forum* 25:735, 1998.

22. Caraceni A, Portenoy RK: An international survey of cancer pain characteristics and syndromes, *Pain* 82: 263, 1999.

23. Caraceni A and others: Gabapentin as an adjuvant to opioid analgesia for neuropathic cancer pain, *J Pain Symptom Manage* 17:441, 1999.

24. Carron AT, Kynn J, Keaney P: End-of-life care in medical textbooks, *Ann Intern Med* 130:82, 1999.

25. Cherny NI, Portenoy RK: The management of cancer pain, *CA Cancer J Clin* 44:262, 1994.

26. Cherny NI: The management of cancer pain, *CA Cancer J Clin* 50:70, 2000.

27. Chin AE and others: Legalized physician-assisted suicide in Oregon—the first year's experience, *N Engl J Med* 340:577, 1999.

28. Cleeland CS: Undertreatment of cancer pain in elderly patients, *JAMA* 279:1914, 1998.

29. Clotfelter CE: The effect of an educational intervention on decreasing pain intensity in elderly people with cancer, *Oncol Nurs Forum* 26:27, 1999.

30. Coyle N, Cherny N, Portenoy RK: Pharmacologic management of cancer pain. In McGuire DB, Yarbro CH, Ferrell BR, editors: *Cancer pain management,* ed 2, Boston, Jones & Bartlett, 1995.

31. Daeninck PJ, Bruerra E: Reduction in constipation and laxative requirements following opioid rotation to meth-

adone: a report of four cases, *J Pain Symptom Manage* 18:303, 1999.

32. Dahl JL: State cancer pain initiatives: a progress report, *APS Bull* 12:5, 1995.

33. Dahl JL: New JCAHO standards from the Joint Commission, *Surg Service Manage* 5:27, 1999.

34. Dalton JA and others: Managing cancer pain: content and scope of an educational program for nurses who work in predominantly rural areas, *J Pain Symptom Manage* 10:214, 1995.

35. Dalton JA, McNaull F: A call for standardizing the clinical rating of pain intensity using a 0 to 10 rating scale, *Cancer Nurs* 21:46, 1998.

36. Derby SA: Opioid conversion guidelines for managing adult cancer pain, *Am J Nurs* 99:62, 1999.

37. de Stoutz ND, Bruera E, Suarez-Almazor M: Opioid rotation for toxicity reduction in terminal cancer patients, *J Pain Symptom Manage* 10:378, 1995.

38. De Wit R and others: A pain education program for chronic cancer pain patients: follow-up results from a randomized controlled trial, *Pain* 73:55, 1997.

39. De Wit R and others: Evaluation of the use of a pain diary in chronic cancer pain patients at home, *Pain* 79:89, 1999.

40. Donner B and others: Long-term treatment of cancer pain with transdermal fentanyl, *J Pain Symptom Manage* 15:168, 1998.

41. Douglas I, Bush D: The use of patient-controlled boluses of local anesthetic via a psoas sheath catheter in the management of malignant pain, *Pain* 82:105, 1999.

42. Duncan SK, Otto SE: Implementing guidelines for acute pain management, *Nurs Manage* 26:40, 1995.

43. Dundee JW, Moore J: The myth of phenothiazine potentiation, *Anesthesiology* 16:95, 1961.

44. Du Pen SL and others: Implementing guidelines for cancer pain management: results of a randomized controlled clinical trial, *J Clin Oncol* 17:361, 1999.

45. Eisenberg E, Carr DB, Chalmers TC: Neurolytic celiac plexus block for treatment of cancer pain: a meta-analysis, *Anesth Analg* 80:290, 1995.

46. Federation of State Medical Boards of the United States, Inc: *Model guidelines for the use of controlled substances for the treatment of pain,* Euless, TX, Author, 1998.

47. Ferrell BR, Ferrell BA: Pain in elderly persons. In McGuire DB, Yarbro CH, Ferrell BR, editors: *Cancer pain management,* ed 2, Boston, Jones & Bartlett, 1995.

48. Ferrell BR and others: The family experience of cancer pain management in children, *Cancer Pract* 2:441, 1994.

49. Ferrell BR and others: The impact of cancer pain education on family caregivers of elderly patients, *Oncol Nurs Forum* 22:1211, 1995.

50. Ferrell BR, Rivera LM: Cancer pain education for patients, *Semin Oncol Nurs* 13:42, 1997.

51. Ferrell, BR, McCaffery M: Nurses' knowledge about equianalgesia and opioid dosing, *Cancer Nurs* 20:201, 1997.

52. Ferrell BR, Juarez G, Borneman T: Use of routine and breakthrough analgesia in home care, *Oncol Nurs Forum* 26:1655, 1999.

53. Fine PG: Low-dose ketamine in the management of opioid nonresponsive terminal cancer pain, *J Pain Symptom Manage* 17:296, 1999.

54. Fins JJ and others: End-of-life decision-making in the hospital: current practice and future prospects, *J Pain Symptom Manage* 17:6, 1999.

55. Fitzgibbon DR, Ready LB: Intravenous high-dose methadone administered by patient controlled analgesia and continuous infusion for the treatment of cancer pain refractory to high-dose morphine, *Pain* 73:259, 1997.

56. Foley KM: Pain assessment and cancer pain syndromes. In Doyle D, Hanks CWC, MacDonald N, editors: *Oxford textbook of palliative medicine,* New York, Oxford University Press, 1993.

57. Foley K: A 44-year-old woman with severe pain at the end of life, *JAMA* 281:1937, 1999.

58. Frank-Stromborg M, Christiansen A: The undertreatment of pain: a liability risk for nurses, *Clin J Oncol Nurs* 4:41, 2000.

59. Grant M and others: Unscheduled readmissions for uncontrolled symptoms: a health care challenge for nurses, *Nurs Clin North Am* 30:673, 1995.

60. Grant M and others: Improving cancer pain management using a performance improvement framework, *J Nurs Care Quality* 13:60, 1999.

61. Grond S and others: Assessment and treatment of neuropathic pain following WHO guidelines, *Pain* 79:15, 1999.

62. Grond S and others: High-dose tramadol in comparison to low-dose morphine for cancer pain relief, *J Pain Symptom Manage* 18:174, 1999.

63. Hester NO: Integrating pain assessment and management into the care of children with cancer. In McGuire DB, Yarbro CH, Ferrell BR, editors: *Cancer pain management,* ed 2, Boston, Jones & Bartlett, 1995.

64. Hill CS: When will adequate pain treatment be the norm? *JAMA* 274:1881, 1995.

65. Holzheimer A, McMillan C, Weitzner M: Improving pain outcomes of hospice patients with cancer, *Oncol Nurs Forum* 26:1499, 1999.

66. Hudzinski DM: An algorithmic approach to cancer pain management, *Nurs Clin North Am* 30:711, 1995.

67. Hunt R and others: A comparison of subcutaneous morphine and fentanyl in hospice cancer patients, *J Pain Symptom Manage* 18:111, 1999.

68. Inturrisi CE, Hanks G: Opioid analgesic therapy. In Doyle D, Hanks GWC, MacDonald N, editors: *Oxford textbook of palliative medicine,* New York, Oxford University Press, 1993.

69. Jacox AD, Carr DB, Payne R: New clinical practice guidelines for the management of pain in patients with cancer, *N Engl J Med* 330(9):651, 1994.

70. Joishy SK, Walsh D: The opioid-sparing effects of intravenous ketorolac as an adjuvant analgesic in cancer pain: application in bone metastases and the opioid bowel syndrome, *J Pain Symptom Manage* 16:334, 1998.

71. Kaiko RF and others: Central nervous system excitatory effects of meperidine in cancer patients, *Ann Neurol* 13:180, 1983.

72. Kettelman KP: Why give more morphine to a dying patient? *Nursing99* 29:54, 1999.

73. Krajnik M and others: Potential use of topical opioids in palliative care—report of 6 cases, *Pain* 80:121, 1999.

74. Kreeger L, Hutton-Potts J: The use of calcitonin in the treatment of metastatic bone pain, *J Pain Symptom Manage* 17:2, 1999.

75. Kwekkeboom K: Postmastectomy pain syndromes, *Cancer Nurs* 19:37, 1996.

76. Levy MH: Pharmacologic treatment of cancer pain, *N Engl J Med* 335:1124, 1996.

77. Levitt SH: Managing pain in elderly patients, *JAMA* 281:605, 1999.

78. Matthew P, Storey P: Subcutaneous methadone in terminally ill patients: manageable local toxicity, *J Pain Symptom Manage* 18:49, 1999.

79. Max MB: Improving outcomes of analgesic treatment: is education enough? *Ann Intern Med* 114:342, 1991.

80. McCaffery M: *Nursing practice theories related to cognition, bodily pain, and man-environment interaction,* Los Angeles, UCLA Students Store, 1968.

81. McCaffery M, Ferrell BR: Influence of professional vs. personal role on pain assessment and use of opioids, *J Contin Educ Nurs* 28:69, 1997.

82. McCaffery M, Ferrell BR: Nurses' knowledge of pain assessment and management: how much progress have we made? *J Pain Symptom Manage* 14:175, 1997.

83. McCaffery M, Ferrell BR: Opioids and pain management: what do nurses know? *Nursing99* 29:48, 1999.

84. McCaffery M, Pasero C: *Pain clinical manual,* St. Louis, Mosby, 1999.

85. McGee JL, Alexander MR: Phenothiazine analgesia: fact or fantasy? *Am J Hosp Pharm* 36:633, 1979.

86. McGuire DB and others: Acute oral pain and mucositis in bone marrow transplant and leukemia patients: data from a pilot study, *Cancer Nurs* 21:385, 1998.

87. Mercadante S and others: Analgesic effects of nonsteroidal anti-inflammatory drugs in cancer pain due to somatic or visceral mechanisms, *J Pain Symptom Manage* 17:351, 1999.

88. Mercadante S and others: Methadone response in advanced cancer patients with pain followed at home, *J Pain Symptom Manage* 18:188, 1999.

89. Merskey H: Classification of chronic pain: description of chronic pain syndrome and definitions of pain terms, *Pain* 3:217, 1986.

90. Miaskowski C, Lee KA: Pain, fatigue, and sleep disturbances in oncology outpatients receiving radiation therapy for bone metastasis: a pilot study, *J Pain Symptom Manage* 17:320, 1999.

91. Mortimer JE, Bartlett NL: Assessment of knowledge about cancer pain management by physicians in training, *J Pain Symptom Manage* 14:21, 1997.

92. Moulin DE and others: Comparison of continuous subcutaneous and intravenous hydromorphone infusions for management of cancer pain, *Lancet* 337:465, 1991.

93. Oncology Nursing Society: *Position statement on the use of placebos for pain management in patients with cancer,* Pittsburgh, Author, 1997.

94. Oncology Nursing Society Position: Cancer pain management, *Oncol Nurs Forum* 25:817, 1998.

95. Paice JA: Unraveling the mystery of pain, *Oncol Nurs Forum* 18:843, 1991.

96. Paice JA, Cohen FL: Validity of a verbally administered numeric rating scale to measure cancer pain intensity, *Cancer Nurs* 20:88, 1997.

97. Paice JA, Toy C, Shott S: Barriers to cancer pain relief: fear of tolerance and addiction, *J Pain Symptom Manage* 16:1, 1998.

98. Paice JA, DuPen A, Schwertz D: Catheter port cleansing techniques and the entry of povidone-iodine into the epidural space, *Oncol Nurs Forum* 26:603, 1999.

99. Parris WCV and others: The use of controlled-release oxycodone for the treatment of chronic cancer pain: A randomized, double-blind study, *J Pain Symptom Manage* 16:205, 1998.

100. Pasero CL, McCaffery M: Avoiding opioid-induced respiratory depression, *Am J Nurs* 94:25, 1994.

101. Pasero C, McCaffery M, Gordon, DB: Build institutional commitment to improving pain management, *Am J Nurs* 99:2, 1999

102. Patterson CH: What new standards are in store for 2000? *Nurs Manage,* 9, December, 1999.

103. Pederson C, Parran L: Bone marrow transplant nurses' knowledge, beliefs and attitudes regarding pain management, *Oncol Nurs Forum* 24:1563, 1997.

104. Pederson C, Parran L: Pain and distress in adults and children undergoing peripheral blood stem cell or bone marrow transplant, *Oncol Nurs Forum* 26:575, 1999.

105. Petzke F and others: Temporal presentation of chronic cancer pain: transitory pains on admission to a multidisciplinary pain clinic, *J Pain Symptom Manage* 17:391, 1999.

106. Portenoy RK: Pharmacologic management of cancer pain. In Yarbro JW, Bornstein RS, Mastrangelo MJ, editors: Chemotherapeutic and nonchemotherapeutic palliative approaches in the treatment of cancer, *Semin Oncol* 22(2 suppl 3):112, 1995.

107. Portenoy RK and others: Oral transmucosal fentanyl citrate (OTFC) for the treatment of breakthrough pain in cancer patients: a controlled dose titration study, *Pain* 79:303, 1999.

108. Portenoy RK, Payne D, Jacobsen P: Breakthrough pain: characteristics and impact in patients with cancer pain, *Pain* 81:129, 1999.

109. Porter AT, Ben-Josef E: Strontium-89 in the treatment of bony metastases, *Important Adv Oncol* 5:87, 1995.

110. Porter J, Jick H: Addiction rate in patients treated with narcotics (letter), *N Engl J Med* 302:123, 1980.

111. Rabow MW and others: End-of-life care content in 50 textbooks from multiple specialties, *JAMA* 283:771, 2000.

112. Riddell A, Fitch MI: Patients' knowledge of and attitudes toward the management of cancer pain, *Onc Nurs Forum* 24:1775, 1997.

113. Ripamonti C and others: Pain relief and sclerosis of bone metastases in a patient with breast cancer treated with tamoxifen, radiotherapy and pamidronate disodium: which treatment helped? *J Pain Symptom Manage* 16:73, 1998.

114. Robison JM, Wilkie DJ, Campbell B: Sublingual and oral morphine administration, *Nurs Clin North Am* 30:725, 1995.

115. Rochon PA, Gurwitz JH: Prescribing for seniors, neither too much or too little, *JAMA* 282:113, 1999.

116. Sallerin-Caute B and others: Does intrathecal morphine in the treatment of cancer pain induce the development of tolerance? *Neurosurgery* 42:44, 1998.

117. Salzman RT and others: Can a controlled-release oral dose form of oxycodone be used as readily as an immediate-release form for the purpose of titrating to stable pain control? *J Pain Symptom Manage* 18:271, 1999.

118. Schmitt Fink R, Gates R: Cultural diversity and cancer pain. In McGuire DB, Yarbro CH, Ferrell BR, editors: *Cancer pain management,* ed 2, Boston, Jones & Bartlett, 1995.

119. Shannon MM and others: Assessment of pain in advanced cancer patients, *J Pain Symptom Manage* 10:274, 1995.

120. Shapiro RS: Liability issues in the management of pain, *J Pain Symptom Manage* 9:146, 1994.

121. Singer PA, Martin DK, Kelner M: Quality end-of-life care: patients' perspectives, *JAMA* 281:163, 1999.

122. Sloan PA, Moulin DE, Hays H: A clinical evaluation of transdermal therapeutic system fentanyl for the treatment of cancer pain, *J Pain Symptom Manage* 16:102, 1998.

123. Smith WB, Gracely RH, Safer MA: The meaning of pain: cancer patients' rating and recall of pain intensity and affect, *Pain* 78:123, 1998.

124. Spross JA: Cancer pain and suffering: clinical lessons from life, literature and legend, *Oncol Nurs Forum* 12:23, 1985.

125. Spross JA, Burke MW: Nonpharmacological management of cancer pain. In McGuire DB, Yarbro CH, Ferrell BR, editors: *Cancer pain management,* ed 2, Boston, Jones & Bartlett, 1995.

126. Spross JA, McGuire DB, Schmitt RN: Oncology Nursing Society position paper on cancer pain. Part I. Scope of nursing practice regarding cancer pain, ethics and practice, *Oncol Nurs Forum* 17:595, 1990.

127. Spross JA, McGuire DB, Schmitt RN: Oncology Nursing Society position paper on cancer pain. Part II. Education, research and list of cancer pain management resources, *Oncol Nurs Forum* 17:751, 1990.

128. Spross JA, McGuire DB, Schmitt RN: Oncology Nursing Society position paper on cancer pain. Part III. Nursing administration, pediatric cancer pain and appendices, *Oncol Nurs Forum* 17:943, 1990.

129. Stevens PE, Dibble SL, Miaskowski C: Prevalence characteristics and impact of postmastectomy pain syndromes: an investigation of women's experience, *Pain* 61:61, 1995.

130. Taddio A and others: A revised measure of acute pain in infants, *J Pain Symptom Manage* 10:456, 1995.

131. Tamakawa S, Iwanami Y, and Ogawa H: High-dose intrathecal morphine to control cancer pain—a case report, *J Pain Symptom Manage* 15:70, 1998.

132. Thomason TE and others: Cancer pain survey: patient-centered issues in control, *J Pain Symptom Manage* 15:275, 1998.

133. Tiseo PJ and others: Morphine-6-glucuronide concentrations and opioid-related side effects: a survey of cancer patients, *Pain* 61:47, 1995.

134. Tumber PS, Fitzgibbon DR: The control of severe cancer pain by continuous intrathecal infusion and patient controlled intrathecal analgesia with morphine, bupivacaine and clonidine, *Pain* 8:217, 1998.

135. Turk DC and others: Adaptation to metastatic cancer pain, regional/local cancer pain and non-cancer pain: role of psychological and behavioral factors, *Pain* 74:247, 1998.

136. Turk DC, Okifuji A: Does sex make a difference in the prescription of treatments and the adaptation to chronic pain by cancer and non-cancer patients? *Pain* 82:139-148, 1999.

137. Twycross RG: *Oral morphine in advanced cancer,* ed 3, Beaconsfield, Bucks, England, Beaconsfield Publishers, 1997.

138. Vallerand AH: A new class of analgesics is introduced, *Pain Management Special Interest Group Newsletter,* Oncology Nursing Society, p. 2, August, 1999.

139. Vanegas G and others: Side effects of morphine administration in cancer patients, *Cancer Nurs* 21:289, 1998.

140. Von Roenn JH and others: Physician attitudes and practice in cancer pain management, *Ann Intern Med* 119:121, 1993.

141. Ward SE, Lin CC, Hernandez L: Beliefs about reporting cancer pain and using analgesics: patients' concerns and misconceptions, *APS Bull* 12:15, 1995.

142. Watanabe S and others: Fentanyl by continuous subcutaneous infusion for the management of cancer pain: a retrospective study, *J Pain Symptom Manage* 16:323, 1998.

143. Weber M, Huber C: Documentation of severe pain, opioid doses and opioid-related side effects in outpatients with cancer: a retrospective study, *J Pain Symptom Manage* 17:49, 1999.

144. Weissman DE: Doctors, opioids, and the law: the effect of controlled substances regulations on cancer pain management: the management of pain in the cancer patient, *Semin Oncol* 20(1 suppl 1):53, 1993.

145. Weissman DE, Dahl JL: Update on the cancer pain role model education program, *J Pain Symptom Manage* 10:292, 1995.

146. Williams-Lee P: Managing pain by the book, *Nurs Manage,* 9, July, 1999.

147. Wolfe J and others: Symptoms and suffering at the end of life in children with cancer, *N Engl J Med* 342:326, 2000.

148. World Health Organization (WHO): *Cancer pain relief and palliative care,* Geneva, Switzerland, Author, 1990.

149. World Health Organization (WHO): *Looking forward to cancer pain relief for all,* International Consensus on the Management of Cancer Pain, Geneva, Switzerland, Author, 1997.

150. Yeager KA and others: Differences in pain knowledge and perception of the pain experience between outpatients with cancer and their caregivers, *Oncol Nurs Forum* 22:1235, 1995.

151. Zhukovsky DS, Walsh D, Doona M: The relative potency between high dose oral oxycodone and intravenous morphine: a case illustration, *J Pain Symptom Manage* 18:53, 1999.

APPENDIX A: STANDARDS FOR MONITORING QUALITY OF ANALGESIC TREATMENT OF ACUTE PAIN AND CANCER PAIN

American Pain Society Subcommittee on Quality Assurance Standards

Summary

Hospital and chronic care facilities in the United States have active "quality assurance committees" that monitor selected outcomes of care, working toward steady improvement in results. In order to harness these existing mechanisms to improve pain treatment, the American Pain Society has drafted a set of standards that embody five key elements for favorably influencing behaviors of patients and clinicians: (1) ensuring that a report of unrelieved pain raises a "red flag" that clinicians cannot ignore; (2) putting information about analgesics conveniently at hand where orders are written; (3) promising patients responsive analgesic care and urging them to communicate pain; (4) providing policies and safeguards for the use of modern analgesic technologies; and (5) monitoring the facility's success in implementing these measures.

Introduction

Undertreatment of acute pain and chronic cancer pain persists despite decades of efforts to provide clinicians with information about analgesics. Traditional educational approaches must be complemented by interventions that more directly influence the routine behaviors of clinicians and patients to ensure that pain is communicated and that treatment is rapidly adjusted to provide relief.

In the United States, virtually all health care facilities have "quality assurance committees" composed of physicians, nurses, pharmacists, other clinicians, and administrators. Each committee chooses a number of clinical objectives that it considers important to monitor. They examine process, that is, whether the appropriate personnel follow the proper procedures in dealing with the clinical problem, and outcome, the result for the patient. Outside organizations, most notably the Joint Commission on Accreditation of Healthcare Organizations (JCAHO), make regular inspections of facilities to assess how well they are monitoring care. Because the economic viability of facilities often depends on successful accreditation, administrators provide strong incentives for professionals to comply.

To support individual clinicians who wish to make pain relief a targeted outcome in their facilities, the American Pain Society developed the following standards with the informal advice of JCAHO staff.

From American Pain Society Subcommittee on Quality Assurance Standards: Standards for monitoring quality of analgesic treatment of acute pain and cancer pain, *Oncol Nurs Forum* 17:952, 1990; and from American Pain Society, *JAMA* 274(23):1874–1880, 1995. Copyrighted 1995, American Medical Association.

American Pain Society Quality Assurance Standards for Treatment of Acute Pain and Cancer Pain in Hospitals and Chronic Care Facilities

Preface (To Be Included with Standards). In the majority of patients with acute pain and chronic cancer pain, comfort can be achieved with the attentive use of analgesic medications. Historically, however, the outcomes of analgesic treatment often have not been satisfactory, largely because clinical care units have had no systems in place to ensure that the occurrence of pain is recognized and that when pain persists, there is rapid feedback to modify treatment. These suggested standards are offered as one approach to developing such a system. Individual facilities may wish to modify these standards to suit their particular needs.

The guidelines are intended both for clinical facilities in which only conventional analgesic methods are used (e.g., intermittent parenteral or oral analgesics) as well as in those using the most modern technology for pain management. In either case, the quality of pain control will be enhanced by a dedicated pain management team whose personnel acquire special training in pain relief. Newer, more aggressive methods of pain control, such as patient-controlled analgesic infusion, epidural opiate administration, and regional anesthetic techniques, may provide better pain relief than intermittent parenteral analgesics in many patients, but they carry their own risks. Should institutions choose to use these methods, they must be delivered by an organized team with frequent follow-up and titration and with adequate briefing of the primary caregivers. Such teams should be organized under one of the recognized medical departments of the facility. Specific standards for such methods, monitored by that department, might well augment the general guidelines articulated here.

I. Acute Pain and Chronic Cancer Pain Are Recognized and Effectively Treated

Required Characteristics (Process)

IA. A measure of pain intensity and a measure of pain relief are recorded on the bedside vital sign chart or on a similar record that facilitates regular review by members of the health care team and is incorporated in the patient's permanent record.

IA1. The intensity of pain/discomfort is assessed and documented on admission, after any known pain-producing procedure, with each new report of pain, and routinely, at regular intervals that depend upon the severity of pain. A simple, valid measure of intensity will be selected by each clinical unit. For children, age-appropriate pain intensity measures will be used.

IA2. The degree of pain relief is determined after each pain management intervention, once sufficient time has elapsed for the treatment to reach peak effect (e.g., 1 hour for parenteral analgesics, 2 hours for oral analgesics). A simple, valid measure of pain relief will be selected by each clinical unit.

IB. Each clinical unit will identify values for pain intensity rating (e.g., greater than the midpoint on the pain intensity scale) and pain relief rating (e.g., < 50% at its maximum) that will elicit a review of the current pain therapy, documentation of the proposed modifications in treatment, and subsequent review of their efficacy. This process of treatment review and follow-up should include participation by physicians and nurses involved in the patient's care. As the general quality of treatment improves, the clinical unit will upgrade this standard to encourage a continuous process of improvement.

Required Characteristics (Outcome)

IC. At regular intervals (to be defined by the clinical unit and the quality assurance committee), each clinical unit will assess a randomly selected sample of patients who have had surgery within the past 72 hours, have another acute pain condition, and/or have a diagnosis of cancer. Patients will be asked whether they have had pain during the current admission. Those who have experienced pain will then be asked about:

1. Current pain intensity.
2. Intensity of the worst pain experienced within the past 24 hours (or other interval selected by the clinical unit).
3. Degree of relief obtained from pain management interventions.
4. Satisfaction with responsiveness of the staff to reports of pain.
5. Satisfaction with relief provided.

II. Information about Analgesics Is Readily Available (Process)

Information about analgesics and other methods of pain management, including charts of relative potencies of analgesics, is situated on the unit in a way that aids writing and interpreting orders. Nurses and physicians can demonstrate the use of this material. Appropriate training to treat patients' pain is available to health professionals and included in continuing education activities.

III. Patients Are Promised Attentive Analgesic Care (Process)

Patients are informed on admission, verbally and in a printed format, that effective pain relief is an important part of their treatment, that their communication of unrelieved pain is essential, and that health professionals will respond quickly to their reports of pain. Pediatric patients and their parents will receive materials appropriate to the age of the patient.

IV. Explicit Policies for Use of Advanced Analgesic Technologies Are Defined (Process)

Advanced pain control techniques, including intraspinal opioids, systemic or intraspinal patient-controlled opioid infusion (PCA) or continuous opioid infusion, local anesthetic infusion, and inhalational analgesia, must be governed by policy and standard procedures that define the acceptable level of patient monitoring and the appropriate roles and limits of practice for all groups of healthcare providers involved. Such policy should include definitions of physician accountability, nurse responsibility to patient and physician, and the role of pharmacy.

V. Adherence to Standards Is Monitored (Process)

Required Characteristics (Structure and Process)

VA. An interdisciplinary committee, including representation from physicians, nurses, and other appropriate disciplines (e.g., pharmacy), monitors compliance with the above standards, considers issues relevant to improving pain treatment, and makes recommendations to improve outcomes and their monitoring. Where a comprehensive pain management team exists, its activities are monitored through the parent department's quality assurance body, which also may serve as the facility's quality assurance committee for pain relief. In a nursing home or very small hospital where an interdisciplinary pain management committee is not feasible, one or several individuals may fulfill this role.

VB. At least the chair of the committee has experience working with issues related to effective pain management.

VC. The committee meets at least every 3 months to review process and outcomes related to pain management.

VD. The committee interacts with clinical units to establish procedures for improving pain management where necessary and reviews the results of these changes within 3 months of implementation.

VE. The committee provides regular reports to administration and to the medical, nursing, and pharmacy staffs.

Example of Patient Outcome Questionnaire (Standard IC) (To be filled out by Interviewer).

1. Have you experienced any pain in the past 24 hours? Yes No
2. On this scale, how much discomfort or pain are you having right now? (Category, numerical [0–10], or VAS scales may be used for questions 3–5.) (record rating)
3. On this scale, please indicate the worst pain you have had in the past 24 hours. (record rating)
4. On this scale, please indicate the average level of pain you have had in the past 24 hours. (record rating)
5. Circle the number below that describes how, during the past 24 hours, pain has interfered with your:
   A. General activity
      0 1 2 3 4 5 6 7 8 9 10
   B. Mood
      0 1 2 3 4 5 6 7 8 9 10
   C. Walking ability
      0 1 2 3 4 5 6 7 8 9 10
   D. Relations with other people
      0 1 2 3 4 5 6 7 8 9 10
   E. Sleep
      0 1 2 3 4 5 6 7 8 9 10
   F. (For postoperative patients) Other activities that are needed to recover from illness (e.g., coughing and deep breathing after surgery; clinician should specify activity).
      0 1 2 3 4 5 6 7 8 9 10
   G. (For outpatients with chronic pain) Normal work, including housework
      0 1 2 3 4 5 6 7 8 9 10
   H. (For patients with chronic pain) Enjoyment of life
      0 1 2 3 4 5 6 7 8 9 10
      Does not interfere
      Completely interferes
6. Select the phrase that indicates how satisfied or dissatisfied you are with the results of your pain treatment overall.

Very dissatisfied   Slightly satisfied
Dissatisfied   Satisfied
Slightly dissatisfied   Very satisfied

7. Select the phrase that indicates how satisfied you are with the way your nurses responded to your reports of pain.
Very dissatisfied   Slightly satisfied
Dissatisfied   Satisfied
Slightly dissatisfied   Very satisfied

8. Select the phrase that indicates how satisfied or dissatisfied you are with the way your physicians responded to your reports of pain.
Very dissatisfied   Slightly satisfied
Dissatisfied   Satisfied
Slightly dissatisfied   Very satisfied

9. When you asked for pain medication, what was the longest time you had to wait to get it?
<10 minutes   >60 minutes
11–20 minutes   Asked for medication, but never
21–30 minutes   received it
31–60 minutes   Never asked for pain medication

10. Was there a time that the medication you were given for pain didn't help and you asked for something more or different to relieve the pain?
Yes   No
If your answer is "yes," how long did it take before your physician or nurse changed your treatment to a stronger or different medication and gave it to you?
<1 hour   5–8 hours
1–2 hours   9–24 hours
3–4 hours   >24 hours

11. Early in your care, did your physician or nurse make it clear to you that we consider treatment of pain very important and that you should be sure to tell them when you have pain?
Yes   No

12. Do you have any suggestions for how your pain management could be improved?

APPENDIX B: RESOURCES

Organizations

American Alliance of Cancer Pain Initiatives (AACPI)
The Resource Center
1300 University Avenue, Rm. #4720
Madison, WI 53706
608-265-4013
608-265-4014 (fax)
www.aacp.@aacpi.org

American Cancer Society, National Office (ACS)
1599 Clifton Road
Atlanta, GA 30329
404-320-3333
888-ACS-5552
www.cancer.org

American Pain Society (APS)
A national chapter of the International Association for the Study of Pain
4700 West Lake Avenue
Glenview, IL 60025-1485
847-375-4715
847-375-6315 (fax)
www.ampainsoc.org

American Society of Pain Management Nurses (ASPMN)
7794 Grow Drive
Pensacola, FL 32514
850-473-0233
850-484-8762 (fax)
www.aspmn.org

City of Hope National Medical Center
Pain Resource Center
1500 East Duarte Road
Duarte, CA 91010
626-359-8111, ext. 3829
626-301-8941 (fax)
www.mayday.coh.org

International Association for the Study of Pain (IASP)
A multidisciplinary professional organization
909 NE 43rd Street, Suite 306
Seattle, WA 98105-6020
206-547-6409
206-547-1703 (fax)
www.halcyon.com/iasp

National Cancer Institute (NCI)
Office of Cancer Communications
NCI/NIH
Bethesda, MD 20892
800-4-CANCER
www.nci.nih.gov

National Hospice Organization (NHO)
Publishes *Hospice* magazine (professional orientation) and *The Hospice Journal* (research orientation)
1901 North Moore Drive, Suite 901
Arlington, VA 22209-1714
703-243-5900
703-525-5762 (fax)
www.nho.org

Oncology Nursing Society (ONS)
501 Holiday Drive
Pittsburgh, PA 15220-2749
412-921-7373
412-921-6565 (fax)
www.ons.org

Professional Publications

APS Journal
Official Journal of the American Pain Society
Harcourt Health Science
11830 Westline Industrial Drive
St. Louis, MO 63146
800-553-5426

Journal of Pain and Symptom Management
A multidisciplinary publication that supports research and
    education in all areas of palliative care
Elsevier Publishing Co., Inc.
Subscription Customer Service
655 Avenue of the Americas
New York, NY 10010
212-633-3950

"Cancer Pain Release"
A publication of the World Health Organization Collaborat-
    ing Center for Policy and Communications in Cancer Care
University of Wisconsin–Madison
1900 University Avenue
Madison, WI 53705
608-263-0727
www.medsch.wisc.edu/WHOcancerpain

"Management of Cancer Pain: Clinical Practice Guideline"
Agency for Health Care Policy and Research (AHCPR)
Publication No. 94-0592, March 1994
"Management of Cancer Pain: Adults. Quick Reference
    Guide for Clinicians"
Publication No. 94-0593, March 1994
U.S. Department of Health and Human Services
Agency for Health Care Policy and Research
Executive Office Center Suite 501
2101 East Jefferson Street
Rockville, MD 20852
800-4-CANCER

"Oncology Nursing Society Position Paper on Cancer Pain
    Monograph"
Oncology Nursing Society (1990)
501 Holiday Drive
Pittsburgh, PA 15220-2749
412-921-7373
412-921-6565 (fax)
www.ons.org

"Oral Morphine in Advanced Cancer" (ed 3, 1995) by R.
    Twycross, S. Lack
Bath, England: Bath Press
(Available through Roxane Laboratories)
P.O. Box 16532
Columbus, OH 43216
800-848-0120
www.roxane.com

"Principles of Analgesic Use in the Treatment of Acute Pain
    and Chronic Cancer Pain: A Concise Guide to Medical
    Practice" (ed 4, 1999)

41-Page booklet
American Pain Society
4700 West Lake Avenue
Glenview, IL 60025
708-966-5595

"Pain: Clinical Manual for Nursing Practice" (1999, 3rd edi-
    tion) by M. McCaffery, C. Pasero
C.V. Mosby Company
11830 Westline Industrial Drive
St. Louis, MO 63146
www.mosby.com

"The Network News"
A newsletter
Memorial Sloan Kettering Cancer Center
Box 421
1275 York Avenue
New York, NY 10021
212-639-3164
www.networkproject.org

Patient Information

Booklets

"Cancer Doesn't Have to Hurt" (1997) by PJ Haylock, CP
    Curtiss
(Book for patients and families)
Hunter House, Inc.
PO Box 2914
Alameda, CA 94501-5592
800-266-5592
510-865-4295 (fax)

"Get Relief from Cancer Pain"
(Booklet in 3 versions—English, Spanish, and large print)
American Cancer Soceity
1599 Clifton Road
Atlanta, GA 30329
800-ACS-2345
www.cancer.org

"Managing Cancer Pain" (Consumer version)
Publication No. 94-0595, March 1994
U.S. Department of Health and Human Services
Agency for Health Care Policy and Research (AHCPR)
Executive Office Center, Suite 501
2101 East Jefferson Street
Rockville, MD 20852
800-4-CANCER

"Oral Morphine: Information for Patients, Families and
    Friends" (1995) by RG Twycross, S Lack
Bath, England: Bath Press
(Available through Roxanne Laboratories)
P.O. 16532
Columbus, OH 43216
800-848-0120
www.roxanne.com

"Questions and Answers About Pain Control: A Guide for
   People with Cancer and Their Families"
National Cancer Institute and the American Cancer Society
(Available through local ACS offices)
"Up-to-Date Answers to Questions About Measuring Pain"
(To help patients living with cancer) (1991)
Purdue Frederick Company
Norwalk, CT 06850-3590
203-853-0123

Cancer Resources on the Internet

Agency for Health Care Policy and Research, www.ahcpr.gov
American Academy of Hospice and Palliative Medicine,
   www.aahpm.org
American Academy of Pain Management,
   www.aapainmanage.org/index.html
American Alliance of Cancer Pain Initiatives,
   www.aacpi.org

American Cancer Society, www.cancer.org
American Pain Society, www.ampainsoc.org
International Association for the Study of Pain,
   www.halcyon.com/iasp
Mayday Pain Resource Center at the City of Hope,
   www.mayday.cho.org
   send e-mail to: mayday pain@smtplink.coh.org
National Hospice Organization, www.nho.org
OncoLink, www.cancer.med.upenn.edu/
Oncology Nursing Society, www.ons.org
Purdue-Frederick, www.partnersagainstpain.com
Resource Center for State Cancer Pain Initiatives,
   www.wisc.edu/molpharm/wcpi
Roxane Laboratories, www.roxane.com
University of Iowa, www.coninfo.nursing.uiowa.edu./www/
   nursing/apn.cncrpian.toc.html
University of Wisconsin Pain and Policy Studies Group,
   www.medsch.wisc.edu/painpolicy
Wisconsin Cancer Pain Initiative, www.wisc.edu/wcpi

Protective Mechanisms

Shirley E. Otto

CHAPTER
31

Numerous mechanisms protect humans from foreign substances and invading organisms. This chapter looks at these mechanisms and their importance to the person with cancer, the nursing process, related nursing diagnoses, and nursing interventions.

IMMUNITY

Immunity is a protective mechanism that maintains the integrity of the body against foreign substances or agents. The study of immunity was based on the study of infectious diseases but cannot be limited to such and now encompasses the areas of solid organ and peripheral blood stem cell or allogeneic bone marrow transplantation (BMT), autoimmunity, blood transfusion, cancer, and genetics.

Four main functions of the immune system include (1) protection—defense against invading organisms; (2) homeostasis—removal of dead "self" cells; (3) surveillance—removal of mutant cells; and (4) regulation—augmentation and depression of immune response.

The major purpose of a fully functional immune system is to distinguish self from nonself. The ability of the body to develop tolerance of self-produced antigens is a part of this function. The two basic types of immunity are *innate* and *acquired.* Innate immunity is a nonspecific immune system function. Acquired immunity is specific and depends on the recognition of self and nonself.[14, 35, 90]

Innate Immunity

Innate immunity is a nonspecific response to any breach of the skin and mucous membranes. This type of immunity is present at birth and is species specific. Innate immunity provides initial protection against foreign substances and invading organisms. The four mechanisms of innate immunity are *mechanical barriers, chemical barriers, fever,* and *phagocytosis* or *inflammation.*[14, 35]

Mechanical Barriers. Mechanical barriers include epithelial surfaces, such as skin and mucous membranes, and their projections along the gastrointestinal (GI), respiratory, and genitourinary (GU) tracts. Intact skin and mucous membranes present an effective physical barrier to the entrance of organisms and toxins. Epithelial surfaces carry receptors for specific antigens on the cell surfaces. These receptors are essential for maintaining the normal microorganism flora of the skin and mucous membranes. Secretory IgA, an antibody, prevents the attachment of pathogenic organisms to epithelial cells. Routine exfoliation of epithelial cells, with loss of adherent organisms, also serves to limit invasion by organisms.[90]

Chemical Barriers. Chemical barriers include such substances as saliva, mucus, tears, sweat, gastric juices, sebum, cerumen, lysozyme products, and numerous other substances secreted by the body. These prevent entry of potentially harmful substances and organisms by various mechanisms such as pH, viscosity, and the presence of other substances with antimicrobial activity that physically inhibits attachment and invasion by organisms.[35]

Fever. Fever (elevated body temperature) is a protective mechanism directed against temperature-sensitive organisms such as bacteria and viruses. These organisms secrete substances that act as pyrogens, elevating body temperature in response to their presence. Temperature-sensitive organisms such as these rarely survive sustained body temperature elevations in excess of 102.2°F (39°C). Warm-blooded animals elevate body temperature by internal means in response to pyrogens such as bacterial toxins and leukocyte products (cytokines) when inflammation or immune response occurs. Fevers of 100.8°F (38.2°C) to 103.1°F (39.5°C) are generally well tolerated. Additional potential causes of fever include drugs, tumor fever, tissue necrosis, and administration of blood product transfusions or biotherapy agents.[8, 11, 90]

Fever is a defense mechanism that has a positive effect on the survival of patients with life-threatening infections. Recent investigations have identified the immune-enhancing effect of fever on antigen recognition and sensitization. There appears to be increasing support for the positive effects of fever and that aggressive antipyresis for low-grade temperature elevations may be detrimental.[8, 11]

Inflammatory Response. The inflammatory response provides immediate but short-term protection against the effects of a local injury or invasion that is initiated when mechanical or chemical barriers of the body are invaded. The type, duration, and extent of the inflammatory response depends on the intensity, duration, severity, size, and duration of exposure to the initiating injury or invasion. This limited, nonspecific response is initiated and mediated by phagocytic white blood cells (WBCs) such as neutrophils, eosinophils, basophils, monocytes, and macrophages. It does not require recognition of self. The process of inflammation is not complete until all invading organisms, dead and dying phagocytic cells, and necrotic cellular debris are removed by macrophages (histiocytes) and tissue damage is repaired by fibroblasts.[11, 14, 35]

Acquired Immunity

Acquired immunity is the body's specific neutralizing response to foreign invaders and their products. This type of immunity is not fully functional at birth. It may take 6 to 7 years for the immune system to mature, and as a person reaches late middle age, its level of functioning begins to decline, as evidenced by increased incidence of autoimmune disorders and cancers. The two main mechanisms of acquired immunity are cell-mediated immunity and humoral immunity. Both use lymphocytes as effector cells.[90]

Lymphocytes. Lymphocytes are small, round, mononuclear cells that make up approximately 30% of the peripheral circulating leukocyte population. Lymphocytes are derived from pleuripotential stem cells found in the bone marrow. Two major subtypes of lymphocytes have been identified: thymus-derived or thymus-dependent lymphocytes (T cells) and bursa-derived or bursa-dependent lymphocytes (B cells [beta cells, B lymphocytes]). Some specific B-cell lymphocytes differentiate to become plasma cells or memory cells that are capable of recognizing a particular antigen at future exposures and produce plasma cells to generate abundant antibodies specific to that antigen. These specific B-cell lymphocytes do not have phagocyte activity.[30, 90]

Cell-Mediated Immunity. Cell-mediated immunity (CMI) uses T cells as the primary effector cells. T cells function as immunoregulatory and cytotoxic cells. CMI provides defense against intracellular bacteria such as

Mycobacterium tuberculosis and *Listeria monocytogenes,* fungi, viruses, and protozoa (Box 31–1). Delayed hypersensitivity reactions are a type of CMI. Transplantation rejection, by both graft and host, is caused in part by the T cell and its ability to distinguish self from nonself. Immune surveillance, or the body's inherent ability to prevent cancers, is also thought to be a function of CMI with the natural killer cell (NK cell or large, granular lymphocyte) being the primary effector cell of surveillance.[30, 90]

Cell-mediated immune deficiencies may be congenital or acquired (Box 31–2). Congenital anomalies include children born without thymus glands and those with poorly functioning thymus glands. Death usually occurs in the first years of life and is caused by infection. Secondary or acquired causes of diminished T-cell function are more common and include acquired immunodeficiency syndrome (AIDS), Hodgkin's disease, allogeneic BMT or organ transplantation immunosuppression, and some autoimmune disorders. Persons who have defects in CMI, regardless of cause, are susceptible to opportunistic infections from a host of bacteria, viruses, fungi, and protozoa and to the development of cancers, particularly those arising from lymphoid tissue.[8, 14, 90]

Humoral Immunity. Humoral immunity is the part of acquired immunity that involves the production of antibodies. *Antibodies* are substances produced by plasma cells (sensitized B cells) in response to specific recognition of an antigen (foreign substance). They are serum proteins called *immunoglobulins.* The five major categories of immunoglobulins are IgG, IgM, IgA, IgD, and IgE. The body has an unlimited ability to produce different antibodies against specific antigens. Antibodies

---

BOX 31–1

Infecting Organisms Associated with Cellular Immune Deficiency

Intracellular Bacteria

Mycobacterium tuberculosis
Atypical mycobacteria
Listeria monocytogenes

Fungi

Candida albicans
Cryptococcus neoformans
Aspergillus species
Histoplasma capsulatum

Viruses

Herpes simplex
Herpes zoster
Cytomegalovirus
Epstein-Barr
Hepatitis B

Protozoa

Pneumocystis carinii
Cryptosporidium
Toxoplasma gondii
Giardia lamblia
Isospora belli

Data from references 11 and 35.

BOX 31-2

Cell-Mediated Immune Deficiencies

PRIMARY IMMUNE DEFICIENCIES

Predominantly T cell

Chronic mucocutaneous candidiasis
Nezelof syndrome
DiGeorge syndrome (thymic-parathyroid aplasia)

Combined T Cell and B Cell

Ataxia-telangiectasia
Severe combined immunodeficiency
Severe combined immunodeficiency with adenosine
   deaminase deficiency
Short-limbed dwarfism
Wiskott-Aldrich syndrome

SECONDARY IMMUNE DEFICIENCIES

Malignant Disease

Acute lymphoblastic leukemia
Chronic lymphocytic leukemia
Hairy cell leukemia
Hodgkin's disease
Mycosis fungoides and Sezary syndrome
Non-Hodgkin's lymphoma
Advanced carcinomas

Therapeutic

Cytotoxic drugs
Immunosuppressive agents
Radiation therapy

Infections

Human immunodeficiency virus
Cytomegalovirus
Epstein-Barr virus
Non-A/non-B hepatitis
Leprosy
Tuberculosis
Histoplasmosis
Cryptococcosis
Toxoplasmosis

Data from references 11 and 35.

---

mune deficiencies, most commonly hypogammaglobulinemias, are often related to lymphoproliferative disorders such as chronic lymphocytic leukemia, non-Hodgkin's lymphomas, and plasma cell dyscrasias such as multiple myeloma and Waldenstrom's macroglobulinemia. Acquired idiopathic hypogammaglobulinemias occur without known cause. Regardless of cause, the person with a defective humoral immune system is susceptible to infection by high-grade (nonopportunistic) encapsulated bacteria, both gram-positive and gram-negative. These infections are often life-threatening and recurrent.[8, 11, 14, 90]

Interactions. The specific immune response requires complex interaction between CMI and humoral immunity. The macrophage (a phagocyte WBC) is necessary for the proper functioning of this response. The macrophage processes and presents the antigen to the T cell for recognition and elicitation of response. The primary responsibility of the T cells is recognition of self. In the presence of nonself antigens, a number of processes are elicited. Among these is the production of lymphokines.

BOX 31-3

Humoral Immune Deficiencies

Primary Antibody Deficiencies

X-linked hypogammaglobulinemia
X-linked hypogammaglobulinemia with growth hormone deficiency
Transient hypogammaglobulinemia of infancy
Common variable unclassifiable hypogammaglobulinemia
Selective immunoglobulin deficiencies (IgA, IgG subclass)
Autosomal recessive hypogammaglobulinemia

Primary Mixed T- and B-Cell Deficiencies

See cell-mediated immune deficiencies listed in
   Box 31-2

Secondary Antibody Deficiencies

Chronic lymphocytic leukemia
Acute lymphoblastic leukemia
Non-Hodgkin's lymphoma—B-cell origin
Multiple myeloma
Heavy-chain disease
Waldenstrom's macroglobulinemia
Thymoma
Nephrotic syndrome
Protein-losing enteropathies
Burns
Splenectomy

Data from references 8 and 35.

---

function by neutralizing toxins, agglutinating and lysing microorganisms and other cells, and serving as opsonins (coating organisms and making them more palatable to phagocytic cells).[14, 90]

Defects in humoral immunity, like those of CMI, may be congenital or acquired (Box 31-3). Agammaglobulinemia and some types of hypogammaglobulinemia may be congenital. These produce lifelong susceptibility to severe bacterial infections. Secondary humoral im-

BOX 31-4

Examples of Cytokines

Monokines

Interleukin-1 (IL-1) or endogenous pyrogen (EP)
Tumor necrosis factor (TNF)
Interferon alfa-2a (leukocyte) (IFN)
Granulocyte colony-stimulating factor (G-CSF)
Granulocyte/macrophage colony-stimulating factor (GM-CSF)
Interleukin-6 (IL-6)
Interleukin-11 (IL-11) oprelvekin (Neumega)

Lymphokines

Macrophage-activating factor (MAF)
Macrophage inhibition factor (MIF)
Interferon, gamma (immune) (IF)
Interleukin-2, T-cell growth factor (IL-2)
Interleukin-3, multi-CSF growth factor (IL-3)
Interleukin-6, B-cell differentiation factor (IL-6)
Chemotactic factor (CF)
B-cell growth factor (BCGF)
Tumor necrosis factor (TNF)
Lymphotoxin (LT)

Data from references 8, 32, 35, 42.

The epidermis, or topmost epithelial layer, functions primarily to conserve water. Pigment-forming cells called *melanocytes* reside within this layer. Constant mitotic activity replaces dead cells. Repair and replacement occur from the bottom up; old cells are lost through wear and tear of daily living and are replaced by new cells developing underneath.[14, 49]

The dermis, or inner layer of skin, determines skin thickness. It is thickest on dorsal surfaces of the body, palms of hands, and soles of feet and thinnest on ventral surfaces including the abdomen and genitalia. The dermis contains blood vessels, lymphatics, and afferent sensory nerve endings. The skin is a multifunctional organ. Its recognized functions include[66, 90]:

Absorbs substances applied directly to the skin
Distinguishes between pain, temperature, and touch
Excretes excess water and electrolytes
Prevents entrance of external gases, liquids, radiation, and pathogens as long as intact thus protects the internal body
Provides nutrition to underlying structures through an abundant blood supply
Regulates body temperature by vasoconstriction and vasodilation
Regulates loss of water and electrolytes

Lymphokines, part of a larger group called *cytokines,* are soluble chemical mediators that facilitate intercellular communication among T cells, B cells, macrophages, and other phagocytic cells. Particular lymphokines (Box 31–4) may cause activation of macrophages, sensitization of other T cells, and conversion of B cells to plasma cells with resultant production of antibodies. T cells are also regulatory cells of the immune system. Helper/inducer T cells (T4 or CD4 lymphocytes) stimulate and promote immune system function, whereas suppressor T cells (T8 or CD8 lymphocytes) inhibit or prevent immune system functioning. T8 or CD8 lymphocytes may also become T cells capable of "cell-to-cell" combat. These cells are "killer" or cytotoxic T cells.[11, 14, 68, 90]

SKIN

Anatomy and Physiology

The skin is one of several mechanical barriers that can prevent the entrance of invading organisms and toxins and maintain homeostasis. The skin is composed of the epidermis, dermis, and assorted derivatives of epidermal/dermal origin, which include hair, nails, cutaneous glands, and teeth.

Pathophysiology

A person with cancer may experience multiple disruptions of skin integrity.

Disease-Related Causes. Disease-related causes of skin integrity disruption include primary skin malignancies such as malignant melanoma, basal cell carcinoma, squamous cell carcinoma, Kaposi's sarcoma, and mycosis fungoides. Premalignant disease-related conditions, such as actinic keratosis, leukoplakia, dysplastic nevus syndrome, may increase the risk of primary skin malignancies for some individuals. Metastatic tumors of the skin, such as chest wall recurrence in breast cancer, and leukemic and lymphomatous infiltrates (leukemia cutis and lymphoma cutis, respectively) may also disrupt skin integrity. Cutaneous manifestations associated with remote effects of malignancy, such as acanthosis nigricans, acquired ichthyosis, dermatomyositis, and exfoliative dermatitis, may cause disruption of skin integrity secondary to scratching and cracking of skin. Thrombocytopenia with resultant petechiae, purpura, and ecchymoses may lead to increased fragility of the skin.[26, 35]

Treatment-Related Causes. Treatment-related causes of skin impairment include those associated with chemotherapy such as drug extravasation, alopecia, hyperpig-

Nursing Management

SKIN INTEGRITY

Nursing Diagnoses

- *Skin integrity, impaired, risk for/actual, related to immobility, malignant skin lesions, infectious skin lesions, nonspecific rashes, irritation from urinary or fecal incontinence, abrasions resulting from scratching and shearing forces, invasive therapeutic procedures, radiation skin reactions, "recall" skin reactions, chemotherapy extravasations, lymphaphatic or vascular obstruction, decubiti, malnutrition*
- *Infection, risk for, related to impairment of skin integrity secondary to any of the contributing factors just listed, surgical incision, presence of long-term venous access device*
- *Pain related to any of the contributing factors just listed, postherpetic neuralgia, pruritus secondary to basic disease process or adverse drug reaction*
- *Body image disturbance related to malignant skin lesions, extremity edema, alopecia*

Outcome Goals

Patient will be able to:

- Identify/demonstrate measures to maintain/promote skin integrity.
- Identify/demonstrate measures to prevent infection related to impaired skin integrity.
- Achieve adequate control of pain related to impaired skin integrity.
- Show evidence of effective coping with body image disturbance related to impaired skin integrity.

INTACT SKIN

Interventions: Assessment

- Inspect high-risk skin areas for color, vascularity, edema, injuries, scars, lesions, nodules.
- Document assessment at least once a shift.[13]

Interventions: Preventive Measures to Maintain Intact Skin

- Reposition, at least every 2 hours, any individual in bed who is assessed to be at risk for developing pressure ulcers.[2, 65, 66]
- Use draw sheet for turning and positioning.

- Elevate head of bed to maximum of 30 degrees except for mealtimes, at which time bed may be elevated more.
- Use footboard to prevent sliding.
- Provide over-bed trapeze to assist in position change.
- Lift patient to change position rather than pulling or sliding.
- Use devices to decrease pressure areas, such as mattress overlays or alternating pressure mattresses (see Pressure Reduction Devices/Specialty Beds on page 922; Dressings and Skin Care Products on page 923, and Support Surfaces, Types and Descriptions on page 924).
- Use heel and elbow protectors.
- Provide meticulous skin hygiene—mild soap, thorough rinsing, patting dry (not rubbing), air drying when feasible, applying lotions to skin over bony prominences.

Interventions: Malnourishment

- Follow general preventive measures.
- Provide adequate nutritional support.
- Assess risk daily.

Interventions: Incontinence

- Follow general preventive measures.
- Offer bedpan and urinal every 2 hours.
- Wash buttocks and perineum after each incontinence; pat or air dry.
- Place waterproof pads between draw sheets rather than next to patient's skin.
- Evaluate need for bowel and bladder retraining program.

Interventions: Immobility[2, 65, 66]

- Follow general preventive measures.
- Use splints and braces to prevent contractures.
- Use dietetic and nutrition consultants.
- Initiate referrals to rehabilitation medicine, social services, and vocational rehabilitation.
- Institute bowel program with stool softeners and laxatives to prevent constipation.
- Provide diversionary activities to prevent boredom.

Interventions: Pruritus[41, 70, 83]

- Follow general preventive measures.
- Maintain hydration of the skin by increasing fluid intake, applying water-soluble emollients to damp skin, and providing a humidified environment.

- Keep fingernails short and smooth.
- Wash hands frequently.[57]
- Use alternative methods of skin stimulation such as pressure, massage, vibration, and cold compresses.
- Avoid inciting agents and tight, irritating, nonabsorbable clothing.
- Prevent vasodilation by providing a cool environment and cool baths and showers, avoiding alcohol- and caffeine-containing foods and beverages, and decreasing anxiety level through use of distraction.
- Institute medical treatment as prescribed, which may include treatment of the underlying malignancy, with antihistamines, corticosteroids, tranquilizers, and topical agents.
- Maintenance of normal skin integrity should be a major emphasis of nursing management. This includes continued assessment, evaluation of risk, prevention of skin breakdown, and specific interventions if impaired skin integrity occurs. Systematic protocols or care plans should be implemented to ensure continuity of care.

Patient and Family Education

Patients and families need to be taught the importance of maintaining intact skin, the fundamentals of assess-

Pressure Reduction Devices/Specialty Beds

Indications for Use	Support Surfaces	Manufacturer	Intended Use
Low risk/prevention: Stages 0–I ulcer	Foam overlay	Bio Clinic Mason Span-America	Used on top of existing mattress; single patient use; least expensive.
	Water/gel-filled overlay	Floatation Systems Mason	Durable; easy to clean; heavy; both may cause high pressure at heels.
Medium risk: Stages I–III ulcer	Static air-filled pressure pad	Gaymar Kinetic Concepts Mason	Redistributes pressure to areas of less pressure.
	Dynamic air-filled pressure pad	Bio Clinic Gaymar Grant Hill-Rom HNE Healthcare Mason	Also called *alternating pressure pads;* pump constantly changes pressure points; requires constant monitoring.
Medium/high risk: Stages I–IV ulcer	Foam mattress; gel and foam mattress	Bio Clinic Hill-Rom Kinetic Concepts Mason Span-America	Provide support and conformity; reduce pressure and shear; may be hospital replacement mattress.
	Low air-loss mattress	Bio Clinic Gaymar Kinetic Concepts	Calibrated to patient's weight; air not cycled—shifts in response to movement.
	Active mattress overlay system	Gaymar Hill-Rom HNE Healthcare Kinetic Concepts	Air cycles continuously; used with standard hospital bed frame and mattress.
High risk: Stage IV ulcer	Dynamic flotation mattress	Bio Clinic Gaymar Hill-Rom HNE Healthcare KineticConcepts Mason	Sensor pad continuously monitors the system.
	Low air-loss bed	Bio Clinic Hill-Rom Kinetic Concepts	On special frame—scales, or CPR quick-release lever.
Ultra-high risk: Stage IV ulcer	Air-fluidized bed	Hill-Rom Kinetic Concepts	For small group of patients who cannot tolerate any pressure.

Modified from Carroll P: Bed selection—help patients rest easy, RN 58(5):44, 1995. Names, phone contacts revised 2/2000.

Bed manufacturers may be contacted as follows: Bio Clinic, 800-388-4083; Floatation Systems Inc, 800-888-8529; Gaymar Industries Inc, 800-828-7341; Grant Airmass Corp, 800-243-5237; Hill-Rom, 800-638-2546; HNE (Huntleigh) Healthcare, 800-223-1218; Kinetic Concepts Inc, 800-531-5346 (KCI); Mason Medical Products, 800-233-4454; Span-America Medical Systems Inc, 800-888-6752. Additional data from references 2, 18, 65, 85, 91.

Dressings and Skin Care Products

DRESSINGS: TYPES WITH DESCRIPTIONS

Absorptives—multilayer dressings that provide either a semiadherent quality or a nonadherent layer combined with highly absorptive layers of fibers, such as cellulose, cotton, or rayon.

Biologicals and synthetic membranes—skin substitutes, artificial skin, or skin equivalents that are placed over a wound and secured.

Collagens—pads, sheets, particles, powders, pastes, or gels derived from bovine, porcine, or avian sources.

Composites—products that combine physically distinct components into a single dressing that provides multiple functions, such as a bacterial barrier, absorption, and adhesion.

Contact layers—thin, nonadherent sheets placed directly on an open wound bed to protect the wound tissue from direct contact with other agents or dressings applied to the wound

Elastic gauzes—bandages that stretch and conform to body contours. They may provide absorption as a second layer or dressing, hold a wound cover in place; apply pressure or cushion the wound.

Foams—sheets and shapes of foamed solutions or polymers, most commonly polyurethane. Small open cells are capable of holding fluids. They vary in thickness and may be impregnated or layered in combination with other materials.

Gauze and nonwoven dressings—sponges and wraps with varying degrees of absorbency used for cleansing, packing, and covering wounds.

Hydrocolloids—wafers, powders, or pastes composed of materials such as gelatin, pectin and carboxymethylcellulose.

Hydrogels: Amorphous—formulations of water, polymers, and other indegredients with no shape, designated to donate moisture to a dry wound and to maintain a moist healing environment.

Impregnated—gauzes or nonwoven sponges saturated with an amorphous gel.

Sheets—three-dimensional networks of cross-linked hydrophilic polymers that are insoluble in water and interact with aqueous solutions by swelling.

Dressings: Impregnated—gauzes or nonwoven sponges saturated with a solution, an emulsion, oil, or some other agent or compound.

Silicone gel sheets—soft sheets of cross-linked polymers reinforced with mesh or fabric, used to improve the appearance of hypertrophic and keloid scars.

Silver technology—products that deliver the antimicrobial effects of silver to a wound while maintaining a moist wound environment; adherent or nonadherent.

Transparent films—thin polymer sheets coated on one side with an adhesive. They are impermeable to liquid, water, and bacteria but permeable to moisture vapor and atmospheric gases.

Wound fillers—powders, pastes, gels, beads, strands, pads, or other devices formulated to fill a wound site.

SKIN CARE PRODUCTS: TYPES WITH DESCRIPTIONS

Adhesive removers—solvents formulated to dissolve adhesives and assist in removing dressings, skin protectants, and tapes.

Antimicrobials/antifungals—agents in cream, ointment, lotion spray, or powder form that may be topically applied to the skin.

Cleansers—solution used to remove urine, feces, contaminants, foreign debris, and exudate from the skin.

Liquid skin protectants—formulations designed to protect vulnerable areas from the effects of mechanical or chemical injury.

Moisture barriers—cream, ointment, or paste preparations formulated to protect the skin from excessive moisture.

Therapeutic moisturizers—cream or ointment preparations used to soothe or soften the skin.

Tapes, closures, and securement products—adhesive or nonadhesive products used to secure or cover dressing, catheters, drainage tubes, or other devices. They may be used to connect lacerated tissue.

Data from references 21, 65, 66, 91.

Support Surfaces, Types and Descriptions

Beds: Powered and air-fluidized—(1) a semielectric or total electric hospital bed with a fully integrated powered mattress with a total height of 3 inches or greater and a surface designed to reduce friction and shear, or (2) a device that uses the circulation of filtered air through silicone-coated ceramic beads creating the characteristics of fluid.

Cushions and seating—powered or nonpowered devices placed on a wheelchair or other seating surface. They may use air, foam, gel, water, wool, or a combination of these.

Mattresses: Nonpowered—devices placed directly on a hospital bed frame. They may use air, foam, gel, water, or a combination of these. They have a durable, waterproof cover.

Mattresses: Powered—devices placed directly on a hospital bed frame that use alternating pressure, low air loss, or powered flotation without air loss. They have an air pump or blower that provides either sequential inflation and deflation or a low interface pressure throughout; an inflated cell height of 5 inches or greater; and a surface designated to reduce friction and shear.

Overlays: Nonpowered—devices placed directly on top of a standard hospital mattress. They may use air, foam, gel, water, wool, or other materials.

Overlays: Powered—devices placed directly on top of a standard hospital mattress that use low air loss, powered flotation without air loss, or alternating pressure. They have an air pump or blower that provides either sequential inflation and deflation or low interface pressure throughout; an inflated cell height of 3.5 inches or greater; and a surface designated to reduce friction and shear.

Positioners—devices used to place, elevate, or support the body or individual parts. They may use air, fiberfill, fluid, foam, gel, water, or other materials.

Protectors—devices used to cover or shield the body or individual parts from insult or injury.

Data from references 21, 65, 66, 91.

---

ing skin, and how to prevent breakdown by proper positioning and padding to prevent pressure points. Patients and families should be taught the signs and symptoms of infection and when and whom to notify on the health care team.

NONINTACT SKIN

Interventions: *Assessment*

- Inspect skin lesions and document: general character, location and distribution, configuration, size (measure), morphologic structure (nodularity, scaling, crusting, erosions, fissures), drainage (color, amount, character, odor), depth of lesion, presence of vital structure in lesion (carotid artery).
- Use National Pressure Ulcer Advisory Panel (NPUAP) staging system for pressure ulcers (see page 925).
- Monitor for signs and symptoms of infection (elevated temperature, tachycardia, tachypnea, change in color and odor of drainage, erythema).[2, 13, 65, 66]
- Evaluate for associated signs and symptoms (pain and tenderness).
- Evaluate patient's physical and psychological responses to lesions.
- Assess patient's and family's ability to care for problem in the home.

Interventions: *General Maintenance*

- Follow general preventive measures.
- Implement infection control measures.

- Implement measures to prevent bleeding and trauma.
- Provide adequate pain control.
- Obtain enterostomal therapy/skin care specialist consult.
- Obtain home health referral well in advance of discharge.

Interventions: *Nonulcerating Lesions*

- Follow general preventive measures.
- Use dry dressings to protect against irritation and trauma.
- Use occlusive dressings with topical medications for increased penetration.

Interventions: *Ulcerating Lesions*

- Cleanse area with antibacterial soap using gentle motion. Rinse well. Prevent cross-contamination if local infection is present.[44]
- Follow recommended protocol for debridement (i.e., cotton swabs, wet-to-dry soaks, continuous soaks, or proteolytic enzymes).[91]

Interventions: *Prevention and Management of Local Infection*

- Irrigate with antibacterial agent as prescribed.
- Use sterile technique.
- Administer systemic antibiotics as prescribed.
- Obtain specimens for culture as ordered or if fever is present.

Staging of Pressure Ulcers

Stage	Description
I	Nonblanchable erythema of intact skin—the heralding lesion of skin ulceration. Reactive hyperemia is the reddening or deepening of skin color that is normally observed once pressure to an area has been relieved. This type of hyperemia is blanchable and will resolve in approximately one half to three fourths the amount of time that the area was exposed to pressure.
I (dark-skinned people)	Use natural or halogen lighting: localized skin color changes at the site of pressure; these colors differ from the patient's normal skin color; a circumscribed area of intact skin at the potential ulceration appears darker than surrounding skin; this area may be taut, shiny, and/or indurated. Stage I ulcer may be developing if area is painful, itching, localized inflammation, and/or edematous.
II	Partial-thickness skin loss involving epidermis and/or dermis. The ulcer is superficial and presents clinically as an abrasion, blister, or shallow crater.
III	Full-thickness skin loss involving damage or necrosis of subcutaneous tissue that may extend down to, but not through, underlying fascia. The ulcer presents clinically as a deep crater with or without undermining of adjacent tissue.
IV	Full-thickness skin loss with extensive destruction, tissue necrosis or damage to muscle, bone, or supporting structures. Undermining and sinus tracts may be associated with stage IV ulcers.

Data from National Pressure Ulcer Advisory Panel: Pressure ulcers in adults: protection and prevention, AHCPR Publication No. 92-0047, Rockville, MD, US Department of Health and Human Services, Public Health Service, Agency for Health Care Policy and Research, May, 1992. Revisions 1994, 1999. Additional data from references 2, 65, 66.

- Apply dry, sterile, nonadherent dressing. Change and cleanse every 8 hours or more often as needed.

Interventions: *Hemostasis*

- Use silver nitrate sticks or styptic pencils as prescribed for mild oozing.
- Apply 1:1000 epinephrine or topical thrombin to areas with moderate oozing as prescribed. Local radiation or application of hemostatic dressings may be used.
- Administer platelet transfusions as ordered for bleeding associated with thrombocytopenia.

Interventions: *Drainage*

- Change dressing as frequently as necessary (as soon as it is wet).
- Use absorbent dressings for small to moderate amounts of drainage or on areas too large to pouch.
- Apply drainage bag or ostomy pouch for copious amounts of drainage. Apply skin protectant to surrounding skin to prevent irritation and breakdown.
- Secure sterile dressings with Montgomery straps, stretchable gauze, or Stomahesive.

Interventions: *Odor*

- Cleanse wound and change dressing as frequently as necessary.
- Obtain culture and sensitivities of wound.
- Apply commercial deodorizing agents to outside of dressings.
- Administer agents such as metronidazole (orally or topically) to control odor caused by anaerobes.
- Place shallow tray of activated charcoal in patient's room.
- Place commercial room deodorizer in room (if room deodorizer is not more offensive than wound odor).

Patient and Family Education

In addition to teaching general preventive measures to maintain intact skin, the nurse should teach the patient/family the signs and symptoms of infection and who and when to notify if they occur. Treatments and procedures should be discussed: clean or sterile technique, handwashing technique, disposal of used/soiled materials and dressings, environmental and personal hygiene practices, measures to prevent cross-contamination, application and expected effects of medications, measures to maintain hydration and nutrition, and measures to control bleeding. The primary caregiver must be instructed how to change the dressing in the home.

mentation, hyperkeratosis, photosensitivity, ulceration, radiation recall reactions, and graft-versus-host disease (GVHD) (skin) related to allogeneic bone marrow transplantation. Skin reactions associated with non-antineoplastic agents include allergic skin eruptions, Stevens-Johnson syndrome, and erythema multiforme. Radiation therapy skin reactions may progress to wet or dry skin desquamation. Surgical incisions and other invasive procedures such as needle biopsies and placement of vascular access devices also disrupt skin integrity.[23, 26, 33, 49, 62, 66]

Complicating Factors. Complicating factors that may interfere with the maintenance of skin integrity include immobility, malnutrition, edema, jaundice, obstruction, infection, incontinence, and pruritus.

Assessment. Skin assessment should include a thorough inspection of all skin surfaces with attention focused on the following: color, vascularity, bleeding (location, type, and amount), lesions (appearance, number, location, distribution, and ulceration), edema, moist areas, and general condition of hair and nails. If lesions are present, the nurse should assess for general characteristics, morphologic structure (nodularity, scaling, crusting, erosions, and fissures), size (measure), drainage (color, character, amount, and odor), associated pain and tenderness, depth of lesions (measure), and presence of vital structures within the lesion (i.e., carotid artery). High-risk areas (chest, abdomen, neck, and scalp) should be palpated with palms of hands for presence of "silent" lesions. Metastatic lesions are generally hard and immovable. Assessment should include attention to any history of allergies, medications, and past or present skin disorders. Risk assessment on a scheduled frequency for pressure ulcers using a reliable instrument such as the Norton scale or the Braden scale is an integral part of the nursing process. Pressure ulcers most commonly occur on the sacrum, coccyx, and the heels; therefore, a continuous reassessment of skin integrity with the specific patient risk factors (i.e., immobility, age, malnutrition) is critical to the patient's recovery process.[13, 17, 21, 61, 65, 85]

Medical Management

Treatment of skin complications may include the administration of antibiotics, antifungals, and antivirals for infection; surgical procedures for incision and drainage, debridement, and skin grafting; radiation therapy for obstructive phenomena; chemotherapy to treat the underlying disease for relief of pruritus; and management of disfiguring, nonhealing, or ulcerating malignant skin lesions. A variety of products are available to treat skin conditions such as pressure ulcers. Products may include skin care protectants, moisturizers, and moisture barriers; multiple varied dressings that protect the skin from moisture, cushion the skin, and absorb wound drainage. Support surfaces include beds, mattresses, seating cushions, or positioning devices to support the body for optimal patient comfort.[2, 18, 21, 85, 91]

MUCOUS MEMBRANES

Anatomy and Physiology

The oral mucosa provides a mechanical barrier to inhibit the invasion of microorganisms. The oral mucosa is composed of three layers: an outer layer of stratified, squamous epithelium; a middle layer, the lamina propria, consisting of fibrous finger-like projections that extend into the epithelium and contain blood vessels, nerves, and glandular tissue; and an inner submucosal layer that varies in thickness with the function at specific anatomic locations. The lamina propria and epithelium are separated by basement membrane. Stem cells of the basement membrane divide and differentiate into the various cells of the surface epithelium. These cells have an estimated life span of 3 to 5 days. It is estimated that the surface epithelial layer of the oral mucosa is replaced every 7 to 14 days. When loss exceeds the rate of replacement, shallow ulcerative lesions occur. Repair continues at a fixed rate, which may leave large areas of mucous membrane denuded of surface epithelium. Intact mucous membranes provide an effective mechanical barrier against harmful exogenous and endogenous organisms. The normal oral flora, mainly consisting of gram-positive bacteria, gram-negative bacteria, and fungi, serve to inhibit the growth of pathogenic organisms. When these barriers are disrupted, bacterial translocation of more pathogenic organisms may occur. Other mucous membrane covered surfaces exhibit similar function with growth and replacement patterns.[8, 9, 58, 59]

Nursing Management

ORAL MUCOUS MEMBRANES

Nursing Diagnoses

- *Oral mucous membranes, altered, related to side effects of chemotherapy or radiation therapy, local infection, tumor*
- *Infection, risk for, related to side effects of systemic chemotherapy or radiation therapy to the head and neck*
- *Knowledge deficit regarding good oral hygiene techniques, side effects of cancer therapy and radiation therapy*
- *Pain related to oral/esophageal mucositis as evidenced by patient's complaints of discomfort, excess or viscous oral secretions, oral lesions leading to discomfort, stimulation of the gag reflex*
- *Nutrition, altered: less than body requirements, related to oral discomfort as evidenced by decreased caloric intake, weight loss of more than 10% of preillness weight, weakness*
- *Communication, impaired verbal, related to oral discomfort, increased or decreased salivation*

Outcome Goals

Patient will be able to:

- Exhibit oral cavity, gums, and lips free of irritation or ulceration.
- Demonstrate knowledge and competency related to prescribed oral hygiene measures.
- Demonstrate relief of pain related to oral mucositis.
- Identify and demonstrate measures to prevent nutritional deficit.
- Achieve adequate verbal communication through the use of pain medications and frequent oral care measures.

Interventions: Measures to Decrease Inflammation of Mucous Membranes

- Avoid exposure to chemical or physical irritants such as commercial mouthwashes, alcohol, tobacco, and hot, spicy, or coarse foods.
- Encourage adequate fluid intake (>3 L/d).
- Use a systematic oral care protocol, which includes oral hygiene measures before and after each meal and at bedtime as a minimum and every 2 hours around the clock when oral mucositis is present.[9, 44, 71, 83, 89]

Interventions: Measures to Increase Comfort

- Use topical protectant and analgesic agents.
- Use systemic analgesics when pain is uncontrolled by topical agents.
- Use safe, effective agents for oral care, which include normal saline (1 tsp/1 L water) and sodium bicarbonate (1 tsp/1 L water) alone or in combination (1:1).
- Facilitate brushing and flossing as the best defense against plaque build-up, but should be discontinued when the absolute neutrophil count (ANC) is less than 1000/mm^3, the platelet count is less than 50,000/mm^3, or mucositis is present. Toothettes or a gauze-wrapped finger may be used instead. Low pressure irrigation set-ups, such as a lavage bag or an IV solution bag with tubing (using 500 mL normal saline), or a bulb syringe may be used to soften and remove debris. Suction equipment should be available for those patients at risk for aspiration.[59, 67, 69, 71, 83]
- Water-soluble lubricants may be used for dry, cracked lips.
- Dentures should be cleaned with a denture brush and an antimicrobial detergent such as chlorhexidine gluconate when oral care is done. Dentures should be rinsed with normal saline or water.[71]
- Dentures should be removed while sleeping and as often as possible to give mucosa a rest. When dentures are not in use, they should be soaked in commercial denture cleanser. Solution should be changed daily.[67, 71]
- Dentures should not be worn except for meals when mucositis is present or when ANC is less than 1000/mm^3 or platelet count is less than 50,000/mm^3 even when no oral pathology is present.
- For mild to moderate mucositis, implement oral care protocol every 2 hours while awake and every 4 hours during night.

- For severe mucositis, implement oral care protocol every 1 to 2 (not to exceed 2) hours during day and every 2 to 4 (not to exceed 4) hours during night.

Interventions: *Measures to Minimize Complications*

- Modify dietary intake to include bland, soft, or liquid food (avoiding acidic foods and liquids) high in calories and protein, served at room temperature or cool, not hot or cold.[40, 53, 89]
- Encourage use of oral hygiene measures before eating.
- Administer topical or systemic analgesics before meals.
- Provide calorie-containing liquids of choice for patient to sip frequently.
- For xerostomia (dry mouth), provide artificial saliva at bedside for patient use. Encourage patient to rinse mouth with water at least every 2 hours while awake. Provide beverages and sauces with meals to help alleviate difficulty swallowing.[59, 76]
- Identify alternative means of communication such as magic slates, notes, cards, and direct, short-response questions.[67]

Interventions: *Medical Treatment*

- Administer antibiotics, antifungals, and antivirals as prescribed.[11, 27, 28, 75, 79]
- Administer analgesics as needed. Patient may require around-the-clock systemic analgesia.[58]
- Administer dietary supplements, enteral nutrition, or parenteral nutrition as prescribed.[5, 48, 76, 89]

- For bleeding from oral mucosa, administer antifibrinolytics and platelets as prescribed, and/or apply topical thrombin and Gelfoam.[32, 37, 39, 83]
- Obtain swabs (specimens) for bacterial, fungal, and viral cultures and sensitivities.
- Nursing management of oral and esophageal mucositis includes systematic assessment and documentation of condition of oral cavity at least once a day, informing the physician of any abnormalities, and using a consistent and safe systematic oral care plan around the clock. Promote comfort through the use of topical anesthetics and systemic analgesics, maintain optimal nutritional status, teach patient/family to use interventions to prevent/minimize oral mucositis, and use precautions when caring for the unresponsive patient to prevent aspiration while administering oral care.

Patient and Family Education

Teaching should include emphasis on the following:

- Importance and technique of daily oral assessment
- Signs and symptoms of mucositis and infection
- Importance of continuing use of a systematic oral care protocol at home
- Importance of fluids and adequate nutrition[10, 36, 40]
- Necessity of dietary changes secondary to the presence or absence of oral and esophageal lesions
- Avoidance of trauma to mucous membranes secondary to smoking, smokeless tobacco, alcohol, extremes of temperature, chemical irritants such as commercial mouthwashes, and physical irritants such as highly seasoned or hard- or sharp-textured foods and poorly fitting dentures.

Pathophysiology

The following terms are defined for the purpose of this discussion:

Stomatitis—a general term referring to the inflammatory reaction and shallow ulcerative lesions occurring on the mucosal surfaces of the mouth and oropharynx 7 to 14 days after administration of certain chemotherapeutic agents and after radiation therapy to the head and neck.

Mucositis—a general term referring to the inflammatory reaction and shallow ulcerative lesions occurring on mucosal surfaces, not limited to the mouth and oropharynx, frequently associated with the administration of certain chemotherapeutic agents and after radiation therapy to mucous membrane-bearing sites. Stomatitis, esophagitis, gastritis, enteritis, colitis, proctitis, and vaginitis are examples of treatment-related mucositis.[58, 59]

Disease-Related Causes. Disease-related causes of the disruption of mucous membranes include primary tumors of the head, neck, GI tract, respiratory tract, and GU tract; agranulocytic oral ulcers; gingival hypertrophy and infiltration associated with acute leukemia; non-Hodgkin's lymphoma or acute leukemia involving Waldeyer's ring; and Kaposi's sarcoma among others. Disease-related immunosuppression may lead to superinfection with herpes simplex virus (HSV), *Candida albicans,* and other opportunistic agents.[8, 26]

Treatment-Related Causes. Treatment-related causes of mucous membrane disruption include chemotherapy-induced mucositis (Box 31–5), radiation-associated mucositis, xerostomia (dry mouth), parotitis (inflamed and swollen salivary glands), osteoradionecrosis of the bone (late destruction of irradiated bone and subsequent loss of teeth), and surgical procedures. Chemotherapy ef-

---

BOX 31-5

Antineoplastic Agents Toxic to Mucous Membranes

Antimetabolites

capecitabine
cytosine arabinoside
fludarabine
fluorouracil
gemcitabine
mercaptopurine
methotrexate
thioguanine
trimetrexate

Plant Alkaloids

etoposide
teniposide
vinblastine
vincristine
vinorelbine

Antibiotics

bleomycin
dactinomycin
daunorubicin
doxorubicin
epirubicin
idarubicin
mitomycin
mitoxantrone
plicamycin

Camptothecins

irinotecan
topotecan

Miscellaneous

hydroxyurea
procarbazine

Alkylating Agents

busulfan
carboplatin
chlorambucil
cisplatin
cyclophosphamide
ifosfamide
melphalan

Taxanes

docetaxel
paclitaxel

Ablative Doses

all antineoplastics

Data from references 15, 32, 42, 62.

---

fects are systemic and widespread and may become a dose-limiting toxicity. Radiation-associated effects are site specific and involve only the areas within the treatment port. Persons undergoing peripheral blood stem cell or bone marrow transplantation are at greater risk for oral complications, related to the intensity of the preparative therapy and manifestations of graft-versus-host disease.[49, 58, 59, 88, 89]

Complicating Factors. Complicating factors include infections, which may become systemic; bleeding from nonintact mucosal surfaces; poor nutritional status; and pain secondary to the lesions. Preexisting dental and periodontal diseases predispose to more severe compli-

cations of disease- and treatment-related mucositis as does chronic exposure to oral mucosal stressors such as chemical and physical irritants (alcohol, heat, and tobacco), other medications associated with drying mucosal surfaces, and oxygen administration. Additional risk factors include age older than 65 or younger than 20 years, inadequate self-care abilities, acutely ill condition, and altered fluid or nutritional status.[14, 40, 83]

Assessment. Numerous oral assessment tools are available in the nursing literature. Most assess the lips, tongue, mucous membranes, gingiva, teeth, saliva, voice, and ability to swallow. The use of an oral assessment guide provides the ability to assign numerical (objective and comparative) scores to the examination. It also provides a common base (language) for ongoing physical assessment and evaluation of patient outcomes.[4]

Oral assessment requires the use of readily available tools including a pair of examination gloves, gauze sponges, flashlight, and tongue depressor. Oral assessment should be done at least twice daily and the findings documented in the patient record. High-risk patients should be identified early, and oral assessments with interventions provided consistently to decrease complications. The patient and family should be taught the techniques of assessment so that they can follow the progress when the patient is home. The patient and family should also be instructed to report any changes in oral sensation or taste and the appearance of lesions.[4, 36, 89]

Rectal and vaginal mucosal assessment in the neutropenic patient should be limited to visual inspection only. This prevents trauma to ulcerated mucosa and decreases the potential for dissemination of infection through manipulation of the rectal and vaginal tissue. The patient should be questioned about the presence or absence of rectal or vaginal bleeding, pain, itching, discharge, drainage, and other discomfort or changes in sensation.[2, 23]

Medical Management

Treatment of complications involving nonintact mucous membranes includes antimicrobials, antifungals, and antivirals for superinfections; platelet transfusion and antifibrinolytic agents for bleeding from mucous membranes; topical and systemic analgesics for pain; and dilation of strictures involving the esophagus and vagina.[38, 44, 48, 53]

Nursing Management

VAGINAL/RECTAL MUCOSITIS

Nursing Diagnoses

- *Tissue integrity, impaired, related to side effects of chemotherapy and/or radiation therapy as evidenced by signs and symptoms of mucositis*
- *Infection, risk for, related to nonintact vaginal and/or rectal mucosa*
- *Knowledge deficit regarding safe sexual practices, good personal hygiene, side effects of mucositis related to cancer therapy*
- *Pain related to mucositis evidenced by the patient's complaints of painful urination, defecation, sexual intercourse*
- *Diarrhea related to gastrointestinal mucositis*
- *Pain related to painful defecation secondary to rectal mucositis*
- *Sexuality patterns, altered, related to decreased energy, potential fear of trauma or infection*

Outcome Goals

Patient will be able to:

- Demonstrate health practices to prevent further impairment and promote integrity of vaginal and rectal mucous membranes.[38]
- Remain infection free related to impaired vaginal or rectal mucositis.
- Achieve adequate pain relief related to vaginal/rectal mucositis.
- Demonstrate measures to control or correct diarrhea.
- Identify and demonstrate strategies to manage or correct alteration in sexuality.

Interventions: *Measures to Decrease Inflammation of Mucous Membranes*

- Avoid exposure to chemical and physical irritants such as tampons, deodorant-containing vaginal pads or liners, deodorant-containing personal hygiene sprays, douches, rectal thermometers and suppositories, and vaginal and anal intercourse.
- Encourage adequate fluid intake.[27, 67]
- Wash perineum with soap and water after each urination and defecation; pat or air dry.

Interventions: *Measures to Increase Comfort*

- Use sitz baths.
- Avoid standing or sitting for long periods.
- Avoid irritating, constricting, nonabsorbent underclothing.

Interventions: *Measures to Minimize Complications*

- Modify dietary intake to minimize diarrhea and constipation.
- Encourage frequent perineal hygiene measures.
- Instruct female patients to wipe from front to back after urination and defecation.
- Avoid trauma to either vaginal or rectal mucosa.
- Monitor patient for signs and symptoms of vaginal infection or rectal cellulitis/abscess; culture as needed; notify physician.[23, 67, 78]

Patient and Family Education

Teaching should include emphasis on the following:

- Personal risk factors for development of mucositis secondary to chemotherapy, radiation therapy.
- Signs and symptoms of mucositis, such as pain, itching, and discharge or drainage, which should be reported.

Measures to Prevent Complications

- Situations that require professional interventions, such as fever, diarrhea, and uncontrolled pain.
- Nursing management of vaginal and rectal mucositis includes frequent, indirect assessment of signs and symptoms of mucositis, prevention of diarrhea and constipation, encouragement of bathing of perineal and rectal areas after each urination and defecation, teaching female patients to wipe front to back to prevent contaminating vaginal and urethral areas with fecal organisms, and teaching sexual practices that minimize trauma and risk of infection.
- Teaching should include the signs and symptoms of mucositis and infection, whom and when to call, and sexual and elimination practices that prevent or minimize the risk of trauma and infection. Vaginal intercourse should be avoided while platelet and neutrophil counts are low and if mucosal ulcerations are present. Intercourse should be permitted and encouraged after recovery of blood counts and mucosa. This may help prevent development of vaginal strictures and webbing, which may occur after pelvic irradiation. Women who are not sexually active may need to use vaginal dilators to maintain vaginal patency after pelvic irradiation. Condoms should be worn by the male partner to prevent transmission of organisms through nonintact mucosa. Adequate lubrication should be obtained using a water-soluble, not a petroleum-based, product. Anal intercourse should be avoided.[38, 59, 83]

BONE MARROW SUPPRESSION

Anatomy and Physiology

The bone marrow is the production site for all formed blood elements: erythrocytes, granulocytes, monocytes, lymphocytes, and megakaryocytes. During early fetal development, hematopoiesis (production of blood) occurs in the liver and yolk sac. By the 20th week of gestation the bone marrow begins to produce blood cells, and by the 30th week the bone marrow has achieved normal cellularity. At birth, active bone marrow is found in all bones of the body. With age the functional marrow space contracts, so that by adulthood active marrow is found primarily in the axial skeleton, sternum, ribs, vertebral bodies, pelvis, skull, and the proximal ends of the long bones.[35]

Bone marrow is a spongy organ made up of a fibrous network of connective tissue called *stroma*. The stroma is supported within the marrow cavity by spicules of bone radiating to the center of the bone marrow cavity from cortical bone. The bone marrow is a highly vascular organ with numerous nutrient arteries and interconnecting venous sinusoids. Poorly understood regulatory mechanisms prevent immature blood cells from entering the venous sinusoids and circulating blood until they reach maturity.[8, 35, 90]

All blood cells arise from a common progenitor cell called the *stem cell*. The stem cell probably resembles and cannot be distinguished by sight from the small mature lymphocyte. The stem cell pool is self-renewing; for every stem cell that enters the differentiation and maturation pool, another cell returns to the stem cell pool. Conditions causing destruction of the stem cell pool lead to the development of marrow aplasia. Stem

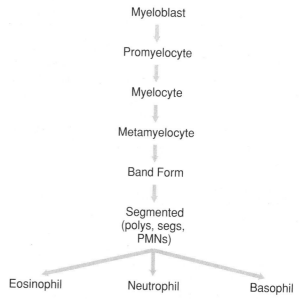

FIGURE 31–2 Myeloid maturation.

cells may be either pleuripotential (uncommitted) or unipotential (committed) (Fig. 31–1).

Once a stem cell has entered a particular cell line, differentiation and maturation occur in a manner characteristic of erythroid, myeloid, lymphoid, or megakaryocytic cells (Fig. 31–2). Residence (maturation) time within the marrow varies from cell line to cell line and with the body's need for the cell type. Some cell lines have storage pools. Once the cells are released into circulation, life span ranges from 6 to 8 hours for the neutrophil to 120 days for the erythrocyte. The marrow is able to respond to increased need for particular cells by permitting early release from the maturation and storage pools.[8, 26, 35]

Stem cells, having entered a designated cell line, mature under the influence of specific hematopoietic growth factors. The first to be identified and the best known of these growth factors is erythropoietin (EPO), a glycoprotein hormone produced by the kidney. EPO acts on specific target cells in the bone marrow to increase the rate of production and release of red blood cells. EPO is necessary for proper differentiation and maturation of erythrocytes (RBCs) and is regulated by the response to changes in tissue oxygenation. The EPO-increased production reflects these changes for oxygen-carrying capacity via hemoglobin.[20, 27, 42, 69]

Substantial research has led to the identification of several other hematopoietic growth factors. Recombinant DNA technology has made it possible to produce large quantities of these growth factors, allowing increased clinical trials. Recently approved is a thrombopoietic growth factor oprelvekin (Neumega) that targets the bone marrow stromal cells, which stimulates

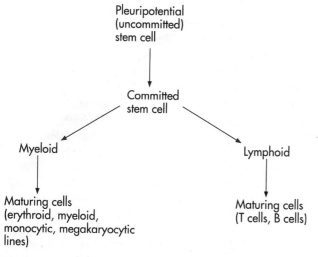

FIGURE 31–1 Stem cell differentiation and maturation.

proliferation of megakaryocyte (platelet) progenitor cells and induces megakaryocyte maturation. Growth factors undergoing trials include, but are not limited to, recombinant erythropoietin (rEPO), granulocyte/macrophage colony-stimulating factor (rGM-CSF), granulocyte colony-stimulating factor (rG-CSF), interleukin-3 (rIL-3) or multi-CSF, stem cell factor (rSCF), macrophage colony-stimulating factor (rM-CSF) and interleukin-11 (rIL-11) or oprelvekin. The target cells of the growth factors both vary and overlap. rGM-CSF, rSCF, and rIL-3 are multilineage in that they stimulate and regulate most of the cell lines of the myeloid series (i.e., granulocytes, monocytes, macrophages, erythrocytes), whereas rEPO, rG-CSF, rM-CSF and rIL-11 are lineage restricted (affecting only the erythrocyte, megakaryocyte, neutrophil, or monocyte/macrophage lines, respectively). rIL-11, rEPO, rGM-CSF, and rG-CSF have received approval from the Food and Drug Administration as supportive therapy for patients undergoing treatment for chemotherapy-induced anemia, thrombocytopenia, or neutropenia; chemotherapy-induced mucositits, in patients with solid tumors, lymphomas, leukemia, myeloproliferative disorders, peripheral blood stem cell or BMT, and human immunodeficiency virus (HIV) infection. Prolonged myelosuppression related to the varied cancer therapies now has a prophylactic approach because the above-mentioned treatments are administered at scheduled intervals to coincide with the response to the specific cancer therapy.[20, 27, 32, 73, 77]

Pathophysiology

Pathologic bone marrow conditions arise from a defect in the stem cell or the marrow microenvironment. The stem cell defect may be intrinsic, as in the leukemias, or extrinsic, as in exposure to stem cell toxins such as benzene or chloramphenicol. Microenvironment problems may occur intrinsically, as in myelofibrosis, a myeloproliferative disorder characterized by replacement of the marrow cavity with fibrous tissue, or extrinsically, as when a nonhematologic malignancy metastasizes to the marrow. Replacement followed by marrow failure may occur. Treatment of malignant disorders by chemotherapy or radiation therapy may alter the stem cell pool and its environment permanently.[20, 27, 35, 77]

Definition of Terms. The following terms are defined for the purpose of this discussion:

Leukopenia—a condition said to occur when the total leukocyte complement is reduced. Leukopenia is a non-specific finding and usually reflects a decrease in all WBCs (Table 31–1).

Granulocytopenia—a condition said to occur when the absolute granulocyte complement is reduced. When granulocytopenia occurs, there is a decrease in neutrophils, eosinophils, and basophils.

Neutropenia—a condition that exists when there is an absolute decrease in the number of circulating neutrophils, usually less than 1000/mm^3. The absolute neutrophil count (ANC) is calculated as follows:

$$\text{Segs (\%) + bands (\%)} \times \text{white blood cell count} = \text{ANC}$$
$$0.10 + 0.10 \times 2000 = 400/mm^3$$

Neutropenia is associated with a profound impairment in the inflammatory response, leading to lack or minimization of the usual signs and symptoms of infection such as erythema, swelling, heat, and pain. Purulence is not present. Neutropenia is the single most important predisposing factor to infection in the person with cancer:

$$\text{ANC} > 1500/mm^3 = \text{normal risk}$$
$$\text{ANC} < 1000/mm^3 = \text{moderate risk}$$
$$\text{ANC} < 500/mm^3 = \text{severe risk}$$
$$\text{ANC} < 100/mm^3 = \text{extreme risk}$$

Neutropenia may be related to basic disease processes such as acute nonlymphocytic leukemia or aplastic anemia. Neutropenia may occur also as a result of myelosuppressive treatment for malignant disease such as chemotherapy or radiation therapy.[78, 90]

Immunosuppression—a condition that exists when lymphocyte function or interaction is suppressed. Immunosuppression may result from either disease process or treatment. Selective immunosuppression may inhibit either cell-mediated or humoral immunity. Immunosuppression may be primary or secondary; secondary immunosuppression is the most common.[75, 78, 84]

Immunosuppression secondary to corticosteroid therapy is the most common secondary or acquired suppression. Acquired immunodeficiency syndrome (AIDS) resulting from depletion of immunoregulatory T cells occurs after infection with HIV. Primary lymphoid malignancies such as chronic lymphocytic leukemia and non-Hodgkin's lymphoma may also cause immunosuppression.

Anemia—a condition characterized by a decrease in hemoglobin level or circulating erythrocytes. Anemia occurs when loss or destruction exceeds production of RBCs. This may occur from acute hemorrhage, replacement of normal marrow elements with abnormal cells, loss of the stem cell pool, decreased or ineffective production of RBCs, and accelerated destruction of RBCs. Anemia may result from both basic disease process and treatment.[53, 67]

TABLE 31-1
Types of Circulating Leukocytes

Type of WBC	% of WBC	Function
Neutrophil	50–70	Phagocytosis, inflammation
Eosinophil	1–4	Chemotaxis, allergies
Basophil	0–4	Anaphylaxis, allergies
Monocyte	2–9	Phagocytosis, inflammation, differentiation into macrophages
Macrophage	—	Circulating and fixed, phagocytosis, antigen-processing and -presenting cell for the T cell
Lymphocyte	20–40	Specific immune response, cell-mediated immunity, and humoral immunity

Thrombocytopenia—a condition characterized by decreased numbers of circulating platelets or thrombocytes. Thrombocytopenia may result from decreased or ineffective production of platelets secondary to marrow replacement by tumor, exposure to marrow toxins or infectious agents, and ionizing radiation. Thrombocytopenia may result also from increased destruction secondary to immune-mediated conditions, such as immune thrombocytopenia purpura (ITP) and heparin-induced thrombocytopenia or thrombosis syndrome (HITTS), or coagulopathies such as disseminated intravascular coagulation (DIC). In some instances platelet numbers may be normal or increased and a bleeding tendency still exist. This abnormal bleeding may result from a qualitative platelet defect. The most common causes of qualitative platelet defects are (1) ingestion of aspirin or similar drugs that interfere with normal platelet function and (2) the presence of abnormal platelets secondary to myeloproliferative disorders.[37, 45, 52, 55, 69]

Pancytopenia—a term used when there is a deficiency of all the cell elements of the blood (erythrocytes, platelets, and all the WBCs [neutrophils, eosinophils, basophils, monocytes, macrophages, and lymphocytes]).

Complicating Factors. Complications associated with bone marrow suppression include increased susceptibility to infection secondary to neutropenia, fatigue associated with anemia, and increased risk of bleeding secondary to low platelet counts.

Assessment
Infection. Daily assessment of the cancer patient should include identification of risk factors for the development of infection, such as neutropenia, lymphopenia, immunosuppressive therapy, nonintact skin or mucous membranes, and the presence of vascular access devices.

Astute observation for the usual signs and symptoms of infection is necessary because neutropenic patients may exhibit little or no inflammatory response. Fever and, occasionally, hypothermia represent serious infection in immunocompromised individuals.[14, 40, 56, 68, 69]

Changes in usual respiratory pattern (rate, depth, breath sounds, sputum production), in GI tract functioning (nausea, vomiting, dysphagia, hiccoughs, abdominal pain, cramping, diarrhea, rectal pain or itching), and in the GU system (dysuria, oliguria, anuria, pelvic pain, vaginal or urethral discharge) are frequently associated with infection. Breaks in the integrity of the skin (head and neck, axillae, intertriginous areas, buttocks, and perineum) and mucous membranes (oral, anal, vaginal) represent portals of entry for infectious organisms and should be duly noted. Sepsis, or blood-borne systemic infection, produces significant morbidity and mortality.

CLINICAL FEATURES
Infection

Temperature > 100.4°F (38°C)
Flushed skin, diaphoresis
Shaking chills
White, cream-colored lesions in mouth
Erythema, swelling, or pain in skin, throat, eyes, joints, perineal or rectal areas
Cough, chest pain, tachypnea, or dyspnea
Changes in character or color of sputum, urine, or stools
Dysuria or frequency of urination
Malaise, lethargy, myalgias, or arthralgias
Skin rash
Confusion, mental status change

Nursing Management

INCREASED SUSCEPTIBILITY TO INFECTION

Nursing Diagnoses

- *Infection, risk for, related to disease entity; side effects of treatment; neutropenia, immune suppression, etc.; disruption of mucous membranes or skin; presence of long-term venous access device*
- *Body temperature, altered, risk for, related to infection secondary to neutropenia, immunosuppression, nonintact skin or mucous membranes*
- *Knowledge deficit regarding basic disease process, treatment, signs and symptoms of infection, neutropenic precautions*
- *Sexuality patterns, altered, related to decreased energy and potential fear of trauma or infection*
- *Social isolation related to therapeutic environment or fear of acquiring an infection*
- *Anxiety related to knowledge of diagnosis, treatment, prognosis*
- *Fear related to discharge concerning home management, self-care, uncertainty about long-term outcome*

Outcome Goals

Patient will be able to:

- Remain infection-free during hospitalization or illness.
- Demonstrate knowledge about diagnosis and disease process, therapy, signs and symptoms of infection, survival skills.
- Report a desire to resume sexual activity.
- Identify reasons for feelings of isolation and identify appropriate diversional activities.
- Relate an increase in psychological and physiologic comfort.
- Express desire for discharge and demonstrate competency in performing self-care activities.

Preventive Measures

Prevention of infection in susceptible individuals is an important nursing measure. Handwashing is the single most important action for the health care professional, the patient, the patient's family, and visitors. The importance of adequate handwashing using running water, soap, and friction cannot be overstated. The health care professional must use good handwashing technique before and after any direct patient contact. Gloves are not to be used as a substitute for good handwashing.

Protective isolation techniques vary from institution to institution. The Centers for Disease Control and Prevention no longer recognizes or recommends protective isolation for persons who are immunosuppressed or neutropenic. Protective isolation can be thought of more as a "mind set" than an actual category of isolation. It must become second nature for the nurse caring for the neutropenic or immunosuppressed patient to be aware of the patient's increased risk and the risk the nurse represents to the patient. Most institutions advocate the use of a private room, good handwashing practices, and an infection-free staff to care for the patient. Dietary restrictions for the neutropenic patient may include an order for "cooked diet" only. Raw fruits and uncooked vegetables are often excluded because of soil contact and repeated handling by dietary personnel during storage and preparation.[49, 58, 59, 63, 81, 82]

Interventions: General Preventive Measures

- Wash hands with soap, water, and friction before and after all direct patient contact.[57]
- Provide private room if possible; if unavailable, ensure uninfected roommate.
- Provide infection-free staff to care for patient.
- Give nursing care to neutropenic patient first to decrease risk of cross-contamination.
- Provide meticulous skin and oral hygiene for patient.
- Provide cooked diet only—no raw fruits or vegetables.[63]
- Do not allow live plants or cut flowers in standing water in room.
- Avoid all sources of stagnant water in room such as water pitchers, denture cups, humidifiers, and respiratory therapy equipment; change daily.
- Screen visitors for illnesses.[56, 75]
- Avoid overcrowded areas such as waiting rooms.
- Use Universal Precautions when caring for all patients.[80]

Interventions: Prompt Recognition of Suspected Infection

- Assume that any change from the ordinary is infection until proven otherwise.
- Assess patient's risk of infection by calculating ANC and reviewing patient history for predisposing factors such as basic disease process, myelosuppressive therapies, immunosuppressive therapies, and antibiotic therapy.

- Assess skin and mucous membranes each shift and document in patient record.
- Assess vital signs including temperature at least every 4 hours and document in patient record.
- Notify physician of temperature elevation to greater than 100.8°F (38.2°C), changes in skin and mucous membrane integrity, lesions, or rashes and any altered level of consciousness.[11]
- Facilitate work-up of suspected infection by obtaining ordered cultures, blood specimens, and radiologic studies in a timely manner.[11, 15]
- Initiate and administer antibiotics as prescribed in a timely manner.
- Observe and assess patient for adverse effects of antibiotic administration.

Nursing management of the infected cancer patient is a complex and challenging task. Infection is the most common cause of death for the person with cancer. Nurses represent a crucial and constant part of the care team—and frequently the difference between life and death for the patient.

Nursing management of infection demands its prompt recognition, which requires the health care professional to maintain a high index of suspicion. Literally anything out of the ordinary could be infection. The nurse's intuitive feelings are frequently helpful in the absence of objective findings of infection. Physician notification and documentation of the nursing assessment in the patient record are essential parts of the nursing process.

The nurse's assistance in the work-up of suspected infection will include timely retrieval of specimens for culture, coordination of radiologic studies, and facilitation of physical assessment by the physician and nurse.

Empiric antibiotic therapy should be instituted within 4 hours of an initial temperature spike, as well as obtaining cultures. It is the nurse's responsibility to provide for timely and safe administration of antibiotics.[11, 12, 28, 47, 72]

Scheduling, timing of infusions, and knowledge of drug toxicities and interactions are also the responsibility of the nurse (see Nursing Implications of Antimicrobial Administration on pages 936 and 937).[33, 43, 49]

Frequent assessment of the patient with suspected infection is essential. Vital signs including temperature should be measured no less frequently than every 4 hours. Other key points of assessment should include auscultation of breath sounds, auscultation and palpation of abdomen, observation of skin and mucous membranes, and assessment of level of consciousness.

Fever management includes administration of antipyretics and the use of tepid baths, cooling blankets, ice packs, and other nonpharmacologic methods of reducing elevated body temperature. Once antipyretics have been instituted and fever recurs, it is often less physiologically stressful to administer them on an around-the-clock schedule to avoid the see-saw pattern of hyperthermia and hypothermia. It is important to prevent shivering, which increases body temperature. Parenteral meperidine or morphine or both may be administered to alleviate rigors.[9, 50, 62]

Early recognition of septic shock is essential to patient survival. Impending sepsis is frequently suggested by the findings of tachycardia, tachypnea, widened pulse pressure, elevated body temperature, hot, dry skin, and altered mental status. Survival is improved if sepsis is recognized before circulatory collapse occurs.

Patient and Family Education

Educational efforts should center on teaching the patient and family the signs and symptoms of infection, which may include any of the following: fever, cough, dysuria, shortness of breath, oral ulcers, diarrhea, nausea, and vomiting. Because of the risk of septic shock associated with neutropenia, it is imperative that the patient and family take any fever seriously and notify the appropriate health care professional. Teaching should be explicit about when and whom to call and include a list of telephone numbers giving the patient and family 24-hour access to the health care setting.

"Survival teaching" should be individualized to each patient, taking into consideration readiness to learn and ability to take charge of his life and illness. Content may include laboratory test interpretation; calculation of an ANC; keeping a journal of dates, drugs, dosages, blood counts, and side effects; neutropenic precautions; handwashing technique; personal hygiene practices; activity; diet; and sexual practices.

Nursing Implications of Antimicrobial Administration

Drugs	Side Effects	Implications
AMINOGLYCOSIDES Amikacin Gentamycin Tobramycin Vancomycin Netromycin	Nephrotoxicity, ototoxicity	Monitor renal function carefully. Monitor for signs of hearing loss, tinnitus, and vertigo. Observe for signs of superinfection. Follow infusion guidelines carefully.
PENICILLINS (β-lactam) Azlocillin Carbenicillin Mezlocillin Piperacillin Ticarcillin	Skin rashes, drug fever, anaphylaxis, hypokalemia, abnormal platelet function	Monitor renal function carefully. Elicit allergy history. Be prepared for possible allergic reaction. Monitor CBC and liver function tests carefully. Monitor serum electrolytes (potassium [K] and sodium [Na^+]). Observe for signs of superinfection.
CEPHALOSPORINS (β-lactam) Cefoperazone Cefotaxime Ceftazidime Ceftriaxone	Skin rashes, drug fever	Monitor renal function carefully. Observe for phlebitis if given peripherally. Observe for signs of superinfection.
Cefepime hydrochloride (Maxipime)	Allergic reactions, phlebitis, nausea, vomiting, rash, headache	Monitor renal function, incompatible with many solutions. Obtain baseline CBC and PTT. Monitor serum glucose, and electrolytes. Observe for anaphylaxis and immediately initiate interventions.
MONOBACTAMS Aztreonam (β-lactam)	Seizures, altered taste, diarrhea, nausea, vomiting, skin rash, superinfection, anaphylaxis	Elicit history of allergies. Monitor liver function. Monitor renal function. Monitor coagulation. Monitor neurotoxicity. Observe for signs of superinfection.

Drug	Side Effects	Nursing Considerations
CARBAPENEM		
Imipenem/cilastin	Seizures, somnolence, hypotension, nausea, diarrhea, vomiting, rash, phlebitis, anaphylaxis	Elicit allergy history. Monitor renal function. Monitor liver function. Monitor CBC and Coombs' test. Observe for signs of superinfection.
FLUOROQUINOLONES		
Ciprofloxacin	Nausea, vomiting, diarrhea, headache, rash, anaphylaxis, nephrotoxicity, phlebitis	Monitor liver function tests. Restrict caffeine intake. Avoid excess sun exposure. Monitor renal function tests. Observe for phlebitis. Observe for signs of superinfection. Observe for anaphylaxis.
Ofloxacin	Skin rash, consider birth control options, photosensitivity, abdominal pain, cramps, allergic reactions, vein irritation	Avoid excessive sun or artificial light. Limit caffeine intake. Monitor hydration, renal, and hematopoietic and hepatic systems. Monitor renal, liver, BUN, AST, and ALT serum levels. Monitor intake and output ratio. Emphasize 3 L/24-h intake.
(Norfloxacin PO agent)	Headache, nausea, constipation, rash	
ANTIFUNGAL AGENTS		
Amphotericin B Liposomal ampho B (Abelcet, Ambisome, Amphotec); fungizone/generic *Monistat (Miconazole) IV mix with NS or D_5W* Diflucan (Fluconazole) prepackaged and prediluted.	Hypokalemia, fever, rigors, phlebitis, nausea, vomiting, headache, nephrotoxicity, ototoxicity, elevated liver enzymes	Obtain baseline, CBC, serum creatinine and electrolytes, BUN levels. Monitor serum electrolytes, liver and renal function carefully. Premedicate with antipyretics, antihistamines, e.g., diphenhydramine, analgesics, e.g., meperidine, IV prior and during infusion. Observe for anaphylaxis and immediately initiate interventions to manage anaphylaxis. Follow manufacture dilution guidelines: D_5W only: DO NOT MIX PRODUCTS with other diluent, drug, or solution in syringe or infusion bag. Monitor patient's temperature at baseline and during infusion. Infuse slowly, preferably with infusion pump. Drug is a colloid; administer with nonfiltered tubing; agitate bag frequently to maintain in suspension. FOLLOW THE MANUFACTURER'S GUIDELINES REGARDING TEST-DOSE REQUIREMENTS FOR ALL PARENTERAL ANTIFUNGAL AGENTS.

Data from references 15, 32, 42.

Assessment for and early detection of sepsis is important in caring for the severely neutropenic patient.[56, 68, 69]

Bleeding. Assessment for bleeding should include the following: examine daily laboratory values for hemoglobin and platelet count; consider medications that may alter platelet production or function; inspect for the presence of petechiae and ecchymoses, prolonged bleeding from venipunctures, minor cuts, or scratches, frank bleeding from any body orifice, and occult blood in excreta and vomitus.[69]

Anemia. Assessment for anemia and its resultant fatigue should include the following: examine daily laboratory values for hemoglobin and platelet count, inspect for presence of occult blood in the excreta of the thrombocytopenic patient, query the presence of frank bleeding from any body orifice, and monitor the pattern of fatigue and its impact on activities of daily living and life-style.

CLINICAL FEATURES

Impending Septic Shock
(Hyperdynamic or Warm Shock)

Mental confusion
Chills and fever
Skin flushed and dry
Blood pressure normal or slightly low
Pulse pressure widened
Tachycardia
Tachypnea
Hypoxemia
Urine output normal to slightly increased

Nursing Management

INCREASED RISK OF BLEEDING

Nursing Diagnoses

- *Injury, risk for, bleeding related to decreased platelet count, basic disease process, cancer treatment*
- *Knowledge deficit regarding thrombocytopenia and increased risk of bleeding, signs and symptoms of bleeding*
- *Sexuality patterns, altered, related to decreased energy, potential fear of trauma or infection*
- *Anxiety related to knowledge of diagnosis, treatment, prognosis*
- *Fear related to discharge concerning home management, self-care, uncertainty about long-term outcome*

Outcome Goals

Patient will be able to:

- Remain free from injury related to bleeding.
- Demonstrate knowledge of signs and symptoms of bleeding.
- Report desire to resume sexual activity.
- Relate an increase in psychological and physiologic comfort.
- Express desire for discharge and demonstrates competency in performing self-care activities.

Preventive Measures

Bleeding should be prevented in the thrombocytopenic patient. Measures should include those that maintain skin and mucous membrane integrity.

Provision of a safe environment falls within the confines of nursing practice. In severely thrombocytopenic patients, bed rails should be up at all times, the patient should be up with assistance only, and the patient who is weak or showing signs of bleeding should be on complete bed rest.

All excreta and vomitus should be tested for the presence of occult blood. The results of each test should be entered in the patient record and the physician notified if the results vary significantly from previous testing.

Laboratory tests should be done as ordered. The nurse should know results and how they are related to the patient's risk for bleeding. The nurse should be able to interpret laboratory results in terms of platelet disorder, coagulation factor deficiency, mixed coagulopathy, and lack of vascular integrity.[15, 20, 83]

Interventions: *General Preventive Measures*

- Limit invasive procedures.
- Provide safe environment (e.g., side rails up, assistance with ambulation).
- Avoid intramuscular injections.
- Avoid aspirin-containing medications or nonsteroidal anti-inflammatory drugs.
- Suppress menses in premenopausal female patients by hormonal manipulation as ordered by the physician.[89]
- Avoid tooth flossing and hard toothbrushes.[58, 71]
- Avoid use of rectal thermometers, suppositories, enemas, and rectal examinations.
- Avoid alcohol-containing beverages.

Interventions: *Assessment of Bleeding*

- Check laboratory values for platelet count, hemoglobin and hematocrit, and any other coagulation studies, such as prothrombin time (PT), partial thromboplastin time (PTT), fibrinogen, and fibrin degradation products (FDP) to assess patient's risk of bleeding.[3, 15, 20, 24, 83]
- Assess skin and mucous membranes for presence of petechiae, purpura, and ecchymoses, document in patient record, and notify physician of any evidence of bleeding.
- Assess for any evidence of frank bleeding (e.g., epistaxis, hemoptysis, hematemesis, hematochezia, melena, hematuria, vaginal bleeding), document in patient record, and notify physician if present.
- Quantitate amount of frank bleeding as accurately as possible, document, and report.
- Hemetest all stools, urine, and emesis for the presence of occult blood whenever the platelet count is less than 50,000/mm^3.
- Apply pressure and/or pressure dressings to venipunctures, bone marrow aspiration and biopsy sites, and other sites of invasive procedures until hemostasis occurs.
- Observe sites of invasive procedures, such as vascular access device placement, for continued hemostasis and notify physician if bleeding is present or recurs.
- Administer appropriate medications to prevent activities that raise intracranial pressure such as vomiting, coughing, sneezing, and straining in stool.
- Report any complaints of headache with or without change in level of consciousness or vital signs.
- Administer platelet transfusions and other blood component therapy as ordered.
- Obtain physician order and administer premedications of diphenhydramine, acetaminophen, and/or corticosteroids to patient with history of transfusion reaction.
- Monitor patient for signs and symptoms of transfusion reaction and take appropriate measures (see Transfusion Reactions below).[39, 64, 86]

Interventions: *Patient and Family Education*

- Assess skin and mucous membranes daily for evidence of bleeding.
- Assess personal risk of bleeding by knowing current platelet count and other pertinent laboratory values.
- Assess for and report any evidence of frank bleeding including petechiae, purpura, and ecchymoses.

Transfusion Reactions

Type of Reaction	Signs and Symptoms	Interventions
Hemolytic	Fever, chills, low back pain, substernal tightness, dyspnea, circulatory collapse, urticaria, flushing, vomiting, diarrhea, hemoglobinuria, renal shutdown, bleeding diathesis	Prevent by proper identification of patient and blood for transfusion. Discontinue the transfusion; send to blood bank and obtain urine and blood specimens per hospital policy for transfusion reaction work-up. Administer saline diuresis, furosemide, and mannitol to prevent acute renal tubular necrosis.
Allergic	Urticaria, itching, bronchospasm, anaphylactoid reactions, no fever	Elicit history of prior allergic reactions. Premedicate with diphenhydramine and/or corticosteroids. If reaction occurs, stop the transfusion; follow hospital policy for suspected transfusion reaction; for anaphylactoid reaction, administer epinephrine, maintain airway and perfusion; administer additional emergency measures as needed.
Febrile (leukocyte antigens)	Fever with or without rigors, tachycardia, tachypnea, hypotension, cyanosis, fibrinolysis, leukopenia, headache	Elicit history of febrile reactions. Premedicate with acetaminophen. If reaction occurs, stop the transfusion and follow hospital policy for suspected febrile reaction. Consider leukocyte-poor RBCs (filtered, saline-washed or frozen) if fever occurs more than once.
Bacterial (gram-negative organisms and endotoxin release)	Fever, rigors, circulatory collapse, mental confusion, septic shock	Maintain proper blood storage and administration conditions. Stop the transfusion immediately. Obtain blood for cultures; return blood to laboratory for culturing. Administer emergency treatment as needed. Administer antibiotics as ordered.

Data from references 32 and 39.

- Avoid all aspirin-containing compounds. Read the label. Do not take any medications unless prescribed by your physician.
- Report any feelings of increased weakness, change in stool color and consistency, emesis, headache, and change in level of consciousness. For nosebleed, apply ice pack across bridge of nose and pressure to nostrils below bridge of nose. If bleeding does not stop within 5 minutes or bleeding is profuse, notify physician. Anterior or posterior nasal packs may be required.

Nursing management of the bleeding patient depends on prompt recognition of the problem so that definitive therapy can be undertaken. Bleeding precautions should be initiated when the platelet count drops below 50,000/mm³. Frequent assessment should be made of vital signs, mental status, skin and mucous membranes, sites of invasive procedures, and all excreta and vomitus for occult blood. Signs of intracranial hemorrhage include decreased level of consciousness, headache, seizures, unequal pupil size and reaction, hypertension, and bradycardia. Administration of antiemetics, cough suppressants, and stool softeners and laxatives when indicated may help lower the risk of intracranial hemorrhage by preventing the sudden raising of intracranial pressure while retching, coughing, and straining at stool.[62]

Platelet transfusion is generally the treatment of choice for bleeding secondary to thrombocytopenia. Indications for platelet transfusion are not always clear. Some physicians may prefer to wait for signs of bleeding before transfusing platelets; others may opt to transfuse with platelets prophylactically when the platelet count drops below 20,000/mm³. Platelet transfusions may be random donor (obtained from multiple units of fresh whole blood), single donor (obtained by platelet pheresis), or single donor, HLA-matched (obtained by platelet pheresis from a related, matched donor). Transfusion reactions occur most frequently with random donor platelets and usually consist of febrile reactions, urticaria, or both. This type of transfusion reaction is most likely to be related to leukoagglutinins and may be alleviated by premedication or leukocyte-poor platelets. Alloimmunization (development of antiplatelet antibodies) occurs after exposure to platelet transfusions. When this occurs, optimal response to platelet transfusions fails to occur and the platelet count remains the same or drops lower. With alloimmunization it may be necessary to reserve platelet transfusions for times of active bleeding.[39, 53, 55, 64, 77]

Patient and Family Education

The educational process for the patient and family should include practical guidelines for the prevention of bleeding, such as using acetaminophen instead of aspirin, always checking the ingredients of over-the-counter medications, not taking any medications unless prescribed by the physician, avoiding trauma, what to do for ecchymoses, when to call the physician if bleeding occurs or is suspected, what is serious bleeding, and how to recognize intracranial hemorrhage.

Medical Management

Infection. The medical management of suspected infection in the neutropenic or otherwise immunocompromised patient includes its prompt recognition with a workup including cultures, radiologic studies, a thorough physical assessment, and the immediate administration of broad-spectrum, empiric, intravenous antimicrobials. Potential sites for infection in the neutropenic patient are the following: *blood, oral cavity, GI and GU tracts, lungs, and skin*. Blood cultures should be obtained from both peripheral and central venous access sites, if present, for aerobic and anaerobic bacteria, fungi, and viruses if indicated. Obtain specimen cultures from body orifices, suspicious lesions, sputum, urine; stools should be tested for *C. difficile toxin* if the patient has significant diarrhea and cerebrospinal fluid cultures should be obtained from patients with obtundation, confusion, or mental changes that suggest central nervous system infection. All cultures and specimen collections should be obtained before initiating antimicrobial therapy. Blood culture specimens should be collected daily from clinical unstable patients or patients with new clinical symptoms. Patients with progressive pneumonia and no confirmed diagnosis should undergo bronchoscopy and bronchoalveolar lavage.[11, 12, 28, 50]

The antimicrobial selected is based on the organisms prevalent in the patient care setting and their antimicrobial susceptibility patterns (Box 31–6). Guidelines prepared by the Infectious Diseases Society of America suggest that antimicrobial therapy should be administered to neutropenic patients for a single temperature of greater than 101°F (38.3°C) orally for more than 1 hour. A regimen should be selected that provides broad-spectrum coverage against gram-positive and gram-negative bacteria. Controversy continues regarding the use of monotherapy with a single broad-spectrum antimicrobial *or* a combination of an aminoglycoside and a single broad-spectrum β-lactam as the best therapy for suspected infection in the neutropenic patient. Factors to consider include severity of neutropenia, presence

BOX 31-6

Infecting Organisms Associated with Neutropenia

Gram-Negative Bacteria

Pseudomonas aeruginosa
Klebsiella and *Enterobacter* species
Escherichia coli

Gram-Positive Bacteria

Staphylococcus aureus
Streptococcus pyogenes

Fungi

Candida albicans
Aspergillus species
Mucorales species

Long-Term Vascular Access Devices

Staphylococcus epidermidis
Corynebacterium

Data from references 35 and 78.

of suspected focus of infection, sensitivity of a particular organism to various antimicrobial drugs, and the patient's clinical features (i.e., presence of unstable vital signs, sepsis, acute respiratory distress syndrome [ARDS], and mucositis).[11, 16, 22, 47]

Antimicrobial coverage may be narrowed when the culture results are available. Antimicrobial therapy usually continues for a minimum of 10 to 14 days or until the patient's neutrophil count recovers to between 500/mm³ and 1500/mm³ (another point of controversy). If the patient continues febrile for longer than 72 hours, it is advisable to reculture and, depending on previous culture results, change antimicrobial therapy. If the patient has a vascular access device and the current antimicrobials do not have good coagulase-negative staphylococcus coverage, therapy may need to be changed to include a drug such as vancomycin. If the patient's clinical course deteriorates or there is reason to suspect the infecting agent may be either fungal or viral, amphotericin B (an antifungal) or acyclovir (an antiviral) or both may be added empirically. When a neutropenic patient becomes febrile, antimicrobial therapy must be administered promptly even though more than half of the febrile episodes are fever of unknown origin.*

Bleeding. Bleeding related to thrombocytopenia may be manifested as petechiae, purpura, ecchymoses, bleeding

---

* References 11, 16, 22, 31, 47, 72, 79, 80.

from a hollow viscus (GI tract, lungs, or GU tract), intracranial hemorrhage, or occult bleeding identified through routine testing of excreta. Work-up of a suspected bleed should include a thorough physical examination, radiologic examination as indicated by the clinical presentation, and laboratory evaluation, including a complete blood count (CBC), prothrombin time (PT), and partial thromboplastin time (PTT), and fibrinogen and fibrin degradation products (FDPs), if indicated. Treatment depends on the cause or source of the bleeding. If the bleeding is secondary to thrombocytopenia or a qualitative platelet defect, platelet transfusions will be of value. If the bleeding results from a coagulopathy such as DIC, platelets and coagulation factors may be replaced, using concentrates, cryoprecipitate, or fresh frozen plasma. Aminocaproic acid (Amicar) may be added to inhibit lysis of the clot by the fibrinolytic system.[11, 15, 39, 41, 42, 46, 77, 81]

Anemia. Symptoms of anemia may occur at variable levels of hemoglobin, depending on the rapidity with which it has occurred, age of the patient, and status of the cardiorespiratory system. Findings may include palpitations, shortness of breath, orthopnea, congestive heart failure with pulmonary edema, angina, fatigue, weakness, intolerance of cold, tinnitus, digestive complaints, difficulty in concentration, and numerous other nonspecific findings. The work-up should include a thorough physical assessment looking for the site of bleeding and the level of cardiorespiratory compensation. Laboratory examination should include CBC, reticulocyte count, lactic dehydrogenase and bilirubin values, and a hemolysis screen if indicated. A trial of rEPO may be administered to improve hemoglobin levels. Transfusion of RBCs is indicated if there is evidence of cardiac decompensation or if low hemoglobin levels are combined with low platelet counts. Transfusion of whole blood is not indicated unless there is massive bleeding and volume replacement cannot be accomplished by other means. Replacement of circulating red cell mass to improve oxygen-carrying capacity should be accomplished by transfusion of packed RBCs. This provides for more efficient use of blood components and less risk of volume overload.[3, 20, 27, 32, 42]

TRANSFUSION THERAPY

Blood component therapy is one of the more common supportive therapies used in the care of the person with myelosuppression. Even so, transfusion therapy must be used with care. Although major mismatch transfusion reactions are rare and usually result from management systems error (the patient received the wrong unit of blood because of improper identification of blood or patient), febrile transfusion reactions are quite common.

Febrile reactions are caused by the recipient reacting to donor leukocyte antigens. This can be discomforting for the patient and may accelerate alloimmunization or sensitization to transfused blood. The alloimmunization risk may be decreased by limiting the number of transfusions or donors and using leukocyte-depleted components or irradiated blood products.[29, 39, 86]

Historically, febrile reactions have been dealt with by the use of premedications that may suppress the response or by the administration of leukocyte-poor blood products. Saline-washed RBCs provided significantly reduced numbers of leukocytes although this is costly in time, money, and loss of RBCs. Early leukodepletion filters required extra processing and cooling of the RBCs. Leukocyte-poor platelets were rarely provided. Recent technologic advances have produced more efficient filters that are both user-friendly and are available for RBCs and platelets. The provision of leukocyte-poor blood components is more important for persons who are expected to require transfusion support for prolonged periods and alloimmunization prevention. Other potential benefits from leukodepletion include (1) decreased risk of blood-borne pathogens that reside in leukocytes, such as cytomegalovirus (CMV), and (2) possible decreased risk of transfusion-associated graft-versus-host disease (TA-GVHD).[33, 39, 86]

Infection with CMV, especially CMV pneumonitis, carries a significant risk for morbidity and mortality in patients who are severely immunosuppressed. CMV transmission may occur when a CMV-negative (CMV$^-$) recipient is transfused with blood from a CMV-positive (CMV$^+$) donor. The virus may remain dormant in lymphocyte for years after active infection. CMV$^+$ persons with normal immune system function are unaffected by the virus, because their immune system keeps the virus in check. Interest is great regarding methods of reducing risk for the CMV$^-$ person. Leukodepletion of blood components may help decrease the risk by removing potentially infectious leukocytes. Another method that is showing promise is the development/identification of a CMV$^-$ blood donor pool. This necessitates screening and designation of CMV$^-$ donors. Not in widespread use, this method is costly and time-consuming, and removes potential donors from the general blood donor pool.[3, 7, 46, 75, 84]

Since the mid-1980s when HIV transmission via blood transfusion was confirmed, potential blood transfusion recipients have shown a great interest in directed donations (the personal selection of one's blood donors). It has been assumed that directed donors would be safer than donors from the volunteer pools, when in fact it has been shown that the incidence of infectious disease markers is higher in directed donor population. A more recent problem with directed donations is TA-GVHD. Although its occurrence is exceedingly rare, TA-GVHD carries a mortality rate approximating 100%. The high mortality rate is associated with bone marrow failure. Persons susceptible to TA-GVHD are those who have Hodgkin's or non-Hodgkin's lymphoma, aplastic anemia, acute leukemia, or a congenital immunodeficiency disorder and patients undergoing BMT or directed donation from first-degree relatives.[34, 88, 92]

Transfusion-associated GVHD has been associated most frequently with directed donations from first-degree relatives such as parents or siblings. TA-GVHD occurs when the transfusion recipient has two nonidentical HLA haplotypes and the transfusion (lymphocyte) donor is homozygous for either of the HLA haplotypes of the recipient. The recipient is unable to recognize the donor lymphocytes as "nonself" while the donor (transfused) lymphocytes are able to recognize the recipient as "nonself." The lymphocyte reaction is essentially the same as that seen after allogeneic BMT. The exception is that the recipient marrow stem cells are a target organ for the graft-versus-host (GVH) reaction, whereas in BMT-associated GVHD, the marrow stem cells are of donor origin and therefore "self" and are not reacted against. The potential for TA-GVHD after directed donation is such that it is recommended that all blood components from first-degree relatives be irradiated before transfusion. The irradiation process destroys the ability of the donor lymphocytes to engraft in the patient. Irradiation of blood components before transfusion is standard procedure for BMT recipients and premature or other immunocompromised neonates. It is possible that leukodepletion filtration may decrease the risk of TA-GVHD, but it is not as effective as ionizing radiation.[34, 86, 88, 90, 92]

CONCLUSION

Protective mechanisms such as skin, mucous membrane, and bone marrow protect the body from foreign substances and invading organisms. The patient with cancer undergoing the various treatment modalities becomes at risk for breakdown of one or all of these protective mechanisms. Nursing management requires prompt recognition of the signs and symptoms of infection, bleeding, and skin breakdown so that definitive therapy can be implemented. Nurses caring for these patients are key members of the health care team at this crucial time.

Nursing Management

FATIGUE ASSOCIATED WITH ANEMIA

Nursing Diagnoses

- *Activity intolerance, risk for/actual, related to anemia secondary to bone marrow suppression; related to decreased tissue perfusion secondary to anemia as evidenced by fatigue, motor weakness, and inability to perform activities of daily living*
- *Gas exchange, impaired, related to decreased oxygenation secondary to anemia (decreased hemoglobin)*
- *Sexuality patterns, altered, related to decreased energy secondary to anemia*
- *Mobility, impaired physical, related to decreased strength and endurance*
- *Knowledge deficit related to basic disease process, signs and symptoms of anemia*

Outcome Goals

Patient will be able to:

- Demonstrate an increase in activity tolerance and a decrease in subjective complaints of fatigue.
- Demonstrate knowledge of relationship of red blood cells, hemoglobin, and availability of oxygen to fulfill needs of body tissue for normal functioning.
- Relate desire to resume sexual activity.
- Identify measures necessary to reduce the risks of injury related to decreased strength and endurance.
- Demonstrate knowledge of signs and symptoms of decreased oxygen availability to tissue.

Preventive Measures

Preventive measures include the following: frequent assessment of skin and mucous membranes for pallor; frequent assessment of cardiovascular system for signs of decompensation such as irregular rhythms, murmurs, changes in blood pressure and pulse rate, peripheral edema, and dyspnea; pulmonary examination for changes in rate and depth of respirations and rales; and neurologic examination for altered levels of consciousness and inability to concentrate. Nurses should be aware of current laboratory values for hemoglobin, hematocrit, reticulocyte count, and platelet count. Persons known to be anemic should be encouraged to monitor their activity closely to prevent overtiring.

Interventions

Nursing management of the patient with fatigue associated with anemia should include teaching energy conservation techniques, helping the patient cope with the changes in life-style that severe fatigue may dictate, providing the time and opportunity for the patient to ventilate anger, frustration, and feelings of depression, monitoring patient activity, planning activities to prevent overtiring, and transfusing packed red blood cells as ordered by the physician. The nurse must be aware of safe transfusion practices, signs and symptoms of transfusion reactions (listed on page 939), and indications for premedication and administration of leukocyte-poor blood.[39, 78]

Patient and Family Education

Teaching plans should include the following instructions:

- Rest when tired—anemia and fatigue are expected and temporary side effects of treatment for cancer.
- Develop a progressive ambulation plan—do not try too much at one time.[73]
- Pace your activities—try to maintain as normal a life-style as possible; plan periods of exercise and rest.
- Seek assistance with such things as child care, meal planning and preparation, laundry, and housecleaning.
- Eat a nutritionally balanced diet.
- Maintain usual patterns of sleep.

PATIENT TEACHING PRIORITIES

Protective Mechanisms

Discuss normal functions of immune system, bone marrow, and barrier defenses.

Discuss relationship between disease process, treatment, and impaired host defenses.

Discuss signs and symptoms to report to physician/nurse.

Plan for management of impaired protective mechanisms.[57]

Obtain culture-sensitive teaching materials.[51, 54]

Discuss complementary therapies and need for communicating with physician.[19, 54, 87]

Discuss availability of community resources—financial, nursing care, durable medical equipment, transportation, support groups.[36, 67, 87]

Chapter Questions

1. The major function(s) of the immune system is:
   a. Excretion, homeostasis, protection, regulation
   b. Fever, homeostasis, regulation, surveillance
   c. Homeostasis, protection, regulation, surveillance
   d. Regulation, surveillance, fever, homeostasis
2. Immunosuppression involves a defect in cell-mediated immunity, humoral immunity, and/or a combination of both; this *combination* occurs most often in the patient with:
   a. Acute myelogenous leukemia 60 days after allogeneic bone marrow transplantation
   b. Autoimmune hemolytic anemia receiving high-dose corticosteroid therapy
   c. Breast cancer, stage III, surgical resection, adjuvant chemotherapy
   d. Non-Hodgkin's lymphoma receiving combination chemotherapy
3. Patients that are at risk for TA-GVHD include:
   a. Bone marrow transplantation, exchange transfusion neonate, Hodgkin's disease, directed blood donation to self
   b. Bone marrow transplantation, exchange transfusion neonate, Hodgkin's disease, directed donation from blood relatives
   c. Bone marrow transplantation, platelet transfusion, breast cancer, directed donation from blood relatives
   d. Bone marrow transplantation, platelet transfusion, breast cancer, directed blood donation to self
4. Chills, dyspnea, fever, headache, hemoglobinuria, and low back pain are clinical features for:
   a. Allergic reaction
   b. Bacterial reaction
   c. Febrile reaction
   d. Hemolytic reaction
5. The major side effects of aminoglycocides include:
   a. Ototoxicity, nephrotoxicity, cardiac toxicity, vertigo
   b. Ototoxicity, nephrotoxicity, tinnitus, vertigo
   c. Ototoxicity, hepatic toxicity, tinnitus, vertigo
   d. Ototoxicity, hypokalemia, nausea, vertigo
6. The description of a stage III pressure ulcer includes:
   a. Full-thickness skin loss involving epidermis and/or dermis
   b. Full-thickness skin loss with extensive destruction
   c. Non-blanchable erythema intact skin, reactive hyperemia
   d. Partial-thickness skin loss involving epidermis or dermis
7. Interventions measures to decrease inflammation to mucus membranes include:
   a. Hydrogen peroxide/water 1:1 solution rinses every 2 hours, provide small frequent meals
   b. Inspect high-risk areas for color, edema, and nodules; provide frequent high-calorie foods
   c. Irrigate mouth with antibacterial agents, change diet to tepid clear liquids
   d. Topical anesthetic sprays, modify diet to include bland foods
8. Potential medication administration for the specified clinical condition include:
   a. Erythropoietin (Procrit, Epoetin Alfa) for neutropenia
   b. Granulocyte/macrophage-colony stimulating factor (GM-CSF) for anemia
   c. Oprelvekin (Neumega) for prevention of chemotherapy-induced thrombocytopenia
   d. Ticarcillin for cytomegalovirus-negative pneumonia
9. Appropriate, Immediate, and Sequential interventions for the neutropenic patient with potential sepsis include:
   a. Administer antimicrobials within 8 hours, Obtain blood and vascular access cultures, and Notify physician
   b. Administer antipyretics, Notify physician, and Initiate antimicrobials
   c. Initiate oxygen therapy, Notify physician, and Administer antimicrobials within 6 hours
   d. Notify physician, Obtain blood and vascular access cultures, Administer antimicrobials within 2 hours
10. Innate immunity is comprised of the following mechanisms:
    a. Cell-mediated immunity, humoral immunity, lymphocytes, and stem cells
    b. Chemical barriers, mechanical barriers, fever, and phagocytosis (inflammation)
    c. Erythrocytes, granulocytes, megakarocytes, and monocytes,
    d. Homeostasis, fever, megakarocytes, and stem cells

BIBLIOGRAPHY

1. Aeschlimann JR, Hersberger E, Rybak MJ: Analysis of vancomycin-intermediate *Staphylococcus aureus, Antimicrob Agents Chemother* 43:1914, 1999.

2. Agency for Health Care Policy and Research: *Treatment of pressure ulcers,* Rockville, MD, US Department of Health and Human Services, 1994.

3. Alcoser PW, Burchett S: Bone marrow transplantation: immune system suppression and reconstitution, *Am J Nurs* 99:26, 1999.

4. Anderson P and others: Testing an oral assessment guide during chemotherapy treatment in a Swedish care setting: a pilot study, *J Clin Nurs* 8:150, 1999.

5. *ASPEN Nutrition Support Practice Manual,* Silver Spring, MD, Aspen Publishers, 1998.

6. Baldwin KM, Ziegler SM: Pressure ulcer risk following critical traumatic injury, *Adv Wound Care* 11:168, 1998.

7. Ball P: Therapy for pneumonococcal infection at the millennium: doubts and certainties, *Am J Med* 107(1A): 77S, 1999.

8. Berger A, Portenoy R, Weissman D: *Principles and practices of supportive oncology,* Philadelphia, Lippincott-Raven, 1998.

9. Berger AM, Eilers J: Factors influencing oral cavity status during high-dose antineoplastic therapy: a secondary analysis, *Oncol Nurs Forum* 25:1623, 1998.

10. Bloch AS: Alternative nutritional regiments targeted to persons with cancer, *Cancer Pract* 7:151, 1999.

11. Bodey GP: Fever in the neutropenic patient. In Abeloff MD, Armitage JO, Lichter AS, Neiderhuber JE, editors: *Clinical oncology,* ed 2, New York, Churchill Livingstone, 1999.

12. Bosi A and others: An open evaluation of triple antibiotic therapy including vancomycin for febrile bone marrow transplant recipients with severe neutropenia, *J Chemother* 11:287, 1999.

13. Bours GJJW and others: The development of a national registration form to measure the prevalence of pressure ulcers in the Netherlands, *Ostomy/Wound Manage* 45:28, 1999.

14. Brophy L: Immunology. In Itano JK, Taoka KN, editors: *Core curriculum for oncology nursing,* ed 3, Philadelphia, Saunders, 1998.

15. Camp-Sorrell D: Myelosuppression. In Itano JK, Taoka KN, editors: *Core curriculum for oncology nursing,* ed 3, Philadelphia, Saunders, 1998.

16. Carbon C, Poole MD: The role of newer macrolides in the treatment of community-acquired respiratory tract infection. A review of experimental and clinical data, *J Chemother* 11:107, 1999.

17. Carlson EV, Kemp MG, Shott S: Predicting the risk of pressure ulcers in critically ill patients, *Am J Crit Care* 8: 262, 1999.

18. Carroll P: Bed selection—help patients rest easy, *RN* 58:44, 1995.

19. Cassileth BR: *The alternative medicine handbook: the complete reference guide to alternative and complementary therapies,* New York, Norton, 1998.

20. Cella D, Bron D: The effect of epoetin alfa on quality of life in anemic cancer patients, *Cancer Pract* 7:177, 1999.

21. Chen LM and others: Interobserver variability in data collection of the APACHE II score in teaching and community hospitals, *Crit Care Med* 27:1999, 1999.

22. Circiumaru B, Baldock F, Cohen J: A prospective study of fever in the intensive care unit, *Intensive Care Med* 25:668, 1999.

23. Conrad KJ: Cutaneous reactions. In Yasko JM, editor: *Nursing management of symptoms associated with chemotherapy,* Bala Cynwyd, PA, Pharmacia & Upjohn, Meniscus Health Care Communications, 1998.

24. Comley AL and others: Effect of subcutaneous granulocyte colony-stimulating factor injectate volume on drug efficacy, site complications, and client comfort, *Oncol Nurs Forum* 26:87, 1999.

25. Dalakas MC: Autoimmune peripheral neuropathies, pathogenesis and treatment, Omaha, Nebraska Health Science Center, Clinical Communications Inc., 1998.

26. DeVita VT Jr, Hellman S, Roseman SA, editors: *Cancer: principles and practice of oncology,* ed 5, Philadelphia, Lippincott-Raven, 1997.

27. Dunphy FR and others: Erythropoietin reduces anemia and transfusion: a randomized trial with or without erythropoietin during chemotherapy, *Cancer* 86:1362, 1999.

28. Engervall P and others: Cefepime as empirical monotherapy in febrile patients with hematological malignancies and neutropenia: a randomized, single-center phase II trial, *J Chemother* 11:278, 1999.

29. Estrin JT and others: A retrospective review of blood transfusions in cancer patients with anemia, *Oncologist* 4:318, 1999.

30. Ferguson NR, Galley HF, Webster NR: T helper cell subset ratios in patients with severe sepsis, *Intensive Care Med* 25:106, 1999.

31. Fisher NC and others: Fungal infection and liposomal amphotericin B (AmBisome) therapy in liver transplantation: a 2 year review, *J Antimicrobial Chemother* 43:597, 1999.

32. Gahart BL, Nazareno AR: *Intravenous medications,* ed 16, St. Louis, Mosby, 2000.

33. Gorski LA, editor: *Best practices in home infusion therapy,* Fredrick, MD, Aspen Publishers, 1999.

34. Grass JA and others: Prevention of transfusion-associated graft-versus-host disease by photochemical treatment, *Blood* 93:3140, 1999.

35. Guyton AC, Hall T: *Textbook of medical physiology,* ed 9, Philadelphia, Saunders, 1996.

36. Haas BK: Focus on health promotion: self-efficacy in oncology nursing research and practice, *Oncol Nurs Forum* 27:89, 2000.

37. Haas S and others: Heparin-induced thrombocytopenia: the role of platelet activation and therapeutic implications, *Semin Thromb Hemost* 25(suppl 1):67, 1999.

38. Haisfield-Wolfe ME, Rund C: A nursing protocol for the management of perineal-rectal skin alterations, *Clin J Oncol Nurs* 4:15, 2000.

39. Harmening DM, editor: *Modern blood banking and transfusion practices,* ed 4, Philadelphia, Davis, 1999.

40. Henry L: Immunocompromised patients and nutrition, *Prof Nurse* 12:655, 1997.

41. Hoban DJ, Zhanel GG, Karlowsky JA: In vitro susceptibilities of *Candida* and *Cryptococcus neoformans* isolates from blood cultures of neutropenic patients, *Antimicrob Agents Chemother* 43:1463, 1999.

42. Hodgson BB, Kizior RJ: *Saunders nursing drug handbook,* Philadelphia, Saunders, 2000.

43. Johnson BL, Gross J: *Handbook of oncology nursing,* ed 3, Boston, Jones & Bartlett, 1998.

44. Jones RD: Bacterial resistance and topical antimicrobial wash products, *Am J Infect Control* 27:351, 1999.

45. Kadidal VV, Mayo DJ, Horne MK III: Heparin-induced thrombocytopenia, (HIT) due to heparin flushes: a report of three cases, *J Intern Med* 246:325, 1999.

46. Kolar M, Latal T, Hajek V: Development of bacterial resistance to the third generation cephalosporins and their clinical use, *J Chemother* 11:260, 1999.

47. Krumpe PE and others: Intravenous and oral mono- or combination-therapy in the treatment of severe infections: ciproflaxin versus standard antibiotic therapy. Ciproflaxin Study Group, *J Antimicrob Chemother* 43(suppl A):117, 1999.

48. Kudski KA, Teasley-Straysburg K: Parenteral nutrition: guidelines for formula selection, administration and potential complications. Enteral and parenteral nutrition. In: Irwin RS, Cerra FB, Rippe JM, editors: *Intensive care medicine,* ed 4, vol II, Philadelphia, Lippincott-Raven, 1999.

49. LaClaire S: Supportive care issues in patients receiving radiation therapy, *Highlights in Oncol Pract* 17:54, 1999.

50. Li RC, Zhu M, Schentag JJ: Achieving an optimal outcome in the treatment of infections, the role of clinical pharmacokinetics and pharmacodynamics of antimicrobials, *Clin Pharmacokinet* 37:1, 1999.

51. Lipson JE, Dibble SL, Minarik PA, editors: *Culture and nursing care: a pocket guide,* University of California, San Francisco, USCF Nursing Press, 1996.

52. Masucci IP and others: Thrombocytopenia, after isolated limb or hepatic perfusions with melphalan: the risk of heparin-induced thrombocytopenia, *Ann Surg Oncol* 6:476, 1999.

53. Matassarin-Jacobs E: Nursing care of clients with hematologic disorders. In Black JM, Matassarin-Jacobs E, editors: *Medical-surgical nursing,* ed 5, Philadelphia, Saunders, 1997.

54. Mayer D: Cancer patient empowerment, *Oncol Nurs Updates* 6:1, 1999.

55. Mayo DJ and others: Serologic evidence of heparin sensitization in cancer patients receiving heparin flushes of venous access devices, *Support Care Cancer* 7:425, 1999.

56. McConnell EA: Infection control: more than a matter of economics, *Nurs Manage* 30:64, 1999.

57. McGucklin M and others: Patient education model for increasing handwashing compliance, *Am J Infect Control* 27:309, 1999.

58. McGuire DB and others: Acute oral pain and mucositis in bone marrow transplant and leukemia patients: data from a pilot study, *Cancer Nurs* 21:385, 1998.

59. Miller SE: Stomatitis and esophagitis. In Yasko JM, editor: *Nursing management of symptoms associated with chemotherapy,* Bala Cynwyd, PA, Pharmacia & Upjohn, Meniscus Health Care Communications, 1998.

60. North American Nursing Diagnosis Association: *Nursing diagnosis: definitions and classification,* Philadelphia, The Association, 1999.

61. Olson K, Tkachuk L, Hanson J: Preventing pressure sores in oncology patients, *Clin Nurs Res* 7:207, 1998.

62. Oncology Nursing Society: *Cancer chemotherapy guidelines and recommendations for practice,* Pittsburgh, Oncology Nursing Press, 1999.

63. Osterblad M and others: Antimicrobial susceptibility of enterobacteriaceae isolated from vegetables, *J Antimicrob Chemother* 43:503, 1999.

64. Pall Medical: *IV filtration: choice or necessity?* Technical Report, Ann Arbor, MI, Pall Medical Corporation, 1999.

65. Panel on the Prediction and Prevention of Pressure Ulcers in Adults: *Pressure ulcers in adults: prediction and prevention.* Rockville, MD, Agency for Health Care Policy and Research, Public Health Service, US Department of Health and Human Services, 1992.

66. Pearce JD: Alterations in mobility, skin integrity, and neurologic status. In Itano JK, Taoka KN, editors: *Core curriculum for oncology nursing,* ed 3, Philadelphia, Saunders, 1998.

67. Perry AG, Potter PA: *Clinical nursing skills & techniques,* ed 4, St. Louis, Mosby, 1998.

68. Peterson PG: Sepsis and septic shock. In Chernecky C, Berger B, editors: *Advanced and critical care oncology nursing,* Philadelphia, Saunders, 1998.

69. Petursson CT: Bleeding due to thrombocytopenia. In Yasko JM, editor: *Nursing management of symptoms associated with chemotherapy,* Bala Cynwyd, PA, Pharmacia & Upjohn, Meniscus Health Care Communications, 1998.

70. Phipps WJ, Sands JK, Marek JF: *Medical-surgical nursing: concepts and clinical practice,* ed 6, St. Louis, Mosby, 1999.

71. Ransier A and others: A combined analysis of a toothbrush, foam brush, and a chlorhexidine-soaked foam brush on maintaining oral hygiene, *Cancer Nurs* 18:393, 1995.

72. Rapp RP: Antimicrobial resistance in gram-positive bacteria: the myth of the MIC. Minimum inhibitory concentration, *Pharmacotherapy* 19(7 part 2):112 S, 1999.

73. Ream E, Richardson A: From theory to practice: designing interventions to reduce fatigue in patients with cancer, *Oncol Nurs Forum* 26:1295, 1999.

74. Rieger PT: Management of cancer in the next millennium: DNA holds the key, *Highlights Oncol Pract* 16:110, 1999.

75. Risi GF, Tomascak V: Prevention of infection in the immunocompromised host, *Am J Infect Control* 26:594, 1998.

76. Rivadenereia DE and others: Nutritional support of the cancer patient, *CA Cancer J Clin* 48:69, 1998.

77. Rust DM, Wood LS, Battiato LA: Oprelvekin: an alternative treatment for thrombocytopenia, *Clin J Oncol* 3:57, 1999.

78. Schafer SL: Infection due to leukopenia. In Yasko JM, editor: *Nursing management of symptoms associated with chemotherapy,* Bala Cynwyd, PA, Pharmacia & Upjohn, Meniscus Health Care Communications, 1998.

79. Shankar SM and others: Pharmacokinetics of single daily dose gentamycin in children with cancer, *J Pediatr Hematol Oncol* 21:284, 1999.

80. Sheff B: VRE and MRSA: putting bad bugs out of business, *Nurs Manage* 30:42, 1999.

81. Shirrell DJ and others: Therapeutic drug monitoring, *Am J Nurs* 99:42, 1999.

82. Todd J and others: The low-bacteria diet for immunocompromised patients, reasonable prudence or clinical superstition? *Cancer Pract* 7:205, 1999.

83. Van Gulick AJ: Anemia. In Yasko JM, editor: *Nursing management of symptoms associated with chemotherapy*, Bala Cynwyd, PA, Pharmacia & Upjohn, Meniscus Health Care Communications, 1998.

84. Wang FD and others: A comparative study of cefepime versus ceftazidime as empiric therapy of febrile episodes in neutropenic patients, *Chemotherapy* 45:370, 1999.

85. Watts D and others: Insult after injury: pressure ulcers in trauma patients, *Orthop Nurs* 17:84, 1998.

86. Weiskopf RB: Do we know when to transfuse red cells to treat acute anemia? *Transfusion* 38:517, 1998.

87. Webster A: Mind/body medicine: self-care skills for persons with cancer, *Cancer Pract* 7:43, 1999.

88. Williamson LM: Transfusion-associated graft-versus-host disease: new insights and a route towards therapy? *Transfus Med* 8:169, 1998.

89. Wilson RL: Optimizing nutrition for patients with cancer, *Clin J Oncol Nurs* 4:23, 2000.

90. Workman ML: The lymphoid system and its role in maintaining immunocompetence, *Semin Oncol* 14:248, 1998.

91. *Wound product sourcebook*, Hinesburg, VT, Green Mountain Wellness Publishers, 1999.

92. Yasuura K, Matsuura A: High risk of transfusion-associated graft-versus-host disease with nonirradiated allogeneic blood transfusion in cardiac surgery, *Transfusion* 38:117, 1998.

Psychosocial Issues, Outcomes, and Quality of Life

Judith A. Shell and Suzanne Kirsch

32 CHAPTER

I wanted a perfect ending so I sat down to write the book with the ending in place before there even was an ending. Now I've learned the hard way that some poems don't rhyme, and some stories do not have a clear beginning, middle, and end. Like my life, this book has ambiguity. Like my life, this book is about not knowing, having to change, taking the moment and making the best of it without knowing what is going to happen next.[78]

INTRODUCTION

All cancer patients and families face challenges during their life cycle; some are sudden and untimely (unexpected death or disaster), whereas others are expected (divorce and remarriage or retirement). The cancer illness in one member of a family will alter the emotional balance, finances, division of responsibility, and social activities of the spouse or partner, as well as the rest of the family.[50] How patients and families become organized, and how they communicate and solve problems together to cope with the threat often foretells their ability to recover. A support network of extended family, friends, neighbors, spiritual counselors, employers, and available community resources will also contribute to the recovery process.

Because many patients, even today, consider a cancer diagnosis as a sentence of impending and painful death, there is a great psychological impact on the functioning of the patient and family. Initially, a psychological crisis is created, which causes many emotions ranging from the anxiety, anger, fear, and depression of the often emotionally paralyzing diagnosis and treatment options, to despair and hopelessness.[49] Following this immediate crisis response, Weisman and Worden's landmark study explains the "existential plight," of the individual during the first 100 days after diagnosis.[91] The patient attempts to address the meaning of the illness and the possible changes in life patterns and the life-altering decisions that must be made; the possibility of dying is also included. Nurses must not underestimate this "plight" because there are a wide range of responses encountered as patients search for and try to make sense of the meaning of cancer. We must caution patients not to consider their responses abnormal or maladaptive because there is nothing "normal" about getting a cancer diagnosis.

Along with these genuine emotional responses, patients experience the sense of a total loss of control. One of the greatest fears that cancer patients often express is that fear of loss of control. Patients are burdened with the need to comply with tests (often on different days at various facilities) or several different doctor appointments (often to receive chemotherapy or radiation therapy), and these obligations cause other losses such as ability to work or care for the family. Schedules and plans are a thing of the past, and patients often focus primarily on the demands of the illness and getting well. As one patient explained, "I just couldn't do anything. I couldn't think. I couldn't read. I couldn't work. And it went on for weeks."[38] Indeck and Bunney report that as patients begin to create meaning in relation to the illness, they experience a sense of victory over the many life-changing events, which leads to an increased sense of some control.[49] As an increased sense of control emerges, patients can think more efficiently and act constructively; they can become active rather than passive in their plan of care.

This chapter will identify psychosocial factors of adjustment for patients and families during the many phases of the cancer trajectory including diagnosis and treatment, after treatment, progressive disease and completion of life, as well as long-term survival. Nursing strategies will be offered for all phases of psychosocial circumstances. Cancer patients and families can have a more positive and empowering experience, and an increased survival rate if good psychosocial management is integrated into their plan of care.[28, 29] There may also be a reduction in problem-oriented physical distresses such as discomfort and side effects, affairs of daily living such as relationship and vocational issues, and a significant reduction in emotional distress such as depression, hopelessness, confusion, anxiety, and avoidance; quality of life will likewise be enhanced.[26, 32, 88] The nurse, then, must recognize signs of psychosocial suffering and also be aware of those at increased risk for distress, such as those with a history of emotional problems, a lack of resources, and advanced disease.[46]

PATIENT/FAMILY RESPONSE ALONG THE CANCER CONTINUUM

Patient Emotional Response and Ability to Cope

On learning of a cancer diagnosis, patients experience new and multiple kinds of distress that they must learn to cope with. Denial, the "it can't be true," is often initially used and is a very adaptive temporary response. In immediate succession come anger (why me?), fear (doesn't cancer mean death?), general anxiety (fear of the unknown), "test" anxiety (waiting for results), and mourning their many losses. They must also be prepared to learn the foreign language of medicine, make choices that are life-changing decisions, and all the while wonder if they are "going crazy" (am I losing my mind?). These are all examples of distress that patients must now handle as a conglomerate, whereas previously they may have encountered them only on an individual basis.[35, 44]

One important factor related to how patients respond to the diagnosis of cancer will depend on how they are told the news. Although, initially, it is usually the responsibility of the primary physician/surgeon to deliver "sad and bad" news to the patient/family, oncology nurses usually participate in this endeavor as well, either by accompanying the physician or by reinforcing what has been said. Recent literature has provided some general principles through which a recommended process was developed (Table 32–1). Fallowfield relates that "professional detachment" can offend the recipient of bad news; therefore, we must develop the skills to deliver information truthfully yet gently that can maintain hope and a sense of reassurance.[27] Other elements (principles) that influence response include developmental tasks and goals according to age, prior levels of psychological and social adjustment to illness, religious and cultural attitudes, the level of social support, the potential for rehabilitation, and the patient's own personality.[20, 35]

Although patients may be informed of the diagnosis in an empathic and appropriate manner, they may still feel overwhelmed with a lost sense of equilibrium that

---

T A B L E   3 2 – 1

Recommended Steps for Breaking Bad News

Steps	Process
1. Privacy and Adequate Time	Provide quiet space. Provide enough time for thought/questions. Ideally, family member should be present.
2. Assess Understanding	Is patient aware of situation and prognosis? Ask patient how much information they want. Be aware of culture, race, religion and social background.
3. Simple, Honest Information	Speak simply and avoid medical jargon. Use the word "cancer." Consider writing information down.
4. Advocate Expression of Feelings	Normalize feelings of numbness, disbelief and anger. Respond with empathy and warmth.
5. Promote a Broad Time Frame	Avoid definite time scale; be realistic. Reassure and provide support to promote comfort.
6. Arrange a Review	Plan a discussion to review the situation soon after the initial consult.
7. Discuss Treatment Options	Clearly relate treatment options and encourage patient/family to participate in final decisions.
8. Offer Assistance to Tell Others	Support communication of diagnosis between family and friends. Promote use of family therapist to help with children.
9. Provide Resource Information	Offer referral to various support services and personnel, e.g., groups, funds, therapists for families.
10. Document Information Given	Document concisely all information given and people involved in consultation sessions.

From Girgis A, Sanson-Fisher RW: Breaking bad news: consensus guidelines for medical practitioners, J Clin Oncol 13:2449, 1995.

---

precipitates a crisis. Adjustment to a chronic illness like cancer can, however, occur more rapidly in those who exhibit more resiliency factors such as problem-solving communication, equality, spirituality, flexibility, truthfulness, hope, family hardiness, family time and routines, social support, and health.[61] Whether or not the newly diagnosed patient adjusts gradually or more rapidly, numerous coping tasks must be managed (Table 32–2).

Role Adjustment and Altered Relationships

Once the patient is projected into the cancer domain, various factors will alter established roles and relationships. The ability to fulfill usual roles and responsibilities will change, new roles will be added, and role relationships with others will operate in a modified manner. The usual functions associated with being a spouse or partner and lover, parent, sibling, child, friend, employer, employee, or any other group will shift dramatically. Changed relationships may manifest themselves by a new separateness, increased concern and kindness, or by distancing and avoidance.[21] The nature of the new

roles and relationships can create feelings of incompetence and discomfort. These people who have become cancer patients are now labeled as "different."

Because the perception may now exist that this person is different somehow, it might be necessary for that person to set the tone for maintaining relationships. This can create a feeling of overwhelming frustration because the patient is also trying to recover and heal. There will often be a new sense of awareness of who will help with household chores, who takes time to be attentive and visit, and who listens when the patient feels like talking about illness. However, troubled thoughts of abandonment may intermittently surface if anticipated support is felt to be lacking.[20]

The wish for privacy can actually cause problems. This is due to the fact that the patient may not wish to share much information regarding the illness with many

T A B L E 3 2 – 2
Typology of Coping Tasks of Chronically Ill Adults

Broad Task Category	Subconcepts in the Category
1. Maintaining a sense of normalcy	Hiding, minimizing illness and/or responding to curious inquiries of others
2. Modifying daily routine; adjusting lifestyle	Living as normally as possible despite daily therapy and obvious symptoms Providing for safety
3. Obtaining knowledge and skill for continuing self-care	Having internal awareness Monitoring effects of therapy
4. Maintaining a positive self-concept	Integrating illness into self-concept Maintaining or enhancing self-esteem
5. Adjusting to altered social relationships	Experiencing loneliness or social isolation Undergoing patient or other initiated disengagement Preserving relationships with friends and family who satisfy dependency needs Maintaining family solidarity
6. Grieving over losses concomitant with chronic illness	Losing physical abilities, function Losing status Losing income and social relationships Losing roles and dignity Dealing with financial losses
7. Dealing with role change	Losing roles—social, work, family Gaining roles—dependent help seeker, self-care agent, chronically ill patient
8. Handling physical discomfort	Handling illness-induced discomfort Handling pain caused by therapy
9. Complying with prescribed regimen	
10. Confronting the inevitability of one's own death	
11. Dealing with social stigma of illness or disability	
12. Maintaining a feeling of being in control	Exerting cognitive control Exerting behavioral control Exerting decisional control
13. Maintaining hope despite uncertain or downward course of health	Experiencing effects of hope Finding meaning in physical changes

From Miller JF: Analysis of coping with illness. In Miller JF, editor: Coping with chronic illness: overcoming powerlessness, *Philadelphia, Davis, 1992. Used with permission.*

people other than immediate family, at least initially. Consequently, isolation may be created when information is kept private. Social isolation not only can be due to privacy factors, but also to the stigma of cancer, to the anger of family/friends because the patient developed the disease, and to the fact that disability has arisen and prevents participation in many social activities. Although family and friends want to help, often by voicing cheery encouragement, the patient should be counseled to ask for what they need by clearly stating how they feel and what would be helpful. Occasionally, friendships that were cultivated before the illness do not remain intact for various reasons; they may need to be discontinued.

Sexual health and the sexual relationship are important aspects of the patient's very being; however, focus is usually centered around the physical well-being of the patient during diagnosis and treatment. As the patient traverses the treatment process and beyond, sexual functioning can be threatened via numerous avenues (e.g., fear of contagion, disfiguring surgery, fertility issues, chemotherapy side effects like fatigue and malaise, nausea and vomiting, pain). (See Chapter 33 for an in-depth portrayal of impact on sexuality.)

Psychological Disorders: Anxiety and Depression

Two of the most frequent and common psychological disorders in cancer patients are anxiety and depression. Given the fact that cancer is an obvious threat to the person's very well-being, these feelings are quite normal. However, many myths and assumptions exist which suggest that "all" cancer patients must be depressed and require psychiatric intervention. In reality, Lesko reports that several psychosocial studies indicate cancer patients do experience illness-related emotional distress; however, they are for the most part psychologically healthy.[53]

Anxiety. Normally, anxiety occurs at different points throughout the course of illness and treatment. Technically, anxiety disorders are classified in the *Diagnostic and Statistical Manual of Mental Disorders* (*DSM-IV*).[2] Although the most common anxiety response in cancer patients is classified in the *DSM-IV* as adjustment disorder with anxious mood (with or without depression), the other types include generalized anxiety disorder, panic disorder, phobias, posttraumatic stress disorder, and anxiety due to medical illness.[2]

Adjustment disorder with anxious mood is commonly referred to as reactive or situational anxiety and is caused by the normal or expected fears that occur after diagnosis and during treatment. They manifest themselves through tension, nervousness, feeling upset, and an inability to sleep.[14] This acute form of anxiety can occur during various phases of the illness, which include:

- Awaiting procedures and tests
- Awaiting test results and diagnosis
- Anticipating major treatment (surgery, chemotherapy/biotherapy, radiation)
- Completion of treatment
- Learning of relapse
- Anticipating more (often more severe) treatment
- During advanced illness
- On anniversary dates of diagnosis, treatments, or other related events[20, 53]

Symptoms of acute anxiety may also surface due to pain, uncontrolled or conditioned nausea and vomiting, hypoxia, treatment withdrawal, and various medications. Although these symptoms create some discomfort, Clark asserts that minimal to moderate levels of anxiety may be motivating for some patients.[19]

Chronic anxiety, which precedes the cancer diagnosis, may exacerbate the generalized anxiety disorders, phobias, and panic states. This creates greater risk for the individual because she may perceive an increased threat from cancer and be overwhelmed with symptoms of fatigue, restlessness and inability to concentrate, irritability and tension, rapid heart rate, losing control, and feelings of "going crazy."[14] As the nurse attends to the patient, McDaniel and coworkers remind us that, "because of the level of anxiety and concern exhibited in most families with sick members, it is especially important to respond to their story with empathy, respect, and a lack of blame and to emphasize the strengths exhibited by the family in their response to this crisis."[64]

Depression. Although sadness and a sense of hopelessness may be considered normal reactions to the cancer diagnosis, other factors can contribute to a depressed mood. They include the disease process (tests, treatment, side effect management), medications (chemotherapy, biotherapy, and steroids), or a biologic depression not necessarily related to the present event. Other risk factors include the severity of the disease, particular disease sites (pancreatic or head and neck), lack of social support, fear of uncontrolled pain, and other stressful life events.[7, 63] Depression, as with anxiety, is diagnosed according to the *DSM-IV*.[2] They stipulate that the patient must experience symptoms of depression for at least 2 weeks, and at least four of several conditions such as anorexia, fatigue, weight loss, and insomnia must be present. Consequently, a diagnosis of depression can be difficult to make due to the fact that these particular symptoms of depression mimic the side effects of cancer and its treatment.

Although it is considered common during the first 7 to 14 days to observe a depressive mood if a preexisting depressive disorder was present (e.g., a bipolar mood disorder), it can be difficult to determine the actual cause of the depression.[45, 53] As well, many times depression is undertreated or ignored because it is not recognized, and it is considered to be customary for cancer patients to be depressed.[1] Whether etiology is from the stressful cancer event, biologic in nature, or from medications, the patient deserves to be treated just as aggressively for the depression as for the cancer or other treatment-related side effects.

Family Emotional Response and Ability to Cope

A cancer diagnosis is perhaps one of the most profound stressors an individual can experience. The physical disease process affects only its host, but the experience of illness and the inherent potential for stress is shared by the entire family. How patients and their families cope with the cancer experience has a profound effect on the perceived level of suffering. Cancer demands new ways of coping for both the patient and the family as they face changes in the way they define themselves personally and as a family unit. A family's ability to cope with the emotional, physical, and relational challenges that the diagnosis and treatment of cancer can impose will be influenced by a variety of factors some of which may be the level of support available to the family, family illness beliefs, the family's sense of agency, degree of hope, and the family's level of communication around their feelings, needs, and wants.

Support. It is not uncommon for patients with serious illness and their families to feel isolated even from close friends and family members. McDaniel and colleagues note the importance of the emotional bonds and a sense of support and being cared for, and loved by a community of family, friends and professionals, and suggest this may be the most powerful psychosocial factor in health and illness.[64] It is one's support network that has the greatest influence on health risk behavior and this upholds the idea of and lends importance to the nurses' partnership with patients and family members.[48] The nurses' role of facilitating a collaborative partnership between the patient, family, and health care team can be instrumental in providing emotional support for the entire family.

Illness Beliefs. Susan Sontag reminds us that "everyone who is born holds dual citizenship, in the kingdom of the well and in the kingdom of the sick" and although some citizens escape personal illness for much of their lives, most will be affected at least indirectly by the illness beliefs of a loved family member.[84] We cannot escape the broad brush of the illness experience and its meaning as it paints confusion, fear, disability, and sometimes death on family and friends. Often, little attention is paid to the impact a prior experience of illness has on the manner in which patients and their families deal with a diagnosis of cancer. Current attitudes, understandings, fears, hopes, ability to cope and so forth are all crafted, in part, by past experiences with serious illness. Each family with its own unique illness story and meaning will be challenged to cope with the plethora of emotional themes that emerge in the face of a cancer diagnosis and its treatment.

Agency. For those families experiencing cancer who walk the illness journey with their loved one, cancer may be the most "out of control" experience they have ever participated in. Loving family members who once were competent protectors, caretakers, and providers can feel helpless in the company of cancer and a health care system that may seemingly wedge themselves between patient and loved ones, and alter the ways in which they are accustomed to experiencing one another. Our health care system is organized, in large part, for the convenience of health care providers and the efficacy of their work; it plays a powerful role in inviting a passive "good patient/family" role and sense of helplessness and loss of agency. Nurses can work to increase a sense of agency for families by helping them accept what they must and to work to change what they can.[66]

Hope. Some have likened the experience of cancer to a roller coaster ride with the unpredictable highs and lows of hope and despair. Beliefs have a significant influence on the way in which people can hold hope during an illness experience. Hope is not the same as desires and expectations and is not exclusive to the wish for a cure; thus, patients and their families can explore the possibility of holding hope for a broad range of physical, emotional, and relational outcomes. The dominant medical system may not address the idea of hope and optimism in the illness experience, yet nurses can gain some understanding of the existence of hope by asking family members their beliefs about the future with the illness. McDaniel and colleagues suggest that patients and their families generally feel discouraged during the early phases of an illness and find it difficult to hold hope.[66] Yet, they also look eagerly for positive stories from those who have had a similar condition. After the illness seems more stabilized, patients and families are often reassured and become more hopeful.

Communication. Most people have not been raised in an atmosphere that fosters awareness of the importance of talking about illness, its challenges, and the feelings that accompany it. Patients and families may experience less anxiety when they are able to communicate honestly with one another; yet, there is a great tendency to try to say the right thing, to cheer one another up too quickly, or to try to protect one another from the real emotions that each is experiencing. A failure to communicate with one another will lead to unnecessary tension, misunderstanding, and suffering that will adversely affect the family's ability to cope with the illness experience. An honest and open atmosphere of communication can convey a sense of trust and respect for each family member's ability to cope with the truth and manage the challenges that lie ahead. Patients and family members will also benefit most from honest and direct communication from the medical/nursing team about prognosis, treatment options, and possible outcomes. Physicians, nurses, and other health care providers vary in what they tell patients and families; this may be in part because they are uncertain about the course the illness may take. The oncology nurse can be instrumental in strengthening a family's sense of agency and connectedness to one another and to the health care team during the time of illness by her role as facilitator of conversation and as collaborator with the entire health care team.

Role Adjustment, Altered Relationships, and Family Organization

Family adaptability is a quality required for well-functioning families but is particularly necessary for families facing serious illness. Illness and its challenges have been said to arrive like an unwanted, demanding, and unsettling guest that requires the entire household to shift and reorganize the ways in which it has been experiencing family routine and relationships with one another. According to Rolland, the ability of a family to adapt to changing circumstances or life cycle developmental tasks is balanced by a family's need for enduring values, traditions, and predictable consistent rules for behavior.[79]

A serious illness can derail a family from its natural life cycle momentum as the family struggles to maintain a challenging balancing act. They must adjust physical, emotional, relational, and financial demands so that they can respond to the needs of their sick member and help implement the treatment plan, while at the same time continue their own lives in a normal fashion. Families may not be prepared for the role shifts and relationship skews that may occur within the domain of serious illness. Changes in family organization will be needed as disorder continues to interact with normal family and individual members' life cycle development.[79]

Stay-at-home moms, who enjoy their role and experience as primary caregivers to their young children, may be required to get a job outside the home when the father becomes too ill to continue to work. Fathers who take pride in their ability to be providers and protectors of the family can experience emotional as well as physical suffering when cancer treatment and its side effects render them unable to be productive in their professions. If a married adult daughter decides to take care of her ill mother, not only must she cope with the stresses

of an additional household member who is ill, but she must also continue to accommodate the needs of her own family. In the family with adolescents or young dependent adults, the serious illness of a parent can impede the completion of the major life cycle task of weaning children from parents. Not only does the parental illness interfere with the adolescents' achievement of independence through the usual rebellion and focus outside of the family, but the adolescent may be called on to act as parental surrogate with siblings, which holds her tightly to the family.[11] Brown further believes that those deaths or serious illnesses whose victims are in the prime of life are the most disruptive to the family function; this may be due, in part, because it is at this phase of the life cycle that the individual has the greatest responsibilities.[10] Illness can also test the role and organization flexibility of the extended family when, for instance, a grandmother becomes sick and can no longer take care of herself. Will the adult children be able to take care of their mother, and will the mother be able to shift her role from caregiver to care-receiver?

Within the context of illness, flexibility and adaptability can help a family better manage the myriad of changes that have the potential to disrupt family organization, values, traditions, rules, and particularly the manner in which family members relate to one another and the roles that each person plays. Family strength requires clear, yet flexible, boundaries and subsystems to mobilize alternative coping patterns when stressed by the challenges of illness and disability.[79]

Facing Cancer with a Spouse

For many couples, there are no family stories about how to cope with life-threatening or terminal illness, and they may be unprepared for the strains of living with serious illness. This illness can have a devastating effect on a couple's relationship in which their dreams have not considered what life together with illness would involve. Serious illness or disability can offer opportunity for growth and understanding in a relationship, but it can also confuse, frustrate, and distance a couple from one another, and can powerfully challenge the relationship rules, boundaries, and family organization of the couple.

Rolland views the dimension of time as a central organizing principle for most couples and families dealing with a long-term condition.[80] He believes that all family members adapt best when they understand the strengths and vulnerabilities connected to their past experiences and, at the same time, are able to integrate these prior experiences with the current illness in a useful way. Whatever a couple's history together, illness will challenge them with a balancing act that juggles maintaining normalcy within the relationship, while at the same time caring for a partner with an uncertain cancer diagnosis.

The spouse has been identified as the most pivotal person within the patient's social support network, and a spouse often uses words to describe his or her own suffering in language similar to that of the ill person; tension, anxiety, depression, loss, grief, isolation, and fear of death or recurrence. In a study of women with breast cancer, marital support was conceptualized as the perceived degree of satisfaction with a spouse's response to emotional and interactional needs during the diagnostic, postsurgical, adjuvant therapy, and ongoing recovery phases.[47] When a spouse learns that his loved one has cancer, a myriad of emotions flood his being, perhaps the most profound being fear and shock. A spouse may wonder what his ill partner needs from him during the time of crisis and how, or if, he will be able to help. The emotional support that a spouse is able to offer will play a major role in how well a patient is able to cope with the disease, and how the disease will draw a couple closer to, or distance them from, one another.

The ill spouse will need both emotional and concrete support in many ways. How well a partner can accomplish this support will depend on the strengths of the relationship, the resources available, the ability of the well spouse to understand what is happening to his partner, and each partner's response to the illness experience. What can a spouse do to help?

Listening is reportedly one of the most supportive ways to help a partner with a serious illness.[66] Illness can be an isolating experience especially when there isn't a safe person to share feelings with. Listening promotes safety and connection, both for the patient and the spouse.

Staying emotionally responsive even when the patient turns inward and takes time to process is important. It can take a great deal of energy to be ill and many patients "recharge" their batteries by becoming introspective at times, but this is not a cue to withdraw from the patient.

Offering physical closeness, while at the same time showing acceptance of the full range of feelings, supports the ill spouse's need for assurance that she is still loved and understood. It can be difficult to maintain optimism while at the same time avoiding the temptation to deny the ill spouse's painful illness experience. This conduct is needed and appreciated and is a way of validating the experience of the ill spouse.

Respect the need of the ill spouse to remain in control of her life. Depending on the stage of the illness, much of what a patient called "normal" may be taken away. A partner can support the patient by understanding her great sense of security and accomplishment in retaining as much of what was "normal" as possible in a very abnormal experience. Concrete

ways in which the spouse can support the ill partner are to help handle daily household/child rearing tasks, and, most importantly, to be able to handle shifts in family roles and activities. Most families can find methods to adapt to changes when open discussion is offered to ease the tensions and fears.

PSYCHOSOCIAL ADJUSTMENT AND QUALITY OF LIFE

Initial Diagnosis and Treatment

Individuals diagnosed with cancer often face uncertainties about their mortality, the future course of their illness, their ability to care for themselves and their families, their physical capabilities, the effects of symptoms, and threatened relationships. The emotional repertoire ranges from denial, anger, and fear, to anxiety, depression, guilt, loss, and loneliness, and is shared and experienced by family members as well as the patient. The initial diagnosis can be one of the most emotionally stressful periods of the cancer time frame, and the patient's need to learn how to go on living in a purposeful way, despite the uncertainty, fear, and worry, can seem an impossible task. Box 32–1 lists several nursing diagnoses associated with psychosocial care.

The primary concern of a newly diagnosed person is life versus death, and it is not uncommon for family members to worry for the patient and for themselves as they grapple with the uncertainty that a cancer diagnosis can bring.[93] Fear during this period can be crippling and is often rooted in uncertainty. During the diagnostic period, the individual, family, and friends can be overwhelmed and unable to comprehend all of the information provided by a nurse or physician. This information often seems vague, expansive, and detached to many patients and families. Many individuals feel numb or shocked and particularly vulnerable in instances when they are told the diagnosis while alone; even greater distress is reported by those told of their diagnosis while in a recovery room or over the telephone.

Patients with cancer can be supported in their efforts to adjust to the stress that accompanies the initial diagnosis by thoughtful and respectful communication practices. If suspicions of cancer are confirmed, it should be the doctor who tells the patient with family present. This experience may give the patient an increased sense of confidence that the truth is being told and that no one is withholding information. This practice also provides opportunity for patient and family members to ask questions and share in the interpretation and understanding of the diagnosis. Some patients have reported a need to have their sense of personal tragedy acknowledged, but without familiar and caring support around them they are often unable to speak honestly about their emotions.[54] However, each individual is unique and

---

BOX 32-1

Nursing Diagnoses Related to Psychosocial Care

Relating

Impaired Social Interaction
Social Isolation
Risk for Loneliness
Altered Role Performance
Altered Parenting

Risk for Altered Parenting
Altered Family Processes
Caregiver Role Strain
Risk for Caregiver Role Strain

Valuing

Spiritual Distress (Distress of the Human Spirit)
Risk for Spiritual Distress

Potential for Enhanced Spiritual Well-Being

Choosing

Ineffective Individual Coping
Impaired Adjustment
Defensive Coping
Ineffective Denial
Potential for Enhanced Community
Coping

Ineffective Community Coping
Ineffective Family Coping: Disabling
Ineffective Family Coping: Compromised
Family Coping: Potential for Growth
Decisional Conflict: Treatment versus No Treatment

Perceiving

Hopelessness

Powerlessness

Feeling

Dysfunctional Grieving
Anticipatory Grieving
Anxiety

Death Anxiety
Fear

Data from reference 73.

---

some patients prefer to have privacy while being told the diagnosis.

According to the National Cancer Institute (NCI), the stress of a cancer diagnosis can cause a wide range of physical symptoms such as increased heart rate and blood pressure, headaches, muscle pains, dizziness, loss of appetite, nausea, diarrhea, trembling, weakness, tightness in throat and chest, and sleep disturbances.[70] Some believe that stress can affect the body's immune system and its role in fighting disease. Oncology nurses care not only for physical needs, but they also are an important source of emotional support at this phase of the illness by attentive and patient listening to the patient's hopes and concerns, and by expressing empathy with what they are going through. Furthermore, education at appropriate moments and helping patients discover and express their needs to other health care providers, family, and friends can sustain emotional stability.

The Crisis and Disruption of Treatment

The rigorous schedule and the side effects of surgery, chemotherapy, and radiation treatment often require the combined efforts of many family members to provide the best physical and emotional support to the patient. Enormous blocks of time are spent traveling to and from clinics, undergoing laboratory tests, standing in doctors' offices, lying in hospital beds, and waiting. The treatments for cancer can interfere significantly with diet, sexuality, life-style, relationships, recreation, and other taken-for-granted activities of daily living. All are exhausting and can create frustration, irritability, fear, and hopelessness.

According to Rolland, the complexity, frequency, and efficacy of a treatment regimen and the amount of home versus hospital-based care required by an illness can vary widely across disorders and will have important implications for individual and family adaptation.[79] To understand more clearly the impact of cancer treatment on the patient and family, one must consider the fit between the demands of the illness and the family pattern of functioning. For instance, a family accustomed to and comfortable with working together toward a goal will probably have less trouble adapting to disorders that involve regular teamwork as part of the treatment care.

Cancer treatment can place demands on the patients' spirit as well as the body. During treatment, it is not uncommon for individuals to grieve the loss of feeling that life is open ended, that health is a given, and that one is in control of one's body. Other feelings that may arise are anger, depression (caused by anger turned inward), anxiety, a sense of being helpless or out of control, and an intense feeling of vulnerability that can be accompanied by feelings of betrayal and unfairness. Help and encouragement for patients to gather wanted information, to take an active part in the treatment process when possible, and to find the support they need to deal with their feelings will all contribute to a sense of well-being during the treatment phase. As patients learn how illness and treatment can affect their bodies and are able to stay informed about the progress of treatment, they may naturally become more engaged in their own treatment and care. Encouraging a patient to ask questions of the physician, nurse, and other members of the treatment team will empower the patient and decrease feelings of vulnerability. Patients can be further encouraged to keep their doctors and nurses informed of their physical and emotional responses to the treatment regimen. Often patients are reluctant to report signs and symptoms of illness or side effects because they do not consider them important enough or do not want to "bother" anyone. Nurses can educate patients of the value in providing this information and can be instrumental in creating a collaborative atmosphere that cares for the emotional as well as the physical aspects of the patient.

It is important for the nurse to observe the manner in which a partner responds to the ill spouse because these reactions are often correlated with how well patients cope and are important to their psychological well-being. One report suggested that a couple's adjustment to changes after diagnosis and treatment of cancer depended on two things.[5] The first was the degree of a spouse's involvement in treatment planning; this suggested that spouses who remain outside this process and offer no help at this stage may have greater difficulty after treatment completion. Second, when the patient was hospitalized for treatment, the extent of the partner's contact with the patient, how often visits occurred, and telephone calls made was an indicator of how easily they were able to become integrated into the new circumstances.[5]

Family physicians, nurses, and family therapists are beginning to recognize that the impact of physical illness reaches beyond biologic processes, and that behavioral/social factors play a role in disease etiology and health maintenance.[95] The recognition of this relationship has led to changes in the way physicians and nurses include spouses, partners, and other family members in decisions around treatment issues. Because of the oncology nurses' close relationship with patient and family, they are often in a position to decide when conversation around illness is appropriate or necessary, and how best to include illness issues into conversations with family members. These decisions can best be made if the nurse is able to understand how family members interact with one another, both in the present and in the past.

Posttreatment Phase

Treatment Followed by Cure. Most patients and families will attest to the fact that nearly all control within their lives is lost during diagnosis and treatment for cancer. However, they now may feel an even greater loss of control when treatment ends due to the fact that they are no longer doing anything active to battle cancer. Some feel that this has truly been the battle of their lives. Many patients report that throughout this struggle, the medical procedures and side effects they endured were just as traumatic as the cancer diagnosis itself.[96] They feel just as triumphant that they have been able to survive the treatment for cancer and consider this an independent victory in itself.

Although the patient's success is now a realistic concept, it is also met with uncertainty and ambivalence. Health has been restored; however, there are many emotional feelings and physical side effects (intermediate and long term) to process. The troublesome and possibly serious physical side effects may include chronic fatigue, lymphedema, psychoneurologic difficulties, disfigurement due to loss of limb or other surgeries, stunted growth, problems with fertility, secondary tumors, and damage to major organ systems.[17, 41, 72] As patients begin to deal with the physical impact of treatment, they begin to understand that a new person has evolved with new physiologic responses and uncertainties. How are these dilemmas resolved? As these intermittent anxieties are encountered, the patient may begin to assign meaning to the experience and incorporate a notion of self as important, significant, and worthy of love and appreciation. Adult survivors confess that to recognize and accept the "new" self, they must grieve the loss of the "old" self as they once knew it.[71] If they fail to successfully overcome the anxiety, discomfort, and disabling physical conditions, healthy psychological growth may be hindered.[46] A review by the physician and reinforced by the nurse of the information originally (at diagnosis) given to the patient and family regarding the possible long-term consequences of cancer treatment can help patients prepare and offset emotional pain caused by not understanding physical responses. Because the focus at the time of diagnosis is the elimination of the malignancy, this information should again be reinforced during routine follow-up examination at the end of medical treatment.

Survival is usually the goal of successful cancer treatment for the patient and the family. The ultimate goal, however, may encompass a "quality" survival that allows the patient to transcend the terror of diagnosis and treatment, create a new life-style congruous with a chronic illness, and renew the practice of accomplishing life goals. This may in part be attained through normalization and recognition by the nurse of patient/family resiliency (strengths) and the hard work it took to triumph over adversity[13, 25] (Table 32–3).

Remission Followed by Recurrence. Once again, the sense of personal control surfaces as we speak about the fear of recurrence. Herold and Roetzheim attribute five possible living outcomes that can contribute to the fear of recurrence and negative stress.[41] They include living without recurrence for many years, living an extended period with no cancer and then surrendering to a quick death from a recurrence or second malignancy, living with alternating intervals of cancer recurrence, living beyond projected death, or dying from unrelated disease or other reasons unrelated to cancer.[41] If patients experience significant negative stressors, this may adversely affect their sense of control and well-being.

TABLE 32-3
Indicators of Family Strengths

Category	Indicators
Values	Commitment to the family as a group
	Respect for and trust in each other
	Investment in improving relationships
	Willingness to seek help for problems
	Value for family rituals and traditions
	Strong sense of spirituality
	Belief in service to others[60–62]
Competencies	Assorted list of problem-solving and coping strategies
	Flexibility and adaptability in roles, especially in times of crisis
	Knowledge and skills used to recognize concerns, identify needs, and specify desired outcomes
	Planning ability to meet goals
	Ability to identify, obtain, and manage resources for meeting the family's needs
	Ability to see positive aspects of life
	Ability to initiate and maintain social support[60–62]
Interactional patterns	Expression of appreciation, warmth, support, and nurturance
	Engage in proactive problem solving
	Positive communication patterns—good listening—sharing ideas—conveying negative emotions creatively and constructively
	Seek opportunity to spend time together
	Engage in leisure time together
	Sense of plan and humor
	Relaxed home environment[60–62]

Once recurrence is identified, patients' feelings range from complete surprise, disappointment, and hopelessness, to relief from the uncertainty of when it would happen.[35] Munkres and coworkers actually found no significant difference in patient mood scores between the original diagnosis and a recurrence.[69] Although the latitude of feelings and fears is widespread, discussions, decisions, and preparation must be made to face this adversary again: discussion of the significance of the feelings and fears, decision regarding treatment options, preparation for treatment, and potential for success or failure.[35]

As the impact begins to affect the patient and family, issues and questions will arise related to how they feel about incorporating cancer treatment again into their lives, and adjustments will again need to be made to the caretaker roles. There may be greater feelings of loss, greater fears, increased hopelessness, and an increased danger of dying. When treatment for the recurrence nears its end, the patient and family will once again need to deal with the results of treatment (test results, success or failure) and decide what their next step will be.[20, 35] Emphasizing personal and family strengths and normalizing the innumerable feelings that surround the significance of recurrence and the termination of treatment for the second time may again assist in restructuring family roles, and in the expression of special needs and concerns of the patient and caregivers. Now that it is certain never to leave conscious awareness, patient and family must learn how to *live* with cancer rather than harboring a focus on *dying*. Even though cancer recurrence is not an unusual event, there is little in the research literature to afford us knowledge regarding how cancer patients express their fears or cope with recurrence of their illness according to Mahon and Casperson.[56] Lavery and Clarke, however, assert that those patients who engage in problem-focused coping strategies, like changing eating habits and seeking more information about cancer, actually report fewer feelings of helplessness and rated their adjustment to living with cancer as excellent.[51]

Progressive Disease and Completion of Life

Daily Living with Illness, Progressive Deterioration, and Providing Comfort. In all phases of cancer, it is important for life to go on as usual, or at least as usual as possible. In the diagnostic stage, the patient and family are usually immobilized by shock, fear, and often denial. In the crisis phase of cancer, a patient and the family may be united in their mission to devote all efforts to fight the disease, but progression to the advanced phase of illness can be particularly difficult. This now means that for most patients who accepted the diagnosis, any lingering hope for a cure is relinquished. The terminally ill patients' attention may be focused zealously on the specifics of their bodily condition that could indicate the signs of worsening disease. However, even in the advanced stages of cancer, there may be spells of improvement, which can cause confusion for patients and families who have already accepted and resigned themselves to the inevitability of death.

As the symptoms of progressive disease begin, the sufferer loses faith in the dependability and adaptability of basic bodily processes that the rest of us rely on as part of our general sense of well-being. This loss of confidence can lead to demoralization and hopelessness. Some patients, at this point, will blame themselves for the advanced disease, because they feel that had their will power or desire to live and ability to fight been stronger, they could have overcome the cancer. Rolland feels that it is important to hold a flexible belief that defines success in terms of active participation rather than in terms of a purely biologic outcome.[80] Those terminally ill patients who have only one acceptable outcome, a cure, and who feel that they have "lost" the battle with cancer will be further burdened with feelings of guilt if they believe that they could have "willed" the cancer away.

Progressive disease may demand even more intense psychosocial adjustment that will best be supported by close family and friends, with additional support coming from nurses and other health care staff, counselors, therapists, and support groups. David Spiegel of Stanford University has shown in a study of women with metastatic breast cancer that participation in a support group can increase longevity and enhance quality of life.[85] The patient may not be able to change the status of the illness, but she may be able to improve how she deals with the illness and its challenges. Being among supportive people who have a similar condition can promote honest communication about the illness experience and can promote emotional healing, lessen feelings of isolation, and encourage the patient to begin to reorder her life and pay attention to what she values most.

A diagnosis of progressive or advanced disease is an opportunity to gain a greater level of appreciation for those aspects of their lives that they can still choose to enjoy, and a chance to redirect one's life in new and productive ways. Many cancer patients say that they never realized how important family is, how much they are loved, how deep their faith is, how emotionally strong they can be, and how blessed they have been in life until they were faced with their own mortality. Although patients with end-stage illness may no longer be able to hope for a cure, nurses can support them in finding other ways to hope that give meaning to their lives. Individuals dying of cancer have learned to hope for acceptance of the illness, dying in the presence of their loved ones, finishing old business before they say

goodbye, taking one last trip to see loved ones, or finishing a simple project.

Human contact and relationships are domains of existence that are valued by all people, healthy and ill alike, and these seem to be of particular importance for those people who have had their relationships threatened by severe illness. Nurses must be mindful that maintaining meaningful relationships with the seriously ill requires continued presence and availability, often in the midst of considerable pain, fear, sorrow, anger, and grief. To give any less than this is to deny the reality of the patient's illness experience. Nurses can provide additional comfort and enhance patient self-esteem by empathic listening and helping the patient maintain as much independence and personal control as possible. Patients can be encouraged to make decisions regarding their own care, establish daily routine and set realistic personal goals, make plans for their future, the moment of death and who they want in attendance, and to participate in their own funeral arrangements. One patient expressed a real feeling of control over her death as she worked with her daughter to plan her own funeral and wake.

Long-Term Survival

Optimally, cancer survivorship would indicate a renewed enthusiasm for and enjoyment of life. Realistically, the cancer survivor experiences concerns related to physical sequelae (second malignancies, organ dysfunction, residual fatigue, disability, and disfigurement) and continuing emotional distress (hypervigilance, chronic anxiety, and depression). Gorman reviews three phases of survivorship: acute survival, extended survival, permanent survival.[35] Acute survival relates to the cancer diagnosis and a goal to survive aggressive medical treatment. Extended survival begins as treatment for cancer ends (remission) and the potential for recurrence is confronted. Permanent survival is related to a "cure," and the likelihood of recurrence is minimal. Long-term survival is not an isolated experience, but rather, within the continuum of experiences and earlier phases of life.[76]

A new group of survivors has emerged and these individuals have come together through various forums to search, explore, and learn together. They attend meetings, share newsletters, and write books. They exchange "war" stories and work together to achieve quality time. They have found meaning and usefulness in the concept of survival rather than cure. The organization called the *National Coalition for Cancer Survivorship* (*NCCS*) was thus formed, and it defines survivorship as a dynamic process of living with, through, and beyond cancer.[40]

An estimated 8 million Americans with a history of cancer share survivorship concerns. In an attempt to call public attention to the survivor's needs, the American Cancer Society (ACS) put forth "The Cancer Survivor's Bill of Rights." These rights address medical care, personal life adjustment, job opportunities, and insurance coverage. The aim is to have society foster a truly normal life span for cancer survivors.

Despite progress in treatment, cancer continues to be associated with negative outcomes. With such a prevailing attitude, often too little thought is given to aggressive rehabilitation. The growing survivorship movement has refocused concern on life after treatment and the rehabilitation needs of cancer patients. The continued struggle of living with residual disease or treatment effects defines rehabilitation needs. The rehabilitation philosophy has become a component of survivorship and focuses on self-care and maximizing potential for wellness.[90, 92]

Interpersonal Difficulties. Effective survivorship skills may influence the patient's management of the inner turmoil of being a cancer survivor as he relates to others on a long-term basis. Working to find spiritual meaning may help to put cancer in its place and to understand other people's discomfort and biases related to the cancer experience. Telling one's cancer story about victory over the illness can reduce the fears and misconceptions that others often carry; this empowers the patient and transforms him from victim to victor.[52] Story telling that gives meaning to the illness may also help with survivor "guilt." This very real feeling arises when other family or friends with cancer do not do as well or die from the disease, while the patient has survived.

A sensitive interpersonal difficulty for survivors involves intimacy, marriage, and reproduction. A study done by Gray and coworkers indicated that survivors reported a higher degree of intimacy motivation than did a control group.[36] At the same time, these survivors were less satisfied with their current relationships than the control group.[36] Another study done by Hays and associates revealed cancer survivors had lower marriage and cohabitation rates than control groups and were older at their first marriage.[39] Researchers suggested that this was due to treatment during late teen years or to the general tendency for survivors to consider decisions that have less certain outcomes more carefully. Finally, changes in reproduction are explained by Herold and Roetzheim as due to decreased fertility, and they report that "fertility rates in cancer survivors range from 40% to 85% of expected rates."[41] These patients will most likely benefit from being informed early (before treatment commences) about possible sterility so they can plan for procedures such as sperm banking or embryo preservation.

Workplace Challenges and Discrimination. Approximately 25% of Americans in the workplace or seeking to enter it experience some form of job discrimination, including demotions, firings, unwanted transfers, social isolation and animosity, and required medical examinations unrelated to job efficiency.[43] Discrimination still abounds due to myths like: cancer is a terminal disease, cancer is contagious, and cancer survivors are more of an economic burden than productive employees.[43]

Employment often means more than a source of income. A job or career may denote feelings of identity and self-worth. Most successfully treated cancer patients are able to resume previous occupations with minor or no alteration in circumstances. Those who do face problems when returning to work cite the attitudes of employers and coworkers as a major concern, and nurses should prepare patients for the possibility of such reactions.[24] Some patients recognize their own attitudes as the obstacle, along with fear of recurrence and fatalism about the disease. Some cancer survivors are hesitant to change positions because of specific concerns about obtaining insurance benefits and feel locked into their present position. Actual discrimination may be difficult to prove because it can be subtle. The Americans with Disabilities Act (ADA) of 1990 requires equal opportunity in selection, testing, and hiring of qualified applicants with disabilities.[3] Under the act, anyone who has had cancer is considered disabled. This law prohibits discrimination against workers with disabilities and is similar to the Civil Rights Act of 1964 and Title V of the Rehabilitation Act of 1973.

The ADA covers discrimination that may occur in hiring, promotion, pay, job training, benefits, and firing. Since 1994, the law applies to any private employer with 15 or more employees, state and local government agencies, labor organizations, religious bodies that are employers, and Congress. A different law covers federal government employees. Individuals who are familiar with these laws can protect themselves from discrimination through preventive strategies. Unless the effects of disease or treatment directly affect the individual's ability to perform the essential functions of a job, there is no obligation to disclose information. It is important not to lie but also unnecessary to volunteer information. The employee should be prepared to educate the employer and to stress specific job qualifications and abilities. The emphasis must be on present ability to perform the job, not on disability or medical history. The Equal Employment Opportunity Commission (EEOC) assumes the federal government role of enforcing the standard. Local government offices can assist in investigations or claims.

Any person with a history of cancer who meets specified job qualifications and can perform the essential functions of the employment position is protected under the ADA. The employer is required to provide reasonable accommodations, which includes retraining, special devices, or a change in part of the job such as flexible scheduling. Thus, said accommodations make the disabled enabled.

When residual effects of disease or treatment alter the individual's ability to continue in the preillness job, vocational rehabilitation intervention may be necessary. Retraining, partial disability, or full disability, however, may be the only alternative. In these situations, a rehabilitation team with programs and services in place is needed to smooth transition from the encounters with acute care and ambulatory care settings to self-care in the home setting. Oncology nurses, along with rehabilitation specialists, can assist in successful reentry.

Finances, Insurance, and the Law. An individual's insurance coverage and financial resources greatly influence access to and quality of care. The uninsured and underinsured are limited to indigent care providers or state and federal programs with limited resources. Limited coverage and services can place individuals in the compromised position of underreporting health problems. This situation fosters delayed diagnosis and treatment, increased acuity, and spiraling of health care costs.

The cost of care adds to the individual's and family's burden of living with cancer. They may be faced with the dilemma of forced choices: limited job mobility, paying medical bills versus living expenses, not reporting symptoms, seeking financial assistance, changing relationships, and insurance limitations. All are a subtle form of discrimination.

Insurance companies can decide the type of insurance contract they will sell and to whom. Contracts are negotiated with employers and with individuals and the cost is determined by coverage limits. The individual with evidence of persistent or recurrent disease may be considered a high risk to the insurance industry. The concept of excess mortality (observed death rates versus standard expected rates) is used in calculating premiums. Private insurance companies can establish waiting periods, deny coverage, and cancel policies based on the provision of each policy.

Currently no federal law guarantees a right to adequate health insurance. Cancer survivors do have the opportunity of keeping the health insurance obtained through their employer even after they are no longer employed. This opportunity is provided through the Comprehensive Omnibus Budget Reconciliation Act (COBRA) and the Employee Retirement and Income Security Act (ERISA). The COBRA plan can provide short-term coverage while the individual is seeking new employment or a new group plan. ERISA entitles the individual to file a claim when benefits are denied through discrimination. ERISA is enforced by the Pension and Welfare Benefits Administration of the United States Department of Labor. Nurses and other interdisciplinary team members can support the individual with financial concerns by sensitively assessing their situation and educating them about rights and resources.

Making Choices and Regaining Control. Long-term survival has created unique challenges for cancer survivors, but has also permitted them to return to their families and perform a wide variety of social roles. There are several opportunities for this population to make positive choices, to regain control, and provide a heightened quality of life. These opportunities take shape through varied approaches, and may include:

- Engaging in positive affirmations to enhance self-esteem
- Rearranging schedules or activities to adjust to residual deficits
- Using makeup, hairstyles, or clothing to disguise scars or defects
- Putting cancer in its place and into the past rather than choosing to be preoccupied with recurrence
- Most importantly, NEVER postponing a pleasure[16]

Many feel an increased sense of control as they reprioritize their lives and activities to include volunteering to help others with cancer or to accomplish a long time goal in a more immediate fashion.[76] Gorman offers that "others may make difficult decisions more easily (e.g., leaving a destructive relationship, completing work towards a longed-for degree) because of a sense of urgency created by having a potentially fatal illness."[35]

As the social climate continues to improve past the year 2000, and more well-known people like athletes and celebrities share and publicize early detection and their positive cancer experiences, the fears and misconceptions will be dispelled. There will be less stigma associated with cancer and more open communication, and people surviving cancer will experience less shame and have less difficulty in relationships, which will promote less isolation from family, friends, employers, and others.

NURSING STRATEGIES

Mobilizing Social Support Systems

During the time of illness, there are a multitude of social support systems for the patient to draw on, and family and friends are customarily the first to offer their assistance. Family members along with others in the social system can play a significant role in how the patient copes and adjusts to this illness.[57, 77] As well, other systems can become involved, especially if family and friends are scarce or unable to be mobilized.

The nurse can be most effective if he or she is cognizant of support services that are available in the community and how to activate them. Another notable task is to convince the patient, who already feels like a burden, that these systems are created to help and will affect recovery in a positive manner. The most common systems to be recognized, along with family and friends, include neighbors, coworkers, and fellow spiritual companions; health care professionals like nurses, physical therapists and community and home care agencies; psychosocial professionals like social workers, clergy, counselors, and therapists.[58]

To activate these systems, it is helpful to include family members and friends, and encourage participation in conferences that plan treatment or when discussion centers around changes in the patient's condition. Families, friends, and even coworkers feel much more like partners when inspired to participate in support group activities or programs like the "We Can Weekend" sponsored by the ACS. Groups such as these help to normalize the cancer experience and validate individual meanings of illness. Fellow group members may be able to model effective coping strategies and concentrate on realistic goals.[40]

When patients require specialized care to attend to physical or psychosocial needs after discharge from the hospital or while being treated as an outpatient, more structured services may be needed to support families in the form of home care nurses or therapists. Other assistance in the form of a homemaker service may also be needed to maintain household responsibilities. A referral list of the various support professionals who specialize in cancer care may be needed to maintain the patient and family system and is a helpful addition for all patients and families seeking support.

In addition to the positive outcomes, negative consequences are reported in the literature as well. Cloutier and Ferral assert that, "invasion of privacy, unkept promises, unwelcome advice, forced dependency, and encouraged noncompliance with treatment are examples."[20] Awareness and monitoring for these possibilities by the nurse will enable the patient and family to use appropriate support systems and benefit from their services.

Maintaining Communication

How does one best talk with someone who has cancer? Families generally do not talk with one another about their illness concerns, yet when family members are able to discuss their needs and desires they generally do better in managing the illness experience.[8, 34] The key to coping with cancer is communication and, because cancer is a chronic as well as an acute illness, the diagnosis signifies a great threat that can only be managed by patient and family members if there is conversation about it.

Generally the ways in which family members have communicated with one another prior to cancer will be similar to the way they will communicate in the midst of illness. If family members have been open with their feelings and emotions, it is likely that they will react in a similar fashion, although this is not always the case. The fear of the unknown can render patient and family unsure of how to speak about what they are feeling. Nurses can enhance open communication with their patients by asking open-ended questions such as, "What are you feeling?" rather than just "How are you feeling?" Open-ended questions have the potential to invite an honest sharing of feelings, to strengthen a family's sense of connectedness, and provide emotional support.

Although there may be just one illness, there is never just one illness story in a family. Each member will have his own unique view about the meaning of the symptoms and the impact of the illness on the family.[64] Within families there is often a desire to protect one another from additional emotional stress and so communication can break down as individuals keep feelings, wants, and needs to themselves. Nurses can help family members realize that different perceptions, meanings, and emotions are to be expected and can encourage them to hear and appreciate the experiences of one another. Respectful listening to one another and an open acceptance of the experience of others can promote empathy within the family. Dakof and Liddle, in their research with cancer patients, found no one particular communication style that was most adaptive for all individuals and couples facing illness.[22] This study showed that the couples who both wanted to talk about the illness did well, and couples who both agreed that they did not want to talk about the illness also did well. This suggests that family members can be supportive of one another without communicating about the illness.

Nurses not only have an opportunity to promote communication within the family, they have a responsibility to maintain honest conversation with the patient regarding prognosis, disease course, and treatment plans. Honest communication provides patients with critical information needed to decide how to respond to the illness and may allow them a greater sense of competency and confidence in their ability to manage the illness experience.[64] Openness, honesty, respect, clarity, responsibility, accountability, and a willingness to listen and learn are qualities that will promote and maintain effective communication between patient and family members, as well as between patient, family, and health care providers.

Promoting the Sense of Agency

The empowerment of the patient and all members of a family is essential to their coping with the crisis of illness.

When patients are able to mobilize all of their physical, emotional, spiritual, and relational resources toward the goal of health and wellness, life is experienced more fully; the patient and loved ones are able to take back some control that cancer and its treatment took from them. Thirty or 40 years ago patients did not know they had options. They were passive, and their role was to follow the physicians' instructions and interventions and to pray, if the patient was so inclined. Today, patients can choose to be an active part of the team working toward their recovery, or they can still choose to be somewhat passive, handing over most of the responsibility for their recovery to the health care team.[9] The choice to enhance the sense of agency has never been more available than it is today. Although there is a choice, there is no right or wrong, no good or bad choice. The patient's choice must be honored because no one knows more about what is good and right than the patient herself.

Each individual is unique and will have coping strategies that work especially well for them and their families. There is no one way to navigate the emotional seas of cancer, but there are some attitudes and strategies that seem to be empowering and promote a renewed sense of agency for many patients. According to Benjamin, patients can help in the fight for recovery by making plans for the future as a way of unconsciously not giving up, fighting unwanted aloneness by communicating to friends and family what is wanted and expected of them, and doing whatever possible to keep relationships and intimacy alive.[9] They can use methods to evoke the relaxation response, regain and maintain as much control of life as is reasonable, become partners with the physician and nurse in the recovery effort, be with other people who have cancer as a way of being validated and understood, and do what can be done to keep hope alive. These ideas are not easy to accomplish, nor is each useful for every patient, but experience has shown that some patients gain a sense of agency, and an improved quality of life when they are able to intentionally incorporate these ideas into their illness experience.

When families are better able to cope with the crisis of an illness, they begin to feel more competent and in control of the illness experience, and if they "do not feel completely entrapped by illness, they have greater enthusiasm for constructing more enriched lives."[64] Nurses may be reluctant to take on the role of emotional teacher, or they may not have the time to do so, but the quality of care is enhanced when patients and families have opportunities to learn more about the disease and discover new and useful coping strategies. Nurses can share information about how others are coping and can encourage patients and families to read and ask questions. Additional possibilities for future change and a renewed sense of agency can be opened as past illness experiences are explored, and a discussion with the nurse examines which illness beliefs constrain and which facilitate the management of illness.[94] An important developmental challenge is to create a meaning for the illness experience that can promote a sense of competency and mastery: an empowering narrative. Rather than viewing competency and mastery in a rigid way that focuses only on biologic outcomes as the sole determinant of success, facilitators can suggest that agency and mastery can be defined in a more "holistic" sense. A "holistic" view will consider involvement and participation in the overall process as a viable and more realistic criteria of competence and agency.[81]

Informational Support to Maintain Independence

It is said that *knowledge is power*, and for the patient and family with cancer, this knowledge can promote the feeling of increased control and independence, especially for the patient. Before illness progresses and treatment begins, patient roles are essentially the same. However, as the continuum proceeds, role responsibilities change dramatically and when the patient is kept well informed, roles may be able to be maintained to some degree.

Patients and families find it most helpful if there are professionals to answer their questions regarding medical issues surrounding the diagnosis, treatment and its options, and side effects.[18] It is our responsibility to assist them to clarify their concerns and articulate their fears and needs so the relationship with their professional caregivers can be maintained or improved. Nurses or therapists can aid with development of specific questions and create role play to effectively respond to closed, uninformative conversation or reports from medical personnel.

Nurses in an outpatient or office setting may determine various technical reasons for patients who do not keep follow-up appointments. Patients may require more information; therefore, the nurse can stress the importance of maintaining appropriate health care. If the patient lacks transportation, has lost medical insurance, has problems with day care, or is hindered by a language barrier, referrals can be made to social service agencies. Many other resources are available and range from audio and videotapes for the illiterate, to teleconference programs, to the computer and the Internet, to community workshops, to national programs, which are illustrated at the end of this chapter. Preserving patient independence via knowledge throughout the cancer experience can improve self-esteem and provide the necessary encouragement, patience, and stamina to continue their courageous fight.

Promoting a Healthy Response to Anxiety and Depression

Anxiety. Assessment will be necessary to determine the cause of the anxiety; reasons for anxiety during the cancer experience have been previously identified. To enable the nurse to construct an appropriate plan of care and intervention, it is helpful to know where the patient is in the course of illness. Commonly, there are two types of intervention, nonpharmacologic and pharmacologic, and either or both will be beneficial at various points along the cancer continuum.[14]

Many techniques are helpful within the nonpharmacologic class. Initially, it is important to demonstrate interest by using open-ended questions, and McDaniel and coworkers suggest several questions to elicit the patient's and family members' illness perceptions.[64] Some examples are:

- What do you think caused your problem?
- What do you think your sickness does to you? How does it work?
- What do you fear most about your sickness?
- What might make healing now a struggle for you?[64]

Once a cause for the anxiety is identified, the nurse can validate the patients' feelings and reassure them that anxiety is quite normal in relation to cancer. The nurse can also reframe (create a different story) the patients' perception of the potential threat, which may also reduce stress and anxiety.[46] Other strategies, cognitive and behavioral, will teach coping skills and help the patient maintain control when anxiety arises. Although cognitive-behavioral therapy is used by psychotherapists as part of a brief therapy model, nurses can also practice some of those techniques while providing other nursing interventions.

A cognitive intervention may be used in an attempt to prevent anxiety or when anxious moments occur. The nurse can help patients reduce negative self-talk, reframe obstacles as challenges, and expand possibilities. A patient with colon cancer can be taught to identify a self-defeating belief (e.g., "No one will ever find me attractive now that I have an ostomy.") and to substitute it with a self-enhancing belief (e.g., "My sexuality is more than just the appearance of my abdomen.").[14] One of the authors' patients was encouraged to experience the pain she was having from thoracic surgery as what was necessary to help cure her of her lung cancer, rather than as a fear that her cancer had returned. This reframing of an obsessive recurrence "phobia" helped to prevent the severe anxiety she felt when she experienced sharp shooting pain within her chest.

Behavioral techniques can offer stress reduction and teach patients coping skills if they are exposed to an anxiety-producing thought or event. Relaxation or distraction using music and techniques such as breathing exercises and yoga, guided imagery, biofeedback, and meditation make up several behavioral components of nondrug therapy.[23, 59] A psychotherapy consult may be appropriate to teach hypnosis and self-hypnosis, and in cases of severe phobias or panic attacks, eye movement desensitization and reprocessing (EMDR) procedures might be considered.

Support groups such as "I Can Cope" and educational services, like those provided by the ACS and NCI, offer emotional and educational information and help reduce anxiety while the patient learns cognitive and behavioral techniques.[49] Many patients and families continue to use these kinds of services even after cancer treatment has subsided. However, individual/family psychotherapy is often a more desirable option in that it provides a safe and professional setting in which to process emotional and private issues inappropriate to support groups or doctor visits.

For cancer patients/families who would benefit from individual or family counseling, a psychotherapeutic model of crisis intervention or brief therapy is advocated by Barbara Anderson.[4] Brief cognitive-behavioral therapy uses:

- Expeditious diagnosis and assessment
- A focus on the present time and current issues
- A limited number of therapeutic goals
- Specific suggestions and guidance from the therapist
- Confrontation and change in perceptions, interpretation, assumptions, and attributions
- Behavioral and practical therapeutic techniques and interventions

Greer and coworkers reported that patients who receive health education, brief, problem-focused cognitive-behavioral psychotherapy, and support services had significantly reduced emotional and physical distress; fewer episodes of anxiety and depression, and other psychological symptoms; a better outlook on life; and more cooperative and realistic involvement with their medical treatment.[37]

Referral by nursing staff or the physician for psychotherapeutic intervention involving the individual, couple, or family can be beneficial to reduce the distress, increase coping styles, and assist in decision-making. These services are most often provided by psychiatric clinical nurse specialists or nurse practitioners, social workers, medical (marriage and family) therapists, or psychologists, and are meant to compliment already existing comprehensive support and educational groups.

Pharmacologic intervention for anxiety is usually accomplished with drugs from the benzodiazepine family; however, stronger antipsychotic medications like phenothiazine can be used if a patient is severely anxious. There are several commonly prescribed benzodiazepines for anxiety in cancer patients. They include the short-acting drugs such as lorazepam (Ativan) and oxazepam (Serax); an intermediate-acting drug, alprazolam (Xanax); and several long-acting drugs such as chlordiazepoxide (Librium), diazepam (Valium), and clorazepate (Tranxene).[53] Because the benzodiazepines can cause respiratory depression, antihistamines can be used for patients with serious breathing impairment. Other drugs can be used such as the tricyclic antidepressants; however, they are usually used to treat depression and anxiety together and will be discussed at a later time. Cancer patients often have underlying pathology that can create agitation and restlessness, and as Bush reports, "careful assessment is needed to ensure that the correct medication is being used to treat the appropriate symptom and that the underlying medical problem is being addressed."[14]

Depression. Assessment, again, is necessary to help identify the depressed cancer patient. A brief, one-page assessment scale that is easily used for screening and to score is the Beck Depression Inventory, Primary Care Version. Factors that contribute to a depressed and hopeless state have been previously identified. As in the anxiety response, nonpharmacologic and pharmacologic techniques can be used to treat depression. Some of the nonpharmacologic methods are identical to those used for anxiety; however, the drugs used to treat depression are generally from the antidepressant family unless the patient suffers from both maladies.

If patients are severely depressed or suicidal, they should be evaluated for potential (do they have a plan?) to do immediate harm to themselves. If a strong potential for self-harm is evident, assistance may be needed to hospitalize them where psychiatric help is readily available.[53] However, many cancer patients suffer from a "situational" depression, which lasts about 2 weeks and can be managed briefly by the oncology nurse, and more consistently by a medical family therapist or a psychiatric clinical nurse specialist/nurse practitioner.[1] Often, the most helpful type of therapy is with the entire family where unresolved issues can be identified and discussed. Family as well as patient may share in the depressed mood due to stress from the illness, and all may have a sense of guilt, shame, and resentment because of these occult feelings. The therapist can encourage verbalization and exploration of these forbidden feelings, and ". . . help families realize that multiple perceptions are to be expected and that many possible responses are acceptable."[64]

During initial conversation with the patient, a validation of feelings is important, while avoiding premature reassurance. Body language can also be significant as a communication tool; effective eye contact, active listening, and a caring touch portray interest and sensibility.

Although reflective interaction can help patients admit and accept feelings, it can also frustrate patients if this type of response is not used skillfully. If a patient simply hears her statement repeated back to her, she may feel as if the interviewer possesses little if any understanding. Open-ended questions encourage patients to express thoughts and feelings. Cloutier and Ferrall caution us that, "depressed individuals can often sense others' reluctance or discomfort when they try to initiate conversation about their depressed mood."[20] Because depression often accompanies anxiety, the relaxation or diversion methods (e.g., music, relaxation therapy, guided imagery) are most useful.

When considering the use of medication for depression, it is important to ascertain whether the depression is severe, recurrent, or experienced with psychotic symptoms. If any are the case, medication is begun immediately with psychotherapy to follow. There are many antidepressant drug families on the market which include the tricyclic antidepressants, the selective serotonin reuptake inhibitors (SSRIs), and the monoamine oxidase inhibitors (MAOIs). The most popular tricyclic antidepressants are amtriptyline (Elavil), doxepin (Sinequan), and imipramine (Tofranil); the SSRIs include fluoxetine (Prozac), paroxetine (Paxil), and sertraline (Zoloft); the MAOIs include phenelzine (Nardil) and tranylcypromine (Parnate). For an in-depth discussion of the pros and cons to each medication, refer to Bush in *Psychosocial Nursing Care Along the Cancer Continuum.*[15] Because the side effects of cancer treatment can mimic depressive symptoms, it is imperative that the oncology nurse be attentive to the signs of depression to ensure proper treatment for this devastating sense of hopelessness.

Assisting the Patient/Family with Goal Setting

At varying stages of the illness experience, patients may begin to prioritize their lives in a way which honors life with illness, gives clarity to what they really value about living, and encourages them to choose intentionally how they will engage each day they live. Patients often will realize how much of life they have been "accumulating" that has not been particularly significant, and will decide to set new goals for themselves that better incorporate more of the meaningful aspects of life that have been neglected. Patients facing a life-threatening illness may at some time begin to realize that "the ultimate value of illness is that it teaches us the value of being alive."[31]

Nurses can encourage patients and families to explore what really matters and what they realistically are able to manage. McDaniel and coworkers stress the importance of helping patients to simplify goals and to notice and appreciate the small achievements that come along.[66] Cancer is stressful and although some stress can be helpful as a means of pushing us to take action, too much stress can harm our health and make us feel like we are losing control.

It is important to consider goals that will support the whole patient: the patient's emotional, spiritual, physical, and relational well-being. Goals should be empowering and appropriate for the patient's stage of cancer, support healthy self-esteem, be measurable and realistically achievable, give joy, and help the patient experience illness not as a tragedy but rather as a different way of living. Because the illness experience is shared in varying degrees by the entire family, the patient may want members of the family to participate in setting goals. Nurses can work with the patient, family, and other health care team members to monitor the progress of the patient and assess the usefulness of established goals. Goals will naturally change over the course of the illness.

Assisting the Patient/Family to Reveal Illness History and Its Meaning

According to Seaburn and colleagues, one of the most important roles that a health care provider can play in the lives of patients and families challenged by a chronic or terminal illness is to be a witness to the stories of their experience and the role that meaning plays in their experience of illness.[83] These stories cannot be told unless someone listens, and although being an audience to the story is not a cure for the illness, it is often a critical source of comfort and healing. Nurses have a unique advantage by the close proximity of their relationship to the patient and family and are therefore in a position to facilitate conversations around illness history and its meaning. A simple question asking, "Has anyone else in your family had cancer?" can open a conversation that may inform a nurse about the patient's understanding of the illness and possible myths they may be holding onto that are not supportive of hope and control.

Rolland suggests that beliefs about what is normal and abnormal, and the importance a family places on conformity and excellence in relation to the average family, will significantly affect the family's ability to adapt to illness.[81] Families desperately want to know that they are doing the best they can under the circumstances. The establishment of a community of families with shared experiences reduces their sense of isolation and helps them realize that their reactions, feelings, and struggles are "normal" for the illness experience.[86] Groups offer the advantage of publicly sharing stories of illness history and meanings with people in similar situations.

Bruner emphasizes meaning-making as a key feature of human experience and suggests that it is by participa-tion in culture that meaning is rendered public and shared.[12] People with cancer and other chronic illness do not often have the opportunity to share the meanings they have made of their situation and therefore are vulnerable to isolation. A patient's and family's capacity to find meaning in their dilemma can greatly impact their ability to cope. Oncology nurses can pose questions that open discussion around the meanings made of the illness. Some suitable questions could be:

- "How often does your family talk about the illness and its impact on everyone's life?"
- "Do you think there is a reason the illness occurred?"
- "How do you approach the future?"
- "Can your illness bring your family closer?"
- "How could it separate you?"

Perhaps one of the most pivotal challenges for individuals with cancer is how to make meaning of senselessness, how to find a reason to live in the face of a chronic illness, and how to really live well with illness. Individuals may be called on to realize that they may not always be cured of illness, but maybe they can strive to be emotionally and spiritually healed and embrace all of their experiences, even illness. As nurses listen to the sometimes agonizing stories of their patients, they can be comforted in the knowledge that it is not only in the physical doing that they care for their patients, but that their best intervention may be just "being" who they are in that precious moment when a patient shares her story and knows that she is heard and understood.

Addressing the Needs of Family Caregivers

Family members, not professionals, are the primary health care providers for most patients.[65] Caregivers have a demanding and exhausting job and may find it difficult to care for themselves in light of their partner/family member's illness. Few people seem to recognize the danger and the losses to the caregiver. Society lacks adequate terms to express the experience of caring, so the experience of caregiving goes mainly unrecognized.[31] Because the obvious focus of concern is on the person who is ill, few recognize the overwhelming sense of anxiety, fear, guilt, depression, grief, and isolation that the caregiver experiences. In a study of mastectomy, testicular, and colon cancer patients, it was found that spouses reported as many and similar psychological problems as did the patients.[6] Nurses can support the caregivers in the family by inquiring about the resources the family has available to them and by informing them of community support systems and counseling services available. Participation in support groups is shown to be most helpful in the support of family caregivers.[89] Studies reveal that caregiving partners with sufficient social support and self-care exhibited significantly better coping skills that can have a direct effect on promoting the highest quality of life for partners and patients.[55, 68]

The Family Life History model, which was designed to be broadly applicable to situations where families are having to cope with physical illness, suggests that a process unfolds in many families with chronic illness in which family life is increasingly organized around illness-generated needs and demands.[87] As the illness is allowed to dictate the parameters of family life, family caregivers as well as other family members' priorities inevitably and increasingly emphasize an illness-centered family organization.

Nurses can support family caregivers by helping them make decisions about the role that the illness should be allowed to have in the family. Families can be advised to take a closer look at current resources available and to consider reallocation of resources in a way that meets the needs of the patient but also the needs of the caregivers and other family members.

Rolland notes the importance of renegotiation of rigid role definitions, the partner's acknowledgment and expression of personal limits, and families engaging in discussions around issues of balance, flexibility, and shared participation of responsibilities.[80] This is seen as crucial to meeting the demands of caring for a chronically ill family member. The National Family Caregivers Association has suggested that some basic principles of empowerment can help caregivers find a sense of direction. Caregiver tips are noted in Box 32–2.

Promoting Hope

Of all the ingredients in the will to live, hope is the most vital; the emotional and mental state that motivates you to keep on living, to accomplish things and succeed. Hope is a component of a positive attitude and acceptance of our fate in life.[82] Hope influences survival, is a source of energy, enables healthy coping, and saves individuals from the pain of an agonizing state.[67] In addition, hope is a prerequisite for effective coping and a significant factor to physical and emotional well-being.[42] When patients are robbed of hope, they feel cheated of the promise of a future and will succumb to depression. When people fall to that low emotional state, their will to live is threatened and their bodies may shut down. The tumultuous illness journey is marked with periods of high hopes and deep despair, neither of which may make sense at the time they present themselves. Although patients can at times feel at the mercy of the highs and lows of emotions, they can often learn to anticipate and cope with them and discover ways to keep the flames of hope burning.

Most individuals, when asked to explain how they have managed to transcend their problems, will report that they have gone through a similar process of emo-

---

BOX 32–2

10 Tips for Family Caregivers

1. Choose to take charge of your life, and don't let your loved one's illness or disability always take center stage.
2. Remember to be good to yourself. Love, honor and value yourself. You're doing a very hard job and you deserve some quality time, just for you.
3. Watch for signs of depression, and don't delay in getting professional help when you need it.
4. When people offer to help, accept the offer and suggest specific things that they can do.
5. Educate yourself about your loved one's condition. Information is empowering.
6. There's a difference between caring and doing. Be open to technologies and ideas that promote your loved one's independence.
7. Trust your instincts. Most of the time they'll lead you in the right direction.
8. Grieve for your losses, and then allow yourself to dream new dreams.
9. Stand up for your rights as a caregiver and a citizen.
10. Seek support from other caregivers. There is great strength in knowing you are not alone.

Reprinted with permission of the National Family Caregivers Association, Kensington, MD, the only organization for all family caregivers. 1-800-896-3650; www.nfcacares.org.

---

tional recovery in the past. Nurses can facilitate the nurturance of hope by helping patients to talk about how they have managed in other situations to transcend difficulties, some of which may have been illness related. Nurses can prompt conversation and exploration of the ways in which the patient and family have managed to keep hope alive in the past, and what were the inherent strengths the family had drawn on to do so.

Being able to find something important yet realistic to hope for is important for patients and their families. Some families experiencing cancer realize that they are able to shift their hope for a cure to the hope of being able to use their remaining times together to the utmost, hope that their loved one does not suffer, or even for a peaceful transition from life to death. In one qualitative study with 30 cancer patients, hope was identified and equated with a person's search for meaning and value in one's life.[74]

In research conducted by Patel, hope-inspiring tools were revealed that related ways in which oncology nurses care for, interact with, and educate patients, families, and other health care team members.[75] They are prayer and faith in God, support from family and friends, and positive relationships with the health care team. These promoted confidence in the treatment plan, spousal devotion for the patient, optimistic attitude, physical presence of loved ones at the patient's bedside, and talking to others. Nurses often influence the spouse and patient's hope objects through the information they provide, and they must be mindful of the professional power they wield in dispensing this information to patients and families.

CONCLUSION

Psychosocial services and psychotherapeutic interventions should be available to and directly involved with the treatment of the cancer patient and their family in conjunction with oncologic medical treatment. Nurses serving the oncology population in all settings have the capability to face unique challenges and the opportunity to affect not only physical deficits, but also to provide all whom they minister to understanding and empathy.

Because the literature reminds us that we are in the earliest stages of learning in regard to the needs of this population, we have the potential to contribute to this literature by recording our work, creating research studies that will reveal and assess strategies, and providing data on successful interventions. In addition, more work must be done in relation to healthy members of the patient's family and increased study of the psychosocial needs and adjustment of cancer survivors. Our challenge is to cultivate patient/family strengths and resources and to improve psychological functioning and adjustment to illness through the provision of strategies, the mobilization of support, and the inspiration of hope.

Chapter Questions

1. Cancer patients rehabilitation needs are legally best addressed by the:
   a. Americans with Disabilities Act (1990)
   b. Title V Rehabilitation Act (1973)
   c. Civil Rights Act (1964)
   d. Patient Self-Determination Act (1991)
2. Initially when a person learns he has cancer, the first psychological circumstance that happens is:
   a. The patient attempts to address the meaning of the illness.
   b. There is a psychological crisis.
   c. The patient falls into an "existential plight."
   d. Nothing. The patient is completely numb.
3. Cancer patients and families can have a more positive experience if which of the following occurs?
   a. Problem-solving techniques are taught immediately after the physician tells the patient of the diagnosis.

   b. The physician and nurse tell the patient first and then the family the "bad news" about the cancer diagnosis and treatment.
   c. The patient is told nothing of the illness, especially if he has a history of emotional problems and a lack of resources.
   d. Good psychosocial management is integrated into the patient's entire plan of care.
4. Breaking the news that the patient has cancer should include all of the following steps *except*:
   a. A message delivered with professional detachment
   b. Simple, honest information
   c. Advocating the expression of all feelings
   d. A discussion of treatment options
5. When the nurse is assessing the patient for acute anxiety, she should:
   a. Assess for panic disorder.
   b. Blame the patient for being ridiculous, because the cancer just isn't that bad.
   c. Watch for symptoms of chronic anxiety, which creates greater risk for the patient to experience acute anxiety.
   d. Disregard the patient's story because that has nothing to do with the symptoms of rapid heart rate, fatigue, and restlessness.
6. It is believed that serious illness in families who are in the prime of life (in their late thirties to forties) are the most disruptive to family function because:
   a. These families most always have teenagers who are in trouble.
   b. These families have no sense of "personal boundaries."
   c. They have rarely experienced illness before.
   d. They are in the phase of life that has the greatest responsibilities.
7. Long-term survival for cancer patients entails:
   a. Little worry about recurrence
   b. Renewed intimacy and anticipation of having children
   c. Returning to their job with no fears of discrimination
   d. Concerns about physical sequelae and continued emotional distress
8. Nurses can best assist patients and families with open communication by:
   a. Asking open-ended questions, which invites the sharing of feelings
   b. Encouraging patients to keep most illness concerns to themselves so they do not worry family members needlessly
   c. Reminding patients that their story is really not unique because they have cancer just like all of the other patients

d. Withholding most information because details will just confuse patients and families anyway

9. Being a witness to the patient's story is important because:
   a. This can help cure the illness because it promotes comfort and healing.
   b. It helps inform the nurse about the patient's understanding of the illness.
   c. It really isn't important to listen to these stories because there are usually more important duties to accomplish.
   d. The nurse should know everything about the patient so she can make the treatment decisions for the patient.

10. Family members who are caregivers should be encouraged and reminded to:
    a. Make sure the loved one's illness or disability always takes "center stage."
    b. Try not to accept help from those who offer because illness is a private matter.
    c. Remember to value and be good to yourself, because your job is difficult.
    d. Try to do the most you can for a loved one because independence is not important at such a critical time.

BIBLIOGRAPHY

1. Albright AV, Valente SM: Depression and suicide. In Carroll-Johnson RM, Gorman LM, Bush NJ, editors: *Psychosocial nursing care: along the cancer continuum*, Pittsburgh, Oncology Nursing Press, 1998.
2. American Psychiatric Association: *Diagnostic and statistical manual of mental disorders*, ed 4, Washington DC, Author, 1994.
3. Americans with Disabilities Act of 1990, 42 U.S.C.A. 12101 et seq. (West 1993).
4. Anderson B: Psychosocial interventions for cancer patients to enhance the quality of life, *J Consult Clin Psychol* 60:552, 1992.
5. Ayers L: *The answer is within you*, New York, Crossroads Publishing, 1994.
6. Baider L, Kaplan De-Nour A: Adjustment to cancer: who is the patient—the husband or the wife? *Isr J Med Sci* 24:631, 1998.
7. Baile WF and others: Depression and tumor stage in cancer of head and neck, *Psycho-oncology* 1:15, 1992.
8. Baker L: Families and illness. In Crouch M, Roberts L, editors: *The family in medical practice*, New York, Springer-Verlag, 1987.
9. Benjamin HH: Wellness: participating in your fight for recovery on the psychosocial front. In Dollinger M, Rosenbaum EH, Cable G, editors: *Everyone's guide to cancer therapy: how cancer is diagnosed, treated, and managed day to day*, Kansas City, Andrews McMeel Publishing, 1991.
10. Brown FH: The impact of death and serious illness on the family life cycle. In Carter B, Goldrick M, editors: *The changing family life cycle: a framework for family therapy*, Boston, Allyn & Bacon, 1989.
11. Brown P: The concept of hope: implications for care of the critically ill, *Crit Care Nurse* 9:97, 1989.
12. Bruner J: *Acts of meaning*, Cambridge, Harvard University Press, 1990.
13. Buckley MR, Thorngren JM, Kleist DM: Family resiliency: a neglected family construct, *Fam J* 5:241, 1998.
14. Bush NJ: Anxiety and the cancer experience. In Carroll-Johnson RM, Gorman LM, Bush NJ, editors: *Psychosocial nursing care: along the cancer continuum*, Pittsburgh, Oncology Nursing Press, 1998.
15. Bush NJ: Coping and adaptation. In Carroll-Johnson RM, Gorman LM, Bush NJ, editors: *Psychosocial nursing care along the cancer continuum*, Pittsburgh, Oncology Nursing Press, 1998.
16. Carnevali DL, Reiner AC: *The cancer experience: nursing diagnosis and management*, Philadelphia, Lippincott, 1990.
17. Carter MC, Thompson EI, Simone JV: The survivors of childhood solid tumor, *Pediatr Clin North Am* 38:505, 1991.
18. Christ G: A model for the development of psychosocial interventions, *Recent Results Cancer Res* 121:302, 1991.
19. Clark J: Psychosocial responses of the patient. In Groenwald SL, Frogge MH, Goodman M, Yarbro CH, editors: *Cancer nursing: principles and practice*, Boston, Jones & Bartlett, 1993.
20. Cloutier A, Ferrall S: Psychosocial aspects of complex responses to cancer. In Barry P, editor: *Psychosocial nursing: care of physically ill patients and their families*, ed 3, Philadelphia, Lippincott, 1996.
21. Cole-Kelly, K: Two families, two stories: courage and chronic illness. In McDaniel S, Hepworth J, Doherty W, editors: *The shared experience of illness: stories of patients, families, and their therapists*, New York, Basic Books, 1997.
22. Dakof G, Liddle H: *Communication between cancer patients and their spouses: is it an essential aspect of adjustment?* Paper given at the American Psychological Association Annual Meeting, Boston, August 12, 1990.
23. Danton WG and others: Nondrug treatment of anxiety, *Am Fam Phys* 49:161, 1994.
24. Dow K: The growing phenomenon of cancer survivorship, *J Prof Nurs* 7:54, 1991.
25. Dunst CJ, Trivette CM, Thompson RB: *Supporting and strengthening families: methods, strategies and practices*, Cambridge, MA, Brookline, 1994.
26. Edgar L, Rosberger Z, Nowlis D: Coping with cancer during the first year after diagnosis: assessment and intervention, *Cancer* 69:817, 1992.
27. Fallowfield L: Giving sad and bad news, *Lancet* 341:476, 1993.
28. Fawzy F and others: Malignant melanoma: effects of early structured psychotic intervention, coping, and affective state on recurrence and survival 6 years later, *Arch Gen Psychiatry* 50:681, 1993.
29. Fawzy FI and others: Critical review of psychosocial interventions in cancer care, *Arch Gen Psychiatry* 52:100, 1995.
30. Fawzy FI and others: Brief, coping-oriented therapy for patients with malignant melanoma. In Spira JL, editor:

Group therapy for medically ill patients, New York, Guilford Press, 1997.

31. Frank A: *At the will of the body: reflections on illness,* Boston/New York, Houghton Mifflin, 1991.

32. Fuller S, Swensen C: Marital quality and quality of life among cancer patients and their spouses, *J Psychosoc Oncol* 10:41, 1992.

33. Gonzalez S, Steinglass P, Reiss D: Putting the illness in its place: discussion groups for families with chronic medical illnesses, *Family Process* 28(1):69, 1989.

34. Gonzalez S, Steinglass P, Reiss D: *Family-centered interventions for people with chronic disabilities: the eight-session multiple family discussion group program.* Washington, DC, Center for Family Research, Department of Psychiatry and Behavioral Science, George Washington University Medical Center, 1987.

35. Gorman LM: The psychosocial impact of cancer on the individual, family, and society. In Carroll-Johnson RM, Gorman LM, Bush NJ, editors: *Psychosocial nursing care: along the cancer continuum,* Pittsburgh, Oncology Nursing Press, 1998.

36. Gray RE and others: Psychologic adaptation of survivors of childhood cancer, *Cancer* 70:2713, 1992.

37. Greer S and others: Adjuvant psychological therapy for patients with cancer: a prospective randomized trial, *Br Med J* 304:675, 1992.

38. Hagopian GA: Cognitive strategies used in adapting to a cancer diagnosis, *Oncol Nurs Forum* 20:759, 1993.

39. Hays DM and others: Educational, occupational and insurance status of childhood cancer survivors in their fourth and fifth decades of life, *J Clin Oncol* 10:1397, 1992.

40. Herbst S: Survivorship: redefining the cancer experience, *Oncol Nurs Forum* 2:527, 1995.

41. Herold AH, Roetzheim RG: Cancer survivors, *Cancer Diagn Treat* 19:779, 1992.

42. Herth K: The relationship between level of hope and level of coping responses and other variables in patients with cancer, *Oncol Nurs Forum* 16:67, 1989.

43. Hoffman B: Employment discrimination: another hurdle for cancer survivors, *Cancer Invest* 9:589, 1991.

44. Holland J, Rowland J, editors: Psychological care of the patient. In *Handbook of Psycho-oncology,* New York, Oxford Press, 1989.

45. Holland J: *Depression in cancer patients is underrecognized, undertreated,* Psychiatric Update Memorial Sloan Kettering Cancer Center, Oncology News International, 1996.

46. Holland J: *Psycho-oncology,* New York, Oxford University Press, 1998.

47. Hoskins CN and others: Social support and patterns of adjustment to breast cancer, *Schol Inq Nurs Pract* 10(2):99, 1996.

48. House J, Landis K, Umberson D: Social relationships and health, *Science* 241:540, 1988.

49. Indeck B, Bunney M: Community resources. In Devita VT, Hellman S, Rosenberg S, editors: *Cancer: principles and practice of oncology,* ed 5, Philadelphia, Lippincott-Raven, 1997.

50. Kaye J, Gracely E: Psychological distress in cancer patients and their spouses, *J Cancer Educ* 8:47, 1993.

51. Lavery JF, Clarke VA: Causal attributions, coping strategies, and adjustment to breast cancer, *Cancer Nurs* 19:20, 1996.

52. Leigh S: Cancer survivorship: a consumer movement, *Semin Oncol* 216:783, 1994.

53. Lesko L: Psychologic issues. In Devita V, Hellman S, Rosenberg S, editors: *Cancer: principles and practice of oncology,* ed 5, Philadelphia, Lippincott-Raven, 1997.

54. Lind S: Telling the diagnosis of cancer, *J Clin Oncol* 7:583, 1989.

55. Lutzky SM, Knight BG: Explaining gender differences in caregiver distress: the roles of emotional attentiveness and coping styles, *Psychol Aging* 9:13, 1994.

56. Mahon SM, Casperson DS: Psychosocial concerns associated with recurrent cancer, *Cancer Pract* 3:372, 1995.

57. Manne S and others: Social support and negative responses in close relationships: their association with psychological adjustment among individuals with cancer, *J Behav Med* 20:101, 1997.

58. Manne S: Cancer in the marital context: a review of the literature, *Cancer Invest* 16:188, 1998.

59. Massie MJ, Shakin EF: Management of depression and anxiety in cancer patients. In Breadboard W, Holland JC, editors: Washington, DC, American Psychiatric Press, 1993.

60. McCubbin HI, McCubbin A, Futrell J, editors: *Resiliency in ethnic minority families: African-American families,* vol 2, Madison, WI, University of Wisconsin, Center for Excellence in Family Studies, 1995.

61. McCubbin HI and others: Families under stress: what makes them resilient? *J Fam Consumer Sci* 2:55, 1997.

62. McCubbin HI and others, editors: *Resiliency in ethnic minority families: native and immigrant families,* vol 1, Madison, WI, University of Wisconsin, Center for Excellence in Family Studies, 1995.

63. McDaniel JS, Nemeroff CB: Depression in the cancer patient: diagnostic, biological and treatment aspects. In Chapman CR, Foley KM, editors: *Current and merging issues in cancer patient: research and practice,* New York, Raven Press, 1993.

64. McDaniel SH, Hepworth J, Doherty WJ: *Medical family therapy: a biopsychosocial approach to families with health problems,* New York, Basic Books, 1992, p 392.

65. McDaniel SH, Campbell TL: Family caregiving and coping with chronic illness, *Families, Systems & Health* 16, 1998.

66. McDaniel SH, Hepworth J, Doherty WJ: *The shared experience of illness: stories of patients, families, and their therapists,* New York, BasicBooks, 1997.

67. Miller JF: Developing and maintaining hope in families of the critically ill, *ACCN Clin Issues Crit Care Nurs* 2:307, 1992.

68. Morse SR, Fife B: Coping with a partner's cancer: adjustment at four states of illness trajectory, *Oncol Nurs Forum* 25:751, 1998.

69. Munkres A, Oberst MT, Hughes SH: Appraisal of illness, symptom distress, self-care burden, and mood states in patients receiving chemotherapy for initial and recurrent cancer, *Oncol Nurs Forum* 19:1201, 1992.

70. National Cancer Institute: *Taking time: support for people with cancer and the people who care for them,* In the National Institutes of Health booklet, 1999, 800-4-CANCER.

71. Nessims S, Ellis J: *Cancervive,* Boston, Houghton Mifflin, 1991.

72. Nicholson JS, Mulvihill JJ, Byrne J: Late effects of therapy in adult survivors of osteosarcoma and Ewing's sarcoma, *Med Pediatr Oncol* 20:6, 1992.

73. North American Nursing Diagnosis Association: *Nursing diagnoses: definitions and classification,* Philadelphia, Author, 1996.

74. O'Connor A, Wicker C, Germino B: Understanding the cancer patient's search for meaning, *Cancer Nurs* 13: 167, 1990.

75. Patel CTC: Hope-inspiring strategies of spouses of critically ill adults, *J Holistic Nurs* 14:44, 1996.

76. Pelusi J: The lived experience of surviving breast cancer, *Oncol Nurs Forum* 24:1343, 1997.

77. Pistrang N, Barker C: The partner relationship in psychological response to breast cancer, *Soc Sci Med* 40:789, 1995.

78. Radner G: *It's always something,* New York, Simon & Schuster, 1989.

79. Rolland JS: *Families, illness, & disability,* New York, Basic Books, 1994.

80. Rolland JS: A journey with hope, fear, and loss: young couples and cancer. In McDaniel SH, Hepworth J, Doherty WH, editors: *A shared experience of illness: stories of patients, families, and their therapists,* New York, BasicBooks, 1997.

81. Rolland JS: Beliefs and collaboration in illness: evolution over time, *Family Systems & Health* 16:7, 1998.

82. Rosenbaum EH, Rosenbaum IR: The will to live. In Dollinger M, Rosenbaum EJ, Cable C, editors: *Everyone's guide to cancer therapy: how cancer is diagnosed, treated, and managed day to day,* Kansas City, Andrews McMeel Publishing, 1991.

83. Seaburn D and others: A mother's death: family stories of illness, loss and healing, *Families, Systems & Health* 14:3, 1996.

84. Sontag S: *Illness as metaphor,* New York, Farrar, Straus & Giroux, 1978.

85. Spiegel D and others: Effect of psychosocial treatment on survival of patients with metastatic breast cancer, *Lancet* 2(8668): 888, 1989.

86. Steinglass P: Multiple family discussion groups for patients with chronic medical illness, *Family, Systems & Health* 16:55, 1998.

87. Steinglass P and others: *The alcoholic family,* New York, BasicBooks, 1987.

88. Tope D, Ashles T, Silberfarb P: Psycho-oncology: psychological well-being as one component of quality of life, *Psychother Psychosomat* 60:129, 1993.

89. Toseland RW and others: Comparative effectiveness of individual and group interventions to support family caregivers, *Social Work* 35:209, 1990.

90. Webster JS: Survivorship issues in post-induction therapy, *Nursing Care Issues in Adult Acute Leukemia* 2:28, 1995.

91. Weisman J, Worden W: The existential plight in cancer: significance of the first 100 days, *Int J Psychiatry Med* 7:1, 1976.

92. Wolfelt AD: *Understanding grief, helping yourself heal,* Muncie, IN, Accelerated Development, 1992.

93. Worden JW: *Grief counseling and grief therapy,* ed 2, New York, Springer, 1991.

94. Wright LM, Watson WL, Bell JM: *Beliefs: the heart of healing in families and illness,* New York, BasicBooks, 1996.

95. Young D, Rosenthal D: Couples' experience of illness: the daily lives of patients and spouses, *Families, Systems & Health* 17:64, 1999.

96. Zeltzer LK: Cancer in adolescents and young adults psychosocial aspects, *Cancer* 71:3463, 1993.

APPENDIX: PSYCHOSOCIAL RESOURCES

Associations/Advocacy Groups

Alliance for Lung Cancer Advocacy, Support and Education (ALCASE): Dedicated to helping people living with lung cancer. Programs include education, early detection, psychosocial support and advocacy issues. 1601 Lincoln Avenue, Vancouver, WA 98660. 800-298-2436. Website: http://www.alcase.org

American Association of Retired Persons (AARP): Services provided include information and supplemental insurance. Fees vary based on policy chosen. 202-434-2277

American Brain Tumor Association: Services offered include free publications on brain tumors, social service consultation by telephone, a mentorship program, support group lists, a resource list of physicians and a pen pal program. 2720 River Road, Suite 146, Des Plaines, IL 60018. 800-886-2282. Website: http://www.abta.org

American Cancer Society (ACS): Programs offered include Children's Camps, Hope Lodge, I Can Cope, Look Good . . . Feel Better, Man to Man, Reach to Recovery, Road to Recovery, and TLC for breast cancer patients. Services offered include education, free publications, support groups lists, and many others depending on the particular state/community. 1599 Clifton Road NE, Atlanta, GA 30329. 800-ACS-2345. Website: http://www.cancer.org

Blood and Marrow Transplant Information Network: Services include a quarterly newsletter for bone marrow, peripheral stem cell and cord blood transplant patients, a book describing BMTs and PBSCTs, an attorney list to help resolve insurance problems, a patient-to-survivor telephone link, and a directory of transplant centers. 2900 Skokie Valley Road, Highland Park, IL 60035. 847-433-3313. Website: http://www.bmtnews.org

Cancer Care, Inc: Services include free professional counseling, support groups, education and information, and referrals for patients and families to assist with psychological and social issues. 275 Seventh Avenue, New York, NY 10001. 800-813-HOPE. Website: http://www.cancercare.org

Choice in Dying: Advocates recognition and protection of individual rights at the end of life. Services include counseling regarding preparation and use of living wills and durable powers of attorney for healthcare. 1035 30th Street NW, Washington, DC 20007. 800-989-WILL. Website: http://www.choices.org

CONVERSATIONS: The International Ovarian Cancer Connection: Services provided include a free monthly newsletter (CONVERSATIONS! The International Newsletter for Those Fighting Ovarian Cancer) and a survivor-to-fighter matching service. P.O. Box 7948, Amarillo, TX 79114. 806-355-2565. Website: http://www.ovarian-news.org

Corporate Angel Network, Inc (CAN): Provides free plane transportation for cancer patients going to/from cancer treatment centers. There are no financial requirements or limits on number of trips. One Loop Road, Westchester County Airport, White Plains, NY 10604. 914-328-1313. Website: http://www.corpangelnetwork.org

Dave Dravecky's Outreach of Hope: Offers encouragement and hope through the love of Jesus Christ to those suffering from cancer or amputation. Services offered include prayer support, correspondence, resource referral and encouraging literature. 13840 Gleneagle Drive, Colorado Springs, CO 80921. 719-481-3528. Website: http://www.outreachofhope.org

International Association of Laryngectomees (IAL): Services offered include pre- and postoperative visits to laryngeal cancer patients, support education for laryngectomees and families, educational materials, and an annual meeting and Voice Restoration Institute at a rotating location each year. 7822 Ivymount Terrace, Potomac, MD 20854. 301-983-9323

International Myeloma Foundation: Services provided include a quarterly newsletter, "Myeloma Today," education about myeloma, and patient/family seminars. 2129 Stanley Hills Drive, Los Angeles, CA 90046. 800-452-CURE. Website: http://www.myeloma.org

Kidney Cancer Association: Services provided include providing information to patients/families and acts as advocate. 1234 Sherman Avenue, Suite 203, Evanston, IL 60202. 800-850-9132. Website: http://www.nkca.org

Leukemia Society of America: Services provided include free educational materials, patient aid, peer support, family support groups, and education regarding leukemia, lymphoma, Hodgkin's disease, and myeloma. 600 Third Avenue, New York, NY 10016. 800-955-4LSA. Website: http://www.leukemia.org

Mathews Foundation for Prostate Cancer Research: Services provided include customized information packages and individual answers to questions about the disease and its symptoms and treatment therapies. 11242 NE 58th Street, Kirkland, WA 98033. 800-234-6284. Website: http://www.mathews.org

Mautner Project for Lesbians with Cancer: Services provided include support, education, information, and advocacy for health issues relating to lesbians/families with cancer. 1707 L Street NW, Suite 500, Washington, DC 20036. 202-332-0662. Website: http://www.mautnerproject.org

National Alliance of Breast Cancer Organization (NABCO): Services provided include information, assistance, and referral, education for the public, and links underserved women to medical services. 9 East 37th Street, 10th Floor, New York, NY 10016. 888-80-NABCO. Website: http://www.nabco.org

National Cancer Institute (NCI): Services provided include a nationwide telephone service that answers questions and free information booklets about cancer. 800-4-CANCER. Website: www.nci.nih.gov

Patient Advocate Foundation (PAF): Services provided include education relative to managed care terminology and policy issues, legal intervention services, and counseling to resolve job and insurance problems. 780 Pilot House Drive, Suite 100C, Newport News, VA 23606. 800-532-5274. Website: http://www.patientadvocate.org

Southwest Airlines: Provides air transportation for medical need with written request and physician letter. 214-904-4103

Support for People with Oral and Head and Neck Cancer, Inc. (SPOHNC): Services provided include support and information addressing the emotional, psychological, and humanistic needs of oral and head and neck cancer patients/families. PO Box 53, Locust Valley, NY 11560. 561-759-5333. Website: http://www.spohnc.org

United Ostomy Association, Inc: Services provided include educational materials (some free of charge) and rehabilitation of all ostomates. 19772 Macarthur Boulevard, Suite 200, Irvine, CA 92612. 800-826-0826. Website: http://www.uoa.org

Well Spouse Foundation: Services provided include support groups and newsletters for partners and caregivers of the chronically ill. 800-838-0879 or 212-724-7209

Y-ME: National Breast Cancer Organization: Services provided include hotline counseling, educational programs, open door meetings for breast cancer patients/families/friends, and a Y-ME Men's Support Line. 212 West Van Buren Avenue, Chicago, IL 60607. 800-221-2141 (24 hour), 800-986-9505. Website: http://www.y-me.org

Financial Resources

Social Security Administration
  Supplemental Security Income (SSI): a federally funded income maintenance program for the aged, blind, or disabled. There are restrictions on amount of income and assets a recipient may have.
  Social Security Disability (SSD): a federally funded program for the disabled and for survivors of a decreased wage earner.
  For the above programs, contact the local Social Security Office or call 800-772-1213.

Community for Agriculture: Services provided include publication of a state-by-state analysis of health insurance programs for high-risk individuals, including plan information and cost. 800-850-3276.

National Insurance Consumer Organization: Services provided include assistance with insurance problems. 703-549-8050

Energy Assistance: Services provided include financial assistance offered by many states to low-income households to help pay energy costs. Contact the local Department of Social Services, local infoline, or local fuel bank.

U.S. Department of Veteran Affairs: Services provided include benefit information to veterans regarding educational assistance, disability compensation, medical care, life insurance, burial benefits, and dependent benefits.

Survivor Services

Cancervive: Assists cancer survivors to face and overcome the challenges of having cancer. 310-203-9232

Coping Magazine: Bimonthly publication dedicated to patients/families/friends involved with cancer. 615-790-2400

National Coalition for Cancer Survivorship: Provides peer support and information to patients/families regarding issues of survivorship. 301-650-8868

The Wellness Community: Services provided include professionally led support groups, education, stress management, and social networking with a focus on health and well-being for individuals recovering from cancer. 35 East 7th Street, Suite 412, Cincinnati, OH 45202. 888-793-WELL. Website: http://www.wellness-community.org

Impact of Cancer on Sexuality

CHAPTER 33

Judith A. Shell

Human beings are sexual from the time of birth until their death, and being sexual is a primary part of being human. If this factor is dismissed by the nurse or physician, patients may perceive themselves as less than human. Until recently, health care professionals were inclined to focus on the physical and emotional aspects of the human being while overlooking the psychosexual. This was especially true with patients who were disabled, chronically ill, or over the age of 62.

Although sexuality remains a sensitive topic, attitudes have changed and sexual rehabilitation is more often part of cancer treatment. Reasons for this change in attitude may include better education concerning human sexuality and a more receptive attitude by society. The standard of physical attractiveness is beginning to change from one of only youth and vitality to include that of the 50- to 60-year-old who is somewhat overweight. Recently, thanks to new legislation, active patient advocacy groups and more sensitive media attention and portrayal, people with impairments are more active and visible and the concept of "normal" is expanding.

Sexuality is a term that can mean different things to different people. The definition Weiss offers best details male and female humanness[83]:

Sexuality isn't really about the things we've been taught to think it is. It isn't about pleasing others, nor is it about owning or controlling others. It isn't about intercourse or having babies. It isn't about competition and beauty contests or proving ourselves more beautiful or sexy than others. It isn't about giving others pleasure so we can feel loved by them, nor is it about trading our bodies for financial, material, or emotional security and comfort. It isn't even only about having orgasms and other pleasurable physical sensations. Sexuality is about connecting our head with our gut through our heart. It's about genuinely caring for ourselves, finding ecstasy in simply being alive, and giving creative voice to our ideas and feelings. It's about bridging physical pleasures with spiritual awareness and serenity. It's about opening ourselves to the sensations of the body and to the joys of the imagination and the heart. It's about sharing and enjoying our sexual selves with partners we feel affectionate and safe with, and it's about loving ourselves and others.

Although nurses often feel a responsibility to address their patients' sexual concerns, many experience discomfort with this role. This discomfort may be because of (1) personal feelings of anxiety regarding sexual topics, (2) embarrassment about obtaining a sexual history, and (3) negative societal stereotypes about sexuality and chronic illness or disability.[20] Increased confidence in sexual assessment and intervention may be attained, however, if specific information and "how-to's" are made available. The Oncology Nursing Society (ONS) and American Nurses Association (ANA) "Outcome Standards for Cancer Nursing Practice" have provided guidelines for the nurse, which include the area of sexuality, and this chapter expands on those guidelines with details of site-specific concerns.

PSYCHOSOCIAL DEVELOPMENT THROUGH THE LIFE CYCLE

Of the many patients faced with a diagnosis of cancer, most experience a life crisis. Although death is often the first fear, the potential for other stressors exists.[40] Surgery, adjuvant therapy (chemotherapy and radiation), the possible spread of malignancy, and an uncertain prognosis are all factors that necessitate life-style adjustments. Changes in role function and an altered body image or self-esteem often threaten the patient with loss of feelings of femininity or masculinity, as well as sexual functioning. As early as 1966, Masters and Johnson explained that almost half of all couples who are physically and psychologically "healthy" have had sexual problems at some time during their relationship.[30] It is reasonable to assume, then, that many cancer patients will have sexual concerns given the added stressors of their disease. In the 1990s, Masters, Johnson, and Koloday continued to espouse the fact that "in cases where passion has turned to indifference, or where a couple is having fundamental problems with unfulfilling sex, it often takes careful orchestration to get things back in tune."[38]

A person's sexual expression varies throughout the life cycle. Although personal beliefs and values are influential, interference with the psychosexual stages of development by an event such as disease may impact sexual function (Table 33–1).[54] For the cancer patient, passage from one stage to the next may be precluded by the disease and its treatment or prognosis. Awareness of these stages will help the caregiver recognize patients at risk for possible sexual dysfunction.

In addition to these stages, various other factors of importance should be considered. As well, the patient's personal reaction to the illness and previous experience with the disease should be explored. If the patient has a significant other, spouse or partner, consideration should be given to the couple's prior strengths and the stability of the relationship. What were their feelings toward sexuality before the disease? If the partners were supportive before diagnosis, they tend to be supportive after diagnosis.[40] Marriage stability after cancer diagnosis and treatment is generally based on the precancer situation.

ANTICIPATION OF AND ADAPTATION TO THE EFFECTS OF CANCER

Once patients are assured of survival beyond the initial diagnosis, the quality of their lives becomes a concern. Will they be able to function as "normal" people do? Taken-for-granted activities like work, recreation, travel, parenting, and sex take on a new importance. While undergoing treatment or in the recovery period, patients will experience fluctuating degrees of fatigue, anorexia and nausea, and discomfort and debilitation. These will affect their level of sexual interest and ability and their sense of adequacy and self-esteem. Depending on the type of cancer and therapy used, specific physiologic and psychological changes can interrupt normal sexual functioning and feelings of femininity or masculinity.[6, 18]

Sense of Adequacy

Femaleness and maleness is not only expressed in the bedroom. Sexuality is a part of all of the activities in which a person engages, such as work, political discussions, decorating one's home, eating a meal or watching

TABLE 33–1
Psychosexual Stages of Development

Stage	Basic Psychosocial Task	Sexual Task
Infancy (0–2 y)	Acquiring basic trust; learning to walk, talk	Gender identity
Childhood (2–12 y)	Acquiring a sense of autonomy versus shame and doubt; entering and adjusting to school	Pleasure-pain associated with sexual organs and eliminative functions; masturbation takes place with resulting shame and acceptance; secondary sex characteristics become evident
Adolescence (13–20 y)	Acquiring sense of identity versus role confusion	Mastery over impulse control, acceptance of conflict between moral proscription and sexual urges, handling new physiologic functions (menses for girls and ejaculate for boys)
Young adulthood (20–45 y)	Acquiring a sense of intimacy versus isolation; vocational effectiveness; interpersonal security, "sexual adequacy"	Sexual adequacy and performance plus fertility concerns and questions related to parenting
Middle adulthood (50–70 y)	Acquiring a sense of self-esteem versus despair; adjusting to diminution of one's energy and competence; "empty nest syndrome" plus care of aging parents or their death; adjusting to change in physique and evidence of aging	For the woman, menopause and resulting vasomotor changes, atrophy of breasts, clitoral size, and vaginal lubrication; for the man, delay on attaining an erection, reduced compulsion to ejaculate, episodic impotence, possible prostatitis
Old age	Adjusting to loss of friends, family, confrontations with old age and dying, painful joint conditions, reduced hearing and visual acuity; adjustment to social stigmatization of being "old"	Reduced vitality, fear of incompetence or injury (coital coronary); fear of being viewed as "dirty old person"; unavailability of a partner (widowhood); limited physical capacity and reduced options

From Schain W: Sexual problems of patients with cancer. In DeVita VT, Hellman S, Rosenberg SA, editors: Cancer: principles and practice of oncology, ed 2, Philadelphia, Lippincott, 1985.

a movie, arguments, child-rearing, and expressions of affection. For some people, the mere process of being ill may cast doubt on their sexual identity and response, which in turn will reflect on their sense of adequacy. Because of the seriousness of their illness, cancer patients are often too embarrassed to raise questions about their sexual concerns. They may feel that worrying about such a relatively unimportant matter as sex is unjustified. It must be emphasized, however, that sexuality is physically and emotionally a source of satisfaction and great pleasure and also the most intimate way we share ourselves with others.

Male and female sexual response is normally integrated into the sexual response cycle (excitement, plateau, orgasm, and resolution). The *male sexual response* (desire, subjective arousal, erection, emission, ejaculation, and orgasm) has separate mechanisms of control and can therefore be affected independently.[38] Although cancer therapy may destroy the capability for an erection, the pleasure of sexual arousal and orgasm often remain intact. This factor is important because men are often worried about whether they can function as they did before. Schover and colleagues present an in-depth explanation of male and female sexual response during the cancer experience.[58] Masters, Johnson, and Koloday also provide a thorough description of the physical changes during the sexual response cycle, a conceptual model of sexual desire, and detailed photographs of the internal and external changes of the penis, vagina, and breast during sexual intercourse.[38]

Female sexual response (desire, subjective arousal, vaginal expansion and lubrication, and orgasm) is less well understood. Women with cancer may lose sexual desire during debilitating treatment, especially if the therapy affects the structure or innervation of the clitoris or vagina. This, along with painful intercourse, are factors that tend to interfere with orgasm. In addition, emphasis is placed on perceived damage resulting from therapy, which women feel may lead to rejection from their partner.[4, 26, 84]

Because the capability of relating sexually is extremely important in our culture, some patients may declare a lost interest in sex just to protect themselves from the embarrassment of lost orgasmic function or erectile failure.

Sexual dysfunction apart from a disability may also be present. This can be caused by "special problems such as alcohol, drug abuse, a history of physical and sexual abuse, or a history of irresponsible sexual behavior."[38] Moreover, added sexual inadequacy that is the result of a potentially fatal disease often leads to a threatened self-image.

Sense of Self-Esteem

Even when there is no organic illness, feelings of unworthiness and incompetence lead to a negative body image. Cancer patients are at much greater risk of having a negative body image because of mutilating surgery and devastating side effects of therapy. Cancer and its treatment can produce considerable loss of economic independence, alter role behavior, change significant relationships, and reduce sexual responsiveness. What follows is fear of abandonment, withdrawal, and sexual dysfunction. To enhance sexual self-esteem, resumption of the ability to function sexually one way or another becomes of paramount importance. This allows the patient to feel more desirable and retain the ability to relate intimately with others.[68]

Gratification and Performance

The feelings of belonging and receiving approval are closely associated with the process of giving and receiving sexual pleasure. Cancer patients often feel undesirable and unattractive and, because they are now typecast as "ill," feel they are not supposed to be sexual. For others, conquering the challenges of the cancer diagnosis and treatment phases is seen as offering a second chance at life and a new appreciation for relationships. It has been reported, however, that patients and their partners retain a continued desire for physical affectionate behavior, but a decrease in the desire for sexual intercourse.[57] One of the authors' patients stated, "I would just love to have the closeness and touching back again." Many times patients feel sexual desires but take it for granted that their partner does not desire them. The partner, in turn, worries that the patient may be too sick to want sexual activity and feels guilty about having a sexual interest in someone who is sick and under treatment. Unfortunately, if these misconceptions persist, patients and their partners are likely to avoid the intimate and sexual contact that might be possible.

Nurses must not fail to see alternatives to stereotypical sexual behavior and must acknowledge each patient's unique sexual identity.[10] It is the nurse's responsibility to be free of fixed ideas and to continue to discuss sexual concerns at all stages of cancer and its treatment, regardless of the patient's circumstances or age. It must never be assumed that the patient who has raised no question has no concerns. Concentrated attention must be given to the issue of sexuality just as it is given to other aspects of cancer care, because sexuality is one of the most fundamental aspects of humanity.

NURSING DIAGNOSES RELATED TO SEXUALITY

The following nursing diagnoses apply to the nursing interventions that are discussed.[47]

Relating

Impaired social interaction
Social isolation
Risk for loneliness
Sexual dysfunction
Altered family processes
Altered sexuality patterns
Altered role performance

Valuing

Risk for spiritual distress
Potential for enhanced spiritual well-being

Moving

Impaired physical mobility
Fatigue
Risk for activity intolerance
Bathing/hygiene self-care deficit
Dressing/grooming self-care
Toileting self-care deficit

Perceiving

Body image disturbance
Self-esteem disturbance
Chronic low self-esteem
Situational low self-esteem
Personal identity disturbance
Sensory/perceptual alterations (visual, auditory, kinesthetic, tactile, olfactory)

SITE-SPECIFIC ISSUES AFFECTING SEXUALITY

Most discussions in the literature related to sexual problems of cancer patients begin with malignancies of the genital organs because cancer in this area is most likely to cause sexual dysfunction. Consequently, head and neck cancers, sarcomas that result in amputation, hematologic malignancies, and lung cancers are frequently overlooked or barely mentioned. Therefore, a nursing approach to these concerns will be addressed first.

Head and Neck Cancer

Physiologic and Body Image Alterations. Although the social significance of youth and facial beauty continues to be profound and is exemplified through movies, television, and magazines, it is beginning to be somewhat less dramatic. However, even a patient is usually portrayed on television as perfectly made up and clad in a beautiful robe, and the few older people portrayed by the mass media are usually fairly attractive. Therefore, the impact of head and neck cancer and its treatment can be particularly devastating because the defects caused by the disease are immediately recognizable. The patient feels grossly unattractive and frequently has difficulty with life's most basic needs, such as talking, eating, and even breathing. Given these fundamental problems, it is not surprising that little or no attention is given to the need for closeness, touching, and genital sexual pleasures.

Sexual relationships may be influenced by the patient's age, smoking and drinking habits, and the general emotional impact of treatment. Many patients are more than 60 years of age at the time of diagnosis and are entering a period of adjustment to a decrease in frequency of sexual intercourse, although desire often remains about the same.[38] The patient may also be an alcoholic, which will influence treatment and the rehabilitation process. Intimacy, trust, and open communication are frequently nonexistent in alcoholic relationships because intimacy is too threatening to the alcoholic individual.[44] Because alcoholic men and women are known to have a low sense of self-esteem, the nurse may have to focus on this issue before moving on to the patient's feelings of masculinity or femininity.[57]

Patients with head and neck cancer often require rehabilitation, which may be accomplished with reconstructive surgery or prostheses or both. It is important to remember that the expectations of the patient may differ from actual treatment results. Consequently, the patient may suffer one or more disappointments, as illustrated by the following anecdote.[16]

A woman had an oral prosthesis made. The match and the appearance were excellent, and she regained confidence and employment and she delighted in sociability. Her praise and gratitude were profuse. However, once when we had lunch together she said, "I have so much to be thankful for and yet . . ." and she turned away and she touched the prosthesis. "When I laugh, this never laughs, and when I take it off I sometimes wonder if I can go on."[16]

Patients with head and neck cancer will necessarily face lingering cosmetic and functional impairments, which will affect their body image and sexuality. Often, presurgical levels of function and aesthetics cannot be restored.[74] Although attempts at prosthetic rehabilitation are noble, the health care professional should remember that the patient's concept is often quite different from the medical concept. Rehabilitation will change the patient's practices and habits. To this patient, a kiss and a hug may be worth a thousand words.

Nursing Management

HEAD AND NECK CANCER

Interventions

- A gastrostomy tube may be placed to rid the patient of nasogastric feeding tube, which interferes with kissing and facial petting.
- Sugarless mints and artificial saliva help to freshen stale breath caused by a dry mouth (from radiation therapy).[17] Artificial saliva (Moi-Stir, Xerolube) also helps prevent tooth decay.
- The patient may have a decreased sense of smell, so that perfumes cannot be appreciated. Candles, scented or not, can provide a relaxed ambience for both patient and partner, though the fragrance is not appreciated by the patient.

- Tracheostomies should be cleaned of mucus and covered lightly during sexual activity. (For information on obtaining tracheostomy covers, see the appendix at the end of this chapter, page 998.)
- Partners should be made aware that the patient's heavy breathing may sound different. If the larynx is removed, a sexy voice, whispered love talk, and other eroticisms will be eliminated.
- Various positions may need to be tried for sexual activity because the partner may be fearful of cutting off the patient's air supply.
- Patients, especially women, may wish to wear a fancy nightgown with a high neck, or other erotic neckwear. Men may wish to wear a dickey.

Sarcomas of Bone and Soft Tissue and Limb Amputation

Physiologic and Body Image Alterations. There continues to be a dearth of information available regarding the sexual adjustment of those with upper or lower extremity amputation. Commonly, concentration is placed on the patient's functional problems during and after prosthetic rehabilitation and reference to sexuality is often omitted.[84]

If major limb amputation is necessary, it can create emotional hurdles for the patient's self-perception, as well as acceptance by their partner (Fig. 33–1). A decrease in self-esteem and a negative body image are common because of the presence of a gross defect that is obvious even when covered with clothes. The man may equate the loss of a limb to the loss of manhood. Some patients may view the surgery as a punishment for past transgressions.[40]

Limb amputation creates several potential sexual problems, which include the simple mechanics of body positioning during intercourse, immobility because of physical isolation, amputee fetishism, associated disease states that can alter sexual function, and phantom pain sensations.[69, 78] Phantom limb pain can be quite disturbing and can in itself impair sexual functioning.

Amputees are admittedly apprehensive about their physical capabilities, but this fear often subsides once they begin prosthetic training, ambulation, or articulation. As patients become more independent, confidence in their sexuality usually returns.[84] Some patients fail to gain satisfaction from a prosthesis. Those patients then resort to using crutches rather than to be restricted by the somewhat awkward movement of artificial limbs. They forfeit a better cosmetic appearance, however.

The life-style of amputees may be profoundly affected, especially if they have been independent and physically active. The range of problems usually depends on the extensiveness of the amputation. For

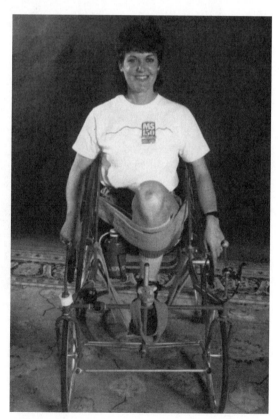

FIGURE 33–1 Lou Keyes, hemipelvectomy patient, in her racing wheelchair. Lou also uses a prosthetic device proficiently and crutches when she is in a hurry.

example, a woman with a shoulder disarticulation may find that simple tasks like styling hair and getting clothing to look good are difficult. Less dramatic upper extremity amputations allow for easier manipulation of a conventional hand prosthesis, a hook prosthesis, or a newer myoelectric-powered hand (Fig. 33–2).

Lower extremity amputees, especially those with hip disarticulations and hemipelvectomies, have a different set of uncertainties with prosthetics.[42] Most prevalent worries are socket discomfort, mobility, and energy expenditure. With an exoskeletal device for disarticulation or hemipelvectomy, the socket area envelops the entire pelvis and adds to hip and waist measurements (Fig. 33–3). One woman stated that she couldn't tuck her blouses in and thought her clothes looked too big. Women often have difficulty wearing sanitary pads dur-

ing menses and may wish to use double tampons. All amputees must deal with undesirable noises produced by prosthetic joints, and even buying a pair of shoes can be disconcerting.

For patients without partners, there may be a support group or sporting activities to become involved in, such as wheelchair racing. These are good opportunities to meet people and share like experiences. The more the patient gets out and regains self-confidence, the easier it will be to meet and interact with other people. (For more information, see Support Groups [LEAPS] at the end of this chapter.)

For those patients with partners, feelings of maleness or femaleness can be regained with the partner's love, support, and understanding. A loving and intimate relationship can help restore self-confidence and determination to adapt to their disability.

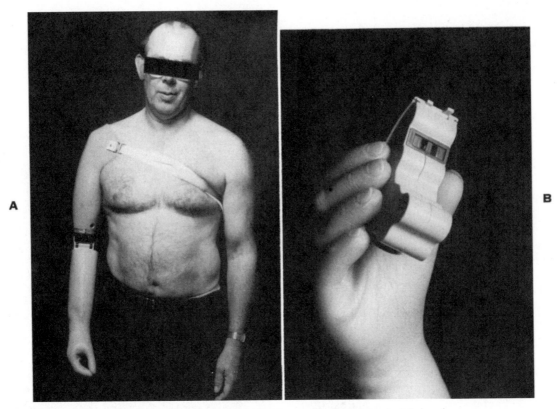

FIGURE 33–2 A, Above the elbow, myoelectric prosthesis. **B,** Myoelectric hand grasping object.

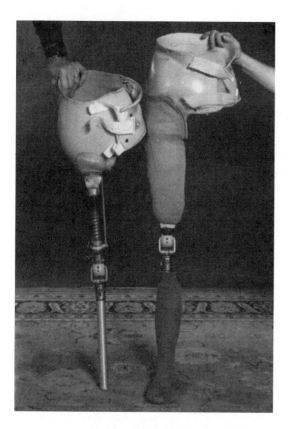

FIGURE 33–3 Prosthesis on left is a hip flexion bias system without a rotator knee and no flexibility in the socket; cost $11,000. Prosthesis on the right is a hip flexion bias system with a rotator knee and partially flexible socket; cost $13,000.

Nursing Management

LIMB AMPUTATION

Interventions

Not only is the amputee's body image and self-concept threatened, but often many taken-for-granted activities are either eliminated or severely hampered. Some suggestions that may be helpful to amputees in resuming an intimate relationship with their partners follow:

- After some experimenting, some amputees find that intercourse can be maintained without any modification or adjustment of positions.
- Some patients may expend slightly more energy, which may result in mild fatigue, but this rarely hampers sexual function.
- If balance and movement are a problem, pillows or other forms of support may be used to maintain a level pelvis.[69]

- Lovemaking does not always have to occur in the bedroom. A sofa or large chair can be used to balance on, or the female amputee can lean against a chair while her partner enters her from behind.
- The woman may need to assume the superior position during coitus.
- An upper extremity amputee may wish to use a side-lying position with the existing arm free to balance.
- Hemipelvectomy patients may have extra folds of skin used to make their flaps. Because these patients may be uncomfortable exposing themselves to their partner, these skinfolds can be held in place by a "compression sock." This sock compresses the folds into a hiplike shape, and the sock can then be modified with an opening in the crotch to allow for intercourse.

Hematologic Malignancies

Impact of Therapy Side Effects on Body Image. Although the diagnosis of lymphoma/leukemia or multiple myeloma can be terrifying, treatment does not comprise surgery or amputation, which can cause disfigurement. What the individual may not realize, however, is that chemotherapy and radiation therapy can be just as devastating to sexuality. Except for multiple myeloma, these diagnoses are often made in young, active people who see themselves as infallible, and they often do not comprehend the impact of the illness until well into their therapy.

Most men and women experience reduced desire for sexual intercourse during chemotherapy treatments, particularly during the first few days after receiving the drugs. This is usually the result of increased weakness, fatigue, and intermittent nausea and vomiting. Also, whether the patient is young or old or male or female, defacement caused by hair loss can destroy self-confidence. Another problem for patients with acute myelocytic leukemia is the prolonged hospitalization during chemotherapy with consequent lack of privacy.

Lack of sexual eagerness can also be induced by an effect on the testes or ovaries due to chemotherapy. Ovarian dysfunction is progressive, and women may experience symptoms such as amenorrhea or irregular menses, hot flashes, decreased libido, and vaginal dryness. Testicular dysfunction occurs more abruptly and results in oligospermia (decreased sperm) or azoospermia (absent sperm), as well as difficulty with erections.[65, 72] Fortunately, these problems are often temporary and hormone levels and sexual desire return to normal after chemotherapy or radiation therapy ends.

Myelosuppression and its consequences can cause fatigue and shortness of breath, which decrease sexual desire. Concern about bleeding and infection will be present because of low platelet and white blood cell/absolute neutrophil counts. A perfect environment for a vaginal yeast infection may be created, which inflames the lining of the vagina and causes itching and burning during intercourse. The male patient's ability to have an erection may also be affected. Creativity will be necessary to promote sexual intimacy.

Many patients will experience moments of anxiety and depression throughout their treatment, and therapy can last for as long as 3 years. The nurse should stress the importance of maintaining involvement in activities and relationships with their friends when they feel good. Patients should be advised on ways to ask for assistance with activities of daily living and should be reminded not to be ashamed to ask for help, as they have most likely often helped others.

A discussion will most likely be needed to assess the feelings of the spouse or significant other. It is helpful to identify ways they can support the patient's feelings of self-worth and masculinity or femininity. They should be encouraged to reassure the patient that sexuality and ability to be loved are not affected by appearance only.

One of the most stressful events for any patient is alopecia.[49] Some patients may feel that hair loss is even worse than amputation, and because of its effect on body image, sexual inadequacy can ensue. Sensitivity should be used when explaining this side effect to any patient, male or female, and patients should be provided with the information presented in Box 33–1.

BOX 33–1

Suggestions for Patients Who Experience Alopecia

Use a mild, protein-based shampoo, cream rinse, and conditioner.

Rinse the hair well and pat dry, *not* vigorously.

Shampoo every 4 to 7 days.

Avoid excessive brushing and use a wide-toothed comb/brush.

Avoid hair spray and hair dye.

Permanents are okay, but if hair loss is expected, it is best to wait until regrowth to perm the hair.

Avoid electric hair dryers and curling irons, clips, bobby pins, barrettes, and pony tails.

Many types of hats and caps are available.

Purchase some kind of head wrap or turban, whether it is winter or summer, because the hair helps to keep the head warm.

Even in warm weather, the head can get very cold if left uncovered in an air-conditioned environment.

Use sunscreen on scalp when outside.

Nursing Management

HEMATOLOGIC MALIGNANCIES

Interventions

- The patient who is neutropenic should be advised against oral, penile/vaginal, and anal sexual manipulation. Remind the patient and partner that gratification may be derived from simply touching and holding. The couple may bathe together. Bubbles, a little candlelight, romantic music, and some wine (in plastic glasses) make for an intimate experience. The couple can share each other intimately without performance anxiety, and the warm water may help ease some of the general aches and pains.
- Intercourse can be planned for after antiemetics are given and when the medications will be most effective.
- Advise patients to avoid the stress of heavy meals and liquor before intercourse.

- To avoid fatigue, a nap before intercourse may be helpful. The supine position or a side-lying position uses less energy. Also, avoid temperature extremes if possible.
- The importance of contraceptive measures during chemotherapy and radiation must be emphasized to all patients. Although chemotherapy will affect sperm count and ovulation, the patient cannot depend on this alone for contraception.[52, 63] Teratogenic effects are seen during the first trimester of pregnancy, especially if the woman is under treatment.[28, 33, 43] Studies are underway to determine possible effects on future generations.[28, 35]
- Encourage sperm banking before initiation of chemotherapy.
- If the patient's complexion is pale because of decreased erythrocytes, encourage bright colors and the use of make-up to enhance appearance.

Breast Cancer

Physiologic and Body Image Alterations. Today's society has idealized the female breast to such an extent that it has become a "sociosexual" symbol of sexuality and femininity.[51] Physiologically, removal of a breast should not decrease sexual desire or activity, but in reality studies have demonstrated high levels of stress in regard to sexual functioning among mastectomy patients.[23, 24] Mastectomy makes an obvious change in the body's contour, which can lead to fears about loss of identity as a woman and a desirable sexual being. The partner's perceived importance of a breast can also affect the woman's perspective should she choose mastectomy, even though reconstruction is more prevalent today. Anxiety is also present regarding the cancer diagnosis.

The patient who is treated with lumpectomy and radiation therapy has concerns about her sexuality as well. Although this patient's breast is preserved, she may experience a skin reaction and increased fatigue while receiving radiation treatment. This can last for several weeks and also lead to decreased desire for sexual activity. Long-term depression and maladjustment are not as likely in this population, but it is just as important to assist these patients with their doubts and anxieties.[55]

A woman's response to treatment for breast cancer and its corresponding threat to sexuality will depend on several conditions[3, 26]:

- Her feelings about her femininity
- The value she bestows on her missing breast
- Her physical discomfort
- The response of her significant other

- The reinforcement she receives from the nurse regarding her sexual identity
- Her sense of self-worth

The status of the patient's preoperative sexual relationships and her interpretation of sexual satisfaction must also be ascertained. Cultural and religious attitudes will also influence "acceptable" sexual practices.

Schover explains that unmarried patients with breast cancer may have increased insecurities related to meeting new dating partners and when and how to tell them about their diagnosis.[64] An excellent resource for this population, as well as for married women, is the Reach to Recovery program (see Support Groups at the end of this chapter). This program tries to pair the patient with a volunteer mastectomy patient of the same race, side of mastectomy, social status (single, married, widowed, divorced), and in some areas, sexual orientation. The volunteer explains exercises for the affected side's arm, tells where to get prostheses and clothing, and gives emotional support.

Rehabilitation may consist of reconstructive surgery, which may be done immediately or several months after treatment is complete. Occasionally, surgical repair must be done before good reconstruction can be accomplished. Although the reconstructed breast will never look like the original breast, some women exercise this option because they feel it looks more natural. These women must be reminded that there is little to no sensation in this breast, which may be particularly disappointing during foreplay. A multitude of breast prostheses are also available; some of them are listed in the Resources at the end of this chapter.

Nursing Management

BREAST CANCER

Interventions

In the recent past, patients and their partners had time to begin to experience the loss of the breast (if mastectomy occurred) together in the hospital. However, with the changes in health care, most women go home the next day with bandage and drain in place, with little time to acclimate emotionally. The partner often has no choice but to assist the patient, and hopefully, a home health nurse will be present to assist with the physical and emotional needs.

Couples may not be sure how to begin to experience the loss of a breast or the reaction of the breast to radiation therapy together. One behavior seen on television is where the woman disrobes in front of her spouse to show him her changed body and the scar. A more reasonable and less threatening activity may be for both members of a couple to stand nude together in front of a mirror and express the thoughts and feelings this elicits. In this circumstance, the patient is likely to feel less vulnerable, because she and her partner are both nude. Of course, not all couples will be able to accept or handle this type of exercise, and they should be encouraged to use their own coping strategies. Because coping mechanisms will vary from person to person and couple to couple, numerous behaviors will be exhibited. These will range from allowing the partner to participate in care and view the mastectomy scar immediately to not allowing anyone but the physician to see the wound. Support is continually needed to promote healthy adjustment by the patient and partner.

When making love, these suggestions may be incorporated:

- Until the woman is ready to disrobe or let her partner touch the wound area, she can wear a fancy camisole or short nightgown. This camouflages the area but is still sexually stimulating for the couple.
- To minimize a direct view of the woman's missing breast, the partner may assume the superior position (missionary position) or use a rear-entry position. *Joy of Sex,* edited by Dr. Alex Comfort, is an excellent reference for positions a couple may use to increase sexual pleasure.
- The couple may make love by candlelight to decrease the impact of the change in body contour.
- Concentration on a certain sexual task (sensate focus) may increase stimulation and reduce appearance concerns. One suggestion is a touching exercise, explained in depth in the American Cancer Society's book *Sexuality and Cancer: For the Woman Who Has Cancer, and Her Partner.* The focus is initially on massaging the extremities and back and ignoring the genital sexual organs, and the result is relaxation and sensual pleasure.[62]
- Because many women derive great pleasure from stroking, sucking, and manipulation of the breast during foreplay, the remaining breast can continue to be stimulated if the woman so desires. Reassure the patient that manipulation will not cause another breast cancer.

Female Pelvic and Genital Cancer

Physiologic and Body Image Alterations. As in breast cancer, the surgery needed to cure women of cancers of the genital organs can be very threatening to a woman's sexuality.[3, 73]

A threat to a woman's capability of being physically sexual can lead to a lost sense of femininity and consequent fluctuations in self-esteem and body image.[4] The female sexual response cycle will most likely be affected if treatment affects the structure and innervation of the clitoris or the vagina.

Surgical resection or radiation therapy for cancer of the cervix, uterus, ovary, vulva, vagina, and bladder can be either simple or extensive. Women faced with this type of treatment have many apprehensions:

- Threat to life
- Feelings of lost femininity
- Concern about what their external region will look like
- Ability to have intercourse and, if so, whether it will be painful
- Fear that along with the loss of fertility will come loss of vitality and orgasmic potential
- Fear of physical aging, diminished libido, loss of vaginal lubrication, and dyspareunia

To prevent extensive morbidity and sexual dysfunction from the concerns just mentioned, early intervention with counseling is imperative for the gynecologic cancer patient.

Nursing Management

FEMALE PELVIC AND GENITAL CANCER

The following nursing interventions apply to radical hysterectomy, partial or total pelvic exenteration, radical vulvectomy, cystectomy, and radiation therapy.

Interventions

Radical Hysterectomy

As discussed in Chapter 11, in radical hysterectomy, the vaginal canal is shortened somewhat (up to one half) but is not believed to be sexually appreciable in all cases. Penile thrusting may be uncomfortable, because the trigone of the bladder and sigmoid colon may be closely associated with the new vaginal apex.

Donahue and Knapp suggest alternate methods of intercourse that can be most helpful (see the box below).[19] Delayed resumption of bladder function introduces an embarrassing problem. If a long-term indwelling catheter is present, vaginal sexual relations can be impeded. Partners may change positions, and rear-entry intercourse can be practiced.[18] To prevent dislodgment, the catheter can be placed up over the lower abdomen and taped into place. Alternate ways of expressing physical love can also be fulfilling and can include oral, anal, and digital expressions.

Vaginal dryness, atrophy, and pain can be caused by various cancer treatments and their side effects. Often, women are advised to use oral estrogen replacement therapy or estrogen creams. Both of these can raise the blood levels of estrogen and this is usually considered dangerous if a woman has an estrogen-sensitive tumor. A new product on the market used to relieve vaginal dryness and atrophy was approved in 1996 and is called the Estring. It is a 2-inch circle of estradiol that is inserted into the vagina like a diaphragm and left in place for 3 months. There is a circle of silicon polymer that regulates the release of estradiol.[85] Whittelsey reports that this may be a safer alternative, because changes in blood levels of estradiol were very small and temporary.[83] However, it has not been tested in breast cancer survivors as yet and cannot be recommended without caution.

Women who have undergone radical hysterectomy may also realize a decrease in sexual desire and "a loss of sensation in the nipples and clitoris, as well as fleeting, barely pleasant orgasms. . . ."[85] This may be due simply to a deficiency in testosterone. Usually this can be easily remedied with a prescription for an estrogen-testosterone supplement. However, if the patient is a breast cancer survivor, it may be necessary for her to have a testosterone product compounded by a pharmacist because no company makes a testosterone only version. The dose of testosterone is very low (1.5 mg/d) and rarely causes masculinizing effects like facial hair growth.[85]

Pelvic Exenteration

Several factors of adjustment may be generated by this particular surgery.[58] These can include adaptation to a urinary conduit, bowel conduit, or both, and this can cause worry about appearance and appliance fit, possible leakage, and odor. The vulva will be extensively denervated, which results in decreased erotic sensations. Creation of a neovagina may also be necessary. Clitoral swelling and pain may occur, requiring a clitoridectomy for relief. It is understandable that many patients report decreased frequency of sexual activity and satisfaction and a loss of sexual self-confidence.

To ensure the most beneficial adjustment psychologically and sexually for the patient and her partner, it is necessary to provide specific alternatives and realistic information before surgery. Unfortunately, some women have been told that sexual intercourse will feel the same and be as good as before the surgery. Many women complain of the inability to voluntarily constrict the vaginal introitus, and for those women with a neovagina, some allege that it is too short or too large or associate it with an increased chronic discharge.[58] Some women maintain the ability to have an orgasm, but others lose it or achieve orgasm only

---

Alternative Coital Positions and Coital Equivalents

Angle of penile thrust can be altered by elevating the woman's hips on 1 or 2 pillows.

Deeper vaginal barrel can be mimicked by enclosing the penis within one or both palms.

Some patients find that vaginal penetration from behind between closely adducted thighs will increase pleasure.

If coitus is not possible, the basic mechanics of cunnilingus (application of tongue or mouth to the vulva) and fellatio (sexual gratification by intromission of the penis into another individual's mouth) should be explained.

From Donahue V, Knapp R: Sexual rehabilitation of gynecologic cancer patients, *Obstet Gynecol* 49:118, 1977. Reprinted with permission from the American College of Obstetricians and Gynecologists.

with extra effort. Also, after reconstruction, vaginal sensation is usually decreased. To promote total healing and the ability to detect early recurrence, a waiting period of 6 weeks to 2 months is advised before resumption of sexual intercourse.[19]

Alternatives to sexual intercourse available to women who have had vaginal reconstruction may include nudity, cuddling, and general pleasuring; auto-eroticism and masturbation with a partner; oral-genital relations and anal love play; and fantasy.

Radical Vulvectomy and Cystectomy

Cancer of the vulva usually occurs in women who are well past menopause, and these older women are often reluctant to seek treatment until the disease has progressed. As a result, the therapy can have a particularly frightful impact on body image and sexual identity.[5]

For early stage disease, patients are usually treated with skinning vulvectomy (a partial vulvectomy of the superficial skin), laser treatment, or wide local excision rather than simple vulvectomy. With a skinning vulvectomy, a split-thickness graft from the inner thigh is often applied to cover the denuded area.[22] This procedure gives an optimal cosmetic and functional result. Laser treatment involves destruction of the lesion by vaporizing the tissue. Healing is excellent with this procedure, but a thorough pathologic review cannot be done of the diseased specimen.[22] Patients have few complaints of dyspareunia or decreased sexual responsiveness with laser therapy.

In radical vulvectomy, the fine sensory perception experienced during foreplay is destroyed and must be compensated for by excitement of other erogenous zones such as the earlobes, breasts, fingers, toes, and inner thighs.[63]

The patient's partner must be included in all education and counseling because of the radical nature of the treatment and long recuperative period after therapy. Patients comment that adequate information is rarely given so they can begin to alter their sexual expectations, and others state that the treatment is embarrassing and creates an isolated feeling.[14]

Little is mentioned in the literature concerning women undergoing cystectomy and the sexual problems that arise from excision of the bladder and more than one third of the vagina. Problems identified are vaginal tightness and dryness and self-conscious anxiety because of the ostomy.[48] Scarring can develop, as well as numbness and lost sensation, because of impaired innervation of the perineum. Recommended remedies may include a vaginal estrogen cream and vaginal dilators to help decrease dyspareunia.[58] Most women like to cover their ostomy appliance with a fabric cover, and feminine lingerie may also be worn during sexual activity. Kegel exercises are helpful to relieve tension and decrease dyspareunia.[14] Positive reinforcement, specific suggestions, and a supportive partner can make an important difference in the woman's achievement of a satisfying sexual adjustment.

Radiation Therapy

Both external therapy and internal radiation insertion can cause irritating side effects, which are disruptive to sexual activity. Diarrhea, skin reaction of the external genitalia, and especially vaginal irritation, stenosis, and dryness are the most troublesome.[9] To prevent a diminished sense of femininity, a discussion with pertinent facts and proposals should precede radiation therapy.

The vagina will react to radiation by becoming shorter and narrower, having adhesions and problems with lubrication. The nurse may suggest the following:

- Continued sexual intercourse during treatment is usually encouraged to decrease possible adhesions and prevent shortening. Sometimes tissues may become tender, or an external skin reaction may necessitate stopping sexual intercourse. It can be resumed when healing and comfort allow.
- A water-soluble lubricating jelly is always needed to decrease vaginal discomfort and can be applied privately or as part of foreplay.[58]
- During sexual activity, the hips may be elevated or the adducted thighs lubricated to emulate a deeper vaginal barrel and improve sexual stimulation for a male partner. The female-superior position allows her more control but is usually not as comfortable. Rear entry is another alternative.
- Vaginal dilators can be used if a woman does not have a sexual partner or is not sexually active. Sexually active women may also use dilators during treatment if intercourse is too exhausting. Normal sexual activity is preferred because some women hesitate to place foreign objects into their vagina, and some are concerned about implications of masturbation. Sometimes dilators are indeed necessary, and the patient's compliance will increase if she is made aware that complete vaginal stenosis will occur, obstructing the physician's view in follow-up, if not used.[9]
- It is important to be sensitive to both the patient and her partner when explaining dilator use.

Male Pelvic Cancer

Physiologic and Body Image Alterations. Societal expectations of men have changed little since the 1980s. They are supposed to be heroes and good providers, to hide their emotions and be strong, not to touch each other unless engaging in sports, and rarely to relate on an emotional level or be dependent on another.[70] Masculinity is also equated with activity and productivity; a man must never admit to possible physical problems and must always be in control.[70] Pertaining to sexuality, the state of a man's penis is always of utmost importance. Consequently, when the male patient experiences a malignancy in the pelvis or genital area, his entire self-image may be threatened. After diagnosis and treatment are complete and the fear of death is no longer uppermost in the patient's mind, he concentrates on the sequelae.[77] The impact on self-image will be even greater if his sexuality is threatened.

When the malignancy involves the prostate, testicle, or penis, there can be a temporary or permanent disturbance in relation to erection, emission, or ejaculation. Orgasm is not as frequently affected and can actually be achieved even when genital function is lost. Table 33–2 provides an in-depth description of common cancer surgeries of the male pelvis and their effect on sexual functioning.[70] To promote adjustment and sexual rehabilitation, support and assistance for the patient and his partner are essential through knowledge and specific interventions.

T A B L E   3 3 – 2

Effects of Surgery on Male Sexual Functioning

Surgery	Direct Effect	Indirect Effect
AP resection	Damage to sympathetic and parasympathetic nervous systems resulting in: 1. Varying degrees of impotence (erectile difficulties) 2. Ejaculatory problems 2.1. Retrograde ejaculation 2.2. Decreased amount ejaculate 2.3. Decreased ejaculatory force	Altered sexual expression as a result of: 1. Physical impairment 2. Body image change 3. Altered self-esteem 4. Fears 5. Pain
Radical cystectomy	As above but to a greater extent 1. May be 100% impotent 2. Retrograde or no ejaculation	As above
Pelvic exenteration	As with AP resection and radical cystectomy	As above
Radical prostatectomy	Stress incontinence (temporary) Varying degrees of impotence	As above
Orchiectomy	Loss of gonads and testosterone resulting in: 1. Sterility 2. Decreased libido	As above
Cord surgeries Paraplegia Quadriplegia (tumor removal, pain control)	As with AP resection	As above

From Shipes E, Lehr S: Sexuality and the male cancer patient, Cancer Nurs *5:375, 1982.*

Nursing Management

MALE PELVIC CANCER

Interventions

Prostate

Surgery for prostate cancer has a definite impact on male sexual potency, depending on how extensive it is. When transurethral resection (TUR) is used in early stage disease, approximately 80% of these patients experience scanty or absent ejaculation, although they are still able to have an erection. Until recently, if radical prostatectomy was the treatment of choice, 85% to 90% of those patients experienced erectile impotence. Now with nerve-sparing surgical techniques, men can achieve erections with better success; however, difficulties remain.[1, 25, 77] Problems can occur when radiation is used in lieu of surgery because of probable fibrosis of the pelvic arteries. Incidental reports of erectile impotence vary from 14% to 46% after treatment with external radiation. Interstitial treatment may be used if the tumor burden is small, and incidence of impotence is reported between 7% and 13%.[58, 79, 86]

Endocrine treatment (castration, estrogen, and/or a luteinizing hormone/regulatory hormone [LH/RH] antagonist [Lupron]) commonly causes difficult and embarrassing problems such as gynecomastia, phallic atrophy, loss of libido, and erectile impotence.[79] Many men experience physical debilitation, depression, anxiety, and pain, all of which may decrease sexual desire.

One of the most important issues in the area of male pelvic cancers may be to help the patient and his partner develop a change in attitude toward sexual intercourse if erection is no longer possible or if it is impaired. The goal of an intimate interlude may no longer be penile vaginal intercourse, but rather one of caressing and fondling each other toward pleasant stimulation with possible orgasm. Even if frequency drops, the potential for sexual arousal remains with the correct stimulus:

- Many men become sexually aroused with erotic books, pictures, or movies.
- Long periods of foreplay, including romantic dinners, showering or bathing together, and using different rooms for lovemaking, may be stimulating. A changed or new environment such as a local motel or house sitting for a friend may bring new excitement.
- If a full erection is not possible, mutual masturbation may allow the patient to reach orgasm and ejaculation. The partner should massage the penis in a downward motion with pressure beginning at the base of the penis. The penis should not be pulled up toward the abdomen or it can lose blood. A female partner can assist erection by inserting a partially erect penis into the vagina and flexing her perineal muscles, like Kegel exercises.
- During ejaculation, semen may be propelled into the bladder, which may threaten the man's sense of masculinity.[46] The partner, however, may enjoy oral stimulation more because she no longer has to experience the taste of semen.
- If the patient has problems with urinary incontinence, he should empty his bladder before intercourse and perhaps wear a condom if this becomes worrisome to his partner. Remind the couple that urine is sterile and will not harm the partner.
- The risks and benefits of penile implants should be explained to the couple. Many urologists recommend waiting 6 months after surgery before installing a prosthesis.[58] The patient and partner may choose from several different types of prosthesis. A comparison of two of the types (shown on page 987) is given on page 988. An excellent resource is *Bio-Potency: A Medical Guide to Sexual Success* by Richard and Deborah Berg.
- Intracavernous injections into the penis using papaverine, 30 mg/mL to stimulate erections is one common treatment.[50] Side effects can include syncope, flushing, hypotension, and transient ischemic attacks. It is contraindicated in cardiac disease.
- Urethral suppositories are another pharmacologic option for men who do not wish to inject their penis. Alprostadil (Muse) is effective in 5 to 7 minutes, peak effect is 19 to 25 minutes, and it lasts for 60 to 90 minutes. Dosage starts at 125 μg and comes in increments of 250, 500, 1000 μg. However, the suppositories are quite expensive ($20–$25 each) and they are not covered by insurance as are other medications.[15] It can also be used as an intracavernous injection.
- Today's most popular medication for impotence is sildenofil (Viagra). Drug onset is usually within 60 minutes and erections last 60 to 90 minutes. Side effects may include headache, flushing, cardiac irregularities and a change in vision (a blue aura).[15]
- Finally, like other cancer patients, this patient may simply need physical closeness and intimacy. Sexual activity is not always what is needed to promote feelings of love and belonging.

Testicle

Not surprisingly, men with cancer of the testicle not only have problems with fertility, but also with their

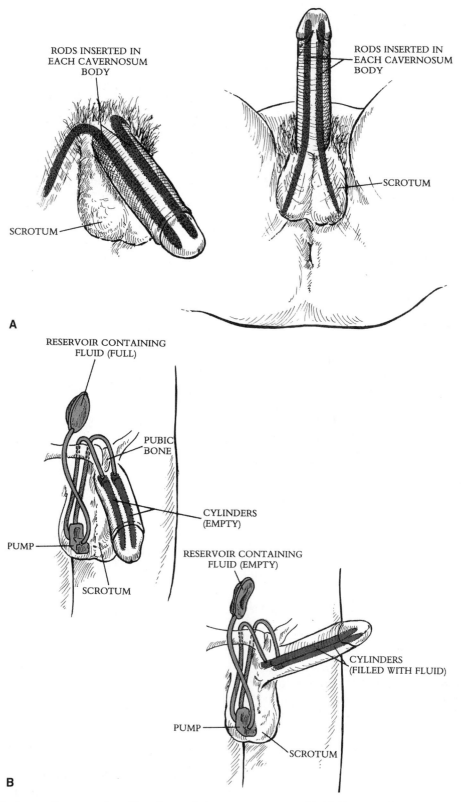

Penile prostheses can be of two types. **A,** In one type two semirigid silicone rods are implanted into the penis. **B,** In the second type two expandable cylinders are inserted into the penis and are connected by a tubing system to a fluid-filled bulb. (From Denney N, Quadagno D: *Human sexuality,* St. Louis, Mosby, 1988.)

Comparison of Inflatable and Semirigid Penile Prostheses

	Type of Prosthesis	
Factor	Semirigid	Inflatable
Ease of concealment	May need special briefs; noticeable in locker room or at public urinal	Little problem, although self-contained version may not lie down completely
Size of erection	Some loss of length and thickness	Normal thickness, some loss of length (self-contained version cannot add thickness)
Function during sexual intercourse	80–90% of patients satisfied	80–90% of patients satisfied
Infection during healing	Occurs in 1–2% of patients	Occurs in 1–2% of patients
Prosthesis erodes through spongy tissue inside penis	In <5% of patients	No problems
Prolonged pain after healing	Rare	Rare
Need to repair prosthesis	Rare	5–15% reoperation rates
Usual hospital stay*	2–4 days	2–5 days
Total costs*	$6,000–$10,000	$10,000–$12,000

*Based on our experiences in 1987 with surgery performed under a general anesthesic.
From Schover L: Sexuality and cancer: for the man who has cancer, and his partner, New York, American Cancer Society, 1988. Additional data from references 58 and 63 and from the web sites listed in the appendix to this chapter.

intimate relationships.[75] This population is generally young (15–34 years old) and in a crucial stage in life, and cancer treatment produces organic problems and sexual anxieties leading to dysfunction. When more treatment than unilateral orchiectomy is necessary, sexual dysfunction increases. Extensive surgery (retroperitoneal lymph node dissection [RLND]), radiation, and chemotherapy may cause erectile and orgasmic dysfunction.[75] To prevent sexual dissatisfaction, the couple should be educated and encouraged with the following information (this does not include fertility information):

- Stress the fact that normal sexual desire and pleasurable sensations, erection, and orgasm will probably continue. If sexual desire is lost, serum testosterone should be checked; replacement therapy may be needed.
- α-Adrenergic-stimulating drugs can increase ejaculation and occasionally the intensity of orgasm for some patients who have had RLND.[15]
- Loss of a testicle can cause embarrassment; however, this can no longer be remedied by a silicone prosthesis because they have been removed from the market.
- Reinforce the fact that the cancer is not contagious through sexual activity and that radiation therapy will not contaminate the partner.
- For those patients with permanent erectile difficulties, see the suggestions under prostate cancer and penile implants.
- Encourage both partners to ask directly for the type of caressing and touching they prefer.[56]

- Remind the patient that often people feel awkward and anxious when resuming sexual activity, but sexual relations, if physiologically possible, may resume about 6 weeks after pelvic surgery.
- If retrograde ejaculation is a problem because of RLND and cannot be reversed, there is a technique that can be used to harvest sperm after orgasm. Postorgasmic urine is immediately voided into a sterile container, and viable sperm cells are centrifuged out. They are then placed in a nutrient solution which prepares them for use in artificial insemination.[60]
- Sperm banking may be an option worth exploring if the number and motility of the sperm are adequate. This is costly, and the success of future artificial insemination is not guaranteed. If the patient is interested, however, sperm banking must be done before chemotherapy begins or between the first and second treatments.

Penis

Penile cancer, although very rare, results in the greatest risk of sexual dysfunction. Partial or total penectomy is usually needed to control the cancer. If partial-penectomy is done, the penile stump usually becomes erect with stimulation and is long enough for intercourse with antegrade ejaculation. If the entire glans penis is removed, a perineal urethrostomy is created behind the scrotum.[71] When it is stimulated to orgasm, ejaculation takes place through the perineal urethrostomy. Counseling for this man and his partner must include reassurance that both can be satisfied in several different ways:

- Some couples may wish to use a phallic-shaped vibrator as a substitute penis for partner satisfaction.
- If total penectomy has occurred, stimulation of the mons pubis, perineum, and scrotum can produce orgasms with pleasurable contractions in the remaining cavernous musculature.[65]
- If partial penectomy has occurred, men report erections and orgasms of normal or near normal intensity with the phallic stump.[71]
- Female partners must be advised (without instilling avoidance of sexual contact) to have a yearly Papanicolaou (Pap) smear, because they may be at increased risk for cervical cancer from exposure to the human papillomavirus.[63]

Cystectomy

Sexual dysfunction after cystectomy is similar to that after radical prostatectomy. The surgery is similar except that with radical cystectomy, urethrectomy may be included, which further damages penile innervation or blood flow. The other major difference is that a urinary diversion must be done, which can result in the need for an ostomy appliance. Many patients choose to have a continent internal urinary reservoir or ileocolonic neobladder, and those men are reported to remain more sexually active than men with appliances.[29]

In addition to the interventions mentioned previously, following are a few ways to decrease anxiety from a urostomy:

- Before intercourse, the appliance should be emptied. Some patients secure the bag with a supportive belt.
- Like women, men may choose to wear a cover over their ostomy bag. Men may also wish to wear provocative underwear (silk boxer shorts) and expose only their genitalia during intercourse.
- To avoid friction on the stoma and pouch, other positions besides the missionary position may be tried.
- Some patients like to have their stomas touched during lovemaking, but they must be reminded that the stoma is fragile and too much rubbing may cause tearing. Objects should not be placed into the stoma.
- Male pelvic cancer patients, like their female counterparts, must be treated with tenderness and understanding during the time of diagnosis, treatment, and long-term adjustment. Although many suggestions for mechanical aids and alternatives have been forthcoming, it is also important to remember the common expressions of affection and love.

Colorectal Cancer

Physiologic and Body Image Alterations. Surgery for colorectal cancer often has a profound effect on body image and sexual responsiveness. Because of the societal taboos centered around eliminative functions, many men and women feel disgusted that their feces are now eliminated through an opening on their abdomen.[68] Women undergo feelings of having been violated, whereas men experience the surgery as castration or mutilation.[29, 68] Some patients report embarrassment because they equate the cleaning of their stomas with masturbation. Others are distressed because they have no "vacation" from stoma maintenance. They must always make sure that there are adequate facilities for cleaning themselves in private; consequently, leisure activities may be compromised.[68]

Regardless of the type of surgical diversion performed (colostomy, ileostomy, or urinary diversion), patients express many common reactions. These reactions may include (1) greater-than-expected fatigue and weakness; (2) feelings of fragility and vulnerability to harm; (3) despair at the initial viewing of the stoma; (4) feelings of invalidism and depression; (5) fear of accidents, odor, leakage, and staining; (6) excessive emotional investment in the stoma; and (7) feelings of lost personal control.[68] Understanding and support from the nurse are important for healthy recovery. If the nurse is not an ostomate herself, the patient may receive great reassurance from a fellow ostomate. Members of the United Ostomy Association will visit the patient on request, both before and after surgery, and substantially reduce anxiety and depression. Rehabilitation is of utmost importance to these patients, so they are able to reenter the mainstream of life with a good self-image and self-confidence.

Nursing Management

COLORECTAL CANCER

Interventions

Many patients with colon cancer are not ready to talk about their sexuality and sexual activity immediately after surgery. Many say that sex is one of the farthest things from their mind. The subject should at least be broached so patients will feel more comfortable thinking about their sexuality and will feel freer to ask questions at a later date.

Sexuality education is more readily available for ostomates and their partners than for many cancers (see Resources in Appendix 33-A at the end of this chapter). The following methods may be useful:

- Prepare the pouch before sexual activity by emptying and ensuring the seal. If the ostomy is dry or controllable with irrigation, a small cover or patch may be sufficient cover.
- Deodorize the pouch (1 or 2 drops of Banish is helpful) and avoid foods that cause gas.

- Test out comfortable positions (e.g., lateral scissors position, rear entry).
- Wear attractive camouflage like a cummerbund or cloth cover for the pouch.
- To protect from leakage, a rubber sheet may be placed under the sheet and a towel on top of the sheet.
- Underwear with an opening up the center is provocative and also provides a cover.
- Men may experience retrograde ejaculation after surgery and should be warned of this to prevent thoughts that "things aren't working quite right."
- Penile implants are an option for men unable to have an erection.
- Most important, a good sense of humor is necessary, because accidents will happen. The couple may even consider rehearsing for when that time comes. Encourage them to "save water and shower with a friend."

Lung Cancer

Physiologic and Body Image Alterations. Unlike many other malignancies discussed in this chapter, lung cancer has a less optimistic prognosis unless it is diagnosed in the early stages and surgery is performed. Even if disease is outside the lung, treatment with chemotherapy and radiation therapy is producing longer intervals of controlled disease.[31] Little is realized in the literature in relation to psychosocial issues and the person with lung cancer. Some researchers are including sexuality issues within their studies (e.g., loss of libido), but there are no specific sexuality studies in relation to people with lung cancer.[27] Reasons for this may be because these patients are often diagnosed with advanced disease that progresses rapidly and their performance status is often very poor.[7] Quality of life is always an important factor in relation to the person with cancer and should be especially important to those with a shortened life expectancy. Because treatment for these people is often palliative rather than curative, it is important to consider their feelings of masculinity, femininity, and self-esteem, along with the basic aspects of care such as pain control. Because of the often rapidly fatal nature of lung cancer, the patient and partner must make sig-

nificant decisions and adjustments, which often affects the patient's sense of self-esteem and worthiness if: (1) the patient has been a smoker, he or she will probably have tremendous feelings of guilt to overcome or deal with; (2) the patient's performance status is poor and remains so as a result of fatigue and weakness, he or she will be unable to continue as a productive member of the family; (3) the patient/partner decide to take treatment (chemotherapy, radiation therapy), energy must be expended to cope with the side effects; and (4) the patient/partner decide not to take treatment, there will be issues to resolve such as coping with an early death and caregiving. In regard to treatment decisions, Bernhard and others explain that, to the person with lung cancer, treatment is often associated with hope. "This allows active efforts in dealing with the course of disease and helps cancer patients manage free-floating anxiety."[8] Given all of these anxiety-producing symptoms, side effects, and treatment regimens to deal with, it is not surprising that Bernhard and others report that patients with lung cancer tend to withdraw socially.[8] All of these factors will have an effect on the relationship the patient has with a partner, and it is no wonder that there may be little time, energy, or desire for intimacy.

Nursing Management

LUNG CANCER

Interventions

The nurse should encourage lung cancer patients and their partners to experience sexual closeness that does not necessarily lead to intercourse, which can exacerbate excessive fatigue and dyspnea. Along with the other interventions mentioned in this chapter, the following suggestions may be helpful:

- When experiencing sexual closeness, the significant other should continue to treat the patient as a partner rather than an invalid. These are the few moments when the patient can feel like a real person again.
- Make sure the significant other can be near to the patient when in an office setting or in a hospital bed.
- Being physically close, hand holding, sharing an intimate moment will enhance feelings of maleness and femaleness, especially when the patient is getting treatment or is hospitalized.

- Soft caressing or light massage with oils or creams is sensual and can help reduce pain and discomfort.
- Mutual masturbation while watching adult movies promotes intimacy and conserves energy.
- Decrease environmental irritants, perfumes, colognes, and hairsprays that can trigger bronchospasm.
- Take extra pillows and covers off the bed to allow the patient to feel less "closed-in."
- Making love on a pad on the floor may help remove the fear of sinking into a soft surface and not getting enough air.
- Avoid long kisses on the mouth, which can create a fear of not getting enough air to breathe.
- Avoid positions that put pressure on the chest and restrict breathing.
- Consider the use of a waterbed. Movement of the water will move the patient without much effort, and reduce exertion during sex.

SPECIAL ISSUES INFLUENCING SEXUALITY

The Gerontologic Patient

Even though much of society finds it difficult to believe that their parents and their elderly grandparents are engaging in sexual activity, Lauman and coworkers report that in a survey of people between 55 and 59 years of age, 42% of 89 respondents were sexually active a few times per month; 17% were having sex two to three times per week. Older people often face a double bias about their sexuality. It is assumed that "old" people are (1) too ill to be thinking sexually and (2) incapable of sexual activity. If attitudes such as these prevail, chances are few that sexual issues will be considered in these patients' general health care.[66]

We must reflect on our own attitudes about sexuality and the aging population and ask ourselves some questions. How do I feel about my elderly parents or grandparents having sex? If I see two elderly people kissing and fondling each other, how do I react? (Fig. 33–4).

When providing sexual counseling for older adults, the nurse should be aware that all couples will not be interested in sexual activity. Respect for this option is necessary. However, the nurse should make sure that the couple is not abstaining because that is what is expected of them.

Various methods of sexual relating besides vaginal intercourse should be discussed with an older couple. For those patients who still have the desire for sexual involvement, the nurse may wish to encourage the following:

- A weak back or muscles can be helped by exercising those muscles. This will also make the person feel more sexually attractive.
- A nutritional diet using the Food Guide Pyramid can prevent depression and apathy, which may decrease sexual performance and interest.
- For the partners to achieve lubrication and erection, longer precoital stimulation may be needed to compensate for slowed physical response.

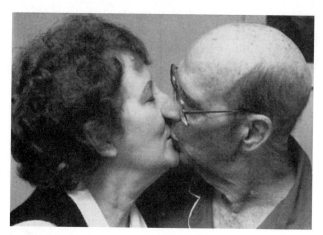

FIGURE 33–4 Henry and Margie share a tender moment.

- Because of musculoskeletal changes, various positions for intercourse should be tried to promote comfort and save energy.[61, 62]
- Both partners may not achieve orgasm; however, sexual pleasuring can still be enjoyed. Also the male may have little or no ejaculate.[38]
- During prolonged hospitalization or nursing home confinement, privacy should be provided for couples to hold, touch, fondle, and have intercourse if desired. This holds true for couples of any age.
- Warm baths, gentle massage, caressing and touching, masturbation, and fantasy all provide a sense of satisfaction and reassurance.
- Cleanliness, skin care (makeup, perfume, aftershave), hair care, mouth care, and attractive clothing can enhance feelings of masculinity and femininity.

The Gay/Lesbian Patient

It must never be assumed that all patients have or wish to have a partner or that all partners are of the opposite sex. It is the nurse's responsibility to be knowledgeable about the entire patient population and not to be judgmental. All patients are entitled to competence and a caring attitude. This is not always easy, however, because the literature that offers information concerning the gay/lesbian cancer population is limited. There are several books on counseling gay/lesbian people/couples; however, few are written specifically in relation to cancer care.[11, 21, 32] It is also not always clear that the patient is homosexual.[67]

The sociocultural structure of gay relationships differs from that of lesbians. Six types of sociosexual relationships have been identified for the male, ranging from one-night stands to stable cohabitation or "marriage."[21] Less is known about lesbian relationships, but there is less promiscuity and more lesbians marry.[11] The gay/lesbian sexual repertoire and erotic positions are similar to those of heterosexuals except when limited by identical anatomy. As with heterosexuals, the precancer sexual relationship has an important effect on the stability of the postcancer relationship. Those gays and lesbians involved in a permanent sexual relationship usually have fewer problems. If the patient has been diagnosed with cancer and still has to "cruise" (look for a sexual partner), it will be as difficult to deal with the new body image as it is for the heterosexual patient. Because of inexperience in the area of sensitivity to behavioral cues, staff may be unsuccessful in obtaining information about sexual orientation because they do not ask the right questions. Rather than asking about a spouse, husband, or wife, the nurse can ask whether the patient is sexually active or has a significant other.[37] Questions about sexual activity may deal with sexual preference such as "Do you prefer sexual activity with women, men, or both?"[67] Mapou tells us that ". . . most clients are not offended by such questions and those who are gay or lesbian are likely to appreciate the candor."[37] The nurse should treat the significant other as a spouse and involve the individual in the treatment process. This is likely to promote self-confidence and self-esteem in both members of the couple.[37]

In a group of gay patients with testicular cancer, one man expressed worry that his homosexuality caused his testicular cancer. Others were embarrassed at the lack of semen at ejaculation and did not know how to explain this to their partner.[59] Gay ostomates may wish to use their stomas as receptacles for intercourse, and they must be emphatically cautioned against this practice. The stoma is fragile and can tear and bleed.

The Patient Experiencing Spinal Cord Compression

All cancers have the propensity to metastasize to other areas of the body including the spinal cord, and most of the cancers dealt with in this chapter can cause problems of this nature. Because the literature on rehabilitative medicine and nursing has dealt extensively with the issue of sexuality and the paralyzed patient, this chapter will not address the topic. The reader is referred to the list of resources in the appendix at the end of this chapter for information.

STERILITY, INFERTILITY, AND PREGNANCY

It has been reported that 5% of new cancer cases occur in patients age 34 years or younger, and this means that each year approximately 5000 or more patients will be treated for cancer during their reproductive years.[5] The patient's age, gender, and stage of development and the type, dose, and duration of therapy are all integral factors in relation to reproductive tissue damage. Many concerns are reported in relation to reproductive damage and future capacity; they include (1) abnormal sexual development, impaired sexual performance, and infertility; (2) potential damage to germ cells producing chromosomal changes; (3) transmission of the cancer-bearing gene to offspring; (4) problems with childbearing capabilities; and (5) likelihood for marriage.[52, 63] Cancer transmission has not been reported except for genetic forms of cancer. Increased spontaneous abortion with combination (radiation and chemotherapy) therapy is known to occur.[52, 63] The young cancer survivor tends to be less likely to marry than the average person.

Generally, male fertility is more susceptible to early damage than female fertility because of the constant mitotic cycles needed for spermatogenesis compared with the relative inactivity of the female oocyte. Testes are more susceptible to injury than are ovaries because rapidly dividing cells are most often affected by cancer therapies. Consequently, many chemotherapy agents alone, and especially in combination, can cause azospermia, oligospermia, or permanent sterility.[15] Alkylating agents such as nitrogen mustard, cyclophosphamide, and chlorambucil cause sterility in the majority of treated male patients. However, depending on the drugs used, drug dose, and length of treatment, fertility may return, and the time frame can vary from 15 to 49 months after completion of therapy.[65, 72] Comparisons of different chemotherapy combinations are reported by Averette and others, and one study showed that 3 of 21 patients in a nitrogen mustard, Oncovin, procarbazine, prednisone (MOPP) regimen had return of spermatogenesis, whereas all patients in an Adriamycin, bleomycin, vinblastine, dacarbazine (ABVD) group showed recovery.[72] "Several reports suggest decreased sensitivity to chemotherapy-induced gonadal toxicity in the prepubertal testes compared with the adult testes."[72] Successful pregnancy is often limited because of abnormalities of the pretreatment sperm specimen. However, with the advent of assisted reproductive technologies (ART) such as in vitro fertilization (IVF), gamete intrafallopian transfer (GIFT), and zygote intrafallopian transfer (ZIFT), men with lower than normal sperm concentration can take advantage of semen cryopreservation.[72]

Again, age plays a role for the woman concerning possible ovarian dysfunction after treatment with chemotherapy because there are progressively fewer germ cells in the aging ovary. Averette and others reported on several studies that used multiagent chemotherapy such as MOPP; 49% of patients experienced ovarian failure, and 34% had irregular ovarian activity, some of which progressed to complete ovarian failure. An age-dependent effect was noted because 89% of the patients with amenorrhea received treatment after age 25.[5]

As with boys, the ovarian function of prepubertal girls seems less susceptible to damage from chemotherapy. One other major concern for women is cancer and pregnancy. Harris reports that 1 in 1800 pregnant women will have cancer and all forms of neoplasms are found during pregnancy, with breast, cervical, ovarian, lymphoma, and colorectal occurring most frequently.[28] In making a decision whether to treat the patient during pregnancy, several factors should be considered: (1) "gestation age of the fetus; (2) maternal and fetal health at the time of diagnosis; (3) mother's prognosis and likelihood of future pregnancies after treatment; and (4) the known teratogenic effects of the drugs to be used."[80] If the administration of chemotherapy is initiated after the first trimester, surprisingly few complications are associated with treatment. Also, pregnancy after chemotherapy is not usually discouraged although some oncologists are concerned about recurrence facili-

tated by hormonal and immunologic changes. Because little scientific data support these worries, women should consider ultimate prognosis and the desire for children.

Finally, the children of patients treated with chemotherapy must be considered. No known studies are available that show an increase in congenital anomalies or other diseases in these children. One study that followed a subset of children up to 12 years (median follow-up, 2.5 years) showed growth, development, and school performance to be normal.[35] If the parent is treated with a combination of chemotherapy and radiation therapy, there appears to be more complications of pregnancy. Wives of male patients have more spontaneous abortions, and female patients have more offspring with a variety of problems. Many scientists feel that prolonged observation must be done to better define the possible mutagenic nature of chemotherapy and radiation therapy in these children.

ASSESSING AND PRESERVING THE SEXUAL HEALTH OF THE CANCER PATIENT

Nursing Assessment Techniques

When performing a sexual health assessment, several elements can enhance both the nurse's and the patient's comfort during the discussion.[36] Key elements that will promote optimal patient teaching can be found in Box 33–2.

There are several different approaches to sexual history taking. Three sets of questions are presented here.

McPhetridge includes assessment of the effects of the illness on sexuality as a part of the nursing history. For our purposes, these questions might read as follows[41]:

- Has having cancer (or its treatment) interfered with your being a mother (wife, husband, father)?
- Has your cancer (or its treatment) changed the way you see yourself as a man (woman)?
- Has your cancer (or its treatment) caused any change in your sexual functioning (sex life)?
- Do you expect your sexual functioning (sex life) to be changed in any way after you leave the hospital?

Kolodny and others recommend general basic questions in the original contacts with patients when it is known that sexuality is likely to be affected by treatment. The focus in this brief sexual history is on sexual functions[30]:

1. Are you sexually active? (If "yes," then 2.)
2. What is the approximate frequency of your sexual activity?
3. Are you satisfied with your sex life? (If "no," then proceed.) Why not?

BOX 33-2

Sexual Health Assessment

Privacy is essential when doing the assessment. If the patient is not in a private room, move to another area if possible. An office, conference room, or a vacant patient room is preferable.

Assure the patient of confidentiality. This tends to decrease the level of anxiety markedly. Usually it is good to include the partner, but it may be necessary to meet privately with the patient at first to establish rapport.

Try to obtain a sexual history early in your association with the patient (see the approaches described in text). This implies that sexuality is an important and natural part of good health. Fatigue and how it can affect the patient's sexual activity may be included during an explanation of chemotherapy side effects. In this way one can introduce the concept, talk about it somewhat, and come back to it without making the patient uncomfortable.

Avoid overreaction in your verbal and nonverbal communication. Wide eyes and an open mouth are not conducive to trust. Also try not to be bored. Listening with genuine interest helps to convey acceptance.

Move from less sensitive to more sensitive issues.

Determine the patient's goals for treatment.

Realize when a problem is too complex to handle or when you do not know enough to be therapeutic and refer the problem on (e.g., clinical nurse specialist, psychologist, sexual rehabilitation counselor).

For Men

4. Do you have difficulty obtaining or maintaining an erection?
5. Do you have difficulty with control of ejaculation?

For Women

6. Do you have difficulty becoming aroused?
7. Do you have any difficulty having orgasm?

For Both Men and Women

8. Do you have pain with intercourse?
9. Do you have any questions or problems?

VerSteeg describes an early assessment approach that is more comprehensive and addresses the following areas[76]:

Couple's relationship. What kind of relationship is it? What are its strengths, resources, coping abilities, degree of closeness, and importance of sexual aspects?

Understanding of cancer and its treatments. What do they understand about the disease and its treatments? What is their understanding of the anatomy and physiology involved? What do they know about changes from therapy, its side effects, and their duration?

Impact on sexuality. What do they understand about the impacts of cancer and its treatment—physically, psychologically, and socially? What do they understand about effects on sexuality and fertility?

Preparation for changes. How do they want to prepare for expected changes? What kind of anticipatory guidance will help them be ready for common initial responses (anxiety and depression)? How can they explore alternatives, plan new responses, and communicate ideas and feelings?

Planning and participation in care. How does the person being treated want to participate in planning for hospital care? What are the mutual expectations between patient and staff for self-care in the hospital and later at home? How will the partner be involved? What is the patient's investment in various facets of care? What is the nature of support needed and how can the partner respond to that need?

Control and optimism will help. What kinds of support will help the patient have a sense of control and optimism or hope regarding self, body, environment, and the unknowns involved in the situation?

Expansion of sexuality. How does the couple want to expand their perceptions of sexuality and potential sexual activities? What are the best avenues of new learning for them, and in what order? Do they want information in printed form? Discussion with the nurse or with others who have had similar therapy? Do they want exercises to explore new behaviors together?

The PLISSIT is a model frequently used for sexuality counseling or a nursing intervention. Each step is taken depending on the nurse's knowledge and comfort level[13]:

P = permission. This promotes discussion and encourages the couple to continue in their present pattern of sexual activity plus suggests some risk taking.

LI = limited information. Includes the permission already given plus some new information specific to their sexuality concerns.

SS = specific suggestions. May include new activities for the couple, which may entail "homework."

IT = intensive therapy. This is when the couple is referred on to a therapist for more intense treatment.

A more complete model has been created by Schain.[53] Her model uses eight letters, PLEASURE, to cue the nurse to the topic area and to represent a good feeling. For a more in-depth explanation of this method, see Schain's article[53]:

P = *partner*. Is there one, how many, what kind of relationship? Problems identified and recommendations will depend on whether there is a partner or not.

L = *lovemaking*. What are the motives for being sexually active? Permission to engage in autoerotic behavior may be helpful.

E = *emotions*. What is the patient's attitude about the illness and sexual problems? If underlying psychological problems surface, referral may be appropriate.

A = *attitude*. What is the "norm" of sexual activity for this patient and what are your own values?

S = *symptoms*. An explicit explanation of the problems in regard to the three phases of the sexual response cycle is needed here.

U = *understanding*. What are the etiologic factors (intrapsychic, physiologic, relationship) contributing to the problem?

R = *reproduction*. What is the desire to have children, and if this ability is eliminated, how does that affect the patient's life goals?

E = *energy*. How does the problem interfere with the individual's overall psychological and sexual comfort, and do they want formalized sexual counseling?

PRESERVING INTIMACY

Today patients survive longer after their treatment for cancer. Survivorship means that the nurse must look with the patient to rehabilitation. In sexual rehabilitation, the nurse's goal of helping to restore the patient's sexual function is followed closely by the goals of restoring self-image and self-esteem. Each patient's sexuality is unique and is reflected in touching, smelling, hearing, tasting, and visual stimulation. These create for the patient and partner their own special intimacy, sense of affection, and physical gratification. Many references have been made and suggestions given in this chapter, but when there are *no* acceptable alternatives within a relationship, it is the nurse's duty to normalize this choice and help the couple use their own coping strategies and strengths. The values and beliefs of the couple are important to the use and success of various alternatives. What may be an acceptable expression for some may not be for others. Sometimes all they need is to be given permission to try something different. Encourage them to take the risk, and be there to support them.

CONCLUSION

As health care professionals continue to struggle to understand and be comfortable with their own sexuality, cancer patients continue to ask for help in dealing with disease- and treatment-related to sexual issues. In this situation it is important to extend our efforts beyond the disease and focus on the whole patient. For all of us, receiving sexual pleasure and closeness is linked to a sense of belonging and worthiness. Being accepted is intimately bound to self-esteem. As one author put it, "self-esteem is the sum total of all our feelings about ourselves . . . it is the reputation we share of ourselves with ourself."[12]

Chapter Questions

1. Once patients are diagnosed with cancer, they may be concerned about several issues related to *sexuality* including which of the following?
   a. Denial of cancer disease
   b. Complexity of chemotherapy regimen
   c. Altered body image, self-esteem, impact on femininity or masculinity, and sexual function
   d. Potential for disease spread or death

2. When people are ill, they begin to doubt their sexual identity. All of the following may impact this feeling *except*:
   a. Embarrassment to raise questions about sexual concerns due to the cancer disease
   b. The effect the illness will have on their ability to respond sexually (male and female)
   c. A wish to belong and receive approval, which is associated with receiving sexual pleasure
   d. Disinterest in sex because it is not important in our society

3. The person who has experienced limb amputation as a result of cancer may face several sexual problems that inhibit a sexual relationship including:
   a. Amputee fetishism
   b. Body position during intercourse
   c. Phantom pain sensation
   d. All the above

4. Potential sexual concerns with long-term effects for the patient with a hematologic malignancy include:
   a. Myelosuppression related to fatigue, infection, and bleeding.
   b. Ovarian dysfunction, testicular dysfunction, potential infertility.
   c. Intermittent nausea and vomiting, increased weakness.
   d. Hair loss related to the side effects of chemotherapy.

5. Patients' sexuality concerns related to reproductive damage include:
   a. Damage to germ cells, transmission of cancer-bearing genes, childbearing, finances

b. Infertility, childbearing, damage to germ cells, finances

c. Damage to germ cells, childbearing, infertility, marriage likelihood

d. Infertility, damage to germ cells, transmission of cancer-bearing genes, pain

6. Older couples are often still sexually active and require the following discussion about sexuality regarding:

a. Longer precoital stimulation and various different positions for intercourse may need to be tried due to slowed physical response and musculoskeletal changes.

b. Exercise and massage will not enhance a sexual relationship at this late life stage.

c. Because either or both partners may not achieve orgasm, sex is no longer important.

d. Privacy is not needed during hospitalization, because couples should not engage in sexual intimacy.

7. Appropriate interventions for sexuality concerns of patients with head and neck cancer include:

a. Use artificial saliva or sugarless mints to freshen stale breath and prevent tooth decay.

b. Use scented candles, perfumes, and aftershaves to enhance sexual intimacy.

c. Use of a fancy nightgown with a high neck or a dickey to cover the tracheostomy site.

d. All the above.

8. Alternate methods to sexual intercourse may need to be tried after surgery for many of the female patients with genital cancer during and after the area has healed. All of the following may be included *except*:

a. Close encounters such as cuddling, nudity (taking a bath together), and general pleasuring with massage

b. The best solution is to give up a sexual relationship with a partner and to masturbate if becoming sexually frustrated.

c. New positions may need to be used, such as female on top to control penile thrusting and comfort.

d. Oral-genital relations, mutual masturbation, and love-play or fantasy may be acceptable to some patients/couples.

9. Men who experience pelvic genital concerns often feel demasculinated and unlovable. Potential intervention(s) to enhance the man's perspective on his masculinity include:

a. Encourage aspects of arousal, intimacy and foreplay.

b. Always wear a condom.

c. Avoid use of penile injection or vacuum devices to provide erection.

d. Limit discussions regarding sexuality concerns.

10. Nursing diagnosis categories related to sexuality include:

a. Coping, moving, perceiving, valuing

b. Relating, valuing, moving, perceiving

c. Comfort, perceiving, relating, valuing

d. Mobility, relating, valuing, perceiving

BIBLIOGRAPHY

1. Aboseif S and others: Role of penile vascular injury in erectile dysfunction after radical prostatectomy, *Br J Urol* 73:75, 1994.

2. Anastasia PJ: Altered sexuality. In Carroll-Johnson RM, Gorman LM, Bush NJ, editors: *Psychosocial nursing care along the cancer continuum,* Pittsburgh, Oncology Nursing Press, 1998.

3. Anderson B, Golden-Kreutz D: Sexual self-concept for the woman with cancer. In Baider L, Cooper CL, Kaplan De-Nour A, editors: *Cancer and the family,* New York, Wiley, 1996.

4. Anderson BL, Woods XA, Copeland LJ: Sexual self-schema and sexual morbidity among gynecologic cancer survivors, *J Consult Clin Psychol* 65:221, 1997.

5. Averette H, Boike G, Jerrel M: Effects of cancer chemotherapy on gonadal function and reproductive capacity, *CA Cancer J Clin* 4:4, 1990.

6. Bello LK, McIntire S: Body image disturbances in young adults with cancer: implications for the oncology clinical nurse specialist, *Cancer Nurs* 18:138, 1995.

7. Bernhard J, Ganz P: Psychosocial issues in lung cancer patients (part 1), *Chest* 99:1, 1991.

8. Bernhard J, Ganz P: Psychosocial issues in lung cancer patients (part 2), *Chest* 99:2, 1991.

9. Brunner DW and others: Vaginal stenosis and sexual function following intracavitary radiation for the treatment of cervical and endometrial carcinoma, *Int J Radiat Oncol Biol Phys* 27:825, 1993.

10. Burt K: The effects of cancer on body image and sexuality, *Nurs Times* 91:36, 1995.

11. Butler S, Rosenblum B: *Cancer in two voices,* Duluth, MN, Spinsters, 1991.

12. Cantor R: Self-esteem, sexuality and cancer-related stress, *Front Radiat Ther Oncol* 14:51, 1980.

13. Cooley M, Yeomans A, Cobb S: Sexual and reproductive issues for women with Hodgkin's disease: application of PLISSIT model, *Cancer Nurs* 9:248, 1986.

14. Corney RH and others: Psychosexual dysfunction in women with gynecological cancer following radical pelvic surgery, *Br J Obstet Gynecol* 100:73, 1993.

15. Crenshaw JL, Goldberg JP: *Sexual pharmacology,* New York, Norton, 1996.

16. Curtis T, Zlotglow I: Sexuality and head and neck cancer, *Front Radiat Ther Oncol* 14:26, 1980.

17. Daeffler RJ: Mucous membranes. In Gross J, Johnson BL, editors: *Handbook of oncology nursing,* ed 2, Sudbury, MA, Jones & Bartlett, 1994.

18. Daniluk J: *Women's sexuality across the life span,* New York, Guilford Press, 1998.

19. Donahue V, Knapp R: Sexual rehabilitation of gynecologic cancer patients, *Obstet Gynecol* 49:118, 1977.
20. Ducharma S, Gill K: Sexual values, training and professional roles, *J Head Trauma Rehab* 5:2, 1990.
21. Dworkin SH, Gutierrez FJ: *Counseling gay men & lesbians: journey to the end of the rainbow,* Alexandria, VA, American Counseling Association, 1992.
22. Eifel P, Berek J, Thigpen JT: Gynecologic tumors. In DeVita VT, Hellman S, Rosenberg SA, editors: *Cancer: principles and practices of oncology,* ed 5, Philadelphia, Lippincott-Raven, 1997.
23. Gantz PA and others: Life after breast cancer: understanding women's health-related quality of life and sexual functioning, *J Clin Oncol* 16:501, 1998.
24. Gantz PA: Sexual functioning after breast cancer: a conceptual framework for future studies, *Ann Oncol* 8:105, 1997.
25. Geary ES and others: Nerve sparing radical prostatectomy: a different view, *J Urol* 154:145, 1995.
26. Ghizzani A and others: The evaluation of some factors influencing the sexual life of women affected by breast cancer, *J Sex Marital Ther* 21:57, 1995.
27. Ginsberg ML and others: Psychiatric illness and psychosocial concerns of patients with newly diagnosed lung cancer, *Can Med Assoc J* 152:701, 1995.
28. Harris B: Issues in nursing care of pregnant patients with cancer. In Lowdermilk D, editor: *NAACOG's clinical issues in perinatal and women's health nursing,* Philadelphia, Lippincott, 1990.
29. Klopp AL: Body image and self-concept among individuals with stomas, *J Enterostomal Ther* 17:98, 1990.
30. Kolodny R, Masters W, Johnson V: *Textbook of human sexuality,* Boston, Little, Brown, 1979.
31. Kris MG: Lung cancer cure, care and cost: let the data be your guide, *J Clin Oncol* 15:3027, 1997.
32. Laird J, Green RJ: *Lesbians and gays in couples and families: a handbook for therapists,* San Francisco, Josey-Bass, 1996.
33. Lamb MA: Effects of cancer on sexuality and fertility of women, *Semin Oncol Nurs* 11:120, 1995.
34. Laumann EO and others: *The social organization of sexuality: sexual practices in the United States,* Chicago, University of Chicago Press, 1994.
35. Li F: Genetic studies of survivors of childhood cancer, *Am J Pediatr Hematol Oncol* 9:104, 1987.
36. MacElveen-Hoehn P: Sexual assessment and counseling, *Semin Oncol Nurs* 1:69, 1985.
37. Mapou R: Traumatic brain injury rehabilitation with gay and lesbian individuals, *J Head Trauma Rehab* 5:2, 1990.
38. Masters W, Johnson V, Koloday R: *Heterosexuality,* New York, Harper Perennial, 1994.
39. Masters W, Johnson V: *Human sexual response,* Boston, Little, Brown, 1966.
40. McDaniel SH, Hepworth J, Doherty WJ: *Medical family therapy: a biopsychosocial approach to families with health problems,* New York, BasicBooks, 1992.
41. McPhetridge L: Nursing history: one means to personalize care, *Am J Nurs* 68:73, 1968.
42. Medhat A, Huber P, Medhat M: Factors that influence the level of activities in persons with lower extremity amputation, *Rehabil Nurs* 15:13, 1990.
43. Meistrich M, Vassilopoulou-Sellan R, Lipshultz L: Gonadal dysfunction. In DeVita VT, Hellman S, Rosenberg SA, editors: *Cancer: principles and practices of oncology,* ed 5, Philadelphia, Lippincott-Raven, 1997.
44. Minarik P: Psychosocial intervention with ineffective coping responses to physical illness: depression related. In Barry P, editor: *Psychosocial nursing,* ed 3, Philadelphia, Lippincott, 1996.
45. Monga U: Sexuality in cancer patients, *Phys Med Rehabil: State of the Art Rev* 9:417, 1995.
46. Nishimoto PW: Sex and sexuality in the cancer patient, *Nurs Pract Forum* 6:221, 1995.
47. North American Nursing Diagnosis Association: *Nursing diagnoses: definitions and classification,* Philadelphia, Author, 1996.
48. Ofman U: Psychosocial and sexual implications of genitourinary cancers, *Semin Oncol Nurs* 9:286, 1993.
49. Pickard-Holly S: The symptom experience of alopecia, *Semin Oncol Nurs* 11:235, 1995.
50. Pierce A and others: Pharmacologic creation with intracavernosal injection for men with sexual dysfunction following irradiation: a preliminary report, *Int J Radiat Oncol Biol Phys* 21:677, 1991.
51. Renshaw D: Beacons, breasts, symbols, sex and cancer, *Theor Med* 15:4, 1994.
52. Schahin MS, Puscheck E: Reproductive sequelae of cancer treatment 2, *Obstet Gynecol Clin North Am* 5:423, 1998.
53. Schain W: A sexual interview is a sexual intervention, *Innovations Oncol Nurs* 4:2, 1988.
54. Schain W: Sexual problems of patients with cancer. In DeVita VT, Hellman S, Rosenberg SA, editors: *Cancer: principles and practice of oncology,* ed 2, Philadelphia, Lippincott, 1985.
55. Schain WS and others: Mastectomy versus conservative surgery and radiation therapy: psychosocial consequences, *Cancer* 73:1221, 1994.
56. Schnarch DM: *Passionate marriage: keeping love and intimacy alive in committed relationships,* New York, Norton, 1997.
57. Schover L, Jensen S: *Sexuality and chronic illness,* New York, Guilford Press, 1988.
58. Schover L, Montague D, Lakin M: Psychologic aspects of patients with cancer: sexual problems of patients with cancer. In DeVita VT, Hellman S, Rosenberg SA, editors: *Cancer: principles and practices of oncology,* ed 5, Philadelphia, Lippincott-Raven, 1997.
59. Schover L, von Eschenbach A: Sexual and marital counseling with men treated for testicular cancer, *J Sex Marital Ther* 10:29, 1984.
60. Schover L: *Sexual problems in men with pelvic or genital malignancies: workshop on psychosexual and reproductive issues affecting patients with cancer,* San Antonio, TX, American Cancer Society, January 1987.
61. Schover L: *Sexuality and cancer: for the man who has cancer, and his partner,* ed 3, Atlanta, American Cancer Society, 1999.
62. Schover L: *Sexuality and cancer: for the woman who has cancer, and her partner,* ed 3, Atlanta, American Cancer Society, 1999.

63. Schover L: *Sexuality and fertility after cancer,* New York, Wiley, 1997.

64. Schover L: The impact of breast cancer on sexuality, body image, and intimate relationships, *CA Cancer J Clin* 41:112, 1991.

65. Shell J, Bell K, Dougherty M: Gonadal toxicities. In Liebman M, Camp-Sorrell D, editors: *Multimodal therapy in oncology nursing,* St. Louis, Mosby, 1996.

66. Shell J, Smith C: Sexuality and the older person with cancer, *Oncol Nurs Forum* 21:553, 1994.

67. Shell J: Do you like the things that life is showing you? The sensitive self image of the person with cancer, *Oncol Nurs Forum* 22:907, 1995.

68. Shell J: The psychosexual impact of ostomy surgery, *Progressions: Developments in Ostomy and Wound Care* 4:5, 1992.

69. Shell JA, Miller ME: The cancer amputee and sexuality, *Orthopedic Nurs,* September-October, 53, 1999.

70. Shipes E, Lehr S: Sexuality and the male cancer patient, *Cancer Nurs* 5:375, 1982.

71. Smith D, Babian R: The effects of treatment for cancer on male fertility and sexuality, *Cancer Nurs* 15:271, 1992.

72. Sweet V, Servy EJ, Karow AM: Reproductive issues for men with cancer: technology and nursing management, *Oncol Nurs Forum* 23:51, 1996.

73. Thranov I, Klee M: Sexuality among gynecological cancer patients—a cross-sectional study, *Gynecol Oncol* 52:14, 1994.

74. Urken MI and others: Functional evaluation following microvascular oromandibular reconstruction of the oral cancer patient: a comparative study of reconstructed and nonreconstructed patients, *Laryngoscope* 101:935, 1991.

75. Van Basten JP and others: Sexual functioning after multimodality treatment for disseminated nonseminomatous testicular germ cell tumor, *J Urol* 158:1411, 1997.

76. VerSteeg M: Options for sexual expression. In von Eschenbach P, Rodriguez D, editors: *Sexual rehabilitation of the urological cancer patient,* Boston, Hall, 1981.

77. Walsh PC, Partin AW, Epstein JI: Cancer control and quality of life following anatomical radical retropubic prostatectomy: results at 10 years, *J Urol* 152:1831, 1994.

78. Walters AS, Williamson GM: Sexual satisfaction predicts quality of life: a study of adult amputees, *Sex Disabil* 16:103, 1998.

79. Waxman E: Sexual dysfunction following treatment for prostate cancer: nursing assessment and interventions, *Oncol Nurs Forum* 20:1567, 1993.

80. Weeks D: Acute leukemia and pregnancy. In Lowdermilk D, editor: *NAACOG's clinical issues in perinatal and women's health nursing,* Philadelphia, Lippincott, 1990.

81. Weijmar Schultz WCM and others: Psychosexual functioning after the treatment of cancer of the vulva, *Cancer* 66:402, 1990.

82. Weiss K: *Women's experience of sex and sexuality,* Center City, MN, Hazelden Educational Materials, 1992.

83. Whittelsey FC: The secrets about sex, *Mamm,* May, 49, 1999.

84. Williamson GM, Walters AS: Perceived impact amputation on sexual activity: a study of adult amputees, *J Sex Res* 33:221, 1996.

85. Zacharias DR, Gilg CA, Foxall MJ: Quality of life and coping in patients with gynecological cancer and their spouses, *Oncol Nurs Forum* 21:1699, 1994.

86. Zinreich E and others: Pre- and post-treatment evaluation of sexual function in patients with adenocarcinoma of the prostate, *Int J Radiat Oncol Biol Phys* 19:3, 1990.

APPENDIX: RESOURCES

Literature

Literature on rehabilitation for the patient with spinal cord compression:

Christina Mumma, editor: *Rehabilitation nursing: concepts and practice,* ed 2; available from Rehabilitation Nursing Foundation, 2506 Gross Point Road, Evanston, IL 60201.

Kolodny R, Masters W, Johnson V: *Textbook of human sexuality for nurses,* Boston, Little, Brown, 1979.

Literature with reference to sexuality issues:

Johnson J, Klein L: *I can cope: staying healthy with cancer,* Minneapolis, MN, DCI, 1988.

Noyes D, Mellody P: *Beauty and cancer,* Los Angeles, AC Press, 1988.

Schover L: *Sexuality and cancer: for the woman who has cancer, and her partner,* ed 3, Atlanta, GA, American Cancer Society, 1999.

Schover L: *Sexuality and cancer: for the man who has cancer, and his partner,* ed. 3, Atlanta, GA, American Cancer Society, 1999.

Literature to recommend to patients:

Altman C: *You can be your own sex therapist: a systematized behavioral approach to enhancing your sensual pleasures and improving your sexual enjoyment,* Casper, 1997.

Barbach L: *For each other: sharing sexual intimacy,* New American Library, 1984.

Rako S: *The hormone of desire,* Harmony Books, 1996.

Richman J: *I'm not in the mood,* William Morrow, 1998.

Good Vibrations/Sexuality Library, "Catalog of Toys." Open Enterprises, Inc, 938 Howard Street, Suite 101, San Francisco, CA 94103-4163. 800-284-8423.

Literature on sexuality education for ostomates is available for a small charge from the United Ostomy Association, Inc, 19772 MacArthur Boulevard, Suite 200, Irvine, CA 92612, 800-826-0826.

Web Sites

The Sexual Health Information Center, www.sexhealth.org.
Medic Impotence Research Center, www.en.com/medic/impotence.html.
ONCOLINK; Cancer and sexuality, http://cancer.med.upenn.edu/psychosocial/sexuality.

American Association of Sex Educators, Counselors and Therapists (AASECT), www.aasect.org.

Power Surge-Information about Menopause, www.power-surge.com.

Support Groups

Support groups for head and neck cancer patients are often sponsored by the American Cancer Society, such as "The Lost Chord" for laryngectomies.

One of the first support groups in the country for amputees was founded in the Kansas City area by Lou Keyes and is called LEAPS. This stands for Lower Extremity Amputees Providing Support; the telephone number is 816-361-3206. This group also has access to information about support groups nationwide.

"Reach to Recovery" is a voluntary group of mastectomy patients sponsored and trained by the American Cancer Society (ACS). The ACS is located in most cities in the United States.

Prostate cancer support groups (ACS). Man to Man.

Personal Articles

Head covers: Headliner, Designs for Comfort, Inc, PO Box 671044, Marietta, GA 30066, 800-443-9226.

Tracheostomy covers may be obtained from Byram Health Care Center, Inc, Tracheo-stoma Bibs, 75 Holly Hill Lane, Greenwich, CT 06380, 800-354-4054.

Breast prostheses:

Capital Marketing, "Nearly Me," silicone-gel; 800-887-3370.

B & B (formerly, Bosom Buddy), all fabric, weight adjustable breast form: PO Box 5731, Boise, ID 83705, 800-262-2789.

Vaginal dilators: Syracuse Medical Devices, Inc, 214 Hurlburt Road, Syracuse, NY 13224, 315-449-0657, fax, 315-449-0756. Cost of dilator: extra small, $7.60; small, $7.40; medium, $8.40; large, $9.40.

Vaginal lubricants/moisturizer:

Astroglide Lubricant and Silken Secret Vaginal Moisturizer, Bio Film, Inc, 3121 Scott Street, Vista, CA 800-848-5900. Professional samples available.

Lubrin Vaginal Suppositories, Bradley Pharmaceuticals, 800-929-9300. Professional samples available.

Glossary

ABO compatibility testing is required for whole blood; red blood cells; testing is preferred for fresh-frozen plasma.

absolute risk the number of specific cancer cases (breast) in a given population divided by the number of people (women) in the population—may be expressed as an average risk for every woman in that group.

accreditation a standardized program for evaluating health care organizations to ensure a specified level of quality, as defined by a set of standards.

acquired immunity specific and depends on the recognition of self and nonself.

active immunotherapy the administration of biologic or chemical products that stimulate the immune system of the host.

adjuvant chemotherapy chemotherapy designed to eradicate microscopic foci of metastatic disease after local control with surgery, radiation therapy, or both.

adoptive immunotherapy (passive immunotherapy) the direct transfer of cells or products of the immune system to a host.

allogeneic having cell types that are antigenically distinct.

allograft a graft of tissue between individuals of the same species but of different genotype, called also *allogenic graft.*

anaphase a stage of mitosis in which the chromosomes begin to move apart toward opposite poles of the spindle.

anaplasia the loss of structural organization and useful function of a cell.

aneuploid having more or less than the normal diploid number of chromosomes.

antibody an immunoglobulin protein produced by plasma cells and B cells in response to antigen, which has the ability to combine with the antigen that stimulated its production.

antigen a molecule that is specifically recognized by antibody and by cells of the adaptive immune system.

assault an intentional act that is designed to make the victim fearful and produces reasonable apprehension of harm.

autonomy is the right of a person to make independent decisions about personal affairs (determine their own course of action, according to a plan they chose).

attributable risk the number of cancer cases in a population that are associated with a given risk factor and that could potentially be prevented by alteration or removal of that factor.

autologous related to self, designating products or components of the same individual organism.

azotemia an excess of urea or other nitrogenous bodies in the blood.

B cells (B lymphocytes) cells derived from bone marrow stem cell in humans, capable of responding to antigen by the production of antibody.

battery the touching of a person by another without permission; any intentional, unwanted, unprovoked, harmful physical contact by a person on another person.

beneficence a person has the duty to take active positive steps to help others; prevent or remove harm.

biological response modifier (BRM) an agent that can modify host reactions against disease, with resultant potential to prevent progression of cancer or metastatic spread; includes, but not limited to, immunotherapy.

biotherapy treatment with agents derived from biologic sources or affecting biologic response.

blast cell an immature form of a blood cell or a normal embryonic cell.

cachexia malnutrition with overall general poor health.

cancer control a term including the entire spectrum of cancer care: prevention; screening; early detection; diagnosis; treatment; rehab; and palliation.

cancer in situ early stage cancer; before the invasion of surrounding tissue; usually implies total cancer removal with surgical incision or biopsy.

capitation a type of risk sharing reimbursement method whereby providers in the network receive fixed periodic payments for health services rendered to plan members.

capillary leak syndrome shift of fluid from the intravascular space resulting in accumulation of fluid in the extravascular space; symptoms include hypotension, tachycardia, and weight gain.

carcinogenesis the production or origin of cancer.

case management a utilization management technique frequently used by third-party and self-insured employers to monitor and coordinate treatment for specific diagnoses; particularly those of high cost.

CD4 cell cell expressing the CD4 protein on its surface, primarily cells of the immune system, particularly T helper cells (T4 cells) and monocytes/macrophages.

CD8 cell cell expressing the CD8 protein on its surface, primarily a subpopulation of T cells, particularly cytotoxic T cells (T8 cells) and suppressor T cells.

cellularity the ratio of hematopoietic (blood-forming) tissue to adipose tissue in the marrow.

cell-mediated immunity involving specifically immune T cells and cells of the natural immune system (natural killer [NK] cells and monocytes/macrophages), particularly important to the body's defense against viral-infected cells and malignant cells.

chemotactic the movement of an organism or an individual cell, such as a leukocyte, in response to a chemical concentration gradient.

cocarcinogen an agent that becomes carcinogenic when it interacts with a cancer-causing agent.

colony-stimulating factor (hematopoietic growth factor) a group of hormone-like glycoproteins that are secreted by a wide range of cells in the body and on which the processes of hemopoiesis depend; substances that stimulate growth or orderly maturation of cells of the hematopoietic system; commitment process by which components of the hemopoietic hierarchy increasingly lose the potential to differentiate into alternative cell lines.

complete carcinogens have initiating and promoting properties, so that exposure to a complete carcinogen can cause malignant transformation without additional exposure to an additional promoter.

confidentiality handling of information in a way that contributes to patient care and does not disclose information.

contact inhibition the growth and movement of a normal cell stops when it comes in contact with another cell.

credentialing the process of checking a practitioner's references and documenting their credentials, including training, experience, demonstrated ability, licensure, and malpractice insurance; to ensure qualified practitioners with demonstrated competence have practice privileges.

criteria relevant measurable indicators of the standards of clinical nursing practice.

culture a set of values, beliefs, and rules for behavior; provides structure for meaning and decision-making.

cytokine a protein hormone of the immune system that is responsible for communication with other cells of the immune system or with cells outside this system.

cytokinesis the changes that occur in the cytoplasm during mitosis, meiosis, and fertilization.

cytostatic suppresses cell proliferation.

cytotoxic able to kill cells.

deafferentation the elimination or interruption of afferent nerve impulses, as by destruction of the afferent pathways.

diaphanoscopy examination with the diaphanoscope; transillumination.

differentiation to develop a specialized shape, character, or function that differs from that of other cells or tissues; usually implies a loss of malignant nature.

diploid an individual or cell having two full sets of homologous chromosomes.

DNA a complex protein of high molecular weight, consisting of deoxyribose, phosphoric acid, and four bases (two purines, adenine and guanine, and two pyrimidines, thymine and cytosine). These are arranged as two long chains that twist around each other to form a double helix joined by bonds between the complementary system. Nucleic acid is present in chromosomes of the nuclei of cells and is the chemical basis of heredity and the carrier of genetic information for all organisms except the RNA viruses.

doubling time is the period of time required for a tumor mass to double in size.

dysphonia difficulty or pain in speaking.

dysplasia disturbance in the size, shape, and organization of cells and tissues.

effector cells cells of the immune system that mediate an immune response.

ELISA (enzyme-linked immunosorbent assay) capable of detecting either antibody or antigen by the binding of an enzyme coupled to either anti-Ig or antibody specific to the antigen; used to detect HIV antibodies.

enzymes proteins that act as a catalyst to induce or speed up chemical reactions inside or outside the cell.

epidemiologic approach examines the frequency of the disease among relatives.

extravasation an inadvertent leakage of blood, drug, from a vessel into the tissues.

felony a crime of serious nature usually punishable by imprisonment for 1 year or longer; or by death; may be prohibited from engaging in an occupation that requires a license.

fidelity an ethical rule that describes a person's duty to establish a mutual and reciprocal relationship.

gene therapy insertion of a functioning gene into a human cell to direct the natural antiviral human cell response; provides a new function to the cell.

genetic approach studies the pattern of disease expression among relatives.

genetics the study of heredity and possible genetic factors influencing the occurrence of a pathologic condition.

genome the complete set of hereditary factors, as contained in the haploid assortment of chromosomes.

genotype the entire set of genes one inherits from both parents.

glycoprotein any of a class of conjugated proteins consisting of a compound of protein with a carbohydrate group.

haplotype the group of alleles of linked genes contributed by either parent.

hematopoiesis the process by which blood cells are produced in the bone marrow.

hematopoietic pertaining to or affecting the formation of blood cells.

hemolytic destruction of blood cells, resulting in liberation of hemoglobin from the red blood cell.

heterogeneous derived from a different source or species; xenograft.

heterogeneity cancer cells that are different cells within the tumor and have different characteristics.

homeostasis the condition in which the external and internal environment of a cell remains relatively constant.

homogeneous composed of similar elements or ingredients; of a uniform quality throughout.

humoral immunity specific immunity activated by antibody found in blood and lymph; particularly important in trapping viral and bacterial organisms that have not yet invaded cells of the body.

hybridoma technology process by which fusion cells, produced by myeloma plasma cells, are introduced into an immunized mouse.

hyperbaric characterized by greater than normal pressure or weight; applied to gases under greater than atmospheric pressure; as hyperbaric oxygen.

hyperplasia an increase in the number of cells in a tissue or organ.

hypoguesic abnormally diminished acuteness of the sense of taste.

idiotype an antigenic determinant present on and characteristic of a certain antibody molecule, usually located in the variable region.

immunity a protective mechanism that serves to maintain the integrity of the body against foreign substances or agents.

immunogenic capable of stimulating an immune response.

immunoglobulin a glycoprotein composed of heavy and light chains that functions as antibody; in humans, the five classes are designated as IgG, IgA, IgM, IgD, and IgE.

immunomodulation alteration of the immune response to induce up-regulation, suppression, or tolerance.

immunosuppression blocking or diminishing the functioning of the immune system.

immunosurveillance a theory that postulates that the immune system plays an important role in the prevention of development of detectable cancer.

incidence the number of newly diagnosed cases of cancer in a specified period of time (calendar year) in a defined population.

indolent slow-growing tumor.

informed consent a person's agreement to allow something to happen: e.g. surgery; 5 basic steps: explanation of medical condition; purpose of the procedure/ treatment; treatment/procedure process; known risks, benefits, alternatives and consequences of not accepting treatment and the right to refuse consent or withdraw consent at any time.

initiation the first step in turning a normal cell cancerous as by drugs, chemicals, or other agents.

interferon (IFN) a class of cytokines originally identified for their ability to inhibit growth of viruses within cells; selectively inhibit the synthesis of viral RNA in infected cells; immunoregulatory functions, including enhancing the activities of macrophages and natural killer cells.

interleukin (IL) a class of cytokines produced by lymphocytes or macrophages in response to antigenic or mitogenic stimulation, which mediate communication among cells of the immune system.

interphase initial phase of mitosis; cells grow in size; chromosomes elongate; replication of DNA.

in vitro within a glass; observable in a test tube; in an artificial environment.

in vivo within the living body.

ionizing radiation a type of radiation that involves gamma rays that penetrate deeply into tissues; this form of radiation may have an enhanced biologic effect on tumors by degrading tumor DNA.

ipsilateral on the same side.

justice a basic ethical principle that describes the duty to give others what is due or owed to them.

karyotype the chromosomal constitution of the nucleus of a cell.

lentivirus any of a group of retroviruses, including those that cause maedi and visna in sheep.

leukoagglutinin an agglutinin directed against leukocytes.

leukocytosis a transient increase in the number of leukocytes in the blood, resulting from various causes such as hemorrhage, fever, infection.

libel written defamation; a false or malicious writing that is intended to defame/dishonor another person.

lymphocytapheresis the selective removal of lymphocytes from withdrawn blood, which is then retransfused into the donor.

lymphokine activated killer cell—effector cell capable of killing tumor cells; activated by cytokines derived from lymphocytes (lymphokine), particularly interleukin-2; has broad activity.

lymphotoxin a product of lymphocytes; lymphotoxin is toxic for certain tumor cells and shares several properties with tumor necrosis factor.

malpractice professional misconduct, improper discharge of professional duties; *failure to meet standard of care of a professional which resulted in harm.*

metaphase the stage of mitosis in which the chromosome becomes aligned between the centrioles.

metaplasia one adult cell type is substituted for another type not usually found in the involved tissue (e.g., glandular for squamous).

metastasis the spread of cells from a primary tumor via the lymphatic system or venous system to distant body parts where such cells give rise to tumor mass.

monoclonal antibody (moab) an antibody produced from a single clone of cells; mAbs recognize a specific antigen.

monocytosis increase in the proportion of monocytes in the blood.

monokines cytokines such as tumor necrosis factor released by mononuclear phagocytes.

morbidity the condition of being diseased or morbid; the sick rate; the ratio of sick to well persons in a community.

morphology the science of the forms and structures of organisms.

mortality the number of deaths attributed to cancer in a specified time period in a defined population.

multipotent progenitor cell an early component of the hematopoietic hierarchy that has undergone some degree of differentiation but still has the potential to develop into any of several of the cell lines and has limited self-replicative ability.

murine pertaining to or affecting mice or rats.

mutagen a substance that alters DNA in a cell.

myelophthisis invasion of the bone marrow by neoplastic elements.

myeloproliferative pertaining to or characterized by medullary and extramedullary proliferation of bone marrow constituents.

negligence the failure to exercise reasonable or ordinary amount of care in a situation that causes harm to someone or something.

neoadjuvant chemotherapy chemotherapy administered before other therapies.

neoplasm an abnormal mass of cells typically exhibiting progressive and uncontrolled growth; classified by the cell type from which they originate and their biologic behavior.

neuropathic functional disturbances or pathologic changes in the peripheral nervous system.

nonmaleficence a basic ethical principal that purports the duty of avoiding intentional conflict or harm.

nociceptive receiving injury.

oncogene a gene involved in the transformation of a normal cell into a malignant cell, or a gene that increases neoplastic properties of a cell.

osteoradionecrosis necrosis of the bone after irradiation.

outcome the result of service delivery including patient, staff, and organizational performances.

passive immunotherapy the direct transfer of cells or products of the immune system to a host.

phenotype the entire physical, biochemical, and physiologic makeup of an individual as determined both genetically and environmentally as opposed to genotype.

pleiotropic the quality of a gene to manifest itself in multiple ways.

plexopathy any disorder of a plexus, especially of nerves.

ploidy the aggressiveness of a neoplasm by analyzing the cellular DNA content.

pluripotent stem cell the most primitive of the blood cells in the hematopoietic hierarchy; these cells, as yet unidentified in humans, are the forerunners of all of the cell lineages; the pluripotent stem cell is characterized by infrequent cell cycling and the ability to self-replicate.

precursor cell a nucleated cell that is morphologically recognizable as belonging to a specific lineage and that gives rise immediately to the mature components of the circulating blood.

prevalence measurement of all the cancer cases, both old and new, at a designated point in time.

primary prevention measures taken to ensure that cancer never develops (e.g., decreasing the number of new smokers).

peer review a system by which colleagues evaluate each other for clinical practice and professional performance.

process criteria descriptions of major sequence of events and activities required to obtain desired outcomes.

process the manner in which service will be delivered; procedures, practice guidelines/protocols, action plans, and documentation systems describe process.

progenitor cells an early ancestor of the mature components of the blood; pluripotent stem cells are called also *common progenitor cells.*

prophase the second phase of mitosis, in which the DNA coils and the centrioles move to opposite poles.

prospective in advance; usually with respect to utilization: admissions and/or payment.

provirus the genome of an animal virus integrated into the genetic material of a host cell.

radiobiology that branch of science that is concerned with the effect of light and ultraviolet and ionizing radiations on living tissue or organisms.

randomized to make random for scientific experimentation.

recombinant DNA technology process by which there is identification of a gene for a specific substance; the gene is then cloned and inserted into a bacterium that then serves as a factory to produce the desired substances (IL-2, TNF, IL-1).

refractory not readily yielding to treatment.

relative risk the incidence of cancer (breast) in a population (women) with a known or suspected risk factor (genetic) divided by the incidence rate of cancer (breast) in a population (women) without that risk factor (genetic).

reticuloendothelial pertaining to tissues having both reticular and endothelial attributes.

retinoid any derivative of retinol, whether naturally occurring or synthetic.

retrovirus a large group of RNA viruses that carry reverse transcriptase.

reverse transcriptase an enzyme that catalyzes RNA-directed polymerization of DNA.

risk management a comprehensive program of activities to identify, evaluate, and take corrective action against risks that may lead to patient or employee injury, property loss or damage; financial/legal liability.

RNA (ribonucleic acid) a part of the messenger system through which DNA controls protein production within the cell.

secondary prevention measures used for detecting and treating early diagnosed cancer while in its most curable stage.

sequestration isolation of a patient; the net increase in the quantity of blood within a limited vascular area.

seroconversion the change of serologic test from negative to positive, indicating the production of detectable, circulating antibodies.

simian pertaining to, characteristic of, or resembling an ape or monkey.

somatic growth factors substances that regulate growth of nonblood cells in the body; this is a more diverse and less well understood system, with positive and negative regulation (insulin-like, epidermal, and platelet-derived growth factors).

standard a written value defining the rules, actions, results, or analyses that are related to the patient, staff, or system and that are sanctioned by an authority.

standard of practice a written value statement that defines the rules, actions, or conditions that direct patient care.

stem cell a cell with unlimited reproductive capacity; daughter cells may differentiate into other cells.

stereotactic pertaining to or characterized by precise positioning in space, said especially of discrete areas of the brain that control specific functions.

stratification the art or process of stratifying; developing different levels.

structure the circumstances under which a service will be delivered; the organization's mission, philosophy, goals, and policies define its structure.

structure criteria descriptions of the environment and resources needed to achieve desired outcomes.

suppressor T cells a subset of T lymphocytes that reduces the activity of other T and B cells.

syngeneic having identical matched cell type.

tachyphylaxis a rapidly decreasing response to a drug or physiologically active agent after administration of a few doses.

T cells (T lymphocytes) thymus-dependent cells that are involved in a variety of cell-mediated immune responses.

telangiectasis the spot formed most commonly on the skin by a dilated capillary or terminal artery.

telophase the final phase of mitosis, in which migration of chromosomes to cells is complete.

tenesmus straining, especially ineffectual and painful straining at stool or in urination.

teratogen a substance causing mutation in a developing fetus.

thermography a technique wherein an infrared camera is used to photographically portray the surface temperatures of the body, based on the self-emanating infrared radiation.

threshold (for evaluation) a preestablished level or pattern of performance related to an indicator at which further evaluation of the quality and appropriateness of an important aspect of care is initiated.

tort a wrong done to another person (civil opposed to criminal) that does not involve a contract.

transcription the normal cellular response of turning a DNA gene copy into messenger RNA (mRNA).

translocation   an interchange in which one segment of a chromosome is transferred to another chromosome, generally the result of breakage and abnormal reattachment.

trending   analyzing the results of numerous studies on the same indicator to identify patterns that may influence the quality of outcomes related to the important aspect of care or service being monitored.

tumor marker   a product produced by a cancer cell or in response to the presence of cancer, which may be released into the circulation or may remain associated with the cancer cell.

tumor necrosis factor (TNF)   produced primarily by activated macrophages; TNF is cytostatic or cytotoxic for some neoplastic cells, induces hemorrhagic necrosis of some tumors, and has a range of activities similar to lymphotoxin.

unipotent progenitor cell   early component of the hematopoietic hierarchy that has undergone further differentiation and is committed to one or two cell lines.

veracity   means telling the truth; give information regarding the nature and prognosis of illness/treatment.

Western blot   an immunoassay used for measuring antiviral antibody responses, useful for distinguishing antibody responses to specific viral proteins; frequently used as a confirmatory test for HIV status.

window phase   the time between the dates of actual exposure leading to infection and development of detectable serum antibodies.

Test	Purpose	Normal Values (Adult)	Nursing Action
Arterial blood gases (ABGs)	Assess respiratory status, acid–base balance.	pH, 7.35–7.45; $Paco_2$, 35–45 mm Hg; Pao_2, >70 mm Hg; HCO_3^-, 23–28; BE, 0 ± 3 mEq/L; Sao_2, >93% Fio_2	Mark laboratory slip as for any O_2 therapy at time sample collected. Send specimen on ice to laboratory immediately. Apply pressure on puncture site for 5 min. Include respiratory rate and O_2 therapy status when reporting ABG results to physician.
CHEMISTRY			
Electrolytes			
Calcium (Ca^{++})	Assess renal, neuromuscular bone status; parathyroid, thyroid function; increased levels with bone metastasis.	8.5–10.5 mg/dL	Observe for increased or decreased neuromuscular activity with Ca^{++} level <7 mg/dL or >13 mg/dL.
Ionized calcium	Serum ionized calcium level is *not* affected by changes in serum protein/albumin concentrations and it reflects calcium metabolism better than total calcium values.	4.4–5.9 mg/dL 2.2–2.5 mEq/L 1.1–1.24 mmol/L	
Chloride (Cl^-)	Assess renal status, acid–base balance.	95–100 mEq/L	Potassium replacement therapy should be accompanied by a 1:1 ratio of potassium to chloride.
Magnesium (Mg^{++})	Assess renal, metabolic, neuromuscular status, GI losses, alcoholism.	1.4–2.3 mEq/L	Assess antacid ingestion. If increased levels, observe and implement seizure precautions.
Phosphorus (P)	Assess renal, parathyroid function, bone status.	2.5–4.5 mg/dL	Assess dietary intake (e.g., starvation).
Potassium (K^+)	Assess renal status, endocrine, cardiac function, acid–base balance.	3.5–5.0 mEq/L	Monitor higher or lower level for potential cardiac toxicity; if increased level, metabolic acidosis.
Sodium (Na^+)	Assess renal status, endocrine function, acid–base balance.	135–145 mEq/L	Monitor fluid intake/output; implement precautionary safety measures if <120 mEq/L; decreased levels with metabolic alkalosis.
Albumin serum Prealbumin	Assess renal and nutritional status. Assess nutritional status.	3.5–5.0 g/dL (20-d half-life) 17–42 mg/dL (short half-life)	Provides an analysis of protein changes during previous 2 d.
Bilirubin	Assess hepatic, biliary tract, or hemolytic function; hemorrhage, drug toxicities, blood transfusion.	Total: 0.2–1.2 mg/dL Direct: 0.1–0.4 mg/dL Indirect: 0.1–0.8 mg/dL	
Calcitonin serum	Assess malignancy of thyroid.	50–500 pg/mL High-risk: Male: 25 Female: 35	
High-density lipoproteins (HDLs)		Moderate-risk: Male/female: 45–55 Low-risk: Male/female: 60–70	
Cholesterol	Assess hepatic, pancreatic, biliary tract, thyroid function. Assess risk of coronary heart disease.	Age 40+: 150–300 mg/dL Age 30–39: 140–270 mg/dL Age 20–29: 120–240 mg/dL	High-fat, high-sugar diet may alter results. Test preparation usually requires a 12–14 h fast after eating a low-fat meal.

Table continued on following page

Laboratory Values *Continued*

Test	Purpose	Normal Values (Adult)	Nursing Action
Copper serum	Assess hepatic function.	70–165 μg/dL	
Creatinine serum	Assess renal and urinary tract function, bone status; ARF profile: Increased BUN, creatinine, potassium; decreased sodium.	0.7–1.4 mg/dL	
Glucose serum	Assess pancreatic, liver, or endocrine status, diabetes mellitus, hypoglycemia, malabsorption, Cushing's syndrome.	Fasting (FBS) 65–110 mg/dL	NPO past midnight before test. Report glucose levels of <40 mg/dL or >400 mg/dL immediately. Eating and specimen collection schedules must be coordinated.
Glycohemoglobulin (Hemoglobin A₁c)	Assess pancreatic, liver, or endocrine status, diabetes mellitus.	2-h postprandial (2-h PP) glucose level should be within normal limits 4.3–6.1%	Provides steady state of blood glucose level over 4–6 wk.
Urea nitrogen blood (BUN)	Assess renal function, hydration status.	10–20 mg/dL	A ratio of BUN to serum creatinine of >10:1 may be suggestive of dehydration, GI bleeding, or decreased cardiac output.
Uric acid serum	Assess renal function; hypercalcemia.	Female: 2.2–7.7 mg/dL Male: 3.9–9.0 mg/dL	Monitor intake and output; observe for elevations with rapidly dividing cell destruction; administer appropriate interventions.
Triglycerides lipid profile test	Assess risk of coronary and vascular disease.	Adult/elderly: Female: 35–135 mg/dL or 0.40–1.52 mmol/L (SI units) Male: 40–160 mg/dL or 0.45–1.81 mmol/L (SI units)	
Guaiac (fecal) or occult blood, Hemoccult	Determine presence of blood that is not visible.	Negative	Instruct patient to abstain from red meats and vitamin C products for 48–72 h before test.
HEMATOLOGY			
Complete blood count (CBC)	Assess clotting status, response to infection and inflammation.	RBC, WBC, platelets	**Do not draw blood sample from same extremity as IV infusion.**
Red blood cells (RBC)	Assess anemias, hydration, oxygen transport; RBC fragmentation, acute leukemia/myelodysplasia.	Female: 4.2–5.5 mil/mm³ Male: 4.4–6.0 mil/mm³ Older adult: 3.5 mil/mm³	
Hematocrit (Hct)	Assess blood loss, hydration, hematologic disorders.	Female: 37–47% Male: 42–52%	
Hemoglobin (Hgb)	Assess blood loss, anemias, dehydration.	Female: 12–16 g/dL Male: 14–18 g/dL	
RBC indices	Assess anemias and polycythemia.		
Mean corpuscular hemoglobin (MCH) (normal color)	Assess chronic blood loss, lead poisoning.	28–34 pg Older adult: 28–32 pg	
Mean corpuscular hemoglobin concentration (MCHC)		30–40% Older adult: 29–33%	

Test	Normal Values	Purpose	Notes
Mean corpuscular volume (MCV) (size of RBC)	82–101 μg^3 Older adult: 90.5–105 μg^3	Assess anemia; bone marrow function.	
Reticulocyte count	Female: 0.5–1.5% of erythrocytes Male: 0.5–2.5% of erythrocytes	Assess amount of infection, inflammation, and healing.	
White blood cell count (WBC)	4,000–11,000/mm³	Determine presence of infection, inflammation, and stress.	Steroid drugs may suppress WBCs.
Differential neutrophils (polymorphonuclears [polys] or segmentals [segs])	42–66% or 3000–7000/μL Older adult: 43–79%		Granulocytes include neutrophils, basophils, and eosinophils. Monitor for neutropenia; implement measures to prevent or minimize infectious process.
Band cells (stabs)	3%	Assess presence of recent infection.	
Basophils	0.4–1.0% or 40–100/μL	Assess status of polycythemia vera, leukemias, Hodgkin's disease, allergic reactions, and stress.	
Eosinophils	1–3% or 50–400/μL Older adult: 0–0.3%	Assess response to ACTH or epinephrine or status of allergy, leukemia, Hodgkin's disease.	
Lymphocytes	25–33% or 1000–4000/μL Older adult: 11–48%	Assess status of infection, especially viral, and stress.	
Monocytes	0–9% or 100–600/μL Older adult: 1–5%	Assess status of bacterial phagocytosis and healing.	
Erythrocyte sedimentation rate (ESR)	Female: 0–30 mm/h Male: 0–20 mm/h	Assess nonspecific inflammation and tissue injury; malignancy, rheumatic fever, and arthritis; acute and/or chronic infections.	
Platelets	150,000–450,000/mm³	Assess bone marrow, clotting status; increases in advanced malignancy.	Monitor for thrombocytopenia. Implement measures to prevent or minimize bleeding. Moderate risk <50,000. Severe risk <20,000; potential for CNS hemorrhage.
Platelet adhesion		Assess platelet function.	
Platelet aggregation		Assess platelet function.	
Platelet volume	8–10 fl 2.5 μm in diameter	Determine platelet size; assess purpura, DIC, anemias.	
Ferritin serum	Female: 5–100 ng/mL Male: 10–270 ng/mL	Assess hematopoietic status; increased levels with neuroblastoma.	
Folic acid serum	4–16 ng/mL	Assess anemias.	
Iron serum	50–100 μg/dL	Assess anemias.	
Total iron-binding capacity (TIBC)	250–400 μg/dL	Assess amount of iron that could be carried if transferrin were completely saturated: anemias, chronic blood loss, and liver disease.	
Ham (acid serum test)	10–50% hemolysis of RBCs	Used to detect paroxysmal nocturnal hemoglobinuria.	
Coagulation factors			
Factor I: fibrinogen	60–100 mg/mL	Assess clotting status, hemophilia.	
Factor II: prothrombin	10–15 mg/dL		
Factor V: proaccelerin	5–10 mg/dL	Assess vitamin K deficiency.	Contraindications: persons with recent blood transfusions. Report abnormal results.

Table continued on following page

Test	Purpose	Normal Values (Adult)	Nursing Action
Factor VII: proconvertin		5–20 mg/dL	
Factor VIII: antihemophilic globin	Assess von Willebrand hemophilia A.	30–35 mg/dL	
Factor IX: thromboplastin	Assess hemophilia B (Christmas disease).	30 mg/dL	
Factor X: Stuart-Prower		8–10 mg/dL	
Factor XI: morphilic		20–30 mg/dL	
Factor XII: Hageman	Assess for DIC.	0 mg/dL	
Factor XIII: fibrin stabilizing	Assess for bleeding tendency.	1 mg/dL	
Coagulation time (Lee-White, clotting time)	Assess coagulation; monitor heparin therapy.	5–15 min	Assess for potential bleeding. Pressure may be required on puncture site for 5 min.
D-dimer	Confirms DIC.	Negative (no D-dimer fragments present); <250 ng/mL or 250 µg/L (SI units)	
Fibrin split products (FSPs)	Assess degree of coagulation.	<4 µg/ml	Monitor/report elevated levels of FSP.
Fibrin degradation products (FDPs)	Assess disorders (e.g., DIC).	<10	Monitor/report elevated levels of FDP.
Fibrinogen	Assess ability to form clots; to assess for leukemia, liver damage, DIC.	160–300 mg/dL Older adult: 470–485 mg/100 mL	DIC profile: decreased platelets, fibrinogen, plasminogen; increased PT, PTT, FDPs report results STAT.
Prothrombin time (pro time PT)	Assess coagulant activity of the "extrinsic" system including factors V, VII, X, fibrinogen, and prothrombin.	100%; also reported in seconds, approximately 11–15; varies with laboratory	Assess for potential bleeding. Pressure may be required on puncture site for 5 min. Report results as ratio of patient to control rather than seconds.
Plasminogen	Assess DIC.	73–122%	
Protamine sulfate	Assess coagulation, DIC.	Negative	
Activated partial thromboplastin time (APTT) or partial thromboplastin time (PTT)	Assess all plasma coagulation factors except VII and XII (e.g., stage II clotting disorders such as hemophilia).	APTT: 30–45 sec PTT: 16–25 sec	
Template B time (Bleeding time)	Assess coagulation, monitor theparin therapy	1–8 min.	
Thrombin clotting time (thrombin time; TT)	Assess factor III clotting.	10–20 sec or within 3 sec of control	
Agglutin febrile	Diagnose infectious disease, e.g., salmonella	No agglutination titers < 1:80	
Agglutin cold	Diagnose pneumonia, influenza, mononucleosis	No agglutination titers < 1:15	
Immunoglobulins	Assess immune system status.	Levels vary with age	Report abnormal results.
IgA	Assess for autoimmune disease.	65–650 mg/dL	
IgD	Assess for multiple myeloma.	0–30 mg/dL	
IgE	Assess for potential allergies.	0–200 ng/mL	
IgG	Assess for multiple myeloma.	600–1700 mg/dL	
IgM	Assess for hepatitis, mononucleosis, autoimmune disease, sarcoidosis	50–300 mg/dL	

ISOENZYMES

Test	Normal Value	Purpose	Comments
Acid phosphatase serum	<4 ng/mL	Assess prostate status, multiple myeloma, parathyroid, or renal function.	Usually done on a serial basis for 3 d. Elevated in 75% of patients with bone metastases.
Alkaline phosphatase (ALP) serum	30–115 mU/mL	Assess status of bone and of renal, hepatic, intestinal, and biliary tract; indicator for GVHD, osteogenic sarcoma.	NPO 8 h before test; food can raise levels up to 25%.
Amylase serum	20–110 mU/mL	Assess pancreatic, renal, or salivary gland.	
CPK serum	CPK: total Female: <51 mU/mL Male: <82 mU/mL CPK-MB bands 3% indicate cardiac damage. CPK-MM bands 97–100% indicate muscle damage. CPK-BB bands 0% indicate brain damage	Assess myocardial, muscle, and brain damage; infectious disease: HIV, hepatitis.	Elevation of MB bands 3–6 h after onset of acute myocardial infarction; peaks in 24 h.
Lactic dehydrogenase (LDH) serum	100–205 mU/mL	Assess hepatic, cardiac, renal, muscular, or RBC status.	Elevation seen 12–24 h after onset of acute myocardial infarction; peaks in 2–6 d; elevation may indicate high-risk leukemia and lymphoma and/or relapse of these diseases.
LDH₁ cardiac	14–26%		A flipped LDH$_1$/LDH$_2$ ratio with LDH$_1$ the highest indicates a myocardial infarction.
LDH₂ cardiac	27–37%		
LDH₃ pulmonary	13–26%		
LDH₄ hepatic	8–16%		
LDH₅ hepatic	6–16%		
Lipase serum	0–190 U/L	Assess pancreas.	
Aspartate aminotransferase (AST) (formerly serum glutamic oxaloacetic transaminase [SGOT])	1–36 U/L	Assess status of many organs (e.g., liver, heart); cellular death (chemotherapy and radiotherapy).	Elevation seen 8–12 h after onset of acute myocardial infarction; peaks in 48 h.
Alanine aminotransferase (ALT) (formerly serum glutamic pyruvic transaminase [SGPT])	5–35 IU/L	Assess status of many organs (e.g., liver); cellular death (chemotherapy and radiotherapy); hepatitis, cirrhosis, mononucleosis.	

OTHER TESTS

Test	Normal Value	Purpose	Comments
Cerebrospinal fluid values	Albumin mean: 29.5 mg/dL + 112 SD: 11–48 mg/dL Bilirubin: 0 Cell count: 0–5 mononuclear cell per mm³ Chloride: 120–130 mEq/L	Assess cerebrospinal system; brain tumor, CVA, meningitis.	

Table continued on following page

APPENDIX B
Laboratory Values *Continued*

Test	Purpose	Normal Values (Adult)	Nursing Action
OTHER TESTS *continued*			

		Glucose: 50–75 mg/dL
		IgG mean: 4.3 mg/dL + 112 SD: 0–8.6 mg/dL
		Protein
		  Lumbar: 15–45 mg/dL
		  Cisternal: 15–25 mg/dL
		  Ventricular: 5–15 mg/dL
			Sterile procedure for specimen collection; send specimen to laboratory immediately. *Do not* refrigerate specimen, because refrigeration may inhibit growth of meningococcus organisms and alter test accuracy.

Estrogen receptor assay	Useful in determining the prognosis and treatment of breast cancer.	Negative: <10 fmol/mg of protein Positive: >10 fmol/mg of protein	
Progesterone receptor assay	Useful in determining the prognosis and treatment of breast cancer.	Negative: <10 fmol/g of tissue Positive: >10 fmol/g of tissue	
Prostate specific antigen (PSA)	Assess prostate disease.	Normal: 0–4 ng/mL BPH: 4–19 ng/mL Prostate cancer: 10–120 ng/mL	
Helicobacter pylori	Detect *H. pylori* infection in gastric mucosa	Negative	

Gastric analysis	Assess gastric function; carcinoma of stomach, pernicious anemia, and gastric atrophy.	Basal
		  Female: 2.0 + 1.8 mEq/h
		  Male: 3.0 + 2.0 mEq/h
		Maximal (after histalog or gastrin)
		  Female: 16 + 5 mEq/h
		  Male: 23 + 5 mEq/h
			NPO 8 h before; requires nasogastric tube insertion to collect specimen. Assess gag reflex after procedure.

Gastrin	Evaluate patients with peptic ulcer disease, Zollinger-Ellison syndrome, G-cell hyperplasia	Adult: <200 ng/L; levels are higher in elderly patients Child: <10–125 ng/L pH: 5.5–7.5 Amylase: over 1200 U total Trypsin: 35–160%	
Duodenal drainage	Assess for duodenal ulcer status.	Viscosity: 3 min or less Negative: usually drawn from different site to coincide with temperature elevation	
Blood cultures	Determine presence of pathogens.	Negative	Implement precaution measures for potential infection. Administer prescribed antibiotics.
Papanicolaou smear (Pap)	Assess cervical tissue for presence of disease.	Color, turbidity: clear	Collect three separate slide specimens.
Urinalysis	Screening tool; assess renal, endocrine status, infection.	Negative for glucose, ketones, blood, bile, protein, bilirubin, crystals, RBC, WBC Casts: not waxy; few hyaline, epithelial, or granular	Urine sample must be fresh for accurate results.
Specific gravity		1.010–1.025 (urine osmolarity should always be higher than blood serum osmolarity)	
pH		5.0–7.5	
Acetone	Levels are affected by vegetarian, fruit, meat in diet.	Negative	

Test	Purpose	Normal Values	Nursing Considerations
Amylase	Assess oncologic status; multiple myeloma.	24–76 μg/mL	
Bence-Jones protein	Assess parathyroid.	Negative	
Calcium		Negative	
Catecholamine	Assess renal system, Cushing's syndrome.	Epinephrine: <20 μg Norepinephrine: <100 μg Metanephrine: <1.3 mg Vanillylmandelic acid: <6 mg	Keep urine container on ice.
Creatinine clearance	Assess renal status.	75–125 mL/min Female: 0.8–1.8 g/24 h Male: 1.0–2.0 g/24 h	Collection container is kept on ice; collect all urine for 24 h.
Culture	Determine presence of pathogens.	Negative or <10,000 organisms/mL	Usually drawn serially from different sites to coincide with temperature elevation.
Urobilinogen urine	Assess GI malfunction.	Up to 1 mg in a 24-h specimen	Collection container is kept on ice.
24-h urine	Assess renal status.	Same as creatinine clearance	
Viruses	Determine presence of virus.		Implement infection precautions for positive virus results; report positive results for all viruses.
HTLV I	Detect T-cell leukemia.	Negative	HIV: 1—Seroconversion—usually occurs within 6 months of infection contact 2—Lymph node involvement 3—Progressive lymphadenopathy 4—a—ARC fever; weight loss b—Neuropathy changes c—Infectious disease d—Malignancy 5—Long-term nonprogression (LTNP); 5% of HIV population is LTNP. Viral load copies (burden) of HIV RNA copies >5000–10,000 copies/mL low-risk clinical progression >10,000–100,000 copies/mL moderate-risk clinical progression >100,000 copies/mL high-risk clinical progression
HTLV II	Detect hairy-cell leukemia.	Negative	
HTLV III	Detect retrovirus (HIV) AIDS.	Negative	
Herpes simplex	Detect herpes simplex virus I or II.	Negative	
Varicella zoster	Detect chicken pox, shingles.	Negative	
Cytomegalovirus	Detect pneumonia.	Negative	
Epstein-Barr	Detect infectious mononucleosis.	Negative	
Rubella	Detect measles.	Negative	
Tumor markers are listed in Chapter 4.			
Hepatitis			
A—Anti-HAV, IgM	Infectious hepatitis.	Negative	
B—HBsAg, HBeAg	Serum hepatitis.	Negative	
C—Anti-HCV	Posttransfusion non-A, non-B hepatitis.	Negative	
D—Anti-HDV	Delta virus.	Negative	
E—No test available	Enteric non-A, non-B hepatitis.	Negative	
G—No test available	Detected in 1–2% blood donors.	Negative	

Normal Term Newborn Blood Values

HEMATOLOGY

Hemoglobin	15–20 g/dL
Hematocrit	43–61%
WBC	10,000–30,000/mm^3
Neutrophils	40–80%
Immature WBCs	3–10%
Platelets	100,000–280,000/mm^3
Reticulocytes	3–6%
Blood volume	82.3 mL/kg (third day after early cord clamping)
	92.6 mL/kg (third day after delayed cord clamping)

CHEMISTRY

Sodium	124–156 mmol/L
Potassium	5.3–7.3 mmol/L
Chloride	90–111 mmol/L
Calcium	7.3–9.2 mg/dL
Glucose	40–97 mg/dL
IEM-PKU (inborn error of metabolism, phenylketonuria)	**<4 mg**
Bilirubin (capillary heel stick)	4–6 mg/dL (Bilirubin level peaks 3–5 d and should not exceed 13 mg/dL.)
Cord blood bilirubin	1.0–1.8 mg/dL

URINALYSIS VALUES

Protein	<5–10 mg/dL
WBCs	<2–3
RBCs	Negative
Casts	Negative
Bacteria	Negative
Specific gravity	1.001–1.025
Color	Pale yellow

Breast-milk jaundice: Bilirubin rises the 4th day after mature breast milk comes in; bilirubin peak of 20–25 mg/dL is reached at 2–3 weeks of age.

Selected Diagnostic Tests

Diagnostic Test	Purpose	Procedure/Preparation	After Procedure
Angiography	Used in various segments of the arterial system to determine vessel patency or the presence of an aneurysm, embolism, or arterial/venous malformations.	Assess for allergy to iodine preparation; NPO past midnight, sedation before procedure, local anesthesia before catheter insertion via fluoroscopy; contrast medium is infused via catheter; serial-timed radiographs are obtained.	A pressure dressing or sandbag may be applied to the entry site; monitor vital signs as ordered.
Barium studies	Assess for evidence of disease, anatomic abnormalities, malabsorption syndrome.	NPO status before test varies; 300–600 mL of contrast medium swallowed by patient for upper GI; lower GI preparation may include clear liquids, bowel prep of laxatives, suppositories, or enemas.	Large fluid intake is encouraged to promote barium excretion and minimize fluid loss.
Bone densitrometry	Determine bone mineral content and density, diagnose osteoporosis, osteopenia, multiple myeloma, and/or unexplained fractures.	Should *NOT* be performed within 10 days of barium studies because barium may falsely increase bone density in the lumbar spine. Remove all metallic objects (belt buckles, zippers, keys, coins,) that might be in the scanning path. Procedure takes about 30–45 min to perform.	Data are interpreted by radiologist.
Bone marrow biopsy	Examine the bone marrow for number, size, and shape of RBCs, WBCs, and megakaryocytes, estimation of cellularity, and determination of the presence of fibrotic tissue.	Aspiration of the marrow from the sternum, iliac crest, anterior and/or posterior iliac spine; proximal tibia in children; local anesthesia.	Apply pressure to puncture site; observe site for bleeding.
Bronchoscopy	Assess strictures, inflammation, or bleeding. Examine or remove pooled secretions and foreign bodies. Perform biopsy for analysis; place radiation beads for unresectable lung tumors.	NPO past midnight, sedation and atropine before procedure; fiberoptic bronchoscope inserted through nares.	Monitor vital signs; NPO status maintained until return of gag reflex.
Chest tomography	Allows visualization of a section ("slice") of lung at any vertical plane, shows characteristics of border, central area, and/or presence of calcification of a lung nodule, lung lesion, cavitation and/or metastasis.	No fasting is required. No special care required. Remove all metal objects.	Data are interpreted by radiologist.
Chest x-ray	Provide visualization of heart, lung, mediastinum, pulmonary vessels, trachea, bronchi, pleura, and diaphragm; assess response to therapy, location of monitoring catheters, pacemaker wires, etc., pleural effusions, neoplasms.	Optimal visualization requires that patient take in and hold a deep breath.	Data are interpreted by radiologist.

APPENDIX C
Selected Diagnostic Tests *Continued*

Diagnostic Test	Purpose	Procedure/Preparation	After Procedure
Cholangiogram IV	Visualization of the biliary ductal system; assess inflammation; presence of stones and/or obstruction.	NPO past midnight; bowel preparation; IV infusion of iodine dye. Assess that bilirubin level is <3.5 mg/dL so visualization is possible; if bilirubin is elevated, procedure may be cancelled.	Observe for allergic reaction from dye.
Colonoscopy	Examine the left, transverse, and right colon and sigmoid.	Clear liquid diet 1–3 d before; sedation and cathartics before exam, NPO past midnight; colonoscope inserted through anus.	Observe for unexpected bleeding.
Colposcopy	Provide direct visualization of the vagina, vulva, and cervical epithelium; to biopsy cervical tissue.	Colposcope is inserted into the vagina and advanced toward the cervix.	Monitor vital signs; observe for vaginal bleeding.
Computed axial tomography (CT scan)	Noninvasive procedure to analyze tissue for density, assess for evidence of disease, inflammation, displacement, or enlargement.	May require NPO status; may be performed with or without a dye injection; CT scanning provides a cross-sectional image.	Data are interpreted by radiologist.
Computed tomography portogram	Evaluate presence of disease in the chest, e.g., tumor, pneumonia, atelectasis, abscess, and/or pleural effusion.	Verify NON-allergy to iodinated dyes. NPO 4 h before test.	Evaluate response to test.
Culdoscopy	Permit observation of the uterus, fallopian tubes, ovaries, broad ligaments, rectal wall, and sigmoid colon from inside the cul-de-sac.	NPO past midnight; local, regional, or general anesthesia; surgical incision is made in the posterior vaginal wall; culdoscope is inserted into the vagina and passed through the incision into the cul-de-sac.	Monitor vital signs; observe for vaginal bleeding.
Cystoscopy	Permit direct examination of the urethra and bladder for strictures or bleeding sites; remove biopsy specimens of the prostate, bladder, and urethra; place ureteral catheters.	May require sedation or anesthesia before examination; cystoscope is inserted into the urethra and advanced into the bladder.	Monitor for urinary retention or bleeding and monitor vital signs.
Echocardiography	Assess congenital ischemic or acquired heart disease, presence of pericardial effusion, structure and mobility of heart.	Gel is applied to the skin, and the transducer is moved along the skin with some pressure. Heart valves and pericardial sac are examined.	Monitor vital signs.
Electrocardiography (12-lead ECG)	Record electrical activity within the heart.	Electrodes are attached to patient's chest and to each of the four extremities.	Observe patient status.
Electroencephalography (EEG)	Assess intracranial pathophysiology and organic brain syndrome and determine presence and type of epilepsy.	From 16 to 32 electrodes are applied to the head with electrode paste.	Assist with hair washing.
Endoscopic retrograde cholangiopancreatography (ERCP)	Assess suspected biliary duct pathology and pancreatic disease. Percutaneous transhepatic cholangiography (PTC) and ERCP are the only methods available to visualize the biliary tree in jaundiced patients.	NPO, sedative before procedure; IV access for medication administration; fiberoptic scope inserted for visualization.	Monitor vital signs; observe for bleeding; NPO status maintained until return of gag reflex.

Procedure	Purpose	Preparation/Procedure	Nursing Implications
Esophagoscopy with gastroscopy	Permit direct visualization of esophagus and stomach. Biopsy specimens, brushings, or washings may be obtained.	NPO, sedative before procedure; local anesthesia. Fiberoptic scope is inserted through the mouth.	Monitor vital signs; NPO status maintained until return of gag reflex.
I-125 fibrinogen uptake	Noninvasive test to identify suspected thrombus formation in the deep veins.	IV access for medication administration.	Monitor vital signs.
Immunoscintigraphy	Detect recurrent metastatic colorectal or ovarian cancer.	No fasting required; injection with radiolabeled monoclonal antibody (radionuclide indium chloride-111). Images are obtained in 48–72 hours; the procedure takes approximately 1 h each day for at least 1–4 d.	Same as nuclear scans. Encourage fluids.
Intravenous pyelogram (IVP)	Provide visualization of the kidneys, ureters, and bladder to determine abnormalities, obstruction, and/or hematoma.	Assess for allergy to iodine preparation; contrast medium is injected IV and concentrates in the urine; NPO for 12 h before examination; bowel prep may be required.	Monitor vital signs; encourage fluid intake.
Laparoscopy	Permit visualization of pelvis and intestines; ovarian biopsy or other surgical procedures may be performed as part of laparoscopy (e.g., lysis of adhesions, tubal ligation).	NPO past midnight; general anesthesia; a surgical incision is made and a trocar is inserted and then aspirated to ensure that intestine or large vessels have not been perforated; nitrous oxide or carbon dioxide may be inserted to create a pneumoperitoneum.	Monitor vital signs; observe for abdominal discomfort and bleeding.
Liver biopsy	Assess liver malfunction or disease.	NPO 6–8 h before; sedative before procedure; local anesthetic; needle insertion to obtain specimen.	Apply pressure to biopsy site; turn patient on right side; observe for bleeding; give vitamin K injection; monitor vital signs.
Lumbar puncture	Assess diagnosis of brain or spinal cord neoplasm, hemorrhage, meningitis, encephalitis, autoimmune disorders of CNS, and/or degenerative brain disease.	Sterile procedure; place patient in lateral decubitus (fetal) position; local anesthetic; obtain 3 sterile specimens.	Explain to the patient that he or she MUST lie still during the procedure; rest in bed (flat position) for 1 h after procedure.
Lymphangiography	Performed for staging purposes with lymphoma or to detect metastasis; to examine lymph vessels for obstruction.	Assess for allergy to iodine preparation: dye injected intradermally to test for allergy. If no apparent reaction, then give dye intravenously; serial-timed radiographs obtained.	Monitor vital signs; observe for respiratory distress.
Magnetic resonance imaging (MRI)	Noninvasive method for assessing tissue function and chemical composition of the body.	May require NPO status; contraindicated for patients with aneurysm clips or pacemakers because of magnetic field.	Ensure return of personal items (e.g., jewelry)
Mammography	Determine presence of benign or malignant breast disease and cysts and to guide needle biopsy.	Breast is placed between the camera and film and compressed for a clear image.	Data are interpreted by radiologist.
Mediastinoscopy	Allow visualization of mediastinum; potential biopsy of lymph nodes; to permit diagnosis and staging of cancer, infection, and sarcoidosis.	NPO past midnight; sedation before procedure; local or general anesthesia before insertion of mediastinoscope via incision at suprasternal notch.	Monitor vital signs; potential for bleeding and dyspnea; NPO status until return of gag reflex.
Myelography	Permit visualization of the subarachnoid space to detect abnormalities of the spinal cord and vertebrae and locate obstruction in the flow of cerebrospinal fluid (CSF).	NPO for 4 h before procedure; local anesthetic; needle inserted into lumbar space; contrast medium injected with timed serial radiographs.	Monitor vital signs and neurologic status; follow postprocedure body position orders.

Table continued on following page

APPENDIX C
Selected Diagnostic Tests *Continued*

Diagnostic Test	Purpose	Procedure/Preparation	After Procedure
Nuclear medicine scans Bone	Detect focal defects in the bone, infection, fractures; to assess disease process.	Assess for previous reaction to contrast media; requires IV access for injection of dye; serial radiographs are obtained; NPO and sedation may be required.	Encourage fluid intake to aid in urinary excretion of radionuclide.
Brain	Delineate subdural hematoma, arteriovenous malformation, thrombosis, abscess, neoplasms, glioma, or other metastatic tumors.	Assess for previous reaction to contrast media; requires IV access for injection of dye; serial radiographs are obtained; NPO and sedation may be required.	Encourage fluid intake to aid in urinary excretion of radionuclide.
Gallium	Determine presence of neoplasms, lymphoma, bronchogenic cancer, Hodgkin's disease, or inflammation.	Assess for previous reaction to contrast media; requires IV access for injection of dye; serial radiographs are obtained; NPO and sedation may be required.	Encourage fluid intake to aid in urinary excretion of radionuclide.
Gastric emptying scan	Assess obstruction, (e.g., ulcer, malignancy); patency of surgical anastomosis.	Patient to ingest "test meal" containing a radionuclide technetium; stomach is scanned until gastric emptying is complete.	Encourage fluid intake to aid in urinary excretion of radionuclide.
Liver and spleen	Detect lesions (e.g., cysts, hematomas, abscesses, adenomas, lacerations, metastasis).	Assess for previous reaction to contrast media; requires IV access for injection of dye; serial radiographs are obtained; NPO and sedation may be required.	Encourage fluid intake to aid in urinary excretion of radionuclide.
Lung	Examine pulmonary vascular circulation and to locate pulmonary emboli.	Assess for previous reaction to contrast media; requires IV access for injection of dye; serial radiographs are obtained; NPO and sedation may be required.	Encourage fluid intake to aid in urinary excretion of radionuclide.
Multiple gated acquisition (MUGA)	Assess indices of ventricular effectiveness, ejection fraction, and ventricular volume of heart.	Assess for previous reaction to contrast media; requires IV access for injection of dye; serial radiographs are obtained; NPO and sedation may be required.	Encourage fluid intake to aid in urinary excretion of radionuclide.
Positron emission tomography (PET)	A unique technique that combines nuclear medicine with precise localization to penetrate body's metabolism by recording traces of nuclear annihilations in body tissue. Designed to measure blood flow and volume, protein metabolism.	Requires more than one IV access (infusion of radioisotope and serial blood samples); no restriction on diet or fluids; no sedatives or tranquilizers should be taken.	Encourage fluid intake to aid in urinary excretion of radionuclide.
Renal	Provide data on kidney size, shape, location, and perfusion.	Assess for previous reaction to contrast media; requires IV access for injection of dye; serial radiographs are obtained; NPO and sedation may be required.	Encourage fluid intake to aid in urinary excretion of radionuclide.
Thallium	Identify myocardial fibrosis and ischemia; perfusion imaging.	Assess for previous reaction to contrast media; requires IV access for injection of dye; serial radiographs are obtained; NPO and sedation may be required.	Encourage fluid intake to aid in urinary excretion of radionuclide.

Test	Description	Patient Preparation	Nursing Considerations
Thyroid	Assess location, size, shape, and anatomic function of the substernal or enlarged thyroid glands.	Assess for previous reaction to contrast media; requires IV access for injection of dye; serial radiographs are obtained; NPO and sedation may be required.	Encourage fluid intake to aid in urinary excretion of radionuclide.
Oximetry	Assess arterial oxygen saturation (Sao_2); shock lung, pneumonia, asthma, mechanical ventilation status.	Place monitoring probe or sensor on the earlobe/fingertip.	Assure patient that test is noninvasive.
Paracentesis	Confirm presence of ascites; specimen analyzed for protein, amylase, RBC, WBC, fat, specific gravity, and cancer cells; fluid may be removed for palliative measures.	Local anesthetic; insertion of trocar, then catheter for drainage; may be continuous flow set-up.	Monitor vital signs; observe and record fluid loss.
Pericardiocentesis	Needle aspiration of fluid from pericardial sac; used for diagnostic or therapeutic purposes; ECG monitoring for localization and position of needle tip.	IV access for keep-vein-open rate; patient in supine position with head of bed elevated 60 degrees.	Observe and monitor vital signs, potential bleeding, and dyspnea.
Proctoscopy	Explore anus, rectum, and sigmoid colon.	Clear liquid diet, laxatives, NPO, enemas till clear before examination.	Observe for unexpected bleeding or sharp pain.
Sella turcia radiography	Screen for pituitary adenomas.	All objects above the neck must be removed.	No special aftercare.
Sialography	Assess salivary ducts (parotid, submaxillary, submandibular, sublingual) and related glandular structures.	Ingestion of contrast medium; x-ray films are taken with the patient in various positions; patient is given a sour substance to stimulate salivary excretion.	Provide fluids or food upon return from exams.
Sigmoidoscopy (flexible)	Examine left, transverse, right, and sigmoid colon with a flexible fiberoptic endoscope; biopsy and removal of polyps may be performed at this time.	Clear liquid diet 1–3 d before, NPO 6–8 h before; cathartics before examination; fiberoptic endoscope inserted via anus.	Observe for unexpected bleeding or sharp pain.
Spinal radiography Patient positioning (cervical, thoracic, lumbar, test sacral, or coccygeal)	Determine traumatic or pathologic fractures, degenerative arthritis changes.	Remove all metal objects. Immobilize patient if spinal fracture is suspected. Patient positioning depends on results.	Data are interpreted by radiologist.
Thermography	Technique by which differences in heat energy emanating from the skin of the breast are photographed using an infrared detector; hot spots may be a tumor, fibrocystic changes, or infection.	Thermoscope is placed over a small area of the breast to determine normal breast temperature; then both breasts scanned with infrared device; no discomfort is associated with the test.	Data are interpreted by radiologist.
Thoracentesis	Obtain pleural fluid for analysis; therapeutic is performed to relieve intrathoracic pressure associated with excess fluid in the lung.	Local anesthesia before insertion of trocar, then chest tubes; needle insertion for biopsy may be guided by fluoroscopy.	Monitor vital signs; observe for respiratory distress, bleeding at entry site, and excessive blood in sputum.
Tomography	Assess nodules or calcification in pulmonary mass or infiltrate.	Radiographic imaging through a predetermined cross section of the body; optimal visualization requires that patient take in and hold a deep breath.	Data are interpreted by radiologist.
Ultrasonography Doppler	Noninvasive procedure using sound waves to assess tissue function, abscess, trauma; determine blood flow velocity.	Gel is placed on the patient and the transducer is moved along the skin with some pressure	Provide skin cleansing items.

Table continued on following page

Selected Diagnostic Tests *Continued*

Diagnostic Test	Purpose	Procedure/Preparation	After Procedure
Venography	Demonstrate nonfilling of a vessel; assess for abnormal valves, thrombophlebitis, or hematoma.	Assess for allergy to contrast medium; inject contrast medium; serial-timed radiographs are obtained.	Monitor vital signs; observe for bleeding at entry site.
Ventriculography	Observe size, shape, and filling of ventricles; detect lesions and/or cerebral anomalies.	Serial x-ray of the skull after air or contrast material is injected via burr holes in the skull. Requires general/local anesthesia, NPO status past midnight; monitor vital signs after procedure every 15–30 min for the initial 24 h; head of bed elevated 10–15 degrees for 24 h.	Observe scalp dressing; monitor pain and administer analgesics. Monitor vitals and return of gag reflex.

BIBLIOGRAPHY

1. Berger A, Portenoy R, Weissman D: *Principles and practices of supportive oncology,* Philadelphia, Lippincott-Raven, 1998.
2. Carroll P: Analyzing the chem 7, *RN* 60:32, 1997.
3. DeGroot-Kosolcharden J: Culture and sensitivity testing, *Nursing* 26:33, 1996.
4. Fried LF, Palevsky PM: Hyponatremia and hypernatremia, *Med Clin North Am* 81:585, 1997.
5. Frizzell J: Avoiding lab test pitfalls, *Am J Nurs* 98:34, 1998.
6. Gorski LA, editor: *Best practices in home infusion therapy,* Gaithersburg, MD, Aspen Publishers, 1999.
7. Harmening DM, editor: *Modern blood banking and transfusion practices,* ed 4, Philadelphia, Davis, 1999.
8. Hazinski MF: *Manual of pediatric critical care,* St. Louis, Mosby, 1999.
9. Intravenous Nurses Society: *Infusion Nursing* 23(65): 2000.
10. Ipolito G and others: *Prevention, management & chemoprophylaxis of occupational exposure to HIV,* Charlottesville, VA, International Health Care Worker Safety Center, 1997.
11. Itano JK, Taoka KN: *Core curriculum for oncology nursing,* ed 3, Philadelphia, Saunders, 1998.
12. Johnson BL, Gross J: *Handbook of oncology nursing,* ed 3, Boston, Jones & Bartlett, 1998.
13. Marx JF: Understanding the varieties of hepatitis, *Nursing* 28:43, 1998.
14. Oncology Nursing Society: *Cancer chemotherapy guidelines and recommendations for practice,* Pittsburgh, Oncology Nursing Press, 1999.
15. Orr ME: Vascular access device selection for parenteral nutrition, ASPEN, *Nutr Clin Pract,* 14:172, 1999.
16. Pagana KD, Pagana TJ: *Mosby's manual of diagnostic and laboratory tests,* St. Louis, Mosby, 1998.
17. Perry AG, Potter PA: *Clinical nursing skills & techniques,* ed 4, St. Louis, Mosby, 1998.
18. Phipps WJ, Sands JK, Marek JF: *Medical-surgical nursing: concepts and clinical practice,* ed 6, St. Louis, Mosby, 1999.
19. Shirrell DJ and others: Therapeutic drug monitoring, *Am J Nurs* 99:42, 1999.
20. Wallach J: *Handbook of interpretation of diagnostics,* Philadelphia, Lippincott-Raven, 1998.
21. Whaley LF, Wong DL: *Nursing care of infants and children,* ed 6, St. Louis, Mosby, 1999.
22. Wong DL, Perry SE: *Maternal child nursing,* St. Louis, Mosby, 1998.

Answers

CHAPTER 1

1.	c	6.	d
2.	b	7.	a
3.	c	8.	a
4.	a	9.	c
5.	d	10.	d

CHAPTER 2

1.	b	6.	d
2.	d	7.	b
3.	b	8.	a
4.	c	9.	c
5.	b	10.	d

CHAPTER 3

1.	a	6.	a
2.	a	7.	d
3.	b	8.	b
4.	a	9.	d
5.	d	10.	c

CHAPTER 4

1.	b	6.	a
2.	b	7.	b
3.	c	8.	c
4.	c	9.	d
5.	a	10.	d

CHAPTER 5

1.	c	6.	d
2.	d	7.	d
3.	a	8.	a
4.	d	9.	b
5.	d	10.	b

CHAPTER 6

1.	a	6.	c
2.	c	7.	b
3.	d	8.	d
4.	b	9.	b
5.	c	10.	a

CHAPTER 7

1.	c	6.	c
2.	b	7.	d
3.	d	8.	c
4.	d	9.	d
5.	a	10.	a

CHAPTER 8

1.	d	6.	a
2.	c	7.	b
3.	a	8.	c
4.	d	9.	a
5.	d	10.	b

CHAPTER 9

1.	d	6.	d
2.	a	7.	b
3.	b	8.	b
4.	c	9.	a
5.	a	10.	a

CHAPTER 10

1.	b	6.	a
2.	c	7.	c
3.	a	8.	b
4.	c	9.	c
5.	b	10.	a

CHAPTER 11

1.	d	6.	b
2.	c	7.	c
3.	d	8.	d
4.	b	9.	b
5.	a	10.	a

CHAPTER 12

1.	d	6.	b
2.	d	7.	c
3.	c	8.	d
4.	b	9.	b
5.	a	10.	a

CHAPTER 13

1.	d	6.	c
2.	d	7.	c
3.	a	8.	b
4.	c	9.	b
5.	d	10.	a

CHAPTER 14

1.	d	6.	c
2.	d	7.	a
3.	c	8.	d
4.	b	9.	b
5.	a	10.	b

CHAPTER 15

1.	d	7.	b
2.	a	8.	a
3.	c	9.	c
4.	b	10.	d
5.	a	11.	b
6.	c	12.	d

CHAPTER 16

1.	d	6.	d
2.	a	7.	b
3.	a	8.	a
4.	c	9.	c
5.	d	10.	d

CHAPTER 17

1.	a
2.	d
3.	c
4.	b
5.	d

CHAPTER 18

1.	a	6.	a
2.	a	7.	c
3.	b	8.	b
4.	d	9.	c
5.	d	10.	c

CHAPTER 19

1.	d	6.	d
2.	d	7.	b
3.	a	8.	a
4.	d	9.	b
5.	a	10.	c

CHAPTER 20

1.	c	9.	d
2.	d	10.	a
3.	b	11.	b
4.	c	12.	d
5.	b	13.	c
6.	a	14.	d
7.	b	15.	b
8.	a		

CHAPTER 21

1.	c	6.	c
2.	c	7.	d
3.	c	8.	b
4.	c	9.	a
5.	b	10.	d

CHAPTER 22

1.	d	6.	c
2.	a	7.	a
3.	b	8.	d
4.	d	9.	c
5.	b	10.	c

CHAPTER 23

1.	a	6.	c
2.	b	7.	a
3.	b	8.	c
4.	a	9.	b
5.	d	10.	d

CHAPTER 24

1.	c	7.	a
2.	d	8.	d
3.	a	9.	b
4.	d	10.	b
5.	c	11.	c
6.	d	12.	a

CHAPTER 25

1.	d	6.	c
2.	c	7.	a
3.	c	8.	d
4.	a	9.	b
5.	d	10.	a

CHAPTER 26

1.	b	6.	b
2.	c	7.	d
3.	d	8.	a
4.	a	9.	c
5.	b	10.	d

CHAPTER 27

1.	b	6.	a
2.	c	7.	c
3.	b	8.	d
4.	a	9.	d
5.	d	10.	b

CHAPTER 28

1.	d	6.	b
2.	a	7.	d
3.	c	8.	b
4.	c	9.	a
5.	d	10.	a

CHAPTER 29

1.	b	6.	a
2.	c	7.	b
3.	d	8.	c
4.	d	9.	a
5.	c	10.	b

CHAPTER 30

1.	c	6.	d
2.	d	7.	a
3.	b	8.	a
4.	c	9.	b
5.	b	10.	d

CHAPTER 31

1.	c	6.	a
2.	a	7.	d
3.	b	8.	c
4.	d	9.	d
5.	b	10.	b

CHAPTER 32

1.	a	6.	d
2.	b	7.	d
3.	d	8.	a
4.	a	9.	b
5.	c	10.	c

CHAPTER 33

1.	c	6.	a
2.	d	7.	d
3.	d	8.	b
4.	b	9.	a
5.	c	10.	b

Index

Note: Page numbers in *italics* indicate figures; those followed by t indicate tables; those followed by b indicate boxed material.

RHODE ISLAND COLLEGE LIBRARY

3 1510 00458 9041

DATE DUE			
GAYLORD			PRINTED IN U.S.A.

NO LONGER THE
PROPERTY
OF RHODE ISLAND
COLLEGE